ISBN 978-0-483-02219-5
PIBN 10006506

American Medicine.

Volume XVIII., Complete Series
Volume VII., New Series
JANUARY — DECEMBER
1912

American Medical Publishing Company,
Burlington, Vt., and New York, N. Y.

CONTRIBUTORS.

ABBOTT, W. C., M. D., Chicago
AGER, LOUIS CURTIS, M. D., Brooklyn
AYRES, WINFIELD, M. D., New York
BALLIN, MILTON J., M. D., New York
BANDLER, SAMUEL W., M. D., New York
BARCLAY, HAROLD, M. D., New York
BEDFORD, EDWIN RAPALJE, M. D., Brooklyn
BERG, A. A., M. D., New York
BLOCK, SIEGFRIED, A. M., M. D., Brooklyn
BOLDT, HERMAN J., M. D., New York
BRAUN, ALFRED, M. D., New York
BRAV, AARON, M. D., Philadelphia
BROWN, SAMUEL HORTON, M. D., Philadelphia
BRUCE, OLIVER, M. R. C. S., L. R. C. P., (London) London, Eng.
BUMSTEAD, REV. HORACE, D. D., Boston
CAMPBELL, WILLIAM FRANCIS, M. D., Brooklyn
CARTER, WILLIAM WESLEY, A. M., M. D., New York
CHETWOOD, CHARLES H., M. D., New York
CISIN, M., M. D., New York
COLCORD, A. W., M. D., Clairton, Pa.
CRUTCHER, HOWARD, M. D., Roswell, N. M.
FRAUENTHAL, HENRY W., M. D., New York
FREEMAN, ALPHEUS M. D., New York
GALLOWAY, D. H., M. D., Roswell, N. Mex.
GOODHUE, E. S., M. D., Hawaii
GRAY, ALBERT A., M. D., Glasgow, Scotland
GREGORY, WM. M., M. D., Berea, O.
HAMMOND, R. L., M. D., Woodsboro, Md.
HAYNES, IRVING S., Ph. B., M. D., New York.
HAYS, HAROLD, A. M., M. D., New York

HELD, R. J., M. D., New York
HELLMAN, ALFRED M., M. D., New York
HOUGHTON, H. SEYMOUR, M. D., New York
HUBBY, LESTER MEAD, M. D., New York
IMPERATORI, CHAS. J., M. D., New York
IRWELL, LAWRENCE, M. A., B. C. L., Buffalo, N. Y.
JOHNSON, C. K., M. D., Burlington, Vt.
KAHN, L. MILLER, M. D., New York
KERR, LEGRAND, M. D., Brooklyn, N. Y.
KILMER, THERON W., M. D., New York
KNOTT, JOHN, A. M., M. D., Ch. B., V. D. P. H., (Univ. Dub.) Dublin, Ireland
LONDON, JULIUS, M. D., New York
MANGES, MORRIS, M. D., New York
MARBOURG, J. L., M. D., Seattle, Wash.
MARX, S., M. D., New York
MEYER, WM. H., M. D., New York
MEYERS, GEORGE, M. D., New York
McLEAN, WILLIAM, M. D., New York
McMASTER, GILBERT TOTTEN, M. D., New Haven, Conn.
MONTGOMERY, DOUGLASS W., M. D., San Francisco, Cal.
MORDEN, LUCETTA, M. D., Brooklyn
MORRIS, ROBERT T., M. D., New York
MULOT, O. L., M. D., Brooklyn
NEUMANN, HEINRICH, M. D., Vienna, Austria
NORTHRUP, W. P., M. D., New York
O'DONNALL, PATRICK S., M. D., Chicago
OPPENHEIMER, SEYMOUR, M. D., New York
PACKARD, MAURICE, M. D., New York
PISEK, GODFREY ROGER, M. D., New York
RAVAUT, P., M. D., Paris, France

ROBERTS, NORMAN, A. B., M. D., Washington, D. C.
ROBINSON, BEVERLEY, M. D., New York
ROGERS, HUGH E., M. D., Brooklyn
RONGY, A. J., M. D., New York
ROSE, A., M. D., New York
ROSS, WALTER H., M. D., Brooklyn
ROTTER, OSCAR, M. D., New York
SCHWARZ, HERMAN, M. D., New York
SHEFFIELD, HERMAN B., M. D., New York
SHERMAN, GEORGE H., M. D., Detroit, Mich.
SHIVELY, HENRY L., M. D., New York
SINCLAIR, D. A., M. D., New York
STARKEY, T. A., M. D., D. P. H., (London) Montreal, Canada
STEINACH, WILLIAM, M. D., New York
STERN, HEINRICH, M. D., New York
SYMS, PARKER, M. D., New York
VAN ZANDT, I. L., M. D., Fort Worth, Texas
VINNEDGE, W. W., M. D., Lafayette, Ind.
VON OEFELE, FELIX, M. D., New York
VOORHEES, IRVING WILSON, M. S., M. D., New York
WALKER, J. T. AINSLIE, F. R. S. M., F. C. S., New York
WAUGH, W. F., M. D., Chicago
WELLS, BROOKS H., M. D., New York
WHITE, JOHN BLAKE, M. D., New York
WILLIAMS, G. R., M. D., Paris, Ill.
WILLIAMS, TOM A., M. B., C. M., (Edin.) Washington, D. C.
WOLBARST, ABR. L., M. D., New York
WOODRUFF, CHAS. E., M. D., U. S. Army, San Francisco, Cal.

INDEX.

American Medicine

H. EDWIN LEWIS, M. D., *Managing Editor.*

PUBLISHED MONTHLY BY THE AMERICAN-MEDICAL PUBLISHING COMPANY.

Copyrighted by the American Medical Publishing Co., 1912.

Complete Series, Vol. XVIII., No. 1.
New Series, Vol. VII., No. 1.

JANUARY, 1912.

$1.00 YEARLY in advance.

The problem of modern pharmaceutical preparations is one that should receive the calm, thoughtful consideration of every thinking medical man. We say "calm, thoughtful" consideration, for the problem has been subjected to so much hysteria and hasty, intemperate condemnation that many cardinal facts have been overlooked or disregarded entirely. No honest man in studying any question wishes to lose sight of any facts or truths that can help him to form correct conclusions. Consequently it is desirable that every topic be approached in a spirit of fairness and in a state of mind that will enable one to grasp not only one but every side of a proposition. Certainly without this fair and honest method of investigating every vital question, no one can expect to arrive at a fair and honest conclusion. Unfortunately, there has been altogether too common a tendency to consider many problems in the light of personal prejudice rather than in that of justice or truth. It is a very human shortcoming to form personal prejudices on insufficient or ill founded information, and as medical men are essentially human, many popular views to the contrary notwithstanding, this shortcoming has been very frequently met in medical circles. Unfortunately, again, this tendency to draw hasty conclusions on insufficient or erroneous data has led the whole profession into many embarrassing positions. We say the whole profession for it has always happened that the few most apt to condemn good things hastily, or to laud worthless things precipitately have been so placed in positions of authority or with such opportunities for expressing themselves as to appear to represent the whole profession. As a matter of fact, and this accounts for the way that the great majority of medical men have so promptly reached a sound position on most questions, those who have presumed to speak for the whole profession have rarely if ever presented other than their own views. Naturally these erstwhile leaders or spokesmen of the profession have had a certain following. The medical fraternity has its sycophants and hypocrites as well as all other callings. But, thank heaven, the average doctor to-day does his own thinking. He makes his mistakes, he lacks much that he ought to have, and in his innermost self he realizes his deficiencies as no one else possibly can. But there is no denying the fact that the average American physician is doing better work for suffering humanity than ever before. He has made himself a better diagnostician, he is a much more accurate observer, and he gets results or at least takes his patient to some one who can, that were undreamed of twenty years back. Just witness his work in preventive medicine! Could the remarkable successes of the past decade have ever been reached but for the country's faithful practitioners? With a devotion to human needs that cannot fail to command respect and admiration, the average doctor has sacrificed every selfish interest and thrown himself into the struggle against disease with but one aim, to do his duty as he saw it. Every one who knows many doctors, country doctors especially, is bound to appreciate the nobility of their work, and realize the absolute truth of the foregoing. These are the men who must calmly and thoughtfully analyze the pharmaceutical questions of the hour. These are the men who must consider not alone the abuses but also the benefits that attend the use of pharmaceutical remedies. Common sense and intelligence will tell them no industry could ever have reached the proportions that the pharmaceutical has unless in response to definite needs and demands. Realizing all this and omitting no relevant fact, medical men will be in a position to weigh the evils that have developed and decide sensibly and conscientiously what their attitude is to be toward modern pharmaceutical products.

We hold no brief for the pharmaceutical manufacturer in these remarks. No one who knows anything about pharmacy and its offspring, the pharmaceutical industry, can deny that grave evils and abuses have been allowed to creep into the manufacture and exploitation of the remedies which have been submitted to the medical profession. That a little learning is a dangerous thing was never better exemplified than in the evolution of many remedial preparations and their introduction to physicians. Enthusiastic and honestly confident of the virtues of a product many a manufacturer has fallen into the error of

making extravagant and exaggerated claims concerning its action. As a consequence, a large amount of pharmaceutical literature has been prepared and distributed to the profession that has been ridiculous. For laymen to prepare literature for the guidance of medical men has been not only the limit of bumptiousness, but positively insulting to the whole medical profession. This, of course, does not refer to literature prepared by chemical or pharmacologic experts, nor compilations and abstracts made by men of literary ability specially trained in chemistry or physiology. Appreciating the situation, many of the reliable houses who have sought professional patronage have never allowed any literature to go to medical men that was not prepared by competent experts or at least carefully censored by some one specially qualified. Indeed not a few firms have employed medical graduates trained in laboratory or pharmacologic work to prepare all scientific literature designed to go to the profession. It requires no argument to show the desirability of having all pharmaceutical booklets, circulars, etc., prepared by those competent to make correct statements and form proper and warrantable conclusions. By the same token it is quite as apparent that literature prepared carelessly or by those who are incompetent, is neither honorable nor decent. As a matter of self protection, if nothing else, one would suppose that every firm would hesitate to submit any statement or offer any advice to medical men without assuring themselves as to its accuracy and authenticity. That there have been plenty of firms who have taken no pains with their literature, except to see that it lauded this, that or the other product to the skies, has been a shame and nothing but condemnation is deserved by such methods. So much for statements based on ignorance and incompetent material. Relative to sophisticated, unwarranted and untrue statements, not a single word of excuse or extenuation can be uttered. The firm or person who for the sake of monetary gain can wilfully claim that a product offered for the relief of sickness or suffering, is what it is not, or contains what it does not, deserves no consideration at the hands of honest men. Dishonesty no matter what its guise, is hateful and disreputable. It can claim nothing but the severest censure and criticism. Frankly and freely we do not hesitate to say that any pharmaceutical product that is dishonest and a sham, in that claims are made for it *that are known to be false and untrue,* should be shunned and avoided by every medical man. Such a statement seems almost superfluous, for no medical man of common intelligence, to say nothing of honesty, would be apt to use any remedy that he knows to be dishonest. In this day of moral progress—of a keener grasp of our moral obligations as members of the social organism—there is no excuse for dishonesty. In no field of endeavor is this more true than in the preparation and marketing of medical and surgical supplies. Honest products of definite worth are bound to live and win their deserved measure of success. Dishonest products on the other hand, with nothing but false and misleading claims behind them, are bound to fail and sooner or later go down to oblivion. It may take time to prove the dishonesty of a product, but the ultimate result in every case is as sure as the working of a natural law. Happily, medical men have become keener, more capable of detecting fraud and consequently more

critical. It behooves every pharmaceutical manufacturer, therefore, to recognize all this and meet the situation fairly and squarely. A considerable number of clean, honorable firms have—to our knowledge—long been hewing to the highest standards. These firms have nothing to fear. There are quite a few other firms, who through ignorance, unwise advice or mistaken views have committed errors in the past, but thanks to various agencies they have recognized their obligations to the medical profession and henceforth their methods will be above reproach. In plain words, they have awakened to the situation, realized their mistakes, "cleaned house" and established standards that command respect. As long as they adhere to the course they have thus set for themselves, they will merit the confidence, esteem and patronage of the profession. If they keep good faith and maintain unfailing integrity in their relations with the medical men of the country, we earnestly believe they may depend on the cooperation and support of the profession. But if they waver, make the slightest concession to dishonest methods, try to use the profession as a crutch to reach the laity, or prove guilty of betraying any confidence reposed in them—they can blame no one but themselves for whatever may happen.

It is a matter, however, for sincere congratulation that so few of the firms dealing with medical men more or less exclusively can be classed as intentionally dishonest. Aside from ordinary reasons of policy and the common sense business methods that have caused the great majority of those who manufacture and market medical and surgical supplies to adhere strictly to honor and honesty, a genuine pride in the quality and efficiency of their products has not failed to give material aid in this same direction. It is a healthy sign when a manufacturer shows pride in his preparations and their efficiency. Honest pride helps to create ideals, and ideals are as valuable in the pharmaceutical industry as they are in any other line of human enterprise. While we do not assume to speak for the medical profession, we believe that medical men generally will be quick to appreciate the growth of ideals in the development, manufacture, exploitation, and sale of everything that they can employ with advantage and safety to their patients, or special convenience and satisfaction to themselves.

In our effort to point out that much rests with the pharmaceutical manufacturers of the country in whatever successes they may win—or good they may accomplish—in the future, we have not forgotten that the medical profession has a reciprocal part to play. All pharmaceutical manufacturers have clear cut duties—so also have all medical men. On one side are obligations to be honest, to tell the truth, to respect and keep inviolate all confidences, to make all possible progress, and to keep good faith; on the other are the obligations to give a fair hearing, to form no hasty conclusions, to respect honest enthusiasm and endeavor, never to condemn without considering all phases of a proposition, and finally, to realize that the physician who neglects to use a product that represents the slightest advance is as false to his trust, as the physician who on insufficient data uses and praises a product that has no merit or value. All in all, the solution of the pharmaceutical problem would seem to rest on a better realization on the part of the interested parties of the honest obligations each owes to the other.

Pharmaceutical abuses unquestionably were responsible for the organization of the Council on Pharmacy and Chemistry of the American Medical Association. When this plan for the correction of abuses and evils in the pharmaceutical industry was definitely launched at the Portland, Oregon, meeting of the Association in 1905, the writer felt that it was a mistake, that it was a dangerous movement, illy conceived, and altogether much more apt to do harm than good. Many and various were the criticisms heard and it was believed by not a few that the whole undertaking was a scheme to drive the specialty manufacturers out of business and further the interests of certain large manufacturing houses. For some time these ideas—supplemented by many wild rumors—held sway, and the harsh, militant methods brought immediately into action all served to strengthen these views. But gradually our opinion concerning the Council on Pharmacy and Chemistry has undergone very great change, and a movement that we viewed with suspicion and regret, we are now free to commend. The creation of the Council was a progressive step, it was opportune, and without the slightest hesitancy we are ready to say that the project is fundamentally good. No honest man who has kept in touch with the work of the Council can deny that much has been done that deserves hearty commendation. But while granting all this, it must be as freely admitted that certain criticisms are merited. The Council, with all the good accomplished, has made its mistakes and shown its deficiencies, just as all other man-made institutions always do, and the man who denies this is as great an enemy to real progress as the man who questions the benefits that have assuredly been obtained. To begin with, more than one real, highly obnoxious evil has been exposed. But not a few things brought forward as vicious evils have been mistakes that have crept in through usage and custom. Tolerance, however, has been seldom exercised, and not a single error or shortcoming has failed to receive its full measure of caustic condemnation. No consideration has been shown for errors of judgment or the mistakes attributable to carelessness or unwisdom. All this is to be regretted. If the Council on Pharmacy and Chemistry has failed, therefore, to accomplish all that was anticipated, this can only be laid to the fact that it has been too destructive in its methods and has shown too little fairness and liberality.

Much as we would like to have our remarks on the Council taken in the earnest kindly spirit they are written, we know they will be misinterpreted and looked upon as ulterior in motive. But it is a common thing to be misunderstood, to have one's most unselfish and honest efforts viewed askance. So we must accept the practical certainty that we shall be charged with selfish purposes, with malicious efforts to belittle the work of the Council and with being an enemy to the Association and what it is doing.

Right here let us say that this is one of the principal criticisms we have to offer of the Council and those who are directing the work of the Association. Every adverse remark, every objection, every honest expression of doubt, immediately damns the individual and wins him the designation of being an enemy to the Association. It is apparently inconceivable that any person can be thoroughly appreciative of the great good that has been accomplished and still see simple details that arouse honest criticism. As we have repeatedly said, few institutions in this great country of ours are as deeply admired and respected as the American Medical Association. If the whole American medical profession felt as the writer does and appreciated as sincerely the genius of those who have made the Association the force it is to-day in American medical affairs, every physician in the country would be a member of the Association and a reader of the *Journal*. The work that has been done in a few years has been remarkable. From an insignificant body made up of a few thousand physicians, the Association has grown under intelligent guidance until it is one of the largest and most powerful organizations in the world. Let no one make the mistake of thinking that the wonderful progress the Association has made has been spontaneous or has resulted from the natural course of events. Hard, conscientious work by a few men who have toiled faithfully and well has brought the Association to where it is. All credit to such work and those who have given so much, cheerfully and uncomplainingly. We would be recreant indeed to every decent instinct if we denied one iota of the honor and credit that belongs to the men who are responsible for the Association's present commanding position.

But having acknowledged the good things, we are entitled to make such criticisms as we deem essential of those details that bid fair to hamper the progress that we and all other earnest members hope and expect to witness.

First is this attitude of intolerance to criticism however kindly tendered. No man or group of men has a monopoly of knowledge, morality or virtue. Every one is open to mistakes and misunderstanding. So in the work of the Council on Pharmacy and Chemistry, conclusive as some of it has been, a large part of it has been opinion, conjecture and belief, and therefore essentially controversial in character. Without the slightest equivocation, we deprecate the nihilistic note that has been so prominent in the comments and conclusions of the Council. It should be remembered that for years *a large part of the income of the Journal came from the same firms whose products are now so severely condemned.* Without the financial support of these very firms, once so eagerly sought and so freely accepted, it is doubtful if the present surplus would have reached its handsome proportions. It does not seem right or proper that the sudden decision of any group of men, however erudite, should be the sole determining factor as to a product's worth or uselessness. If a preparation or a number of preparations have been fit to use for many years, without the slightest question as to their quality or efficacy, does it seem reasonable that on the instant say-so of a few men they become valueless, lose every virtue and become harmful to employ? Such a conclusion is little short of ridiculous, and while it was eminently proper to establish fixed standards which each and every product should conform to to secure admission to the advertising pages of the *Journal,* to make failure to conform to these standards the sole reason for discontinuing the use of a product does not leave very much to a physician's knowledge or intelligence. If a preparation really deserves such sudden rejection, one may be very sure that few intelligent medical men have been employing it for a long time, while on the other hand if physicians

have been using a product right along with more or less satisfaction, its sudden rejection is pretty apt to be unfair and unwarranted. The point we would make is that the standards of the Council are arbitrary rules laid down by the pharmacists, chemists, laboratory experts, and non-practitioners of medicine, who constitute the Council. These standards as a result are debatable, their very origin makes them subject to controversy, and the physician who denies their accuracy in toto has as much right to his opinion as the one who accepts them without question. Dragging in the National Formulary "substitutes" for original preparations was a grave mistake, for many a physician has asked with all propriety how, if some product advertised for years in the *Journal* must be suddenly rejected, it can be wiser, safer or more ethical for him to employ a very palpable substitute? To state it as it appears to us it all depends on the view point of the individual doctor. If a physician prefers to use a "substitute" for any original product or preparation, that is entirely a matter for him to decide. He is the arbiter of the question and the responsibility of the decision rests on him alone. After all that can be said concerning these various matters, the fact that persists is that *the individual physician is the court of last resort.* He is the one to decide what he can or cannot, will or will not employ, in his work. It is right for the Council and the *Journal* to supply him with all the information available that will help him to arrive at correct conclusions concerning the value of different preparations. The Council of Pharmacy and Chemistry is essentially an investigating or examining body whose proper province is to ascertain and present facts concerning all pharmaceutical and drug products, everything in-

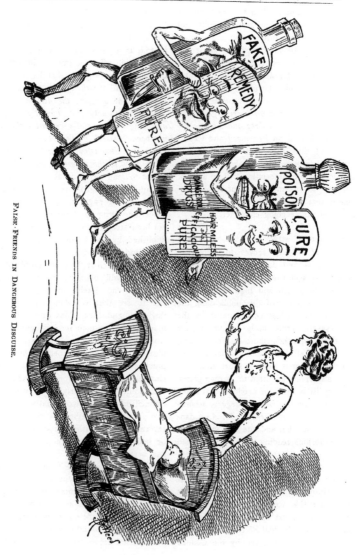

FALSE-FRIENDS IN DANGEROUS DISGUISE.

deed that is employed in the treatment of disease. The more accurate, definite and unprejudiced such information is, the more helpful it will be and the greater aid it will offer in solving these pharmaceutical problems, which, after all, are only incidental to the great, big, burning question that confronts the profession as never before, *how best to utilize every useful agent with greatest degrees of safety and success.*

If the Council on Pharmacy and Chemistry will thus direct its efforts to the broader questions of clinical therapy it is certain that the Association will do a work not only for its members, but for all humanity that cannot fail to bring results of the most far reaching character.

The recent attack on the American Journal of Surgery serves to emphasize all the evils and dangers of a policy of destruction and ruin. Although freely admitting the worth and high character of the reading pages of this publication, the *Journal* nevertheless condemns it in the most severe terms, hotly taking to task all those who contribute to its reading pages, and all because it carries the advertisements that only a short time ago were also freely admitted to its own pages. A long list is given of products that make the *American Journal of Surgery*, according to the *Journal of the A. M. A.*, a dangerous publication and one that in spite of its meritorious reading pages medical men should avoid, boycott and turn from generally. We have too great faith in the American physician to believe he will tolerate such unfairness. With a few exceptions the worst that can be said against any product in the list of those advertised in the *American Journal of Surgery*, is that it has not been approved by the Council

of Pharmacy and Chemistry! To make this "approval" the touchstone of honesty and therapeutic efficiency, is not only ridiculous, it is a perversion of right, and if it prevails will offer the greatest impediment to therapeutic progress that has ever appeared. *Will the thoughtful physician accept without question the dictum that he cannot honorably or honestly employ any drug or remedial preparation that has not been "passed" by the Council of Pharmacy and Chemistry of the A. M. A., a corporation of the state of Illinois?* Will he refuse to read any journal that appeals to his intelligence and interest simply because its advertising pages carry announcements concerning drugs and products that have not been accepted for inclusion in the book published by the Council and known as New and Non-Official Remedies? We doubt very much if the rank and file of the profession will submit to any such domination, for no intelligent physician can fail to see that valuable and useful as the work and conclusions of the Council may be, they are none the less open to controversy and change. The preposterous idea of taking our therapeutic morals and practice from the Council's deductions exclusively is apparent from more than one standpoint. For nearly seven years the Council has been at work and yet the last two years has witnessed the acceptance of several well established products. Can it be believed that any intelligent physician has been kept from using such products by the tardiness of the Council to accept them? Again not a few useful preparations have had their acceptances delayed by prolonged controversies as to some real or fancied fault in their nomenclature, labels or literature. Months in many instances have passed before these details have been arranged to suit the Council. Not a doubt has existed relative to the therapeutic efficiency of these products. *Should the physician have denied himself the service of these remedies while they were held up solely by technicalities?* Finally, quite a goodly number of products that have enjoyed the Council's approval, and graciously been allowed to advertise in the *Journal* have recently been cast out into outer darkness. For one reason or another such as objectionable name, uncertain utility, and so forth, these preparations are no longer acceptable to the Council. In passing it may be remarked that they are no different than they were at the time they were "passed" and admitted to the inner circle. In connection with their original acceptance they conformed to every requirement and made all changes demanded of them. But alas, the Council is revising its standards, altering its opinions, and viewing matters in a far different light than at the outset, for products supposedly fixtures in New and Non-Official Remedies have been rudely and ignominiously withdrawn from the book. While these acts of the Council may be praiseworthy in that they show an admirable independence, *the all important fact for the practitioner and every interested person to note is that the Council's conclusions are by no means absolute.* Its work shows beyond all doubt that the whole problem is ambiguous, that there are no fixed values and that standards are essentially open to change. All this means what we have repeatedly said that *the whole question is in its controversial or debatable stage.* Until ideas and opinions are more settled and standards more certain and fixed, the *Journal* outrages every instinct of fairness and right when it makes an onslaught such as that on the *American*

Journal of Surgery. Its conversion and "redemption" are too recent and its vaunted surplus represents too much of the same money it accuses independent journals of seeking, to justify a "holier-than-thou" attitude toward a publication that is serving the medical profession as faithfully as is the *American Journal of Surgery.*

Our position is just this. We are thoroughly appreciative of the good features of the work the Council has been doing. But we are as sensible of its failures and shortcomings as we are of its successes and unquestionable possibilities. It would be a calamity for the Council to discontinue its work. As an examining and investigating body it can supply the profession with facts of the utmost value. But having supplied those facts its obligations cease. *It is up to the medical profession to weigh these facts, study them intelligently and liberally, and then be guided by them just so far as each man's individual judgment dictates.* We have found some, yes much of the Council's findings of the utmost help. Other findings have left us in doubt, while not a few of their deductions have seemed wholly and absolutely wrong. As repeatedly stated we have regretted the too great prevalence of the spirit of intolerance, as we have also the too great tendency to consider all criticism as borne of enmity and animosity. We have regretted that instead of fostering friendly cooperative relations with the independent medical press of the country, the apparent object has been to belittle every effort and question every motive. AMERICAN MEDICINE does not have the slightest intention of restricting its advertising pages to only such products as are in good odor with the Council on Pharmacy and Chemistry.

The medical men responsible for AMERICAN MEDICINE are perfectly able to establish standards that will meet every requirement of the honest physician. The pharmaceutical problem is subject to too much controversy and there is too much uncertainty on every side to justify any medical publication, aside from the *Journal* and possibly the state journals, accepting *the arbitrary dictum of a body that freely admits it may repudiate to-morrow the action it takes to-day!!* Again, too many of the findings of the Council have shown the bias of individual members, and too much happens to be known concerning certain of its "passes" as well its "rejections" to warrant AMERICAN MEDICINE—or any other independent journal—accepting them without question..

There is a mistaken idea that medical journalism is exceedingly profitable. This is indeed wrong and no independent medical publication run in behalf of its readers can ever become rich and opulent. This is borne out by every one of the high grade journals that are honestly and fearlessly contributing their part to the uplift and progress of contemporary medical journalism. But happily there are other rewards than those measured in dollars and cents and we know we are stating the exact situation when we say that every physician or group of physicians at the helm of every independent medical journal that is justifying its existence seeks something prized a great deal more highly than money. This something is the knowledge of faithful service, a realization that one has been a factor in a constructive undertaking, even though it may have been small and insignificant. The faith and confidence we have in the American doctor, and an unfaltering belief that right always

wins in the end, leave no doubt as to the ultimate outcome. AMERICAN MEDICINE is going on striving to serve its readers and the medical profession to the limit of its opportunities and the ability of those directing it. Honesty, integrity and a square deal in every transaction shall be our constant aim. Service, clean honorable service, shall continue to be our watchword. In every way we shall conscientiously strive to protect our readers against imposition, fraud or dishonesty not only in our reading pages but equally in our advertising pages. We shall exercise our discretion as to accepting articles which mention pharmaceutical products. *The slightest suspicion of collusion between an author and a firm will be sufficient to lead us to take the most drastic action.* On the other hand if a physician whose integrity is unimpeachable sees fit to mention a preparation, we shall not insult him by cutting out such mention. It matters not whether his mention is favorable or derogatory. The author is the one responsible for his statement and the journal has nothing to do with it after assuring itself as far as possible that the statement is a clean and honest expression of opinion. Pharmaceutical manufacturers have ever been ready to criticise a journal that refused to allow physicians of even the highest standing to mention pharmaceutical products by their proper names. That we henceforth leave the matter to the discretion of each author will probably gratify those manufacturers who have complained so bitterly when the names of products have been eliminated by a zealous editor. But in this connection we want it distinctly understood that adverse opinions will likewise have no restrictions. If a manufacturer wants a journal to be independent and liberal enough to print the full and literal statement made by any honorable physician who may chance to speak favorably concerning any honest pharmaceutical product, he must be big enough to acknowledge the justice of printing no less readily the comment of the honest physician who may happen to speak unfavorably. This is simply in line with AMERICAN MEDICINE's efforts to merit not only the respect but also the confidence of every honorable medical man. Those who guide its course and direct its policies have no doubt that mistakes will be made in the future, just as they have been made in the past. But we shall make as few as possible, and try our best never to make the same one twice. In closing, let us say that we regret exceedingly having devoted so much space to these matters of policy and purpose. We feel, however, in view of the attitude of the *Journal of the American Medical Association* toward the independent medical journals of the country that it is due to the thousands of honorable physicians who have given AMERICAN MEDICINE their support during the past five years, to come out into the open and state our position exactly as we understand it. Having done so we are perfectly willing to leave the verdict to the physicians of America. We brook no fight with any one. The victories we hope to win are those of honest, constructive endeavor. That there is a place not only for AMERICAN MEDICINE but a goodly number of other purposeful medical journals, is proven by the success and standing that so many have achieved. Every one of the reputable independent medical journals of the country would be glad to cooperate with the great official organ of the American Medical Association. Every one of these journals would be glad to work along consistent lines for the abolition of every well defined evil that threatens the usefulness of the medical profession. Every one of these journals would be glad to have the splendid resources of the Association employed to point the way to better things. But not one of these journals wants to see this work, however urgently it may be needed, undertaken with a spirit of intolerance, animosity or revenge. Not one of these journals will suffer coercion, *especially by those who know nothing of the problems of the practising physician*. And finally not one of these journals is ready to concede that the establishment of a series of arbitrary rules and regulations gives the *Journal of the American Medical Association,* or any other journal however estimable, a monopoly of virtue, aspiration or morality. The opportunity to unite the medical profession, to marshal every active force, and to make the whole American profession a genuine fraternity, is within the immediate scope and power of those who are at present in control of the Association. The opportunity is passing. It may never come again. Will it be seized and taken advantage of? Are those in command able to grasp the situation and create a united, harmonious and splendidly organized profession that shall have its destiny in its own hands, and not as our British brethren now find theirs—in the talons of the politicians? We cannot say. We do not know. We can only hope. But this we can say with all the earnestness at our command and a thorough appreciation of the gravity of existing conditions, and that is aspiring medical men expect something a great deal more uplifting from their leaders than an acrimonious warfare on the independent medical journals of the country.

A little patience, and the few evils that still exist will be overcome. Permanent and lasting reform always takes time. Vast improvement has been made by every "worth while" independent medical journal and the whole movement is upward and forward. But if warfare is the program and annihilation the object, as is presaged by the attacks already made, one thing is certain it will not be a one-sided struggle. And after the smoke and noise of battle has cleared away, one fact will stand forth and that will be that those who prosecute a holy war need to be all that they claim, or they may have to pay a cost in damaged reputations and broken halos that will be out of all proportion to the victory won.

Heart strain in the aged has lately become of considerable importance, although it is an old subject in the medical world. The Surgeon General of the Army in his last annual report has called attention to the damage done to old hearts by endurance tests, and taken in conjunction with the sudden deaths alleged to have been due to the tests, this report leaves no doubt that the human frame cannot possibly endure such strains after it begins the downward course after 45 or 40 years of age. Even 35 years, weakens some of the tissues so that they are dangerously strained by pressures harmless to the boy of 15 or 20. Hard daily training to keep in "condition" for muscular feats is therefore to be condemned after 35 or 40, but the exercise must be gradually lessened to keep below the danger line of tissues which are weakening as nature intended them to. Endurance lessens and we cannot keep it. Our efforts only lessen it. The strenuous life after 40 is unnatural and dangerous, and after 60

is out of the question, except for a very few exceptional men who ought to be in better business anyhow.

———

A study of mistaken diagnosis is the title chosen by Dr. R. C. Cabot of Boston for an article (*Jour. A. M. A.,* Oct. 15, 1910) comparing his clinical findings with the subsequent autopsy in 1,000 cases during the past ten years. The title is ill-chosen, for it gives the impression of failure whereas it illustrates the rapidly increasing accuracy of modern scientific diagnosis. In view of the fact that so many concurrent pathologic processes give little or no sign of their presence, it is little short of amazing that so few are overlooked. Furthermore, the signs in many diseases are so often obscure or paralleled by other conditions, that it is highly gratifying there are so few errors of commission. No typhoid was overlooked—a remarkable record in view of the fact that in the early stages no one can make a diagnosis. Three cases of general septicemia and two of miliary tuberculosis were wrongly considered typhoid, but they merely show how closely some infections imitate others. It is curious to note how rapidly we are raising our ideal of perfect diagnosis, and perhaps we always will raise it and never attain it. That is, in the future we will not be satisfied with discovering the main trouble, but will be disappointed if unable to find all the secondary or concurrent ones. Dr. Cabot has summarized his long experience in eighteen short conclusions, which are so valuable that it would be well for every physician to memorize them, and then have them printed on a card and pasted on his desk to avoid forgetting them—or keep them in his hat.

ORIGINAL ARTICLES.

PENETRATING WOUNDS OF THE EYE LEADING TO ENUCLEATION; PRESENTATION OF SPECIMENS.

BY

WILLIAM McLEAN, M. D.,
Assistant Surgeon to New York Ophthalmic Hospital.

New York City.

In this article the illustrations are from specimens removed because of various conditions, resulting principally from penetrating wounds.

material is carried into the eye a panophthalmitis usually occurs. An injured eye which has escaped infection but never has become quiescent, or is subject to attacks of inflammation, especially those involving the uveal tract, should be looked upon with apprehension as it may at any time cause sympathetic trouble in its fellow. (One of the specimens here shown is an illustration of the above statement).

The specimens presented are all anteroposteriorly sectioned and are mounted in gelatine. That you may get a fairly accurate conception of the intraocular structures of the eye, I will present a specimen having the various structures intact.

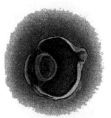

Specimen No. 1.

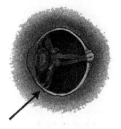

Specimen No. 2.

Penetrating wounds of the eyeball, it is needless to say, should always be looked upon as serious and should in consequence receive very careful attention from the moment of the injury. If seen shortly after the accident, the injured eye may be saved; or, if it is not possible to preserve useful vision, the necessity for an enucleation may be prevented. In the absence of special attention the eye may remain a menace to its fellow, or its removal may be necessitated.

Not all of the eyes injured by penetrating objects become infected, nor do they all result in loss of vision, but where infective

This specimen has been sectioned in the horizontal plane and shows the cornea, iris, crystalline lens, retina, choroid, sclera and entrance of the nerve in their proper relations. The nucleus of the lens shows very prettily in this specimen.

Specimen No. 2 was enucleated from a young man. He was a machinist and while at work at his lathe a small metal shaving struck him in the eye. The piece of metal could not be located by his fellow workmen. The eye did not seem to give him any trouble except that it became red and remained so for two weeks, when the redness gradually disappeared. After a short period the vision became gradually diminished until sight was entirely gone. Not until the vision was gone did he consult an oculist. Then an ophthalmoscopic examination revealed a detached retina and on the nasal side a reddish brown mass which subsequently proved to be the piece of metal.

There was a peculiar congestive zone in the sclera surrounding the cornea and an enucleation was advised. In the specimen the retinal detachment is evident, and the reddish brown mass which was discovered at the time of the ophthalmoscopic examination is now visible in the specimen.

Specimen No. 3 was removed from a man who was an iron worker. While at work with a riveting machine a piece of the tool broke and struck him in the eye. He was at work in another city when the accident occurred and was hurried to a hospital where the wound was dressed. The services of an oculist could not be obtained there at once, so he was advised to come immediately to New York, but it was three days before he acted on this advice, and when I saw him at the expiration of this three day period the eye was very painful and decidedly congested. The vitreous chamber was cloudy and appeared to contain

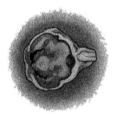

Specimen No. 3.

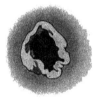

Specimen No. 4.

This is a type of one condition where retention of the eyeball is a constant source of danger and it may at any time cause sympathetic trouble, yet aside from the peculiar congestive zone the eye to all outward appearances was as good as its fellow. Had this man sought the services of an oculist immediately after the injury, the eye might have been saved by removing the foreign body through an incision in the tunics of the eyeball immediately over the lodgment of the foreign body. The location of this intruder could have been determined by the use of the ophthalmoscope, the transilluminator, or the Roentgen rays.

pus. In his statement of the injury he said the piece of metal that hit the eye was quite large and he saw it fall after it struck his eye.

Measures were instituted to stop the advance of pus formation but without success. Panophthalmitis resulted and a large incision of the eyeball had to be made to allow drainage. A piece of steel was found within the eyeball. As soon as the inflammatory process was controlled the eye was removed. On section it was found that the retina and choroid were nearly obliterated by the inflammatory process and the eyeball is filled with fibrous tissue.

This is a type where retention of the eyeball in its orbit, while possible to produce future trouble, is not as dangerous as the condition in the preceding case.

In Specimen No. 4, we have a condition following injury, similar to the preceding case and one where the danger from sympathetic trouble would appear to be greatly lessened, yet it did produce sympathetic trouble and the man became totally blind. He was a strong healthy stone worker. A blast over which he was working in the stone quarry prematurely exploded. One eye was injured and the sight lost. When recovery was attained the eye was a sightless shrunken member.

during the process of maturing his vision would be getting less and less; that it would be necessary for him to be blind for a short period before the cataract would be ready for removal. This could have been considered a consoling statement had it been true. After the third attack I saw him. The eye was then soft, vision reduced to about 15/100, iridodonesis plainly visible, also a slight cataractous condition of the lens and a state of ocular degeneration was present.

On palpating the sightless eye, considerable tenderness to pressure was elicited at the upper inner portion and because of this tenderness the injured eye stump was re-

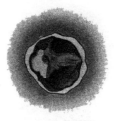

Specimen No. 5.

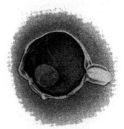

Specimen No. 6.

The other eye was uninjured and the vision was good. About three years later he had an inflammation in the good eye. This was diagnosed as iritis by an oculist and he was put in the hospital for treatment. A few months after this had cleared he had another attack which was treated in the same way. After the second attack he noticed that his vision was not as good as formerly.

The oculist who had treated him through these two attacks explained the loss of vision as due to a commencing cataract, which would necessarily have to become mature before it could be removed, and

moved in the hope of arresting the inflammatory attacks in the other eye. It was some months after the operation and we were beginning to have hope that the process had ceased when he had another flare up and one after another has followed until his sight is now gone completely.

It is often very difficult to control these processes when they once become firmly established.

Text-books advise that where there is any vision in the injured or exciting eye it is better to retain that eye as when the inflammatory process ceases there may be better vision in that eye than the irritated one possessing the sympathetic trouble. In this case we had nothing to lose and everything to gain as the irritating eye was sightless.

Specimen No. 5 was removed from a man who while chopping wood was injured by a chip of wood being catapulted upward and hitting the eye. A laceration of the sclera above and close to the cornea occurred. The iris was protruding through the wound, and its appearance was that of a preliminary iridectomy minus the clipping off of the protruding iris.

He was placed in the hospital and the accidental partial iridectomy was completed. Appropriate treatment was admin-

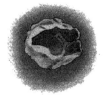

Specimen No. 7.

istered. There was no direct infection but a traumatic irido-cyclo-choroiditis set in and the vision was lost. In the specimen may be seen the retinal detachment, and newly formed tissue in the ciliary region.

Specimen No. 6 received an injury to the cornea and an infection followed. Probably he had a perforating ulcer of the cornea and the iris became involved, as there was keratoconus with complete anterior synechia and glaucoma when I first saw him. The specimen also shows a dislocated lens. On account of the complete loss of vision, even to imperception of light resulting from the glaucoma and complete anterior synechia, also a conspicuous unsightly keratoconus, an enucleation was advised.

Specimen No. 7 was removed from a carpenter. While he was using the hammer it chipped, and a piece of steel which was thin and sharp entered the eye at the limbus. In twenty-four hours the eye was full of pus. As soon as the inflammation subsided the eye was removed. In the section it may be seen that all intra-ocular structures have been obliterated by the inflammation.

Specimen No. 8 does not belong to this class of injuries; its removal being necessitated by the pain from persistent inflammatory glaucoma. When first seen the glaucoma had had some weeks duration and vision was obliterated by the constant intra-

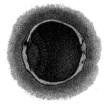

Specimen No. 8.

ocular pressure on the optic nerve at the lamina cribrosa.

An iridectomy was advised and a good generous slice of the iris was removed, care being taken to excise close to the base of the iris. This controlled the pain for a short time only and on a recurrence of the increased tension and its resulting pain, a posterior sclerotomy was done, allowing a small portion of the vitreous to escape. The second operation held the process in check for a time, but the pain gradually returned and an enucleation was advised. To this the patient willingly acceded and the eye was removed. The specimen shows the lens pushed forward producing the shallow anterior chamber. The scar in the sclera of the iridectomy also the paracentesis of the posterior sclerotomy may be seen.

Specimen No. 9 is a melano-sarcoma of the eye. This case presented all the prominent symptoms of acute inflammatory glaucoma and in addition gave a history of a sudden loss of vision in the lower half of the field nine months previously. There was at that time no pain or other symptoms. An oculist whom she consulted gave a diagnosis of detachment of the retina due to a probable tumor. Questioning brought out

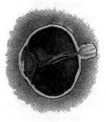

Specimen No. 9.

the facts that the patient had had a tumor of the breast removed and later an hysterectomy for uterine fibroma. Both of these growths, however, were diagnosed by the pathologist as fibromata. In view of all these facts and because forty-eight hours of treatment failed to alter the glaucoma in any way, an enucleation was advised. The pathologist's report was melanotic, small and large round and spindle celled sarcoma.

In the specimen may be seen the detachment of the retina also the tumor about the size of a large pea occupying about one-fourth of the vitreous chamber.

391 West End Avenue.

SCROFULOSIS.

BY

HERMAN B. SHEFFIELD, M. D.,

Instructor in Diseases of Children, N. Y. Post-
Graduate Medical School and Hospital, etc.,
New York City.

With the discovery of the tuberculin reaction the tuberculous nature of the symptom-complex embraced under the term "scrofula" has been fully established. The disease is nowadays generally described as "Tuberculosis of the skin, mucous membranes and glands." It usually attacks children with undermined constitution who are poorly fed and housed and exposed to tuberculous infection. Various skin eruptions or injuries, exanthemata, decayed teeth, and diseased tonsils or adenoids serve as portals of entry to the tubercle bacilli. The immediate result of the tuberculous infection is hyperplasia, and the more remote effect, caseous degeneration of the parts primarily involved and quite frequently also secondary infection of the adjacent structures.

Clinically, scrofulosis is characterized by simultaneous or successive involvement of the skin, mucous membranes and lymphatic glands. Like tuberculosis of the bones it runs a chronic course and shows a great tendency towards slow, spontaneous recovery, or gradual transition into general tuberculosis. The skin is ordinarily first involved, forming the seat of a nodular or pustular eruption, which resists simple local treatment, extends to the subcutaneous tissue, breaks down and forms slowly discharging abscesses or indolent ulcers. The lesion is most frequently situated upon the back and nates, but is found also upon the scalp and face—probably carried from one part of the body to the other by scratching with infected fingers.

Scrofulosis of the mucous membranes is manifested chiefly by chronic nasopharyngitis. The nasal mucous membrane is red and swollen and discharges a seropurulent secretion which produces yellowish green crusts within and around the nares and excoriation of the upper lip. A similar acrid discharge is usually observed also from the ears. Both the nasal as well as the aural discharge may become purulent and fetid, by implication of the periosteum, cartilage, and bony structures of the nose and ears and lead to permanent deformities and functional defects, e. g., ozena, deafness, etc.

Scrofulosis of the eyes, the so-called *strumous ophthalmia,* usually begins with redness and swelling of the palpebral mucous membrane, and in a great number of cases is soon followed by involvement of the cornea in the form of *phlyctenular keratitis* with strong lacrimation, pain and photophobia, with a great tendency to corneal ulceration and opacities.

The lymphatic glands are affected either early in the course of disease or late—secondarily to the inflammation of the skin or mucous membranes. They often undergo caseation and suppuration, and unless completely extirpated, open spontaneously and continue as pus-discharging fistulae or indolent ulcers. The course of the disease depends greatly upon the vitality of the patient and the mode of treatment. It is always chronic. Children removed from the obnoxious surroundings and placed under suitable constitutional as well as local treatment frequently recover completely. Otherwise the tuberculous process is prone to spread to the osseous system and the internal organs. Spina ventosa, osteomyelitis and spondylitis form frequent sequelae,

and transition into general tuberculosis is not uncommon.

Characteristic as the symptom-complex of scrofula seems to be, errors in the diagnosis are nevertheless very apt to be made. The perplexity is often great in differentiating it from inherited syphilis with which affection scrofula has many symptoms in common. In all such doubtful cases we must, on the one hand, employ the tuberculin reaction and examine the discharges for tubercle bacilli, and on the other hand, resort to Wassermann's reaction or administer mercury and the iodids. One should not be too hasty in pronouncing a case as "scrofulosis" because of the so-called "torpid habitus" of the child (i. e., pale, flabby, puffed face, thick nose, swollen and excoriated lips, etc.) as this appearance may be met also with hypertrophied tonsils and adenoids and local infections by other micro-organisms, especially the streptococcus and staphylococcus. In fact, it is this group of cases which most frequently leads to diagnostic errors and tends to abnegate the existence of true scrofulosis, i. e., local tuberculosis.

Scrofula like other forms of tuberculosis demands early and energetic treatment. The patient should be removed from the obnoxious surroundings, well nourished and kept outdoors the greater part of the day. Cleanliness of the body, especially of the skin, hair, nose, throat and ears, are of greatest importance. Diseased foci, such as large tonsils and adenoids, decayed teeth and caseated glands, should be removed without delay and open wounds or simple skin eruptions should be carefully protected against infection. The patient's finger nails should be kept closely clipped and scrupulously clean to prevent scratching of the diseased parts and further infection of healthy structures. Complications should be treated vigorously in accord with modern methods. Internally the syrup iodid of iron with compound syrup hypophosphites and cod liver oil, continued for several months, will be found to act admirably. On another occasion (in my treatise on "Modern Diagnosis and Treatment of Diseases of Children") I called attention to the great value of small, gradually increased doses of tuberculin, especially in incipient cases.' Since then I have been able to convince myself of its signal benefit also in protracted cases.

127 West 87th Street.

THERAPEUTIC IMMUNIZATION WITH BACTERIAL VACCINES.

BY

GEORGE H. SHERMAN, M. D.,
Detroit, Mich.

As a result of extensive research experiments on lower animals conducted by numerous investigators, many . of the changes taking place in the animal body during an infective process while establishing an immunity have been quite accurately worked out. Buchner, Nuttall and others found that fresh normal blood serum has a bactericidal power, dissolving many kinds of germs to a limited extent. Park showed that 30,000 germs per c. c. of fluid by adding 0.1 c. c. of normal blood serum and incubating at 98.1 for 27 hours, all the germs will be destroyed but by adding 100,000 germs to the same amount of serum, the number of germs will be very much diminished during the first and second hours of incubation, but if incubated for 27 hours the number of germs would be materially increased, the remaining live germs having multiplied. This shows that normal blood serum contains something that is consumed while destroying germs and that if there are any germs left after this substance is consumed they will begin to multiply.

Ehrlich and Morgenroth found that this bactericidal power of fresh serum is due to the presence, in very small quantity of a variety of substances they call inter-bodies which combine with another substance complement, present in comparatively large amount. These inter-bodies fit a large variety of organisms, but when an animal is immunized to some specific organism the inter-body corresponding to that organism becomes enormously increased, becoming the immune body while the amount of complement present remains practically stationary. Since the germ destroying power depends on the combination of the immune body with complement it can readily be seen that in cases of advanced infections the immunizing process may be retarded from a deficiency in complement.

Longscope (*University of Penn. Med. Bulletin,* 1902, XV 331), in an investigation of the complement-content of the infectious diseases in general has found that the complement is constantly low and is diminished still more when septic complications intervene.

Gay, Perkins and Thompson (*Journal Med. Research,* 1903, X 196) found a diminished bacteriolitic complement constant in variola. Wasserman suggested (Immune Sera by C. F. Bolduan, 1911, page 81) that the curative power of many bactericidal sera might be increased by the simultaneous injection of the sera of certain normal animals in order thus to gain an increased amount of complement.

In infections caused by the diphtheria or tetanus bacilli distinct antitoxins are formed as the principal immunizing factor. From infections caused by endotoxic organisms of which the pus group, streptococci, pneumococci, staphylococci, colon bacilli, and typhoid bacilli are the most important, the immune body or amboceptor expresses itself in the form of agglutinins, lycins, precipitates, etc. Metchnikoff found that the white corpuscle plays an important part in the immunizing process as phagocytes or "devouring cells" having the power to take up germs and destroy them by a process of digestion.

Sir A. E. Wright, following up Metchnikoff's work found that the phagocytic power of the white corpuscles was very slow or almost negative unless the corpuscles are suspended in blood serum and that when suspended in blood serum obtained from previously immunized animals the phagocytic power is specific, it only taking place when the same kind of germs are used in the experiment that the animal was immunized with.

From these investigations Wright concluded that the blood serum contains a substance that has a sensitizing effect on the invading organism and that this substance is materially increased during the immunizing process. This bacteriotropic substance has been termed an opsonin (Latin, opsono, I prepare the food for). It was this phagocytic power of the blood as demonstrated in the incubated test tube that led Wright to make extensive investigations as to the opsonic power of the blood in man under various conditions.

From this brief review of the immunizing process it becomes apparent that the process is somewhat complicated and no doubt many other important factors exist which have not been worked out. Which one of these various immunizing methods is the most important is difficult to determine, except in diphtheria and tetanus where distinct antitoxines are produced, and even here it has been found that opsonins are formed during immunization.

Immunity may be natural or acquired. Natural immunity consists in some species being able to withstand pathogenic microorganisms that will attack others. Acquired immunity is one that is established as a consequence of successfully eradicating an attack of disease producing bacteria. When an infection once exists it is evident that the individual is not immune to that particular organism and to eradicate the infection it is essential to establish an immunity at the earliest possible moment. In treating diphtheria this is accomplished by injecting under the skin diphtheria antitoxin, a ready prepared antibody obtained from the blood serum of some highly immunized animal. An immunity thus established is known as a passive immunity because the individual does not necessarily play an important part in its production.

The successful treatment of diphtheria with the serum method at once created the hope that other infectious diseases could be just as effectively treated with the same method, but on account of an inherent difference in the immunizing process of these organisms, it has been found that animals cannot be immunized to a sufficient intensity to make their serum available for immunizing purposes.

Serum therapy, not being efficient for treating infections caused by the pus group of organisms, quite naturally attention was directed towards hastening the establishment of an active immunity by bacterial inoculations. While Koch, Pasteur and others treated infections with bacterial products before Wright, yet it was his work by using sterile standardized bacterial suspensions, so the dose could be accurately measured, that placed bacterial inoculations as a therapeutic measure on a practical substantial basis. By means of the opsonic index he conclusively showed that the germ destroying power of the blood was materially increased within one or two days after inoculating a sufficient number of sterilized bacteria in cases previously infected with a corresponding organism. This clearly demonstrated the value of bacterial inoculations for therapeutic purposes. He accounts for this action of the vaccine on the ground that immunizing substances are formed in the tissues where the inoculation was made and from there absorbed in the general circulation.

Abundant clinical experience shows that the best results with bacterial vaccines are obtained when treatment is started early in the course of the disease. This can be readily accounted for from what is known concerning the problem of immunity. When an infection takes place the immunizing mechanism is called into activity for the production of immunizing substances. If the infection continues to spread it is evident that the immunizing mechanism is not responding adequately. If now a sufficient number of killed germs of the same kind causing the infection are injected under the skin an occasion for an additional stimulation of the immunizing faculty is created. The germs being dead no harm can be done because they cannot multiply. Furthermore, experience shows that in many instances a progressive infection is distinctly toxic with very little immunizing influence while a dose of vaccine is distinctly immunizing without any toxic effect. Why this should be so may not be so easily explained. It has been supposed that the toxic element in an infective process is the

one that is essentially instrumental in stimulating the defense organs. If this contention were correct, the time would be reached in all infective processes when the immunizing apparatus would be stimulated enough to bring about any immunity, but in many instances, instead of the patient becoming immune he dies of toxemia. We find that in very toxic cases the infection spreads most rapidly. This in itself would indicate that other factors besides the toxic element are essential in the immunizing process.

In typhoid immunization, experience teaches that old nontoxic cultures answer the best purpose. The proteid and not the toxic radical of the organism possesses the immunizing influence. In explaining the toxic character of infection, Prof. Leary suggests (*The Boston Med. and Surgical Journal*, Oct. 6, 1910, page 529), "It is possible that there is some selective action in absorption so that certain beneficial stimulating substances may not be taken up by the lymph stream from the focus of injection." In severe localized infections the toxic element usually causes intense swelling of the surrounding tissues and it is probable that this swollen condition, associated with devitalized tissue cells hinders the absorption of the necessary substances to stimulate the immunizing mechanism. On the other hand when a vaccine is used, dead organisms are injected under the skin and being dead, practically no inflammation is produced, leaving conditions such that free absorption of immunizing substances can take place. In most cases of toxic localized infection produced by streptococci the effect of a dose of streptococcus vaccine is none less than marvelous, the temperature dropping, and swelling subsiding within 24 to 36 hours. This cannot all very well be ascribed to the immunizing substances absorbed from the point of vaccine inoculation. It is more reasonable to suppose that when the swelling in the infected area subsides as a consequence of using the vaccine, additional antibodies are absorbed from the infected tissues.

Some writers contend that bacterial vaccines are contraindicated in general infections, on the theory that giving vaccine to such cases would be simply adding toxic material to a system already overtaxed with toxemia. This contention looks quite plausible, but in actual practice it does not work out. Experience is a good teacher. The unquestionable good results obtained in general staphylococcus infections, pneumonia, typhoid fever, and the early stages of streptococcus infections is quite conclusive evidence that a vaccine consisting of a sufficient number of dead germs, corresponding to the infecting organism, when injected under the skin has a special immunizing influence during the course of an active infection. Why this should be so may not be so easily explained. A series of experiments conducted by Hektoen (Journal of Infectious Diseases, VII, 319), on animals showed that antibacterial substances are not formed in the blood but in the tissues. When giving vaccines in general infections we should also consider that as a consequence of an existing infection the tissue cells in all probability are to a certain extent prepared to produce immunizing substances when met with the stimulating influence of the vaccine. It is also necessary to consider that while the tissues are building up an immunity against the infecting organism the germs are also busy surrounding themselves with defense substances. Prof. James G. Collison (Medical Record, June 24, 1911, page 1137), in attempting to

explain this special immunizing influence of a vaccine in general infection suggests that: By subcutaneous inoculations of dead organisms these bacterial proteids are brought in great concentration into contact with those connective tissue substances which seem to be most active in the production of antibodies, and that the tissue-cell energy under the stimulus of these dead germs is expended in the production of antibodies, while in the progressive infection much of the cell energy is used up in combating the living organism.

Deaver, DaCosta and Pfeiffer (Congress of American Physicians and Surgeons, Vol. VIII, 1910, page 199), in part sum up their results thus: "Specific vaccine treatment in our hands has not proved of benefit in the later stages of streptococcic septicemia." "Staphylococcic septicemia has been treated with most favorable results at all stages."

"Septic intoxications without demonstrated blood invasion in a majority of the cases display general and local improvement under the use of vaccines if given early; the later the treatment the less certain and satisfactory the result."

Prof. Timothy Leary of Boston (Boston Med. and Surgical Journal, Oct. 6, 1911, page 529), says on this subject: "The objections to the use of vaccines in infectious conditions seem to focus themselves against their use in general infections. They will, therefore, be considered here. The general harmlessness of vaccines is indicated by two cases of infection in which, through error, 10 ccm. of staphylococcus pyogenes aureus vaccine containing 10,000,000 organisms were injected at one time as the initial dose. In one case no untoward symptoms appeared. In the second, there was a temporary collapse, with prompt response to heat and stimulation. There are few powerful drugs in the pharmacopeia which could be used with such disregard for dosage without serious results."

"The most obvious objection to the use of vaccines in general infections is that the patient is undergoing extreme intoxication. I have called attention to our theory of muscle immunity, and to the fact that physiological doses of vaccines are not followed by a toxic (negative) phase. The dose of vaccine used in pneumonia, for example, contains fewer organisms than will be found in a few out of the myriads of infected air sacs of the lung in this disease. The dosage is so infinitesimal, and its toxic effect is so slight, if any, that it is not measurable. As evidence that even much larger doses are at least harmless, I might cite the case of a child of seven years undergoing an infection with pneumonia, with a temperature of 103 and extreme meningeal symptoms, into whose body was injected, as an initial dose, 1,600,000,000 pneumococci. This child received sixteen times the adult dose of vaccine. The standard dose for adults is 8 minims, or 100,000,000 pneumococci. A second child with pneumococcus meningitis showed prompt diminution in the cerebrospinal fluid, and sharp amelioration of symptoms accompanying the use of four to eight times the standard adult dose of pneumococcus vaccine."

Prof. J. G. Adami says (*Journal A. M. A.* June 11, 1910, page 1922), "The good results obtained in these cases can no longer be questioned, and what is interesting is that the system evidently benefits from the slight temporary added rise of temperature which shows itself during the six hours or so immediately following the vaccination. ... Time forbids me to do more than note this curious paradox that often such vaccination converts a disease like typhoid fever, that ordinarily recovers by lysis, into a recovery by crisis, and vice versa, time and again cause a disease like pneumonia culminating in crisis into one healing by relatively slow, but favorable lysis."

Dr. W. H. Waters of Boston (*The New England Medical Gazette,* Sept., 1910, page 408), has this to say on this subject: "In general septicemia of streptococcus origin, we have frequently observed distinct amelioration following the hypodermic administration of bacterial emulsions, both autogenous and stock. This is by no means universal, however, some apparently hopeful case finally succumbing to the disease. In even these fatal cases we can usually note clinically an increased degree of resistance on the part of the patient with a correspondingly prolonged fight before finally overcome. It is puerperal septicemia, however, in which some of our most satisfactory results have been obtained."

Russell says: "Vaccination during the disease (typhoid fever) fails to reveal any evidences of a negative phase."

As regards my own experience with bacterial vaccines, I wish to say that it has been quite extensive both in acute and chronic cases, having given over 7,000 doses during the past five years. In addition, I am constantly in consultation here in Detroit, over the 'phone and otherwise, with physicians as regards the progress of their cases being likewise treated. From these observations I find that the vaccine treatment is the best treatment at our command for treating infectious diseases, the most satisfactory results being obtained when given early. From all my experience I have never seen a bad result that could be attributed to the vaccine, nor have I seen a case reported where it was claimed that vaccines given in cases of advanced acute

24   AMERICAN MEDICINE
Complete Series, Vol. XVIII. }   ORIGINAL ARTICLES { JANUARY, 1912.
New Series, Vol. VII., No. 1.

general infection did any harm, from clinical appearances, but on the contrary all claim that such treatment was either harmless or beneficial.

Many advocates of vaccine therapy give the impression that autogenous vaccines are so much better than stocks that autogenous vaccines should always be used where possible. I have had much experience with both. Extensive clinical evidence by many observers shows that in staphylococcus infections properly prepared stock vaccines are just as efficient as autogenous.

Gilchrist (*Congress of American Physicians and Surgeons,* Vol. VIII, 1910, page 164), on the use of staphylococcus vaccine in skin infections says: "Autogenous vaccines were made at first, but later it was found that stock vaccines acted just as well, so the former were not often used." Martin F. Engman (*Congress of American Physicians and Surgeons,* Vol. VIII, page 191), in reference to the use of staphylococcus vaccine says: "Stock suspensions we have found very reliable and can be used in most instances............Autogenous suspensions are indicated where 'stocks fail.'" It is now quite generally admitted that in gonorrheal infections, stock vaccines answer every purpose.

In typhoid infections experience shows that carefully selected old cultures make a better vaccine for treating typhoid fever than autogenous vaccines.

The successful treatment of streptococcus infections is very important because of the danger involved, especially in puerperal fever, infected wounds and erysipelas. Here experience shows that the early use of streptococcus vaccine is of utmost importance. This necessarily implies the use of stock vaccines to obtain the best results

because it takes too long to prepare autogenous vaccines to gain the advantage of early treatment. Many advocate the use of stock vaccines in such cases until an autogenous vaccine can be prepared. Such procedure at once recognizes the value of a stock vaccine and if with this method a patient progresses favorably under the preliminary stock vaccine, how are we to know that he will do better with an autogenous preparation?

The same condition presents itself in treating pneumonia where stock vaccines are of unquestionable value when used early, the earlier the better.

Dr. Wm. A. Repp, one of the staff surgeons in St. Mary's Hospital, Detroit, informs me that he has treated 10 successive cases of perpetual sepsis, using a mixed streptococcus and staphylococcus stock vaccine with uniform good results.

Dr. J. M. Van Cott (*New York State Journal of Medicine,* July, 1911, page 320), after giving tabulated results of 74 cases treated with a mixed streptococcus, staphylococcus and colon bacillus vaccine says: "Analysis of the table results in the following conclusions:

First.—Proper use of the polyvalent vaccine described above is not only harmless, but it is also of positive value in many cases of infection.

Second.—A stock vaccine containing virulent strains has the advantage over the autogenous vaccines of saving valuable time, and being available at any moment for physicians who lack the facilities for procuring autogenous vaccines.

Third.—Vaccination is useless, if the patient be already swamped with toxine. The only hope in such cases is to eliminate the toxine by catharsis, and the Murphy drip, or, where the infecting organism is known, by the use of an anti-serum in conjunction with the vaccine.

Fourth.—Early vaccination offers the best prospect of success."

From my observations, stock vaccines should be used in the early stage of all acute infections, and autogenous vaccines should be made in treating cases where bacterial examination shows an unusual organism present and where stock vaccines have not given the desired results.

As regards the size of the dose required, extensive experience has resulted in adopting approximate standards. It is well to start treatment with an average dose and children should be given from one-quarter to one-half as much. The opsonic index to determine when to repeat the inoculation is not much employed, clinical symptoms being quite as accurate. In acute infections, especially those caused by streptococci and pneumococci, inoculations should be made at comparatively short intervals, varying from 1 to 3 days, while in subacute and chronic cases the interval should be from 3 to 7 days.

The operation of these vaccines being specific the question of making a diagnosis to determine what vaccine to give naturally is very important. In this connection it should be remembered that while clinically we have a large variety of diseases, biologically we have comparatively few. Diseased conditions are usually recognized by the part of the body involved, rather than by the cause of the trouble. Thus we may have a bronchitis, iritis, neuritis, mastoiditis, tonsillitis, endocarditis, arthritis, cystitis, appendicitis, peritonitis, lymphangitis, otitis, erysipelas, septicemia, or even gangrene, all caused by the streptococcus. Clinically these conditions are all different, yet biologically they can only be the same.

The pneumococcus, staphylococcus, gonococcus, colon bacillus, tubercle bacillus and other organisms may cause an equal variety of diseases by attacking different parts of the body. Mixed infections of two or more of the organisms are commonly met with.

In treating diseased conditions with vaccines, the treatment is directed at the cause of the trouble regardless to what part of the body may be involved. Thus the same vaccine is given in a case of rheumatic iritis that is used in a streptococcus infected wound. If diseased conditions were recognized by the causative organism instead of the part of the body involved much confusion would be avoided. In infections where the germ causing the trouble can be procured a positive diagnosis may be obtained by making a bacterial examination. In many cases, however, it is very difficult or impossible to procure a specimen to make a bacterial examination, as for instance in iritis, otitis media in the early stage, in a penetrating wound, such as being caused by tramping on a nail, an appendicitis, etc.

Ordinarily a diagnosis made from clinical symptoms is sufficient for the administration of the vaccines when certain general characteristic symptoms produced by various organisms are observed. In this connection it should be remembered that infections caused by the streptococcus, staphylococcus or pneumococcus are the ones most commonly met with. Of these, infections caused by the streptococcus, are the most dangerous and should be constantly guarded against. Where infections have a tendency to spread rapidly leaving red chains, they may safely be regarded as streptococcic, while those caused by the staphylococcus are more confined near the point of infection. The characteristic picture of erysipelas is easily recognized. Lobar pneumonia by its spectacular ushering in with chill, fever, rapid pulse and respiration and pain in lung while coughing up bloody mucus could not very well be mistaken for any other disease.

Follicular tonsillitis may safely be classed as a streptococcus infection, while pharyngitis and bronchitis are more often mixed infections of the pneumococcus and streptococcus with the staphylococcus coming in as a secondary invader. In appendicitis the colon bacillus is nearly always found, while streptococci or pneumococci when present are very dangerous. Puerperal infections are so dangerous that no one will pass them by lightly and even here where a bacterial examination, by taking a culture from the uterine contents, is possible, it is not advisable to delay the vaccine treatment until a bacterial diagnosis can be made. Time in these cases is a very important factor in getting the system immunized against the invading organism. The streptococcus being the most probably dangerous germ, the patient should be given a dose of streptococcus vaccine at once. In this way the immunizing faculty of the system will be stimulated and an immunity established before the infection has extended sufficiently to do much harm. In puerperal infections we also often have staphylococcus and colon bacillus infections. For this reason it is advisable to give a mixed vaccine containing streptococci and staphylococci. The colon bacillus causes a foul odor to the discharge, and in such cases streptococcus and colon bacillus combination vaccine should be given.

In this connection it is well to consider the question of giving mixed vaccines and what effect such vaccines have if no corresponding infection exists to all the organisms presented in the vaccines. In this regard it should be realized that the dose of vaccine given for therapeutic purposes is small and will make no noticeable impression even if given in health. No one can know how harmless a dose of vaccine is, until he has tried it on himself. In this way only can its harmless character and curative value be thoroughly appreciated.

From these general considerations the tremendous advantages of the vaccine treatment as compared with ordinary medication can readily be seen. The use of medicine ordinarily only gives relief while nature effects a cure. These vaccines, however, are real curative agents. They stimulate the immunizing mechanism and thereby hasten the establishment of an immunity, and a very important factor is that an immunity thus established is an active immunity effecting a permanent cure.

FUNNEL BREAST DEFORMITY (TRICHTER BRUST) CONSIDERED ESPECIALLY IN ITS RELATION TO TUBERCULOSIS OF THE LUNGS AND OTHER DISEASES OF THE CHEST.

BY

HENRY L. SHIVELY, M. D.,
New York City.

Funnel breast deformity was first carefully studied by Ebstein in 1882, but a remarkable case was reported by an anonymous author in the *Gazette des Hôpiteaux* as early as 1860 of a congenital case in which the excavation was the size of an infant's head. C. T. Williams also described in considerable detail a case in 1872. Since then there have been numerous other examples reported, especially in Germany, and the condition is not so rare as was at one time supposed. The acquired form of funnel breast was mentioned as frequently occurring in shoemakers and other artisans by Laennec as long ago as 1825 in the introduction to his treatise on diseases of the chest.

Funnel breast is a singular and striking deformity possessing interest alike for the embryologist, the anatomist, orthopedic surgeon, neurologist, obstetrician, path-

tal angle. The depression resembles an inverted cone, the apex at or near the xiphoid cartilage. The open base is usually circular or oval in outline or may be rhomboid or lozenge shaped in the extreme type of the deformity. There is also a somewhat characteristic alteration in the shape of the entire thorax which is flattened and broader than the normal chest, and the shoulders are often thrown somewhat forward. This is well shown in the cyrtometric tracing in Figure 1.

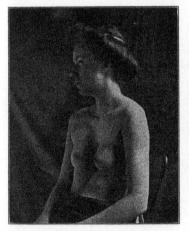

Figure 1. M. K. described as Case IX in text.

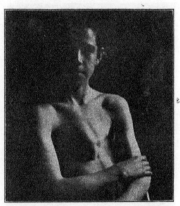

Figure 2. Pigeon chest in brother of patient shown in Figure 3.

ologist, and specialist in diseases of the chest. It is also not without interest for the alienist and pediatrician. In its characteristic and typical form it may be described as a pronounced depression in the anterior thoracic wall of varying depth, corresponding to the body of the sternum or junction of the body with ensiform cartilage. It is limited above usually by the lower border of the manubrium, laterally by the costal cartilages and ribs, and below by the abdominal wall beyond the cos-

Various and rather unsatisfactory explanations as to the etiology of this malformation have been made. Ebstein believed the condition to be due to an early embryological defect and arrest of development of sternum. Eggel ascribed it to a nutritional disturbance which renders the sternum more flexible and capable of being depressed by atmospheric pressure. Schiff and Flesch believe that an abnormal length of the ribs was one of the etiological factors. Hagmann suggested loose chrondro-sternal articulations as a cause. Von Hueter and Niemeyer regarded it as a manifestation of fetal rickets. Against this etiological theory, however, is the opinion of most authorities that rickets is always an acquired disease due to malnutrition. Marfan, however, contrary to the opinion of most of his countrymen, has in the second edition of his authoritative work on rickets abandoned the contention that rickets is never congenital and has gone over to the views of the German and Aus-

fact. A number of cases were reported by him and also by Ribbert in which the chin of the newborn child exactly fitted into the deformity. In other cases an adducted knee or elbow, or in the case of twins, the head of one child impinging upon the breast bone of the other may be the cause. Ribbert suggested that a deficiency of liquor amnii may be a predisposing factor in the production of this pressure effect upon the soft fetal tissues. Raubitschek has recorded an interesting case of tem-

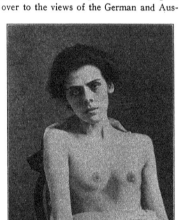

Figure 3. L. L., Case VIII, marked funnel breast in tuberculous patient.

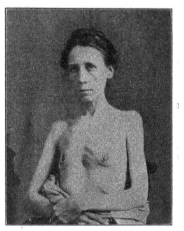

Figure 4. Shallow funnel breast with tuberculosis of lungs. Described as Case VII.

trian authorities that there are undoubted cases of congenital rickets. Gaucher, Crouzon and Fournier have regarded many cases of Trichter Brust to be due to hereditary syphilis.

A number of French observers, including Marie and Ramadier and Sérièux have pronounced it one of the numerous stigmata of degeneracy. Many cases are undoubtedly due to intrauterine pressure. Zuckerkandl was the first to emphasize this

porary funnel breast in a recently delivered twin in which the deformity disappeared within two weeks. Hagmann has considered one of his cases to be due to the continued pressure of the heels of the child upon the breast bone in a breech presentation. Heredity is an undoubted factor in some cases. In three cases reported by Klemperer, two were brothers. Vetlesen described a case in which he thought the deformity had been produced by the pressure of the thumbs upon the thorax in vigorous and successful efforts to resuscitate an asphyxiated, newborn child.

The malformation is frequently associated with other deformities, scoliosis is not infrequently present, sometimes club foot and hammertoe. Hoffa and Chlumsky have described it in association with congenital dislocation of the hip. It is occasionally associated with knock knees or bowlegs, which would suggest a rachitic origin, although pigeon breast is the typi-

and retraction of the chest wall. Osler believes that some cases in young children are caused by enlarged tonsils and adenoids. Landouzy and Déjerine have described a number of cases of acquired funnel breast occurring in patients with progressive muscular atrophy. The cyrtometric tracing shown in Figure 10 was taken from a patient with progressive muscular atrophy of the facio-scapulohumeral type. This patient had the exophthalmos, the thick lips, immobility of

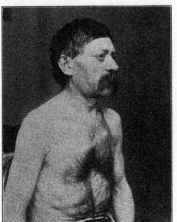

Figure 5. Well marked trichter brust in a case of aneurism of aorta.

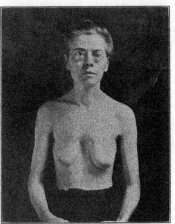

Figure 6. Deep funnel breast without chest symptoms.

cal thoracic deformity in rickets. In this connection is shown in Figure 2 a typical and extreme example of pectus carinatum, the patient a younger brother of the girl shown in Figure 3 with a strikingly marked funnel breast deformity, the abnormal projection in the former equaling the deep excavation in the latter. Jacobi of New York has seen cases which he considers to be due to inflammation of the mediastinal and bronchial glands producing adhesions

expression, and winged scapulae so characteristic of this affection. He also had a displaced and dilated heart.

Funnel breast is also reported by many French writers as a somatic anomaly occurring along with ogival palate, prognathism, adherent ear lobules, faulty implantation of the teeth, syndactylism, supernumerary digits, imperfectly developed or absent metacarpal bones, cryptorchidism, strabismus, vitiligo and other stigmata of degeneracy of the mentally defective, imbeciles, insane and epileptic. Rieder has described cases of Trichter Brust in which portions of the pectoralis major and minor muscles were wanting. In the ascendancy of many patients a history of tuberculosis, alcoholism, syphilis or epilepsy is found. Chapard relates a case which was due to the retraction of a mediastinal metastasis of sarcoma of the testicle. Not infrequently the xiphoid of the sternum is absent or undeveloped.

Neurologists have frequently observed funnel breast deformity in connection with such psychoses as melancholia, hypochrondriasis, hysteria, convulsions, tics and stut-

Funnel breast deformity in the majority of cases is to be regarded merely as a pathological curiosity of little clinical significance and not requiring treatment. In some cases of marked degree such as is shown in Figure 1, the condition may be possibly one of great gravity if with the deformity a left sided pleurisy with effusion should occur. In at least one such case the heart action was seriously embarrassed on account of the organ being incapable of shifting its position to the right, as usually occurs in a pleurisy of the left side. The heart imprisoned in the left chest by the extreme deformity of the thoracic wall and subjected to pressure by the

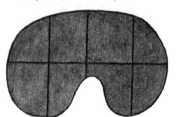

Figure 7. Cyrtometric tracing of Case IX, Fig. 1.

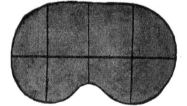

Figure 8. Cyrtometric tracing of Case XIV.

tering, and pediatricians have remarked upon its not infrequent occurrence in defective and backward children, who are late in speech and walking, associated with asymmetries of the face, inequalities of the limbs on the two sides and hyperextensibility of the joints.

E. Testart reports an interesting case of acquired Trichter Brust consecutive to a pleurisy in a patient who had tuberculosis of the lungs. Béclèrc reports a case of Trichter Brust occurring in a patient with empyema. Marie observed a case associated with stenosis of the aorta and a lesion of the tricuspid valve.

large accumulation of pleuritic fluid, became extremely rapid and weak in action; the patient suffered from dyspnea and symptoms of syncope, and was only saved from impending death by a prompt aspiration of the pleuritic fluid. G. Rosenfeld has described a case of marked displacement of the heart downward and to the left, with palpitation, dyspnea, and inability to lie on the left side, due to well marked Trichter Brust deformity.

As treatment Chlumsky has even suggested a plastic operation where the heart and lung function are seriously impeded. In congenital cases and in young children with soft flexible thoracic walls, much may be accomplished by manual exercises and lateral compression with the hands upon the thorax. Deep breathing exercises and blowing upon a trumpet against resistance have also been suggested as measures to overcome the deformity. Hoffa has suggested a traction treatment by means of strips of plaster attached to the depressed portion of the chest and fastened to a band about the thorax. In young children suction by a vacuum apparatus may be applied to draw out and expand the retracted portion of the chest wall.

Mühlhauser reports a case with only three inches between the breast bone and

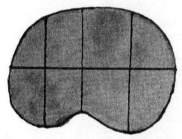

Figure 9. Cyrtometric tracing of Case XII.

the vertebral column. In the cyrtometric tracing of M. K., Figure 7, the antero-posterior diameter of the chest measured opposite the deepest portion of the excavation was 12 c. m. which allowing for the soft parts shows even a greater degree of deformity than in Mühlhauser's case.

Eichhorst in an examination of 14,000 patients found only six cases of Trichter Brust. He reports thirty cases in which there is a much greater incidence of the deformity in men than in women, twenty-three men to seven women, 76.7 per cent. to 23.3 per cent. Ebstein collected 97 cases of whom 87 were men and ten women.

Goesche in his series of twenty-four cases reported nineteen men and five women.

Following are brief notes of the histories of sixteen cases of well marked funnel breast deformity seen by the writer in the past five years at the Presbyterian Hospital Tuberculosis Clinic, at St. Joseph's Hospital for Consumptives and in private practice. None of these cases has previously been reported.

Case I. G. B., aet. 62, a native of Armenia, proprietor of a restaurant. No history of deformity or hereditary disease in his family. His health has been good until two months ago when his appetite failed. He began to cough, had purulent sputa, pain in chest, shortness of breath, chilly sensations and fever. These symptoms have continued to the present time.

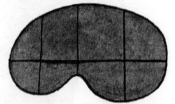

Figure 10. Cyrtometric tracing of Case XVII.

Physical Examination: Poorly nourished; the heart is normal and there are no positive morbid pulmonary signs. There is revealed however, a remarkable deformity involving the lower third of the sternal region and the upper part of the abdominal wall included in the costal angle. There is a marked "Trichter Brust" depression, the deepest point corresponding to the junction of the xiphoid and body of the sternum. The size of the excavation would about correspond to that of the closed fist, as indicated in sketch. Patient did not return for cyrtometric tracing or measurements. Figure 11 shows very well the degree of deformity.

Case II. W. M., aet. 23. Machinist. No history of tuberculosis or deformity in his family. Has had a cough for five weeks, mucopurulent sputa, hemoptysis, pains in chest, chills, fever, night sweats, loss of flesh and strength.

Physical Examination: Well nourished and not anemic. Well marked dulness, bronchial breathing over both upper lobes. Patient presents a well marked funnel breast, circumference of which is oval in outline, the greatest depth of the depression corresponding to tip of xiphoid appen-

side and dyspnea on exertion. Menstruation is irregular.

Physical Examination: Excessively pale; heart and lungs are normal. Presents a marked funnel breast deformity.

Case IV. May D., aet. 32, saleswoman. Has had several attacks of acute articular rheumatism, one of which at the age of fifteen was very severe. Since then she has

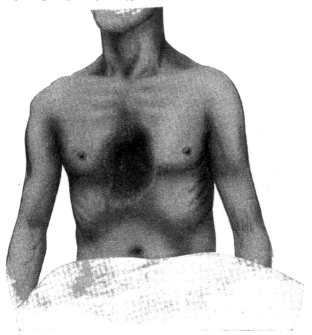

Figure 11. Drawing of Case I.

dix. He thinks he has always had this peculiar chest formation, and no other deformity is present.

Case III. Simple anemia. M. G., aet. 21, housemaid. Family history negative. A year ago was operated on at the German Hospital for a right sided pleurisy with effusion. For two months she has been feeling badly, has lost flesh and is easily fatigued. Complains of pain in her right

had palpitation and pain about heart, dyspnea on exertion, cough and hemoptysis and poor appetite.

Physical Examination: Emaciated, pale. Cardiac area enlarged downward and to left. To the left of the ensiform cartilage is heard a murmur of moderate intensity, presystolic in time and not transmitted. A thrill is felt at the apex. In second space to left of the sternum is heard a double murmur, the systolic element transmitted upward and to the right, the diastolic can be followed down the sternum. Pulse 90, regular. This patient presents a marked Trichter Brust deformity.

Case V. J. W., aet. 25, native of Ireland; clerk. No history of tuberculosis or deformity in family. For six months patient has had cough, purulent sputa, loss of flesh and strength, fever, night sweats and poor appetite.

Physical Examination: He is pale and emaciated and lungs show dulness and increased breathing over both upper lobes. Temperature 99.8 F. At lower end· of sternum there is a rather shallow but typical·funnel breast deformity.

Case VI. L. C., aet. 36, native of Ireland, laborer. Family history negative as to tuberculosis and deformities. For fifteen months has had a cough, muco-purulent sputa, pain in side, loss of flesh and strength, poor appetite. On physical examination there are dulness, increased breathing and fine râles over both apices. Temperature 99.2. Comprehending lower half of sternum and extending laterally to costal cartilages there is a well marked funnel breast of a circular outline.

Case VII. K. L., aet. 34. Housewife. No morbid family history of significance, no deformity, no tuberculosis. She has had a cough for twelve years, purulent sputa which is blood streaked at times, loss of flesh and strength; chills, fever, and sweats, pains in chest, scanty menstruation. On physical examination is pale and ill nourished. There is dulness, increased vocal fremitus, bronchial breathing and whispering broncophony over both upper lobes. Temperature 100, weight 100½, a year ago, 110. Tubercle bacilli present in sputum. Lower third of sternum is marked by a depression showing a grooved or gutter type of "Trichter Brust" deformity, (Figure 4) which patient has had as long as she can remember. The cavity of the depression will hold six fluid drams of water.

Case VIII. L. L., aet. 18, skirt binder. Father died of "bronchitis"; a brother has a marked pigeon chest deformity. Cough for a year and a half, muco-purulent sputa, hemoptysis, pain in chest, loss of flesh and strength, poor appetite, indigestion, chills, fever, night sweats, dyspnea, scanty menstruation.

Physical Examination: Poorly nourished, excessively anemic. Chest is broad and flat, short antero-posterior diameter, and presents a typical deep conical excavation involving lower third of sternal region and abdominal wall between cartilages of false ribs. The superior circumference of the de-,pression is of a somewhat rhomboid or lozenge shaped outline (Figure 3). There is marked dulness and increased breathing over both upper lobes. Temperature 101, weight 106½, a year ago 126. She is the fourth of ten children. So far as she knows she has always had her chest deformity.

Case IX. M. K., aet. 21, cook. Family history negative as to tuberculosis or deformity. Scarlet fever and diphtheria when two years old. Has had a cough, which is worse in the winter, since the age of fourteen. The sputum is purulent, and there was slight hemoptysis two days ago. There has been considerable loss of flesh and strength, she is short of breath on slight exertion. Appetite is variable and digestion poor. She has had no night sweats, has frequent chilly sensations and fever afternoons, and complains of pain in chest. Menstruation is scanty. On physical examination she is tall and rather poorly nourished, chest is broad and rather flat and presents a remarkable malformation. The entire anterior chest wall looks to be pushed back in a deep excavation of a conical form, the deepest point of which is 7 cm. from the undepressed surface (Figure 1) of the chest. The cyrtometric tracing (Figure 7) gives a good idea of the extent of the deformity which is attributed by her mother to the attack of scarlet fever and diphtheria she had when two years old. She was born with a well formed chest. There is dulness and increased breathing over right upper lobe and left apex. Temperature 99½, pulse 90; respiration 20. Weight 121 pounds, six months ago 131. Was admitted to Stonywold Sanitarium Dec. 4th, 1908, where she made a very good recovery from her tuberculosis.

Case X. Mrs. R. D., aet. 48; married, housewife. Family history negative. No important previous illnesses. Mother of three children. Cough for three years, muco-purulent sputa, occasional hemoptysis, loss of flesh and strength, chilly sensations, fever afternoons. Has had a few night sweats, appetite and digestion poor.

Physical Examination: Very much emaciated, pale, sallow. Marked dulness, bronchial breathing and whisper over both upper and right middle lobes, over the entire chest subcrepitant râles. Temperature 99.8, pulse 114. From the junction of the manubrium and body of the sternum there is a considerable excavation and depression shared in by the abdominal wall included in the costal angle and bounded laterally by the costal cartilages of the fourth, fifth, sixth and seventh ribs. This depression is of a general oval contour and its maximum depth is half an inch below the level of the nipple line and corresponds to the union of the ensiform cartilage and gladiolus. From this point there extends a vertical groove or sulcus one and one-half inches in length which is gradually lost in the abdominal wall above the umbilicus. This marked deformity developed subsequent to her tuberculosis and has gradually increased. There is no scoliosis or other malformation and no history of similar deformity in her family.

Case XI. E. F., aet. 29, stenographer. Her father died of hasty consumption, also a brother and both paternal grandparents. Had an attack of mucous colitis at the age of sixteen and has had attacks at intervals since until a year ago when they ceased. She has had a cough for eighteen months. Purulent sputa, no hemoptysis. Marked loss of flesh and strength, chilly sensations, fever afternoons, pain in the chest, slight night sweats, menstruation scanty and irregular. Appetite poor. Suffers from indigestion.

Physical Examination: She is ill nourished and has a poorly developed flat chest with a typical funnel breast deformity, the greatest depth of the concavity corresponding to the tip of the ensiform cartilage. Dulness, bronchial breathing and whisper, fine râles over both upper and right middle lobe, more marked over the right side. Temperature 99½, pulse 120, weight 95½, a year ago 116.

Case XII. C. C., aet. 12, school girl; family history negative as to tuberculosis, chest or other deformities. She has had measles, whooping cough and an attack of pneumonia when five years old. Came under treatment December 27th, 1909. For three years she has had a winter cough which has been much worse for the past three weeks. Muco-purulent sputa, fever afternoons, loss of flesh and strength, pain in the back, night sweats for a week, chills, dyspnea on exertion. Appetite and digestion good.

Physical Examination: She is tall for her age but slight, she has a fair white skin, arched eyebrows, long eyelashes, tapering fingers, a good example of the romantic type of tuberculosis. She has a well marked and typical funnel breast deformity which is shown in the cyrtometric tracing in Figure 9. There are dulness, increased vocal fremitus, exaggerated whisper and breathing over right upper lobe, and in the left axilla and below the scapula an area of dulness and moist râles. Temperature 99.6, pulse 88, respiration 20, weight 88 lbs. No tubercle bacilli in the sputum.

Case XIII. Marion M., a girl aet. 7 whose mother died of pulmonary tuberculosis and who from the age of two has been an inmate of St. Joseph's Hospital. Has always been a delicate child, has frequent attacks of vomiting and indigestion, and had measles nine months ago. Has had a hacking cough from infancy. On physical examination is pale and ill nourished, cheeks are flushed, cervical glands are enlarged. There is dulness, bronchial breathing and whisper over the right upper lobe, percussion note high pitched over left apex. The chest is asymmetrical, poorly developed, and shows a well marked funnel breast deformity, the point of deepest depression corresponding to the junction of the xiphoid and body of the sternum.

Case XIV. Mary O., aet. 34. Family history negative, as to tuberculosis and deformities. Has always been well. Cough for three weeks; muco-purulent sputa, pains in chest. On physical examination no morbid pulmonary or cardiac signs, but presents a well marked funnel breast which begins nine centimetres below the sternal notch, the point of maximum depression corresponding to the ensiform cartilage. The cyrtometric tracing is shown in Figure 8. She has no other malformation and no stigmata of degeneration.

Case XV. The patient with aneurism of the ascending portion of the arch of the aorta shown in Figure 5.

Case XVI. Mrs. O. B., with no chest symptoms. A patient of Dr. John B. Solley, to whom the writer is indebted for the photograph (Figure 6), and permission to include the case in this paper.

Case XVII. A case of Trichter Brust occurring in a boy aet. 18, with progressive muscular atrophy of the Landouzy-Déjerine type. Cyrtometric tracing shown in Figure 10. This patient also had a greatly dilated heart.

In the cases here reported only well marked examples have been shown. In any chest clinic where many patients are examined there are numerous cases presenting slight gutter like or shallow depressions with asymmetries of the chest which merge by insensible gradations into the characteristic and typical forms of funnel breast.

It is somewhat remarkable that in this series of seventeen cases, eleven are in women and but six are in men. As already noted a much greater incidence of the condition in men than in women has hitherto been reported. That ten of these cases were seen in patients with tuberculosis of the lungs is largely accounted for by the fact that the majority of them occurred in a tuberculosis hospital service. It is quite conceivable, however, that in its extreme forms funnel breast deformity by limiting the normal respiratory movements of the thorax, and thus preventing the full expression and development of the lungs may be a predisposing cause of tuberculosis of some significance.

303 Amsterdam Ave.

BIBLIOGRAPHY.

Gazette des Hôpitaux, Jan., 1860, p. 10.
Ebstein, W., Deutsch. Archiv. f. Klin. Med. 30 XXX, 1882, p. 411.
Noica et Haret, Bull. de la Société Anatomique de Paris, 1899.
Goesche, H., Ueber Trichter Brust Inaugural Dissertation, Berlin, 1895.
Hoffa, Lehrbuch der Orthopädischen Chirurgie, 5th Ed. Stuttgart, 1905.
Eichhorst, H., Erworbene Trichterbrust Beutsch. Archiv. f. Klin. Med. Bd. 48, pp. 613-618.
Thèse de Paris. Le Thorax en Entonnoir dans ses Rapports avec l'hérédo, Syphilis, 1907.
Dubreuil, Chambordel, Malformations Cardio Thoraciques, etc., Bull. et Mém. Soc. d'Anthrop. de Paris, 1907—55, VIII, p. 409.
Bystrow, P., Ueber die Angeborene Trichterbrust Archiv. f. Orthop. Wiesbaden, 1907, VI, pp. 10-28.
Preleitner, K., Wien. Klin. Woch., 1906, XIX, p. 1499.
Renzi, Mitt. aus den Grenzgeb. d. Med. u. Chir. Jena, 1906, XVI, p. 562.
Testart, E., Contribution à l'étude du sternum infundibuliforme, Paris, 1906, p. 58.
Rehn, H., Die Wichtigsten Formveränderungen des Menschlichen Burstkorbs, Wien, 1875.
Allison, S. C., Depression of the upper and anterior aspect of the thorax, etc., London Jour. of Med. 1851, 3, p. 1070.
Chowne, Congenital malformation of the chest, Lancet, 1851, II, p. 229.
Coulson, W., Deformities of the chest, London Med. Gaz. 1829, IV, p. 69.
Eggel, Archiv. f. Path. Anat. Berlin, 1870, XLIX, p. 230.
Flesch, M., Archiv. f. Path. Anat. Berlin, 1873, LVII, p. 289.
Hagmann, N. Jahrbuch f. Kinderheil. Leipzig, 1880, XV, p. 455.
Langer, Zuckerkandl, Allg. Wien. Med. Ztg. 1880, XXV, p. 514.
Rees, G. A., London Med. Gaz. 1839, Vol. I, p. 557.
Williams, C. T., Congenital Malformations of the Thorax. Tr. Path. Soc. London, 1872, XXXIII, p. 50.
Ebstein, Samuel, Klin. Vortr. n. f. Inn. Med. No. 167-8, Leipzig, 1909.
Rosenfeld, G., Festschrift des Stuttgarter, Arzt. Vereins 1897, p. 115.
Fabre, Thèse de Paris, 1899.
Larrabee, F. W., Phila. Med. Jour. Vol. IV, p. 884.
Picqué et Colombani, Revue d'Orthopèdie, 1900, No. 3, p. 157.
Chlumsky, Zeitsch. f. Orthopäd. Chir. 1901, Bd. 8, p. 465.
Gaucher, La Semaine Médicale 1901, p. 359.
Judson, Medical News, 1901, LXXVIII, p. 643.
Preleitner, K., Zentralblatt Klin. Med. 1907, I p. 26.
Raubitschek, F., Archiv. f. Orthopäd. Mechanotherapie, 1906 Bd. 4, p. 87.

36   AMERICAN MEDICINE }
Complete Series, Vol. XVIII. }   ORIGINAL ARTICLES   { JANUARY, 1912.
{ New Series, Vol. VII., No. 1.

Arneill, J. R., Philadelphia Med. Jour. 1899, p. 559.

Fisher, T., Deformities of the chest in children, Brit. Jour. of Children's Dis., London, 1906, Vol. III, p. 7.

Moreau, Gqz. Méd. de Centre, 1906, XI, p. 104.

Saint Martin, Gaz. Med. de Nantes, 1906, XXIV, p. 53.

Silberstein, Zeitsch. f. Orthop. Chir. 1905, Vol. XV, p. 24.

Variot, Rev. Gen. de Clin. et de Therap., Paris, 1906, XX, p. 23.

Béclèrc, Bull. de la Soc. Méd. Jan. 18th, 1895.

Flesch, M., Virchow's Archiv. Bd. 57, p. 289.

Fournier, Thèse de Paris, 1897.

Clement, Thèse de Paris, 1905.

Ramadier et Sérièux, ·Bull. de Soc. de Anthrop., May, 1891.

Chapard, Thèse de Paris, 1896.

Marie, P., Jour. de la Soc. Med. des Hôpitaux, 1895, p. 808.

Appert, Bull. de la Soc. des Med. Hopit. 1899.

Klemperer, G., Deut. Med. Woch., July, 1888, p. 732.

Woillez, Union Médicale, 1860.

Mühlhauser, Deutsch. Archiv. 1883 Bd. 33, p. 98.

Ribbert, Deutsch. Med. Woch. 1884, p. 533.

Kundmüller, Deutsch. Archiv. 1885, Bd. 26, p. 543.

Vetlesen, H. G., Zentralblatt f. Klin. Med. 1886, No. 43, p. 745.

Frey, Deutsch. Med. Woch. 1887, No. 27, p. 645.

Herbst, E., Archiv. f. Klin. Med. 1887, Bd. 41, p. 308.

Déjerine, J., Compt. Rend. de la Soc. de Biologie, 1891, p. 508.

Féré, C., et Schmid, Jour. de l'Anat. et Phys., Paris, 1893, Tome 29, p. 564.

Marfan, A. B., Rachitisme in Maladies des Os, Brouardel et Gilbert, Paris, 1912.

INGROWN NAIL.

The removal of a wedge of skin (*American Journal of Surgery*) at the side of an ingrown nail, as in Cotting's operation, is rarely necessary and usually objectionable. Granulations disappear quickly when the nail segment is withdrawn; if they are exuberant they may be snipped or burned off.

ACUTE NEPHRITIS.

Unless dropsy is present (*Medical Standard*) the patient may be given to drink freely of a beverage consisting of a dram or two of potassium bitartrate added to a pint of boiling water, flavored with lemon juice and a bit of lemon peel. The mixture should be allowed to cool before drinking.

THE PREVENTION OF ANAPHYLAXIS.

BY

O. L. MULOT, M. D.,

Brooklyn, N. Y.

The role that sera are destined to play, in the treatment of acute infectious diseases, must be evident to everyone who has intelligently followed the efforts and results along this line. Simply because wholly satisfactory products have as yet not been realized for all diseases in which serum treatment is logical and the justified hope, is no ground for pessimism. Some slight modification of technique, today not thought of, may tomorrow bring the realized hopes.

But beside the optimism of serum treatment stands, like a grim forbidding spectre, anaphylaxis; mocking and taunting us that though we may cheat death of some of its immediate victims, we do so at the risk of prematurely throwing others in the arms of the Grim Reaper. By using the rectum as the way for administrating the curative serum, it is true we can ignore the danger of anaphylaxis, but this security is purchased at the expense of a much slower absorption; nor is this slower absorption the only drawback to this mode of procedure, but we also sacrifice some of the potency of our dose. There are cases and times, as in meningitis, when the delayed action due to slower absorption and a loss of the full effect of the dose, may seriously threaten the success of our therapeutics.

In another class of cases, as in acute tuberculosis, in which anaphylaxis is particularly prone to be encountered, the loss of the full potency entails the use of more serum and so adds materially to the cost of the treatment.

These things, taken all in all, are indeed sufficiently important to stimulate a search for means to overcome this danger. It was long held that the phenomena of serum disease were due to some error, some defect, or deterioration of the serum administered, but as both Hallion and Besredka point out, that this is most frequently encountered when the second administration of serum occurs, such a theory is based upon error. Further, this point is of capital importance to the practitioner; he continually sees cases of diphtheria or pseudo-diphtheria in which only the microscope will give the positive diagnosis, but these cases may be of such apparent severity that the physician does not feel justified in waiting 24 or 36 hours for a report from the laboratory before injecting antitoxin. Now, if at some previous time that patient has had an immunizing or therapeutic injection, the doctor must be prepared for and may expect anaphylaxis. The severity of these phenomena may vary from a trifling urticarial rash to the severest and most distressing symptoms of collapse and impending dissolution—even death has frequently occurred—against all of which our efforts and means are largely if not entirely impotent. Since we have no means of foretelling when we may be brought face to face with serum disease in its worst form, every conscientious physician administers a serum injection with considerable trepidation and he that does not, to him applies the quotation about, "Fools rush in, etc."

It has been sought to avoid these accidents by addition of various substances to the serum, but all such attempts have only resulted in failures. Besredka, of the Paris Pasteur Institute, convinced that nothing was to be gained by further search along that line, attacked the problem from an entirely different point. Previously anaphylactized guinea pigs, he chloroformed, and while they were under narcosis, injected them with serum; no anaphylactic symptoms followed. He next administered a large dose of alcohol and after the period of excitement was passed, he injected the serum without untoward results. From a purely scientific point, these results were very instructive but for clinical purposes entirely unavailable. Now the same investigator had observed that, when a guinea pig had successfully withstood a dose of serum, and had recovered from anaphylactic phenomena, it then was in an antianaphylactic state or we may describe it as having been vaccinated against anaphylaxis; taking his hint from this he began by injecting very small doses of serum. If a series of guinea pigs showed an anaphylaxis to a dose of 1/10 of a cubic centimeter, he injected 1/50 or even less, 1/100, then an half hour later a dose of 1/10 c. c., then a little later he injected 1 c. c., a dose ten times greater than the one at first fatal. The rapidity with which this anti-anaphylactic state was established, differed very much according to whether the vaccinating injection was made into the peritoneum, or subcutaneously, or intra-venously. Thus, four hours were necessary for the establishment of anti-anaphylaxis after a subcutaneous injection; from one to two hours when the injection was made into the peritoneum or into the cerebro-spinal canal, while if made intravenously, it occurred after half a minute, and may be considered almost instantaneous. Thanks to Besredka, we have but to observe his technique, to avoid, what under certain conditions may give rise to most deplorable results. By making our serum injections into veins, first a drop, a half a minute later a few, then after a little time some more and so on, we may safely inject any size of serum dose without fear; the whole not requiring more than five minutes more than we now give to the same operation. The increased safety is well worth the extra time.

424 Halsey St.

CERVICAL MYOMA; REPORT OF A CASE; OPERATION; RECOVERY.

BY

M. CISIN, M. D.,
New York City.

The case I wish to report because of its somewhat unusual character gave the following history:

Female, age thirty-five years, and single. Family history negative. In her early life she suffered from a severe form of rachitis resulting in a dorso-lumbar curvature of the spine (or kyphosis) and a flat pelvis with contraction in all its diameters. Her menstruation appeared at the age of fourteen years, and has been regular and painless until about two years ago. At that time she began to suffer from dysmenorrhea. The first few months the pain was not very severe, coming on one day before, and lasting through the first day of menstruation. At this time the pain was relieved by ordinary anodyne treatment, and there were no symptoms during the intermenstrual periods. Later on, however, the suffering became more severe and of longer duration. About three months previous to my first visit, she was compelled to remain in bed throughout a whole period suffering from a persistent, intense dysmenorrhea with a cramp-like and boring pain in the hypogastrium; the flow was scanty, but constant; she was very anemic and nervous and her general health was notably depressed.

The abdominal pain was so severe that even the free use of morphine hypodermatically only partially relieved the suffering.

On bimanual examination, the vaginal portion of the cervix was found to be very much enlarged, filling the upper part of the vaginal canal; through the os which was dilated the size of a cent, thus admitting the tip of the examining finger, the smooth surface and firm consistency of the bulging tumor could be easily felt. The attenuated cervical wall tightly stretched upon the tumor produced an impression similar to the beginning of labor in a primipara. Upon these characteristic physical signs, I based my diagnosis of submucous fibro-myoma of the cervix; excluding the possible mucous polypus which is usually oval in shape, often lobulated and of softer consistency. The body of the uterus was much enlarged and in retroposition. For obvious reasons, removal of the tumor through the cervix by morcellation, or by the way of a vaginal hysterectomy was out of question. My advice of abdominal hysterectomy was accepted. By reason of the convexity of the posterior aspect of the body, caused by the spinal curvature, the abdomen presented a deep concavity between the thorax and pubes, similar to a Turkish saddle, rendering the abdominal walls lax, and flabby and the distance between those prominences comparatively small. Consequently, any incision in the median line, although extended above the umbilicus was necessarily insufficient for satisfactory manipulation. Indeed, the general enfeebled and anemic condition of the patient in addition to her deformity was not of the kind to encourage even a man who does hysterectomies many times a week.

I frankly admit my apprehension, when confronted with the fact that a case of this nature was under my care in the private ward of the Beth Israel Hospital. Nevertheless, realizing the urgency of the operation it was undertaken as soon as her condition warranted. A median abdominal incision was made and the uterus lifted out of the incision. It presented an oblong mass of two distinct tumors, separated by a constriction at the level with the internal os.

Both ovaries were undergoing cystic degeneration and the bladder was firmly adherent to the cervix. The usual procedure was then followed of ligating the ovarian vessels, and round ligaments, as well as the detachment of the vesico-uterine fold, after which smooth sailing was naturally effected.

Not so, however, with the separation of the firmly adherent bladder; especially embarrassing, in fact almost impossible was the ligation of the uterine vessels. The large cervical myoma filled the lower pelvis to such an extent that there was actually no space to reach the wedged in uterine vessels.

Following the suggestion of Dr. Louis J. Ladinski (to whom I wish to express my warm thanks for his kind assistance and excellent advice), I bisected the body of the uterus in the median line down to the internal os, and extracted the exposed cervical myoma with a Musseau forceps. This helped to reduce the bulk of the cervix, and I was enabled to complete the operation in the usual manner.

The patient made a good recovery, and left the hospital after three weeks perfectly well.

The interesting points in this case are, viz.:·

In the first place, while it is true that tumors in the cervix are of frequent occurrence, they are mostly of the mucous polyp variety, or myomata that have had their origin in the body of the uterus and slowly descend into the cervix by uterine contractions. In the case under discussion, however, indisputable evidence leaves no doubt that this myoma was originated and developed in the cervix, in spite of the statements of many observers, especially of Prof. Winter of Berlin, that pure cervical myomata are rarely seen.

In conclusion, I wish to mention the fact, that in such and similar cases, where all the landmarks are obliterated and the danger of secondary hemorrhage is so great, the method of procedure cannot follow exactly the same routine plan as in the simpler forms of hysterectomy. The procedure advised by Dr. Ladinski seems to me, is at once the most advisable, and the safest.

And lastly, this very case should serve as an important warning that in all cases of prolonged and severe dysmenorrhea, we must not rely upon drugs without investiga-

tion to ascertain the underlying cause, even in virgins. The same week this patient went to the hospital, she was already prepared by another colleague for a simple curettage at her home.

THE USE OF A NEW OPIUM PREPARATION BEFORE ANESTHESIA —A PRELIMINARY NOTE WITH A REPORT OF 50 CASES.[1]

BY

ALFRED M. HELLMAN, M. D.,
Anesthetist to the German and Har Moriah Hospitals.

The drug that I have been investigating, though much employed on the European continent has never before been dealt with in this country. The great deluge of new pharmaceutical preparations that is steadily sweeping down upon the physician and crying for his attention makes an explanation necessary before calling on him to consider still another.

· My ever-increasing dissatisfaction with morphine before anesthesia and my realizing in common with other anesthetists and most surgeons, the need of making the induction stage of anesthesia easier for the patient, and the need of lessening the quantity of anesthetic used, made me at once wish to try pantopon after my attention had been called to this drug and I had read among other articles those of Sahli and Brustlein.

Let me briefly state my objections to morphine so that we may consider afterwards whether pantopon does away with all or even some of them. Shallow, insufficient respiration, inactive or absent corneal re-

[1] Read before the Clinical Society of the German Hospital, May 13, 1911.

flex, contracted inactive pupil and an abnormally slow pulse during anesthesia, and an occasional morphine collapse, no effect on the post-operative vomiting, but afterwards restlessness, constipation and lessening of the secretions.

Pantopon, first introduced by Sahli in 1909, is an opium preparation containing the total alkaloids of opium in readily soluble form, and suitable for hypodermic injection in sterile solution. It is obtainable in tablets or compressed powders of $\frac{1}{6}$ gr. or in solution $\frac{1}{3}$ gr. in each glass vial. This using of the total alkaloids is contrary to the modern therapeutic tendency, which is to use as much as possible only chemical principles, but, as Sahli says, "it is nevertheless justified so long as the secondary alkaloids of opium in their pure state are difficult to isolate and their action has been insufficiently studied (particularly on human beings) and perhaps even not all of them are known."

The dose of pantopon is gr. $\frac{1}{6}$ to gr. $\frac{1}{3}$ hypodermatically and may be repeated with safety. The method of investigation generally used in the following fifty cases was to give every case that came along, some children excepted, one injection of gr. $\frac{1}{3}$ pantopon combined with 1-100 atropine as nearly $\frac{3}{4}$ hours before operation as possible. This was difficult, for, as cases are operated one after another in a general hospital, some would receive the injection too early when the previous operation took longer than expected and the effects would wear off too soon, and others received their injection at the last moment and not until near the end of the operation did the effects become manifest. The anesthesia was administered by the house staff in the regular course of their duties and I made and tabulated the observations. The anesthetics were ether and anesthol on an open mask.

In all cases the pulse was steadied and but slightly slowed. Respirations were shallow, but less so than with morphine. Pupils contracted but as a rule able to react. Corneal and other reflexes remained active and no collapse of any kind was noticed.

We see from a careful perusal of the fifty cases that not one was harmed by the injection—there was nothing resembling a collapse.

Case 17—Where operation started 5 minutes after injection, there was no effect from drug noted throughout. The patient was very alcoholic, and was having bullets removed from knee and chest.

Case 22—A bad phlegmon in an alcoholic where morphine and scopolamin were likewise ineffectual.

Case 43—An interrupted anesthesia for ulcer of tongue was unaffected by the drug.

All other cases at some time during the course of the operation showed some beneficial effect from the injection. The induction was noted as not being especially quiet in only eleven cases, of which in three the injection was given within 10 minutes of onset of anesthesia; in five others only 35 minutes or less had elapsed; in one, 60 minutes; in one, 80 minutes; and in one, 2 hours. The operations ranged from curettage to hysterectomy and from phlegmon to a Kraske.

The quantity of anesthesia was little for the length and nature of the operations and the method of administration. It could have been less had the men realized how much they could depend on the pantopon when the patient was seemingly superficial.

Thirty-one cases did not vomit, of which four had no anesthesia. Eleven vomited only once, and a small amount; eight vomited twice or more.

That takes up the main points. Now let us compare these findings with our morphine. With pantopon, as with morphine, the respiration is made shallow but to a less degree, and it is never insufficient. The corneal reflex was not affected by the drug. It was not made inactive, and did not disappear as with morphine. The pupil was contracted, but never rendered entirely inactive. as with morphine. The pulse with morphine is made abnormally slow. Here it is steadied and if I were dealing with the drug from any point other than as an anesthetic, I would tell you how I have seen brilliant results in heart cases from using this drug when morphine had failed. As to collapse, we have not had one since we started with pantopon.

Now in regard to post-operative vomiting, pantopon certainly allays this more than any drug we have before tried, and I believe post-operative vomiting will be rare when this is properly administered, and the anesthetic quantity thereby reduced. There was no noticeable constipation or lessening of the secretions and the patients in general awoke from the anesthetic quietly and free from pain, and the post-operative narcotic was given later than had been the custom previously.

The results of using as safe a drug as pantopon before anesthesia are obviously better than those obtained when no preliminary hypnotic is administered. For, as you see, pantopon properly administered shortens the induction period, renders both it and the anesthesia quiet, with a minimum of anesthetic. It steadies the pulse and tends to lessen the post-operative vomiting and restlessness.

The two slightly unpleasant features of pantopon are the shallow respiration during anesthesia, when pantopon has been previously given, and the contracted pupil. They are less objectionable with pantopon than with any other drug I have seen used for this purpose.

I have started further experiments on slightly different lines which promise even better results. I have left off the atropine, for it is not needed and only adds another poison.

The new experiments now in progress can be classed under five heads, and I wish others would work along these lines so that large clinical results would be at our disposal.

Following are the five lines along which I am making further observations on this drug.

1. Give pantopon gr. $\frac{1}{3}$, three-quarters of an hour before operation.

2. Give it three-quarters of an hour before and repeat just before operation.

3. Give the first dose with hyoscine gr, I-100.

4. In selected cases even repeat the hyoscine with the second dose of pantopon.

5. In the above cases when necessary after operation to give an hypnotic or sedative, use pantopon instead of morphine for pain and possible vomiting.

Brüstlein, of Berne, has already tried it successfully in some of these ways. He has frequently operated without any anesthetic.

In conclusion I can only repeat that while formerly I thoroughly disliked morphine before anesthesia, I feel that in pantopon I have a safe and reliable aid.

I must thank the surgeons and gynecologists of our hospital for so willingly placing these cases at my disposal, and the house staff and nurses for their many courtesies.

2 West 86th St., New York City.

CASE No.	SEX AND AGE.	OPERATION.	INJECTION.	TIME BEFORE OPERATION.	ANESTHETIC.	QUANTITY USED.
1.	F. 53	Femoral hernia	Pant. 1/3 Atrop. 1/100	15 mins.	Anesthol Ether	80 cc. 10 cc.
2.	M. 43	Tbc. Testicle and cord	Pant. 1/3 Atrop. 1/100	1 hr. 20 mins.	Anesthol Ether	25 cc. 400 cc.
3.	F. 29	Ectopic	Pant. 1/3 Atrop. 1/100	45 mins.	Anesthol Ether	5 cc. 125 cc.
4.	F. 29	Ectopic	Pant. 1/3 Atrop. 1/100	45 mins.	Anesthol Ether	5 cc. 125 cc.
5.	F. 22	Ovarian abscess	Pant. 1/3 Atrop. 1/100	1 hr.	Anesthol Ether	10 cc. 125 cc.
6.	F. 28	Hysterectomy	Pant. 1/3 Atrop. 1/100	20 mins.	Anesthol Ether	15 cc. 70 cc.
7.	M. 40	Hydrocele (Winkler)	Pant. 1/3 Atrop. 1/100	1 hr.	Anesthol	30 cc.
8.	M. 3	Cervical adenitis	Pant. 1/12	1 hr.	Ether	35 cc.
9.	F. 26	Ventral suspension	Pant. 1/3 Atrop. 1/100	½ hr.	Ether Anesthol	75 cc. 10 cc.
10.	M. 29	Colostomy	Pant. 1/3 Atrop. 1/100	45 mins.	Anesthol Ether	15 cc. 400 cc.
11.	F. 29	Curettage	Pant. 1/3 Atrop. 1/100	10 mins.	Anesthol	20 cc.
12.	F. 32	Curettage	Pant. 1/3 Atrop. 1/100	45 mins.	Anesthol Ether	10 cc. 30 cc.
13.	F. 21	Ectopic	Pant. 1/3 Atrop. 1/100	(?)	Anesthol Ether	20 cc. 200 cc.
14.	F. 28	Curettage	Pant. 1/3 Atrop. 1/100	No anesthesia—	patient quiet, experienced no pain	
15.	F. 32	Hyterectomy	Pant. 1/3 Atrop. 1/100	35 mins.	Anesthol Ether	10 cc. 250 cc.
16.	F. 48	Plastic ventral suspension	Pant. 1/3 Atrop. 1/100	1 hr. 30 mins.	Anesthol Ether	10 cc. 150 cc.
17.	M. 28	Removal of bullets from chest and knee	Pant. 1/3 Atrop. 1/100	5 mins.	Anesthol Ether	25 cc. 100 cc.
18.	M. 9	Appendicitis	Pant. 1/3 Atrop. 1/100	40 mins.	Anesthol Ether	25 cc. 70 cc.
19.	F. 25	Appendectomy	Pant. 1/3 Atrop. 1/100	40 mins.	Anesthol Ether	30 cc. 10 cc.
20.	F. 17	Appendectomy	Pant. 1/3 Atrop. 1/100	40 mins.	Anesthol	25 cc.
21.	M. 40	Double inguinal hernia	Pant. 1/3 Atrop. 1/100	50 mins.	Anesthol Ether	20 cc. 100 cc.
22.	M. 46	Phlegmon	Pant. 2/3 Magn. 4/u iv Scopol. 1/120	5 mins.	Anesthol	30 cc.
23.	F. 26	Trachelorrhaphy	Pant. 1/3 Atrop. 1/100	15 mins.	Anesthol Ether	20 cc. 75 cc.
24.	F. 28	Curettage	Pant. 1/3 Atrop. 1/100	5 mins.	Ether	100 cc.
25.	F. 44	Goitre	Pant. 1/3 Atrop. 1/100	2 hrs.	Effect entirely worn off	
26.	F. 53	Ventral hernia	Pant. 1/3 Atrop. 1/100	1 hr.	Anesthol Ether	5 cc. 200 cc.
27.	M. 61	Gastrostomy	Pant. 1/3 Atrop. 1/100	50 mins.	Anesthol	40 cc.
28.	F. 38	Ventral hernia	Pant. 1/3 Atrop. 1/100	1 hr. 20 mins.	Anesthol Ether	100 cc. 60 cc.
29.	M. 25	Inguinal hernia	Pant. 1/3 Atrop. 1/100	35 mins.	Anesthol Ether	5 cc. 60 cc.
30.	M. 36	Suprapubic cystostomy	Pant. 1/3 Atrop. 1/100	45 mins.	Anesthol	75 cc.
31.	F. 58	Hysterectomy	Pant. 1/3 Atrop. 1/100	45 mins.	Anesthol Ether	20 cc. 45 cc.
32.	F. 33	Abd. Inc. and drainage	Pant. 1/3 Atrop. 1/100	45 mins.	Anesthol	50 cc.
33.	F. 34	Curettage and abortion	Pant. 1/3 Atrop. 1/100	40 mins.	Anesthol	25 cc.
34.	F. 36	Expl. for brain tumor	Pant. 1/3 Atrop. 1/100	45 mins.	Chloroform Oxygen	20 cc.

LENGTH OF ANESTHESIA.	INDUCTION.	POST-OPERATIVE VOMITING.	REMARKS.
1 hr. 25 mins.	Easy	Once next morning	Pulse steadied. R. slightly shallow. Pupils contracted.
1 hr. 10 mins.	Noisy	Vomited once	Patient very alcoholic — took ether well, anesthol badly. Pulse once poor. R. as above, comfortable all night.
40 mins.	Induction quiet; anesthol 5 cc., no excitement stage, patient drowsy	None	Pulse good. R. good and quiet. Patient superficial — quiet; no retching, no vomiting. Patient awoke during skin suture. Felt
35 mins.	at onset	None	no pain.
50 mins.		None	
1 hr. 20 mins.	Induction not affected, as injection was too late	None	About 45 minutes after injection drug showed its effect. Little more was needed. Though reflexes were active and patient superficial she was quiet and seemingly undisturbed by the operation.
20 mins.	Induction drowsy; 5 cc. anesthol	None	Nothing special noted during operation. Quiet and no pain after operation.
45 mins.	Unaffected	None	Toward end of operation patient quiet. Shortly after operation was playing with other children and complained of no pain.
45 mins.	Quiet	None	Everything satisfactory.
1 hr. 45 mins.	Quiet	Once	Everything satisfactory.
25 mins.	No effect	None	Everything satisfactory.
25 mins.	Quiet	Several times	Nothing of note.
1 hr. 10 mins.	Quiet	None	Everything satisfactory.
1 hr. 20 mins.	Unaffected	Once	1 hour after injection drug began to work and patient carried along on occasional drop of ether on open mask.
1 hr. 25 mins.	Very quiet	None	Everything satisfactory.
50 mins.	1 bag of gas	After operation allowed water & vomited twice	Very alcoholic. No effect.
50 mins.	2 mins. 5 cc. anesthol	None	Everything satisfactory.
40 mins.	5 cc. anesthol	Twice	Everything satisfactory.
35 mins.	Quiet	Several times	Everything satisfactory.
35 mins.	Quiet	None	Everything satisfactory.
25 mins.	Very wild	None	No effect from drugs.
40 mins.	Quiet	Several times white mucus	Everything satisfactory.
20 mins.	Not affected	Once	Everything satisfactory.
		Several times	
2 hrs.	Quiet as a baby in natural sleep	None	Weight 250 lbs.
45 mins.	Quiet	None	Everything satisfactory.
1 hr. 15 mins.	Quiet	None	No further hypo. Slept well. Everything satisfactory.
1 hr. 10 mins.	Quiet	None	Everything satisfactory.
1 hr. 35 mins.	Quiet	Once	Some blueness, probably due to position.
1 hr. 10 mins.	Quiet	Once	Vaginal reflex very active, otherwise everything satisfactory.
50 mins.	Quiet	Twice	Everything satisfactory.
40 mins.	Quiet	None	Everything satisfactory.
1 hr.	Quiet	None	Everything satisfactory.

44   AMERICAN MEDICINE }
Complete Series, Vol. XVIII. }   ORIGINAL ARTICLES   { JANUARY, 1912.
{ New Series, Vol. VII., No. 1.

CASE No.	SEX AND AGE.	OPERATION.	INJECTION.	TIME BEFORE OPERATION.	ANESTHETIC.	QUANTITY USED.
35.	F. 37	Nephrotomy	Pant. 1/3 Atrop. 1/100	1 hr.	Anesthol	30 cc.
36.	M. 43	Excision of ulcer of tongue	Pant. 1/3 Atrop. 1/100	30 mins.	Chloroform Anesthol	35 cc. 10 cc.
37.	F. 27	Posterior Vag. incision	Pant. 1/3 Atrop. 1/100	30 mins.	Gas Ether	1 bag 50 cc.
38.	F. 37	Goitre	Pant. 1/3 Atrop. 1/100	30 mins.	Anesthol	80 cc.
39.	M. 20	Undescended testicle	Pant. 1/3 Atrop. 1/100	1 hr. 50 mins.	Anesthol	40 cc.
40.	F. 58	Exploratory, appendectomy	Pant. 1/3 Atrop. 1/100	45 mins.	Anesthol	20 cc.
41.	F. 24	Curettage	Pant. 1/3 Atrop. 1/100	25 mins.	Anesthol Ether	40 cc. 10 cc.
42.	F. 51	Exploratory and appendectomy	Pant. 1/3 Atrop. 1/100	45 mins.	Anesthol Ether	200 cc. 10 cc.
43.	M. 50	Necrosis of tibia	Pant. 1/3 Atrop. 1/100	20 mins.	Anesthol	30 cc.
44.	M. 37	Ing. hernia	Pant. 1/3 Atrop. 1/100	1 hr.	Anesthol	55 cc.
45.	M. 29	Removal of rectum	Pant. 1/3 Atrop. 1/100	1 hr. 15 mins.	Anesthol Ether	60 cc. 100 cc.
46.	M. 54	Occlusion of common carotid (Matas)	Pant. 1/3 Atrop. 1/100	1 hr. 25 mins.	None	
47.	F. 56	Umbilical hernia	Pant. 1/3 Atrop. 1/100	25 mins.	Not measured	
48.	F. 35	Cholecystectomy	Pant. 1/3 Atrop. 1/100	1 hr. 25 mins.	Ether Anesthol	10 cc. 70 cc.
49.	F. 40	Curettage	Pant. 1/3 Atrop. 1/100	30 mins.	None	
50.	F. 30	Curettage	Pant. 1/3 Atrop. 1/100	20 mins.	None	

BIBLIOGRAPHY.

DR. H. SAHLI.—Ueber Pantopon. (Thera-
peutische Monatshefte, Januar, 1909).

DR. JULIUS HALLERVORDEN.—Ueber die
Anwendung des Pantopon (Sahli). (Sonder-
Abdruck aus Therapie der Gegenwart. Jahr-
gang, 1910, Heft 5).

DR. FRITZ HEIMANN.—Klinische Beobach-
tungen über die Wirkung des Pantopon. (Sonderdruck aus der Münchener Medizinischen
Wochenschrift, No. 7, 1910).

DR. W. H. BECKER.—Pantopon, ein Ersatz-
mittel des Opiums und seine Verwendbarkeit
in der Irrenpflege. (Sonderabdruck aus Reichs-
Medizinal-Anzeiger, 1910, No. 18).

DR. H. SAHLI.—Ueber Pantopon. (Sonderdruck aus der Münchener Medizinischen Wochenschrift, No. 25, 1910).

DR. G. BRUSTLEIN.—Ueber die Scopolamin-
Pantoponnarkose. (Sep.-Abdruck a. d. Cor-
respondenz-Blatt für Schweizer Aerzte, 1910, No.
26).

DR. ERNEST GRAFENBERG.—Die Bedeu-
tung des Pantopons (Sahli) für die Gynäkologie und Geburtshilfe. (Sonder-Abdruck aus
der Deutschen Medizinischen Wochenschrift,
1910, No. 34).

ROSE WERTHEIMER-RAFFALOVICH.—Experimentelle Untersuchungen über die Panto-
ponwirkungen. (Sonder-Abdruck aus der Deutschen Medizinischen Wochenschrift, 1910, No.
37).

DR. THOMAS PERTIK.—Ueber das Sahlische
Pantopon. (Sonder-Abdruck aus der Deutschen
Medizinischen Wochenschrift, 1910, No. 36).

DR. C. A. EWALD.—Das Pantopon-Sahli.
(Sonder Abdruck aus der Berliner klin. Woch-
enschr., 1910, No. 35 u. 42).

DR. HERMANN HAYMANN.—Pantopon in
der Psychiatrie. (Sonderdruck aus der Münchener Medizinischen Wochenschrift, 1910, No.
43).

DR. OSCAR JAEGER.—Versuche zur Herab-
setzung des Wehenschmerzes bei der Geburt.

LENGTH OF ANESTHESIA.	INDUCTION.	POST-OPERATIVE VOMITING.	REMARKS.
45 mins.	Quiet	Once	Everything satisfactory.
25 mins.	No effect	Once	No effect.
30 mins.	Quiet	None	Everything satisfactory.
1 hr. 30 mins.	Unaffected by drug	Several times	
1 hr.	Quiet	Several times	
30 mins.	Quiet	None	Very quiet.
35 mins.	Quiet	None	Everything satisfactory.
1 hr. 20 mins.	Quiet.	None	Everything satisfactory.
30 mins.	Difficult	None	Everything satisfactory.
1 hr.	Quiet	None	Everything satisfactory.
1 hr. 55 mins.	Quiet	None	Everything satisfactory.
			Cocain and Schleich intra and subcutaneous, none in the deeper tissues. Patient felt slight pain but was quiet. No pain after operation.
1 hr.	Quiet	None	Everything satisfactory.
1 hr. 5 mins.	Quiet.	None	Weight 230 pounds.
			Slight pain on one side.
			Very nervous before. Had had one operation.

(Zentralblatt für Gynäkologie, Sonderabdruck aus Nr. 46, 1910).

DR. A. LOEWY.—Ueber die Wirkung des Pantopons auf das Atemzentrum. (Sonderdruck aus der Münchener Medizinischen Wochenschrift, No. 46, 1910).

DR. WALTER BERGIEN.—Ueber die Beeinflussung von Atmung und Zirkulation durch Pantopon. (Sonderdruck aus der Münchener Medizinischen Wochenschrift, No. 46, 1910).

DR. EMIL DOBELI.—Ueber die Empfindlichkeit verschieden alter Tiere gegen die Opiumalkaloide. (Separat-Abdruck aus der Monatsschrift für Kinderheilkunde, IX, Bd., Abteilung Originalien 1, 1910).

DR. WALTER BERGIEN.—Ueber die Beeinflussung von Atmung und Zirkulation durch Pantopon. (Inaugural-Dissertation, Bern.).

DR. C. L. LEIPOLDT.—Remarks on Pantopon Anesthesia. (The Lancet, London, Feb. 11, 1910).

DR. TOMASCHNY.—Ueber die Anwendung des Pantopons in der Psychiatrie. (Separat-Abdruck aus Neurologisches Centralblatt).

DR. P. RODARI.—Klinische Erfahrungen über das Pantopon (Roche). (Separat-Abdruck aus der Schweizerischen Rundschau für Medizin, No. 4, 28 Januar, 1911).

DR. JOH. RUD. HANI.—Ueber die Verstärkung der Wirkung verschiedener Narkotika, speziell des Pantopons, durch Skopolamin. (Sonderabdruck aus der Therapie der Gegenwart, Februar, 1911).

SOME REMARKS ON OTITIC PURULENT LEPTOMENINGITIS AND BRAIN ABSCESS, WITH REPORT OF A CASE.

BY

ALFRED BRAUN, M. D.,
New York City.

It is a well known fact that by far the most common cause of brain abscess is disease of the middle ear. The most common form of middle ear disease responsible for this condition, is the chronic suppurative form with cholesteatoma formation. Brain abscess rarely complicates acute middle ear suppuration, the spread of infection to the cranial cavity, in these cases, being so rapid, that a diffuse meningitic or encephalitic process results. Cholesteatoma, which consists of desquamated epithelial cells and cholesterin crystals, causes a gradual erosion of the bone by pressure, and forms a very good culture medium for infective organisms. The spread of the infection is so slow, in these chronic middle ear conditions, that the dura becomes adherent to the brain, and the infective intracranial condition is circumscribed in character. But sometimes chronic middle ear disease results in diffuse meningitis, and on the other hand, occasionally, acute middle ear disease results in brain abscess.

Neumann has laid down the following postulate in regard to the occurrence of these complications:

"Infection via pre-existing tracts (with the exception of the aqueductus vestibuli) tends to meningitis, whilst infection by way of tracts not previously existing, inclusive of the aqueductus vestibuli, results in circumscribed extradural and cerebral abscess." By pre-existing tracts, are meant the labyrinth and internal auditory meatus, and aqueductus cochleae.

The various means by which infection may travel from the middle ear and mastoid to the interior of the skull, are the following:

1. By a preformed channel, as the labyrinth and internal auditory meatus.

2. By destruction of bone.

3. By infective thrombi in the veins which pass through the bone from the middle ear to the interior of the skull.

4. By the lymphatics which accompany the vessels passing through the bone.

5. Through the inner wall of the lateral sinus, in infective processes within the sinus.

Otitic brain abscess occurs in one of two locations; either in the temporo-sphenoidal lobe, or in the cerebellum; rarely, in both locations together. According to Neumann, it is twice as common in the temporo-sphenoidal lobe, as in the cerebellum. Abscess in the temporo-sphenoidal lobe occurs as the result of extension of the disease through the roof of the middle ear and antrum, into the middle fossa of the skull. Abscess in the cerebellum occurs as the result of extension of the disease from the mastoid through the inner plate into the posterior fossa of the skull, through the internal auditory meatus, or through the inner wall of the lateral sinus, in infective processes within the sinus.

The abscess cavity in the brain may be directly continuous with the abscess in the middle ear or mastoid, there being a fistula in the dura; or the dura may be intact, and a considerable thickness of normal brain tissue may be present between the brain abscess and the dura. Rarely, the abscess may even be located in the opposite hemisphere to the diseased ear, as the result of metastatic infection. When the abscess lies a considerable distance from the surface, the chances of finding it at operation, are very much diminished. Abscesses in the cerebellum are usually located in the mesial portions of the lateral lobes, near the central lobe, this being the portion of the cerebellum, which is in relation to the petrous portion of the temporal bone. Cerebellar abscesses are often multiple.

A brain abscess may exist for months or even years, without giving rise to any symptoms. If left untreated, it will eventually break into the ventricles, or onto the surface of the brain, giving rise to a purulent meningitis. There have been a few cases reported, where a brain abscess has evacuated itself through the middle ear, and occasionally we hear of a case, where, in a very small abscess, the pus has become absorbed, and the abscess healed, without operation. But these are very rare exceptions, and we can state, as a broad general rule, that, unless operated on, all brain abscesses are fatal.

The symptoms of brain abscess are often indistinguishable from those of the middle ear and mastoid disease. In many cases, there is no temperature. Sometimes, the temperature is subnormal. The pulse is usually very slow. There may or may not be an optic neuritis.

A diagnosis can only be made, when a part of the brain is involved, whose function we know. Destruction of such an area causes focal symptoms. In abscess of the left temporo-sphenoidal lobe, we have aphasia, and in abscess of the cerebellum, we have nystagmus, vertigo, vomiting and ataxia. Abscess of the cerebellum is sometimes difficult to differentiate from suppurative disease of the labyrinth. The

diagnosis is based principally upon the fact that in disease of the labyrinth, the hearing is destroyed, while in cerebellar disease, it is unaffected. In disease of the labyrinth, the symptoms usually clear up at the end of a week or two, whereas, in cerebellar abscess, they persist, or grow worse. The character of the nystagmus, and the direction of falling, may help to a certain extent. But in a certain proportion of cases, the two conditions co-exist, the cerebellar abscess being caused by the labyrinthine suppuration. In these cases, the diagnosis of cerebellar abscess can only be made, when the symptoms persist, in spite of extirpation of the diseased labyrinth.

In some cases of brain abscess, as in the present case, there are no symptoms pointing to intracranial disease, until the abscess has ruptured into the ventricles or onto the surface of the brain, setting up a meningitis.

The only treatment for brain abscess, is operative. The statistics of operations for brain abscess, compiled by various observers, vary from 25% to 50% of recoveries.

Operations for abscess in the temporosphenoidal lobe, may be performed in one of three ways:

1. Through the mastoid.

2. Through the squama of the temporal bone.

3. Combined route, through the mastoid and squama.

In operating by way of the mastoid route, we have the advantage of removing the original source of infection of the brain abscess, and following up the abscess along the probable path of infection. We may find a fistula in the dura over the roof of the middle ear and antrum, which leads directly into the abscess. On the other hand, if the dura is healthy, and the abscess is some distance from the surface, we have the disadvantage of going through the dura in an infected region, and probably carrying infection into the meninges or brain. There is also the disadvantage that only a small area of dura is exposed on removal of the roof of the middle ear and antrum.

In the second method, that is, by operating through the squama, a large area of dura is exposed, with consequent freedom of manipulation, and the brain is entered through an uninfected region. It has the disadvantage, however, that the primary source of infection in the middle ear and mastoid, is left untouched.

The ideal operation is by the third or combined method, in which the operation is done through the mastoid and squama. This eradicates the primary focus of infection, gives a large area of exposure, and allows through and through drainage, which is a very important factor in the successful healing of a brain abscess.

The operation is performed as follows: The usual post-auricular incision is made for the mastoid operation. If we are dealing with an acute middle ear condition, we do a simple mastoid operation. If there is a chronic middle ear suppuration, we do a radical mastoid. The inner table, constituting the roof of the antrum and middle ear, is removed by means of a rongeur, exposing the dura over the under surface of the temporo-sphenoidal lobe of the brain. The skin incision is then extended upward for about an inch and a half and then forward another inch and a half or two inches, and the soft tissues and periosteum retracted from the underlying bone. In this way, the entire squamous portion of the temporal

bone is exposed. With a broad rongeur, the squama is removed, being careful not to tear the dura. This exposes a large portion of the dura covering the lateral surface of the temporo-sphenoidal lobe. The entire operative field is now carefully disinfected, by washing out with alcohol followed by saline.

Two or three vertical incisions about an inch apart, and half an inch in length, are made through the dura, over the outer surface of the brain, and another incision over the under surface. Some operators prefer to wait a day, before incising the brain, in order that inflammatory adhesions may take place between the dura and surface of the brain at the site of the dural incision, so that the pus, when it escapes from the abscess, should not infect the pia. But if the symptoms are very urgent, the brain must be incised at once. The knife should never be plunged into the brain through an intact dura, for two reasons. First, because infection may be carried into the brain from the outer surface of the dura, and second, because, if you strike the abscess, the pus, in escaping, is much more likely to spread itself over the surface of the brain, under the dura.

A long narrow-bladed knife is used in searching for the abscess. An aspirating needle is of no use, because the soft brain tissue is very apt to occlude the lumen of the needle, and the pus is often too thick to pass through. A clean incision with a narrow bladed knife inflicts no appreciable injury to the brain. The knife is plunged into the brain in various directions, through the various dural incisions, to a distance of an inch and a half or two inches. When the knife is inserted to this depth, the blade is slightly rotated about its long axis, so as

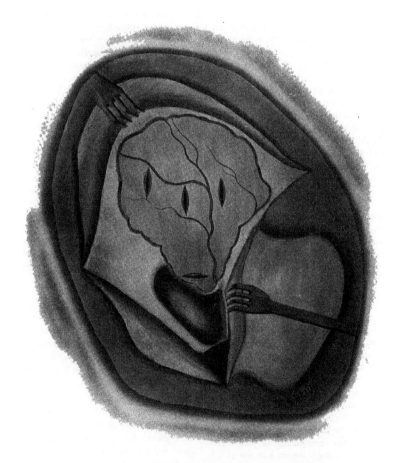

Fig. 1. Operation for abscess of temporo-sphenoidal lobe of brain.

to make the wound gape, and facilitate exit of the pus. In this way, eight or ten incisions may be made.

When the abscess is reached, all of the pus and necrotic brain tissue is allowed to escape. The cavity should not be irrigated or mopped out. The brain should be handled as little as possible.

It is very difficult to secure proper drainage for a brain abscess, especially if it lies some distance from the surface. The best results are obtained from the use of incollapsible drainage tubes, either rubber, or preferably decalcified bone. The tubes should have fenestrae at the sides. Through and through drainage should be obtained, the tubes passing through an opening on the outer surface of the brain, through the abscess, and emerging from an opening on the base. The mastoid wound is lightly packed with iodoform gauze, covered with sterile gauze fluff, and a bandage applied. Where the abscess is near the surface, and where the walls of the abscess are fairly firm, one drainage opening is usually sufficient. The frequency with which the drainage tubes should be changed, depends upon their effectiveness. Usually once a day is sufficient. If there is much damming back of pus, the tubes must be changed twice a day, or even three times. The drainage tubes are gradually shortened, until they can be dispensed with, altogether.

Very often, a hernia of the brain occurs into the wound. An attempt should be made to replace it by a pressure bandage. If this fails, the hernia must be excised.

Cerebellar abscess may be operated on through the outer surface of the occipital bone, or through the mastoid wound. It is preferable to operate through the mastoid wound, because the abscess is usually situated near the median lobe, in direct relation with the posterior surface of the petrous portion of the temporal bone.

The operation is performed as follows: A radical mastoid operation is done. The inner plate is then removed over the anterior portion of the lateral sinus. The inner plate is then removed beyond the sinus, anteriorly, until the posterior semicircular canal is reached. This exposes the dura over a triangular area of the cerebellum, the base of which is above, and is formed by the angle between the middle and posterior fossae of the skull, the posterior border is formed by the anterior border of the lateral sinus, and the anterior border, by the posterior semicircular canal. In cases where the labyrinth is diseased, the entire internal ear is exenterated, exposing the dura as far forward as the internal auditory meatus. The dura is incised in this triangular area, and the knife passed into the cerebellum in various directions, until the abscess is reached. The abscess is drained by means of decalcified bone or rubber drainage tubes.

Otitic leptomeningitis occurs in one of three forms; serous meningitis, circumscribed purulent meningitis, and diffuse purulent meningitis. The prognosis of serous meningitis is very good. Almost all of the cases recover. The prognosis of the circumscribed purulent form is fairly good, if the primary source of infection is removed, and early adequate drainage instituted. The prognosis of the diffuse purulent form is very bad. It is extremely rare for a patient to recover from this form. Some authors even claim that there are no recoveries. The reported cases of cure are claimed by them to have been cases of circumscribed purulent meningitis.

Otitic meningitis may follow acute or chronic middle ear suppuration, without mastoiditis. It may follow middle ear suppuration with mastoiditis. It may follow labyrinthine suppuration. It may follow infective sigmoid sinus thrombosis. It may follow brain abscess.

Lumbar puncture shows a clear sterile cerebro-spinal fluid, under considerable pressure. These cases usually get well. However, this may be the first stage of a purulent meningitis. A second lumbar puncture, made several days later, may show cloudy fluid.

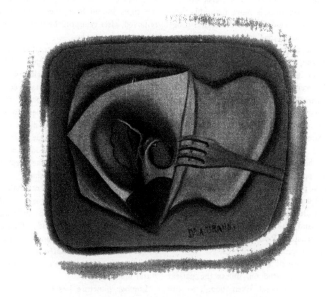

Fig. 2. Operation for cerebellar abscess.

In serous meningitis, the diagnosis can only be made by lumbar puncture. The subjective symptoms are the same as in purulent meningitis. There is some temperature, with an irregular rapid pulse, stupor or irritability, hyperesthesia of the skin, headache, rigidity of the neck, strabismus, with inequality of the pupils, optic neuritis, Kernig's and Babinski's signs, retracted abdomen, and tâche cerebrale.

Circumscribed purulent meningitis shows a cloudy cerebro-spinal fluid, containing large numbers of polynuclear leucocytes and a few lymphocytes. There may or may not be bacteria present. The tension of the fluid may or may not be increased.

In diffuse purulent meningitis, the onset is usually sudden, the symptoms very severe, and death often comes on within a day or two. The cerebro-spinal fluid is very turbid, containing large numbers of polynuclear leucocytes and bacteria. There are cases in which no bacteria have been found, in which the diagnosis of diffuse purulent leptomeningitis has been confirmed by autopsy. The tension of the fluid may or may not be increased.

In the cases in which bacteria are absent, the prognosis is more favorable. The more turbid the fluid, the worse the prognosis. Alexander has reported several cases of brain abscess without meningitis, in which the cerebro-spinal fluid was cloudy and contained no bacteria.

It is sometimes possible, at the time of the operation, to judge whether we are dealing with a case of circumscribed or diffuse meningitis. If we can trace an inflammatory tract from the interior of the mastoid to the dura, and we find a circumscribed inflammatory area on the dura at this point, we will usually have to deal with a partial, encapsulated, or circumscribed meningitis. This condition is sometimes called subdural abscess. If, on the other hand, the dura adjacent to the affected mastoid looks normal, we are apt to have a general meningitis.

Every case of otitic purulent meningitis should be operated on, unless the patient is actually moribund. Even though we can only save an occasional patient, it is worth while, for if we do not operate, the patient will surely die. Even in the cases which eventually die, the operation often improves the symptoms for a time. Death is scarcely ever due to the operation itself.

In the cases of serous meningitis it is sufficient to remove the primary source of infection, by doing a simple or radical mastoid. In the cases of purulent meningitis, the primary source of infection should first be removed. A simple or radical mastoid

should be done, as the case may indicate. If the labyrinth is diseased, it should be exenterated. If the patient's condition allows, it is wise to test the labyrinthine functions, before operating, in order to determine whether the labyrinth is diseased. If there is a brain abscess it should be evacuated and drained. If there is a sinus thrombosis, the sinus should be opened, and the clots removed, after tying off the internal jugular vein.

In addition to these procedures, the subdural space should be drained. This is done by making several incisions in the dura. As the meningitis usually starts in the middle and posterior fossae, the incisions should be made in these locations. Two or three incisions, each about half an inch in length, should be made in the dura over the temporo-sphenoidal lobe, and two incisions in the dura over the cerebellum, one in front of, and one behind the lateral sinus. There is usually an encephalitis accompanying the meningitis, as a result of which, the brain tissue is immediately pushed into the dural wound. This interferes considerably with drainage. Drainage might possibly be facilitated by introducing a short thin wick of gauze into the subdural space.

Lumbar puncture has only a diagnostic value. No cases have been cured by lumbar puncture. Recently, a few cases have been reported cured by the intrathecal injection of urotropin, and the administration of urotropin by mouth, about 30 grains daily. However, it is possible that these cases might have gotten well without the urotropin.

The following case is of interest on account of the complete recovery following an operation done when the patient seemed to be almost moribund.

Michael D., a laborer, 24 years of age, was admitted to Dr. Berens' service at the Manhattan Eye, Ear and Throat Hospital on September 6, 1911, with the following history:

The patient had always been well until four years ago, when he had pain in the left ear, and discharge, which recurred at intervals, up to the present attack. The present attack began on July 28, six weeks before admission, with pain in the left ear, followed by discharge. On September 6, he came to the hospital, with some pain in the ear, and slight headache. Temperature was normal. Most of the left drum-membrane was gone, and there were some granulations in the middle ear. There was slight tenderness over the left mastoid. Blood examination showed 15,000 leucocytes, with 90% of polynuclears. The patient did not look very sick. His ear was irrigated with hot bichloride solution, every 2 hours, and he was kept under close observation.

On September 9, three days after admission, Dr. Asch, the house surgeon, called me up at 10 o'clock in the evening, and informed me that the patient had just had a convulsion and had become comatose, his temperature going up to 104.2° F., pulse 108, and respiration 32.

We could not get into communication with the patient's family in order to get permission for an operation, until the following morning. When seen at 11 o'clock the next morning he was very deeply comatose. His temperature was 104.6° F. There was rigidity of the neck, and divergent strabismus. The pupils were dilated, and unresponsive. There was no Kernig's sign. The eye-grounds were normal. He had had several more convulsions in the course of the night.

He was immediately brought to the operating room. A lumbar puncture was done, showing a thick turbid cerebro-spinal fluid, under considerable pressure. About 20 c. c. were drawn off. The fluid was so turbid, that on standing for an hour, there was a sediment an inch thick at the bottom of the test-tube. Smears from the cerebrospinal fluid showed abundant pus cells, but no bacteria. A culture of the fluid showed no growth. A blood culture taken at this time was negative.

The mastoid was opened. After going through a thick, dense cortex, the antrum was found full of pus under pressure. The pus welled out, with a pulsating rhythm. The middle ear was found full of granulations. The posterior canal wall and outer attic wall were taken down, and a complete radical mastoid was done. It was found that the roof of the antrum and middle ear was gone. The dura of the middle fossa, covered with granulations, bulged down for about half an inch, into the antrum and attic. A portion of the squama was removed, until healthy dura appeared on all sides. No fistula could be found in the dura. After carefully sterilizing the field, the dura was incised over the lower surface of the temporo-sphenoidal lobe, for a distance of ¾ inch. It was found that the brain-cortex was adherent to the dura at this point. The knife was passed directly upward into the brain, and at a distance of about ½ inch from the surface, pus was encountered. The knife was rotated laterally, and considerable thick, foul-smelling pus was discharged. A bivalve nasal speculum was then introduced into the abscess, and the blades separated, and some more pus and necrotic brain-tissue were evacuated. In all, about ½ ounce of pus was obtained. The interior of the abscess cavity could now be seen through the speculum, and it was found that the cavity had a fairly firm wall. For this reason, and because the abscess was so near to the surface, it was decided that through and through drainage would not be necessary. Two rubber drainage tubes, about 2½ inches long, and ½ inch thick, with perforations at the sides were introduced into the abscess, and the mastoid wound was lightly packed with iodoform gauze. I did not attempt to irrigate the abscess. When the patient left the table, the pulse and respiration were better than before the operation.

Cultures from the brain abscess and mastoid showed the Friedlaender bacillus.

On the day following the operation, the temperature dropped to 102° F. The patient was conscious, and answered questions rationally. He complained of severe headache. On removing the drainage tubes, about two drachms of pus gushed out. The tubes were cleaned and reintroduced. The next day, the temperature had dropped down to 101° F. His headache had diminished somewhat. On removing the drainage tubes, no pus came out, showing that the tubes were doing their work properly. At the end of a week, the temperature was normal, and the patient felt perfectly well. The drainage tubes were gradually shortened, until on October 5, three and a half weeks· after the operation, they were removed altogether. On October 7, the abscess had entirely filled up. A meatal flap was then made, and the mastoid wound sutured. The middle ear cavity epidermatized over completely, at the end of five weeks. He has had no mental symptoms of any kind since the operation. He is now attending to his work again.

616 Madison Avenue.

A PHYSICAN'S VISIT TO SAO PAULO AND THE INSTITUTION FOR PREPARING ANTIDOTAL SNAKE SERA AT BUTANAN, BRAZIL.

BY

DOUGLASS W. MONTGOMERY, M. D.,

Professor of Diseases of the Skin, University of California.

While in Rio de Janeiro, we ran up the government railroad, a distance of 497 kilometers, to Sao Paulo, the most progressive city in the most progressive state of Brazil. We paid twenty-five milreis, or about eight dollars and thirty cents for sleeping accommodations for one night for each person. The train was called a "train de luxe," although there was nothing luxurious about it but the price. We slept on benches with stiff wire bottoms over which sheets were thrown. Another folded sheet and blanket, and a couple of pillows represented the entire furnishing of the simple bed. We thought we were expected to undress as in Europe and America. Not at all—the Brazilians, as we found afterwards, rolled themselves, as they were, in the sheet and blanket, and addressed themselves to sleep, and they were wise, for, toward morning it grew to be bitterly cold. I finally arose, gave my blanket to my companion, and dressed myself. It was the wretched damp cold of the tropical winter, and at one of the stations I saw a poor devil, barefooted and clad in thin cotton, going along hunched up with that peculiar "cold dog" gait, that is the very attitude and eloquent mark of chilliness and self retraction. My boots were not blackened, my clothes were not brushed, my bed was not made, the car was neither cleaned nor heated, and to cap all, the week kneed son of perdition that acted as conductor and porter combined, allowed a man to occupy the women's dressing room. I have rarely got so little for my money, and this was on a state owned railroad. Many of the stations along the route seemed much too large, and too expensively built for the size of the towns they served. In spite of there being so many fine stations we got coffee in the morning in a wayside shed at a standup lunch counter. This is one of the frailties of government ownership. The fine buildings represented the man that had "pull." There was a varied assortment of beggars at many of the stops. At one of the towns one fellow, just outside the station grounds, was lying in a bed or bier on wheels, covered with a canopy. He sent two little boys to collect his toll from the passengers.

The tropics are almost always poor, as nearly everything they use or consume such as flour, much of the meat, books, machinery, and almost all manufactured articles are imported. Brazil also imports her coal and petroleum. The flow of money out of the country is therefore immense, but in spite of this the crop of the state of Sao Paulo is so abundant, and so valuable that enough is left over to make it prosperous. The crop is coffee. Coffee is seen everywhere, and everyone talks coffee, and a visit to a coffee hacienda is an interesting experience.

The town of Sao Paulo enjoys a temperate climate, at 426 meters above the sea level. As a contrast to Rio almost all the inhabitants are white, and they. look vigorous, busy, are well dressed, and the town has a neat, well kept appearance. A feature of the town in contrast to Rio, is the large number of book stores. I was in at least five well stocked ones during my short stay, and was able to get one book in Sao Paulo, that we hunted for in vain in Rio. There is, however, the same curious lack of city directories as in Rio. Or it may be, that as they construct their directories on the same plan as those of Rio, where they index them on the basis of the Christian name, and find them unserviceable, they do not use them. In looking up the address of a man to whom I had a letter of introduction, a Sao Paulan and myself wandered from business house to business house until we attained our object. No one thought of consulting a directory.

A COFFEE PLANTATION.

Early on a sharp cold morning we left Sao Paulo, to go several miles by rail to Campinas to see a coffee plantation. On reaching Campinas we had to drive still farther to attain our object, and after the usual haggling with a cab driver we set out over the stone paved streets of a town, that, as far as appearances were concerned, might just as well have been situated. in southern Europe, and then on out into the country over a clay road, so cut up by

teams as to give us lots of jolting. This clay is red, and in some places almost vermilion, and it is in this red clay that the coffee plant grows so well. Nor does it need any shade as in hotter countries, where each plant is sheltered by a mulberry bush. Finally we turned through a gate into a field with coffee bushes on either hand as far as we could see.

The machinery for cleaning, hulling, and separating the beans into different grades is both extensive and expensive. The beans are carried from place to place, and separated into different grades by streams of water. For instance the lighter beans float on the surface of the stream and are carried into one chute, and the heavier, finer beans are carried along near the bottom, and enter another chute. In this way the beans are also cleaned of sand and gravel; the green beans are separated from the ripe ones; and the large fine ones from those that are small and light.

The coffee from such a plantation is put into bags of one hundred and thirty pounds each, and sent down to Santos, the sea port, whence it is shipped to all parts of the world.

SANTOS.

Santos is the great coffee port of the world, as over fifty percent of the world's product is shipped through it. When we passed through Santos we were told by one of the largest dealers that there was very little coffee on hand, only one million three hundred thousand bags that day. This was enough, one would think to put the whole world on a "coffee jag."

Some years ago the cultivation of coffee was very profitable, and this naturally led to overproduction. Instead of allowing this state of affairs to right itself, the queer paternal government stepped in, and became a heavy buyer. The result was more coffee, with its ultimate, inevitable fall in price. Then production naturally fell off, and in addition to this the government again stepped in and restricted the planting of coffee. The price is now remunerative and the government has been able to unload some of its stored product, and it is said at a profit. Naturally I asked the question if the government would not still be a loser through insects, through rodents, and from deterioration. It appears, however, that neither insects, nor any of the lower animals attack the coffee bean, and that instead of deteriorating, the bean improves with age.

Through the kindness of a friend we visited a coffee broker, and while we were present a number of sellers of coffee presented themselves. Each came with a sample enclosed in a small round tin box, marked with the number of bags he had for sale. The broker poured out the contents of the box on a piece of stiff black paper, and with a sweep of the hand spread them out into a thin layer, and on this inspection reached his conclusion as to the grade of the sample and the price it would command. He said that misrepresentation by sample was very rare, and one can readily see that the inconvenience of this form of cheating would necessarily make it unfashionable.

It is an interesting sight to watch the stevedores carry the coffee from the warehouses to the ships. Each man takes a bag across his shoulders, and with bowed head and hurried step, ascends the gang plank, throws down the bag, and trots back for another. If you cross such a line they will run against you like blind men. You then realize that they work like insects, neither hearing nor seeing anything that passes around them. Like bathing girls their clothing was more an accentuation than a concealment of their nakedness.

Santos harbor is less beautiful than that of Rio, but of the same type. It is a depression among the coast hills, opening out to sea, and the long narrow channel called the river, is not a river at all, but a sinuous valley. Santos itself is built on an island in the harbor.

As the bay of Santos is much smaller than that of Rio, and the outlet to the sea long and narrow, fouling of the water, in the moisture-laden hot atmosphere under a tropical sun, takes place much more readily than at Rio. There are cool balmy days in winter, for we were there in one of them, but the summer must be swelteringly hot, and favorable to the pullulation of fever germs. As, however, the contest with the infectious diseases is a commercial fight, it is successfully carried out, and what was once a death trap, is now free from yellow fever.

THE INSTITUTION FOR PREPARING ANTIDOTAL SNAKE SERA AT BUTANAN.

While in Sao Paulo we drove to Butanan to see the institute for making antitoxins, and antidotal serums. Those antidotal to snake poisoning were particularly interesting, and the Director, Dr. Vital Brazil, took infinite pains in explaining them to us.

This country is rich in venomous reptiles, and there seems to be no difficulty in getting material for studying them. The mere study of venomous reptiles is apt, however, like that of other branches of natural history, to degenerate into academic, nebulous, pointless, observation. Dr. Brazil, however, has the practical proposition before him of saving life by the preparation of antidotal serums, and this gives definiteness to his work and makes it correspondingly interesting. He goes still further than this, and is studying the habits of serpents in order the better to combat them, and, as we shall see, is making decided advances in this direction.

Three kinds of antidotal snake sera are prepared in this institution. One kind, the anticrotalic, is to be used when bitten by a snake called the cascavel; another, the antibothricopic, is injected when the victim is poisoned by any of the Lachesis group, such as the uratu, the cruzeiro, or the lachesis atrox; yet another serum is prepared to be used when the kind of snake is unknown. This last is therefore polyvalent, and is called antiophidic serum. It is an interesting fact, especially dwelt upon by Doctor Brazil, that there is enough difference in the poison of different species of snakes to render the serum that is antidotal for one kind, useless when employed against poisoning by another kind. Should a man, therefore, be bitten by a species of snake unknown to him, polyvalent serum may be used, although it is not nearly so effective as either the antibothricopic or the anticrotalic.

A great deal is being done to teach the people to distinguish between the different kinds of serpents, and whenever a man brings a poisonous snake to the institution, he is told its distinguishing marks, and is given a bottle of the serum antidotal to its venom. This is the very best kind of practical lesson, as it conveys special information in regard to this particular venomous serpent to the man who comes in contact with it.

We were first shown many kinds of snakes preserved in Keiserling fluid or in alcohol, and so mounted as to demonstrate the anatomy. The females that were split open to show the eggs were very interesting. The eggs looked like preserved apricots, and many of them contained embryos.

We then went into an enclosure in the rear of the building, where the living snakes were kept in concrete wells resembling ash bins. For demonstration the snakes were taken out with an iron hook, on which they just naturally twisted themselves. One fellow clothed in an ash colored velvety coat, and looking like the father of all evil, was so vicious that he bit himself. His women folks, as ancestresses, had not done the decent thing by him, in either liking to look pretty themselves, or in choosing handsome consorts. According to the theories of Charles Darwin, if they had been more particular, their descendant would have been a handsomer fellow. Vicious appearances are however, sometimes deceptive, and this was not a poisonous snake.

The doctor had an ingenious method of handling the snakes. A sliding metal loop at the end of a stick was slipped over the animal's head, and then drawn snugly about the neck so as to prevent its squirming around. It could then be grasped with the finger and thumb behind the neck without fear. To get the virus a Petri dish was now presented to the snake, and he did not lose time in biting it, and the glass rang under the vigor of his jaws. The long upper fangs hooked over the edge, and the poison flowing down them fell into the dish. To get still more virus the situation of the poison glands was vigorously stroked or milked forward. The virus itself was a clear glairy substance like white of egg. Some years ago Mrs. Montgomery visited Haffkin's Laboratory in Bombay, and there a piece of rubber dam was stretched like a drumhead over a precipitating glass, and on the serpent biting through the rubber, the poison ran down his great fangs into the sterilized cavity of the glass. Dr. Brazil considered this precaution unnecessary as the poison in no case could be obtained sterile on account of the microorganisms in the mouth.

A price is paid for every snake delivered to the institution, and when a venomous one is brought, a flask of the proper antidotal serum is given to the man with instructions how to use it. Each transaction therefore constitutes a very valuable practical lesson, both as to the kind of snake handled and as to serum. In this way this serum is distributed to the very people who are exposed to the danger of being poisoned by those snakes.

Other valuable information is given to the public about these animals. For instance there is one kind of snake, a beautiful, graceful, dark iridescent creature, about three feet long, whose only food is other snakes. It will not attack man, and is not venomous. It is highly necessary, therefore, as a prophylactic measure, that this snake should not be killed. The doctor took one of them out of its lair, and stroked and petted it quite lovingly, and it laid its head in his palm, and tried to insinuate its head into the opening of his vest. It seemed to enjoy petting like a cat. As before mentioned this snake feeds on snakes. It appears these animals are very selective in their diet, some living on toads, and others on birds, and so on. Furthermore, they can go long spaces of time, even a year, without eating.

In order to still further study the nature of these animals, there was being constructed in the grounds an extensive area, enclosed by a wall and by a ditch lined with concrete. Here the snakes will be al-lowed to live as in nature, and many a fact in their life history, either interesting in itself, or interesting in regard to their relations with man, will be observed.

Some men, who are deeply interested in this subject, labor under the disadvantage of working with old virus transported a long distance, as from India to Paris for example, while still others who have Doctor Brazil's opportunities, take only a languid interest in their work. Doctor Brazil is enthusiastic, and he has the material, but he labors under one serious drawback; his native language, the language he speaks and writes most easily, is Portuguese. Portuguese is even worse than Spanish as a medium for communicating with those who are in sympathy with him. It is sad to think that these two nations that once occupied such a prominent place in the world are now so far removed from the highway along which ideas travel. Anything written in Portuguese finds a pitifully restricted audience. Surely it will not always be like this, for although Portugal is dead and the greater part of Brazil is either savage or moribund, yet the great state of Sao Paulo is alive. We have previously had occasion to speak of the well stocked book stores of Sao Paulo, and as another evidence there is this antidotal serum institute at Butanan. These indicate the beginnings of enlightenment. This state is large enough, rich enough, and has a temperate enough climate to form a center of culture for itself.

HEMOPTYSIS.

In hemorrhage of the lungs (*Medical Standard*) in phthisis pulmonalis, lycopus virginicus is one of our best remedies. It has the property of quieting cough and irritation of the lungs, and the expectoration becomes checked.

CORRESPONDENCE.

DR. MELTZER REPLIES.

To the Editor
American Medicine:—

The issue of American Medicine for December, 1911 (p. 631) contains an editorial which picks out a statement of mine to illustrate the sin of premature conclusions on insufficient evidence. It quotes from an editorial in the *N. Y. State Journal of Medicine* of October, 1910, in which I said that "606" "sterilizes the entire infected body with one single injection in less than 24 hours"—though there was not a particle of evidence on which to base such a conclusion, says the editorial in American Medicine. It quotes me further as stating that "physicians should not forget that this brilliant new remedy * * * came from theoretical laboratory studies." "We won't forget it," says the editorial in American Medicine, "and ask Mr. Pritchett to take note of it." The editorial then winds up with some uncomplimentary remarks about research workers in general some of which were apparently intended in particular for the present writer. I hope that, for the sake of truth and justice, American Medicine will publish my reply to this editorial.

My editorial which was published about 15 months ago, was prepared at the request of the editor of the *N. Y. State Journal of Medicine*. It presented a brief discussion of the principles underlying the action of "606" and of the results as they were reported until that time. It dealt with the experimental work of animals in the laboratory and with the reports of the "practical men" on human beings. As to the first, Ehrlich and Hata established the fact by numerous experiments that in diseases of animals produced by spirilla, like relapsing fever, framboesia, syphilis and chicken spirillosis, 606 "sterilizes the entire infected body with a single injection in less than 24 hours." Not a single doubt was raised against this conclusion in the medical literature of the entire civilized world. Furthermore in the observations made by physicians upon human diseases this statement was found to hold good also

for European and African relapsing fever, and probably also for yaws. *These undisputed facts served as a basis for my above quoted statement.* That the editorial writer of American Medicine should say nevertheless that there was not a particle of evidence on which to base such a conclusion is rather astonishing, but is perhaps a good illustration of the truth of the contention of that writer that "premature conclusions on insufficient evidence have always been the curse of medicine." As to the use of "606" in human syphilis, I only said there that "it is of immense practical value in syphilis." This conclusion was based upon observations of *many leading clinicians and dermatologists made on a material of 8,000 to 10,000 cases.* The reports on these cases came from "practical men" and not from "laboratories." Obviously it matters very little that six months later Dr. Gottheil, "on the strength of actual trial in 44 cases," assumed a cool attitude towards the remedy, as it mattered very little that Buschke, another otherwise meritorious dermatologist, gave up the remedy after an actual trial on six cases. I may also point out that in the same article I said that "Without doubt the remedy has its limitations. It will take the ripened, critical experience of many years to establish definitely the indications or contraindications of this remedy." Fifteen months passed since I wrote that incriminating article. Did the further development of the knowledge of our subject demonstrate that I was wrong in any of my statements? The writer in American Medicine seems to believe so; then he holds up the "scientist" to scorn for expressing an opinion without waiting for facts. However, there is sufficient "legal evidence" that the familiarity of that writer with the development of the subject of which he offers positive opinions is not too great. He says, for instance, "we must not use it (the remedy) intravenously as first advised from the laboratory." Everybody who has a modest knowledge of the subject *knows that the reverse of this statement is true.* In the laboratory (Ehrlich) intramuscular injections were used practically exclusively. It was not until several months after the introduction of the remedy in medical practice that, on the initiative of the such "practical" physicians as Iverson, Schreiber and Weintraud, the method of intravenous injections of the remedy was tried. At the risk of being held up to scorn again, I venture to state that after an accumulated experience of 15 months the great majority of informed practical medical men hold today that salvarsan is a brilliant discovery and that "it is of immense practical value in syphilis" where, however, it has its limitations. That is exactly what I said in the criticized article. As to the uncomplimentary things said in the editorial about "research workers" and "scientists," in so far as they refer to present writer, I find no fault in that. If a man who spent more than a quarter of a century in an extensive active practice is called in the fall of his life a research worker, a scientist, he ought to feel complimented, even if it is meant as an abuse. What I am sorry for, is the avowed tendency of the editorial writer to create an antagonism between the research workers and practical men in medicine. For years I tried to contribute my share to making the bridge connecting the followers of the sciences and the practice of medicine as short and as easily passable as possible. The close union will benefit both parties and help to make medicine an efficient science. It was this motive which made me say that practitioners should remember that the brilliant remedy was discovered in the laboratory.

S. J. MELTZER, M. D.

The Rockefeller Institute for Medical Research.

————

(While we cannot blame Dr. Meltzer for taking exception to the editorial he refers to, we wish to disavow any desire or intention on the part of any member of the editorial staff of AMERICAN MEDICINE to offer the slightest affront to Dr. Meltzer or to cast the slightest reflection on his work. We regret that the writer of the editorial objected to, is away and prevented by the force of circumstances from making adequate explanation of his remarks to Dr. Meltzer. We promise, however, that such explanation will be forthcoming at the earliest opportunity. In the meantime may we ask Dr. Meltzer to accept in good faith our earnest disavowal of any intentional attack on himself or his work?)—EDITOR.

ETIOLOGY AND DIAGNOSIS.

The Diagnosis of Smallpox.—Owing to the quite considerable increase of smallpox throughout the country, the editorial discussion of diagnosis in the current issue of the *Medical Era* is of more than passing interest. As is well said, the confusing and conflicting opinions which prevail among physicians in the differentiation of smallpox and varicella are due to the variety of forms in which both of these diseases express themselves.

We are too apt to overlook the fact that smallpox and chicken-pox, like other diseases, are liable to present typical and atypical forms. This is most apt to occur when they coincidently invade the same field and commingle their operations. Each disease now assumes to a certain extent the livery of the other, which, in a measure, changes the characteristics of both, and often renders their identification difficult. Divergent opinions will continue to confuse the medical mind until the causes of smallpox and varicella are definitely ascertained. The most experienced observers are yet divided on the question of relationship between these diseases. American authorities are inclined to ascribe them to separate and distinct forms of virus, while many English and German writers recognize varicella as a modified form of variola. Erasmus Wilson, Hebra, Kaposi and Kassowitz have adopted the latter theory, and their opinions are entitled to great weight; but the fact that chicken-pox often prevails where there is not a single case of smallpox to be found, and presents an entirely different history, affecting mostly children, while smallpox finds its most favorable soil for proliferation in the adult, weakens the position they have taken. It is possible that their opinions have been formed from their observation of varicella as it develops in connection with smallpox. Here it assumes some of the outward forms of smallpox, but these forms do not mature. They do not produce the grave symptoms of smallpox. They complete their work in from eight to fourteen days, while smallpox requires four weeks or more. Chicken-pox differs also from varioloid in many respects. Varioloid passes through all the stages of variola, but they are milder in type and shorter in duration. Varicella runs its course, as above stated, in from one to two weeks; varioloid requires from three to four weeks, and variola from four to five weeks. The constancy of their separate histories would seem to bar a unity of origin in variola and varicella. We are too apt to base our opinion of chicken-pox on the common vesicular form in which it expresses itself, but this form is only constant when chicken-pox operates independently of smallpox. When it follows in the wake of smallpox the initial lesion assumes the cone form and is described by some authorities as "varicella coniformis." It is this borrowed element of chicken-pox with which we are not familiar, that often leads us to confound it with smallpox. If we bear this in mind we will have less trouble in distinguishing one from the other.

While it is difficult to recognize smallpox before the eruption appears, the following symptoms will lead us to prepare for its advent: A severe chill, persistent vomiting, pain in the loins of a marked character, and high fever. The appearance, in about three days after these symptoms have developed of papules on the forehead, face, hands and wrists, gradually extending to other parts of the body, which inside of twenty-four hours are converted into umbilicated vesicles and later pass into pustules, will leave no doubt on the mind concerning the nature of the disease. In connection with these manifestations, if the fever has subsided after the appearance of the papular eruption and reappeared on the development of the pustular stage, our evidence of the disease is complete. It is readily distinguished from measles, scarlatina and syphilis, and we have only to bear in mind its different degrees of virulence, due to the potency of the virus and the sanitary environment of the patient, to differentiate it from varicella in all of its various forms.

Chronic Appendicitis.[1]—After a critical study of the post-operative end results in 100 cases, and a review of the literature the writer arrives at the following conclusions:—

(1) The majority of patients suffering from chronic appendicitis give a history of having had one or more attacks of abdominal illness, with a sequence of symptoms recognizable as those of an acute appendix attack, viz., sudden severe abdominal pain, usually beginning in the epigastrium or mid-abdomen, accompanied by nausea and vomiting and followed by a period of pain and tenderness in the right lower quadrant.

(2) "Appendiceal dyspepsia" has been characterized by symptoms strikingly analogous to the earliest symptoms of acute appendicitis, viz., attacks of epigastric or mid-abdominal pain, or distress, only rarely accompanied by subjective symptoms referable to the region of the appendix. During these attacks the pain or distress is nearly always increased by food intake.

(3) Pain confined chiefly to the right lower quadrant and not associated with attacks of epigastric pain and nausea is seldom due to the appendix, and before making a diagnosis of chronic appendicitis in these cases every other possible condition should be excluded.

(4) The majority of failures have been in patients complaining of right inguinal pain associated with chronic constipation. At operation these patients have presented an unusually long or dilated cecum, usually accompanied by other evidences of enteroptosis. In the future a certain proportion of these patients may be cured by some such operation as that advocated by Wilms, but appendicectomy alone does not cure.

(5) Unless the diagnosis is absolutely certain, the gall-bladder, stomach, and right kidney should be explored, and the possibility of a Lane's kink excluded in all cases operated upon for chronic appendicitis.

Diagnosis of Scarlet Fever.[1]—The writer states that too little attention is given to the condition of the mouth, nose and throat, in respect to diagnosis. Most text-books say there are three varieties: simple, toxic and septic throats.

The characteristic appearance of the throat, whether mild or toxic, is red, shiny, glazed and angry looking, with minute points of injection on the tonsils, uvula and palate.

There may be swollen tonsils, general edema and no exudation. With such a throat and the so-called pulse temperature ratio, we may expect a rash.

In the septic forms an exudation is present and the diagnosis lies between diphtheria and scarlet fever, and the nonscarlatinal tonsillitis.

In the severe septic forms, tonsillar swelling is great, with ulceration, discharge and perhaps otitis media.

In the mild forms of mixed infection we may have simple scarlet fever plus follicular tonsillitis.

With a definite false membrane, an appeal to the bacteriologist is imperative.

The association of diphtheria and scarlet fever causes much trouble. The author regards post scarlatinal diphtheria and diphtherial scarlet fever as preventable while coincident infection may be common.

Apart from membranous and ulcerative throats, other exudative conditions are to be seen, and sometimes the ordinary appearance of follicular tonsillitis.

The transient nature of the rash in scarlet fever should lead to the ability to diagnose a case without seeing the eruption. Bacteriologists may later give us a simple test, but at present we must rely on clinical observation, (a) before the appearance of the rash is likely, (b) while present, (c) and when absent and no longer expected.

The first period is brief, yet the sudden onset should put one on the alert, and the acceleration of the pulse and temperature greatly aids. The strawberry tongue is regarded as a sign of recession, if not convalescence.

The absence of sweating and high temperature may lead us to expect pneumonia, but the pulse-respiration ratio of the latter as compared with the pulse temperature ratio of scarlet fever, enable us to differentiate.

With a child ill less than 24 hours and definite red papules on the face, behind the ears, and appearing on the body, it is probably "German measles."

[1]E. M. Stanton, M. D., *Annals of Surgery*, Oct., 1911.

[1]P. C. Cruikshank, M. R. C. P., *London Practitioner*, Nov., 1911.

62   AMERICAN MEDICINE }
Complete Series, Vol. XVIII. }   TREATMENT   { JANUARY, 1912.
New Series, Vol. VII., No. 1.

If there is a rash it is first seen on the second day; one seen for the first time on the third or fourth day of an uncomplicated?—?

The typical rash is punctuate, not papular and brick red in color, the tint varies from pink to a deep scarlet. It is seen first over the clavicles and sternum, then down over the trunk, back and limbs, the legs last, disappearing in the same order, and vanishes at the end of the first week, leaving, if severe, a greenish discoloration. The more severe the case the more intense the rash.

With a rash we have to exclude certain acute specific diseases, drug and enema rashes, septic rashes: influenza, diphtheria and food poisoning. Copaiba poisoning may perfectly mimic fever, but does not accelerate the pulse above 100. Belladonna is distinguished by dilation of the pupils. Enema rashes are urticarial. With serum rashes there is intense irritation. It is usually wisest to treat doubtful cases as scarlet fever.

Scarlet fever frequently occurs with but three of the four classical symptoms—rash, throat, tongue and pulse—and may be diagnosed with but two.

In the second week, if called to suggest, confirm or discredit a diagnosis of scarlet fever we should take a culture, especially if severe, staining marked, and desquamation present.

The characteristics of scarlet fever desquamation are: First. Fine powdering on the cheeks, first week. Second. Delicate scaling over the clavicles. Third. Pin holes or worm holes. Fourth. Large scales leaving red tender skin. Scaling is in full swing in the second week with face and neck clear.

TREATMENT.

The Treatment of Acute Rheumatism.[1]—The chief indications in the treatment of acute articular rheumatism, says Yeo and Phear, are as follows:—(1) To endeavor to cut short the course of the attack and thereby to lessen the danger-period during which there is the risk of cardiac complications. (2) To relieve the joint pains and other distressing symptoms. (3) To meet any complication which may arise, and specially to be ready with the promptest treatment in the event of hyperpyrexia. (4) To guard against the danger of relapse by prolonging treatment beyond the period of symptoms and by special supervision during convalescence.

The first step to be taken in the practical application of these principles is to order the patient to bed and to maintain absolute rest in bed during the acute stage and for a considerable period after the subsidence of all acute symptoms. The patient must not be allowed to leave his bed for any purpose whatever. The clothing should be arranged with a view to minimising the inconvenience caused by the profuse and repeated sweats which are a constant feature of acute rheumatism. The night-dress should be of soft thin flannel, and made to open down the whole length in front in order in facilitate the frequent changes that are required. The patient should lie on a soft blanket, and the bedclothes should be as light as is consistent with warmth. The weight of the clothes may be raised off the swollen and painful joints by means of a cradle, and a small cushion or air-pillow placed below the knees with the object of supporting the joints in a slightly flexed position will lessen the tension of the distended joints and contribute to the comfort of the patient. A dose of calomel followed by a saline purgative is given as an initial step in the treatment, and a regular action of the bowels should be maintained.

During the acute stage the diet is rigidly restricted to fluids, and should consist of milk, suitably diluted. At least five ounces of milk should be given every two hours, and more if the patient is willing to take it. In this way three or four pints of milk are given in the 24 hours. If the patient is asleep, it is a mistake to rouse him for the special purpose of taking food, as there is usually no difficulty in making up the quantity missed in subsequent feeds. The milk should be diluted with an equal volume of boiled water, which may contain either sodium bicarbonate or sodium citrate, thirty to forty grains to the pint; when milk forms the staple nutriment for a prolonged period, there are advantages in using the citrate solution as a diluent. The fluid taken may be warm, cool, or iced according to the preference of the patient.

Variety may be introduced by an occasional feed flavored with tea or coffee; but, as a rule, the tongue is coated, the sense of taste is lost, and the patient is indifferent to flavors. As a result of the continued drain of moisture from the skin the patient suffers from thirst, and the urine becomes scanty, concentrated, and highly acid, with a copious deposit of urates on cooling. The loss of fluid may be made good by alkaline drinks consisting of unsweetened lemonade or barley-water, to which bicarbonate of potassium is added, twenty or thirty grains to the pint. This may be taken freely in the intervals between the feeds of milk, and will be found considerably to increase the comfort of the patient. Beef-tea and broths should not be given, except in the case of those who have difficulty in taking milk. Meat extracts are undesirable, and the use of alcohol should be reserved for special circumstances.

Attempts have been made to treat acute rheumatism with antitoxic sera and vaccines; but up to the present no satisfactory result has been obtained by this method. In the absence of any remedy which is specific in the strict bacteriological sense, it is fortunate that in the various salicyl compounds we possess a group of remedies, which, if suitably administered, give results in articular rheumatism not unworthy of comparison with the effects of vaccines or antitoxic treatment in other diseases. The rheumatic process is in fact so rapidly and completely controlled by the ex-

[1] I. Burney Yeo, M. D., and A. G. Phear, M. D., *The Practitioner*, January, 1912.

hibition of salicylates in appropriate doses that the therapeutic influence of these substances may be fairly compared with that of quinine in the case of malaria, and mercury in the case of syphilis. The earliest effect of salicylates is on the pain, which is lessened within a few hours of the first dose, and may be completely relieved in the course of two days. At the same time the inflammatory swelling subsides, and there is a steady fall of temperature, which may be reduced to the normal within three or four days of commencing treatment. The rapidity and completeness with which relief is provided may in itself constitute a difficulty in the management of the case, as a considerable amount of persuasion may be needed to convince the patient of the necessity for the long and tedious period over which treatment must be continued.

The object to be aimed at in the adminfstration of salicylates is to bring the patient under the full influence of the drug as rapidly as possible, and to this end it is desirable to begin with large doses given at frequent intervals, and to continue the full dose until either the symptoms of the disease are relieved, or indications of intolerance arise. In either event the dose must be reduced. The earliest evidences of an excessive dose are buzzing noises in the head with headache and deafness; later effects consist of nausea, vomiting, dimness of vision, and hematuria; and if the drug is continued, in full doses the result may be delirium and a train of symptoms similar to those associated with the acetonemia of diabetes; it is hardly necessary to say that the earlier symptoms should suffice as an indication for a reduction in dose.

In an attack of moderate severity initial doses of 10 grains of sodium salicylate may be given every two hours. If the attack is severe, it is desirable to give larger doses—15 or 20 grains every two hours, representing a total quantity of three to four drachms in the 24 hours. In the absence of undesirable effects this dose should be continued until the acute symptoms have yielded to the treatment. After two days it is generally feasible, by increasing the interval between doses to four hours, to reduce the total amount given by one-half. If the advantage gained under the larger dose is maintained and the patient remains free from pain and fever, the reduced dose may be contiued for a period of four to five days, and at the end of that time the amount may be further reduced to 15 or 20 grains three times a day, best spread over equal eight-hourly intervals. It is a point of the greatest importance that the remedy should be continued for two whole weeks after the disappearance of all acute symptoms; many relapses arise from a neglect of this rule, and, more serious than relapse, the origin of a cardiac lesion, leading to crippling of the heart for life, may depend on a too early discontinuance of the salicylate treatment.

The unpleasant taste of salicylates may be covered by syrup of orange or of ginger, or the drug may be dissolved in water and given with milk.

In striking contrast to the controlling influence of salicylates over the synovial lesions of rheumatism is the indecisive character of their action in the cardiac complications of the disease. Not only do most cases of cardiac rheumatism appear to run their course unmodified favorably by salicylates, but there is a risk of the heart being adversely influenced through the depressing effects of the drug on the cardiac muscle, and the existence of recent cardiac complications may be taken as a contraindication to the use of such large doses of salicylates as are desirable in the treatment of the uncomplicated articular form of the disease. The value of salicylates from the point of view of cardiac rheumatism is chiefly preventive, and depends on their effect in shortening the course of articular rheumatism, thereby minimizing the risk to which the heart is subjected.

A number of allied drugs with similar properties, such as salicin, salicylic acid, salophen, aspirin, have from time to time been advocated in place of sodium salicylate; but, with the exception of salicin and possibly aspirin, none of them equals the salicylates in efficacy. Aspirin has gained a great reputation in the treatment of rheumatic affections, and it has been claimed for it that, while possessing all the virtues of sodium salicylate, it is remarkably free from the bad effects which occasionally follow treatment with salicylates. As a result of numerous observations with the object of comparing the two remedies, we conclude that in the treatment of acute rheumatism in adults aspirin, while of admittedly great value, possesses no advantage over the salicylates, and indeed is relatively less efficient in the rapidity and thoroughness with which the disease is brought under control. In children and in the milder forms of articular rheumatism there may possibly be some advantages in the use of aspirin; but in all cases with severe joint symptoms we should not hesitate in our preference for the salicylate compound.

Salicin is a less depressing drug than sodium salicylate, and may be administered freely with a smaller risk of producing toxic symptoms. It is scarcely, if at all, inferior in its specific effects, and the value of this remedy in the treatment of rheumatism has hardly met with the recognition it deserves. It is decidedly preferable to salicylates in the treatment of weakly individuals, and should be given a trial in all cases where undue susceptibility to the effects of salicylates is present. It may be given in initial doses of 15 to 30 grains, combined with half the quantity of potassium citrate, every two or three hours, the dose to be reduced as soon as acute symptoms are relieved. The solubility of salicin in cold water is but slight, but it readily dissolves in hot water, and should always be given in solution.

The use of alkalies in the treatment of rheumatism, originally based on the hypothesis of a general morbid acidity of the fluids of the body, fell for a time out of fashion on the introduction of salicylates. It is a mistake, however, to assume that alkalies have no place in the

64   AMERICAN MEDICINE }
Complete Series, Vol. XVIII. }   SOCIETY PROCEEDINGS   {   JANUARY, 1912.
{ New Series, Vol. VII., No. 1.

therapeutics of this disease, and in our opinion the best results are obtained by a combination of the two remedies. It has been claimed that the free administration of alkalies lessens the risk of cardiac complications; but, without entering on a discussion of this difficult question, there is reason to believe that in the presence of alkalies it is possible to give larger doses of salicylates without risk of symptoms of acetonemia than would otherwise be the case, and that their administration has at least the indirect advantage of enabling salicylate treatment to be developed to its full extent. A solution of sodium bicarbonate or potassium citrate may be used as a diluting fluid for the milk; or, as an alternative, 30 grains of potassium bicarbonate may be added to each 20-grain dose of sodium salicylate, and dissolved in at least 2 ounces of water; if desired an effervescing mixture may be obtained by the addition of a dessertspoonful of lemon juice. An increase in the flow of urine, and a change of reaction, indicate that a sufficiency of alkali is being given, and the dose may then be reduced to the point at which an alkaline reaction is just maintained.

The relief afforded by salicylates is usually so prompt that no special local treatment of the joints is called for beyond a loose wrapping of cotton-wool and the use of a cradle to carry the weight of the bedclothes. The application of a warm alkaline lotion containing twenty grains of sodium bicarbonate and one drachm of laudanum to the ounce of water is soothing and may be employed for the purpose of easing pain in the initial stage before there has been time for remedies given by the mouth to produce their full effect.

An opportunity for the local use of methyl salicylate may be found, on the other hand, in the later stages of rheumatism; in cases where some local pain and swelling persist and are refractory to the internal use of salicylates about half a drachm of methyl salicylate may be applied with a brush and allowed to dry on the exposed surface; or the remedy may be diluted with an equal quantity of olive oil and gently rubbed into the skin over the painful joint; excessive friction should be avoided and no wrapping should be applied to the joint. In other cases of protracted local symptoms the condition yields to counter-irritation by means of blistering paper, which should be applied in strips, one and a half to two inches wide, just above and below the affected joint. The method of local counter-irritation may be advantageously combined with the internal administration of potassium iodide in five-grain doses with potassium bicarbonate in ten or fifteen-grain doses three times a day.

A Method of Curing Corns.—In the method to be described, says the *Medical Summary*, the writer depends upon the macerating power of ordinary adhesive plaster to effect the result sought. A strip of this material from three-eighths to one-half of an inch in width and four to six inches long is to be applied in spiral fashion to the affected toe, covering the digit from neck to nail. The degree of tightness of the application deserves consideration to avoid compression. However, the feelings of the patient when stepping upon the foot will serve as an adequate guide in this matter. Given instructions to cut through the plaster lengthwise or to soak off the entire dressing by immersion in hot water foot bath afford ample protection in cases of undetected microbic infection. Soaking the foot from ten to twenty minutes in water at a temperature of 100 degrees with gentle removal of rubbing with a piece of sterilized pumice stone or forceps of the crown of hardened epidermis shortens the time of treatment. Properly applied the plaster strap dressing described should afford relief from the moment of its application and may be worn continuously for from one to six or eight weeks—bathing seeming to unaffect the adhesive properties of the plaster after having once set. Removal of the dressing at the end of an adequate time reveals the cornus completely freed, when it may be picked out entirely by means of a dressing forceps or after an additional soaking. A wisp of absorbent cotton held on by means of a narrow adhesive strip may be subsequently worn for a few days.

SOCIETY PROCEEDINGS.

THE EASTERN MEDICAL SOCIETY OF THE CITY OF NEW YORK.

Stated Meeting, January 12th, 1912.

EXECUTIVE SESSION.

The reports of officers and standing committees for the past year were presented.

The officers for the ensuing year were inaugurated.

Dr. S. J. Kopetzky, in his inaugural address, after thanking the members for the confidence reposed in him, took up for consideration three important economic problems of interest to the medical profession in general.

He called attention to the tendency of the Health Department to extend throughout the city the new Dispensary System, and while he commented favorably on the excellent work of the department in checking the spread of contagious and communicable diseases, he questioned the authority of the department either to practice practical medicine or to engage in the manufacture or sale of drugs. In his opinion the department should use to its utmost capacity the institutions already in existence in the city, instead of starting a new system as they seemed minded to do. He hoped that co-operation would take place between the profession and the Department of Health in discussion, as to the advisability and wisdom of their plans.

He endorsed the stand of the Board of Education on the question of school hygiene, believing it an advantage to have medical experts attached to and under the supervision of the head of the Educational Department in the Board of Education, to study hygiene of the school from the standpoint of the *healthy* child. The system of medical inspection now in vogue under the Board of Health takes cognizance mostly of the sick child, and a reference to Superintendent Maxwell's reports would show the necessity of the suggested reform.

On the question of dispensary abuse in general, he held that continuation of the present conditions, while it added factors towards the curtailment of the younger medical men's income, worked its most serious harm in preventing the proper medical care of the worthy poor, for whom primarily this charity was instituted. He held that pride in the character of the work done and the knowledge that it had administered to those really in need of it should be the desired end, rather than a report of the large numbers treated. He showed that the present system of investigating those applying for treatment was inadequate, and recommended that a law be placed on the statute books which would make the institution found guilty punishable by a fine for each offense; such fine to be paid from the surplus earned by the dispensaries, their reports usually showing that they do earn profits. A statute such as this would at once curtail the evil, because the institution would at once institute an investigation, for fear that among those applying for treatment would be some one gathering evidence against them.

Regarding contract medicine, he said that men were actually bidding to handle large numbers of people at most insignificant fees, and younger graduates were entering the field of work taking contracts at progressively cheaper rates. He warned the young graduate who takes up such work, that if he stayed in it for any length of time he would become a marked man and his medical progress would cease, as there is not one incentive to do conscientious work in the system, and even his employers look askance at him. He regretted that the evil had passed unnoticed by the powers that should have strangled it in its infancy, and commented on the fact that either the senior members of the profession deemed the consideration of this problem beneath their dignity, or had no idea of its extent and character.

He recommended cooperation between representatives of regular medical societies and these employers of medical men. He suggested that a uniform system of contract be adopted, mutually agreeable, in which a minimum rate of fee should be established and a limit be put upon the number of those treated for a given fee.

Finally he desired that only such men should be eligible to hold these contracts, whose character, medical ability and conduct would be approved by the medical societies. He thought that the last provision would force many who were now outside of the breastwork to come in and join some representative medical society.

In order to give sanction to this form of practice, the principles of medical ethics should be made to conform with conditions as they exist. The code should not only afford this status recognition, but should make it unethical and unprofessional and punishable by proper means, for a physician to bid, or have bid, in his name for any contract, in any lodge society, insurance company, or any other organization at a figure lower than his predecessor in office. Furthermore, it should be made unethical and punishable for any physician to use unfair means to take from another in good professional standing the position he occupies. Some such amendment to the code, in his opinion, would ameliorate the conditions almost wholly, as it would legalize and control the situation; and from information in his possession, obtained from those employing medical men, some such plan as this seems to find favor with them too.

Finally he recommended the appointment of committees to carry out and make effective these plans.

Following was the Scientific Program of the evening:

1. Presentation of cases.
   - A. Fracture and dislocation of the second cervical vertebra.
   - B. Fracture of the spinous process of the second cervical vertebra.
                              Dr. Henry Keller.
2. Papers:—Symposium on practical features of diseases of the genito-urinary tract.
   - A. Transperitoneal operation on the bladder.
         Dr. Parker Syms, (By invitation).
   - B. Renal lithiasis.
                              Dr. Winfield Ayers.
   - C. Early diagnosis and treatment of renal tuberculosis.
                           Dr. Maurice Packard.
   - D. Hydronephrosis.
   Dr. Charles H. Chetwood, (By invitation).

This symposium will appear in full in another portion of AMERICAN MEDICINE.

The discussion was of great interest but was necessarily curtailed owing to the lateness of the hour.

ITEMS OF INTEREST.

The Western Issue of the American Journal of Surgery.—The January number of the *American Journal of Surgery* contains a wealth of valuable material. Written by men whose work is recognized the world over, the papers which appear in this issue are notable contributions to the various subjects considered.

The following list of the articles which appear will give an excellent idea of their character and scope:

The Operation of Gastroenterostomy, by William J. Mayo, Rochester, Minn.

Operative Treatment for Graves Disease, by George W. Crile, Cleveland, Ohio.

Colonic Intoxication, by J. E. Binney, Kansas City, Mo.

Practical Points in the Surgical Treatment of Exophthalmic Goitre, by A. J. Oschner, Chicago, Ill.

Treatment of Foreign Bodies in the Esophagus, by E. Fletcher Ingals, Chicago, Ill.

Brain Surgery Technique, by J. Rilus Eastman, Indianapolis, Ind.

Treatment of Abscesses and of the Necrotic Foci Resulting from the Use of Salvarsan, by A. Ravogli, Cincinnati, Ohio.

Treatment of Prostatic Obstructions, by E. O. Smith, Cincinnati, Ohio.

Artificial Tendons and Ligaments in the Surgical Treatment of Paralysis, by Nathaniel Allison, St. Louis, Mo.

Uterine Cancer, by John C. Murphy, St. Louis, Mo.

Arthritis Deformans, by Leonard W. Ely, Denver, Colo.

Acute Angulation and Flexure of the Sigmoid, as a Causative Factor in Epilepsy with Special Reference to Treatment, by W. H. Axtell, Bellingham, Wash.

The issue is profusely illustrated and in every way shows the conscientious, untiring effort that has been expended to produce a number creditable not alone to Western surgery, but to American surgery. No one can read this splendid number without appreciating the forces that have entered into its production. Work that is so evidently honest, clean, and constructive is bound to count, and those responsible for what the *American Journal of Surgery* has been doing and will continue to do for the medical profession may rest assured that their labors have long been appreciated by many of their fellow workers.

The New Medical Review of Reviews.—We have before us the first issue of the *Medical Review of Reviews* under its new era. Having read the prospectus of this issue—which prospectus by the way was indeed a masterpiece—we perhaps are not as surprised at the notable improvements that have been made, as we might have been, had our expectations been less whetted in advance. In every way, however, this excellent publication has been improved and if this first issue is any indication of the future, it is sure to take high rank among the well established, high class medical journals of the country. To say that this initial number is interesting, readable and possessed of a literary value far and away beyond any preceding copies is to state the obvious. Well printed, and presenting its interesting material in departments that preserve a balance of topics especially deserving of commendation, it is evident that not the least of the factors which have produced this first issue is the ideal back of it all. In spite of the hustle, hurry and struggle to get ahead, ideals count as much today as ever, and if the *Medical Review of Reviews* achieves the success we confidently expect it to, no small part of the credit will belong to the ideals that are so apparent in this initial number prepared under and by the direction of its new owner, Mr. Frederic H. Robinson. Mr. Robinson has organized a new editorial staff of medical men whose medico-literary talents are well known.

Starting its new regime at a time when the ideals and aspirations of medical journalism were never higher, the sense of journalistic responsibility that characterizes the present management, assure results that cannot help but prove uplifting and progressive. It is needless to state that we wish every good thing for the *Medical Review of Reviews*. Nothing will give us keener pleasure than to see it win the success that this first issue promises. More power to every effort, and aspiration is our earnest wish.

Successful Medicine.—One of the most unique, and yet we believe one of the most desirable publications that have recently appeared is *Successful Medicine.* Devoted to the economic phases of medical practice it aims to make doctors better business men. That this is "a consummation devoutly to be wished for," hardly anyone will deny. Physicians have been notoriously bad business men, simply because they have allowed themselves to become victims of the all too common idea that to use business methods in practice is to commercialize medicine. Nothing could be more ridiculous. Of course, it is easy to subordinate everything in medicine to dollars and cents. This is medical commercialism at its worst. But such is not the object of *Successful Medicine.* On the contrary, this breezy, interesting little journal aims to teach the physician to keep careful records, to make proper and definite charges, to render accounts regularly and properly, and in every way, to conduct on a business basis the practice on which he and his family necessarily depend for their livelihood. In plain words, *Successful Medicine* aims to make the doctor's credit better by helping him to get what he earns somewhere near the time when he earns it.

Every issue contains a large amount of material giving different doctors' methods of protecting their interests, and no one can read these experiences without obtaining many new valuable ideas. Edited and published by Dr. Henry R. Harrower (Schiller Bldg., Chicago, Ill.), we understand that the circulation of this exceedingly useful journal already runs way up into the thousands. Its subscription price is only 25 cents per year, and no American physician should fail to have it come to him regularly.

American Medicine

H. EDWIN LEWIS, M. D., *Managing Editor.*
PUBLISHED MONTHLY BY THE AMERICAN-MEDICAL PUBLISHING COMPANY.
Copyrighted by the American Medical Publishing Co., 1912.

Complete Series, Vol. XVIII., No. 2.
New Series, Vol. VII.. No. 2.   **FEBRUARY, 1912.**   **$1.00** YEARLY in advance.

The perfect protective power of revaccination does not seem to be as widely known as it should be and there is urgent need of more publicity of the facts, now that there is a recrudescence of the anti-vaccination delusion. Some of this opposition comes from unbalanced people who are against every constituted system be it religious, political or scientific. They are "born that way," and as there will always be people "born that way," we might as well make up our minds to a perpetual irrepressible anti-vaccination propaganda. It will never be very vigorous because so many of the leaders, who are honest even if deluded, die of smallpox, but there will always be other illogical men ready to take their places. Besides, there are always some *un*moral people who, though vaccinated, join the crusade for ulterior motives —even scoundrelly physicians have done so. Our professional duty is clear, we must institute a perpetual system of public education by demonstrations of the absolute protection afforded by a revaccination.

A primary vaccination causes only an evanescent immunity in many cases and it is this fact which has been used so effectively by anti-vaccinationists to convince the unreasoning that there is no immunity at all. There are no data by which we can estimate how long the immunity will last, and we are much to blame for not having carefully investigated the thousands of cases of smallpox following one vaccination, with the view of determining the time elapsing between the vaccination and the smallpox, for each year of age at vaccination. About the only thing statisticians insist upon is the greatly reduced mortality rate in this class of cases, to show that some protection exists even when complete immunity wears out. The enormous number who escape smallpox, though vaccinated but once in their lives, should convince any one that the chances of lifelong immunity are very great, and that in only the minority does the immunity diminish sufficiently to allow of infection. Unfortunately, the exceptions appeal to such minds. It is now necessary to enlarge upon the fact that a successful revaccination after an interval of some years, so reinforces the diminishing immunity of the first, that smallpox cannot be acquired. As far as we know there are no recorded cases of smallpox in which there is perfect evidence of two successes, one in infancy and one in adult life, and there is reason to believe that reinforcement by revaccination after only five years is permanently protective.

Spurious vaccinations should be carefully eliminated from all such discussions, and only a normal scar be taken as proof.

It is a matter of common knowledge that a coincident infection may be mistaken for the vaccine process, and many people are told that their vaccinations are successful whereas they are not protected at all. These cases, when they do contract smallpox, are also used to prove that vaccination does not protect. We must be more careful. Indeed there is a suspicion that many if not all the fatal cases of smallpox in the "vaccinated" are of this spurious class. Another danger is the use of lymph which has become sterile or "attenuated" by age. When there is no result, we are prone to assert that the patient is immune, whereas we should suspect the lymph used. Moreover a partial result from attenuated old lymph may prevent a proper vaccination for some months or years and during all this time the person is liable to contract the disease and even die of it. It is highly essential then that only fresh material be used and that it should be so stored as to retain its vitality. Besides all this, the infections from poor lymph have created the impression with a few opponents that the operation is unduly dangerous. We can prevent these complications, but of course we cannot prevent the infections due to the patient's scratching into the abrasion with dirty fingers and even causing tetanus. Those cases in dirty families will always occur but we can reduce their number by careful instruction to each mother. We will never be able to stop the cases due to failure to get revaccinated but we can reduce their number by giving the greatest publicity to the fact that the operation must be repeated every few years until a second perfect result is obtained, whereby a permanent immunity is secured, obviating the necessity for any further trials.

We must diminish anti-vaccinationism for it does seem that our own professional shortcomings are partly responsible for much of the opposition, and that if we ourselves become as immaculate as our human nature permits, the anti-vaccinationists will have so few facts to distort that their crusade will be comparatively harmless. Let us therefore put our own house in order and then continue the fight for public health. But, as previously explained, we must not expect to convince all anti-vaccinationists for they exist even in countries where compulsory vaccination has completely eliminated smallpox. In this democracy, they claim the right to resist and we must allow them to kill themselves this way if they so desire, but we ought to lessen the number of their dupes, though, to be sure, people who are duped by such illogical reasoning, are not worth preserving. As far as the eugenic evolution of the race is concerned there is much in favor of the theory that the welfare of society demands that we allow the fools to kill themselves—and the sooner the better. Still it is our duty to educate those who are educatable. So let us get at it. Let us reach a stage wherein we may assert that if a man gets smallpox it is his own fault, and give him no sympathy—perhaps even punish him after recovery, for having become a burden to others!

The number of normal vaccine scars seems to determine the degree of immunity. At least, in those countries where babies are vaccinated at three or four places on each arm, it is exceedingly difficult to cause a second success in adult life and the subjects rarely if ever contract smallpox. It is well to inquire therefore whether we are right in our practice of vaccinating in only one place. We do know that irrespective of the times or numbers of vaccinations, it is a fact that the greater the number of scars the fewer are the cases of smallpox. The disease is practically unknown in those with six normal scars, three on each arm. This matter is so important that it seems public vaccinators should be compelled to make at least three insertions.

The eventual disappearance of private practice seems to be accepted as a matter of course, if we are to judge by the tenor of certain addresses by physicians of an observing and predicting turn of mind. The basis for the opinion is the gradual increase in the number of specialists as well as general practitioners who are under salary; investigators, teachers, pathologists, laboratory clinicians, hospital employees, life insurance directors, public health officers, military and naval officers, physicians to the poor, medical journalists, medical writers, advisors and investigators for pharmaceutical and chemical manufacturers, physicians to beneficial associations, missionaries, and we wish we could add public lecturers to teach hygiene and sanitation to laymen. There have been many references to the fact that the poor are beginning to think that, when they are ill or hurt, they are entitled to free treatment, including housing, clothing and food for themselves as well as money to support the wife and babies. Whether it is right or wrong, they seem to be getting what they think their rights and as we have frequently remarked, society seems to be drifting to a socialism in which all doctors are salaried servants of corporations or society.

The future purpose of medical education is the point brought up by recent addresses on the decay of private practice. Medical colleges were first created to prepare students to enter private practice, but medical education has already become very largely a preparation for public practice or for something else. The teachers must adjust themselves to the new conditions or retire. Students must be prepared for a host of callings, and the colleges themselves must supply the demand and not train students for private practice and then turn them loose to learn how to do the special work which modern civilization demands. Let us wake to the conditions at once, and recognize that a large and increasing percentage of students must be trained to other ways of earning a living than by private fees for advice to the sick. The welfare of society already demands that many should be specially trained to prevent sickness—and injury too, for all accidents have had a medical bearing ever since we found out that they were mostly due to fatigue. Let the medical curriculum be arranged so that early specialization is possible, and men are trained to take up these new lines of work.

The overcrowded medical curriculum is receiving long needed attention at the hands of the Council on Medical Education of the American Medical Association. We have frequently called attention to the fact that we are forcing into the course more than the brain can hold, and now a great variety of suggestions are being made to standardize the colleges by establishing a minimum which each student must learn, no matter what his subsequent career. It is an age of minute division of labor and specialization. Physicians, willy-nilly, find themselves confined to very limited spheres of activity. The keynote for reform is not multiplication of studies for all, but specialization after the minimal rudiments are learned. Now let us get at a reasonable estimate of what these minimal rudiments should be. They will be merely a foundation for the later studies, which will and must assume the role of the technical training in engineering for instance. A mining engineer is not the less efficient in his sphere, if he is ignorant of ship building, and a refractionist need know little of obstetrics.

The Hospital Saturday and Sunday Association, in its last annual report, presents some very interesting figures. Under the auspices of this organization, forty-five hospitals rendered 1,235,524 days of free treatment during the past year, at an expense of over $1,500,000 more than the income derived from invested money, appropriations, or the patients able to pay.

The report shows that during the last twelve months, $115,959 was collected, which represents an increase of 28% over the amounts received the year before—and yet, so extensive has the work and needs of the Association become, that the total receipts are far below the sum required. Private contributions to the fund are the means by which it becomes necessary to supply the deficiency and a strong appeal is being made to the public for donations, however small.

The money collected is divided among the hospitals of the Association to carry on free treatment of the deserving poor who are cared for, irrespective of race, color or religious beliefs. It is a most worthy form of charity and one that should meet with the greatest success.

The financial condition of this particular association, is more or less similar to that of all organizations of its kind and very aptly recalls the thought so often expressed, that it is not what is earned so much as it is what is spent, that governs in a great measure, the resources of the individual or the institution. Undoubtedly, the Hospital Saturday and Sunday Association disburses the means at its command in most effective and advantageous manner and it is to be lamented that it hasn't much more to spend; but from a business as well as professional standpoint, there exists a seemingly small detail which is being lightly passed over by all institutions directly concerned in the free treatment of patients, and which are dependent upon such charitable organizations for money to carry on their work. This is the imposition placed upon all free dispensaries and clinics, by a class of people who are able to pay, at least something for treatment, but who present themselves for the beneficence and privileges primarily devised for the real poor and deserving. There are many, therefore, who dishonestly avail themselves of these gratuitous ministrations, thus necessarily curtailing the benefits received by, and rightfully belonging to the truly indigent.

If the out-patient departments of the city hospitals and clinics were more particular to limit their services to people who are really unable to pay for medical care, there would be more money and requisites left for the deserving. Donations would go farther and greater good would be accomplished.

This brings up the old question of *abuse of the privileges of free treatment,* as offered to the public by the various institutions. We have discussed this subject at previous times—as has most everyone else —and the imposition remains—as no doubt it always will.

To any physician connected with this work, the true state of affairs is most apparent. He is the one person coming into close and intimate contact with these patients. In the course of his work, he learns the truth in many instances and he cannot but feel the injustice of a system which allows the impostors to freely avail themselves of privileges not intended for them, and thus offer so great a hindrance to the dispensing of real charity to the ones who are actually in need.

The word "free" is perhaps the most alluring one in our language. It suggests unlimited possibilities and directly appeals through a fundamental weakness of human nature, namely to get something for nothing. Free medical treatment is most enticing to clinic habitués who frequently become really domineering and impertinent in their manner. From their point of view however, the situation seems most natural. Believing that charitable institutions were established for their especial personal benefit, they mean to profit thereby.

Daily instances are always to be observed, wherein dispensary privileges are abused. A woman—far from really poor— recently brought her boy to a large clinic for an examination and operation. She felt and plainly showed that she was not of the "common class," for she did not take to the idea of waiting her turn, or of sitting among the more shabbily dressed patients. Because of her very appearance and manner, she was diplomatically and most politely asked if she was unable to pay her own physician for doing the work. Impertinently expressed was her reply—"yes, I can pay something but I think I would be very foolish indeed to pay out money for having this done, when I can get it for nothing."

There is much more that might be said upon the subject, but we refrain. Entirely aside from the standpoint of the physician, who of course is thus hindered in his work of carrying on the necessary regular routine of dispensary treatment, what about the direct imposition upon the organizations and institutions which are endeavoring to provide, as they think, for the poor? What about the wrong toward the truly indigent, whom the dispensaries in allowing impostors to consume the time and money set aside for them, are forced to overlook?

Just a few suggestive questions—Would not a more careful and systematic inquiry of every one of the patients applying for free treatment, by the admitting force of charitable institutions aid a little in reducing expense? Or at least would not the exclusion of impostors from the clinics leave more for the legitimate patients, and wouldn't the resources on hand go farther?

It may appear as a very trivial matter— but is it not good business combined with the real aim of humanitarianism to give the best we have where it is most truly needed and deserved? Surely this is always the physician's ideal endeavor. This state of affairs most truly exists—the proof is not wanting.

A Pure Air Law, or act, should be instituted and enforced through municipal action. We are more or less protected by a food and drug act, which guarantees the quality of food and medicine taken into our digestive tract, and since it is obvious that what we take into our respiratory system, or what we breathe, is as important to our good health as what we eat, why should we not be assured of protection against impure and contaminated air?

As an etiological factor in the causation of many acute and chronic affections, defiled air is now of recognized importance. Numerous diseases are known to take origin within the respiratory passages which naturally offer marked facilities for rapid absorption of pathological organisms into the system. Within the lungs, the delicate vascular network permits direct and ready contact of the blood with contaminated air; the poisonous material is absorbed and carried throughout the body, to locate finally at the point of least resistance or lowered vitality, where it promptly sets up symptoms indicative of definite disease.

Ventilation is no new problem, but it is one that bears emphatically upon the state of good health.

Within our homes, we generally recognize the necessity and value of free outside air, and as a rule, employ measures to insure sufficient ventilation. Obviously however, we are not always at home but more frequently in places where there is overcrowding, bad hygienic surroundings, often personal uncleanliness, and most certainly, poor ventilation; where we are entirely dependent upon others for the purity of our air supply. In the struggle for the almighty dollar, we are of necessity continually herded together, and forced to breathe and re-breathe impure air.

Offices, factories, workmen, railway cars and similar modes of conveyance, are nearly always insufficiently ventilated and generally overheated. Many writers upon the subject have pointed out that although carbon dioxide and related end products of respiration are distinctly harmful, the presence of dust, finely divided particles of refuse, smoke, vapors and gases, as well as the dried elements of expectorated material and other germ containing matter, are even more deleterious.

Take for example our places of amusement where many people are often closely gathered together, and which are intended to serve as means of recreation and physical relaxation. It is an old story. They are always poorly ventilated and overheated— and just because we frequent such places for the very purpose of relaxation, releasing muscular tension and permitting more or less complete inaction of the physical defences against disease, we render our bodies more susceptible to contaminating surroundings.

There are at present 12,000 moving picture theatres in the United States. They are, of course, primarily all business enterprises—running to full capacity and with the sole object of "making money." The majority of these "theatres" are of the makeshift variety—the buildings were not originally intended to house a number of people, consequently provision for proper ventilation, cleanliness and heating, were not included in the building plans. Sanitary laws provide a little protection and here and there, holes have been cut in the roof or sides to allow entrance of *some* fresh air; or a circular ventilating fan may have been installed; but in comparison to the amount of air required and that supplied, it is safe to say that little if any outside air ever passes the ticket taker.

Fresh outside air in motion is the only effective means of obtaining proper ventilation—and how many of these places have a continued entrance of such air?

Sunlight is a distinct foe of the motion picture—from a business standpoint—and above all things the "theatre" must be kept dark. Incidentally, the same forbidden sunlight is one of the best, if not the most effective antagonist of contamination—and certainly it *never* enters the building.

The cheaper grade of motion picture houses, and even the upper balconies of the better class of buildings, are excellent breeding places for disease. The low price of admission is in direct ratio to the sanitary condition. Besides, a poorer and more careless class of individuals are necessarily to be found here and in conjunction with dirty and unsanitary surroundings, the factors of personal cleanliness, hygiene, and slovenly habits, such as expectorating upon the floor, violent and unrestrained coughing, grimy clothing and even bodies, add greatly to the danger.

We listen with open mouths and widened eyes to the recital of the story of the Black Hole of Calcutta—yet because the box office is flashily gilded and the entrance is of marble and attractive decoration, we do not hesitate to enter the Black Holes of the Photoplay! And crowding into the first available empty seat, we remain for hours and breathe and re-breathe the impure and germ-laden atmosphere—and usually, when the entertainment becomes especially interesting, with open mouths; most aptly predisposing our respiratory tract to the full action of the polluted and germ-laden atmosphere.

A guarantee of the purity of our food and medicines is now stamped upon most everything coming under this head. It would not be any less reasonable to have all places wherein many people are frequently gathering under suspicious sanitary surroundings, inspected by competent experts at proper intervals, and made to place a guarantee upon the entrance to the effect that "This building has been inspected under the Pure Air Law."

———

The educational unrest is getting worse and we hope it will become more so, for it is an indication that the results of our stupid methods are now causing so much pain that relief measures are imperative. Laymen have been saying of medical education a lot of things, about which doctors have long been growling, and we feel mean enough to call attention to the gruelling criticism of universities at the hands of Prof. David Starr Jordan, in his address on "The Making of a Darwin." (*Science*, Dec. 30, 1910). Of course Darwins and Agassizs are born, not made, but our own Osborn states that even if such a genius would wander into an American university, he would be extinguished by modern methods. It must be remembered that Darwin, Pasteur, Koch, Newton, Franklin and all other great discoverers owe their eminence to the fact that they were not in any university, but were free to do as they pleased with their facts, and free to hunt what facts they pleased. Paul Ehrlich, the latest of the long list, could not even graduate, and, horror of horrors, in chemistry he was worst of all. He was always trying to do things differently than his teachers who had never done an original thing themselves and were merely teaching him what had been taught to them. He was considered a failure as a student at the very time he was the best student of his decade.

74   AMERICAN MEDICINE }
   Complete Series, Vol. XVIII. }   EDITORIAL COMMENT   { FEBRUARY, 1912.
   { New Series, Vol. VII., No. 2.

If education is merely pouring facts into the pupil's skull with a funnel as the majority of teachers practice it, then we are training the memory alone, but if it is to be a real drawing out of mental faculties, then the graduate may be permitted to be as ignorant of old useless facts as Ehrlich was—and the world profit by it. Let us think a bit over this matter and then realize that we want workers and thinkers —not memorizers. Our examining boards might take a hint, for while they must exclude the unlearned they are suspected of asking too much learning and really rejecting some good men. Nothing but good can come of the present critical spirit, so let it continue to the end that education will fit the man and not man the education.

The Death of Lord Lister removes one of the world's great men. Unquestionably to him more than to any one else, the present status of surgery is due. While it is true that antisepsis has been superseded to a large extent by asepsis, it cannot be denied that Lister's comprehension of wound infection laid the foundation for modern surgical technique. To him, then, all credit belongs for the epoch-making studies which paved the way for the remarkable successes of present day surgery. It is given to few men to witness the triumph of their ideas as Lister did. But in spite of the general adoption of his methods, and the complete affirmation of his original views on the role of germs in the causation of suppuration, he never showed the slightest pride or self-appreciation. Although he must have realized the part he had played in the evolution of surgery, he never by word or deed, gave any reason to believe that he expected any glory or credit for his achievements. Honors, to be sure, did come to him and he lived to see his name and work esteemed by all mankind, but he never changed his manner and to the last remained the humble, reserved and gentle physician, proud only of his profession and grateful for the opportunities it offered him to serve his fellow beings. Although in his 85th year when he died his life was still an active one at once an example and an inspiration to his colleagues.

Joseph Lister, the pioneer of antiseptic surgery, was born at Upton, in Essex, in 1827, his father, Joseph Jackson Lister, F. R. S., being the inventor of the achromatic microscope. He was educated at a Quaker school in Tottenham, and lived from childhood in an atmosphere of scientific research. He received the degree of M. B. at the London University in 1852, and in the same year took the F. R. C. S. Eng.

After holding office for a time as a resident assistant in University College Hospital, Lister went to Scotland, where he remained, first as a supernumerary dresser under Mr. Syme, and afterwards as his house surgeon. On resigning his post, in 1856, he married Mr. Syme's daughter, and was soon afterwards appointed Assistant Surgeon to the Edinburgh Royal Infirmary. In this position he began to teach, as a private lecturer on surgery recognized by the University, and continued to do so until his appointment to the Chair of Surgery in the University of Glasgow in 1860. He had already contributed a series of important papers to the Royal Society, papers chiefly based upon microscopical research; and in 1860 he was elected a Fellow. In 1863 he was appointed by the

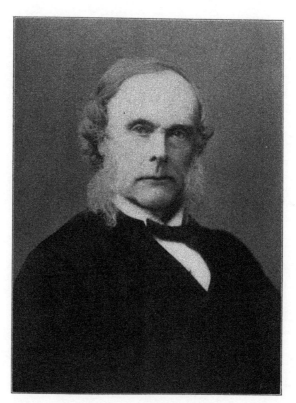

Joseph Lister

February, 1912.
New Series, Vol. VII., No. 2. }   EDITORIAL COMMENT   { American Medicine
Complete Series, Vol. XVIII.   75

Society as Croonian Lecturer, and selected as his subject "The Coagulation of the Blood." About the same time he was a contributor of the articles on "Anesthetics" and on "Amputation" to "Holmes' System of Surgery"; and had written other. papers of very considerable merit.

Quoting from the *Medical Press and Circular:*

"In the early 'sixties Lister became acquainted with the work of Pasteur, whose two great hypotheses—that putrefaction is caused by the agency of living germs, and that these germs are not spontaneously generated—Lister made his own and converted to unthought-of uses, with what results are well known, not only to the whole medical profession, but also to the whole civilized world. Focussing his giant intellect upon the one great object, how to protect wounds from germs of inflammation, he devised the carbolic spray and carbolic gauze, or the Listerian bandage, as it was then called. The effects upon surgical mortality were striking and immediate, no such curative results having been previously obtained. In consequence, operations of much greater magnitude were undertaken with confidence by surgeons which formerly none would have dared to perform. The system soon spread, and was speedily taken up in Germany as well as in this country. Another great advance in surgical art is also associated with Lister's name—the use of the absorbable catgut ligature, which he introduced as a substitute for the silken or flax thread hitherto exclusively used. The work, which had been commenced in Glasgow, was transferred to Edinburgh in 1869, Lister in that year succeeding his father-in-law, Professor Syme, in the Chair of Clinical Surgery in the University of the last-named city. In 1877 an opening

was made for him at King's College, London, and he consented to go there as Professor of Clinical Surgery, a post which he held until 1893, by which time his work was practically done, and the splendid service which he had rendered to mankind could no longer be questioned or concealed. The honors that awaited him were perhaps of little importance compared to his high services, but they were never more justly bestowed. On Mr. Gladstone's recommendation he was, in 1883, made a baronet, and in 1897 he was raised to the peerage. In 1902 he was appointed a member of the newly instituted Order of Merit as well as a P. C. From 1895 to 1900 he was President of the Royal Society. He was Sergeant-Surgeon to Queen Victoria and to King Edward, and has been President of the British Association for the Advancement of Science." His other scientific distinctions are too numerous to give in this brief outline of his career.

As some one has said it has fallen to the lot of no other man of recent times to exert such a profound influence on the welfare of all humanity. Through the introduction of his methods and the subsequent researches which his announcements opened up, Lister has not only saved countless lives, but he has reduced human suffering to a wonderful degree.

With his passing, therefore, much as every one must regret the closing of his career, there comes a feeling of heartfelt gratitude that a man whose life has meant so much to humanity lived in our age and time.

Although ennobled by a grateful sovereign, his work and the fruits thereof gave a nobility to Lister's life that will be remembered long after his title has been forgotten. Indeed as long as men shall live, the memory of Lister will endure as the one who freed mankind from the tyranny of germs—the bondage of infection. May he know the peace—and rest—that passes all understanding!

The possibility of lengthening human life seems to be accepted by nearly everybody, even physicians, but there is remarkably little evidence that we can add a day to it. The whole effort of the medical profession is to keep people alive until worn out, but so far we see no way of preventing senility at the usual time. We are lengthening the average life quite appreciably by preventing early deaths, but not one of our patients is able to live longer than men did some centuries ago when avoidable factors killed so many young people that the average age at death was but 15 or even 10 years. There is some evidence that we save weaklings who can not possibly live to be sixty, and that as time progresses there will be a progressive increase of mortality of men in the 5th, 6th and 7th decades. Formerly if a man was so robust that for 40 years he could resist the factors killing all the weaklings, he was moderately certain to attain a ripe old age, but nowadays his expectation of long life at 40 or 50 is quite reduced. The modern increase of deaths in middle life is therefore a quite normal phenomenon, and a proof of our ability to save children formerly allowed to die. Formerly a man with a large family nearly always lived to see all his children married, but nowadays there is an increasing number of fatherless young people. Orphaned children also seem to be more numerous than in the days when weaklings died too soon to marry. That is, we are prolonging average life but not the maximum. Whether we will ever realize Metchnikoff's dream of postponing senile changes is extremely doubtful, for our tissues seem to be evolved for only a short period of strain, after which they decay in spite of all we can do. The percentage of very old men is about what it always has been and the oldest of them live about as long as those of some centuries back. This condition is likely to continue indefinitely, and all the talk of a future race living 150 years has no basis in fact. We are not built that way.

Vital statistics are uninterpreted by our economists and sociologists. If we were to judge by the lengthening of life in the last half century, it would not be long before we averaged sixty years, which is manifestly absurd, as the ordinary accidents of life would end the careers of most of us before that. The average length of life has been kept down by the enormous infant mortality with a large birth rate, and the great reduction of the birth rate has merely furnished fewer children for this slaughter as the proportion who die before five years of age is still appallingly large. The average life is longest in those countries from which there is a large migration of the young who ordinarily keep the death rate high and average life low. If a man reaches 25 he has every expectation the world over of living about fifteen years, more or less, and generally more, so the average age at death of the stay-at-homes would naturally be high. The average age at death has remarkably lengthened in America too, how much we do not know as we have no vital statistics, but we have proof here and there that modern sanitation is saving many. Since many of these are weaklings who have not the tissues to stand seventy years of strains, they are bowled over in middle life as shown by the enormous increase of deaths from heart, kidney and nerve lesions. Moreover many of these are preserved long enough to marry and beget children, so that there is an increasing percentage of babies congenitally unable to survive seventy years. It is quite likely therefore that after a temporary increase of average life, it will actually diminish. There is no evidence that the maximum life is increasing and much evidence that it may decrease, so that we should not accept the rosy predictions of a time when we average fifty and many live to 100. Even the present figures of 50 or over for the average in Scandinavians are open to suspicion.

The "mania of power" is receiving a lot of academic attention, but it is a more practical matter than our psychologists and historians have been willing to admit. As a rule, the extreme egotism of monarchs and their strong delusions of infallibility and "divine right," have been considered peculiar to them alone and the main reasons why hereditary chieftainship is the worst form of executive government a democracy could devise. "Monarchy," by the way, no longer has a literal meaning. It has been assumed that an elected executive with a limited term is far better as there is not sufficient time for the mania of power to develop. Nevertheless, the British "muddle" along very nicely indeed, and never bother much as to what the King thinks. They have the comforting satisfaction that if he does not act the way they think right they can elect another who will, though it is a rather bloody process not undertaken lightly. He is in fact elected by common assent, and as it is a first class job to leave

to one's son, English Kings are by all odds the most circumspect of men, compared to whom some of the new world elected presidents have been monsters of iniquity. Since the acts of Porforio Diaz which brought us so near to war, are generally conceded to have been partly the result of this pathological egotism as well as his senile feebleness, it is quite evident that we are not so free of the ills of monarchy as we thought— Mexico having been nearer a true literal monarchy, than any government in Europe. The recent election was like medieval English ones—with swords as ballots. Then there are further south all the other petty monarchies with would-be monarchs by divine right, who give us all sorts of bother. It certainly is a practical matter, and our psychologists might suggest remedies.

The mania of officialism is the special form of the mania of power, from which we must guard ourselves, though not any more so than in Europe, where it is equally harmful. Long tenure of office invariably produces a mental condition similar to that of the mania of power, and the official not only considers his own ideas the best, but in time begins to look on those with different ideas as something akin to traitors to our institutions or dangerous revolutionists. Progress is obstructed and inefficiency is the rule. So we used to have periodical housecleanings, to "turn the rascals out," but we found the cure worse than the disease. Only by life tenure of office can we get the most efficient and faithful, so our present problem is to prevent the injury of the "mania of power." Whether this is possible is a question, but that it is the minor of two evils is no reason for tolerating it, if remedies are possible. Here again our psychologists may mix up in politics to the public

78   AMERICAN MEDICINE }
Complete Series, Vol. XVIII. }   EDITORIAL COMMENT   { FEBRUARY, 1912.
{ New Series, Vol. VII., No. 2.

weal. As we are all in glass houses we should throw stones with great circumspection. Our professional record of the obstruction of officialism is about as black as can be—indeed it is perfectly natural. What we should aim at is the evolution of a system which will save us from ourselves. This is a rather large contract, but the whole course of civilization is to eliminate the "personal equation" which warps judgment—mania of power being the greatest of them, official conservatism the least. We may feel flattered at the adulation of copyists but should not permit that feeling to cause us to kick every man with a new idea.

The criminal ancestry of the McNamara brothers will probably be the subject of much discussion now that it has been discovered that their father had served a term in prison and that he never lived with his family after his conviction. It will doubtless be said by certain enthusiasts that if the criminal tendency had been discovered soon enough and sterilization performed, we would have prevented the outrages and wholesale murders which have shocked the whole world. Yet, as far as known, he was a perfectly respectable man when these boys were born, but later something in his struggle for existence broke down the inhibitions to crime which had been strong enough before. It must first be found out why he fell,—why he became unfit and antisocial so suddenly. It may be discovered to be due to causes which successfully tempt much stronger men, even bankers. As for the boys, their portraits show no signs of degeneration—merely a cynical expression which would not be ordinarily noticed. We are not justified, so far, in any other opinion than they were injured by their environment, and taught to be criminals like many fatherless boys who are necessarily more or less neglected.

The respectable ancestry of the murderer Beattie must be discussed at the same time we condemn the poor bringing up of the McNamaras. As far as known, his family is one of the very best in the land, and it should be possible to find out why this particular individual went wrong. He seems to have had every advantage of heredity and environment which by common consent are supposed to make good citizens, yet something happened to him. Our students of heredity and modifications due to unknown environmental causes, must find out what it was that could thus bring more than sorrow to his relatives. Someone or something has been at fault to prevent the boy developing the morality his due by heredity. We cannot speak of sterilizing bankers because so many of them go wrong, but this case emphasizes what has so often been said in these columns; most criminals have respectable parentage, and there are black sheep in every fold. Very few criminals have criminal parents, but every one of them must have undesirable relatives as in the case of citizens who never commit crime. The whole subject of the cause of criminality is thus entirely too complex for the off-hand judgments which have crowded the literature of penology. These two awful examples of the failure to make good citizens of every boy show that we must revise many of our theories. Wherein are parents neglectful if at all? How are we to be sure that a low moral sense of some remote bad ancestor will not suddenly appear as a reversion? There is an enormous amount of research needed before we can answer such ques-

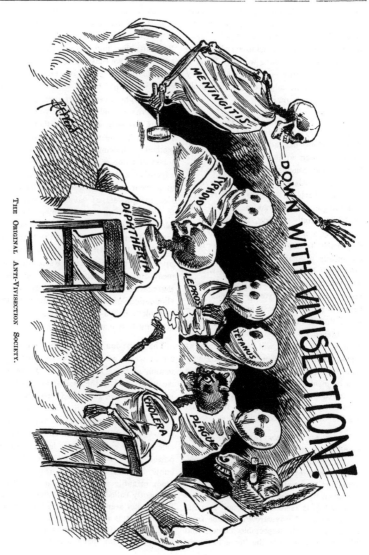

THE ORIGINAL ANTI-VIVISECTION SOCIETY.

80   AMERICAN MEDICINE ⎱
Complete Series, Vol. XVIII. ⎰   EDITORIAL COMMENT   ⎰ FEBRUARY, 1912.
⎱ New Series, Vol. VII., No. 2.

tions. Why should the Goldsborough family, also one of our best, develop the murderer of David Graham Phillips? Why should the young Massachusetts clergyman so foully murder a young woman? There is no family or profession in which every member is impeccable but why should peccability go so far?

The study of wayward girls made in New York by the Episcopal Church Mission of Help, has added more proof to what has been known since long before Lombroso so conclusively showed that they were the female counterpart of the male criminal. Each class comes from respectable families as a rule and as each is more or less mentally lacking, the problem is essentially a medical one to find out why they depart from parental type. The causes are mostly pre-natal, but the environment after birth has a great deal to do with it. The reformatories have proved a thousand times over that the young criminal who through sheer weakness has bent to the evil influences of his environment can be straightened up if properly managed soon enough, and that he will keep straight, as a rule, when he is given this new strength, though of course there is no cure for his lack of mental development. The workers in the female field report equal success with wayward girls who are nearest the normal but the worst are incorrigible.

The causes of waywardness are so profound that it will not do to go into the matter superficially. Society is more interested in the prevention of the birth of such weaklings to avoid the necessity of guarding them from the harm which normal boys and girls resist. It is found that the vast majority of wayward girls come from abnormal though respectable homes, and this may indicate that the home has been the chief factor in their undoing, but it also shows that they are weaklings born of parents unable to make a normal home. We must then find out what has hurt the parents, and we thus get back to the old, old story of the prevention of every other disease—we must begin with the grandparents. The investigators must go deeper still perhaps, and this is a vital matter. Nature has been at work for thousands of years eliminating the unfit by a very brutal method of allowing them to eliminate themselves, but our new civilization finds it too expensive and the decree has gone forth to prevent the weaknesses. We have carried the process of saving the weaklings to such an extent that something like three percent are public burdens and the taxpayers are frantically calling on the Eugenists for relief. We must answer, as the medical profession has the facts. Racial development must not depend upon expensive segregation of the weak in place of nature's elimination of them. Prevention is the shibboleth now-a-days in this as in every other medical matter.

The nutrition of the young is a matter to which we would like to call the attention of these investigators. There is a wealth of data in the case of lower organisms that if we only feed them properly they develop normally in spite of what appears to be fatal adversities. Man himself is no exception, and it is an axiom of medicine that the well fed infant has a resisting power almost beyond conception. We all know of weaklings whose troubles date from infantile malnutrition, and we have frequently called attention to the fact that they do not seem to be able to recover lost ground. It is not at all unlikely that the baby is frail from poisoned nourishment before birth, for many investigators have shown that the weakling in a family of sturdy brothers and sisters, is due to a maternal infection during or just before pregnancy. Tuberculosis has a dreadful effect. So too, a starved mother cannot breed well. Similarly a wayward girl may owe her weakness to any one of a thousand causes afflicting her grandparents—and bad nutrition from ignorance or poverty is one of them, perhaps the greatest. We can prevent the ignorance perhaps and then it will be entirely in order to discuss whether matrimony will be permitted to those unable to provide proper food for a few babies even if they know what is proper.

———

Reinfection with syphilis may be expected with more frequency now that it seems probable that one attack does not confer immunity. When the first reports of salvarsan were published, a few commentators were led to take a rather gloomy view of the effect on morals if the fear of contagion were removed. They have thus been answered much sooner than expected, for if a patient really is promptly cured, he may, in a short time, be just as liable to another attack as he ever was, and the check upon unbridled license is therefore undiminished. Indeed, there is nothing known yet as to the effect of repeated infections. It is entirely possible that cures may be more difficult in such cases and until we do know let us take it for granted that they will be. The disease has taken so long to cure, that the cases of reinfection have been very few, and that has led us to believe that in the process of cure a real immunity to extra infection has existed as a result of treatment. Now that the active organisms can be destroyed before the body cells have taken on any kind of adjustment to their presence, we are confronted by an entirely different proposition. Even the blood tests now so popular may not show the presence of organisms which

are practically hibernating, and we must go slow in the interpretation of positive or negative results. The whole matter of cure and subsequent susceptibility is so new and so involved that it will take a decade or two to clear it up. Twenty years hence, these "cured" cases may be the subjects of extensive investigations by our alienists and neurologists, just as those "cured" by other means are now under observation and restraint. No! Morality won't suffer at all by salvarsan. That drug has made a deservedly big splash even if it doesn't cure a case, but the ripples are already quieting down. The immoral life is just as dangerous as ever.

———

The tramp problem seems to be in process of solution if we may judge by the enthusiasm with which everyone approves the plan for a colony where these sick people can be segregated, studied and cured. The old theory that they were perfectly healthy men too lazy or vicious to work has been definitely and permanently abandoned as untrue. To be sure we all feel the grind of work and long for periods of rest and recuperation, but this does not alter the other fact that a healthy man takes to work like a duck to water. Any one who elects to endure the frightful sufferings of vagabondage when by a little industry he can make himself comfortable, is by the very act proved to be abnormal. He simply cannot work—and that's the end of it. The old plan of forcing him, in his enfeebled state, to do hard labor for which he has to go to the limit of his physique, being given neither the muscles nor energy, is as brutal as compelling an old bank clerk to work as a stevedore. Besides, it merely increases the basic neurasthenia. The modern way is correct because it has succeeded in every place in Europe where it has been tried. Each case is taken to the colony, fed, clothed and rested so that he can build up and do work as will not exhaust but strengthen him. In the meantime he is studied by experts to find out what broke him down, and whether he is such a congenital weakling that severe strains are wholly out of the question. Curiously enough some of these sufferers are men of considerable intelligence with powers of concentration which tempted them to work beyond their limit of daily recuperation. They used up their capital instead of living within the vital income. Some have exhausted themselves in sedentary work involving nerve strain, which we now know is a very serious matter. Hobo printers and barbers must be advised to abandon their old trades and taught new ones involving no strains which cannot be recovered from by the night's rest and sleep.

The cure of vagabondage is a scientific matter involving considerable neurological knowledge. It will not be trusted to a farm superintendent who is a good slave driver because he has more muscle than brain, for he will do more harm than good. These are the present plans as far as we can gather and we earnestly hope they will be promptly carried out. The movement has already been inaugurated on proper lines and will progress of its own momentum. We have referred to the subject every little while and propose to refer to it every little while in the future, for we are quite sure the dreadful social loss of health, life, property and money due to vagabondage can be prevented, and even if permanent confinement of the few incurables is necessary, we can prevent future cases from becoming incurable. Incidentally we would suggest to the workers in this field, that they make careful ethnic studies of these sick men to determine if certain immigrant types are unduly affected by our climate and customs, and if so how many years or generations it takes to show serious results. It is a huge unworked field with

several hundred thousand subjects to study. We would also like to suggest that there be similar studies of prostitutes, as it has been frequently asserted that they have the same nervous defects preventing labor, and would willingly be tramps in preference to prostitutes if they were physically strong enough.

————

Sunshine as a contributing cause of pellagra has been more than suspected both in Europe and America, but chiefly because the skin lesions do not appear on parts of the body shaded by clothing, and it is not a disease of cloudy climates being mostly found in countries blessed with plenty of God's sunshine. Whether it afflicts the least pigmented types the most is doubtful, because the basic cause is evidently a systemic poison affecting all in equal degree, but it would be interesting to know whether the skin lesions are worst in the blondest. Perhaps there are pellagrous negroes without skin lesions. Raubitschek (*Wien. Klin. Woch.*, June 30, 1910) reports some highly important experiments with white rats fed on buckwheat. Those kept in the dark remained healthy but those exposed to sunlight developed a disease more or less resembling pellagra. All albino animals are killed by a sun exposure harmless to those protected by pigment and their natural home must be dark, but this is the first time anything resembling pellagra has been produced. In the case of guinea-pigs and white rabbits the most recent experiments show that if infected with tubercle bacilli, they live longer in the laboratory if it is kept like outdoors in respect to cold and ventilation. Now that the results with some kinds of men are better if treated in a London hospital than in the country open air, physicians ought to realize that sunshine can be so injurious as to cause disease, prevent recovery or hasten death.

ORIGINAL ARTICLES.

DIAGNOSIS AND TREATMENT OF RENAL TUBERCULOSIS.[1]

BY

MAURICE PACKARD, M. D.,

Adjunct Professor of Internal Medicine, New York City Polyclinic Hospital and Medical School.

Recognizing the difficulty of presenting anything new on renal tuberculosis, my principal aim in this discussion is rather to place the various symptoms vividly before your mind, so that this condition will not, as frequently happens, go unrecognized, and thus the best chances for a cure be lost.

My second object is to detail certain facts, corroborated by statistics and authenticated cases, which may assist us to determine what should be done for these patients. But, before taking up the consideration of the diagnosis of this disease, let us review briefly a few salient points of the morbid anatomy upon which the clinical evidence rests.

Most authorities are agreed upon the following general propositions:

(a) That although in the strict sense of the term, it is questionable whether there is ever a primary renal tuberculosis, still, for all practical purposes, the kidney may be the primary organ to be involved.

(b) That although in about 50% of the cases, the disease is bilateral, probably due to its unrecognized condition, both kidneys are not affected to the same degree.

(c) That the process occurs most frequently between the ages of 16 to 46, and that there is very little difference as to its frequency between males and females.

(d) That the most common form is the condition of caseous disease of the kidney, with capsular involvement. It usually begins in the papillae and in the pyramids of the kidney, and from there spreads through the entire cortex and capsule. Just as in pulmonary tuberculosis, the tubercles become confluent, necrosis takes place, and caseous nodules appear. Liquefaction may set in, and the process, in extreme cases, may go on, until the kidney is nothing more than a sac, filled with pus and cheesy material.

(e) That tuberculosis of the kidney may be a part of acute general tuberculosis, the kidney showing numerous miliary tubercles, scattered about the parenchyma. This usually affects children under ten years of age. The signs of such lesions are almost impossible to detect, and are usually masked by symptoms of a general infection.[1]

Diagnosis.— As stated previously, chronic tuberculosis occurs most frequently between the ages of 16 and 40, and is not so uncommon as some of you may think. Fullerton of Belfast found it in 6% of all his cystoscopic examinations.[2] It may go on for years, unsuspected, and be discovered only on the autopsy table. The first symptoms that bring the patients under observation are increased urination, hematuria, renal or vesical pain.

The desire to urinate, especially at night, may be due to reflex irritation in the pelvis of the kidney, or to a coexisting bladder infection. The urine, being acid and highly concentrated, 1020-1035, would naturally cause some vesical pain, which would be ac-

[1]Read at a meeting of the Eastern Med. Soc., Jan. 12, 1912.

[1]Here, the author showed several specimens of kidney tuberculosis in the various stages of caseous nodules, liquefaction, and an extreme case, showing the kidney as a sac filled with pus. These specimens belonged to Dr. Chetwood.

[2]British Medical Journal, July 9, 1910.

centuated later by an ulcerated bladder. Albuminuria, without casts. is the rule. Pus is usually present, but in varying amounts. With this albuminuria, in contradistinction to chronic nephritis, the blood pressure is low, and the heart is not hypertrophied.

The blood is intimately mixed with the urine, giving it the usual smoky appearance. It may be abundant, or recognized only by the microscope. Like pulmonary tuberculosis, it may be the first sign of the disease. It does not, like calculus or tumor, bear any relation to the activities of the patient.

Pain, with tenderness in the loin, may be out of all proportion to the pathological findings. Sometimes, with very little involvement, suffering may be intense, and again, with marked destruction of the parenchyma, there may be an entire absence of pain. It is chiefly due to distension of the capsule, but if the pelvis or ureter become occluded with cheesy pus, intermittent hydro or pyonephrosis, with true colicky pain, may result.

It is well to remember that the pain is often referred to the undiseased kidney, especially when lying upon the healthy side.

The disagreeable sensations which occur in the bladder and urethra consist chiefly of a painful desire to urinate, and burning pain before and after micturition. It is because of this fact that so many patients are treated so long for cystitis. This vesical irritation is peculiar, inasmuch as irrigations of silver have a tendency to make the patient worse. If the disease goes on for any length of time, and the patient empties his bladder at every inclination. contraction of this organ will undoubtedly ensue.

An examination of the kidney by palpation may show an enlargement, but whether this is the healthy hypertrophied organ or the diseased one can only be settled by the cystoscope.

These tuberculous kidneys may not be enlarged at all, but if enlarged, they may be drawn up by adhesions under the costal arches, so that the size of the organ cannot be definitely determined.

Again, an enlarged kidney, after hemorrhage, may empty a tubercular focus in the pelvis, and become smaller.

The healthy kidney may compensate and become hypertrophied, thereby causing not only enlargement, but by capsular distension, may even give pain and soreness in the loin.

The x-ray may help us in differentiating from a calculus and pyelography from a pyelitis, by the demonstration of a pyonephrosis or a cortical abscess.

The most important point in diagnosing chronic renal tuberculosis is to demonstrate the tubercle bacilli in the urine, and to exclude any other organ but the kidney as their source. The latter can be done only by the trained surgeon, and therefore I will not attempt to describe a method in which I am not proficient.

Tubercle bacilli in the urine may be found after the use of the centrifuge, by cultivation, or by inoculation. A quick method of inoculation is described by Bloch, who injects 1 cubic centimeter of urine in the thigh of a guinea-pig, massages upwards, injures the inguinal glands, and then removes the same glands after 10 to 12 days.

If a cultural examination of the urine is made, and if the same is sterile, and if the gonococcus can be ruled out, it is usually tubercular.

I believe it is wise to consider every chronic cystitis which resists treatment to be the effect of a tubercular kidney until it is proven otherwise.

The general tuberculosis tests, as the Von Pirquet or tuberculin injections might be employed. Positive reactions would only show the presence of tubercle somewhere in the body, but pain and swelling of the kidney after tuberculin injections would be more conclusive.

The general health may not be affected, although the disease may be present for a number of years. I have a patient who complained of painful urination and hematuria just 17 years ago, and who first came to see me 4 years ago, stating that he had suffered from time to time with these attacks ever since. Diagnosis of tuberculosis of uro-genital canal was made, by the demonstration of tubercle bacilli in the urine. When this was reported to him, he left my care and became the patient of a very prominent surgeon. The diagnosis was corroborated, and by cystoscopic examination it was proved that not only the kidneys, but the bladder, as well, was affected. Under the best hygienic surroundings in the Adirondacks, and with a three weeks' course of treatment yearly at Countreville, he is better at present, as concerns appearances and subjective symptoms, than at any time during his illness. I cannot state positively that he had tuberculosis 17 years ago, but from his history it is certainly at least a probability.

The general health, in my opinion, is not affected until a secondary infection, with the colon bacilli, gonococcus, or some other pyogenic germ takes place. It seems that the tubercle bacilli's viciousness is not thoroughly aroused until a companion germ acquaints him of their combined strength.

It must not be overlooked that a gonorrheal condition may not only be superimposed upon a tubercular lesion, but vice versa, tuberculosis may be secondary to an old gonorrheal affection. Nor must it be forgotten that a calculus may be present along with tuberculosis, either due to the tuberculosis or merely coexisting.

You will note that I have placed before you only the general symptoms of renal tuberculosis, but one of the most important questions to be decided, especially as regards treatment, is whether one or both kidneys are diseased. This can be determined only by catheterization of the ureters and the examination of the separate specimens of urine for tubercular bacilli.

Unfortunately, the second kidney may be diseased, and still show little or nothing abnormal. It is not my province to dwell on the various tests to determine the functionating power of the kidney. That these tests are all-important, no one will deny; but lest we grow too enthusiastic, it is well to remember the words of that master of urology, Nitze, who said that these tests, after all, are unavailing, as they do not teach us "whether the remaining kidney after nephrectomy is alone capable of eliminating the metabolic products."[1]

Treatment.— In discussing the management of a case of renal tuberculosis, there are several points to be taken into consideration. Severe pyelitis or abscess of the kidney means nephrotomy, and I believe the surgeons are united in considering this a palliative measure, or the first step in a two-stage nephrectomy.

To remove a kidney is apparently safe. The mortality in the hands of the best sur-

[1]Martin Ware diagnosis, *N. Y. Med. Jour.*, Jan. 4, 1908.

geons is from 2 to 4 per cent. But at the same time, it deprives the patient of one-half of the total supply which is necessary to life. It is stated by competent physiologists that two-thirds of the entire kidney substance may be destroyed and still the remaining one-third will be able to carry out the functionating activities, so that life will be maintained. In other words, if nephrectomy is done, you must have two-thirds of the other kidney absolutely healthy, or else your patient will die of renal insufficiency. It must also be remembered that even a diseased kidney may have some functionating power, probably just enough to help out the other kidney in carrying out the necessary allotted work.

If such is the case, nephrectomy, after all, is a grave problem.

The best way, though, to draw any conclusions, is to weigh the results of the surgeons, and compare them with cases that have not been operated. The only results worth estimating are in those cases that have been followed for a number of years.

I have been able to gather statistics regarding 250 nephrectomies for renal tuberculosis, which have been observed for ten years, and I find that the direct mortality of the operation is about 4½%.

The greatest mortality is during the first ten months after the operation, about 80% of the total; and the total mortality is about 22%.

These statistics are taken from Kronlein, von Stoffman, Czerny and Broeckel, in Europe, and several American surgeons. The results are so nearly alike that I will not give the individual statistics.

To offset this, let us consider the medical aspect.

There are a number of authenticated cases of spontaneous healing reported, but with the following results:

In 21 cases that came to autopsy for some other condition, it was found in some that the kidney lost its entire parenchyma by sclerosis; in others, the ureter was obstructed by cicatrization, and hydronephrosis resulted, while at the same time some other organ, as the bladder, lung, etc., was secondarily infected. Yet, in spite of these facts, the prognosis under medical care is not nearly as hopeless as you would gather from the above records.[1]

Dr. James Pedersen[2] reports two cases cured with tuberculin injections. I hardly believe that Dr. Pedersen has followed them long enough to report cures; "temporary cure," or "improvement" would be the better title.

I have observed five cases, and am very much impressed with the periodicity of the symptoms. Just as in tuberculosis of other parts of the body, there may be a subsidence of signs. One girl was free from all symptoms, several times, for periods of months, but just as soon as some intercurrent disease, as an ordinary cold, was ushered in, the symptoms would reappear. It is now 6 years since I first saw her, and although she has pulmonary tuberculosis as well, she is able to do considerable work during the year.

I would like to relate to you the story of her case. Eight years ago she complained of burning micturition. Her urine was found to contain pus, and although the physician found an intact hymen, and absolutely no inflammation of the vulvo-

[1] Another specimen of Dr. Chetwood's was shown by the author of "so-called" spontaneous healing.
[2] N. Y. Med. Jour., Feb. 25, 1911.

vaginal glands or of the cervix, he gave her to understand that she was suffering from gonorrhea, and treated her accordingly.

Sedatives seemed to help her, but she was never entirely cured. Two years later, on account of a severe hematuria, she come to the Polyclinic Hospital. I found a tender and enlarged right kidney, together with positive signs of tuberculosis of both lungs. Tubercle bacilli were found in the urine with very little difficulty.

Another case is well, with the exception of a contracted bladder. This bladder will not hold more than 1 or 2 ounces, and in order to insure undisturbed sleep, the patient wears a large rubber bag tied around his urethra.

Still another went through pregnancy several years ago, but I have lost track of her, and do not know whether or not she is alive.

Sanatoriums claim excellent results from climatic conditions.

When we look over the surgical statistics, we note that the greatest mortality was recorded in the first year. It was due, in all probability, to a bilateral infection, where the disease was not discovered in its early stage. The treatment, therefore, will depend upon how early the diagnosis is made.

As there is no specific for tuberculosis, I will not take up your time enumerating the different agents which have been used to combat the condition. Tuberculin holds out the greatest promise, but still, in my experience my patients did as well without this agent as with it. There have been a number of cures reported after its use, and it certainly should be tried.

Although, theoretically, urotropin should not be given when the urine is acid, clinically it has proved to be the best drug.

In summing up the treatment, I would deduce that if one kidney alone is involved, nephrectomy should be done. But you must not stop with this, as general hygienic and dietetic measures should be instituted.

If both kidneys are affected, general treatment must be depended upon to improve the strength and powers of resistance, plus tuberculin injection and urotropin. If there is a secondary infection, urotropin and vaccine treatment should be employed to combat the offending secondary microorganisms, followed by tuberculin. Tuberculin, in my hands, has proven of inestimable value in tuberculosis of the glands, but as soon as there was a secondary infection, it was of absolutely no worth.

Although operation may be out of the question, under favorable circumstances, life may be prolonged in comparative comfort for a number of years. In conclusion, let me state that removal of a kidney, after all, requires serious consideration, and involves grave risks; and it is because of the easy recourse to nephrectomy that I have brought forth these facts, and I wish to urge upon you the courage to state to your surgeon that when your case has more than a unilateral infection, it wears the placard of "nolli vel tangere."

———

I the Lord will hold thy right hand, saying unto thee: Fear not; I will help thee. —*Isaiah xii., 13.*

———

The law of the harvest is to reap more than you sow. Sow an act and you reap a habit; sow a habit and you reap a character; sow a character and you reap a destiny.— *George D. Boardman.*

———

Chaste and immaculate in every thought. —*Shakespeare.*

TRANSPERITONEAL OPERATIONS ON THE BLADDER.[1]

BY

PARKER SYMS, M. D.,

Attending Surgeon to the Lebanon Hospital, New York City.

In bringing this subject to your attention, I know that I am suggesting nothing new and that I am really adding nothing to surgical literature. But I feel that I have an excuse for writing this short paper in the fact that I shall be urging the more frequent employment of a very useful method of operating and one that has been singularly neglected heretofore.

Another motive that prompts me is the fact that the proper credit has not always been given to the proposer of this procedure. I refer to Dr. Francis Harrington of Boston. As far as I know, Dr. Harrington was the first to propose and describe this operation as a definite surgical procedure. In 1893, in an article entitled, "On the Feasibility of Intraperitoneal Cystotomy," he very definitely and concisely described the steps of the operation and detailed a case in which he had employed this method. He advocated this operation as suitable in cases of tumors of the bladder, in cases of enlarged prostates, etc. And he pointed out the fact that it has many important points of superiority as compared with operating through any of the other routes. Before he performed and described this operation, he had worked it up carefully by experimenting on the cadaver. So it was a very deliberately planned and elaborated procedure as far as Harrington was concerned, and he and he only is entitled to the credit of having originated and described it.

[1] Read at a meeting of the Eastern Med. Soc., Jan. 12, 1912.

Notwithstanding the fact that this operation is so valuable a one and one whose merits are now fully appreciated by a few, it remained almost completely ignored, for many years. In 1904, Dr. Albert Berg brought it into prominence and added some valuable suggestions as to the radical removal of the lymphatics in cases of carcinoma. In 1908, Charles Mayo wrote a paper showing his appreciation of the merits of this operation and in the same year Dr. Charles Scudder and Lincoln Davis conjointly wrote a paper not only extolling the advantages of the method but also giving due and proper credit to Dr. Harrington.

The usual methods of approaching the bladder have been by the urethra, by the perineum, by the vagina in females, and by the suprapubic, extraperitoneal route. Of the first three of these I need not speak in this connection. Each one has had its special advocates and each one has some special advantages and also some special disadvantages. It is rather with suprapubic cystotomy that we should compare this method.

For many years surgeons have been agreed that there were certain cases and certain conditions which could best be reached by a suprapubic cystotomy. I think the time has come when we should feel that suprapubic cystotomy has a very limited field and that the transperitoneal route is the one of choice in nearly all of those conditions which we had assigned to the suprapubic operations. In a general way I may enumerate these as the various tumors of the bladder, certain cases of enlarged prostate, bladder stones too large or unsuitable for crushing, and cases of stone at or near the vesical orifices of the ureters.

For my own part I have always found and thought that suprapubic cystotomy was a very unsatisfactory operation. I have not based this opinion on unfortunate experiences of my own. I have based it on theoretical reasoning partly, but more to be done blindly and in a more or less haphazard manner. The dangers of the operation are grave, for the cellular space (the space of Retius) is very prone to infection and is so situated that it is a difficult region to protect while operating and a

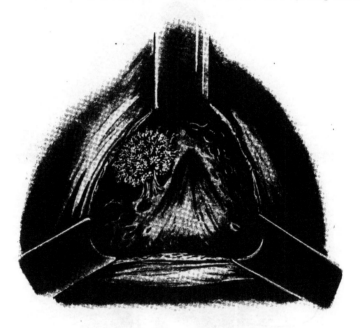

FIGURE I. (After Charles Mayo).
Bladder widely opened: showing papilloma.

particularly upon my knowledge and observation of unfortunate results which have been produced by men who are addicted to this particular form of surgery. The suprapubic approach to the bladder is a very unsatisfactory one in many respects. In most instances the exposure of the diseased area is not good, and much of the work has very difficult one to drain and treat when once it has been infected. The suprapubic route possesses many positive disadvantages, and negatively, it is lacking in many actual advantages as compared with the transperitoneal route.

Transperitoneal cystotomy is in itself an ideal operation. It gives the best possible

means of exposing, of inspecting, of palpat- in almost any other intra-abdominal opera-
ing, of reaching and of operating upon the tion. After the main operation has been
interior of the bladder. It should always completed (such as removal of a tumor, or

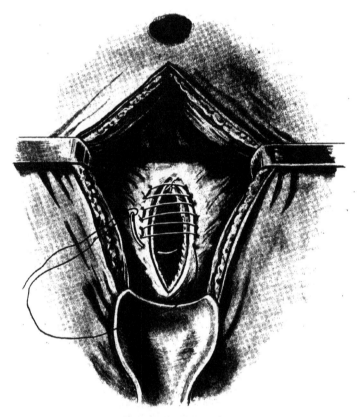

FIGURE II. (After Charles Mayo).
Continuous suture passing through all the coats.

be safe as far as infection is concerned, for of a stone) the closure of the bladder and
one should be able to protect the peritoneum of the abdomen should be effected without
much more satisfactorily than can be done drainage. Of course I mean as far as the

abdominal route is concerned. If some condition has been found which makes one feel that the bladder should be drained, this should be accomplished by an external perineal urethrotomy.

the pubis, care being taken not to carry the incision to the vesical reflection of the peritoneum. In other words, we want to operate entirely within the abdomen and we want to be careful not to open the pre-

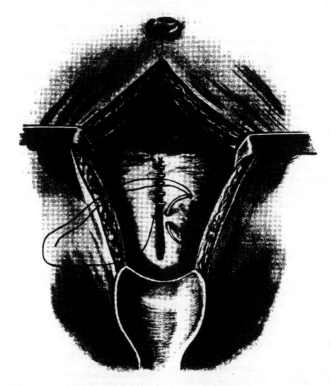

FIGURE III. (After Charles Mayo).
Cushing's suture closing the peritoneal coat.

The operation of transperitoneal or intraperitoneal cystotomy is performed as follows: The abdomen is opened in the median line from the umbilicus nearly to

vesical space. Having completed the abdominal incision, the patient is placed in extreme Trendelenberg position, and the intestines and omentum are pushed upward, well away from the bladder region. This whole region must be thoroughly protected by laparotomy pads and then the bladder should be opened by a longitudinal section in the middle line. This opening may be made as freely as one finds necessary for satisfactory exposure of the bladder interior. It is remarkable what a perfect exposure is obtained and how satisfactorily one may proceed with and accomplish what he has undertaken to do. In the removal of a tumor one may be able to estimate the size of the base, to determine whether. or not he is making his excision through normal tissue and at a sufficient distance from the site of the tumor itself. Should the diseased area involve the orifice of the ureter, the ureter may be resected or transplanted to another portion of the bladder. Diverticuli of the bladder may be accurately estimated and they may be operated upon by this means in a much more satisfactory manner than would be possible through a suprapubic cystotomy. Extensive resections of the bladder may be made with competent closure of the viscus and, as Dr. Berg has pointed out, this is the only way in which we may expect to do a radical operation in cases of cancer of the bladder. For we can not only remove all of the apparent growth itself, but we can continue our dissection behind the peritoneum and thereby remove all the lymphatics as far as the bifurcation of the common iliac artery.

Having completed our work within the bladder, we close the incision exactly as we would close an incision in the stomach. We should first make a complete continuous suture passed through all the coats of the bladder. This should be done with very fine chromic catgut, using as small a needle as possible. We supplement this with a continuous suture of fine silk or celluloid linen involving the peritoneal coat only. The Harvey Cushing method of suture is the best.

Having accomplished this satisfactorily we need have no fear of leakage. If we have succeeded in operating without soiling the peritoneum we may close the abdominal wound without drainage and without fear of infection. This is very different as compared with a suprapubic cystotomy, where ideal closure of the bladder is not always successful or possible and is often a menace to the patient when attempted.

If this brief paper will have stimulated an interest in this method of operating, I shall feel that it has been well worth the writing, for this is a most important surgical procedure, and it is one that has been strangely neglected heretofore.

BIBLIOGRAPHY.

Francis Harrington, *Annals of Surgery,* 1893, XVIII, p. 408.

Albert A. Berg, *Annals of Surgery*, 1904, XL, p. 382.

Chas. Mayo, *Annals of Surgery*, 1908, XLVIII, p. 105.

Chas. L. Scudder and Lincoln Davis, *Annals of Surgery*, 1908, XLVIII, p. 862.

540 Parke Ave.

————

A man's ingress into the world is naked and
    bare,
His progress through the world is trouble
    and care;
His egress out of the world is, nobody
    knows where.
If we do well here, we shall do well there;
I can tell you no more if I preach a whole
    year.
            —*John Edwin* (1749-1790).

————

The surest way to get a larger place is to make our service fill and overflow the place we occupy.—*Josiah Strong.*

RENAL LITHIASIS.[1]

BY

WINFIELD AYRES, M. D.,
New York City.

Agglutinations of crystalline or amorphous sediment of the urine are called urinary calculi. Calculi vary in size from smaller than the head of a pin to masses three or four inches in length. The smallest ones may give very little trouble, but the larger are extremely annoying and often dangerous to life.

Conditions which produce urinary calculi are, first, the presence of crystalline material in the urine and, second, the presence of some substance to catch and cement the crystals together. Some writers think the cement substance is a colloid, but the majority believe it to be mucus thrown out by inflammation or congestion. Crystals in the urine is accounted for by faulty metabolism, intestinal indigestion, etc. It is possible the crystals in the urine produce sufficient irritation of the delicate structure of the kidney to cause an excess secretion of mucus; and it is also possible that the faulty metabolism or what not which produced the crystals so change conditions in the kidney as to make the formation of calculi easy. Faulty drainage of the renal pelvis is said to be a contributing cause of renal calculus, but in those cases of floating kidney and high attached ureter the writer has studied, only a small proportion was found to be complicated by calculus.

The nucleus of a calculus may form in the substance of the kidney and unless infection occur it will stay there, slowly growing; or it may begin on the wall of the renal pelvis and if it is not passed shortly after its formation as what is commonly

[1] Read at a meeting of the Eastern Med. Soc., Jan. 12, 1912.

called "gravel" will reach appreciable size. While still small it may engage in the mouth of the ureter and slowly or rapidly work its way into the bladder, or perhaps become lodged at some point in the ureter. A calculus which remains in the renal pelvis may take on fantastic shapes, sending prolongations into the calices of the pelvis. But should infection occur the kidney is slowly destroyed and the calculus increases in size, sometimes becoming as large as an orange.

Calculi may be located in the renal pelvis or ureter for years and give no symptom of their presence. On the other hand minute concretions, not large enough to be easily found in the urine may cause the most intense suffering. The cardinal symptoms of renal or ureteral calculus are pain, nausea and vomiting, chill, blood or pus in the urine, and disturbance of urination.

Pain.—A severe renal colic is one of the most painful afflictions to which the human flesh is heir. It must be remembered, however, that it is simply a spasm of the muscular wall of the ureter and is by no means pathognomonic of calculus. Passage of an ureteral catheter, a blood-clot, kinking of the ureter may cause colics of greatest severity. The smaller stones are more prolific of colics than those of sufficient size to prevent their engagement in the ureter. Large calculi in the pelvis give rise to annoying, nagging pains and occasionally, when their position changes so as to press on more sensitive parts, to colics—usually not very severe. The seat of pain in these cases is the kidney, but often there are radiations down along the course of the ureter, even to the testicle or penis, and in the female to the vulva. A fact which must not be overlooked is that all symptoms may be referred to the opposite side from the seat of trouble. Accompanying the colic there may be nausea and vomiting and perhaps a chill.

Pus and blood in the urine may be entirely wanting, but usually in those cases where pain is a prominent symptom, one or both are present. The quantity varies from a microscopic amount to sufficient to form a heavy sediment. When blood is present it is usually diffused through the urine, but may be in the form of thin clots.

Disturbance of urination.—The most serious is suppression. In nearly all cases in which this occurs a calculus has plugged one ureter and the opposite kidney stops secretion from sympathy. In one of the writer's cases calculi had plugged both ureters. Increased frequency of urination is by no means a constant symptom. A calculus lodged high is less apt to cause irritability of the bladder than one low down in the ureter. One lodged within the lower two inches of the ureter is very apt to cause all the symptoms of stone in the bladder, even to pain at the head of the penis at the end of urination.

Renal and ureteral calculus must be differentiated from kinking of the ureter, tubercular kidney, pyelitis, appendicitis, disease of the gall-bladder, hypernephroma and so-called essential hematuria. Any case in which a suspicion of renal calculus is entertained should, as a first step in making the diagnosis, be subjected to the x-ray. Even a small stone will show in nine cases out of ten, but a pure uric acid stone will not cast a shadow. The cystoscope and ureteral catheter are of the greatest aid in determining the presence of ureteral or pelvic stones. With the plain catheter one may often recognize the presence of a foreign body by the feel as the catheter passes up the ureter, but the hardened and roughened feel of a tubercular ureter must not be mistaken for calculus. If a wax-tipped catheter be passed and it comes in contact with a calculus, the wax will be found to have been scratched. This method is very difficult in the male and is often impossible. An ureteral catheter may be passed easily, but when an attempt is made to pass the wax-tipped, many difficulties are encountered and in the author's experience failure has occurred in 33% of the cases. An indirect cystoscope is useless for the wax-tipped catheter. Not infrequently an x-ray photograph shows a shadow in the lower abdomen which may and may not be a calculus in the ureter. If a second picture be taken with a lead catheter in the ureter, much valuable information may be obtained.

The management of a renal or ureteral calculus depends on its location, its size, and the amount of disturbance it is causing. A small stone is usually forced along the ureter by the vermicular action of that organ, but sometimes we find minute particles exceedingly slow in their passage and all the while producing intense irritation. Others after causing more or less severe colics become quiescent through the calculus slipping back into the pelvis or becoming lodged somewhere between the kidney and bladder. The ureter is of sufficient size to allow a calculus .0015 m. in diameter to pass and occasionally we find a ureter with a much larger caliber—one that will force out a calculus of .002 m. in diameter. If we know there is a small calculus either in the ureter or renal pelvis we should wait for a time in hope the patient will himself expel the foreign body, but a great deal will depend on how much disturbance the calculus is causing and any patient who suffers severely from renal colic should immediately have some surgical interference. Calculi of .002 m. or more in diameter usually require removal by the knife. Suppression of urine demands immediate operation. The ureters should first be catheterized to locate the calculus (it is usually impossible to pass it) and the obstruction cut down upon and removed. It is impossible in a short paper of this character to describe the different operations for removal of calculi in the various parts of the upper urinary tract.

The most distressing symptom of small calculi is pain. The steady boring pain should be endured without anodynes, but the colics are so exhausting they must be relieved and morphine is the agent usually employed. Periodic muscular contractions of the ureter occur to force the urine into the bladder. When a calculus engages in the ureter muscular action increases in an attempt to expel the foreign body. Overmuscular contraction causes pain known as renal colic. A severe spasm of the ureter defeats its own purpose in that such a contraction holds the calculus wherever it happens to be, but a mild colic forces the stone onward. It is, therefore, our purpose to lessen the pain, but not entirely check it. There is no need to dwell on the dangers of morphine habit likely to follow its injudicious administration, but another danger from this drug which is not so well recognized is that of sudden death. A patient who has been suffering for some time from renal colic receives a large dose of morphine, pain suddenly subsides and the patient goes into collapse. It is much better to give as the initial dose a very small amount of morphine and instead of sitting quietly waiting for the drug to take effect, apply heat over the kidney and along the course of the ureter. Hot cloths are beneficial, but the therapeutic lamp is much more effective in checking spasm. The small dose of morphine combined with heat applied externally will probably accomplish the result desired, namely, relief of spasm of the ureter, making suffering endurable, and yet not entirely paralyzing muscular action of the ureter. Thus pressure is still active in forcing the calculus through the ureter. By following this plan the foreign body is gradually forced onward into the bladder in favorable cases.

It occasionally happens that very small calculi stay lodged in the ureter for months, causing repeated and severe colics. Passage of an ureteral catheter is all that is required to cause their almost immediate expulsion. Larger calculi, say .0015 m. in diameter, are not so easily dislodged. If such a calculus is in the renal pelvis it may sometimes be so disturbed by a large ureteral catheter as to cause it to engage in the ureter and be forced through. If the stone is lodged in the ureter at some distance from the bladder, an injection of oil above the obstruction hastens its journey. If it is lodged low down it is often impossible to pass a catheter by it, but massage of the lower portion of the ureter usually sufficiently changes its position to cause it to be expelled in a few hours. We sometimes find an accumulation of very small calculi in the lowest portion of the ureter and on account of the swelling of the orifice a catheter cannot be passed. These cases also are quickly relieved by the finger in the rectum or vagina.

The writer has by these methods dislodged one calculus from the renal pelvis; six from the middle portion of the ureter; and sixteen from the lower extremity of the ureter.

To illustrate what may be accomplished without the knife, the following histories have been incorporated.

CASE I. Mr. C., 21, medical student, came to the office on June 8th, 1898. He had had renal colics in 1893 and 1895 and after the latter he had passed a small calculus. In January, 1898, he had three severe colics and then quiescence until early in March, when he began to have great frequency of urination with pain at the head of the penis as the bladder emptied. He had been repeatedly examined for stone in the bladder and his urethra had been examined for stricture. In the course of my routine examination, a small nodule was discovered apparently at the tip of the left vesicle. In trying to make out what this was it disappeared. When the patient urinated in a glass after rectal examination, he passed a small calculus. No further examination was deemed necessary. He was entirely relieved of his symptoms until 1903 when he again presented himself suffering as before. He had had no colic. On rectal examination nothing was found, but the lower extremity of the left ureter was massaged. The cystoscope showed a pouting left ureteral orifice, but the catheter could not be induced to enter. The patient passed a small calculus the following afternoon.

CASE II. Dr. O. passed a calculus in 1903 without previous colic or pain. Early in 1908 he had several severe renal colics and for a period, no symptoms. In October he began to have indefinite pains in his left groin and he was troubled with increased frequency of urination. He came to me in February, 1909. Cystoscopic examination showed a pouting left ureteral orifice through which a catheter could not be passed. The finger was introduced into the rectum and the lower extremity of the left ureter massaged. Six hours later he passed a calculus .0025 by .0015 m.

CASE III. Mr. F., 28, came to me on May 23rd, 1908. He had had pain over the right kidney since he was 12 years of age, but had had no colics. He had had numerous x-ray pictures taken, always with negative results. A wax-tipped catheter detected a calculus in the renal pelvis and on July 7th I removed a large irregular stone by pelvotomy. On April 1st, 1909, he came to the office suffering intensely from a renal colic. He was given an injection of morphine and so soon as his vomiting ceased a cystoscope was passed. The right ureteral orifice was normal in appearance, but the catheter encountered an obstruction at ¼ inch. After the cystoscope was removed the lower end of the ureter was massaged. On reintroduction of the cystoscope a calculus was seen projecting from the ureter. Again the ureter was massaged and this time the patient voided a small calculus as he emptied his bladder. Thinking his obstruction had been removed he was allowed to leave the office. The following day he returned with three small calculi which he had passed after reaching his home.

CASE IV. Mr. F., 34, came to the office March 10th, 1905. From 1902 to the above date he had had many renal colics and had passed many calculi, some of which he brought with him. They were pure uric acid, the largest being .0018 m. in diameter. He had a constant pain over the right kidney and a diagnosis of pelvic calculus was made. An x-ray by Dr. Caldwell was negative, but the wax-tipped catheter was decidedly scratched. On account of the friability of the specimens he had passed; the negative result of the skiagraph; and the short duration of his trouble, it seemed probable the calculus was a small one. His ureter was dilated to take a No. 11 catheter and a No. 11 Albarran was passed to the pelvis. With this one could feel the calculus. The tip was pushed into the pelvis several times and withdrawn. Two days later he began to have renal colics and at the end of ten days the calculus was passed. It was .0022 m. in diameter. The patient has had no urinary symptoms since.

CASE V. Mr. M., 64, was brought to me five years ago by the late Dr. Littlejohn of New Haven. For twenty years he had passed a calculus nearly every spring. The renal lithiasis was indicated by severe renal colics and a calculus would be passed in from two to four months, during which time the patient suffered severely from colics. The largest calculus he ever passed was not over .0005 m. in diameter. In In 1905 he had had a prolonged siege of colics on the left side, covering a period of six months. The colics suddenly ceased, but he did not find the calculus which had caused them. In the spring of 1906 he experienced a severe colic on the right side and two weeks later was brought to me. On cystoscopic examination I could see a calculus projecting from the left ureteral orifice and with the tip of the ureteral catheter so loosened it that it dropped into the bladder. The right ureteral orifice was normal in appearance and an ureteral catheter passed smoothly to the renal pelvis. The pelvis and ureter were flushed with boric acid. Two days later the patient had a very mild colic on the right side and within a few hours passed four small calculi. The stone found in the left ureteral orifice was probably the cause of the colics in 1905—it having been caught at that point by its irregular shape. The patient's diet was regulated and he has not had a colic since.

In conclusion:

1. A renal colic does not necessarily mean calculus.

2. A diagnosis of small renal or ureteral calculus having been made the patient should be treated expectantly for a time unless severe symptoms are caused by the foreign body.

3. It is better to attempt to cause a small calculus to pass by local manipulations than to at once resort to the knife.

4. A calculus of .002 m. in diameter or over is usually best removed by the knife.

5. Immediate operation is demanded when suppression of urine occurs as a complication of calculus.

616 Madison Ave.

———

There is an ancient saying, famous among men, that thou shouldst not judge fully of a man's life before he dieth, whether it should be called blest or wretched.— *Sophocles.*

HYDRONEPHROSIS: ITS ETIOLOGY, DIAGNOSIS AND TREATMENT.[1]

BY

CHARLES H. CHETWOOD, M. D., LL. D.,
New York City.

Professor of Genito-Urinary Surgery, New York Polyclinic Medical School and Hospital; Attending Surgeon to Bellevue Hospital; Consulting Surgeon to J. Hood Wright Hospital and St. John's Hospital, Long Island City.

A definition of the condition known as hydronephrosis depends upon the point of view from which it is considered, that is to say, whether it is regarded from a clinical or mechanical aspect. For hydronephrosis *per se,* which is an abnormal retention of urine in the pelvis of the kidney (otherwise spoken of as uronephrosis, hydrorenalis, cystonephrosis, etc.) is in reality a symptom, not a malady; a consequence, not a cause; but as it is the essential feature of its underlying cause, this term fittingly describes the malady in question. The general term, hydronephrosis, implies different varieties and degrees of the condition under consideration, most of which will not be dwelt upon here.

To appreciate the meaning of hydronephrosis, it must be borne in mind that the pelvis of the kidney is not like the urinary bladder, intended as a reservoir for the urine, but is simply a funnel-shaped expansion of the upper end of the ureter in which to receive the excretion of urine from the various renal pyramids and direct the course of these different urinary streams into the excretory duct from the kidney to the bladder. Under normal conditions, the flow is unimpeded and even under a certain amount of resistance, the kidney is still able

[1] Read at a meeting of the Eastern Med. Soc., Jan. 12, 1912.

to overcome this back-pressure without damming of the flow; but when the resistance becomes excessive from any cause within or without the urinary channel, it acts as an obstruction producing a retention in the pelvis of the kidney which, if incomplete or intermittent, causes gradual distension from the point of obstruction upwards and this distension increases so long as the obstacle exists. The result is gradual accumulation of retained urine, continuous in the case of a permanent obstruction, or it may from time to time be emptied out if the obstacle is one of an intermittent character. On the other hand, if the obstruction is complete and permanent, as in the case of a ligature of the ureter during a surgical operation or congenital occlusion of the ureter, the result is not a hydronephrosis but a gradual destruction of the secretory functions of the organ and its final atrophy.

The occurrence of hydronephrosis, its degree and variations are governed by mechanical conditions. As stated the kidney is capable of sustaining a certain amount of back-pressure; when the amount is exceeded, the accumulation or retention of urine in the pelvis occurs with a subsequent distension. If the obstruction is slight, the accumulation is slight; if the obstruction is great and continuous, the accumulation is proportionately greater and the distension more rapid. If on the other hand, the obstruction is intermittent, the effect is temporary and the accumulation is slow. Finally, if it is continuous over a prolonged period and after it exceeds a certain point or becomes complete, total destruction of the kidney may result with an enormous sac of retained fluid or if complete and sudden, total destruction of the kidney is produced without the resulting cystic accumulation.

This description embraces all forms of hydronephrosis which, as will be understood, may be small or large, continuous or intermittent and the causes thereof are spoken of as *congenital* or *acquired.* In any case, however, the obstruction, if permanent, is incomplete or if complete a temporary one.

A variety of causes are generally mentioned as responsible for *congenital* obstruction in the ureter, amongst which are alteration in the lumen, valvules and stenosis, kinks, anomalies of the kidney and misplacement of the ureteral attachment to the pelvis, anomalies of the blood vessels and other organs. One of the most common of these agencies is the persistence of fetal valvules and folds of the mucosa. These valvules of the mucosa perform such a constant role in the fetal urinary apparatus that it is not unlikely that they remain as congenital defects more often than is appreciated and form a basis for the gradual development and the explanation of hydronephrosis in later life.

Of the conditions within the ureter given as a cause of *acquired* hydronephrosis, that of displacement of the kidney and consequent bending and kinking of the ureteral tube is one of the most commonly ascribed causes. It must be admitted, however, that the *bending alone* of the tube *may be insufficient* to produce the obstruction whereas the additional existence within of a constriction or valvule, an anomalous pelvic ureteral departure or periureteral adhesions often furnish the determining causative factor. There has been considerable discussion on this point amongst medical authorities and while the consensus of opinion seems to be that renal prolapse is a prevalent cause of the production of hydronephrosis, it is justly questioned as to whether in many instances, there has not

progressive cause for incomplete renal drainage and consequent retention and might induce gradually an undue mobility of the organ finally culminating in hydro-

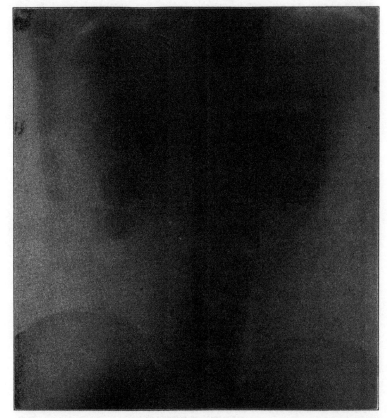

FIGURE 1. Radiograph showing a comparison of the abnormal and normal pelvis by injection with argyrol.

pre-existed one of these congenital defects of the lumen or fixed distortion of the course of the tube. Such abnormality would act after birth as a slow but

nephrosis. However, we may accept undue mobility of the kidney as one of the causes of acquired hydronephrosis when it is demonstrated that an operation for the fixation of the kidney following the existence of such a condition has resulted in complete relief. Yet, on the other hand, it is an important caution to bear in mind that in all cases operated upon for movable

of complete relief.

A case in point of recent experience is one of a young man 24 years of age who was operated upon for movable kidney which was successfully fixed in place

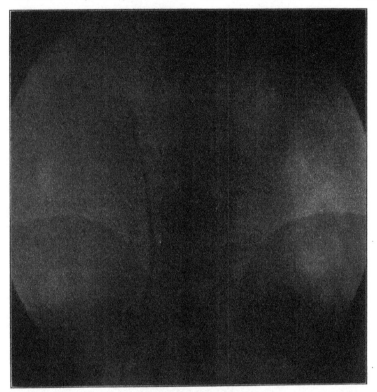

FIGURE 2. Same case as Fig. 1 showing entrance of leaded catheter into affected kidney at same point as opposite side.

kidney in which hydronephrosis has been a symptom, the point of departure of the ureter from the renal pelvis and the calibre of the ureteral canal should be investigated always; otherwise the operation may fail

between three and four years ago; he had had, previous to the operation, attacks of paroxysmal pain which, according to the clinical history given, are suggestive of hydronephrosis, satisfactory x-ray plates having been obtained which showed no calculi. For over a year following the operation, he was free from pain but, since then, there has been a gradual recurrence sists during the attack. The urine is perfectly clear, and the kidney is not palpable.

Cystoscopy.—Both ureters are normal in appearance. Right side contracts regularly;

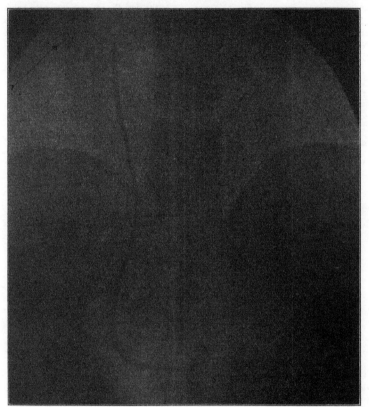

FIGURE 3. Affected kidney following injection of argyrol, showing sacculation below entrance of catheter.

of the pain increasing in intensity and in duration, with shortening intervals between the paroxysms. These paroxysms last as long as 24 hours. The location of the pain is in the left lumbar region, where it per-

no contractions noted on the left or affected side.

Both ureters catheterized, the catheter being advanced without difficulty 28 cms.

Radiography.—(1) Plates taken of vesicorenal regions on both sides, which give negative findings, there being no suspicious shadows.

(2) Plates following ureteral catheterism and injection or argyrol. (Fig. 1). 2 cc. of 50% argyrol injected into the right side and 30 cc. injected into the left side. Note.—Pelvis of right kidney is apparently normal in contour and location. The left

the previous plate, the same sacculated condition and the entrance of the catheter into the kidney on the same level as on the opposite side. (Fig. 3).

At the time the catheter enters the pelvis and before injection, a specimen of urine is obtained which is perfectly clear and flows continuously and not in jets, bearing evidence of existing renal retention.

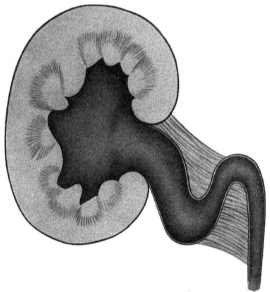

FIGURE 4. Partial prolapse of kidney with fixed distortion of the ureteral course.

kidney outline is lobular in form and shows a large distended area.

(3) Plate of left kidney, following the introduction of a leaded catheter, taken upon a subsequent occasion, shows entrance of the catheter into the pelvis of kidney. (Fig. 2).

(4) Plate following injection of 8 ccs. of 50% argyrol shows to a lesser degree than

The result of this observation would seem to indicate that the lumen of the ureter is perfectly open and that there is at the present time no evidence of infection of the kidney. There is, however, a distinct renal retention which is shown, first, by the flow of urine that comes freely at the time of catheterization and secondly, by the pyelography with argyrol injection giving an unusually large and lobulated outline. Finally, as shown by the leaded catheter, the point of departure of the ureter from the pelvis is far above the most dependent portion of the existing sacculated condition thereof.

It is probable that a plastic operation upon the pelvis at the time of the nephropexy might have avoided the recurrence of symptoms.

The question is sometimes asked why movable kidney is not always accompanied by symptoms of hydronephrosis. The answer can only be that the existing conditions are not of sufficient degree to overcome the intrarenal pressure to the extent of causing pronounced hydronephrosis which, however, may develop at a later date as a result of prolonged back-pressure, while in other cases, the obstruction of the ureter is variable in degree and the symptoms in consequence appear at irregular intervals.

This brings us to the consideration of the so-called "intermittent" hydronephrosis, a term that has been objected to on the part of some authors and not without reason as it suggests that the underlying condition is of a transitory character whereas it is distinctly progressive; yet, as already stated, the cause of its production may be a continuous, incomplete occlusion of the canal and an incomplete or complete temporary one, any of which causes produce progressive dilatation and consequent morbid intrarenal changes; and, in certain cases, where, owing to the mobility of the kidney, or other changing mechanical conditions, the extent of the obstruction varies in degree, there is, as a result, an ebb and flow in the hydronephrosis and the symptoms resulting therefrom necessarily occur at intermittent intervals.

An incomplete obstruction of the ureter together with a movable kidney may become completely obstructed temporarily by movement of that organ and entirely overcome the intrarenal tension which may right itself again by changing position. A pronounced bend of the ureter fixed by adhesions, may exercise a permanent resistence to renal drainage and by a valvular formation, the degree of closure may from time to time become greater or less according to the amount of retention within the kidney. Such a case I have operated upon and in this instance, the patient suffered from paroxysmal pain in the kidney region which came on slowly and gradually increased to a high degree of intensity, then persisted for a varying period and gradually subsided. The pain started in the left lumbar region and was reflected down as far as the corresponding testicle. The attacks increased in intensity and in duration. During the intermediate period between attacks, excellent x-ray pictures were obtained showing all the anatomical landmarks but no evidence of calculi.

Cystoscopy.—Bladder negative; ureteral mouths negative; both ureters catheterized easily.

Right renal pelvis, capacity 16 cc. Left renal pelvis, capacity 32 cc. at which point pain characteristic of the attack is induced. There is a very slight difference between the specimens obtained from the two kidneys.

The patient is submitted to a left nephrotomy and it is found at this time that the ureter, after leaving the pelvis of the kidney, makes a sharp turn upwards and again downwards and that this intervening loop is fastened together by adhesions and the efferent ureter is adherent to the distended pouch of the pelvis. Fig. 4. Under ordinary circumstances, the resistance to the flow was not enough to interfere with the passage of the urine but at certain times, with changing position of the kidney, bending or drooping, there resulted a compression of one or both arms of the syphon with accumulation either within the pelvis or in the loop of the ureter. This valvular obstruction would remain in force until the distension became sufficiently great to open the sluice through the lumen of the loop or changing position of the kidney produce sufficient alteration in the valvular compression to allow a drainage of the accumulated secretion.

Relief of the symptoms then occurred until another period of similar character brought a repetition of the painful crisis. By releasing the adhesions of the ureter, and replacement of the kidney in its normal position, complete relief resulted to this patient. Here again, the ureteral distortion was an important factor.

Such, in brief, is a description of a variety of hydronephrosis to which I desire to direct attention and the report of two cases bearing upon this condition with a view of emphasizing the importance of seeking some interior or exterior structural defect of the ureter as a cause for renal retention whether or not associated with undue mobility of the kidney.

There is a comforting reflection in this connection that with the development of urological proficiency along certain lines, namely, special cystoscopic technic involving differential and functional urinary tests, combined with radiography or pyelography, it is possible to recognize this malady as well as renal lithiasis or renal tuberculosis and that errors in diagnosis may be avoided with such means at our command.

25 Park Avenue.

THE USE OF FATS IN DISORDERS OF THE STOMACH.[1]

BY

ALPHEUS FREEMAN, M. D.,

Physician to Presbyterian Hospital, O. P. D.

The use of olive oil in the treatment of diseases of the stomach is by no means a recent procedure, but has been advocated at times for the last twenty years. Still most American text books on diseases of the stomach make very slight mention of this subject, and it has only appeared in our literature within the last few years. The Germans, however, have not been so behindhand and their writings are fairly well interspersed with experimental work and clinical reports. Formerly the belief prevailed that all dyspeptics and especially those suffering from any form of gastric trouble which brought about excessive gastric acidity should avoid all fats, except perhaps in very small quantities. Fats were regarded as decidedly harmful in acid dyspepsia, the idea being that they would cause further lowering of functional activity and possibly might be a source of furnishing the injurious acids themselves. Any deviation from the normal in the functional activity of the stomach was considered in the direction of deficiency and it was believed that the subjective manifestations of such deviation depended upon organic acids and gaseous fermentation initiated as the immediate consequence of deficiency in the antiseptic hydrochloric acid and stagnation of the stomach contents from deficient motor power.

The Germans later on declared that these ideas were erroneous and pointed out that in acid dyspepsia the high degree of acidity in the stomach was caused by the hydro-

[1]Read before the Lenox Medical and Surgical Society, Nov. 25th, 1911.

chloric acid itself and not by the organic acids. While this opinion is now generally sustained by a majority of observers, some well known authorities still adhere to the existence of an acid dyspepsia caused by organic acid fermentation. For a long time the suspicion had existed that in some unknown manner the presence of fats in the stomach retarded digestion in this organ and Penzolt was one of the first to confirm this. He noticed that after drinking coffee with cream the gastric acidity was lower than with coffee alone. In 1886 Ewald and Boas showed that when starch oil mixture was introduced into the empty stomach very little if any secretion of hydrochloric acid occurred in the first half hour. They also noticed that when bacon fat was added to their test breakfast, stomach digestion was retarded and there was a great diminution in the amount of free hydrochloric acid found in the gastric contents. Twelve years later, in 1898, Strauss and Adler used liquid fats in patients afflicted with various conditions associated with gastric hyperacidity. Cream, butter, almond and pure olive oil were given and the results were said to have been very satisfactory. About the same time Pawlow and his associates experimented on dogs with gastric fistula and furnished valuable information regarding disorders of functional activity. They appear to have shown that olive oil, liquid fats and cream do not exert any stimulating effects on gastric secretion when introduced into a dog's stomach and that on the other hand they exert an inhibiting influence on the secretory processes excited by other foods. In 1900 Bachmann conducted a series of experiments on human subjects and claimed to reduce free hydrochloric acid on an average of 19% by butter and as much as 42% by cream. A little

later Cohnheim reported the case of a patient he had been treating eight months for gastric ulcer but without improvement. The man then left the hospital and returned to his home in North Germany where he took olive oil several weeks and then presented himself again to Cohnheim in apparently healthy condition. Inquiry showed that olive oil was a much used household remedy in that part of the country. Cohnheim then employed olive oil with good results in a number of cases of hyperacidity and concluded that it fulfilled four conditions.

1. Relief of pain.
2. Reduction of friction.
3. As a food.
4. For the inhibition of acids.

Ewald, and later Blum, stated that frequently the oil caused nausea and vomiting, which contra-indicated its use in ulcer, but this is not surprising as at that time two, three, and four ounces of pure oil were given at a single dose. In 1909 Moore and Ferguson in a paper published in the London *Lancet* called attention to the frequent occurrence of hypersecretion of the gastric glands in certain forms of indigestion and demonstrated that fats had a depressing action on the activity of the normal flow of gastric juice. In addition to the diminution of gastric acidity they obtained relief from the associated subjective discomforts and a promotion of the general nutrition of the patient. They made further researches and conducted a number of investigations.

Among the diseases in which the treatment was tried were ulcer of the stomach and duodenum, carcinoma of the stomach, nervous dyspepsia, atonic dilatation of the stomach, alcoholism, constipation and miscellaneous cases. They made tests with an ordinary test breakfast and then on alternate days with an oil test breakfast and compared the results. The oil test breakfast consisted of an ordinary test breakfast but one-half hour before taking it ʒi of almond oil was given and then they determined the total acidity and free hydrochloric acid in the stomach contents. The greatest diminution in acidity was found in those cases that showed the highest acid values after the plain test breakfast and as appeared comparing them with the average results in the patients with gastric and duodenal ulcer and nervous dyspepsia, whether there was any lesion of the stomach or not.

The averages and also the majority of the individual observations further showed that the absolute diminution of the total acidity exceeded that of the free hydrochloric acid—a result difficult of interpretation since it apparently depends on a diminution of other factors than the hydrochloric acid free or combined, which contribute to the total acidity of the stomach contents and which it might be anticipated would be increased by the liberation of fatty acids in the splitting of the neutral fat by the hydrochloric acid and the possible gastric lipase. In quite a number of their cases it was found that the pepsin in the gastric juice was also diminished along with the acid values and digestive power.

These authors regard this as partly due to the deficiency of hydrochloric acid and also to a real diminution of the peptic content. In very simple forms of hyperacidity due to slight hypersecretion, they found that giving considerable cream and butter and diminishing the starches was all that was necessary to relieve the disagreeable complaints. They further state that in all cases the oil has been well borne and in no in-

stance found objectionable. Many, however, will take exception to this statement, for certain patients with hyperacidity exhibit a marked aversion to the oil and find it so disagreeable that they would rather endure their discomforts than take it any longer.

As to the exact manner in which the oil causes reduction of acidity in hyperchlorhydria, opinions differ. Boldereff showed by experiments on dogs that the introduction of oil into the stomach caused a regurgitation into that organ of the duodenal contents consisting of bile, pancreatic and intestinal juice. This is now a well recognized phenomena and is often made use of where it is desirable to obtain a specimen of trypsin. It is difficult to explain just how the oil causes the regurgitation, but some have suggested that it may be partly caused by a smoothing out of the folds of the pylorus and duodenum. Moore and Ferguson consider that it is still doubtful whether the acid reduction following the ingestion of oil is due to a true depression of gastric secretion or to dilution and neutralization by regurgitation of alkaline duodenal contents.

To determine if the oil might act in a mechanical way, they used petroleum in some patients, but in no case was there any diminution of acid values. However, petroleum is considered an irritant by some and this perhaps was not a fair test. Pawlow says fats inhibit the secretion of acids of the stomach by reflex stimulation of the inhibitory nerves on the glands or the inhibitory centre of these nerves. Cowie and Munson, on the other hand, while admitting this may be partly true, hold that the mechanical effect of the oil is much more important, that the food coated by the oil, does not so readily stimulate the gastric nerve endings, which are at the same time covered with oil.

There have been many excellent results reported from the use of olive oil in gastric and duodenal ulcer. It is now generally admitted that persistent hyperacidity of the gastric contents is an important factor, if not in the production of acute gastric ulcer, at least in the recurrent chronic form. If the oil is only given for a short time, in ulcer of the stomach the inhibition of acids by the oil is not permanent, and even if omitted for one or two meals, the acidity immediately rises. But after a long continued use of it there is often no recurrence of gastric symptoms. Lutz thus explains this: "The majority of patients with hyperacidity and gastric ulcer give a history of loss of weight, lowered nutrition, chronic constipation and secondary anemia. These cases under pure olive oil, a liberal diet, and a regulated mode of life, gain steadily in weight. Symptoms of anemia partly disappear and constipation ceases. So long as these patients retain their normal weight, no symptoms of hyperacidity appear." Could it not be possible, he asks, that the hyperacidity, which at the present time has an unknown etiology, is due to a so-called vicious circle—the hyperacidity preventing normal digestion and assimilation with chronic constipation, anemia and poor nutrition as resulting conditions; while these same conditions in their turn act as exciting factors in keeping up the hyperacidity. "By holding in check the excessive acidity for the time being, the oil permits of a more liberal diet, as soon as pain and tenderness are ameliorated."

The oil treatment is considered by many preferable to antacids because of its caloric value, providing the maximum of nourishment in the minimum of bulk, more than double what would be contained in the same weight of dried carbohydrate or protein. It also lessens the peristaltic activity of the stomach for the time being which is another point in favor of its use in gastric ulcer. Some authorities state that even during hemorrhage it may be safely administered combined with bismuth and that it possesses an advantage over nutrient enemata. Lutz says that in ulcer cases, even the administration of nutrient enemata causes secretion of gastric juice, so that gastric juice is present in the stomach without anything to neutralize its action, but when oil is given little or no hydrochloric acid is produced.

Permanent cures have been reported from the oil treatment in cases of spastic stenosis, fissure and erosion of the pylorus, ulcer, and gastritis. Hyperchlorhydria is frequently the cause of pyloric spasm, in which case treatment of the spasm should consist of proper measures to counteract the hyperacidity.

The same treatment is often efficacious in stenosis of the cardia and cardio spasm. Amelioration of symptoms from the use of oil has been reported even in cancer of the stomach. In hypermotility it usually acts well and may be given before, during or after a meal. In doses of ℥ss to ℥iii it has been known to relieve obstinate jaundice and it has been suggested that possibly the discomfort associated with gall-stones was sometimes gastric in origin and associated with hyperchlorhydria and that by diminishing the secretion of hydrochloric. acid the oil relieves the discomfort. During its use patients may pass lumps of white fat composed of undigested palmatin.

Pure oil can usually be given in doses of ℥ss to ℥i t. i. d. but sometimes it is necessary to begin with small quantities, even a few drops and then gradually increase the amount. Using a good mouth wash after each dose is sometimes efficacious in preventing disgust. Some who cannot use olive oil find almond oil palatable and take it successfully. Others do better with cream, which is rich in fat and produces less hydrochloric acid than milk. It can be given in ℥i doses t. i. d. and increased to ℥iv. Then later on oil may be gradually mixed with the cream till pure oil is being taken. Mayonnaise or some good emulsion of olive oil is found agreeable by some and readily taken.

The use of cotton seed oil has been recommended by Block and others, and H. W. Wiley states that one unit of it will furnish over twice as much heat and energy as the same quantity of sugar or starch, and that it is more easily digested than olive oil.

Some persons can take oil better if it is warmed. A suspension of bismuth in oil or five per cent. sodium carbonate have each been considered to possess advantages in certain conditions. When retching or vomiting is caused by the oil, this is generally considered a contra-indication to its use, although some only vomit once and it is not repeated.

In gastric stasis and persistent slow evacuation, oil is contra-indicated.

According to Moore and Ferguson, "If the idea is correct that hyperacidity is more often caused by excessive secretion of the stomach glands than by deficient activity of the same, then the use of oil to neutralize the excess of acidity seems to be well founded."

It is positive that fats depress the activity of normal stomach secretion and it appears to be true that the depressant action exerts a good influence on hyper-acidity. Therefore we may state that fats are indicated in patients exhibiting this condition. The reports of results so far are certainly encouraging enough to justify us in trying this treatment in cases of nervous dyspepsia and gastric hyperacidity from many causes. Moreover we can feel that it is simple and harmless.

975 Lexington Ave.

STOMATITIS IN CHILDREN.

BY

LEGRAND KERR, M. D.,

Visiting Pediatrist to the Methodist Episcopal (Seney), Williamsburgh, Bushwick and Swedish Hospitals, in Brooklyn; Consulting Pediatrist to the Rockaway Beach Hospital, the Industrial Home for Children, the E. N. Y. Dispensary, etc.

Acute catarrhal stomatitis is the commonest affection of the mouth during infancy. It is a part of, or precedes, nearly all other forms of stomatitis. It may evidence itself by a general hyperemia and hypersensitiveness of the membranes, or there may be considerable inflammation with pain, tenderness, and increased secretion.

The usual course in infancy is at first a reddening of the membranes of the tongue and gums (sometimes of all of the mucous membrane of the mouth). Salivation is invariably present and the secretion may be so acid that the lip becomes inflamed. The tongue has white furry coating which becomes gradually darker, then disappears piecemeal.

The infant refuses to nurse after several attempts have been made to do so. The general symptoms are restlessness, slight rise of temperature, and possibly diarrhea of a mild type.

In older children, in whom the disease is much less frequent, there may be added to the usual symptoms of pain, salivation, fever, and coated tongue, a decided swelling of the tongue, with indentures along its side from pressure against the teeth. If any odor is present, it is very faint and never disagreeable. When present, it is worse in the morning and is readily removed by washing out the mouth.

This type of stomatitis arises from various causes; retention of particles of food in the mouth may result in their decomposition, and the irritation caused thereby may be the starting point for the invasion of microorganisms. If the child happens to be in a state of malnutrition or poor health, or there is any factor which diminishes the flow of saliva, the growth of bacteria is favored. When they once gain a foothold, the products of the inflammation tend strongly to produce or invite secondary infections.

Certain drugs, used either locally or internally, may produce it (acids, mercury, strong alkalis, etc.).

Stomatitis mucosa (Thrush, Sprue, etc.) This is a parasitic form of stomatitis. The spores of this causative fungus may be found in the mouth of the healthy infant, and in fact they are everywhere prevalent. All that is needed for their development is the favorable soil, and this may be produced by simple neglect of the mouth. Finding suitable soil, they multiply until they appear upon the surface of the mucosa of the tongue, the posterior surface of the lips and of the cheeks and gums in the form of small white flakes. In some instances there is an extension of the disease into the throat and esophagus.

The flakes are entirely white, and at first are firmly attached to the surface, so that forcible removal leaves an abraded and perhaps a slightly bleeding surface. Later in the disease they separate from the surface spontaneously. Immediately around each spot the mucosa looks drier than normal. When neglected several of these spots may coalesce. The disease is of itself painless, but the accompanying catarrhal stomatitis may cause considerable distress.

This is essentially a disease of the first weeks of life, and while it may develop in children who have passed the early suckling period, it is then associated with other disease which has exhausted the system. Occurring under these circumstances it is a late happening and a serious one.

The diagnosis is made by the mode of development and the nature of the spots, whose chief and constant characteristic is their entirely white color and difficult removal early in the disease.

The general symptoms are those of inflammation, and added to these or modifying them are the symptoms of the associated disease.

Stomatitis unaccompanied by odor or ulceration. Gonorrheal stomatitis is only liable to occur when there has been an injury to the mouth which has removed the epithelium. Subsequent exposure may produce it, but this is unusual. Yellowish-white patches are formed on the tongue and the hard palate and the gonococcus is found in the exudate. There is but little inflammation and tenderness, so that further than a mild remonstrance at first, the infant does not object to being placed at the breast. It is very rare that the condition exists alone in the mouth, but is generally associated with other evidences of gonorrheal infection.

Stomatitis with ulceration and no offensive odor: (Stomatitis aphthosa, canker, sore mouth).. This is characterized by the formation upon the mucous membrane of the tongue, cheeks, and lips of small, shallow, rounded ulcers which usually appear in successive crops. Sometimes the first appearance is of a solitary vesicular lesion upon the tonsil. It does not take long for the eruption to develop, for usually within twenty-four hours it has spread well over the parts. At first the ulcers are about one-eighth of an inch in diameter and covered with a yellowish exudate. The ulcers rapidly coalesce forming large patches which may resemble a diphtheritic exudate. As the ulcer ages it assumes a dirty grayish color, or may be of a dirty yellowish hue, but in either case surrounded by a reddened zone.

Salivation is excessive and excoriation of the lips and chin is the rule. One of the characteristics of this type of ulceration is the entire absence of fetid breath. Another is its common occurrence at the time of the first teething.

The general symptoms are much the same as in the catarrhal form, but much intensified. Pain is much more of a feature in this form than in the simple catarrhal form. The duration of the disease is between one and two weeks.

In diagnosis a distinction has to be made between the disease and ulcerative or diphtheritic stomatitis, as well as from the lesions of variola and varicella as they appear in the mouth. The situation of the ulcers and the entire absence of fetor will exclude ulcerative stomatitis. The early appearance of salivation and the early disappearance of the coalesced patches tend to prove the non-diphtheritic nature of the disease. The history of contagion and the generally severe character of the initial symptoms of variola would help to differentiate it, while from varicella the distinction would be very difficult, and one might have to wait until the true nature of the disease was exposed by the subsequent skin eruption.

Syphilitic stomatitis: This is most frequently observed during the relapses. There are patches formed which are whitish and slightly elevated, with a papillary structure, and this feature is usually so decided that one may see several thickly crowded papillae tops forming the patch. They are situated upon the mucous membrane of the mouth, especially at the angles, and upon the lips, tongue, soft palate and tonsils. Fissures of the lips and of the angles of the mouth are more distinctive of hereditary syphilis when they occur during the first weeks of life; later than that they may appear without syphilis being the cause, and then they are usually the result of fever.

Aphthae of the palate should be mentioned as it may prove misleading; usually appears as a double lesion of the mucous membrane, but on opposite sides of the mouth where the hard and soft palates join. The ulcers are generally symmetrically located and are superficial and circular. They are of a grayish yellow hue.

They are in evidence for about three weeks and then gradually disappear. In abortive children they may spread and the two lesions may coalesce and others be formed, and under these circumstances the duration of the affection is from six to eight weeks. The condition is peculiar to the first few weeks of life.

Stomatitis with ulceration and offensive odor: In this class of cases it is first necessary to determine the source of the odor, for even in the presence of ulceration within the mouth the odor may depend upon some associated condition and be entirely distinct from the ulceration.

When the tongue is considerably coated, there is apt to be more or less disagreeable odor, which is readily removed by mouth washing. A decayed tooth or the presence of decaying food in the mouth will give rise to some odor, but washing removes the smell for a time at least, and in any instance while the odor may be unpleasant, it is not offensive. Rhinitis is one of the most frequent sources of odor and this can be distinguished from other causes by the fact that it is most noticeable during expiration through the nose.

Other causes of offensive odor may be catarrh of the stomach with eructations of foul smelling gas, bronchiectiasiae with fetid contents, and gangrene of the lung.

Stomatitis ulcerosa: This condition may develop at any time of life, but is very unusual before the eruption of the teeth and after the ninth year. It depends largely upon a depraved condition of the general nutritive processes, and in rare instances may be directly traceable to metallic poisons, especially mercury and lead. During scorbutus it is by no means uncommon.

The lesions may occur upon any part of the mucous membrane of the mouth, but usually the very first point of invasion is at the junction of the tooth and gum. The intense offensive odor of the mouth is generally the first thing noticed, then the ulceration is discovered. This is shortly followed by swelling of the gums and they become intensely congested and somewhat friable, bleeding readily from slight pressure. The margins of the gum rise toward the crown of the tooth both internally and externally. The disease may continue until the soft and congested gum falls away from the tooth and pus forms in the intervening spaces or burrows through the alveolar process. Then two things may occur; the teeth become loosened and fall out, or the jaw may become necrotic. The ulcerative process may spread to the buccal mucosa, so that there is soon formed an ulcerated strip of a dirty yellow color, which soon breaks down, leaving an open ulceration with a foul bottom and undermined and broken edges. Associated with this the whole cheek may be greatly swollen and the submaxillary glands enlarged. The tongue may be swollen and indented from the teeth. The general symptoms are unusually mild, unless sepsis occurs.

Stomatitis gangraenosa (noma): This is the most severe type of stomatitis as it occurs in childhood, and is fortunately not common. The time at which it is most likely to occur is during the interval between the first and second dentition. It is usually preceded by a catarrhal stomatitis which occurs in a child whose general nutrition and vitality are not up to standard.

The gangrenous odor of the mouth is usually the first thing noticed, and then the ulcer is discovered. In the commencement the ulcer is a small spot of inflammation which appears upon the cheek, usually after two days of indefinite illness (slight fever, tender sub-maxillary and cervical glands, salivation). This red spot of inflammation rapidly deepens in color, so that it may soon become blue, purple, or black, and it rapidly increases in area as the necrosis spreads over the face. The destruction of tissue is rapid and very widespread, and if the unusual occurrence of spontaneous resolution takes place, the child is terribly deformed by the cicatrix. The general symptoms are severe and the cases usually result in early teeth.

The diagnosis is made from anthrax by the history and the character of the ulcer; in anthrax there is at first a small pustule, which is rapidly formed into a solid but .odorless scab, surrounded by new pustules or vesicles, and then only does a tumor of the soft parts appear. .

Stomatitis with formation of membrane. (Stomatitis membranosa): A pseudo-membrane may form in the mouth and upon the lips during the course of the acute infectious fevers or as the result of irritants. These membranes are generally due to bacterial growth, and may be the forward extension of a croupous angina.

In very rare instances the condition seems to be primary. There is at times a very considerable systemic disturbance. The membranes may assume a darker color from exposure to the air, and this is especially true if any hemorrhage has taken place from fissures in the mucosa. Under treatment or with the exercise of ordinary cleanliness the membranes gradually disappear, leaving the mucous membrane somewhat reddened and denuded of epithelium.

The diagnosis from diphtheria depends entirely upon the absence of the Klebs-Loeffler bacilli. From stomatitis mycosa the diagnosis is made by the absence of the characteristic thrush fungus.

42 Gates Ave., Brooklyn, N. Y.

ULCUS SERPENS.

A 2 per cent. ointment of picric acid in eczematous blepharo-conjunctivitis, lime burns, traumatic keratitis, and ulcus serpens, is excellent. It promotes rapid healing and disappearance of the micro-organism.

DICHOTOMY, OR THE DIVISION OF THE FEE BETWEEN PHYSICIANS.

BY

W. W. VINNEDGE, M. D.,
Lafayette, Indiana.

The practice of the division of the fee between physicians employed in a given case is comparatively new in the profession. It does not mean an equal division of the fee, as my title might suggest to someone, but a transaction between honorable men and women, according to the necessities and requirements of each individual case— a fair division between two or more physicians and the patient, or the latter's "next of friend." The new practice, or the division of the fee by and between the physicians in a given case, appears to me to be a distinct improvement over the old way. This idea means that the physicians on the one hand, the patient, his agent or friend on the other hand, definitely decide as to the fee—as I understand it. An open understanding and agreement in advance of any professional undertaking whenever praticable, cannot be otherwise than advantageous to all parties concerned. These statements do not comprehend the *abuse* of the division of the fee; that is another matter. Every self-respecting physician, whether family physician or specialist, will frown on any division of the fee that makes a commodity of the patient. The division in the way of rebate or on a percentage basis belongs to a low standard of professional morals; it comes under the head of *secret* or questionable practices. Since there is much diversity of opinion as to dichotomy or the division of the fee, is it not plain that correct practices ought to be defined to the whole profession in advance of steps looking towards discipline? I believe so. The legal profession furnishes us an example as to the best way to dispose of the fee question. As I understand it the division of the fee between attorneys in a given case is almost uniformly the subject for consultation and agreement; such action is in the interest of the client and all of the attorneys as well. If the practice commends itself to honorable attorneys having much judicial training why is it not equally wise and fair in the medical profession?

I will try to make my position plainer from personal observations and experiences. About twenty-five years ago, late in December, I had as a patient a young married woman, about 28 years old, the mother of three promising children, the youngest being two years old. This patient had bilateral laceration of the uterine neck, pronounced, together with recurrent uterine hemorrhage of about two months' duration. She was beautiful, educated, gentle, the daughter of a manufacturer—well-to-do. I was doing the best I could for my patient and at the same time conducting microscopic tests as to the question of possible malignancy in the case. Here a neighbor physician asked me to administer an anesthetic while a surgeon whom I knew personally, from a distant city, did an important surgical operation for a young female patient of his. I did this, and the two doctors took luncheon with me afterwards; they were my seniors many years. I told them of my troublesome case, and with the consent of the patient and her husband, both agreed to go with me to see her, Two hours later an examination and consultation was had in the patient's home. The surgeon from abroad was certain the disease was malignant, so was my neighbor, though less positively so, and both advised an immediate operation. I argued that my

patient was anemic, weak from loss of blood already, making the operation proposed—amputation through the uterine neck—too hazardous. I suggested further rest in bed and that other steps be taken to try to recruit her forces—then the operation. My associates thought differently and my patient terminated the debate by suggesting laughingly that I wished to enjoy my Christmas. The operation was done the following morning. Probably half of the somewhat enlarged uterus was cut away—hollowed out so to speak—by means of a strong vulsellum forceps and curved scissors. The patient survived the operation less than three days. With reaction there was a return of hemorrhage. She died from exhaustion.

Immediately after the operation the surgeon received a *cheque* for $200. My neighbor received the customary $10 for administering the anesthetic. At the end of the next quarter I sent a statement of my account, a pittance, by mail to the bereaved husband, as I had done previously; he did not respond. Several months later I called on him in his office. Nothing of moment was said, but he passed his *cheque* to me through the wicket, saying "that is the hardest bill I ever paid." It is needless to say I never did any other professional work for that family. I bore the greater burden of responsibility and all the loss in the case, while the surgeon bore the fee away. I do not complain—only state the facts.

Take a rather recent experience. A bright German Lutheran boy, four years old, suffered a chill followed by coughing and high fever; his ailment soon declared itself to be acute circumscribed pleurisy with exudate which in a short time became purulent to exploratory test. A professional neighbor, who is a surgeon and partial general practitioner, resected a rib, while another physician in the family, gave the anesthetic. The man who gave the anesthetic received $15.00, while the operator settled with the father for $50.00. This made it difficult for me to make a fair settlement and retain my patients. The boy recovered his health. It would have been much more satisfactory for all concerned in this case for the physicians to have met and agreed upon the fee for all the work, and its division, than for each of us to undertake a difficult settlement with the father, as we did do—under the old rule.

These statements reflect actual happenings; they furnish the more salient facts as to fees in the cases they recite. The participants in this work were gentlemen. There was never at any time during the conduct of the cases other than the best of feeling between them. This much seems necessary in order that I may declare that human nature holds its place in the acts of the physician, to wit, that self professional preservation is the first law in practice; the specialist will in the majority of instances look out for his professional and financial interests before considering that of any one else, and thus. it behooves the family physician to take care of his interests in advance of work; otherwise he will frequently be forced to assume serious responsibilities with little if any financial return; he may place himself at a pronounced disadvantage as to fee if this is not arranged for in advance if possible.

Present prevailing professional conditions are so well known and have been so ably and so accurately described by current writers that I need hardly refer to them otherwise than briefly here. Besides the high cost of living and the over-

crowded state of the profession by qualified and unqualified men and women, many of the latter from medical colleges having low standards, the schemes for obtaining practice and fees are varied and numerous. Then the craze for operating is undoubtedly one of the principal causes for the division of the profession into two camps as to work —the specialist and the family physician. Antiseptic surgery appeals to young physicians. As a student and an interne I recall that the surgical clinics were crowded while the medical clinics were meagerly attended. The results in surgical cases are more apparent, more striking, the work more spectacular, and the fees larger, and the more direct way to this work is to become a specialist. Thus this class of physicians is becoming so numerous that the supply exceeds the demand, and the struggle for professional and social existence has become extreme. Will not these undesirable professional conditions have to cure themselves?

What are the remedies against the abuse of the division of the fee? May I suggest that education is the primary remedy. I wish some plan might be advanced by which the doors of commercial medical colleges might be closed permanently. They are the original, if not the chief offenders against the welfare of the profession.

The division of the fee has to do with physicians socially and economically. For this reason the general practitioner in the profession would the more certainly resent interference by organized medicine with his efforts in behalf of his patients, his family, and himself; and if driven to it would probably elect to prosecute his professional work outside of medical organizations rather than accept dictation and discipline from his rivals and competitors, for these are the persons who usually make ethical outcries in medical societies.

The effort to cure little alleged ethical infractions in medical societies through charges and discipline, scandalizes and demoralizes the profession as a whole more than anything else; it rarely cures the alleged offender and at the same time it brings ridicule on the profession at large. It helps the irregulars to persuade statesmen that the regular profession is a *trust* whose scheme is to monopolize the offices and practice of medicine and surgery throughout the country. It helps to lodge in the public mind the idea of *intolerance,* if not bigotry in the profession. In illustration, in the court room on the witness stand, I have had an attorney ask in no friendly tone—"That's against the code of medical ethics, isn't it?" This of course was said to discredit the medical witness with the court and jury.

The majority of physicians—family physicians I mean—know little and care less about medical ethics. In the absence of authority to enforce the attendance and replies to questions on the part of witnesses, the effort to secure justice, fairness and benefit to the majority through this channel is questionable in the majority of instances. Rather the profession should seek to promote a tolerant judicial sentiment in its ranks. Supposed offenders ought to be met and shown the right way in a fraternal spirit. The cause of professional morals cannot be advanced successfully by the use of a club, that is by coercion, especially as to debatable questions.

I wonder if the opponents of a division of the fee are wholly consistent? It is well known that manufacturers of surgical instruments and supplies openly rebate physicians—20% to 25% without the knowledge of the patient. In this way physicians by indirection become the agents of the manufacturers of proprietary medicines. For lavish supplies of "samples" of "strictly ethical preparations" (often with the name of the firm and alleged remedy blown into the bottles) they prescribe these expensive (to the patient) goods—thoughtlessly, carelessly. One of these firms kindly furnished me from its books a tabulated statement (see table in my paper in *American Medicine,* Vol. IV, No. 3, pp. 105-107) of its distribution of "free samples" to physicians by its travelers. Besides samples to medical conventions it distributed 53,597 bottles to physicians in 34 states which sold at wholesale at 60 cents each. The firm was and is prosperous. Some one paid for these "samples." It was not the firm. The sick people did it—many of whom were doubtless poor. And this was only one firm's experience in one year! Why should the profession tolerate the "free sample" and surgical instrument and appliances rebate and hesitate at a proper division of the fee? Is not the patient the commodity in every instance?

Finally, a more enlightened, judicial sentiment should permeate and control in the profession than that urged in the matter of the division of fees. Phariseeism ought to be relegated to the rear, while tolerance, instruction, and persuasion should in my judgment be brought forward as remedies for undesirable existing professional conditions.

———

Sex does not play so important a role in syphilis now, says Breakstone, as it did years ago; but as a rule, women are much less infected with syphilis than men, this being due probably to the greater morality existing among women.

DIGITALIS OR DIGITALIN?

BY

WILLIAM F. WAUGH, A. M., M. D.,
Professor of Therapeutics, Bennett Medical
College, Medical Department Loyola
University, Chicago, Ill.

The question as to the best preparation of the foxglove is of such vast import that the constant recurrence of discussion is intelligible. In France the crystallized digitalin of Nativelle has been employed for more than forty years, with such satisfaction that the profession there has declined to make use of any of the constantly appearing newer forms of the drug. This in itself is good evidence of the value of this one. It may be noted that the French applications of digitalis are based on this, which consists of true digitalin, almost or altogether chemically pure. Digitalin, true, is a powerful heart tonic and a no less effective vasoconstrictor. Hence the French application of it is as a remedy in cardiac failure and the dropsies thereon dependent. Fraenkel called attention to the extreme slowness of digitalin in getting into action, as thirty hours elapse before the effects of a dose begin to be manifest. Hence we find the French administering this remedy in doses widely separated, and in cases where urgency is not a feature of the indication.

Digitoxin resembles digitalin, but is more powerful as a heart tonic and even more so as a vasoconstrictor; its effects according to Fraenkel only becoming evident in sixty hours after administration. It is therefore to be exhibited with caution.

Digitalein forms the principal constituent of the Germanic digitalin. It is a good heart tonic, but possesses little of the vasoconstrictor influence. Its activity commences well within half an hour of administration and is over at the end of four hours.

Digitonin, the saponin-like fourth principle of this plant, is a powerful cardiac depressor and relaxant of vascular tension, opposing the other three glucosides in both respects. Its activity begins to be seen within two to five minutes after administration, and is over within an hour. It is present in varying proportions in the German digitalin. We find that this is largely employed in febrile maladies in conjunction with aconitine, strychnine and veratrine. Digitoxin and digitalin being soluble in alcohol and not in water, are present in the tincture of digitalis; while digitalein and digitonin being only soluble in water, are present in the infusion, and they alone.

We now hold the key to the digitalis preparations and the varying preferences for them manifested by different users. The French would not find the Germanic digitalin satisfactory for it is a different body from that they use, and would not fulfil the same uses. Those who employ digitalin Germanic in fevers would not get the effect they are accustomed to from the French digitalin. We see why Niemeyer preferred the tincture as a heart tonic, and the infusion in certain cases where quicker action was desirable, and where too great vascular tension interfered with renal action, by constricting the renal arteries and cutting off the supply of blood from the kidneys.

When a dose of digitalis in powder is given, within five minutes we get the heart depression and vascular relaxation of digitonin. If patients fall dead within a brief time after taking this drug, this is the cause. Within half an hour this action begins to subside, and is replaced by the cardiac toning and slight vascular tensing of digitalein, which prevails up to four hours. In thirty hours the pulse begins to stiffen and the heart to manifest force from the beginning of digitalin action; and in thirty more the tremendous power of digitoxin increases both activities. If dropsy is due to degeneration of the relaxed capillary system into a swamp, relief is experienced as the blood channels are thus canalized—provided the dose is so accurately fixed as to exactly meet the need. If excessive, we have an obstacle placed before the heart in an undue constriction of the terminals of the arterial system—the outlets.

But digitalis is usually given in doses repeated every four hours, so that when the effects of the digitoxin in the first dose begin to be manifest, the patient is taking his sixteenth dose; and we have following a cumulation of the slower glucosidal activities, that may result in the spectacle of a heart lashed to fury, vainly exhausting itself in the effort to drive the blood through arterioles impermeably constricted by the death clutch of digitoxin. *Delirium cordis* or exhaustion is the consequence.

That this does not occur more frequently is due to two causes, the minute doses often used—too small for therapeutic effect, let alone toxic action—and the miserable quality of the drug often supplied by the markets. But that it does occur sometimes is shown by the trenchant expression of the great French clinician, Peter, at the Paris Academy of Medicine, when he said emphatically: "In the treatment of heart diseases, the fear of digitalis is the beginning of wisdom."

These be our reasons for preferring in fevers and heart diseases the water-soluble digitalein, quick to act, and well away out of the system within the time usually elapsing between doses—four hours; safe and effective for what we want—a heart tonic. But in cases of dropsy with relaxed vascular tension we prefer the slow but enduring true French digitalin, or even the still more powerful digitoxin, giving one full dose once a week. If hypertension develop we relax it with digitonin for quick action and veratrine for more permanent effect. These will then act as diuretics, releasing a freer supply of blood to the kidneys. I am unable to surmise any pathologic condition that demands the exhibition of digitalis as a whole.

CORRESPONDENCE.

MEMBERSHIP IN THE AMERICAN MEDICAL ASSOCIATION.

ROSWELL, NEW MEXICO.

To the Editor
AMERICAN MEDICINE:

The editorial in the July 1911 issue of AMERICAN MEDICINE on membership in the American Medical Association, calls attention to conditions that should interest every one who has at heart the welfare of the organization. I think I can offer an explanation of what is happening in the ranks and is likely to continue for some time to come, inasmuch as certain personal experiences have emphasized the dangers.

The organization of the American Medical Association is at fault and until that is changed, I do not believe it can look for anything like the success which we all hope for it and which is possible for it to reach. I will give a concrete example which will explain what I mean. I am a physician who was in good standing in the Chicago Medical Society and in the American Medical Association, in both of which I took great pride and great interest. I left Chicago and moved to the southwest and located in this place, a town of about six thousand inhabitants. There are here, at all times, twenty-five to thirty-five practicing physicians of various schools. The county society consists of from ten to fifteen members, at the present time; to be exact, I believe there are fourteen members. I immediately joined, and all went well until I began to get some of the business; immediately there was trouble. On four separate occasions I had charges of unprofessional conduct filed against me before the local medical society; these charges were childish to a degree that is hardly believable. I will not enter into the nature of them here, as that does not concern the subject of this letter.

Finally, I was called to a surgical case by a homeopath, who did no surgery, and *for this I was expelled from the society.* This expulsion was welcomed by me, however, because it relieved me from being subjected to charges of unprofessional conduct every time I honestly disagreed in diagnosis when called to consultations that would otherwise have been farcical. I am still, however, a member in good standing, of the Chicago Medical Society.

Now I am coming to the point. I called on a member of the Chaves County Medical Society to administer an anesthetic for me. He did so, and was also expelled as being guilty of "unprofessional conduct." An old-time Chicago professional friend, who was a member of the Chicago Medical Society and the A. M. A., located here, and he was refused admission to the local society because he assisted me in my work!

The local situation, then, is this, fourteen of the physicians are members of the county society, and of these there are seven who are not members of the A. M. A. Five of the present members of the county society by combining (two-thirds vote necessary to elect) can absolutely prevent the election of any one to membership, so that should this town increase in size to twenty-five thousand inhabitants, and should seventy-five more members of the A. M. A. move into this county, they could all be forced to lose their membership in that body because five of the present members objected to them.

I find on referring to the American Medical Directory that seven of the fourteen members of the Chaves County Medical Society are not members of the A. M. A. By further examination of this list I find that I was expelled from the American

Medical Association *by the votes of five men who were not members* of that body and that without their votes I could not have been expelled. Dr. Phillips was expelled on the same basis, and I am informed that Dr. Crutcher has been notified by the secretary of the A. M. A. that he must forfeit his membership in that body unless he joins the Chaves County Society!

Who ever heard of such an anomaly?. A scientific society dependent for the election of its members on the acts of people who have no connection with and no interest whatsoever in that society, and precious little, if any, in science in any form! Is it not a ridiculous situation that five men who are not members, who have no interest in the A. M. A., and are antagonistic to its principles can absolutely control membership in that body in this entire county?

You will probably find, if you investigate, that this condition of affairs prevails in many other parts of the United States. You may say that a man could appeal to the State and National Societies, but such an appeal is worse than a farce. I found it absolutely impossible to get a hearing from the officers of the Territorial Society, and when the secretary spent two days in this town, he made several engagements to meet me but fulfilled none of them, avoided me and the question in every way.

A complaint filed with the officers of the A. M. A. was answered by referring me to the Territorial Medical Society, which completed the vicious circle and made any action or redress impossible.

Respectfully yours,
D. H. GALLOWAY, Ph. G., M. D.

[We print the above communication with considerable satisfaction, since it substantiates the views we have so long held and have so frequently expressed to the effect that the present system of organization is a serious handicap to the growth and progress of the great American Medical Association. Under the present plan the non-member has as much power as the active member. How that power can be used to the detriment and serious injury of the Association is well shown in Dr. Galloway's communication. We do not happen to have the pleasure of knowing Dr. Galloway personally, nor are we prepared to express any opinion *pro* or *con* concerning the purely local or personal phases of the events he recites, but we do know Dr. Crutcher, and if Dr. Galloway can claim him as a friend, that is all the recommendation we need as to the honor, integrity and professional standing of our correspondent.

It is certainly a preposterous condition that election to membership in an organization—affiliation with which means so much to the ambitious physician—should ever depend on the votes of non-members, or by the same token that deprivation of such affiliation should ever be possible by the same influences. Dr. Galloway's experience furnishes much that requires careful thought. The present anomalous situation must soon be changed—and we speak with all respect and regard for an institution that deserves the earnest co-operation and support of every medical man in the country—or the splendid work of the Association will suffer irreparable injury. We can readily understand the colossal efforts that have been needed to bring the organization to where it now is, and it seems a shame that the splendid possibilities of the Association along constructive lines should be jeopardized by the retention of certain conditions that have no advantages—in fact nothing but drawbacks. Membership in the Association should carry real distinction, but it cannot as long as members have no more voice in the affairs of the Association than non-members.—EDITOR.]

ETIOLOGY AND DIAGNOSIS.

Etiology of Appendicitis.[1]—Robertson says a close and careful investigation of the subject has led him to a positive conclusion as to the exact etiology of the disease. He then describes in detail the minute anatomy of the appendix and gives as the reason for the infrequency of the disease in women as compared with men, which is in a proportion of two women to three men, being due to the occasional small branches of the ovarian artery which traverses the appendiculo-ovarian ligament. He sums up his paper with the following conclusions. From the foregoing study the following conclusions may be definitely drawn:

1. The muscles of the colon and appendix are an entity.

2. Muscular contraction in the colon and cecum, whether of the circular fibers or of the longitudinal bands, must be associated with a simultaneous contraction of the muscular walls of the appendix.

3. This contraction is induced by nerve stimulation, the stimulant being presented by the various tabulated predisposing factors as enunciated by many observers, all of which can be accounted for in this one general cause.

4. While the normal muscular contraction and relaxation of the appendix act only to support circulation, when spasmodic in nature it overdoes the matter and produces vascular disturbances.

5. Owing to the peculiar anatomic structure of the appendix, all that tissue within the circular muscle fibers, being spongy in nature, becomes during the abnormal contraction a veritable dam in which the blood is retained until released by the subsidence of the spasm.

6. According to the intensity of the spasm will depend the degree of mucous membrane varicosity and edema, and thus will be determined the varying degrees of inflammatory action.

7. If the spasm be of the mildest degree only, then appendicular colic will result; if of the maximum intensity, gangrene will follow.

8. It may, therefore, be concluded that atrophy, degeneration, hyperemia, congestion, hyperplasia of connective tissue and thrombus formation occur *before*, and not *after*, bacterial invasion of the walls of the appendix.

The Diagnosis of Chronic Interstitial Nephritis.[1]—The beginning of chronic interstitial nephritis is insidious, says Stewart. The early symptoms, while suggestive to the diagnostician, rarely lead the patient to suspicion the onset of a serious malady. If he consults his physician he does so apologizingly or simply seeks a remedy for a mere symptom of the disease. He may complain of lassitude, headache, insomnia, shortness of breath on exertion or the inconvenience of having to get up at night to void his urine. The urine, very early in the disease, will be found to present conditions which point to a diagnosis. When freshly passed it is acid in reaction, light in color, copious and of low specific gravity. Traces of albumin are found, but early in the disease may not be constant. The sediment is scanty and in it are found a few hyaline or granular casts.

Increased arterial tension is a constant symptom in chronic interstitial nephritis. The pulse is hard and not easily compressed. If the disease has existed long, the vessels will be found exceedingly fibrous and beyond the point of compression may be readily felt beneath the examining finger. A normal vessel examined in this manner can not be differentiated from its surrounding tissue. Hypertrophy of the heart occurs, as already shown, the direct result of toxic material in the blood stream, and also follows an effort to overcome the resistance offered in the contracted arteries. The apex is displaced downward and to the left and the impulse is notably increased. Finally, the hypertrophy fails, the heart dilates, there is lessened secretion of urine and edema develops. As a result of the cardiac lesion there may be present dyspnea, palpitation of the heart and dizziness. The increased arterial pressure may cause a sudden, fatal termination of the disease in apoplexy. Dickerson is quoted as saying that of the fatal cases of apoplexy one-half are preceded by interstitial nephritis.

---

[1]J. W. Robertson, M. D., *Surg. Gyn. and Obst.*, Oct., 1911.

[1]W. E. Stewart, M. D., *Western Med. Review*, Feb., 1912.

Hemorrhages in other locations may follow the same diseased condition of the blood vessels, as in the retina and from the nose. I had a patient in my own practice a few years ago who suffered from excessive hemorrhage of the stomach from this cause, vomiting no less than two quarts of blood at one time. Any hemorrhage in the middle aged should give rise to suspicion of the existence of chronic nephritis. In consequence of hemorrhage into the retina sudden blindness, as well as dimness of vision, due to retinitis albuminaria is a symptom which may present itself.

In every case of renal insufficiency there is more or less a condition of uremia. Tyson says nearly all the patients he has seen die in the extreme stage of atrophied kidneys, sank under the symptoms of uremia. It may be said that often the first suspicion of the existence of chronic nephritis is in the development of symptoms of uremia.

The onset is so gradual, the early symptoms give rise to so little inconvenience, that by the time the patient presents himself for examination the diagnosis of interstitial nephritis is usually easy. In a patient with increased arterial tension, the apex of the heart dislocated to the left, the second aortic sound ringing and accentuated, the urine increased or at least not decreased in quantity, low specific gravity, traces of albumin, delicate hyaline or granular casts, the diagnosis of chronic interstitial nephritis is certain.

Osler says: "Of all the indications, that offered by the pulse is the most important." If there is any doubt regarding the character of the pulse the blood pressure may be very easily and accurately ascertained by means of the sphygmomanometer. Janeway places much dependence in the use of this instrument. He says: "Given a systolic pressure of over 200 millimeters the diagnosis of contracted kidney must be disproved by repeated examinations before it is abandoned." Tyson, on the other hand, gives greater diagnostic value to the condition of the urine. If, however, the disease really exists, careful examination will reveal the presence of both circulatory and urinary symptoms.

A New Finger Sign.[1]—A new diagnostic sign of organic hemiplegia is described by Gordon, who remarks that among the new discoveries of this kind very few have been pointed out in the upper members. Although it is usually easy to recognize isolated brachial monoplegias of cerebral origin, there are sometimes cases met with that are somewhat puzzling. The sign here described is as follows: "The forearm of the patient's affected limb is elevated and the elbow is placed on a table. The support of the elbow is, however, not essential. The patient's wrist is then lightly embraced by the examiner's hand, with the thumb against

[1] Alfred Gordon, M. D., Phila. Journ. A. M. A., Nov. 11, 1911.

the pisiform bone and the other fingers on the dorsal surface of the wrist. Or one of the examiner's hands may be placed against the back of the patient's wrist and the thumb of the other against the pisiform bone. Pressure is then produced with the thumb against the pisiform body, and especially on its radial side. Care must be taken not to produce pressure on the dorsal surface of the wrist where the extensor muscles are located. The fingers are then seen to extend and sometimes also to spread in a fan-like form. . . . In some cases the extension is observed only in the last two fingers; in others all five fingers extend, and in still others the thumb and the next two fingers. The extension is sometimes more prompt and more distinct when the ring finger is slightly raised before the test and kept raised during the test. This finger must be supported very gently and in a semiextended position." In old hemiplegias, in which the contraction of the fingers is pronounced, this phenomenon is not always prominent. Whether it is constant in hemiplegia the author is not able to state, but if it can be confirmed on a large number of cases its importance, he says, is manifest.

TREATMENT.

The Treatment of Colds with Vaccines.—Hitchens says that the determining factor in simple catarrhs is a bacterial infection of the mucous membrane and its secretion. It is primarily a surface-infection, and the bacteria with their poisons are present in such quantities that they are able to overcome the resistance of the tissues. The methods used to dry up the secretions are efficacious only in the early stages of the cold, and they act really by removing the culture-medium. Frequently such methods merely postpone the attack. Revulsive measures such as purging and sweating reestablish the nervous equilibrium, relieve the local stasis, and restore a more vigorous and healthy circulation locally, thus using the antibacterial power of the blood to the best advantage of the local tissues. Local antisepsis is obviously of little value either theoretically or practically. Later, when the cold has reached the subacute stage, the proper treatment is to apply measures to improve the quality of the blood by building up the general health. Medicinal tonics and personal hygiene are commonly used to accomplish this. What actually happens is that the normal resisting power of the blood is restored, and as it nourishes the overworked cells it is able to offer them greater assistance in neutralizing the toxic substances attacking them; when this happens the cold rapidly disappears. If it is possible for the patient to take a vacation the locality selected should be one free from street dust and other sources of reinfection.

With these facts before us the rationale for the use of bacterial vaccines in catarrhs of the respiratory passages is plain. The proper bacteria are injected in suitable dosage beneath the healthy skin. The usual reaction takes place, resulting in the production of specific antibodies which find their way into the blood and tissue juices. There is no difficulty in bringing the blood of better quality to the infected surface (except possibly in the hypoplastic stage of chronic catarrh) on account of the characteristic blennorrhea which constantly demands more fluid. The ideal condition is present. The focus of infection is being constantly flooded with fresh lymph, and much of that used up does not get back into the body, but is thrown off.

The kind of bacteria to be used as the vaccine is important. A few years ago many attempts were made to determine the particular organism responsible for colds. We now believe that there are many germs pathogenic to the mucous membrane of the respiratory passages, and that any one of them, or a combination of any or all, may be responsible. That different types of colds are caused by different bacterial species there can scarcely be any doubt. Further study may identify the exact relationship. It has been said that certain individuals are more susceptible to one type than another. However this may be, the thought suggested itself to me long ago that the attempt to immunize persons against common colds by the use of special single vaccines was inadequate. Each individual is probably at periods susceptible to the whole list, and if we wish satisfactorily to immunize him against catarrhs we should immunize him to all the more common germs known to be pathogenic to the mucous membranes. And until such a plan is adopted immunization against colds will be inadequate and unsatisfactory.

With this conception of the pathogenesis of and recovery from catarrh in mind, it was decided to make a mixed vaccine and use it for the treatment of an acute catarrh in a person who had had chronic catarrh for twenty years. The results were so encouraging that similar treatment has been started in several other persons suffering with acute and chronic catarrhs, and I am offering this preliminary communication as a suggestion for the routine specific treatment of acute and chronic catarrh.

The vaccine used contained in each cubic centimeter the following bacteria, which were chosen as representing those species most frequently found in the infected respiratory mucous membranes:

Staphylococcus aureus ......150 million.
Staphylococcus albus ....150 million.
Streptococcus .... 50 million.
Pneumococcus .... 50 million.
Members of the Micrococcus
    catarrhalis group .... 50 million.
Members of the bacillus of
    Friedländer group .... 50 million.

In robust persons in the chronic stage of the disease the initial dose of this vaccine has been from 0.25 to 0.5 c.c., administered subcutaneously, generally about the insertion of the deltoid muscle. The subsequent doses have been given at five-day intervals, and the amount has not been increased above 0.5 c.c. A few persons receiving the initial dose during the acute stage were given 0.25 c.c., and this dose was repeated at shorter intervals.

It has been noted that on the third or fourth day after the injection of the vaccine the absence of the usual secretion makes the nose feel very dry. In such conditions an oil spray has been agreeable.

Following the injections there are the usual redness and slight swelling at the point of injection. A few patients have had slight symptoms of a negative reaction on the day following the injection, but this has in no case been severe.

In conclusion, it is my belief that the treatment of catarrh of the respiratory passages by a mixed bacterial vaccine is simple, direct, and specific. To get the best results the vaccine should contain those organisms most commonly pathogenic to the respiratory mucous membranes. The treatment must necessarily include the removal or other surgical treatment of obstructions and growths of various kinds between attacks. It is certain that a number of patients will be found who will not be benefited beyond a certain point by the mixed vaccine. In such cases the mucus should be examined bacteriologically, and the mixed vaccine supplemented by the other pathogenic organisms found.

Gingivitis in Diseases of Metabolism.[1]—Crottan, in his thoughtful paper on the gingival manifestations of certain disorders of metabolism, refers particularly to the gingivitis that accompanies Bright's disease, diabetes, non-diabetic acidosis, and the "uric acid diathesis." In diabetic cases the following formulae are found useful:

(1) For bleeding and painful gums—Tr. opii, 20 parts; chlorate of potash and bicarbonate of soda, of each 10 parts; decoction of marsh mallow, 1,000 parts. Make a mouth-wash,. to be used from time to time.

(2) For excessive fetor—Beta-naphthol, one part; sodi. biborate, 100 parts; Aq. Menth. Pip, 1,000 parts, and distilled water to 5,000 parts. Make a mouth-wash for frequent use.

The Treatment for Pellagra.[2]—If the assumption as to etiology here presented is correct, recurrence is prevented by excluding the oil from the diet or sending the patient to a cold climate. It is unfortunate that some of our renowned authorities are at present very active in asserting in the daily press that there is no cure for pellagra, and that when relieved it

[1]A. F. Crottan, M. D., Dental Cosmos, Dec., 1911.

[2]G. C. Mizell, M. D., Amer. Journ. Clin. Med., Nov., 1911.

will return. One of the most discouraging duties a physician has to face is a hopeless case. Those who have given up hope should not discourage others.

Mild cases will recover without treatment when linolin is excluded from the diet and the patient is kept out of the sun. Because of this fact, many remedies have been credited with being effective. As indicated above, sulphur is practically if not positively a specific. Administered in absorbable form to saturation, together with proper attention to the impaired digestion, it will be effective in every case that has not passed the bounds of medical aid. Calcium sulphide is the most effective form in which sulphur can be gotten into the blood. It is best administered in 1/6-grain granules of reliable make, 3 every three hours or only three times a day, according to the severity of the attack.

The Treatment of Flatulence.[1]—Burnet says that in most cases the diet will have to be carefully chosen and somewhat restricted. A rather dry diet will be found to suit best in nearly all cases—little liquid being allowed with meals. This excludes all soups and broths at the beginning of a meal and allows of only a small quantity of fluid toward the close of the meal. What the special drink should be has to be decided in each particular case. Some will do best with plain water, others may require a little stimulant—alcohol in some form. We have to consider carefully in these cases whether alcohol is necessary, and if so what form is best. If given it should be prescribed with caution, more especially in the case of women suffering from dyspepsia, for oftentimes the temptation to seek temporary relief by its means from discomfort and flatulent distention, and the lassitude accompanying these conditions, is very great. From such beginnings a dependence upon alcoholic stimulants sometimes becomes established. If alcohol has to be given the amount should be clearly defined and given with or just after meals. Effervescing waters are often forbidden, but in the writer's opinion, if taken in strictly limited amount, they are helpful rather than otherwise, owing to the stimulus given by the gas they contain. The light white wines and clarets are of doubtful value, but sometimes a glass of dry sherry seems to aid digestion. Champagne is rarely required, but in some cases where there is much prostration it is useful for a time. Ales and stout are not as a rule well borne. No alcohol in any form should be given on an empty stomach.

Tea must be limited in quantity and must be freshly made. The stewed decoction called tea, so dear to the heart of the hospital out-patient, is a fruitful source of these digestive troubles and of the "spasms" so graphically described by the frequenters of hospital out-patient rooms.

[1]C. Burnet, F. R. C. P., *The Practitioner*, London, Eng., Oct., 1911.

Distention and disturbances of digestion are not, however, by any means confined to the class of persons who come under treatment at hospitals, and as a source of flatulence the excessive use of tea amongst well-to-do people should be always borne in mind.

Animal food is, as a rule, best digested by these patients; it must be carefully selected and well, though plainly, cooked—under rather than overdone; tender beef and mutton, chicken and other birds, game, and fresh white fish. Pork, veal, goose, duck, etc., should be forbidden. It will be often found best at first to limit the meat meals—luncheon and dinner—to practically one course, light tender meat and a little vegetable, with a biscuit and butter to follow. Much green vegetable will usually not be well borne, and what is given should be rubbed through a sieve—cooked as spinach is served. Often it is best to forbid potato for a time, and to substitute toast or second day's bread. Farinaceous foods have to be given carefully and the effect watched, but where digestion by the stomach is chiefly at fault starchy foods, as they are dealt with chiefly in the intestines, may be given in greater amount. The contrary holds good where digestion goes on best in the stomach; then meats are most satisfactorily digested. Ripe fruits have to be taken in great moderation, and raw vegetables, salads, etc., are not usually allowable in the earlier stages.

Whether meat preponderates in the dietary or farinaceous foods, the absolute necessity for slow eating and complete mastication of all solids should be strongly and repeatedly impressed upon the patient. It is always well to ascertain the condition of the teeth, and not infrequently some repairs have to be carried out by the dentist before complete and comfortable mastication can be attained by the patient.

Nux vomica is one of the most useful remedies in these cases and it may be given in tincture, or in pill with a quarter of a grain of capsicum and a couple of grains of compound rhubarb pill. Bismuth is of use in many instances, with an alkali such as bicarbonate of sodium, and columba or other bitter infusion. Salicin is not used so much as we believe it might be, and given in five or ten-grain doses in water before meals is often very helpful. Pepsin seems distinctly indicated, but it is often disappointing, and at the best it must be looked upon more as a palliative than anything else. Pancreatin, too, does not give the relief in all cases that we should expect from it. Salicylate of sodium with liquor pepticus, nux vomica, and spirits of chloroform seems useful in a certain number of cases. Extract of malt given with or just after meals helps in those cases in which the digestion of starchy foods is obviously difficult. A few drops of dilute hydrochloric acid in water shortly after meals is often decidedly beneficial. In some cases iron and quinine seem to be indicated, and in many cases we prescribe them only to find how difficult it is to get them to agree, especially in the earlier stages. When improvement has set in they may be tried with more confidence.

A pill which is often well borne consists of a grain of reduced iron, with extract of nux vomica, quinine, and pil. rhei comp. It acts as a tonic and also as a mild aperient. It may be varied by a grain of pepsin and a twentieth of a grain of arsenous acid in place of the quinine, and it is useful in anemic subjects. Calomel in very small fractional doses, given twice daily for a few days at a time, has often a very good effect, and where there is a sluggish action of the liver a grain or two of blue pill with the pill colocynth and hyoscyamus, or the compound rhubarb pill, should be given occasionally and followed, if necessary, by a mild saline in the morning, but anything like strong purgation should be avoided.

Where the distention is chiefly in the bowels salicylate of bismuth, beta-naphthol, and salol, in cachet, give at least temporary relief.

Lavage is not usually needed in the cases we are considering, but where there is much accumulation of mucus it is very helpful by clearing the stomach and thus giving a fair start to other treatment.

In acute attacks of flatulence hot water, with aromatic spirits of ammonia and spirits of chloroform with perhaps a teaspoonful of brandy, often relieves the tension and spasm. Sometimes a drop or two of oil of cajuput in mucilage has a very good effect.

In cases in which it is possible for the patient to follow such advice we may recommend riding on horseback or traveling, sea-bathing for young subjects, or a voyage, as the best means for completing the cure and preventing a recurrence of the symptoms.

The Biological Treatment of Peritonitis.[1]—

Success in the treatment of peritonitis often depends on how far we understand the natural processes by which the body defends itself against peritoneal infection, and in how far we aid and support these processes and not in any direct assault on the invading bacteria. In a peritoneal infection there is first of all an absorption of bacteria and their toxins which stimulates the formation of antibacterial and antitoxic bodies. There is then an effusion of serum and cells into the peritoneal cavity to combat the local infection. The treatment now almost universally adopted in cases of peritonitis is to establish drainage of the peritoneal cavity, to supply large quantities of saline solution to the body through some channel, and possibly to flush out the peritoneum with saline solution. The great hindrance to efficient drainage is the deposit of fibrin between the intestinal coils gluing them together. The ideal conditions in a case of generalized peritonitis would be a copious secretion of serum by the peritoneum, no adhesions and free drainage.

The writer advocates a method of treatment which he believes goes far towards establishing these ideal conditions. It consists in the introduction into the peritoneal cavity of a moderately concentrated solution of glucose in saline solution. Glucose tends to inhibit the growth of most bacteria, to inhibit their formation of proteolytic ferments and above all to interfere with the deposit of fibrin. The hypertonic solution of sugar excites a very free osmosis of serum into the peritoneal cavity, and makes the patient wash out his own peritoneum. By supplying saline subcutaneously in large quantities a very vigorous outpouring of serum may be kept up and very free drainage will be obtained.

———

Treatment of Tetanus.[1]—Baccelli says that antitetanic serum has proven a great disappointment in the treatment of tetanus, no matter which way it is introduced into the system. Carbolic acid, given subcutaneously in sufficient dosage, is still the best remedy at our disposal. A 2 to 3 per cent. watery solution is employed. At first about 0.3 to 0.5 Gm. of the acid are injected daily to test the tolerance of the patient. If the urine remains free as much as 1 to 1.5 Gm. may be given during the 24 hours. Larger doses should only be used cautiously in very severe cases. According to the author's statistics, the mortality in severe cases could be reduced from 100 per cent. to 2.12 per cent., in very severe cases from 100 per cent. to 18.5 per cent. In a large percentage of the worst cases less than one gram daily was injected, so that the statistics here are no proper criterion for the action of the drug. If desired, the acid may also be injected dissolved in sterile oil.

———

The Treatment of Influenza.[2]—With regard to treatment proper, says Allan, there are some definite rules which can be unhesitatingly laid down. Rest in bed is essential. In the ordinary acute case there will not be much difficulty in having this carried out, for the patient is so sore and helpless that he is glad to remain in bed. In the mild cases, however, it may be difficult to persuade a patient to keep in bed, and yet it ought to be insisted on, because a judicious rest in bed for two or three days will often prevent the occurrence of secondary effects. Patients should be kept warm and quiet, but it should be pointed out that warmth is not to be obtained at the expense of proper ventilation. The patient should be well protected from cold, but the room should be efficiently ventilated, and open windows day and night are favored by some. There is no specific drug for influenza, but many drugs are useful. Among such may be mentioned quinine, phenacetin, antipyrine, sodium salicylate, acetylsalicylic acid, salipyrine, etc. The late Sir William Broadbent's usual prescription was one drachm of ammoniated quinine, and two

———

[1] D. Kuhn, M. D., *Munch. Med. Woch.*, No. 38, 1911.

[1] L. Baccelli, M. D., *Berl. klin. Woch.*

[2] John Allan, M. D. (Edin.) *The Prescriber*, Dec., 1911.

drachms of liquor ammoniæ acetatis every hour for three hours and then every four hours. Personally I favor the salicylate group, and I have great faith in acetyl-salicylic acid. The following prescription, which combines some of the above groups of drugs has been recommended:—Quin. sulph. gr. ii.; caffein. citrat. gr. i.; salol, acetanilid., aa. gr. iiss.—ft. "cachet"; mitte tales xii, Sig.—"One cachet every three hours." Campbell Stark prescribes sodium salicylate, and he believes that in the common type of influenza the following cuts short the disease in two days:—Sod. salicylat. gr. x.; potas. bicarb. gr. x.; tinct. nuc. vom. m. x.; aq. chloroform, ad ʒi. Treatment by purgation formerly attained a great reputation, but it is now seldom employed. Calomel and castor oil were the usual purgatives prescribed. Except in the gastrointestinal form it is rather difficult to imagine how laxatives and intestinal disinfectants, especially calomel, could possibly exert an abortive action in the disease. Calomel certainly ought to be administered with caution. It still, however, finds favor in some quarters. Of intestinal antiseptics or allied drugs which have from time to time been praised may be mentioned carbolic acid, creolin, creosote, oil of cinnamon, salol, sulphocarbolates, calcium sulphide, etc. Cory advises the following:—Quin. disulph. gr. ¼; acid. hydrobrom. dil. m. viiss.; acid. carbol., glycerin, aa gr. ¼ to ⅓; tinct. hydrastis m. viiss.; aq. ad. ʒi. For adults give two tablespoonfuls every three or four hours, one hour after food. Lung cases sometimes do better with: ammon. carb. gr. ii.; glyc. ac. carbol. m. ii.; spt. aeth. nit.; tinct. cinchon., aa m. viiss.; aq. ad. ʒi, every three or four hours. Every case, if taken in time, recovers.

Certain side symptoms may call for special treatment. Heart weakness may be prominent, but this generally occurs if the patient has not rested in bed or has got up prematurely. In the early acute stages this symptom is best treated with strychnine and diffusible stimulants such as ammonia and alcohol. Any undue or violent exertion must be prohibited. Cardiac weakness during convalescence or later is again treated with strychnine, but arsenic, iron, and hypophosphites are also of service.

Neuralgic pains are best treated with antipyrine. Phenacetin also acts well, but acetanilide is less reliable. Salipyrine, a combination of salicylic acid and antipyrine, is also good. Headaches may be treated on similar lines.

For sore throat the local application of tannic acid, or potassium chlorate in the form of a gargle, may be tried, while a few doses of acetyl-salicylic acid or sodium salicylate may help to give relief.

Pyrexia is seldom so alarming that energetic treatment is called for. The cautious use of antipyretic drugs is indicated, the minimum dose required to produce the necessary effect being used. Cold water treatment, so useful in many infectious diseases, is contraindicated in influenza, and as a rule produces exaggeration of the various symptoms.

Cough is often troublesome, and a sedative cough mixture is the best remedy. Heroin hydrochloride is a suitable drug in doses of 1/32 to 1/16 grain every three or four hours. The elixir acetomorphin. co. (B. P. C.) is an elegant preparation. One to two teaspoonfuls occasionally of the following linctus often has a marked sedative effect on this symptom:—Tinct. camph. co., oxymel scillæ, syr. tolu., of each equal parts.

Insomnia rarely requires active treatment. The attack of the disease as a rule only lasts for two or three days, and so it is inadvisable to prescribe active hypnotics. Thirty grains of acetyl-salicylic acid at bedtime will often act as an excellent hypnotic.

The diet in influenza should be nourishing and easily digested. At first milk and egg-albumin water only are given, but this is soon increased by adding egg-flip, chicken broth, beef-tea, etc. Later eggs and chicken, sweetbreads, fish, and finally roast joints may be allowed. Alcoholic beverages may prove useful in the latter stages. Alcohol in the acute stage is prone to increase headache, etc., and unless called for by reason of some special symptom it ought to be withheld.

Convalescence is often prolonged, and post-influenzal debility is often difficult to treat, and for many months the patient may experience attacks of extreme weakness. Rest, change of air and scene, healthy surroundings, and general hygienic living are essential. Time is an important factor, and complete recovery cannot be hastened. Good nourishing diet should be enjoined, and tonics such as glycerophosphates or hypophosphites, with strychnine, are useful. The period of convalescence is an important time for the patient, and every effort should be made to enable him so to build up his system as to withstand effectually another attack.

THERAPEUTIC NOTES.

The Value of Ergot.[1]—Hoyt asks how many of us in general practice think how old our ergot is, or from whence we obtain it, or what knowledge do we have that the product we are using is active, at all. For use by the mouth he thinks the most practical preparation is still the old fluid extract. It is best to obtain it in small amounts direct from some reliable manufacturer and physiologically treated. The idea that ergot is limited in its action in producing tonic contractions of the pregnant uterus is pretty generally believed, but a glance at the later literature on this subject would soon widen this view. Ergot is a powerful vasomotor stimulant acting very much as does adrenalin, namely stimulating the sympathetic vasomotor nerve endings. While its action on the circulation closely resembles adrenalin, it differs in this, that while adrenalin is extremely fugacious and almost immediately destroyed in the body, ergot acts much longer, is probably active when given by the mouth and therefore rationally indicated in conditions of failing circulation. Practically ergot is becom-

[1] D. M. Hoyt, M. D., Med. Council, Nov., 1911.

ing more and more useful in conditions of low blood pressure due to central depression, as in circulatory failure from acute infectious fevers, in delirium tremens, surgical shock, etc. Ergot is a very old remedy in chronic types of diarrhea and deserves a renewed trial here. One of the most interesting phases of the physiological action of the active pressor substances in ergot, is the resemblance to adrenalin, in the difference between their action on the pregnant, and non-pregnant uterus. This has been largely shown by Dale, Dixon, and Cushny, and has a most important clinical bearing. Ergot is commonly used in uterine hemorrhage from many different causes, but in functional types of dysmenorrhea it is generally thought to be contraindicated; from the experimental evidence, however, it should have a fair trial in this direction, and he knows that ergot for some time back has been used empirically for this purpose. He emphasizes, first the importance of having a fresh and active preparation; second, the value of the drug as a powerful vasomotor stimulant; third, its possible value as a uterine sedative.

Treatment of Acne Vulgaris[1]—The face should be thoroughly bathed at least twice a day with hot water and an alkaline soap, followed by copious douches of cold (preferably rain) water. Sulphur internally is of no use. Sulphur externally is not of much value and is liable to cause dermatitis. The author has, however, met with more success with a new form of the drug, known as collodial sulphur. The important point in the treatment consists in utilizing the antiseptic and penetrating properties of alcoholic solutions of iodine. A one percent. solution of iodine in rectified spirit would appear to be the best, and the solution ought to be freshly made. Any seborrhea of the scalp should be suitably treated. [Colloid sulphur is prepared by precipitating sulphur from polysulphides with an acid in the presence of albumin. It is said to excel ordinary precipitated sulphur as an antiseptic.—AB-STRACTOR.]

Hiccough.—The remedies recommended and employed to suppress obstinate attacks of hiccough are multiple, says *The Universal Medical Record*, and any and all of them may fail to give relief in any particular attack. It is worth while, therefore, to put on record some more recent measures that have been adopted and found efficacious. The object aimed at in some of the methods of treatment is to obtain mechanical pressure on the diaphragm. With this view, Dr. Kanngiessen, of Bramfels, conceived the idea of distending the stomach with carbonic acid gas. The patient was an old man who developed an attack of hiccough which failed to yield to all known means of treatment. He administered five grammes of citric

acid and immediately afterwards an equal quantity of sodium bicarbonate. The hiccough ceased at once, and the patient had several hours' sleep. The following day the hiccough returned and the same remedy was applied, but without effect. Dr. Jödicke, of Stettin, has tried to obtain the same effect—mechanical pressure on the diaphragm—by another method. He makes the patient draw up both legs so as to be fully flexed at the knees and hips, and then holds them pressed hard against the abdominal wall, so as to push the viscera as far as possible up against the diaphragm. He has tried the remedy in several cases and has always obtained immediate relief. Dr. Rélby resorts to the measure originally suggested by Nothnagel of applying prolonged compression along the whole length of the vertebral column.

Wounds Without Scars.—Schantz claims that when a healing wound has a slight irritation it heals with the least width of scar. (*Med. Summary.*) He paints a healing wound on the third and on the fifth day, with tincture of iodine. Large wounds he paints once daily, and claims almost thread-like scars.

Treatment of Bromidrosis.[1]—In treating cases of bromidrosis the author takes the patient into hospital. Every pair of his socks is soaked for an hour in bichloride solution 1 to 2,000 and then carefully washed. His shoes are painted on the inside with a solution of one ounce of salicylic acid in four ounces of alcohol. The feet themselves are washed, dried, and painted with this solution, special attention being paid to the interdigital clefts. The entire skin surface becomes white from the deposition of the salicylic acid, after the alcohol has evaporated. Clean socks are then put on and the next day the painting is repeated. Permanent cure, he says, follows two treatments, cleanliness of feet and footgear alone being necessary to maintain it.

Sodium Citrate for Boils.[2]—The writer's treatment of furuncles in the first stage consists in applying a Bier's cup, and scraping off the central vesicle with a scalpel, and sucking out as much as possible of the exhausted serum and blood. A dressing of plain sterilized gauze which has been wrung out of a solution of normal saline and sodium citrate should be applied. Sodium citrate, 1 per cent. solution, precipitates the calcium salts in the lymph and ensures a comparatively free outlet of the lymph discharge. The sodium chloride by osmosis sets up a flow of lymph through the walls of the furuncle, the citrate maintaining the fluidity of the serum. Thus there is

[1]C. W. Hale, M. D., *Progressive Med.*, Sept., 1911.

[2]P. G. Skillen, M. D., *Jour. American Med. Assoc.*, Sept. 16, 1911.

[1]A. R. Gunn, M. D., *Practitioner*, Nov., 1911.

brought about a continuous flow of lymph of high antitrophic power from the congested blood-vessels through the wall of the furuncle and out through the wound.

SOCIETY PROCEEDINGS.

THE EASTERN · MEDICAL SOCIETY OF THE CITY OF NEW YORK.

REGULAR MEETING, FEBRUARY 9th, 1912.

The meeting was called to order at the usual hour, with the President, Dr. Kopetzky, in the chair.

The members present discussed the Antivivisection Bill now pending and voted to send a delegation to Albany to oppose its passage.

Following the executive session the scientific program was taken up as follows:

1. Presentation of Cases.
   A. Case of Streptococcus Tonsilitis followed by Acute Nephritis, Dr. Otto Glogau.
   B. Case of Hernia of Appendix into Subcaecal Fossa, Dr. A. E. Isaacs.
   C. Case of Hernia of Appendix into Subcaecal Fossa.
      Case of Inflamed Hemorrhoids due to Foreign Body, Dr. Leo. B. Meyer.
   D. Case of Pancreatic Calculus, Dr. G. A. Friedman.
2. Symposium on the Differential Diagnosis, in Diseases of the Heart, Stomach, Liver and Pancreas. Papers:
   1. Heart Disease and Epigastric Symptoms, Dr. Morris Manges.
   2. Significance of Epigastric Pain, Dr. Ludwig Kast.
   3. Functional Diseases and Neurosis of the Stomach, Dr. Jacob Kaufman.
   4. Gall Stones and Pancreatic Affections, Dr. John F. Erdman.
   5. Subphrenic Abscess, Dr. Robert T. Morris.

The discussion of these papers was participated in by many prominent surgeons and physicians and was of great interest.

After the meeting a collation was served, as usual, to the members and guests.

ITEMS OF INTEREST.

Comparative Birth-Rates of Large Cities.— The birth-rate in New York City in 1911 was over 27 per 1,000 inhabitants, a figure which is approximately equal to that of Naples, and which among the large cities of the Occident is surpassed only by Moscow, in Russia, which has a birth-rate of over 31 per 1,000, and by Breslau, in Germany, which has a birth-rate of nearly 29 per 1,000. It is hardly necessary to point out that the high rate in New York is due solely to its overwhelmingly foreign population. The birth-rate of London in 1911 was somewhat over 24 per 1,000, that of Amster-dam, Dresden, Milan and Rome somewhat less than 24 per 1,000, that of Vienna about 22, that of Berlin 21.6 and that of Paris only 17.6.

Medical College Graduates.—In 1880 there were graduated 3,241 physicians from all schools. In 1904 the number graduated was 5,747—perhaps the high water mark. Ever since, possibly because of more stringent supervision of standards, the number has decreased, till last fall it reached 4,273. In 1880 there were for every 100 graduates, 82 regulars, 12 homeopaths and 6 eclectics. In 1911 there were for every 100 graduates, 94 regulars, 3½ homeopaths and 2½ eclectics. The homeopathic colleges graduated 380 in 1880 and only 152 in 1910. The reduction in the eclectic graduates has been from 188 to 110. The physiomedical has ceased to exist. This shows the trend of medical education.

Highest and Lowest Death-Rates.—From the director of the census we learn that among a group of 18 cities in the less than 100,000 population class recording high rates of mortality in 1910, Charleston, S. C., shows the highest rate per 1,000 population, namely, 29.7; followed by Raleigh, N. C., with 27.9; Lackawanna, N. Y., 27.2; Savannah, Ga., 26.9; Petersburg, Va., 26.5; Montgomery, Ala., 26.4; Middletown, Conn., 25.6; Cranston, R. I., 25.4; Pontiac, Mich., 25.2; Augusta, Me., 25.1; Ogdensburg, N. Y., 24.5; Norristown, Pa., 24.4; Middletown, N. Y., 24.3; Biddeford, Me., 24; Bakersfield, Cal., 23.8; Morristown, N. J., 23.6; and Taunton, Mass., and Ann Arbor, Mich., 23.3 each. West Orange, N. J., returned the lowest death-rate, 8.5, of all cities mentioned in the bulletin. Next came Aberdeen, Wash., with 8.7; Norwood, Ohio, 9; Berkeley, Cal., 9.2; Bellingham, Wash., 9.4; Evanston, Ill., 10.1; Winthrop, Mass., 10.2; Medford, Mass., and Walla Walla, Wash., 10.4 each; East Orange, N. J., 10.7; West Hoboken, N. J., and Lancaster, Ohio, 10.8 each; and Torrington, Conn., 10.9.

A Means of Emptying the Bladder.—Dr. Edward Anderson (*Charlotte Med. Journal*) emphasizes the fact that the bladder, when partially paralyzed from parturition, or any other cause, can always be made to empty itself perfectly by throwing a large amount of very warm water into the bowel, thereby doing away with the necessity of using a catheter—a most important consideration, particularly when the patient lives at a distance from the doctor. After difficult and protracted labors I have been obliged to use the catheter every day for weeks at a time, which was annoying to the patient and inconvenient to myself. Since using the above recommended plan I have had no trouble in this direction, the bowel and the bladder emptying themselves at the same time.

American Medicine

H. EDWIN LEWIS, M. D., *Managing Editor.*
PUBLISHED MONTHLY BY THE AMERICAN-MEDICAL PUBLISHING COMPANY.
Copyrighted by the American Medical Publishing Co., 1912.

New Series, Vol. VII., No. 3. Complete Series. Vol. XVIII., No. 3.	MARCH, 1912.	$1.00 YEARLY in advance.

The medical side of disarmament should be carefully studied by those physicians who are taking the altruistic duties of their profession so seriously that they are joining in the fashionable peace movement. There are many military physicians who are so patriotic as to believe that their main duty is to their country in the way of assisting the authorities to make the soldier a more efficient fighter. They even believe that the main reason for curing the sick and wounded is to get them back in the ranks in the shortest time possible, and though, of course, ordinary humanity to the disabled is a large element, it sinks into insignificance in comparison to national welfare and the protection of all. Those provisions of the international conventions which state that sanitarians can not be held as prisoners of war, but must be grouped with all who cannot do anything towards increasing military efficiency, take the bold stand that sanitation is worthless. This would be insulting were it not the result of an ignorant and absurd retention of rules made before sanitation was born. Now we know that armies cannot exist to repel invasion unless sanitarians are with it to apply the newest sanitary rules for preventing such sickness as occasionally destroyed the greater part of military expeditions. To exempt these experts from capture is as absurd as to exempt the experts in ammunition and other warlike supplies. As physicians then, we do have a vital part in preparing the nation's defenses, and we must abandon the degrading attitude of unpatriotic neutrals when our firesides are threatened.

The appalling results of unpreparedness for war are the main points for physicians to study. We have a traditional hatred of standing armies as somehow inimical to civic liberty, and yet in those countries that have the greatest forces, the professional soldiers are almost entirely excluded from civil positions. In a remarkable report by General Emory Upton on our military policy (*Govt. Printing office,* 1907) written in 1880, but buried for over a quarter of a century, the awful cost in life and money of unpreparedness, is detailed with sickening monotony. What concerns us is the fact that so certain are we that our resources in men and money constitute military strength, that we pay no attention to preparation of that strength to make it effective. We think it requires no preparation at all. Consequently every war witnesses an appalling amount of preventable sickness and subsequent pensions. Von Moltke would not read of our battles because the study of the slaughter by "armed mobs" gave no information as to the management of real armies, which would do the work at far less cost of life. Yet, nowadays, the most valuable lessons are being drawn in Europe from these same battles, and we witness an increasing number of works of medical interest. Curiously enough the whole tenor of all comments is to the effect that disease is the main enemy of untrained troops, and there is an increasing volume of appreciation of the modern preventive systems devised in the Army of the Potomac by Tripler and Letterman of the regular Army Medical Staff. These men are almost unknown at home, but are considered great men abroad. If the medical profession wishes to do its best by the country, it will join in the movement to prepare for war and not the one to disarm and repeat the frightful history we have made. The systems now being adopted in Europe are all based on Letterman's, and his method was evolved to end the unspeakable conditions of 1861 and 1862, brought about by the people who think that it is only a matter of a few days to make an army from raw recruits and a medical department from civilian doctors.

The alleged superior perceptions of lower races has been accepted on faith so long that it is amazing it was not put to the test years ago, but happily the work is now done and it positively disproves the theory that savages, as a whole, possess phenomenally acute vision, hearing or any other sense. Indeed the theory of evolution should have shown us that the complex processes of civilized industries require keener perceptions to carry them on, and that the higher nervous development would naturally cause greater variability of sensitiveness, but somehow the idea became fixed that by reason of our intelligence we were more or less independent of our senses which were becoming dulled from disuse. The error probably arose from travellers' tales of lower races who would naturally perceive familiar things which the stranger would ignore. Prof. R. S. Woodworth of Columbia University (*Science,* Feb. 14, 1910) has described numerous comparative tests, including his own at the St. Louis Exposition, which lead him to the generalization that "on the whole, the keenness of the senses seems to be on a par in the various races of mankind."

The greater variability of civilized perceptions seems to be the law which will explain the apparent discrepancies which Woodworth finds. A low stage of culture requires greater similarity of men, and variations perish which in civilization are carefully preserved as useful. We know that there are very stupid white laborers who are far inferior to savages, while we also produce many types of genius never found among primitive people. The variability of civilized skulls and uniformity of ancient ones in any locality, are long known facts, and it should have been assumed that the same law applies to every other characteristic. Thus, Woodworth found overlapping in every perception, but that of vision, inasmuch as no lower races had any men who equaled the best records in the German Army, and that of hearing, for whites were found superior to savages. The few tests of smell show that lower races are not possessed of any greater ability, while the tactile sense, determined by the points of calipers, did not differ noticeably though the pain sense may have been less. Moreover while the color sense is much the same the world over, whites have a generally superior ability in match-

ing colors,—a matter of extreme importance in a great variety of trades. We can
now understand why it is that when white
men learn what to look for in hunting,
fishing or finding their way in the wilderness, they generally equal the savage and
often surpass him.

**Negroes and Indians cannot possibly
compete with white men** in many of the
callings which have been created by civilization. Of course lack of intelligence renders a negro mechanic less efficient than a
white man, but his failure is partly due to
inability to perceive phenomena which are
perfectly evident to us. It is quite clear,
then, why the present efforts to educate
our lower types to become the economic
equals of "white men" are bound to fail,
as they have always failed in the past. It
does seem that schools for negroes set an
unattainable ideal before the students and
only increase their bitterness when failure
comes. The usual complaint has been that
the lower races,—negro in particular, have
not been given a chance, indeed are dis-
criminated against, though as a fact they
are being constantly tried but found wanting. If a black man can repair watches
better than the white competitors of a
town, he will get all the watch repairing
to do, but his senses are too blunt for such
delicate work, his intelligence too limited
and his judgments defective. We refer to
the real negro—not the more intelligent
half-castes.

The education of lower types is bound
to be put on a different foundation by these
epoch-making observations of the senses.
Pedagogs too often assume that training
is all that is necessary—they must now
know that the material to be taught is to

be considered. The old idea that all men
are equal, or can be made equal by a few
generations of education, is gradually being abandoned now that we know the brain
does not change so rapidly. There is less
and less effort to train minds to do things
hopelessly beyond their capacity, but the
new point is that we can not expect to
make even efficient workmen of lower
races,—except in a few lines or a few
cases. It has long been known that
illiteracy in Europe is not so much due
to lack of opportunity as lack of ability,
and we must moderate our ambitions as
to the education of the lower races now
migrating here in such a flood. Perhaps in
time, it will be possible by psychologic and
physiologic tests, to determine exactly a
child's capacity and educate it accordingly. Our present system of running all of
them through the same mill is a folly which
medical men, particularly physiologists,
can end if they will only continue these
investigations. The welfare of the nation
demands so much more of this work that
extensive investigations by the existing bureaus of the General Government are needed. The Ethnological service has largely
devoted its time to aborigines, now let it
take up the still lower types flocking
here from Europe and Asia, and find out
whether we can make them over into safe
voters, or whether most of them for their
own good should not be disfranchised as
uneducable—or kept out entirely.

The cause of variations still bewilders
the biologists and though the vast majority
are in accord with the medical profession
which cannot conceive of a causeless departure from the normal, yet there are a
few who take the opposite view. Curiously
enough the last word said on the minority

side is the work (*Descendenz und Path-ologie*) by the pathologist, D. von Hanse-mann, who states that a tendency to vary is a fundamental property of living proto-plasm and that it is therefore a waste of time to look for causes of variation. Such an extreme view need only be stated to show its absurdity and it is well that no physician in active practice should think like Hansemann. Success in treatment and prevention depends upon an unremitting search for causes of every abnormality, and the great medical advances of recent de-cades are due to the logical belief that nothing happens without a cause. If there is absolutely no change in the environ-ment, children closely resemble ancestors, though by Mendel's law, they do not neces-sarily resemble the parents or even the grandparents; but when something en-tirely new appears, it is time to look for a disturbing factor in the environment. When Oliver Wendell Holmes suggested beginning treatment with the grandparents he stated a great biological truth which has far more practical value than its whimsical tone implies. Children are not only injured after birth by unhygienic nur-ture, but also during gestation by parental bad habits or infections, and the injury may be so great as to interfere with the propagation of the next generation. We are in a position to detect these causes of mal development and we must do so in-stead of supinely referring it to the will of God. Then avoidance of the discovered causes will prevent the distressing in-stances of degeneration found in almost every normal family. This kind of racial improvement is now called negative eugenics and it is the fundamental reason for the existence of the medical profes-sion.

The impossibility of eliminating quack-ery is fully recognized in Europe, yet America which has suffered the most seems bent upon its total suppression. Germany, which is held up as a model of all things medical, makes no attempt to suppress it. Anyone who pleases may employ quacks, but they are forbidden by law to assume a title they do not possess. They must make it known that they are not legally qualified to give advice, but the State does not restrict the citizen's personal liberty to buy advice from any source. The title of doctor or "learned" can be obtained by any one who submits any proofs that he is learned, but woe be-tide him if he calls himself doctor with-out having his learning tested. Similarly the one who professes to impart his learn-ing, cannot call himself professor unless he is legally appointed to such a position. Yet quacks abound in Germany and no one worries over it. If any of them com-mit downright fraud, they are suppressed like any other swindlers, but no account can be taken of giving ridiculous advice without stepping on the toes of the swarms of doctors at the health resorts, who are noted for their unbounded faith in the mystic properties of the "waters."

Should quacks be permitted to treat the sick? is the title of an address to the Brooklyn Philosophical Association, by Dr. W. J. Robinson of New York City (*Amer. Jour. of Clinical Medicine*). As long as the majority of the people want the quacks, it is not evident how a small minority can prevent the practice, and we are afraid Dr. Robinson has set an unat-tainable ideal. Our past efforts have given rise to the two most serious objections to all medical practice acts, interference with personal liberty and the creation of a medical trust which will stifle progress by making it criminal to advise or use new things not approved by the examining boards. We have seen no harm follow the omission of therapeutics from State examinations. Indeed everyone predicted that if a candidate for a license proved himself learned enough to make a diagnosis, he could be trusted as to the rest. So the State has already established the precedent, that it has no concern as to how the sick are treated, if no fraud is practiced. Would it be too big a step to imitate Germany and other countries, and remove all our present restrictions? Would it not be a tremendous step forward if those who sell medical advice or labor be compelled to keep their licenses on view or tell each patient that they have none? Would it not diminish if not eliminate the advertising evil, if it were a crime to offer to sell advice or labor or drugs without the words "not legally qualified and licensed to practice medicine or sell drugs or appliances?" Prosecutions of Christian Science practitioners for murder does not lessen the demand for them, and we have long acknowledged that we must wait for that delusion to die a natural death like all its predecessors. They may be assumed to be honest people for they do not sail under false colors. Similarly, the prosecutions for practicing without a license do not touch the quacks, so why not try the German way of restricting an evil which only despotism could eliminate?

———

The annual toll of the railroads in human lives is appalling. Hardly a day goes by that the newspapers do not record some railroad accident attended by loss of life. Recently the calamities that have oc- curred on several of the large railway systems, generally considered the best in the country in equipment and management, have furnished new food for thought on the subject. The trains wrecked were supposed to be the finest in the world. Every detail and device that would assure safety were being utilized. Nothing that the human mind could suggest to prevent accident had apparently been neglected. And yet in spite of every precaution, without warning, these trains have crashed into others, run off the tracks, or broken apart with the most frightful results. In the twinkling of an eye valuable lives have been snuffed out, leaving families bereaved and homes desolate. In addition many individuals have been maimed and made helpless cripples. Naturally the question arises, if trains representing the acme of American railroading, on lines that we have every right to expect the most from, in management and in regard for the interests of the public, continue to be wrecked with such startling frequency, where does the responsibility rest? Who or what is to blame for these terrible catastrophes? Are they preventable, and if so, how?

These queries concern every person who travels at all, and the enormous loss of life that must be charged to the railroads, make their careful consideration and answer imperative. It is intolerable that several hundred (217 passengers, 715 employees) lives should be sacrificed in this county in one year, while less than fifty were lost in Great Britain (23 passengers, 9 employees). There must be some fundamental cause that is responsible for the fact that during 1910 American railroads killed nearly thirty times as many as the English! Can one doubt, moreover, that there is a definite reason why in the United States over 6,500 railroad employees were injured in 1910 and only 113 in Great Britain? There is a cause, and the most superficial study will show that it is our present day mania to get from place to place in the shortest possible time. In other words, the spirit of impatience has been allowed to pervade every walk of life, every industry, every enterprise, with the result that everything is subordinated to haste. The railroads in their competition with each other, have taken advantage of this speed mania of the people, and run their trains with regard only to developing the shortest possible schedules. Safety and all other considerations have been sacrificed, until to-day we witness our railroads, to which we are pleased to credit much of our national progress, standing before the world as one of the leading destroyers of human life. A beneficent industry, a product of civilization ostensibly fulfilling a high and noble mission—but at an annual cost of over one thousand lives and 6,791 injuries! Can this long continue?

The American people are speed crazy. To nothing else can the frequency of railroad accidents be attributed. In the effort to meet the hysterical desire of the traveling public to reach its destination with least delay, train after train is being run at the most dangerous speeds. With increase of weight and size of modern coaches, and the development of longer and heavier trains, it has been necessary to build larger and larger locomotives. Unfortunately the evolution of road beds, including rails and methods of fixing them, has not kept pace with the changes in the character of the rolling stock.

Obviously there is a definite ratio between the rolling stock and the road bed and rails, which admits of speed up to a certain point with practical safety, eliminating, of course, all structural defects. But any great increase in the weight and character of the train units without corresponding increase in the size and character of the road bed and rails, is bound to change the ratio of safe speed. It will be apparent to every thoughtful person that while trains have grown mightily in length, size and weight, the tracks and rails have only changed slightly. And yet the speed of these trains has been fearfully increased. Can any one doubt that the limit of safe speed has been far exceeded? Can one with ordinary common sense possibly believe that an eighteen-hour train between New York City and Chicago—a necessarily heavy train with a massive engine running over ordinary rails and road bed at seventy and eighty miles an hour—can ever be safe? The accidents that are continually befalling these trains ought to convince railroad officials of their impracticability under present conditions. But with fatuous disregard of the harm they are doing to the people, they go on running these trains with the smug statement that the public demand them and that they represent the last word in railroad progress! Heaven forbid the term, for such progress is purchased at too great a cost in human lives and limbs.

Safer railroad travel is going to be demanded by thinking people in the very near future. Just as soon as the public realize the price they have been paying for eighteen-hour trains between New York and Chicago, and their expresses at seventy miles an hour, there will be a revulsion in sentiment. Already many persons are shunning the eighteen-hour Chicago trains.

Three or four, or even ten hours, are not much to pay for the certainty of reaching one's destination alive and· with all the limbs with which one started. As a matter of fact, these fateful trains would never have been developed, if our laws placed responsibility for resulting accidents on the person or persons who ordered them. This is the secret of making our American railroads safer, to create laws that will place responsibility on individuals. A railroad official will hesitate long before he will order a train run at speeds that he knows— in view of his technical information concerning rails, road beds, etc.—are dangerous and unsafe. Then when officials, conscious of their personal responsibility, very properly refuse to run trains at speeds that jeopardize their own welfare—and liberty —they will quickly take steps to educate the public to the advantage of safe rather than swift travel.

At the present time there are innumerable trains being run on schedules that are impossible to adhere to. This is done to fool the traveling public, for railroad officials know that people at present will invariably take trains that are advertised to get them to their destinations in quickest time. The public may not know that these trains are always late or else run at unsafe speeds. This shortening of schedules to impossible or dangerous limits is an abuse that must be stopped. When the people awaken to the manner in which they have been hoodwinked or their lives jeopardized by trains run on time schedules that cannot be made, without sacrificing safety or disregarding signals, we shall see a prompt change in the situation. It is to be hoped that this awakening will come in the near future, for existing conditions are a sad reflection not only on the honor and principles of our railroad heads, but also on the intelligence and common sense of the people. It is a national disgrace that a premium should be placed by the American people on speed and haste, when we know these entail such a waste in lives and limbs. We cannot hope to achieve true greatness as a nation until we have learned to cherish human life more dearly. This applies to every American industry. We have held life too cheaply in our industrial development and every individual is paying the price to-day by the greater danger he is forced to run of meeting a sudden or violent death. While the medical profession have been prolonging human life, industrial development has been reducing it. It is a topic that should engage the earnest attention of medical men.

Laws must regulate the time tables of our railroads. Certain speeds for trains of certain length and weight are permissible on our present road beds and rails. Greater speeds are unsafe, not only for a train itself, but also because of the injury that may be done to rails, switches, etc., especially in the winter. Thus a train with a mammoth locomotive and running at terrific speed, may break a rail and yet pass on without accident. But the next train, though run well within safe limits, may strike the broken rail in such a way that a frightful wreck ensues, with the loss of many lives. Consequently, laws should define the speed at which a train of a given size and weight should be allowed to run on a given road bed. Disregard of these regulations should carry severe penalties for the person or persons responsible therefor. Time tables should be carefully censored and schedules lengthened to conform to the truth and the legal speeds allowed to the various trains.

Inspection not only of rolling stock, but of the road bed of every railway should be required and standards of intelligence and qualification for those who do this work should also be established by law. At the present time, with so much depending on the keenness and ability of the men who inspect the rails and road bed of our leading railroads, it is left too often to ill-trained, ignorant, obtuse and incompetent foreigners, who walk the tracks—and that is about all. Conversation with some of the track inspectors of the Hudson River Division of a road as well managed as the New York Central left little room for surprise that only recently a broken rail went undetected until a serious wreck occurred. Intelligent, capable inspectors cost more money. Is that a satisfactory reason for trusting road bed inspection to incompetent men? One wreck may entail a loss that would pay the slight differences in salary between good men and worthless men for many years. But these matters should not be left to the railroads themselves. The lure of dividends is too great and the desire to make a laudable showing in operating expenses too strong, to trust these questions to the disposition of officials who may have selfish interests.

When the state or national government steps in, as soon one or the other must, and regulates railroad speeds and time schedules, establishes standards for proper inspection, and places responsibility for every accident, by imposing penitentiary sentences on the individuals who ordered or sanctioned the conditions that led to it, railroad travel will become infinitely safer, much needless waste will be avoided, and the American people will realize that just as certainly as the spirit of impatience often leads to dire catastrophe, so the spirit of patience usually goes far to avoid it. More than this, cultivating patience never fails to create a poise and peace of mind that develop personal powers that the impatient never have.

Respect for our fellow-workers is one of the finest of human virtues. On the other hand there is hardly anything that robs life of more happiness and throws more gall into the cup of our being than some sneering word, ugly innuendo, or significant shrug of the shoulders. Why are there so many men who can never see any clean motives in the work and efforts of their fellows? Why are there so many who discredit and besmirch the deeds and undertakings of their colleagues and co-workers? Such methods never mean a step forward, nor aid the slightest in advancing the success of the defiler. If it served some purpose or brought a single benefit, it would be comprehensible. But it never does, and the man who decries and meanly slurs his fellow-beings, tagging their efforts or remarks, however sincere and earnest they may be, with motives and meanings undreamed of, simply like the viper he is shows the venom and spirit that rules him. Such a man never, perhaps, does the real harm he would like to do, or that he is credited with. But he is assuredly a thief of happiness, and his kind have not only been with us from the day that human aspiration first began to express itself, but he will be with us as long as the world shall last.

But frankly, is it not a pity that so many men are prone to see the ulterior in every act or word, so apt to invest one's simplest and most innocent statements with hidden intentions? Possibly, as some one has said, suspicion is a matter of jealousy or "bilious-ness." Be that as it may, no one who has ever had an ideal and tried to reach it in working out his ambitions and aims can deny the depressing effect of unkind, spiteful criticism. That many a life has been utterly discouraged and brought close to despair by the carping criticism of some cowardly critic whose only purpose has been to destroy and tear down, is alas too true. Medical men have always been credited with harboring petty spites and jealousies to a considerable degree. But this is not so, at least not to the extent commonly believed. Naturally following a calling that is so dependent on opinion and experience, it is not strange that medical men have often disagreed in their views. Controversy and discussion have been rife, but this has been salutary, for medicine has ever progressed through interchange of opinions. But when it comes to the last analysis physicians will be found as ready to stand by and help each other as any men on earth. There are assuredly no men more ready to acclaim good and skillful work on the part of their fellows. No physician who makes a brilliant discovery or performs any noteworthy act ever lacks for a substantial following. Obviously, a profession that draws from every walk of life as the medical does, must have its full quota of narrow, ill-natured and unkind individuals. But, as we have repeatedly said before, there is something about the practice of medicine that brings out whatever good and noble there is in a man. Whether it is the frequent drafts on his sympathy, the broader comprehension of all that life and living mean, particularly for womankind, or the constant contact with defeated effort and purpose, it is hard to say, but there are no men who are kindlier, friendlier or more unselfish in their dealings with each other or the people at large than physicians. Surely no men are happier and no men do more to lighten the woes and afflictions of humanity. Once in a while, there is a doctor whose manners, methods and deeds lead him far astray. He is an element of discord wherever he is found. In his societies, in his community, in his home, he is a disturbing, destructive force. He sees no good, no worthy effort, no sincerity in any one, and as a consequence ever remains a hurtful influence. Happily his kind are few, and he can well be forgotten in the countless others who dispense hope instead of despair, good cheer instead of unhappiness, aspiration instead of discouragement, and a hearty word of commendation instead of hateful criticism.

"Hasty condemnation," we said some time ago, "is the thing from which we all suffer." Why it is so, it is hard to say. It brings no booty and serves no purpose. Yet it goes on adding to the world's unhappiness, tears and sadness. Some part of the preceding comment has been suggested by the way our earnest, sincere remarks on pharmaceutical abuses and kindred matters in our January issue were received generally. Hundreds of letters were received that were friendly in tone. Many were in accord with our views, others were the reverse. A goodly number took up parts of our editorial and amplified our ideas. Still others who believed differently gave their opinions for so doing. The point to emphasize is that all of these gave us credit for honesty of belief and purpose. We asked nothing else. We certainly do not expect everybody to agree with our views on any subject. What we are constantly trying to do is to present various topics in as interesting light as possible and bring them to the attention of our readers for intelligent study and discussion. That so many of our readers, even those disagreeing with us, realized our sincerity was gratifying beyond expression. Such an attitude was not only a compliment which we thoroughly appreciated, it was also a testimonial to the kind, broad minds of our correspondents.

There were two "gentlemen" who saw in our remarks an attack on the Association, and as they never, no never, could countenance such sacrilege, "off with our heads," i. e. "excise their honorable cognomens from our subscription list." Needless to say we performed the operation (without an anesthetic, let us say in passing), and the patient rallied well with almost no shock.

A number of our journalistic brethren took our remarks in good faith and at the present writing we know only one editor who has seen any unkind or ulterior motive in the statements. Although editing a very creditable and praiseworthy publication in the great Northwest, one that we have long esteemed, he held our editorial up to ridicule with the sententious opinion that it was the most amusing "attempt to straddle the question" that he had seen! God pity a man who can see nothing in our comment but an "attempt to straddle the question."

Such comment concerning a colleague's earnest efforts is a reflection on an editor's state of mind. To place an editorial pen in the hand of such a man is like giving the baby matches to play with, for while he may do a lot of harm to valuable property, it is himself who is most apt to suffer injury. We have a pretty firm conviction that the great bulk of the readers of a scientific journal have an aversion to any evidence of smallness or petty meanness on the part of an editor. This is why those responsible for AMERICAN MEDICINE never allow any malice or unkindness to creep into any honest criticism it may seem wise to make. We never intend to let any word of ours, if we can help it, add one jot or tittle to human unhappiness. If we criticise we shall be as ready to commend. It was this effort to point out the things we took exception to in the Council on Pharmacy's work and at the same time to record our genuine appreciation of the benefits the profession had received, that doubtless led our critic to take us to task for both criticising and commending the Council!

Such a narrow and ill-natured attack is particularly discouraging, coming from sources that one has looked to for bigger things. The physicians of the great Northwest whom we know are all men with great noble minds, far above hasty or malicious criticism. They can disagree with a colleague and not hate him or wish to injure him. This almost leads us to believe that our critic cannot have long enjoyed the broadening influences of his present environment.

We commend these words of Dr. R. B. Leach to him and every other man who has not learned to give others credit for being as honest as himself:

Let us resolve that during Nineteen Hundred Twelve we will so respect one another, and so trust the sincerity of speech and honesty of purpose and of act of one another, that, while each holds steadfast to his own convictions, he is willing to confess that his fellow-citizen is no less earnest and sincere than he is himself in adhesion to what is thought to be the truth.

Discoveries in leprosy are being made in many parts of the world and we can scarcely believe that it is only a matter of months since we learned to cultivate the bacillus.

Progress should be very rapid now that we have so many research workers. An obscure student in some out-of-the-way place, thinks out a theory or stumbles upon a fact which everyone else had seen without seeing, and within a few weeks a thousand other brains will be studying it. That is why the work in the leprosy of the lower animals is racing along since we found the disease in San Francisco rats. Duval and Gurd of New Orleans (*Jour. of Experimental Med.*, Aug. 1, 1911) have now found that practically all the laboratory and farm animals are susceptible to the infection if a sufficient number of bacilli are inoculated or if the animal is first "sensitized" by a preliminary small dose of either living or dead bacilli. This is probably an epoch-making discovery, for it is the opposite process of what is found in most other infections. It may explain why man rarely gets the disease until after long and intimate contact with a leper by whom he is repeatedly infected, but after each recovery he is more sensitive to the next dose. There is some doubt of this explanation, as it is equally logical to suppose that in endemic territory, the "contacts" may really get it from a common source.

A vaccine cure for leprosy seems to be within reach. Major Rost and Captain Williams of the Indian Med. Service (*Scientific Memoirs by officers of the Med. and Sanitary Departments of the Government of India, 1911, No. 42*) both report encouraging progress, Rost stating that of ten treated, two have recovered, two have only slight remnants of the disease and the other six are remarkably improved. These results followed promptly and could not have been spontaneous cures such as occasionally occur, so the outlook is very bright along this line. Nevertheless the theory does not quite agree with what is known of sensitizing the lower animals, and we must not be over-sanguine as we had similar hopes in numerous other "cures" in both leprosy and cancer. In addition, it has been assumed that as the bacilli are found in cells as though they were intrenched invaders and not taken in by phagocytosis, they are able to multiply because they produce proteins which protect them from any poisons in the blood serum. If so, vaccines can not be as effective as in other infections.

The fugu or fuku treatment of leprosy is the newest contribution from Japan, but as the work is secret we may not know anything definite for some time and must be content with rumors. It seems that there is a poisonous fish called *fugu* or *fuku*, which, at certain seasons, kills many people who are driven to eat it through abject poverty. A Japanese physician has conceived the idea that a serum could be made from the poison. He probably has copied the process of making antivenene from snake venom, as this serum created quite an excitement some years ago by its apparent cures of leprosy. There is still a belief here and there that it is successful, and we may expect a repetition of these hopes from Japan. But in the Orient things are seldom what they seem and we cannot judge of this remedy until we know how to make it ourselves.

Leprosy in cold blooded animals has been discovered by Couret (*Jour. Enper. Med.*, 1911, 576) and we thus instinctively fall back on the old fish theory. Indeed, Filipinos believe that the disease is contracted from river bathing, but as they all bathe in rivers, this may be only the uncultured way of putting sequence for result. Since the bacilli are found within cells and also invade ameba, a possible source of contagion is some cold blooded animal of low organization. Thus the prevalence of leprosy among marine peoples becomes significant. The cases in America are either on the seaboard or importations. There is but little known as to whether any of our lepers have ever infected anyone, and it is also possible that the transfer may require an insect not common in America, though the bed-bug has been accused. Brinkerhoff and Reincke (*Bull. 33, Marine Hospital Service*) report that among Hawaiian lepers the males are almost twice as numerous as the females. This suggests that the men do not get it at home, for if the sick were the source the women nurses should be more infected. It has been stated before that the disease seems to prefer those who handle raw fish, and inoculate themselves in the nose.

The relation of fish to disease must be studied more extensively, not that we have any large hopes for the *fugu* cure, but to emphasize what has so often been said though unheeded—it is a great field which the pathologists and pharmacologists have neglected too long. The Japanese are ahead of us even if they do not succeed with fugu. The work is urgent in view of Sambon's theory that pellagra is carried to us from some cold blooded animal by the sand fly (simulium) of certain streams. It attacks only country people who frequent the streams in the fly season, city dwellers escaping. This may be why the Jews have so far furnished no cases. Surely some such generalization is possible in leprosy. The whole subject is involved in many apparent contradictions which may be harmonized by some little fact now before our eyes waiting to be seen.

The heredity of leprosy is another idea long held by the more primitive races and now taking hold of other observers most unaccountably. Japanese so firmly believe it to be a family taint, that they ostracize all the leper's relatives. This is one explanation of the remarkable class of pariahs in Japan—the *etas*, who are still outcasts socially even if their political disabilities have been removed. To save the family from ruin, the facts are concealed, so it is hard to elicit information, but it is now claimed that by long patient search, some blood relatives will always be found. The disease may skip a generation to appear in cousins. It is quite common for a leprous father to have leprous children, and the mother escape infection; and, most curious of all, if both parents are lepers, the children may escape. The difficulty of contracting the disease has been used to bolster up the idea of heredity, and cast discredit upon the bacillus as the sole cause; but then, we did the same to the bacillus of tuberculosis many years after its discovery whenever we were puzzled over the source of infection in any case. It is strange that those who are most convinced of the heredity of leprosy and the harmlessness of the leper, are the most strenuous in insisting on isolation of the harmless man to protect a community already safe. We might be entirely too brutal in our quarantines and we earnestly commend the matter to those in endemic territory. It seems amazing that so little has been published as to the previous habits of lepers. Surely there must be a common factor waiting discovery—perhaps it is right before us, unnoticed. The heredity believers must acknowledge that the beginner of a line of lepers must have contracted it from some other source.

ORIGINAL ARTICLES.

FURTHER EXPERIENCES WITH THY-
ROID MODIFICATION AND
THERAPY.

BY

HEINRICH STERN, M. D.,
New York.

In compensatory therapy there are no drugs of greater importance and wider range of application than the preparations of the thyroid gland; notwithstanding this, however, their employment is still a very limited one. But very few physicians have added the thyroid to their armamentarium, and those who have done so are in most instances not cognizant of its entire scope of usefulness. They restrict its administration to instances of obesity, myxedema and allied conditions, and do not know, or forget, that thyroid insufficiency, or perversity, may evince itself by dozens of intermediary phenomena or conditions. One must not lose sight of the fact that myxedema and cretinism are remoter expressions of hypothyroidism in the same sense as Graves' disease is one of the ulterior manifestations of hyperthyroidism. The lesser exhibitions of thyroid insufficiency are at least as amenable to compensatory therapy as are the pronounced syndromes. An examination by the manager of one of the better drugstores in New York City of the last two thousand prescriptions compounded in his shop showed that there were but six orders for a thyroid preparation all of which but one emanated from the writer of these remarks. Is there a more conclusive proof that thyroid therapy is still in embryo?

Compensatory medication tends to supply or regulate certain deficiencies or perversities of internal secretion. The compensating substance should therefore be analogous in its general characteristics to the normal secretion for the deficiency or anomaly of which it is to exert vicarious activity. In the face of a proper diagnosis thyroid therapy, if pertinently executed, is the most typical example of compensatory medication. With the customarily employed thyroid preparations, however, an exact compensating effect cannot be obtained for the simple reason that there is no parallelism between the composition of the sheep's thyroid, preparations of which are those commonly administered, and that of the human gland. I have shown for instance (*American Medicine*, January, 1910) that there is about sixteen times as much arsenic contained in the human as in the sheep's thyroid. Of course, the physiological activity of the thyroid is only in part due to its arsenic content, but there is a distinct increase in the activity of the commercial thyroid when arsenic in a certain proportion has been added to it. This may be readily demonstrated clinically. An observation which I soon made after I started with the employment of thyroarsenical therapeusis was that considerably smaller doses of thyroid thus combined would yield as good or better results than when given alone in the usual massive amounts. The added arsenic, which is only mechanically admixed with the thyroid, naturally does not enter into the composition of the colloid substance, but it enhances and regulates the thyroglobulin or iodothyrin activity. I have never seen any untoward effects of thyroid medication when a preparation of arsenic was given together with physiologically efficient but small doses of the glandular substance.

It does not make any material difference which preparation of arsenic is employed for purposes of thyroid modification. For many years I made use of arsenious acid (*Journal American Medical Association,* February 15, 1902); about three years ago I started to employ sodium dimethyl arsenate (sodium cacodylate) as a corrective and enhancer of thyroid activity. The cacodylates exhibit all the therapeutic qualities of the alkali arsenites but are decidedly less toxic and may be administered in medicinal amounts for protracted periods without interruption. Such untoward phenomena as gastrointestinal irritation, headache, inflammatory conditions of the upper respiratory tract, thirst and restlessness not infrequently following the exhibition of therapeutic doses of the ordinary arsenical preparations, supervene only in exceptional instances when cacodylates are being given in their place. It is for the very reason that the cacodylates are better borne, and may on this account be administered for longer periods than the commonly prescribed preparations of arsenic, that they are more efficient stimulants of general metabolism than the latter.

The cacodylates are to a degree also stimulating cardiac activity but not as much as to overcome an eventual depressing influence of the thyroid medication. Moreover, in many instances in which thyroid therapy is indicated the condition of the heart is below par. For this reason and inasmuch as a rational thyroid therapy must be continued for prolonged periods, it is of advantage to combine the thyroid-sodium cacodylate with one or the other cardiac stimulant. Adonidin, a glucoside of adonis vernalis, has been my choice of a heart tonic for over 15 years; its prohibitory price, however, forced me to look for another, if possible still more efficient, general cardiac stimulant which could be administered in conjunction with the thyroid compound.

Kothe has stated, and other clinicians have supported his contention, that "epinephrine is the strongest analeptic which we possess at the present day." The therapeutic value of epinephrine is due to its powerful vasoconstricting properties in the presence of deficient blood-current intensity. In vasomotor paralysis and cardiac insufficiency, epinephrine is therefore the rational remedy. Vasomotor paralysis as well as cardiac weakness occasions a decline of arterial pressure and consequently deficient nutrition of the nerve centers. Epinephrine causes constriction of the vessels in the engorged splanchnic vascular system which, in course, raises the blood pressure and tends to regulate blood distribution. By stimulating the vagus center and slowing cardiac activity it does not only exert a decided tonic influence upon the myocardium but acts also as a direct physiological antidote to thyroid preparations. The internal administration of epinephrine has been abandoned to a large degree for the reason that the usual doses have not yielded satisfactory clinical results. While it is undoubtedly true that medicinal doses taken by the mouth cannot compare in intensity of action with its intramuscular or intravenous administration, it is equally true that, when given by the mouth, epinephrine is hardly ever exhibited for sufficiently long periods. Irrespective of the manner in which it is administered, the effect of an insufficient number of doses of epinephrine will always be a transitory one. It is probable that lasting effects can never be produced by epinephrine, but I have observed that its prolonged oral administration gives rise to what—in contradistinction to cumulative action—I may be permitted to designate as "reenforced activity." By this term I wish to express that drugs like epinephrine, given by the mouth and continued in the same amount for long periods, will sooner or later exert a more perceptible influence without accumulating in the system or occasioning untoward manifestations. The oral administration of preparations of the suprarenal glands should therefore be reserved for chronic conditions in which they may be exhibited for a comparatively long time. On this account epinephrine appears to be a rational heart stimulant in all those cases in which the thyroid-cacodylate compound is indicated. The average dose of epinephrine which I order to be taken by the mouth is one milligram (1/60 grain).

The unit of the thyroid compound which I employ at the present time, is the following:

Desiccated thyroid gland substance, 5 centigrams (1 grain).

Epinephrine, 1 milligram (1/60 grain).

Sodium cacodylate, 0.5 milligram (1/200 grain).

In the absence of any determinable local cause or systemic disorders like enteric fever and syphilis, imperfect nutrition or denutrition of the hair upon the scalp and premature baldness have for many years been considered by me as being due to a state of hypothyroidism in a large proportion of the cases. Hypothyrosis in its milder forms is a very frequent condition not only in women but also in men. Its presence is, of course, mostly overlooked, because one involuntarily associates the manifestations of the relatively infrequent myxedema of adults with those of the mild

hypothyrotoxic phenomena. The milder types of hypothyroidism, however, have little in common with myxedema at the bottom of which there often stands complete athyroidism. The symptoms of the milder forms of hypothyrosis are less pronounced and less persistent than those of myxedema. They consist in the main of a dry and rough skin, defective nutrition of hair and nails, bleeding of gums, headache, general lassitude and decline of body temperature at irregular intervals. These symptoms are aggravated in cold, decidedly ameliorated in warm weather.

Thyroid medication often yields surprisingly good and quick results even when certain denutritional changes have already ensued in the hair follicles, the epidermis and corium. So long as the papillae of the hairs are not completely destroyed one may at least expect some beneficial influence from the administration of thyroid. At any rate, the imperfect state of nutrition of the hair yields more unfailingly and readily to thyroid medication than to topical stimulants. Local applications may be combined with a course of thyroid therapy; the observer, however, will soon notice that it is the thyroid ingestion and not the so-called stimulating lotion which occasions increased nutrition of the hair follicles. Thyroid medication often causes quicker effects in the warm than in the cold seasons; in fact, smaller doses may accomplish the same results in the summer than larger ones in the winter. The dose usually employed by me in instances of falling hair or alopecia is from one to two (of afore specified) units three times a day. The medication is continued for not less than from eight to ten weeks. If after this period no definite results have been obtained, it may be concluded that hypothyroidism does not stand at the foundation of the imperfect nutrition of the hair follicles.

Besides a goodly number of instances of premature denutritional changes in the hair-bottom, I had occasion to employ the thyroid-cacodylate compound in a case of coalescent alopecia areata. In less than three months a new, healthy crop of hair of natural color and lustre had appeared.

While bleeding of the gums has been recognized by some as a likely manifestation of hypothyroidism, I believe that I was the first to point out the possible etiologic connection between deficient or perverse thyroid function and Fauchard's or Riggs' disease. As far back as 1902 on the occasion of a series of lectures on disorders of catabolism to post-graduates in medicine I maintained that neither local causes nor the usually assigned systemic affections as diabetes, gout and rhachitis, but an incomplete myxedematous condition was one of the principal causative factors of pyorrhea alveolaris (interstitial gingivitis, Riggs' disease). I have held this view ever since, no matter to what fanciful causes others have tried to fasten the gingival process. Of course, there are local conditions which favor the production of interstitial gingivitis, or aggravate it in case it is already existent; and there are systemic affections, especially syphilis which may be accompanied by Riggs' disease. In the vast majority of instances, however, the local circumstances of pyorrhea alveolaris are of a distinctly secondary nature which is again proved by the fact that topical treatment alone has hardly ever effected a complete cure of the usually very stubborn affection. Moreover, most cases of syphilis do not exhibit pyorrhea alveolaris, and it is an open question whether, when it has ensued, it is

of syphilitic or mercurial origin. Besides, I am convinced that most instances generally considered to be Riggs' disease of syphilitic causation, in reality are not cases of this affection at all but the end-results of mercurial stomatitis. True enough, the so-called constitutional diseases are not infrequently found associated with interstitial gingivitis, but it is equally true that they concur at least as frequently with deficiencies of one or the other internal secretion. Is it not rational, therefore, to assume that a perversity of an internal secretion may occasion a constitutional affection as well as the gingival process, and that the latter belongs either to the syndrome of the former or is a direct manifestation of a disturbance of internal secretion? As far at least as hypothyroidism is concerned in the production of interstitial gingivitis I have abundant clinical and therapeutic data to prove my contention.

I have not kept any special notes of the cases of interstitial gingivitis which I have seen. Nobody consults me on account of his gingival condition which, for many years, I have considered as nothing but an incident in the course of a systemic disorder. Roughly speaking I must have recommended the administration of thyroid extract in cases in which gingivitis was one of the features in not less than 400 or 500 instances. Limiting myself to consulting work, the great majority of these cases was not seen by me beyond the period of diagnostic observation, and for this reason I have no definite information concerning the influence of thyroid ingestion upon the gingival phenomenon in most of the pertaining instances.

However, while I kept no notes of my cases of interstitial gingivitis per se, I have the records of 52 cases of hypothyroidism which were under my continued observation for from two months to nearly two years. Of these 52 cases, 28 showed no gingival symptoms at all; in 10 cases there existed mild affections of the gums (not of a pyorrheal nature and unaccompanied by atrophy, etc.), while in the remaining 14 cases there had ensued more or less pronounced gingival manifestations. These 14 cases had received more or less local care at the hands of dentists which, however, had not availed much in a single instance. (It is nevertheless essential that the teeth and gums be kept in as healthy a condition as possible, that the tartar be removed and local treatment instituted when the circumstances call for it. At the same time too much reliance must not be placed upon the removal of possible local irritants or defects). Administration of from three to nine units per day of the thyroid-cacodylate compound for from six to fourteen weeks was followed by a complete cure of the gingival process—for the time being—in 3 instances, a distinct improvement in 5 others, and a slight improvement in an additional 2 instances. The remaining 4 cases were not ameliorated at all after from three to four months' administration of the drugs. One case of the last group, however, became markedly better when a second attempt at thyroid compensation was undertaken some time later. The fact that out of 14 cases of hypothyrosis with gingival symptoms 10 were beneficially influenced shows conclusively that these manifestations were due to an insufficient thyroid secretion and that the thyroid-cacodylate furnished the compensating means.

In all instances of hypothyrosis, thyroid administration must be continued for protracted periods. When improvement has supervened, the medication may be entirely stopped or its dosage and frequency of administration may be diminished for some time. It stands to reason that the gingival process may again manifest itself together with a recrudescent hypothyroid state. For this reason we can only speak of a cure of hypothyroid gingivitis or denutrition of the hair in the same sense as we speak of a cure of the hypothyrotoxicosis itself.

———

IMPRESSIONS OF THE PANAMA CANAL.

BY

DOUGLASS W. MONTGOMERY, M. D.,
San Francisco, Cal.

The Canal Zone is the strip of territory ten miles wide and about forty-five miles long, rented in perpetuity by the United States from the Government of Panama, and through which the Canal passes like an alimentary tract, and like the alimentary tract the Canal has Colon near one end, and La Boca, or the mouth, at the other. Although Col. Goethals furnished me with a guide I was unable to locate the appendix.

For ages the Isthmus has been considered unhealthy because of its climate. This view in the light of modern science has to be corrected. It is true that the climate is well adapted to the development and transmission of two diseases, malaria and yellow fever, that are particularly destructive to man, but when these are mastered and good food is obtainable, the average of health is well up to the normal. In fact when Mr. Le Prince, the Chief Sanitary Engineer, first went to the Canal Zone immediately after its purchase by the United States, he predicted that Ancon, situated at the southern extremity of the Canal, on the Pacific Ocean, and enjoying a comparatively dry climate, would eventually become a health resort. People thought him daft. Now there is in Ancon a large hospital, the Ancon Hospital and a large hotel, the Tivoli. It was thought sanguine to build such a large hotel, but in December when we were there it was absolutely full, and a large new wing was in course of construction. Further than this, many patients from Colombia and other South American countries now come to the Government Hospital at Ancon, because of the efficiency of the hospital staff, and the good results obtained in treatment. It therefore looks as if Mr. Le Prince's prediction had already come true.

square meals a day, slept eight solid hours without a break, grew fat, round and well favored, took a cold bath every morning and then did not wish to do a d—n thing.

This torpidity is the salient feature here, and must be allowed for in order to keep in good condition. With this torpidity comes acerbity of temper at being disturbed. You would thank your neighbors to let you alone. Therefore the principal danger to health, other than the tropical diseases above referred to, is in laziness of the life functions. The organs slacken in their activity, bringing about what Bouchard would

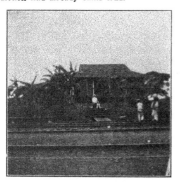

FIG. 1. AN INDIVIDUAL CANAL ZONE HOUSE PROVIDED WITH WIRE MOSQUITO SCREENING.

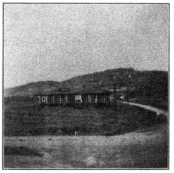

FIG. 2. A CANAL ZONE BOARDING HOUSE PROVIDED WITH WIRE MOSQUITO SCREENING.

The temperature at the Canal Zone is not high, about 85° F. the year round. Heat stroke is unheard of. This temperature, however, and the great humidity of the atmosphere, make people lazy and disinclined to exertion. Perspiration is profuse, dissolving and sticky. .It is the land of the lotus eaters, where it is always afternoon. Like Sidney Smith, you feel like taking off your flesh and sitting in your bones. A doctor told me of a man who was disgusted with the country. He said he ate three

call a slowing down of the nutritional processes. Women who as a class are naturally averse to muscular effort, and those men who are engaged in clerical work, and are therefore enforcedly sedentary in their habits, quickly degenerate. The torpidity of the tropics descends upon them. On the other hand children, who are essentially active, and men engaged in active work look thrifty and robust. I met one man who had taken his child from New Mexico to the Canal Zone on account of its health, and the result justified the measure.

Another feature leading to inactivity is the restricted area of the Zone. It is true it is ten miles wide, but only a narrow strip on either side of the canal and railroad is available for pleasurable activities; a step or two beyond is the dense tropical jungle;

decidedly dryer, there is a pleasant drive along Las Sabanas Road, and a very good bathing beach. In the different towns along the Canal the Young Men's Christian Association is doing excellent work in furnishing gymnasiums, libraries and amusements.

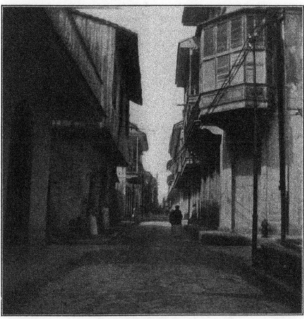

FIG. 3. A STREET IN PANAMA.
The bow window and the shutters are characteristic. Observe that the street is well paved and clean, although in a poor quarter of the town.

"the mansions of the devil—his original estates." The first days of residence one may walk or ride along the roads beside the works, but this soon grows monotonous. The monotony is increased by the unvarying foliage of the even climate, permitting almost no seasonal change. At the Panama end of the Canal, where the climate is

In passing along the Canal the most noteworthy feature is the colossal work accomplished, and the fewness of the people employed. It looks almost as if the machines were running themselves. The curse of the Garden of Eden is now changed. It reads "And thou shalt earn thy bread by the steam of thy engine." Dynamite is used lavishly and everywhere. It is desired for instance to unload a large stone that cannot be rolled off by tipping the platform of the car, as in that case it would take the car and everything with it down the bank. A negro carefully places some sticks of dynamite, and then creeps *under* the car; and off she goes. The labor saving machines and devices have much to do with the health conditions of the Isthmus, as· because of them the men are not over-worked. Besides

the peculiar circumstances under which they attempted to construct the Canal.

The absence of husbandry is remarkable; I don't recall a farm or a garden along the line. In speaking of this to a resident he said, the vegetation, although luxuriant, was coarse and poor, and the soil was thin. Take for instance the palms that make such a brave appª arance. Once I had occasion to chop one down, and imagine my disillusion when my axe sank to the eye in the

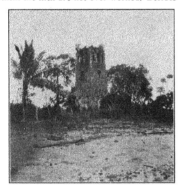

FIG. 4. RUINS OF OLD PANAMA.

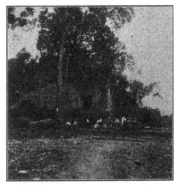

FIG. 5. SCENE IN THE RUINS OF OLD PANAMA.
Old Panama is abandoned, and is overgrown by the tropical jungle. This shows a group of prisoners engaged in opening up the old road, part of the Camino Real, leading from Las Sabanas road to the ruins.

they are well fed, they are guarded from disease by excellent hygienic measures, and they have the best of hospital care. In many of these respects the French worked at a disastrous disadvantage. They had no general system of sanitation, or of water supply, and their hospital system was defective in that the contractor had to pay a dollar each for every day any of his men were in the hospital. Consequently he allowed a sick man to die in the jungle rather than incur the expense. The mortality, therefore, under the French will never be known. This high mortality was not entirely their fault, but was largely due to

trunk as it would in elder pith. The tree was nothing but a weed. The horses fed on the Panamanian grasses are wretchedly poor, meager, little creatures that puff and pant on the least exertion. Dr. Deeks of the Ancon Hospital had a fine large horse with legs that moved like steam pistons, but it was from the United States, and was fed on imported American hay. The cows, if they wish them to give good milk, have also to be fed on imported hay. At one time the Isthmian Canal Commission paid the laborers in full, and allowed them to board themselves. This had to be discontinued as the men lived on tropical food, such as bananas, and could not do their work. "Eat well is work-well's brother" on the Canal as everywhere else. The Canal Zone is in fact a striking example of how essentially poor the tropics are, as nearly everything they use has to be imported.

The most interesting medical subject on the Canal is the fight with the mosquitoes carried on by Dr. Samuel T. Darling and

he is, and besides he is interested in his work. It is from such actions that we get the true meaning of the Kilbarchan weaver's prayer, "Lord, send us a gude conceit o' oursel'!" They have named a species of mosquito, anopheles gorgasi, only one specimen of which has been found, and some one remarked that the reason for finding only one is easily explained, as there is only one Gorgas.

Mr. Le Prince, who is not a doctor but a civil engineer, entered on his work in a

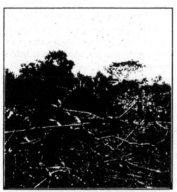

FIG. 6. LA PUENTE DEL REY, NEAR OLD PANAMA.
Ruins of la Puente del Rey, the King's Bridge, on the Camino Real, the King's Highway, between Portobello on the Carribean Sea, and Old Panama. It was along this road and over this bridge that Morgan marched in his raid to take Old Panama.

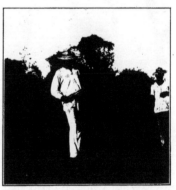

FIG. 7.
Native with a machete in his hand. The blade is like that of a sword, but there is no guard at the hilt. It is a poor mowing instrument, but a fairly good weapon.

Mr. J. A. Le Prince under the leadership of Col. Gorgas, and it is difficult to tell who of them all is most enthusiastic, as all of them have that in their countenance that Alphonse Daudet describes as characteristic of men who love their work. Their attitude may be seen from that of their chief, who refused a better position at a higher salary in the United States, because he thinks he can serve his country better where

peculiar way. He was sent to Havana, Cuba, in the days when it was thought the chief source of the unhealthiness of that city lay in its filthy harbor, and that the main problems were those of the engineer. It soon developed that mosquitoes were the trouble bearers, and Mr. Le Prince turned his attention to them and more especially to the stegomyia, as the distributor of the yellow fever germ. One of the local doctors in Havana was a consistent and industrious

148   AMERICAN MEDICINE }
Complete Series, Vol. XVIII. }   ORIGINAL ARTICLES   { MARCH, 1912.
New Series, Vol. VII., No. 3.

opponent of the view that the stegomyia could be exterminated, and his own home was a ready example, for although visited again and again by the health authorities the pest continued, and the doctor was immune and triumphant. Furthermore the doctor lost no opportunity of "rubbing it into" Mr. Le Prince. One day Mr. Le Prince and his assistants visited the house, and found the doctor absent. This was their opportunity. They started in the attic and worked down, searching every-

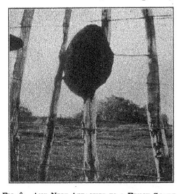

FIG. 8. ANT NEST ATTACHED TO A FENCE STAKE.

thing narrowly. Finally in the cellar they found a barrel containing some old books, and an old can of water with stegomyia larvae in it. After this there was no more trouble from that house, but the doctor never spoke to, or forgave Mr. Le Prince. His self-love had been too deeply wounded.

The climate of the Canal Zone is just suited to the mosquito. It can breed the whole year through in the warm even temperature, and the humidity and heat furnishes an abundance of low vegetable life that is its chief diet. In order, however, for the ova of the female to develop properly a blood meal, according to Dr. Darling,

seems to be necessary, and therefore this sexual impulsion is likely one of the main reasons why they are so bent on attacking man. It having been found that the mosquito was the bearer of the two terrible destroyers of the tropics, yellow fever and malaria, the life history of the mosquito about which almost nothing was known, had to be studied. Not alone this, but the life history of the different species of mosquitoes had to be investigated in order to carry on an intelligent war against them.

The stegomyia, the bearer of the yellow fever germ, is a town dweller, and does not live in the country, while the anopheles albimanus, the principal malaria carrier, is a dweller in the country, and comes to habitations in the evening and at night to get a blood meal. The stegomyia is a shy, timid creature, that bites you behind the ears and around the elbow tips. It is needless to try to strike it with your hands, you wave your hands and slap yourself in vain, as it is away before the blow falls. It breeds in roof gutters, cisterns and in old cans in and around houses, and a little warm water and a green leaf are ideal for it. It was at one time customary to rest the feet of the bedsteads in cans of water to prevent ants getting into the beds. A better breeding place for the stegomyia could not be devised. As mosquitoes are busiest at dusk and at night, people learned that this was a dangerous time of day, and became afraid of the "night air," and put up the shutters and closed the houses securely to exclude it. The sly stegomyia went around in the welcome darkness satisfying its appetite and spreading disease. Now that it is known that mosquitoes are the noxious agents their breeding places in the house are broken up and the air from the outside is allowed to enter freely through copper screens that strain out the mosquitoes. The people, therefore, have the benefit of fresh air without the evil that goes with it. These screens are seen on all the American habitations throughout the Zone and give a curious appearance to the architecture. They are practical but not pretty.

ually in tanks to last over the dry season. These tanks became infested with amebae that caused, when the water was drunk, amebic dysentery. The water was blamed for the evil, and not that which was in the water.

When Mr. Le Prince arrived at Panama

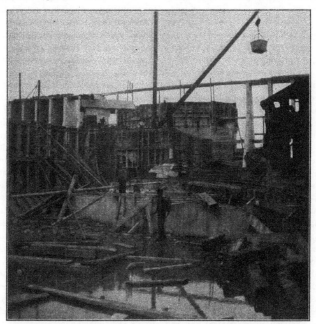

FIG. 9. SPRINKLING LARVACIDE ON STAGNANT WATER IN THE BOTTOM OF THE GATUM LOCKS.
The knapsack-like affair on the boy's back is a can containing larvacide. In his left hand he holds the sprinkler nozzle, fed by a tube from the tank; with his right he works a pump that forces the fluid out of the nozzle.

Folk-lore and medical tradition are always based on truth but it is marvelous how frequently the main point is missed. The supposedly evil effects of night air is only one example. Another relates to the noxiousness of water. Previous to American occupation water was stored individ-

he lived in the French Hospital on Ancon Hill. The first morning at breakfast a tempting dish of fresh fruit, decorated with the American and French flags, was placed in the center of the table. Mr. Le Prince began to eat some, and the waiter returning with the rest of the breakfast, nearly dropped what he had in his hand and rushed from the room. The Mother Superior of the French Sisters then appeared, and told Mr. Le Prince emphatically that if he ate any of that fruit he would surely be dead the next day. It had been placed on the table only as a decoration. The reason for the bad repute of fruit if eaten by recent arrivals lay in the fact that sailors on landing would naturally not be immune. They would first eat large quantities of the cheap and plentiful fruit, then they would fill up on rum, and afterwards would visit quarters of the town where there were plenty of stegomia and other infections. They would catch yellow fever and die quickly, and the fruit was blamed for it. In every instance folk-lore or common sense, had seized on one thing as the poisonous agent, either the air, or the water, or the fruit, and in every instance common sense was wrong. As we learn more facts our idea of common sense changes. The wisdom of today is the foolishness of tomorrow.

In talking to these mosquito hunters it is amusing to hear them unconsciously personify and speak of the mosquitoes' mental attitude as if they were human. The stegomyia, for instance, is shy and timid, while the anopheles albimanus, the malaria carrier, is predatory, fierce and has its own very decided ways of thinking. Kipling in his poem forgot to mention the female mosquito. She will make straight for you across a room. She will do even more, she will make straight for you against the wind across a field. This fact of this mosquito flying against the wind has, Mr. Le Prince told me, been recently elicited, and is of importance as it entails taking special care of breeding places on the windy side of a habitation or settlement. It is wonderful that such a light, frail creature can fly against a breeze. Probably the very highly developed proboscis of the mosquito is able to detect, as borne by the wind, the scent of the human being for a very long distance, and she knows that by flying against the wind she will ultimately reach her victim. The anopheles is so determined to enter a house, that it can be caught in traps set in the ventilators. As soon as caught a wireless seems to be sent to the ant family, that hastens up the studding to the traps, and proceeds to inter the mosquitoes alive in their hungry bowels, leaving nothing but legs and wings.

The proboscis of the mosquito is a wonderful wind instrument and in the multiplicity of its utilities reminds one of those street musicians who go about playing all sorts of different instruments at once, such as drums, pipes, and cymbals. Besides being a respiratory and olfactory organ it is able with surprising speed to penetrate the very resistant horny covering of the skin to reach the nutritious blood stream beneath. In addition to all this Dr. Darling has found that the proboscis is a musical instrument giving rise to the Chinese opera music she entertains you with before settling down to her meal. And it is through this wonderful proboscis that she sucks up *cito et jucunde* two-thirds of her weight in blood into her pesky little body. A mosquito without her proboscis would feel quite at a loss.

To try to kill mosquitoes by striking with a wire brush used for killing flies was found to be as ineffective as slapping them with the palm. That led to using a naturalist's bottle, which is cylindrical, has no neck, and is stoppered with a large cork. Some absorbent cotton is put in this bottle and chloroform poured over it. The mouth of the bottle is placed over the mosquito when at rest, and it falls dead, overcome by the chloroform. An expert can catch a great number in this way.

Dr. Darling keeps many mosquitoes in captivity in glass lantern chimneys. The upper opening of the chimney is covered with gauze, and the lower end is set in a dish, in which is placed food. In the bulging part of the chimney a ring of paper is introduced on which the little beasties can roost. He finds that they get along famously on dates and raisins with an occasional blood meal. The blood meal is given by placing the open lower end of the chimney against a human arm. If the mosquitoes do not attend to business the doctor urges them toward the arm by blowing through the gauze covering the other end of the chimney. It is interesting to know that if a mosquito is fed on bananas instead of dates or raisins and then given a blood meal it becomes constipated with the production of ferments and dies.

The most effective way of battling with the anopheles, as with the stegomyia, is by carrying the war "into Africa" and attacking it in its home breeding places in the swamps and streams. Swampy places may be drained and rendered perfectly innocuous, but in draining, the greatest judgment and knowledge of conditions must be used, such as the advisability of using an open drain, a rock drain or tiling. All of these things, and the different grades are of importance in a country where vegetation is so luxuriant. I was shown a home that had been abandoned because of its insalubrity, that was corrected by draining a small adjacent swampy bit of ground at a cost of one dollar and a half.

Larvacides are also largely used, and are found most effective. It is true that they also destroy the fish that feed on the larvae, but they destroy much more larvae than the fish do, and are therefore preferable. The difficulty with the fish is that the larvae are hidden and protected in algae and under stones where the fish cannot get at them. The best larvacide is made of crude carbolic acid, resin, and caustic soda. The proportions of these ingredients have to be varied according to the amounts of phenols and cresols in the carbolic acid, and a sample of every barrel is first sent to the laboratory in order to ascertain these points. As this larvacide is of such general interest the formula for its preparation is given in detail as follows:

One hundred fifty U. S. gallons of crude carbolic acid of a specific gravity not greater than 0.96 and containing not less than 15% of phenols and cresols is heated to the boiling point of water, when 200 pounds of resin is added and constantly stirred until dissolved. Then 30 pounds of caustic soda is added. The mixture is kept at the boiling point of water and stirred until it is a solution, when tests of a small portion in a test tube are made with water until perfect emulsion is attained. The larvacide is then ready for use.

Cans containing this larvacide are placed along streams, and allowed to trickle out on the surface of the water. We also saw pools of water in the Gatun Dam being sprinkled by darky boys who carried the larvacide on their back in tin reservoirs provided with a pump and a sprinkling nozzle. (See Fig. 9.)

It will be seen by the above that the control of malaria is a fight between man and the mosquito; one brain is pitted against the other, and the mosquito is by no means brainless. The contest becomes as fascinating as fishing, and it only needs an Isaac Walton to make it fashionable.

Of the two diseases, yellow fever and malaria, the latter is the more important, but less dramatic. It is not infrequent to hear people joking about malaria, and it is marvelous how little fear they seem to have for it. Mark Twain said a chill was the best way he knew to take involuntary exercise. Whole civilizations have, however, been killed out by it, as probably those of Greece and Rome. In fact in the old days in Panama, much of the malaria was called yellow fever on account of the yellow complexion of the patients. It is by far more widespread than yellow fever, as yellow fever is confined to the towns, while malaria infests both town and country. In the hospital at Ancon, for example, the Colombians, no matter where they come from, are found so regularly to have an enlarged malarial spleen that it is called "the Colombian spleen."

The importance of the work of the sanitary staff of the Canal Zone cannot be overestimated. The above constitutes only a few notes on what is being done. This work has not alone made possible the building of the Canal, but it serves as a model for sanitation in the tropics. One cannot converse for half an hour with these men without becoming aware of their high minded enthusiasm, and with their untiring industry in eliciting interesting and useful facts and adapting them to the work in hand.

HEART DISEASES AND EPIGASTRIC SYMPTOMS.[1]

BY

MORRIS MANGES, M. D.,

Professor of Clinical Medicine in the University and Bellevue Hospital Medical College; Visiting Physician to Mount Sinai Hospital.

In considering the diagnostic significance of epigastric symptoms it is eminently proper that the greater part of the discus-

[1] Read before the Eastern Medical Society, Feb. 9, 1912.

sion should be devoted to the study of the local lesions since, after all, they play the most important part in the etiology of epigastric symptoms. It is wise, however, to include some reference to the relations of the heart and the circulation, since now-a-days the overshadowing importance of obliterative appendicitis and other lesions in the right iliac fossa as being the cause of reflex epigastric symptoms has led practitioners to neglect the relations of the circulation, organic nervous diseases, renal and pelvic disorders, etc., for these epigastric phenomenon.

The possibility that epigastric phenomena might be due to circulatory disturbances has been especially neglected these days. This is due to the fact that the study of cardiac diseases is so fully occupied in the instrumental investigation of extra systoles, arhythmias, fibrillation, etc., that scant attention is paid by teachers and physicians to the symptomatology of cardiac lesions. Not that these evidences are unknown or unproven. On the contrary, they are taken for granted and are either neglected or overlooked in the hunt for new and so often unproven signs. The popular conception which constantly appears in the daily press when some distinguished financier or politician dies suddenly of his cardiac condition as being due to "acute indigestion," possibly reflects to some degree, at least, the pathological conception in the minds of not a few practitioners.

The close connection between the heart and the epigastrium and its viscera was well known to the old writers and what they taught has been confirmed by the recent work of physiologists and clinicians, more especially by Head and Mackenzie. The connection between the heart and the skin and viscera of the epigastrium is a very

close one in spite of the intervening diaphragm, the vagus and the sympathetic
systems uniting them very closely. Then,
too, in the corresponding segments of the
spinal cord the centrifugal and the centrip-
etal impulses are so intimately intermin-
gled, as shown by Head and Mackenzie, that
referred sensitiveness must necessarily produce very confusing clinical pictures, in
which at times it may be very difficult and
even impossible to distinguish the primary
cause from the secondary phenomena.

Besides the nervous causes of referred
sensitiveness of cardiac symptoms to the
epigastrium there are three other groups:

(1) The mechanical, such as the downward pressure of a very large heart or large
pericardial effusions. Pericardial adhesions
and capsular thickening of the liver which
occur in Pick's disease or multiple serosities
may give rise to marked epigastric symptoms.

(2) The results of venous stasis in the
liver and stomach, infarcts of the spleen,
etc.

(3) The presence of the same lesions in
the stomach and the abdominal aorta and
its branches as exist in the heart or thoracic
aorta. I refer especially to atheroma of
the vessels of the stomach, the celiac axis
and the mesentery which may lead to claudi-
cation and severe epigastric pain, the explanation of which may be very difficult unless we bear these possibilities in mind. In
cases with very high blood pressure where
the hypertension is not due to renal diseases
it is well to think of this possibility where
there are obscure severe attacks of epigastric or abdominal pain.

The lack of time and the fear that I may
trespass upon the time of those who are
to follow will cause me to be very brief in
my remarks and I shall therefore limit

myself to the more important considerations of epigastric symptoms and cardiac
diseases.

1. Organic diseases.
2. Angina pectoris.
3. Pericarditis.

1. The organic diseases of the heart
present epigastric symptoms at some time
or other during their course, and may even
be the first manifestation of them. These
symptoms are so well known that no time
need be spent in detailing them. It is surprising, however, how often these symptoms are either overlooked or falsely interpreted and hence improperly treated. In
aortic disease, angina pectoris and myo-
carditis these symptoms are most important, especially in angina pectoris as will be
shown a little later on. In mitral disease
there may be a curious referred pain in the
left part of the epigastrium along the floating ribs, a symptom to which Dr. Albert
Kohn has called my attention in a few cases.

2. In true and pseudo-angina pectoris
epigastric symptoms play a leading part; indeed in pseudo-angina they are more pronounced than they are in true angina. In
the latter they are often etiological, and
they may precede the onset of the cardiac
symptoms. When present during the attack
they are usually only a part of the referred
and radiating pains in the chest, upper extremity, epigastrium or even hypogastrium.
The interpretation of these radiating pains,
especially those in the epigastrium cannot
be discussed here. However, when confronted by problems of this kind I would
urge that it is always wise for the physician
to assume that there is an organic cause
either in the heart or in the blood vessels,
until repeated careful examinations have
eliminated the possibility of their existence.
Erroneous diagnoses of gastralgia have

been made where the pain is situated in the epigastrium with associated symptoms of flatulence and dyspepsia. Osler[1] quotes Leared, who has described a series of cases in which the heart affection was so strangely masked by that of the stomach that nothing in the statements of the patients had any bearing on the primary disease. Huchard even goes so far as to describe a special type, the pseudo-gastralgic form of angina.

The epigastric symptoms play an important part in the differentiation of true from false angina, a task which may test the skill of the clinician to the utmost. Fortunately we are not confronted with these cases as often as in France where, to judge from the writings of Potain and Huchard, pseudo-angina must be more prevalent than it is with us.

Of far greater importance than entering into any discussion of these differentiations, interesting though they be, is the emphasizing of the great importance of studying the epigastric phenomena in all cases of suspected angina whether of the true or false varieties. One will be repaid for his efforts not alone in the diagnosis, but what is more beneficial to the patient, in the treatment and the relief of the cardiac symptoms. Attacks may be warded off for even years by the careful regulation of the diet, and some writers, among whom I may quote Daland[2] especially, claim even to have cured angina in this way.

3. Pericarditis. The symptoms of onset and the fully developed disease are exceedingly varied and often misleading. I do not refer to the physical signs for these are constant and, after all, the only sure means of making the diagnosis. I mean the general symptoms and especially pain and

tenderness. They are not infrequently absent especially in children, and when they are present, they are very often not referred to the cardiac region at all. The epigastrium is a favorite site, usually in one or the other costal angles; upward pressure, respiration and bodily movements increase the pain. Somtimes the epigastric pain precedes the cardiac; at other times it follows it, appearing when the effusion is at its height.

Two cases may be briefly referred to, to show these variations in the pain in pericarditis, both of which had very large effusions. One is a case of tubercular pericarditis which I published three years· ago,[1] in which the pericardial cavity was tapped twice, an embolic hemiplegia occurring four days after one of the aspirations. In this case a man, 25 years old, the symptoms of onset were most confusing, since the chief pain of which the patient complained was a severe colicky pain in the region of the liver. This pain associated with the fever, marked rigidity, abdominal distension and a leucocytosis of 25,000 led me to make the diagnosis of cholecystitis or gall-stones. The real diagnosis was not made till routine examination of the chest on the 14th day revealed a loud pericardial murmur which was soon followed by a large effusion. With the appearance of the latter, the liver pain at once disappeared; at no time did the patient complain about any pain in his heart.

The second case is equally instructive. The only symptoms of which this patient, a man 50 years old, complained at the onset were severe burning pains in the nape of the neck with a moderate fever. These were the only symptoms for two days when a pericardial murmur appeared. A very large

[1]Angina Pectoris and allied states, 1897, p. 61.
[2]Transactions of American Climatological Association, 1908, Vol. 24.

[1]New York Medical Journal, Sept. 19, 1908. ·

effusion developed rapidly; the pain in the neck persisted for some time; the pain in the precordium which appeared with the effusion was always moderate and was very variable in its presence.

Another type of epigastric pain associated with pericarditis may also be referred to, even though these cases are very rare. In adherent pericarditis (Pick's disease, *Zuckergussleber*) there is never any pain in the precordium; the attacks of pain of which these patients complain are always in the epigastrium, either over the liver or above the ensiform cartilage. I can well recall how severe these attacks of epigastric pains were in a case of this kind which I had under my care 10 years ago. Indeed, throughout the long course of nearly two years which the disease lasted these attacks of severe epigastric pain, which were sometimes accompanied with high fever, were the only pains of which the patient ever complained.

THE COMMITMENT OF THE INSANE.

BY
WILLIAM STEINACH, M. D.,
New York.
Formerly Asst. Physician at Willard State Hospital; Instructor in Nervous Diseases, University and Bellevue Medical College.

In many diseases with which the physician comes in contact the patient frequently becomes irresponsible through delirium or coma but even in the absence of a near relative or friend, the physician frequently takes it upon himself to temporarily restrain the patient until such time as the faculties return. No one questions the right of the physician or relative to prevent a delirious typhoid or pneumonia patient from getting

[1]Read at the regular meeting of the Yorkville Medical Society, Feb. 19, 1912.

out of bed, or jumping out of the window, even if the patient must be restrained to such a degree as to be tied down. However, these conditions fortunately being of short duration the necessity of such restraint soon passes away. In the case of psychoses however, the period of irresponsibility is of longer duration and the public, ever jealous of the liberty of the individual, has prescribed certain legal steps which must, as a matter of necessity be complied with, before the patient can be restrained of his liberty even though it be for the patient's own good or for the protection of the public.

What might be called the technique of commitment varies in different countries and even in the different states of this country. I shall confine my discussion mostly to the method of procedure in New York State, merely touching on that pursued in the neighboring States of New Jersey and Connecticut.

The procedure for commitment to a hospital or sanitarium for the insane is really a legal matter but as the problem nearly always comes under the notice of the physician, and usually the family practitioner, a knowledge of its details is highly important so that when he is consulted some intelligent directions can be given.

Our insanity, like most of the common law is a heritage from the English law, which has been exceedingly jealous of the liberty of the person and has hedged the patient, as it does the defendant in a criminal action, with a number of safeguards, to prevent the detention of a person against his will unless it be done with due process of law. For this reason it often seems to the doctor that the matter of the commitment of the patient is needlessly complicated. While no doubt in the great majority of patients this legal procedure would hardly be necessary and the patient would be willing to stay wherever he is sent without much show of intelligent resistance, however, many patients, especially paranoics, whose consciousness is perfectly clear but whose judgment is so distorted that they cannot appreciate the necessity of their being deprived of their liberty, frequently make every effort to get away from the institution in which they are confined. They have frequent recourse to the writ of habeas corpus which is one of the fundamentals of our liberties, dating back to the Magna Charta, and which gives everyone who is deprived of his liberty the right of appearing in court and having the charge on which he is held, reviewed by a judge. So stringent and jealous is our law on this point, that a judge is subject to a heavy fine if he refuses to grant a writ of habeas corpus when the application is made in proper form. This enables the patient, if he or his friends have the means, to appear in court before a justice of the supreme court, where every technical point of the commitment is reviewed, as well as the mental condition of the patient is enquired into, and if, in the opinion of the judge, the patient is not insane, or there is any technical defect of the commitment, the justice may free the patient. However, I am pleased to say that most of our judges are to a great extent guided by the mental condition of the patient, and I think would hesitate to discharge a dangerous lunatic on a mere legal technicality unless forced to do so by some glaring error which invalidated the commitment.

For obvious reasons then, the technical procedure of the commitment of an insane person is an important duty which must be properly done.

Prior to 1874, a patient could be committed to an institution for the insane in New York State, on the mere order of the superintendent or overseer of the poor. After this however, the law was changed so that it required an examination of the patient by two physicians, who stated what the patient said and did in their presence and gave their reasons for supposing the patient insane. Such certificate had to be approved by a justice of a court of record within five days of the admission of the patient to the hospital or sanitarium and the examination must have been made by the physicians within ten days of the date of the judge's approval.

This procedure remained in force until July 1st, 1896, when the present law covering the commitment of the insane became operative.

An insane person can only be committed to a state hospital, a duly licensed sanitarium or if not dangerous, to the custody of a relative or committee. The manner in which the commitment is to be made is carefully prescribed by law.

The commitment may be made only upon a blank supplied by the State Commission, and consists of a petition, the certificate of the judge relating to personal service, the certificate of the two medical examiners, the order for a hearing if there be one, and the order of commitment.

I shall now take up each one of these parts of the commitment in detail. The petition may be made by a mother, father, brother, sister, husband, wife, or child of the patient, the person at whose house he resides or may be, or the overseer of the poor of the town or superintendent of the poor of the county and in the City of New York the Commissioner of Charities.

Notice that an application for commitment is about to be made must be personally served upon the patient at least one day before the application is made. However, the judge may dispense with such personal service, if it appears to him that such service would excite and harm the patient, or if it be dangerous to serve a violent and homicidal patient. If personal service is dispensed with the judge must state his reasons for dispensing with the service and this forms part of the commitment papers. If the application be made by a superintendent or overseer of the poor or by the Commissioner of Charities such notice must in addition be served upon the husband or wife, father or mother or next of kin if there be any residing within the county and if not, upon the person with whom the alleged person resides or at whose house he may be. The judge may dispense with service entirely or designate some other person upon whom such substituted service may be made.

In this city, in public cases, service is made in all cases on the patient and if there are relatives they are requested to sign a waiver dispensing with service upon them or if they refuse to do so service is made upon them as well as the patient.

The petition which must be sworn to before a notary public, commissioner of deeds or other officer of proper authority, must state the residence of the petitioner, his official position or relationship to the alleged insane person, the residence or whereabouts of the patient, the irrational acts that the petitioner has noticed, that he further believes it for the best interests of the alleged insane person that he be committed to an institution for the insane and the name of the institution to which it is desired to send the patient.

The medical portion of the commitment which most concerns us, must be made and sworn to by two duly qualified examiners in lunacy, who have made a joint examination of the patient within ten days of the date of the judge's order, and must state therein that they have found the patient insane. Such examiners in lunacy must be residents of the state, graduates of an incorporated medical college, have been in the actual practice of their profession for at least three years, whose qualifications have been certified to before a judge of a court of record, who are registered as examiners in lunacy at the office of the State Commission in Lunacy and have received an acknowledgment of such registration, who are not related to the patient or the petitioner and who have no financial or other connection with the institution to which it is desired to send the patient. They must state in the certificate the residence of the patient, his age, sex, nativity, color, occupation, civil condition, birthplace of mother and father, number of previous attacks, duration of present attack, whether previously an inmate of an institution for the insane; whether the attack was sudden or gradual in onset; the patient's physical condition; the presence of any accompanying diseases; the personal habits of the patient, whether filthy or cleanly; his tendencies, whether violent, dangerous, destructive, excited or depressed; homicidal or suicidal; whether suicide or homicide has been attempted or threatened; the supposed cause of the insanity; the patient's heredity and consanguinity of the parents; and the presence of drug and liquor or other habits. The physicians must state the facts on which they base their opinion that the patient is insane and must state what the patient said and did in their presence as well as his manner and appearance. They also add such other facts which indicate insanity and may include what has been told to them by relatives and friends together with any change in disposition, habits, character, etc. The medical certificate must be sworn to as well as the petition and the date of the joint examination is the legal date of the certificate.

The petition, the medical certificate of the examiners with the affidavit of service on the person alleged to be insane are presented to a judge of a court of record which means practically a justice of any court higher than our magistrate's or municipal district courts, who may sign the order of commitment adjudging the patient insane and order his commitment to a state hospital or a duly licensed private institution for the insane. The judge may require more evidence than that given in the certificate or petition or may on his own motion, or that of a relative or friend order a hearing before himself or a referee at some later period not more than five days distant from such order. If there be a hearing the decision of the judge as a result of such hearing must accompany the papers and there is a blank form in the commitment papers for this purpose which is omitted if there is no hearing.

When the patient is committed to a state hospital a statement of the financial condition of the patient signed by the judge must accompany the paper.

If personal service has been made upon the patient the affidavit of such service must be presented to the judge before he will sign the order of commitment. If the judge is satisfied that such personal service would be dangerous or that it would be harmful to the patient, he may. dispense with personal service and must sign a certificate giving his reasons for dispensing with personal service or direct that substituted service be made on some relative or friend, whom he designates. Such certificate must accompany the papers and becomes part of the commitment.

For several years past the Appellate Division of the Supreme Court of the first department—meaning New York County— has required in addition an affidavit made by some relative or friend or other person who is in position to know, that the patient alleged to be insane is not confined upon a criminal charge, that he is not out on bail pending the determination of a criminal charge against him and is not in official custody for the reason of ascertaining his condition after a criminal charge has been made against him.

If the person alleged to be insane is confined upon a criminal charge or out on bail the District Attorney must have ample notice before the order of commitment can be signed. In most of such cases the procedure comes under the criminal courts and the patient is usually sent to the Matteawan State Hospital.

When the patient is sent to a state hospital, the regulations of the State Commission in Lunacy require that he be in a condition of bodily cleanliness and must be provided with new clothing including an overcoat or shawl and gloves during the winter months.

The patient alleged to be insane may be committed directly from his home to the state hospital which receives patients from that portion of the state. When the papers are ready the institution is notified and will send attendants to remove the patient to the hospital. In the Boroughs of Manhattan and the Bronx patients may be sent to the Manhattan State Hospital on Ward's Island or to the Central Islip State Hospital at Central Islip, L. I. Brooklyn patients are sent to the Long Island State Hospital at Flatbush, or to King's Park State Hospital.

If the relatives of the patient desire that he receive homeopathic treatment he may be sent to the Middletown or Gowanda State Hospitals, which are under the direction of homeopathic physicians. Whenever the friends desire that the patient be sent to a state hospital other than the one which receives patients from the district in which the patient resides they may send him to such other hospital if the State Commission in Lunacy issues a special order permitting the admission of the patient. This order will usually be granted if the reasons for such change are of sufficient weight.

If the patient is sent to a private sanitarium the statement of the financial condition, as well as the requirement regarding new clothing is unnecessary.

The patient must be admitted to the hospital within five days of the date of the judge's order, otherwise the institution cannot legally hold him against his will.

In certain cases, "where the condition of the patient is such, that it would be for his benefit to receive immediate care and treatment or if he is dangerously insane so as to render it necessary for public safety that he be immediately confined, he shall be forthwith received by a state institution authorized by law to care for the insane." Under these circumstances, the patient may be received on the regular petition and medical certificate without the judge's order, but in the certificate of the medical examiners, they must state adequate reasons why the patient should be immediately received. These must accompany the patient to the institution a copy of the

verified petition and medical certificate which must remain at the hospital until the original papers with judge's order of commitment are received. Upon the above papers the patient may be held for a period not exceeding five days, during which the judge's order must be obtained. The superintendent of the institution however, may refuse to receive the patient without the judge's order if he deems the conditions not sufficiently urgent.

Instead of committing a patient who is quiet and harmless to an asylum or sanitarium, the judge may commit him to the custody of a relative or committee. In this case, it is necessary for such person to file a copy of the commitment papers in the county clerk's office, transmit one copy to the office of the State Commission in Lunacy at Albany and retain another copy for himself.

A person may be received as a voluntary patient in a state hospital or sanitarium but he must sign a voluntary commitment promising to obey the rules and regulations in the presence of a witness and must give five days' notice in writing before leaving without the permission of the superintendent.

However, before a patient can sign a voluntary commitment his mental condition must be such as to enable him to know what he is doing, otherwise it will be necessary to commit him in the regular way.

Only insane patients may be committed to our state hospitals or sanitaria and this does not include idiots, imbeciles, epileptics, alcoholics, drug habitués or dotards who are not in addition insane.

I have outlined above the procedure necessary to commit the patient directly from his home to a state hospital or sanitarium. Frequently, however, it is necessary to commit persons who have no home or whose relatives have not the means to care for them until they can be committed. In such cases the public authorities must attend to the details, bear the expense of commitment and new clothing which must be provided before they can be admitted to a state hospital.

In places outside of New York City, the superintendent of the poor of the county, or the overseer of the poor of the town must care for the patient in a suitable place, other than a jail and appoint medical examiners who are paid by the town or county.

In New York City this matter falls upon the Commissioner of Public Charities. For Manhattan and the Bronx the Psychopathic Wards of Bellevue Hospital are provided, while in Brooklyn the Kings County Hospital serves in similar capacity. In these institutions, the patients alleged to be insane are examined and committed to the state hospital if insane and discharged if not and the expense of commitment and clothing is borne by the city.

It occasionally happens that an insane person has no relatives who are able to bear the expense of his commitment or who is so dangerous that he cannot be cared for at home until the formalities can be complied with or in other cases the patient may be a troublesome paranoic who has been annoying a stranger and whose relatives refuse to have him committed. In such cases the physician is often called in for advice. I shall briefly refer to the method required in such cases.

If the patient is acting in a manner which would be disorderly in a sane person, an officer may be called in and if he see the patient acting in such a manner he may arrest him and call an ambulance to take the patient to Bellevue.

If the patient is acting in an irrational manner and the relatives are able and willing to bring him to Bellevue and if he makes no intelligent protest at being kept against his will he is held, on an order of the superintendent of the outdoor poor and may so be confined for a period not exceeding ten days.

If however, he refuses to stay, an officer is called and if the patient is manifestly insane he may arrest the patient and hold him as a prisoner, against whom there is the charge of insanity. If on the other hand, the patient acts in an orderly manner and refuses to go to the hospital or if brought to the hospital, refuses to stay it is necessary to go before a city magistrate and the relatives make affidavit before him that the patient has been acting in an irrational manner and specify more particularly what he has done. If the evidence satisfies the magistrate, he issues a warrant for the apprehension of the alleged insane person. The patient is arrested as soon as he can be found and brought before the magistrate, who may then send him to the Psychopathic wards of Bellevue for a period not exceeding five days, during which the alienists must either present the papers to a justice of the supreme court asking for his commitment, if he is insane, or discharge him if he is not insane. All the details outlined above, as to petition, examination and commitment must be gone through as if the patient were committed from his home. The petition is made by the Commissioner of Public Charities or his deputy and service is made both on the patient, and his next of kin or on the person with whom he resides or at whose house he may be, or any of the above designated individuals are requested to sign a waiver of service. New clothing is provided at the expense of the city and the patient is transferred to the state hospital by the attendants of the latter institutions.

As has already been intimated, only patients who are insane can be committed to a state hospital, but there come under the observation of the physician a large number of patients who while not insane within the meaning of the statute, are mentally deteriorated as a result of alcoholic or drug habituation and most urgently need care and treatment in an institution. Such patients often refuse to go to an institution. While at times they might technically be committed to an institution for the insane their pronounced mental symptoms soon pass off and they must then be discharged before they can receive any benefit from treatment which should extend over months and should endeavor to reclaim the alcoholic and again make him a useful member of society.

Recently a step has been taken in the right direction and a Farm Colony for Inebriates is about to be organized to which alcoholics may be committed for a sufficiently long period to effect some permanent good.

Only in the case of women alcoholics or drug habitués, an application may be made to a judge of a court of record or a city magistrate for the commitment of such a patient to St. Vincent's Retreat, at Harrison, N. Y., and the procedure is similar to that provided for in the commitment of the insane, but personal service must in every case be made at least three days before the application and if the patient resists the commitment it results in unenviable notoriety which the relatives and friends naturally dread and in the great majority of cases causes them to prefer not to avail themselves of the law which authorizes the procedure.

The laws of our adjoining State of Connecticut permit a more liberal treatment of the alcoholic and drug problem and allow the commitment of patients who indulge immoderately in alcohol or narcotic drugs and in this wise we can frequently reclaim some patients who would otherwise be lost.

Under the laws of Connecticut an alcoholic morphine or cocaine habitué can be committed either by a voluntary commitment which holds the patient for a definite period such as a year or six months and is binding on the patient just as an involuntary commitment for the whole period, or if the patient refuses to sign any such commitment on the complaint of a friend or relative made to a judge of a Probate Court. The judge appoints two physicians to examine the patient. These examiners must not be related by blood or marriage to the patient or complainant and not have any connection with any asylum for the insane. Personal service must be made upon the patient. In the case of insane patients they may be held for forty-eight hours merely on the complaint of a relative or friend until the patient can be examined and the judge's order obtained.

In securing the commitment of an alcoholic or drug patient the words immoderate use of alcohol or narcotic drugs are substituted for the word insane in the commitment papers.

In the commitment of a person alleged to be insane in New Jersey the procedure is modeled after the New York method, but the physicians must have been in the actual practice of their profession for at least five years and the patient may be taken to the state hospital before the judge approves the papers and kept for a period of ten days. During this period the papers must be submitted to the judge of the court in which the hospital is situated and he may require further testimony if he deems it necessary.

The discussion on Dr. Steinach's paper was opened by Dr. Thornton, who agreed upon almost all points brought out by the reader of the paper, and one of the things emphasized particularly was that the insane were sick persons and should be treated as such and not as criminals when it becomes necessary to commit them to an institution.

CHOLECYSTITIS.

BY

WALTER H. ROSS, M. D.,
Brooklyn, N. Y.

A complete resume of this condition in a single paper of ordinary length is an impossibility. Consequently no such attempt will be made. The object of the writer will be rather to direct attention to the importance of the subject and to a rational treatment based on the underlying factors in cholecystitis with or without gall-stones. The prevalence of instances of gall-stone disease renders the subject one worthy of careful consideration by the general practitioner just as much as by the gastroenterologist and the surgeon. In fact the disease is essentially a medical one. Even those cases in which resort to surgery is necessary are dependent on medication for permanent good results. The lack of appreciation of the number of cases and the want of a rational treatment has caused this fact to be overlooked. Until very recent years the diagnosis of cholecystitis immediately placed the physician in a quandary. If he owned up to comparative

helplessness he lost his reputation and his patient; on the other hand if he promised relief he was gambling on chances and was self-consciously a fakir. A few statistics on the prevalence of gall-stones must be of interest. Autopsies disclose the presence of gall-stones in 25% of all subjects over 60 years of age, and in from 3-10% of all cadavers. Many of the subjects never had a single classical symptom to direct attention to that portion of their anatomy.

Seventy-five per cent. are parturient women from 30 to 60 years of age. Those are the figures for gall-stones in cadavers. Next let us examine a few percentages in cholecystitis. MacCarty in his extensive research and compilation has found that in acute catarrhal cholecystitis 69% have gall-stones, in chronic catarrhal cholecystitis 76% have gall-stones, while in chronic cholecystitis the percentage is 93.

Gall-stone disease is not purely a disease due to a foreign body but is primarily a hepatic disorder. The removal of stones is but the mechanical beginning of treatment as will be appreciated by a consideration of the underlying causes.

Causes.— The disagreement over the cause of cholecystitis is due to the fact that there is no one cause. The condition is the result of all the causes that have been seriously advanced. The oldest theory that gall-stones are the result of biliary deficiency in the sodium salts is as true as it ever was. For many years Nauym's theory of infection has prevailed. Recently Aschoff and Bacmeister after considerable research work and many autopsies have assigned stasis as the essential cause. All are probably true causes, conjointly but not individually.

Stasis may be due to pregnancy (90% of all cases are parturient women) sedentary habits, gormandizing, tight lacing, kinks, anomalies of form or situation of the liver, general ptosis, or external pressure from misplaced organs or of growths or of anything else which prevents the emptying of the gall-bladder by the action of the diaphragm and the abdominal organs.

Infection seems to be an essential factor, at least it is always present. It comes from the portal circulation and an abnormal liver or else extends upward from the duodenum. True the duodenum when healthy does not contain the bacillus coli communis or the bacillus typhosis. But if due consideration be given to the history of every case it will be seen that all cases are preceded by a gastroduodenal catarrh of long duration. In cholecystitis this catarrh has extended by the way of the common duct to the gall-bladder. The consequent excess of mucus changes the composition of the bile and a good medium is thereby provided for bacteria. In those cases where the infection comes from above improper functional activity of the liver has already deteriorated the bile and the effect is the same. While bile pure and undefiled is practically aseptic it is not as was formerly believed, antiseptic. Diluted bile has no germicidal power whatever. Given these conditions it is only natural that gall-stones are the logical sequel.

Next let us consider the composition of the stones. Whether there is one large or one thousand small stones, careful analysis always shows 70 to 80% cholesterin. What is cholesterin? Where does it come from? Where does it go? Whether it is an intermediate product of metabolism or a waste product of digestion is still an open question. Nerve tissue always contains an appreciable amount, the gray matter of the brain yields 20% cholesterin. It is in atheromatous arteries and a little is present in the blood. It is a constituent of pus and all exudates and abnormal collections of fluid.

The properties of cholesterin are of especial interest from a therapeutic standpoint. It is insoluble in water, dilute acids, dilute or concentrate alkalies and cold alcohol. It is soluble in ether, chloroform, benzole and most important of all in volatile fatty acids. It is held in solution in the bile by the bile acid salts. With these facts in mind as a working basis what treatment is to be instituted? The considerations of emergency treatment and differential diagnosis are not within the scope of this limited paper. The condition is cholecystitis. Whether a mild case complaining merely of indigestion, heavy feeling after eating, and general lassitude but with a tender spot on pressure at the tip of the 10th rib (such a case is often diagnosed indigestion and dosed with pepsin and hydrochloric acid or papain) or whether a severe case with colic, palpable gall-bladder, and the many other symptoms the condition varies only in degree.

Treatment.— Complete obstruction of the duct or virulent infection demand immediate operation. Otherwise it is safe to follow the lead of Kehr and Moynahan, who in their exhaustive treatise advise medical measures in all cases for a period of six weeks before deciding definitely that operation is necessary. Whether the case be operative or non-operative the conditions are twofold. In general there is an overloaded and deteriorated system for which tonics, limited diet and stimulation of all the emunctories are indicated. Specifically there are an abnormal liver, a diseased gall-bladder full of bacteria, a debased bile and a gastrointestinal catarrh. For the catarrh, calomel

164   AMERICAN MEDICINE }
Complete Series, Vol. XVIII. }   ORIGINAL ARTICLES   { MARCH, 1912.
New Series, Vol. VII., No. 3.

and salines are indicated, especially sodium phosphate ℥i to ii daily, for the liver we use cholagogues. This method of treatment builds up the system and allays inflammation. But we must remember that the cholecystitis and perhaps the stones are still there. Unless these are removed future attacks are inevitable. To successfully treat this condition it is essential to remember the existence of the stasis and to find and remove its cause, to remember that cholesterin constitutes 70 to 80% of any stones and that it is soluble in volatile fatty acids and is held in solution by the bile salts, also to remember the lack of sodium salts and the presence of bacteria. Former treatment with olive oil, sodium benzoate, saline, glycerine and Durande's drops did not affect these conditions. The modern rational treatment is directed at the underlying causes. Sodium salicylate which is excreted by the epithelial cells of the hepatic duct is valuable for relieving congestion of the mucous membrane as well as for its antiseptic power. Hexamethylene-tetramine is excreted by the liver and the pancreas as well as by the kidneys and is a useful antiseptic in these cases. Acid sodium oleate is useful as a solvent through its excess of oleic acid. It acidifies the bile, keeps it fluid, prevents formation of gall-stones and aids in dissolving them if present. Iron succinate is a cholagogue of thirty-five years standing. Sodium succinate is of more recent origin. Both lessen spasm and aid in emptying the gall-bladder of bile and small stones. Sodium glycocholate and sodium taurocholate act as direct solvents of cholesterin in addition to their physiological action. Each and all supply sodium.

Physiological experiments have proven that these drugs are eliminated at least in part by the liver. They furnish the neces-

sary action where it is needed. Cholecystitis can usually be cured by the intelligent exhibition of the above mentioned remedies combined with a rational mode of life. For successful permanent results whether the case be operative or non-operative, the treatmust must be vigorous and not only the physician but also the patient must be sufficiently impressed with the long duration of the underlying conditions and the consequent necessity of persistent continued and not spasmodic treatment even long after all active symptoms have subsided.

215 Jefferson Ave.

MORBIFIC PROCESSES CONTROLLED BY THE HYPODERMIC USE OF ASEPTIC CHEMICAL SOLUTIONS.[1]

BY

JOHN BLAKE WHITE, M. D.,
New York City.

In the broad field of therapeutics there is no fact better established today than the prompt and energetic absorption of vegetable and mineral substances, administered by way of the skin, their rapid distribution throughout the human economy—and their resultant frequent favorable resolution of disease.

Since the practice of hypodermic medication, first introduced by Dr. Alexander Wood of Edinburgh, a certain limited number of physicians and notably Dr. Charles Hunter of London, appreciating the value of the method, became interested in the subject; but the practice was confined especially to the administration of morphia for the relief of neuralgia. Hunter alone did, however, actively push the practice further;

---

[1] Read before the Greater N. Y. Med. Assoc., Dec. 19th, 1910.

using other remedies from time to time as occasion required, and published his experience with the results in a number of very instructive essays.

Quite a dispute arose at this time over the necessity for localization of the injection and it became a veritable *quaestio vexata,* but I believe it is now pretty generally conceded that the benefit is realized quite as speedily and fully without regard to the special site of the hypodermatic administration, except in some rare instances when direct injections are deemed advisable.

Wood's method did originally have for its object, the local treatment of local affections in this way, but it naturally limited the sphere of its usefulness and its action to various forms of neuralgia, to sciatica, and to such cases as were alone within reach of the hypodermic needle.

Hunter, on the contrary, took the firm stand that localization of the injection even in neuralgic cases was both wrong in theory and unnecessary in practice.

We are living in times when quick results in medicine, as in every pursuit in life, are demanded and expected, and the method of administering remedies for the purpose of safely meeting these conditions cannot fail to secure the utmost attention of the thoughtful physician.

There is far less need, it appears to me of new therapeutical agents than a much better knowledge of the value of those we already possess and the acquirement of superadded judgment and skill in utilizing them.

The fault is, not with the well stocked materia medica but rests, as often asserted, with our own deficiency in appreciation of the therapeutic value of the many good remedies afforded us and the best manner of using the materials at hand in order to obtain the full benefit which is desired.

I have an abiding faith in our ability to overcome many morbific operations with the remedies within our grasp if we only give the time for investigation and exercise the patience required to establish the germs of true value which are realized in the proper administration of these remedies so as to secure speedy results, and to accomplish the purposes for which they are prescribed.

The divine art of healing is fast approaching, if it has not already attained that point in therapeutics when an assurance can be felt, that by a judicious selection and skilful use of remedies employed hypodermatically, diseased action can be summarily checked in many instances. There never was in the history of medicine a time, like the present, when greater caution is required to avoid being misled by popular clamor in favor of some pretentious antitoxins.

The Italian specialist, Tomasoli, claimed remarkable healing results with hypodermic injections of a medicated solution of common salt and bicarbonate of soda, and without referring to other similar reports by reputable authorities the question may be very naturally raised, how much if any of the alleged virtues ascribed to some animal serums may not be justly attributed to the active antiseptic agency of their intermixed saline ingredients if not to the presence of the very antiseptics used for their preservation.

Are we not so zealously seeking for specifics, that we are losing sight of rational therapeutics, doomed at last to find disappointment in the elusive claims of some new drug or exploited serum?

All of the different avenues open to the administration of useful remedies have not been so fully explored that we can assume, without further consideration, the limit of investigation to have been attained.

The credit of opening this new path by hypodermosis to the treatment of disease generally, and of nonlocal affections especially has been justly accorded to Hunter by Scanzoni, Ogle and a few others who have furnished the journals with their experience in trials of this method.

Though the effects are most marked in affections involving the nervous system, there are many other affections referable to blood diseases which furnish decided evidence of the superiority of hypodermatic medication.

An important application of its usefulness was brought to notice by Dr. Moore, of the Bombay medical service in the treatment of malarial fevers, wherein quinine was administered successfully in one-fifth the dose that would have been required by the stomach and with much more positive results. This is very easily understood when we reflect how rapidly morbific processes progress and note the progressive changes which are superinduced and so greatly intensified long before the slow effects of remedies taken by the mouth, to antagonize them, can be absorbed and assimilated.

It must be conceded then, that the hypodermatic method is far superior to the stomachic, rectal, or so-called endermic modes of administering medicine, particularly in emergent cases, where the indications are for anodynes, analgesics, antispasmodics, or when it is desired to arrest the absorption of some septic matter.

There is not much certainty about the stomachic dose so liable to be rejected, and if retained is only partly, or wholly absorbed in so slow a manner, as to do no real good.

In the critical moment of the absorption of deadly toxins, no physician wishes to rely on the administration of antidotes in dilatory doses, by the stomach, if he knows that certain pure chemical substances, whose physiological action has been well ascertained can produce by some antiseptic counter inoculation, results that will positively annul inimical influences and insure speedy convalescence.

What the particular mode of action is however, whereby chemical compounds introduced hypodermically to antagonize disease act, remains still obscure, though physiology and her sister science, pathology, continue to diffuse their searchlights over the mysterious processes of life, in both health and disease. Some explanation may be ventured, in the view advanced, that certain simple antidotal influences are brought about upon somatic poisons, which threaten to derange the blood and tissues, by destroying the toxins in which certain pathogenic germs flourish. Recent researches also seem to demonstrate that they often act as reinforcing allies to the phagocytes, in their friendly efforts to destroy every nidus in which menacing microbes develop and multiply, sending out hostile forces to attack the component materials of the body.

Some reinforcing effects have been observed a number of times from the hypodermic injections of a combination of chloride of gold and sodium with manganese iodide and arsenite of strychnia in tuberculosis and some forms of persistent anemia, due to other causes, after other remedies extolled for such conditions have signally failed to produce any benefit when administered per orem. I have continued to practice this method of treatment in tuberculosis with gratifying success. I did not cast around the composition of the solution, suggested by myself, a veil of mystery as was practiced by a professional brother of a distant city, who catching the cue from my publications on the subject,[1] originated another formula with similar ingredients and derived from it a handsome royalty from a manufacturing chemist. With ordinary human characteristic the profession saw no mystery in the solution which I frankly divulged, so it prescribed generally and continued to recommend the proprietary combination, to the exclusion of the original but less mysterious solution that I advised. It has tritely been said that if you surround anything with mystery it immediately assumes an importance far beyond its merits.

Interest in endermic medication dates far back to 1804 when a treatise was presented by Christien on the intraleptic method, which was translated into German by Bischoff.

Lambert in 1828 and Richter in 1835 discussed the endermatic method in more or less elaborate essays, which were soon followed by the work of Madden of Edinburgh in 1838, who styled his treatise "Experimental enquiry into the physics of cutaneous absorption." Lafargue published results he had accomplished by insertion of morphia into the skin along the trajectory of the nerve affected with neuralgia and inserted a needle trocar whereby he could effectually deposit morphia in form of paste into the skin. He very curiously attributed the curative results of this practice to the pustules that formed at the site of the in-

oculations, and studied very carefully their development and structure.

Vallieux, Cazenave, Malgaigne, Hayem, and others in France; Langenbeck, Bertrand, and Von Bruns in Germany; Rynd in Dublin, and Washington and Taylor in New York repeated the practice of Lafargue, though in some instances modified the method employed. In 1839 Washington and Taylor inserted morphia in solution instead of in a paste, using for the purpose an Anel syringe. In 1859, Scanzoni of Wurtzburg, Oppolzer of Vienna, Von Graefe of Berlin and a number of others, in different localities, adopted the method and reported favorably upon its usefulness. In 1865, Lorent of Bremen published a brief treatise on the subject followed in 1866 by Erlenmeyer, who wrote an elaborate monograph which passed through three editions, so great was the interest manifested in the method. A second elaborate work was published by Albert Eulenberg in Berlin in 1867, in which he referred to two hundred and twenty articles in various languages, chiefly German, that appeared since 1855.

As late, however, as 1868, Anstie wrote that the method was still very much unappreciated in England.

It is said that our countryman the late Fordyce Barker was presented when in England with a hypodermic syringe by Prof. Simpson, which he used on his return to America and was credited as the first in this country to practice hypodermatic medication as used at the present day.

The two methods essentially designated as hypodermatic are the subcutaneous or cellular and the deep or parenchymatous. The former however is the only one that will admit of consideration in this paper, and which is referred to in Bartholow's

[1] N. Y. Med. Rec., Dec. 27, 1890, and March 21, 1891. The Medical and Surgical Bulletin, April 1, 1894.

elaborate work of 1891, 5th edition on "Hypodermatic Medication," wherein he refers to certain additions that became necessary because of the greater importance of the method since the germ theory of disease has so closely occupied the etiological field, and adds that it is only by such means that pathogenic organisms can be promptly and effectually overcome. He declares the important advantages over other methods of treatment are the certainty of the results and if judiciously and skilfully used prove both curative and permanent. No gastric disturbance is likely to follow and the administration can be made to those who are either unwilling or unable to swallow. Further, the remedy given in this way is not modified by the condition of the stomach, nor will it undergo change in structure or chemical constitution by the gastrointestinal juices as it is very likely to do, when given by the stomach.

Neither time nor space will admit of a detailed reference to the various remedies which may be employed hypodermatically, generally and specifically, with advantage, but I will, if I may claim your attention a little longer, give some interesting illustrations of my own experiences on these lines. One's judgment and experience in prescribing will of course suggest suitable remedies in proper form and dose for hypodermic application and fit the remedy to the case. An admirable classification however, of remedies to meet particular conditions will be found in Bartholow's Manual of Hypodermatic Medication.

The public is not yet sufficiently educated to the appreciation of the full value of this method of receiving medicine and as they know of only one remedy which is used in this way, are apt to look upon every hypodermic dose with suspicion as necessarily an anodyne and are therefore often averse to submitting to treatment in this way. So fixed is this idea in the minds of some very impressionable persons that I have noted instances where the patient fell asleep after a hypodermic injection which contained nothing whatever of a soporific nature.

Having used this method very extensively for over fifteen years I could not help being impressed with its importance, and sometimes I have been amazed at the prompt and certain results achieved with remedies that have hitherto failed when administered by the mouth. With a large number of convincing proofs of the utility of hypodermatic medication it is not remarkable in the least that I unhesitatingly advocate its more general adoption and prefer to use rather solutions of pure chemical substances than the less understood animal serums so much flaunted at the present day. It is without fear of proof to the contrary that I am ready to record the assertion that no benefit can be obtained from animal serums which cannot be realized from well selected and prepared chemical solutions administered in like manner for the same purposes.

Many eminent surgeons tell us that the antistreptococcus serum has often disappointed them when used to combat septic conditions, whereas the solution of carbolated sulphoborate of zinc, which I have employed on several occasions will check the progress of pathogenic germ absorption with a degree of certainty that is often surprising.

This treatment was tried in propria persona when septicemia threatened following a wound of the finger acquired while operating on a septic patient. I had headache, fever, the glands of the axilla grew tender and swollen, and the usual reddish line, indicative of septic absorption, extended from the seat of the wound to the axilla, along the chain of the lymphatics. Physical depression and edema of the hand and forearm combined to present alarming evidences of developing septicemia. In the space of an hour after I received the hypodermic of the above mentioned antiseptic solution I experienced such marked relief that I fell asleep, subsequently awoke almost devoid of pain, and all the other associated symptoms had ameliorated. Before the hypodermic was received I had been restless, wakeful, with a sense of fever and general uneasiness, all of which disappeared after three or four administrations of the solution and the improvement continued to a permanent recovery. The lymphangitis with the axillary involvement gradually diminished and finally disappeared.

It was most interesting to note that *pari passu* with each hypodermic medication an unmistakable degree of mitigation was progressively manifest in each one of the urgent symptoms; but the more remarkable evidence of retrogression of the septic influence from the center to the point of invasion was quite perceptible. Just as the septic absorption had advanced before the injections from the periphery toward the interior, so its advance was promptly met and the evidences of its presence gradually receded from the center back toward the original site of its reception. The axillary glands first lost their tender and tumefied condition; next the inflamed course of the lymphatics lessened in hue and gradually faded away from the distal point toward the seat of the primary lesion and finally the edema about the forearm and hand entirely disappeared.

A man of 35 while obtaining some ice from his ice box managed to pierce the palmar surface of the left hand with the point of the ice pick. Soon the hand as well as the forearm became much swollen and painful and the indications of threatening suppuration were very apparent, but the condition and symptoms all promptly yielded to a few antiseptic hypodermics of the nature described and the patient convalesced without his condition advancing to suppuration and demanding incision with drainage.

I have noticed this same happy termination follow this line of treatment in a number of other cases but will not consume more time in similar illustrations as the two instances described will serve in a general way to demonstrate the value of the hypodermatic medication in such emergencies.

It will be noted, moreover, what considerable power to lower the temperature when fever is present that these antiseptic hypodermics possess.

There is no doubt that there are many defects in the manner of administering remedies per integumentum but they are of minor consequence and not beyond correction.

In selecting remedies for hypodermatic use it is of first importance to secure those which are readily soluble and are least likely to cause any irritation to the tissues. The relative therapeutic dose must be carefully determined and the effects always closely watched to guard against the manifestation of idiosyncrasy which some persons show respecting some drugs. For the menstruum, sterile water is always the best when procurable, otherwise the purest spring water obtainable will do. Freshly prepared solutions are always the best to use since most of those which are kept for a long time will undergo decomposition, though it is possible with antiseptics added to overcome this tendency for a limited period.

A word about the hypodermic syringe will not be out of place at this juncture. It should be an instrument so constructed that there would be no possibility of carrying any contaminating material into the system through its agency. Various hypodermic syringes have been brought to notice, every new one showing the regard for antisepsis which the inventor had in mind. There is a new metal syringe made with a solid piston that is an admirable instrument, and another of glass throughout with glass piston also serviceable and safe to use, and they are easily cleansed. I am still devoted to a syringe of my own invention presenting every claim of an antiseptic instrument, which I have on previous occasions shown to those interested in this subject.

The advantages of importance which are claimed for this[1] over other instruments of its kind will be manifest at a glance. The great science of bacteriology has made in its marvelous advance peremptory demand for the institution of proper safeguards around the direct introduction of agents into the blood by subcutaneous injection.

The next matter deserving of our consideration is the quantity of fluid to be used, bearing in mind that too large an amount will not only cause pain but so distend the areolar space as to occasion rupture of small vessels, resulting in hemorrhage and consequent inflammation, followed by suppuration. Sometimes a large amount can be safely introduced, if the injection is care-

fully and slowly made, but no such bulk of fluid is ever required. The slow admission of the injected solution permits of its ready diffusion. Usually not more than ten or fifteen minims of a solution carrying the necessary medication is advised.

The selection of the tissue and site for the operation demand some attention and the best localities, I regard, as those where there is abundant cellular tissue under loose integumentary structure. Such places better accommodate the injected liquid and promote its more rapid diffusion and these sites are found in the lateral lumbar regions or about the abdominal walls.

The arm, forearm, thighs and legs do not present such eligible sites for hypodermics, because the very close relation of the fasciae of muscles and their adjacent tendons affords greater resistance to the insertion of the needle, produces more pain and renders absorption of the fluid much less active.

To properly administer a hypodermic injection the skin should be firmly pinched up between the left forefinger and thumb and the needle pushed quickly, well through the integument into the cellular tissue beyond. Care should be taken not to place the injection between the layers of the skin for the pressure of the fluid, however small in amount, or non-irritating in effect, would certainly occasion unnecessary pain.

To wipe off the seat of the contemplated hypodermic with a clean piece of absorbent cotton saturated with some of the many antiseptic solutions or with alcohol, is always a proper procedure when practicable, and an additional treatment of the spot with ether, insures some degree of insensitiveness of the surface of the skin. This last expedient it is well not to overlook, when dealing with very nervous subjects or such

[1] *Journal of Cutaneous and Genito-Urinary Diseases*, March, 1892.

as are particularly apprehensive of being hurt. Usually no bleeding follows the operation, but if a few drops of blood should exude when the needle is withdrawn it is well to bathe the part with an antiseptic wash and apply slight pressure over the bleeding part.

I have administered as many as a hundred and fifty or more injections to the same subject, selecting different sites for the operation, though I have made some.injections in close proximity to each other, without observing the slightest indication of any local irritation.

In many thousand such operations extending over a period of many years I have never noticed the appearance of an abscess. Occasionally however, some slight inflammation has followed the puncture, but it never progressed to suppuration and this demonstrates, not only the care exercised in the administration of the injections, with the accompanying antiseptic precautions advised, but affords a good additional illustration of the advantages of the hypodermic instrument which I have constantly in use.

1013 Madison Ave., N. Y.

THE DETECTION OF URETERAL AND RENAL CALCULI BY RADIOGRA-PHY: DESCRIPTION OF A NEW TECHNIQUE.

BY

PATRICK S. O'DONNELL, M. D.,
Chicago, Ill.

The value of skiagraphy for diagnosing renal disease has been acknowledged by the leading specialists in genito-urinary work all over the world. With the advancement of the technique of taking radiographs for detecting renal calculi and ureteral calculi, the differentiation of phleboliths from ureteral calculi becomes necessary, because at times it is practically impossible—using ordinary methods—to tell one from the other, especially if the small phleboliths should show somewhere in the line of the ureter.

As an aid to diagnosis many means have been adopted. Usually, passing a ureteral catheter containing lead fuse wire or fine steel is the preliminary procedure. The radiograph is then taken, and should the shadow of the metal lined catheter show in the line of the suspected calculi, it leaves little room for doubt; if entirely away from the shadow of the metal lined catheter, it is usually some calcareous deposit in the smaller veins.

To locate the pelvis of the kidney the passing of the lead line catheter is the only procedure that will give accurately the position, but the objection to this method is that in the removal of the cystoscope, the catheters are so often pulled down slightly that it is never certain the end of the lead line catheter is in the kidney.

A technique that has been adopted by many radiographers and which I find much in vogue, especially among some of the leading genito-urinary specialists, is to discard the lead line catheter entirely and after passing the catheter through the ureter, to inject some silver salt solution. It has been found that this method gives infinitely better results, for even if the catheter is pulled down considerably in removing the cystoscope, some of the silver solution will invariably reach the pelvis of the kidney and thus give a magnificent demarcation outline of the calyx.

Many different silver salt solutions have been used, but the objection to most of them has been that they set up severe irritation and renal colic if used in sufficiently strong solutions. If this irritation is to be avoided the solution has to be weak, possibly not more than 10%, at the most not over 15%, and as a consequence the shadow is so faint that it is practically valueless from a diagnostic standpoint.

A silver salt, cargentos, was introduced to me some time back by the H. K. Mulford Co., Philadelphia, which I have used for some time with gratifying results. I have found it to be absolutely nonirritating, even when used in a 50% solution, and when it is used in this strength, the shadows are equivalent if not more sharply defined than those of the metal line catheters. It is always advisable to take one radiograph of the ureter and kidneys before any catheters have been passed or any silver salt injected. This procedure is of undoubted value in differentiating hydronephrosis and cystic kidney.

In locating deep sinuses a solution of cargentos is again of undoubted value and superior to Beck's bismuth paste. I do not mean from a therapeutic standpoint, but solely for showing a clear demarcation of the extent and depth of the sinus. It has the special advantage that it runs into the cavities better than bismuth paste, and even in ulcerating wounds 50% solution may be used without causing irritation.

In conclusion I may mention that even weak solutions of cargentos, as low as 5 or 10%, give very good shadows in the less dense portion of the body, such as the bladder. Some of my fellow radiographers, who have used the salt claim that the weaker solution does not give good shadows, possibly because they have altered the character of the solution by boiling it; in my opinon this boiling is entirely unnecessary, as I am quite convinced that it is thoroughly bactericidal.

ETIOLOGY AND DIAGNOSIS.

A New Sign in the Diagnosis of Scarlet Fever.—C. Pastia, according to *Pediatrics*, describes a sign which he considers of value in the diagnosis of atypical cases of scarlet fever. It consists of a continuous linear eruption localized in the folds of flexion of the elbows. These lines are at first of a rose color, then become a deep red, and usually assume an ecchymotic appearance. The eruption may take the form of a single line, but is usually multiple, two to four lines being present, and between them the ordinary eruption of scarlet fever may be observed. The sign appears at the beginning of the eruptive period and persists to its close and is then replaced by a linear pigmentation which is visible for some time.

The presence of this linear eruption, or the pigmentation which succeeds it, should give rise to the suspicion of scarlet fever, even when the eruption is scanty on other parts of the body or has already faded. A similar condition may occasionally occur about the axilla, but is less marked and of short duration. This sign was found in 94 percent of the cases of scarlet fever in the wards of M. Grosovici, of Bucharest, as well as in a large number of cases in Paris, but it was absent in measles and various conditions simulating scarlet fever.

The Causes of Perineal Laceration.—In a complete and scholarly paper read at the February meeting of the New York County Medical Society, Dr. Edgar considered the factors which bore directly and indirectly upon the causation of pelvic floor lacerations under four major classes, namely: 1. Anomalies of the expulsive forces. 2. Anomalies of the soft parts. 3. Faulty presentations of the fetus. 4. Faulty posture of the mother. In regard to the fourth factor, he stated that long observation had convinced him that extraction of the head at the outlet with the patient in the exaggerated lithotomy position conduced to unnecessary injury of the pelvic floor. At the moment of extraction or expulsion of the head, the patient's thighs should be brought down into the ordinary dorsal or "cross bed" posture. Moreover, the delivery of the head through the pelvic outlet with the forceps still applied was usually unnecessary and favored laceration. After considering the time when it was advisable to repair these lacerations and the technique that he employed, the writer concluded as follows: 1. More attention should be given to the causes and prevention of perineal lacerations as in this way many perineorrhaphies would be avoided. 2. Broadly speaking, all lacerations were best closed at the time of labor, but in those accompanied by bruising, edema, and swelling the best results were obtained by waiting a few hours or a day or so until conditions were more favorable. Tears involving the rectum should be treated more deliberately, due time being given for the nutrition of the parts to improve, for the patient to recover from the shock of labor, and for the securing of assistance and conveniences. 3. In all cases before suturing the torn surfaces should be cleansed and the edges coapted with tenacula in order to determine their proper relationship. 4. The sutures should not be drawn too tight as they would cut through the tissues. 5. Chemical antiseptics should be avoided. 6. An assistant should be procured to administer the anesthetic; ether should not be entrusted to a nurse unless she was trained in its use. Ether should be used and not chloroform. 7. In rectal tears, sutures knotted in the rectum gave better results, the wound being less likely to become infected than when buried sutures were knotted on the vaginal side of the laceration. 8. In primary perineorrhaphy interrupted sutures for the vaginoperineal lacerations gave better results than the buried layer suture. As to the after treatment, the knees should be loosely bound together and the use of the catheter should be avoided, if possible. Thorough cleanliness of the external genitals should be maintained, but no douche should be used unless the lochia become putrid. The bowels should be made to move after the second day by an injection of oil and an enema should be entrusted only to an experienced nurse. In the passage of a vaginal or rectal tube, the greatest care should be exercised not to disturb the sutures.

TREATMENT.

Treatment of Gastroptosis.[1]—A modification of Rose's adhesive plaster bandage has given Soper much satisfaction, particularly in thin subjects whose abdomens are so depressed that a serious obstacle is presented to the adjustment of a proper support to the displaced viscera. The modification consists in the use of narrow (2 inch) strips. The pubic hair is thus avoided, and much less surface is covered than by Rose's bandage. The patient is therefore more comfortable and enjoys more freedom of movement. The method of applying the bandage is as follows: The patient sits on a couch, the adhesive strip is fastened to the dorsal vertebrae and follows the right lower rib margins; the patient now lies down, the lower abdominal contents are pushed upward with the operator's left hand while the bandage is carried across the abdomen and attached to the left side at Poupart's ligament. The patient again sits up and a second strip is applied to the other side in exactly the same way as the first one. Finally a third strip is attached across from one superior iliac spine to the other, the patient lying down. The bandage can be worn comfortably for two weeks. Bathing is not interfered with. It is easily removed by gasoline and benzine, or by oil of wintergreen. The bandage may be reapplied immediately, or in the event that irritation of the skin occurs, an interval of several days may elapse before replacing it. Special exercises of the abdominal muscles, accompanied by proper breathing, must be at once instituted. The diet should be as nutritious as possible, but in no class of cases is more individualization required. The food should be adapted to the patient's digestive powers.

The Treatment of Gonorrheal Urethritis.[1]— The first principle, says Breakstone, in the treatment of gonorrhea is, as in all inflammations, REST. By "rest," in this case, we mean both urinary and urinary rest. Of course, it is impossible to get urinary rest, so we must be content to limit our efforts in this regard to sexual rest (although we may minimize urinary irritation); and so I instruct my patient to avoid any erotic influences, to sleep in a cool room on a rather hard mattress, and always to lie on his side. Sometimes it becomes necessary for me to instruct him to tie a towel around his waist, with a knot at his spine, so that it will be impossible for him to sleep on his back with any degree of comfort.

The measures named nearly always are sufficient to procure sexual rest. However, in obstinate cases (and I wish to emphasize here, that in some cases the sexual passion is increased in gonorrhea), to avoid chordee, I prescribe, in addition to the measures I have already mentioned, a capsule made up of 2 grains of powdered camphor and one of powdered opium, to be taken on retiring. This dose should be repeated in case any tendency to chordee develops during the night. The patient should always be instructed to empty his bladder before retiring.

The next step in the treatment is to lessen the acidity of the urine, and thus avoid any further local irritation. This is best done by a mixture of the following composition: Copaiba, drs. 6; liquor potassae, drs. 2; camphor water, oz. 1. Label: A teaspoonful, followed by two glasses of water, three times a day, after meals.

Diuretics.—The best diuretic is water, and this is the only one that I ever use. I instruct my patient to drink from eighteen to twenty glasses of water a day. This dilutes the urine and renders it less acid.

Antiseptics.—The only urinary antiseptic that I use is hexamethylenamine. It can be demonstrated that formaldehyde is found in the urine within half an hour after taking this drug. Hexamethylenamine has no effect on the gonococcus, but it keeps the urine aseptic and prevents a mixed infection.

Urinary Sedatives.—The only remedy of this nature I use is the time-honored copaiba, as shown in the prescription just given. This drug has been used for this disease for more than five hundred years, and we still go back to it today. At the Vienna Allgemeines Krankenhaus, which has the largest venereal clinic in the world, the attending physicians prescribe copaiba exclusively. They have printed prescriptions ready to hand out to their patients.

[1]H. W. Soper, M. D., *Jour. of the Missouri State Med. Soc.*, Dec., 1911.

[1]Benj. H. Breakstone, M. D., *Am. Jour. Clin. Med.*, Jan., 1912.

There are cases, it is true, in which copaiba produces a bad effect on the stomach. In such, I substitute cubebs or buchu, or I just give potassium acetate with no other urinary sedative. On the whole, the bad effect that copaiba has on the stomach is rather a good thing in most patients, since this will decrease the appetite and therefore limit the amount of food eaten. It must also be remembered that in a few instances copaiba will produce a rash, which quickly subsides on the withdrawal of the drug.

It is very important to instruct a patient as to diet. All stimulating things must be prohibited. Anything that will increase the acidity of the urine, such as meats and other nitrogenous food, should be very strictly limited. Spices, tea, and coffee should be allowed in but very small quantities. Vegetables, milk, and such like bland foods may be taken in abundance. Overfeeding should be carefully avoided, as in this, the same as in any other infection, we should be careful not to introduce more food than is necessary. In this way it is in our power to limit the local congestion. Above all, everything containing even the smallest quantity of alcohol must be absolutely prohibited. Lemonade, sodawater, pop, ginger ale, and all carbonated waters may be allowed in abundance.

THERAPEUTIC NOTES.

Drugs in Rheumatic Conditions.[1]—Salicylic acid, Stockman says, is undoubtedly the most powerful antirheumatic drug known to us, and the action of all salicyl compounds depends on the extent of their conversion into it in the body. Of these compounds salicin, acetylsalicylic acid, salol and methyl salicylate are of most clinical importance. Salicin has a bitter taste, and is much less nauseous than sodium salicylate, and can be conveniently given dissolved in hot water in which it is fairly soluble. It only yields 43 per cent. of its weight of salicylic acid, and hence the amount required is at least double that of sodium salicylate, 20 to 30 grains every hour or two hours until 1 ounce has been given and then in smaller doses according to the circumstances. Acetylsalicylic acid is very active and has a marked analgesic effect It cannot be prescribed with alkalis which decompose it, and hence it is apt to bring on nausea and vomiting if given continuously. Methyl salicylate is also very apt to irritate the gastric mucous membrane, but in 10 to 20 minim doses up to 60 or 90 minims per day, given in emulsion, or on sugar, or in milk, it acts powerfully, and externally applied it is unrivaled for its analgesic action in rheumatic conditions. Salol and salicylate of quinin are antirheumatics only to the extent of their salicylic acid content, which is roughly about one-half in each case; their value in acute conditions is therefore small. Sodium benzoate has the

[1]R. Stockman, F. R. C. P., *London Practitioner*, Jan., 1912.

same specific effect as the salicylate, but exerts a less powerful and decided influence. On the other hand it is practically nonpoisonous and has no disturbing side-effects. It can be given in 20 grain doses every two or three hours with satisfactory results in cases of uncomplicated rheumatic fever, but its practical usefulness is merely as a substitute for the more powerful salicylate when the latter cannot be tolerated.

GENERAL TOPICS.

Property Rights vs. Public Health.[1]—A New York dealer in drugs was recently prosecuted for counterfeiting the trade-mark of Carter's Little Liver Pills and for selling goods bearing this counterfeit mark. He was found guilty and, although it was the first offense, the court refused to impose a fine, but sentenced him to four months' imprisonment in the penitentiary at hard labor without the possibility of commutation for good behavior. Counterfeiting, of course, is a serious crime and as such should be punished. Nevertheless, there are more serious crimes, such, for instance, as adulterating foodstuffs, selling putrid material for good or dispensing dangerous habit-forming drugs, like cocain, in the shape of soft drinks. All these crimes are crimes against the person—against the public health—against the very lives of the people. Although the government officials have brought evidence sufficient to convict over 1,300 firms or individuals of violating the federal Food and Drugs Act, and although this act provides that its violation may be punished by imprisonment, yet in not a single instance has the court imposed any sentence more severe than a fine. And the majority of the fines have been trivial to a degree. A Canton (Ohio) concern was convicted of selling a soft drink containing cocain. The court considered a $25 fine sufficient punishment. A St. Louis house sold a powder for infants that was said to make "teething" easy; it contained opium. A $10 fine was sufficient punishment. An "agreeable and efficient tonic" was found to contain cocain, although the presence of this drug was not stated. In this case, the court suspended sentence! Some day, possibly, a court may be found that will consider the crimes of making drug fiends of young people, of poisoning babies with opium mixtures or of killing women with headache powders as more serious offenses than the counterfeiting of the label of a fraudulent "patent medicine." Apparently, that time is far off.

Astounding Fecundity.—It is said that a man and his wife in Boynton, Okla., are parents of eleven children born in three years. Triplets one year, triplets the next year, and five the year after. The oldest child is fourteen and then come twins five years old, then the

[1]Editorial *Jour. A. M. A.*, Mar. 9, 1912.

eleven, as given above. At this rate of geometrical progression the parents would better call a halt or they will exhaust their bank account in a few years.

Boils in Diabetes.—Boils in diabetics, when seen early (*Med. Summary*), may often be aborted by rubbing in a 2 per cent. ointment of the yellow oxide of mercury in lanolin. Where they persist, tonics, vaccine, antiseptics, free drainage, and sometimes excision are valuable. After healing, bathing of parts several times daily for two weeks with an antiseptic solution may prevent further infection of the area.

SOCIETY PROCEEDINGS.

THE YORKVILLE MEDICAL SOCIETY.

A meeting of the Yorkville Medical Society was held at the New York Turn Verein Hall, No. 1253 Lexington Ave., Feb. 19th, 1912. The President, Dr. Sidney Jacobson, in the Chair. There was an attendance of about 75 members and visitors.

At the Executive Session, Dr. Samuel Floersheim of No. 808 Lexington Avenue was elected to membership. The report and recommendations of the Committee on Economic Research were presented by its chairman, Dr. O. Rotter, as follows:

"Two subjects were taken up for discussion and action. The abuse of Dispensary charity by patients able to pay for medical services and the growing invasion of the field of private practice by the supplying of free treatment, in many cases without discrimination on the part of the Board of Health. Of various measures discussed to bring about an enforcement of the existing law, restricting free treatment at Dispensaries to the really poor and to keep the therapeutic activity of the Board of Health equally within the restriction of this law the following two plans were adopted and decided upon:

First, to address to the Department of Charities a petition to establish some efficient system of control to carry out the spirit and letter of the Dispensary law, such control to be exercised by the Department of Charity in the interest of a wise and conscientious expenditure of public funds, the physician in private practice, and last but not least, the Dispensary physicians who give their time and services to the community without compensation.

Second, to address a petition to the Board of Health requesting it to restrict its therapeutic activity at the public schools, at its Dispensaries or at the homes of patients, to the poor only.

Dr. L. H. Schwartz, as corresponding secretary of the committee was accordingly instructed to draw up letters of petition to the Department of Charity and the Board of Health.

Dr. Grosse had received information that a certain woman whose husband is established in business on 5th Ave. was receiving free treatment at the Dispensary of the German Hospital. Dr. Grosse notified the superintendent of the hospital to this effect, such notification implying the request to exclude the person named from the benefits of free treatment. Receipt of this letter of protest was duly acknowledged and action promised.

The address delivered before the Professional Club will appear in the next issue of "*American Medicine*." That there is an awakening interest in medico-economic questions in medical circles all over the country is proven by the fact that Dr. Rotter's address before the Yorkville Medical Society on "The Economic Problem as it affects the Medical Profession" was reprinted from the "*Critic and Guide*" by the "*Oklahoma Medical News-Journal*," Oklahoma City, in its January issue.

The following letters were read. Thereafter a motion was made and carried by an unanimous vote to mail them to their respective addresses.

NEW YORK CITY, March, 1912.
Commissioner of Public Charities,
  New York City, N. Y.
Dear Sir:
  Many patients in a position to pay for medical services are treated daily in various dispensaries and hospitals gratis. This is a violation of Section 718 of the Criminal Code, which makes it a misdemeanor to obtain medical aid upon false representations.

Will you kindly inform the members of this society who is responsible for the enforcement of this law, in order that we may stop the abuse or at least lessen it?
      Very respectfully yours,
        OSCAR ROTTER, M. D., 217 East 79th St.,
        Chairman, Committee on Economic
        Research, Yorkville Medical Society, N. Y. City.

NEW YORK CITY, March, 1912.
Board of Health,
  City of New York, N. Y.,
Gentlemen:
  The members of the Yorkville Medical Society wish to call your attention to the fact that a large percentage of patients suffering from pulmonary tuberculosis, summer diarrhea, contagious diseases and various conditions of the eye, ear, nose and throat, treated gratis by the Health Department physicians and nurses, are in a position to pay for such services. We therefore request and urge the Board of Health to restrict its therapeutic activities to the poor and that others be directed and required to consult a physician. We also beg you to instruct your nurses and doctors not to direct children with physical defects to the dispensaries, unless the parents are too poor to have the same attended to outside of these institutions.
      Very respectfully yours,
        OSCAR ROTTER, M. D., 217 East 79th St.

The scientific session began with the presentation of a case of Double Congenital Dislocation of the Lens in a boy of 6 years, by Dr. A. Nettle; also a case of Glaucoma cured by operation, Dr. A. Nettle.

The papers of the evening were:
Commitment of the Insane, by Dr. W. Steinach (see page 155).

A New Remedy for Tuberculosis, by Dr. Fritz Neumann.

Chemical Basis for Treatment of Cancer by Selenium, by Dr. F. von Oefele.

Discussion of Dr. von Oefele's paper was opened by Dr. Eugene Kessler, who said: While Dr. von Oefele has spoken mainly of the theoretical part of the subject of selenium and the chemistry of it, I would add a few words regarding the practical application of selenium in the treatment of carcinoma.

When examining urine for the state of metabolism, the sulphur or, to be exact, the preformed sulphuric acid, is regularly found deficient in carcinoma or in all malignant growths. For the correction of that abnormality the element selenium suggested itself. A number of such cases (inoperable) were treated with preparations of this element; in some of these cases aniline was used in addition.

And here I might say, that I pride myself upon being the first physician to treat a case of human carcinoma with a selenium preparation.

Among a number of cases of carcinoma that I have treated, permit me to cite a typical case.

A. T., 60 years old, unmarried; .15 years ago was operated upon for cancer of the breast.

Status praesens: At the time of my examination, she was cachectic, weight 109 pounds, with an arterial tension of 150 by the Riva-Rocci sphygmomanometer, heart and lungs negative. The liver extended to the umbilicus; surface nodular.

Examination of the urine showed, that the sulphuric acid had been reduced to 38% of the normal amount, and the chlorides increased.

The history of the patient, the general impression and the reduction of the sulphuric acid, led me to the diagnosis of carcinoma of the liver.

From July 27, 1910, on she received t. i. d. 1 mg. selenic oxide (Se O₂). A month later she had gained 2½ pounds and the liver shrunk 2 fingers' breadth. On September 27, the examination showed an improvement of the sulphur metabolism, which had risen to 51% of the normal and by October 20th the sulphur output had risen to the normal or above it (103%). On December 10, her weight was 116 pounds.

January 28, 1911. Steady improvement; weight 119 pounds. From now on 1 milligram sodium selenio-cyanate (Na Se CN) was given t. i. d.

February 11. A slight edema of the wrist. Urine next day showed traces of seralbumin and

hyaline casts. The treatment was stopped. This was probably due to a too rapid elimination of the products of degeneration and a consequent renal irritation.

May 3. Edema gone, weight 121½ pounds.

June 3. The sodium selenio-cyanate was again given in ½ milligram doses with occasional interruptions, and from June 3, 1911, until within a few months ago, when I last observed the patient, there was no indication of disease, and the patient felt well; during that time the sulphur metabolism was within narrow limits of the normal.

The paper was also discussed by Drs. Heckman and Dittrich.

Dr. Neumann did not read his paper and explained the omission by stating that the new remedy of which he desired to speak was lately exploited in such an inethical manner that he had concluded not to speak of the matter at all. His attention was called to this breach of etiquette, by the firm selling this product, only this very day.

A general discussion followed. After a generous collation the attendance dispersed about 11.30 p. m.

THE EASTERN MEDICAL SOCIETY OF THE CITY OF NEW YORK.

Stated Meeting, March 8th, 1912.

The Executive Session was devoted to the transaction of routine business, reports of committees, election of new members, etc.

At the Scientific Session the following papers were presented:

1. **Presentation of New Instruments.**
   A Duodenal Catheter for Infant Feeding, Dr. Alfred F. Hess.

2. **Presentation of Cases.**
   (a) *Tuberculous Glands of Neck, cured by application of X-ray,* Dr. Max Strunsky.
   (b) *Unusual General Infection, by Vincent's Bacillus and Spirocheta—Fatal Termination,* Dr. R. Johnson Held.
   (c) 1. *Vaginal Caesarean Section for Eclampsia;* 2. *Case of Pubiotomy,* Dr. Abraham J. Rongy.
   (d) *Two Cases of Fracture of the Carpal Bones,* Dr. Maurice J. Sittenfield.

3. **Papers.** *Symposium on the Practical Features of the Influenza Infection, especially in regard to Infants and Children.*
   (a) *Characteristics of Influenza in Infants,* Dr. Herman Schwarz.
   (b) *Pulmonary Complications,* Dr. William P. Northrup.
   (c) *Influenza Meningitis,* Dr. Godfrey R. Pisek.

(d) *Complications affecting the Ear, Nose and Throat*, Dr. Seymour Oppenheimer.

The papers were discussed by Drs. Henry D. Chapin, Henry Heiman, Nicol M. Mandl, T. S. Southworth, Abraham Hymanson, Henry M. Stark and Israel Strauss.

The Society then adjourned to take part in the usual collation.

The papers composing the symposium will appear in their entirety in the April issue of AMERICAN MEDICINE.

LITERARY NOTES.

Sociology and Modern Social Problems.— Formerly medicine was a purely personal service to an employer, but it is now recognized that the growth and evolution of the profession was due to its indispensable social role of preserving valuable lives. The reduction of the death rate reflexly caused the reduced birthrate which is now found to be so useful in racial advancement through the better physique and training of the smaller intelligent families, which otherwise would not survive at all. The last century has created public medicine to serve the mass, so that it is now part and parcel of the modern machinery for survival. For these reasons, sociology—the laws of group phenomena—has become a practical matter which every physician should study so as to understand his own relation to the social organism he serves and which in turn preserves him.

Until quite recently, sociology could scarcely be called a science. It was a mere collection of phenomena, which no two writers seemed able to interpret the same way, but now it is recognized as a branch of biology whose general principles explain all the phenomena or at least allow us to classify them better; and this is another reason why the medical profession is interested. To be sure, the laws regulating the conduct of a group of contiguous cells, are not exactly the same as those governing a social group of non-contiguous men, and there will be errors made by applying known biological laws too exactly, but it is far worse not to apply them at all.

We are, therefore, glad to see the present tendency of sociologists to base all their work on proved biological principles. Unfortunately the latest work on the subject, that by Prof. Chas. A. Ellwood, Prof. of Sociology, Univ. of Missouri (*Amer. Book Co.*) makes many statements which are not in accord with medical experience nor accepted by modern biologists. Indeed he does not seem to have grasped the very basis of the evolution he describes—the birth of more than can be fed—a rule which is absolutely universal in both plant and animal life. There are the usual pedagogic exaggerations as to what education can do, and how it could make a silk purse of a sow's ear. In racial matters he does not sufficiently emphasize the law of averages and variations, which fully explains how a few of the superior men of a lower race, overtop many of the inferior of a higher, and this befogs the real issue as to the effect of a high average and many superior variations.

The greatest social and racial problem of the day is not explained—the enormous preponderance of great works per million people in northern Europe as compared to the dearth of discoveries in America or the Mediterranean basin. The statements as to poverty and unemployment being remediable are not in accordance with the latest evidence either in philanthropy or biology, and there are many other evidences of the use of archaic ideas. We presume that the book would be useful to one who is thoroughly aware of the last words in human biology—if such an expression is allowable—but to ignorant students it is dangerous in that it inculcates many false biologic ideas, as well as gives the impression of too many sociologic vagaries—such as what is desirable is possible. Many laws are inoperative because they express what people should do, and not what they can and will do.

Still, it is a beginning in the right direction, and all such beginnings are good work. Sociology is undergoing such a tremendous change that in another decade or two, it will not be comparable with the present form. Every existing work will have merely historic interest, as so many of them are basically wrong and contradict each other.

The physician very frequently needs, for instant reference, a book which gives the best methods of treatment in any given case. Many books have been offered for this purpose, but they consisted only of collections of miscellaneous prescriptions and formulas, totally unrelated to each other, with no rules or reasons to guide in their use, and almost useless to the physician with any independence of thought or scientific bent of mind.

This book[1] gives a condensed intelligent discussion of the best methods of treatment, based on scientific principles, with a well-tried reliable formula occasionally to illustrate the application of the principles. The author gives many modes of treatment far in advance of the present text-books. An ingenious method of indicating relative dosage is to print the name of the drug in CAPITAL LETTERS for large doses, in ordinary type for medium doses, and in *italics* for small doses. An exhaustive "Table of Large, Medium and Small Doses" is given in the book.

[1] BLAIR'S POCKET THERAPEUTICS: A Practitioner's Handbook of Medical Treatment. By Thomas S. Blair, M. D., Neurologist to Harrisburg, Pa., Hospital; Author of "A System of Public Hygiene," "Blair's Practitioner's Handbook of Materia Medica," Member of the Harrisburg Academy of Medicine, American Medical Association, etc.; 373 pages, special Bible paper; bound in limp leather; price, $2.00 Published by The Medical Council Co., Forty-second and Chestnut Streets, Philadelphia, Pa.

178   AMERICAN MEDICINE }
Complete Series, Vol. XVIII. }   LITERARY NOTES   { MARCH, 1912.
{ New Series, Vol. VII., No. 3.

The diseases treated are divided into related groups, each group occupying a chapter, according to the following classification (a copious alphabetical index provides for instant reference to any particular disease):

Chapter I. Diseases Incidental to Birth. II. Essential Diseases of Childhood. III. Essential Diseases of Environment. IV. Diseases of Occupation. V. Infectious Diseases. VI. Diseases of the Pericardium. VII. Diseases of the Heart. VIII. Diseases of the Blood Vessels. IX. Diseases of the Bronchi. X. Diseases of the Lungs. XI. Diseases of the Pleura. XII. Diseases of the Mouth, Salivary Glands and Esophagus. XIII. Diseases of the Stomach. XIV. Diseases of the Pancreas. XV. Diseases of the Intestines. XVI. Diseases of the Rectum. XVII. Diseases of the Liver and Gall-Bladder. XVIII. Diseases of the Spleen. XIX. Diseases of the Peritoneum. XX. Diseases of the Uropoietic System. XXI. Diseases of the Lymphatic Vessels. XXII. Diseases of the Thyroid Gland. XXIII. Nutritive Disorders. XXIV. Diseases of the Blood. XXV. Mental Diseases. XXVI. Diseases of the Brain and Meninges. XXVII. Diseases of the Spinal Cord. XXVIII. Diseases of the Peripheral Nerves. XXIX. Diseases of the Muscles. XXX. Animal Parasites. XXXI. Alcoholism and Drug Addictions. XXXII. Diseases of the Skin. XXXIII. Diseases of the Hair and Nails. XXXIV. The Principal Diseases of the Eye. XXXV. Diseases of the Ear. XXXVI. Diseases of the Nose. XXXVII. Diseases of the Tonsils, Pharynx and Larynx. XXXVIII. Obstetrical Therapeutics. XXXIX. Non-Surgical Gynecology. XL. Surgical Therapeutics. XLI. Essential Diseases of Old Age. XLII. Treatment of Poisoning (arranged Alphabetically as to the Different Poisons). The Appendix gives very many necessary tables for quick reference, followed by an exhaustive Table of Doses, closing with a General Index.

In order to get all this within the compass of a book for the pocket, a very thin, tough Bible paper has been used, so that it is really a much larger book than it looks.

This book will be a useful pocket companion to the physician in his daily work.

———

The object of this book[1] is to encourage more accurate observation and study of cases by supplying a convenient form for a condensed record of each important case, in pocket size, so that the practitioner can have it always with him, and so arranged that the necessary data can be written down in the briefest possible time—preferably while the examination is actually being made.

Thoroughness of examination is encouraged by means of a Syllabus, detailing all the points that should be considered in each case.

The blank for the first thorough examina-

[1] THE TAYLOR POCKET CASE RECORD. By J. J. Taylor, M. D., 252 pages, tough bond paper; red limp leather: $1.00. Published by The Medical Council Co., Forty-second and Chestnut Streets, Philadelphia, Pa.

tion, diagnosis and treatment is followed by spaces for sixteen subsequent visits. The book provides for 120 cases.

———

This is the first regular edition of the Annual New and Nonofficial Remedies,[1] and it contains a list of the remedial preparations approved by the Council on Pharmacy and Chemistry of the American Medical Association. Instead of adhering strictly to an alphabetic arrangement a classification has been adopted which permits an easy comparison of remedies of similar origin and properties. Mixtures are to be found in the appendix and a number of nonproprietary preparations have been added which, for various reasons, have not been admitted to the Pharmacopeia. The descriptions in the appendix have been made as brief as possible and the articles are classified under the names of the manufacturers. Therapeutic indications are not given, as it is assumed that the physician is able to apply his knowledge of the pharmacologic properties of the ingredients without aids from either the Council or the manufacturer. The non-proprietary remedies admitted to the body of the book are described as accurately and carefully as a painstaking search of the literature would permit.

The descriptions of processes of preparations, chemical and physical, and of the physiologic action contain much information which can not fail to be of immense value both to physicians and to pharmacists.

Over 200 different remedies are described, and after mastering the Pharmacopeia the practitioner and the student should become thoroughly familiar with this presentation of the newer materia medica.

———

SURGICAL HINTS.

A severe sore feeling in the throat is frequently complained of by nervous individuals. Close inspection will show numerous fine white spots surrounded by a red areola—herpes.

———

Pressure from a mediastinal tumor or enlarged tubercular glands will often give rise to an irritative condition of the throat which can in no way be relieved by local measures.

———

Severe neuralgic pain over the bridge of the nose indicates pressure on the anterior ethmoidal nerve probably due to a high deviation of the nasal septum.

[1] NEW AND NONOFFICIAL REMEDIES.—Articles Which Have Been Accepted by the Council on Pharmacy and Chemistry of the American Medical Association, Prior to January, 1909. Chicago: Press of the American Medical Association, 103 Dearborn Avenue. Paper, 25c; cloth, 50c.

American Medicine

H. EDWIN LEWIS, M. D., *Managing Editor.*

PUBLISHED MONTHLY BY THE AMERICAN-MEDICAL PUBLISHING COMPANY.

Copyrighted by the American Medical Publishing Co., 1912.

New Series, Vol. VII., No. 4.
Complete Series, Vol. XVIII., No. 4.
APRIL, 1912.
$1.00   YEARLY in advance.

The Titanic horror fills everyone with an indescribable sadness. Hardly any great calamity in recent years has been so startling or has exemplified so fully that "in the midst of Life, we are in Death." Imagination runs rife and the scenes that picture themselves on the tablets of our minds are almost too terrible to describe. Here was the last word in boat construction, a masterpiece from every standpoint —size, convenience, equipment, luxury and safety. With apparently every known device for protection against every force of the sea, if there was ever a boat that was unsinkable, the Titanic was the one. Representing the length and breadth of man's latest knowledge of ship building, the prevailing estimate of this great vessel's fitness to triumph over every danger is shown by the fact that it was insured to the full extent of its enormous value *at the lowest rate ever given a transatlantic steamer.* And this by those considered the most critical, most discriminating experts on insurance in the world! Proudly this great floating hotel put out to sea. Manned as she was by officers and seamen picked for their ability and experience, had any one suggested the possibility of her going to the bottom of the sea in less than three hours, he would have been laughed to scorn. The Titanic sink? The largest, strongest, staunchest, finest ship in the world? Worth over 7,000,000 dollars,

with a cargo reaching well over 3,000,000 dollars, a crew of over 900 trained followers of the sea and a passenger list of nearly 1,500, including many of the leading men and women of two continents, such a boat sink? Impossible. Even the idea was ridiculous. And so she sped along. Making splendid time and with every promise of a quick, delightful trip, one can easily imagine the general admiration felt for the beauties and comforts of this great monster and the satisfaction that arose from having had the good luck to be with her on her maiden trip. Good luck! What a mocker Fate truly is! With her thousands of twinkling lights, a happy throng on deck or in the cabins, hundreds sleeping with all the confidence that they would have had in their own homes, the hand of destiny suddenly struck, without an instant's warning. With hardly a perceptible shock owing to her enormous size and weight, she received her death blow and probably a large part of her supposedly impregnable double bottom of steel was cut away as with a knife, opening bulkheads and in an instant rendering useless all her elaborate defence against the sea. For nearly an hour, hardly any one except possibly the ship's officers, had a suspicion of danger. Even when the orders to put on life preservers, and embark women and children went forth, the whole thing was considered rather of a lark. Not a few were delighted at the break in the monotony and eagerly welcomed the situation as an experience to remember. Without a single doubt hundreds of people went down sleeping peacefully in their cabins with never a warning of their fate. But soon unmistakable evidence of the seriousness of affairs became apparent to those on deck and they knew the terrible truth. The Titanic, the unsinkable boat—the ten million dollar floating palace—with her population larger by far than that of most of the towns and villages of Great Britain or America—was doomed —*she was going down!*

Confusion must have reigned for a few moments. Here were men and women, wealthy and famous, with everything to make life sweet. Husbands speeding home to expectant families, wives looking forward to a return to their husbands and homes. Here were men of great affairs, captains of enterprise with thousands in their service. But instantly all proportions were lost. In that last short period men and women were divested of every material value and rich, powerful and famous were thrown back to just human beings. Some unquestionably believed it impossible for the Titanic to sink, and secure in their confidence preferred to remain on board rather than risk their lives in the life boats. But many knew the truth and left a picture of heroism to the world that time can never destroy. Men whose lives and manner of living had been far removed from hardship or conditions ordinarily looked upon as developing fortitude and courage took their stand side by side with soldiers and sailors trained to meet death bravely. With a heroism that was sublime in its renunciation of self, husbands and fathers kissed their loved ones good bye and with

brave smiles on their faces watched them row away. No one can read the accounts of the survivors without swelling with pride that manhood and womanhood can ring so true at the supreme moment. Tears of sadness will fill our eyes, voices will break and anguish almost overpower us, but still there is an exaltation, a sense of inspiration, that comes from thinking of the nobility of the Titanic's heroes, that cannot help but lift and buoy us up in the face of this greatest calamity of modern times. Let no carping critic of mankind croak again that the flower of chivalry is dead, that men have grown weak or that courage and bravery have been destroyed by our civilization. Let no pessimist tell us the world is going to the bad, that men and women have lost their instincts of honor and self denial through the struggle for wealth and position. Let no one say that mankind has lost any part of its nobility or strength as the years have come and gone. No, when the traducer of humanity tells us that the days of heroism, devotion and unselfish love are no more, we have only to point to the Titanic and that last scene that will never be blotted from the memory of man—a great ship—the largest in the world—going down, hundreds waving good bye and throwing kisses to their loved ones, while the band with unbelievable fortitude was playing that grandest of hymns, Nearer, My God to Thee! In the dark of night, with all the depressing effect of severe cold, over 1,500 souls met their end, and went forth to meet their God. The picture of that tragic moment beggars description. No words can do it justice and each and every one of us must shape it for ourselves in our own consciousness. But terrible indeed as the disaster surely was and bereft as it leaves the world and countless families, humanity cannot fail to gain from the chastening effect it must have on every sentient being, and the aspiration that every true man must feel that his own end shall be as near as possible to that of those "who died like men." As we bring this to a close we cannot refrain from quoting a verse of Abraham Lincoln's favorite poem which has been in the writer's mind constantly since the fatal news was received.

"O why should the spirit of mortal be proud
Like a swift fleeting meteor—a fast flying cloud,
A flash of the lightning—a dash of the wave,
Man passes from life to his end in the grave."

What is the lesson? This is after all the great problem. Without doubt we have grown arrogant from our progress. We have felt ourselves conquerors of the sea and the elements with our monster ships. We have magnified our pigmy strength and minimized the gigantic powers of Nature. In our rush and hustle we have sacrificed safety for speed. Restlessness and impatience have controlled us. We have subordinated care and precaution for haste and hurry. Without sense or judgment we have made foolish drafts on luxury, excitement and the sensational. And now when we have to pay and the collector appears—we find that it is Death! Is it not time to call a halt, to alter our ideas and readjust our values? Is not safety preferable to size and speed? Is it not infinitely preferable to reach our destination a few hours later—but with life and limb intact? Are "four day boats," "eighteen hour trains" and countless things of the same character worth the price we are paying?

As Charles M. Hays, a great railroad man and one of the Titanic's heroes, said only a few hours before his death "some great disaster is sure to come if the fearful attempts at haste and speed are not curbed." Little did he know the prophetic character of his remark. The Titanic was sacrificed to false values, the exaltation of size, speed, luxury and everything appealing to humanity's love for beauty and greatness, at the expense of safety and sensible precaution. Dashing onward at 21 knots an hour (about 26 miles), the danger of icebergs though fully recognized was never heeded and her pace was never slackened. She was "to get in on time." Secure in her great size and with blind confidence in her power to triumph over every accident, lifeboat equipment for less than one in three of her passengers and crew was provided. To reduce the distance and reach her destination quicker, she was following a course that is known to have its constant dangers of icebergs and floes. Admitting that she was in the usual lane of steamship travel, *the fact remains that it was not the safest.* And so we are brought face to face with the grim truth that not the ship builders, not the White Star management, not the captain or his assistants are to blame except incidentally for this awful catastrophe. The culprits are the people at large, those who have encouraged these things—in fact forced their adoption by turning their backs on the cautious and conservative, and patronizing only the swiftest, most daring and most spectacular. Big business is bound to give the people what they want. If a premium in the form of patronage is given to safety, conservative methods and common sense, the public will get just these things. But we have given our support and encouragement to the risky, the daring and the sensational. Consequently we the masses are culpable and common decency should make us realize it. We have ignored the substance for the shadow and it is wrong, cruelly wrong to curse and condemn those who have given us what we wanted. It is only human nature to make some one "the goat," but is this fair? Is it right to make those who do our bidding —the officials and subordinates—bear the burden of our own indifference or neglect? Surely not and that spirit which we proudly call the American spirit of fair play should enable us to be just and generous in this hour of our anguish and remorse. Let us investigate and study the situation in all its aspects, and seek as honest, thoughtful men to reach conclusions and decisions that shall correct conditions and prevent a repetition. But let us take a lesson from our hero dead and with respect for their nobility and unselfishness, refrain from making the small petty mistake of condemning any one—or any group of men—without the fullest hearing and consideration for their actual responsibility. In other words, here is the moment for humanity to rise to new heights of fairness, justice and generosity. We owe it to our dead—but above all to our own manhood and womanhood.

The psychology of courage is interesting but the manifestation of this mental attribute is so interwoven with other mental or psychic forces that it is extremely hard to place it and give it its true value. There are plenty of facts that go to show that courage or bravery in the face of sudden or violent death is most uncertain. Many men who have lived lives and given abundant reason to lead us to anticipate the highest courage from them have proven at the end the veriest cowards. On the other hand there are plenty of those whose character, temperament and environment have led them to appear weak, vacillating and ignoble, but who at the crisis met their fate with the most sublime and splendid courage. Bravery, therefore, is a most uncertain quantity, and can never be predicated on the usual mental qualities or customs of an individual. Love, pride, trust in God, the psychology of the moment, the surroundings, the physical condition and many other factors are all woven into the fabric of courage and heroism, just as fear, despair, lack of control, and some of the same factors that under certain conditions give rise to courage, will cause the most arrant cowardice. No man knows just how he will act at such times until they come. Certain it is, though, that we all hope we can have the curtain rung down at the close and leave behind as clean, noble and uplifting a scene as that enacted by so many men as the Titanic made her last plunge. The doctors on the Titanic seem to have been true to the best traditions of our profession. Medical men with few exceptions have always died well. And after all that is said or done can one have a better or finer epitaph than "Death found him unafraid"? But we who live have our work before us and this calamity emphasizes certain important features. The medical profession is striving with all its strength and knowledge to save and prolong life. Does it not behoove us while we are driving back the hordes of disease to devote more thought and time to pointing out and urging greater efficiency in preventing needless accidents? In other words what is the good of saving countless lives from disease if they are only going to be sacrificed to the Moloch of carelessness and industrial negligence? In all sincerity we believe medical men should give this matter more thought and devote more attention to arousing humanity from its indifference or ignorance of physical danger.

————

The deterioration of the farming class is so frequently asserted that it would be interesting to look into it a little to see if the charge is true that we are evolving a peasantry too stupid for our form of government. There is no doubt of course that the income of farmers is so small that everyone who has ability to make more, generally goes to town where there is great demand for men who have more intelligence than needed to run a farm indifferently well. So too, the man whose active brain cannot stand the dulling monotony of isolation, will abandon farming even if he makes a poorer living with the crowd. Then again the farmer who does succeed is very prone to retire to town and rent his farm, so that there is already a large and rapidly increasing percentage of our best farming lands in the hands of tenants who as a class are not the best farmers by any means. Poor land is generally cultivated by its owner because he cannot make enough to get away, and besides he is generally a man of a lower order of intelligence who has been elbowed out of better places by better men. As intelligence and morality are closely allied, there may be some ground for the frequent assertion that the ideals and conduct in cities are now far above those of the country. The vote sellers of Adams county, Ohio, who constitute the respectable element seem to point to low standards at least there.

Rural immorality seems to be so widespread as to warrant considering it an universal phenomenon. We certainly are having a hard time convincing farmers of the iniquity of selling us dangerous foods. They certainly have killed an awful number of us with typhoid fever, and our sanitary inspectors are in constant danger of assault or worse. Is it possible that we have reversed matters, and the least moral are now in the rural districts? The best farmers of Europe do not come here, —they are too contented at home. We get the failures now and we cannot expect them to do any better than they did in Europe. Fifty years ago they stumbled on good western lands which they immediately despoiled and became rich. Some of these are wandering into Canada to repeat the process, leaving our farms to still worse. On the other hand, the returns of intelligent scientific farming are so great, and abler men are succeeding so well, that an opposite selection is going on by elbowing out those too stupid for modern ways, and who become hired hands. Will these new farmers be able to sustain a higher moral code than the failures have? Time only can tell, but now we must sorrowfully confess that the countryman is not as good as he used to be, so that city vice is largely supported by visitors from the country, bent on a "fling," but who are steady church-goers at home. All bunco and gold-brick swindles are based on the immoral greed of a country victim and should not be blamed on the city exclusively. Cities have enough to shoulder, goodness knows, and in all fairness ought to shift some of the blame on the country.

————

At the very time of Lord Lister's funeral the Antivivisectionists in England could not withhold their sacrilegious hand from an endeavor to make capital out of the occasion. On Feb. 12th, (Lister died on Feb. 10th and was buried on the 16th) there was issued a circular addressed to the editors of various newspapers and entitled, "Lord Lister's Discoveries." It opens as follows: "When so great a surgeon as Lord Lister passes away, none would wish to say a word in detraction of his memory, but, as Carlyle has pointed out the necessity for 'Honoring the right man,' truth compels those who know it to resist the attribution of any reform to one who did not make it. There is a very common impression that modern surgery owes its safety to the practice of antisepsis as Lord Lister understood it. This impression is false." The writer of the circular then attempts to draw an impassable gulf between the details of the early "antiseptic ritual" and modern aseptic surgery, disregarding the fact that it is the establishment of the principle of germ infection of wounds as the cause of surgical disaster that was Lister's great work, not the elaboration of any unalterable "ritual" for overcoming or preventing that infection. The writer of the circular is one "W. R. Hadwen, M. D., J. P., President of the British Union for the Abolition of Vivisection."

It is admitted in the circular that Lister was "a great surgeon." It is, of course a matter of indifference whether some obscure medical man admits that truth or not. No more eloquent or overwhelming testimony could be accorded to it than the throngs of scientists and savants of worldwide reputation who filled Westminster Abbey, that historic Fane wherein England's sovereigns are crowned and England's greatest dead are accorded burial as the highest honor their country can pay to their remains. At Lister's funeral service on Feb. 16th the pall bearers were Lord Rayleigh, representing the Order of Merit, to which Lord Lister belonged, Lord Rosebery, representing the University of London, Lord Iveagh, the Lister Institute; Sir Archibald Geike, President of the Royal Society; Sir Donald MacAlister, Principal of Glasgow University; Sir Watson Cheyne, representing King's College London; Mr. R. J. Godlee, President of the Royal College of Surgeons of England, and Prof. F. M. Caird, representing the University of Edinburgh. King George was represented by Sir Frederick Treves, F. R. C. S., and the Dowager Queen Alexandra by Sir Francis Laking, M. D. The German Emperor sent a magnificent wreath of orchids and lilies, which was placed on the coffin by the German ambassador while it lay in St. Faith's Chapel, the Ambassadors from Austro-Hungary, France, Germany, Italy, and Russia, and the Ministers from Belgium, China, Greece, Sweden, Norway, and Portugal, with the Servian Chargé d'Affaires, paid the homage of their respective countries by their presence. The French Academy of Sciences, the Institut Pasteur of Paris, the French Academy of Medicine, the German Congress of Surgeons, the Société de Chirurgie of Paris, the Medical Association of Amsterdam, the Swedish Academy of Sciences, the Norwegian Society of Science, the Academy of Medicine of Madrid, the Accademia dei Lincei of Rome, and the Imperial Academy of Sciences of St. Petersburgh sent, some their presidents, others high officials or professors, to represent them, while every university in Great Britain and Ireland, many learned societies, medical schools, hospitals and infirmaries, in the persons of their official delegates paid

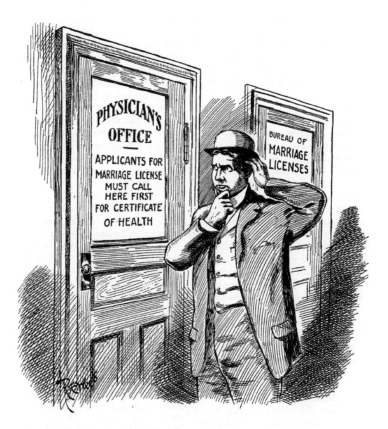

MEMORIES THAT WILL NOT DOWN!

the last tribute of sorrow and respect to the great dead. Noblemen and persons of social degree, with distinguished medical men and scientists, not called on to act as official representatives, filled the choir of the Abbey in their private capacities, while outside the official circle the public at large, rich and poor, assembled to do honor. to one who has been acclaimed as "the greatest Englishman of the Nineteenth Century."

And why was this "Great Surgeon" so honored? A great operator in his day he had assuredly been, but we do no disparagement to him when we say that there have been in many countries, and are now living today, many just as great, possibly even not a few greater. Most assuredly it was not to his mere personal skill as a surgeon that all the world assembled to do honor. It was because of the fact that by his long years of patient observation and thought, aided by experiment, he was led to enunciate and demonstrate in practice beyond question the great principle of the nature and cause of wound infection, and to place in the hands of the surgical world the knowledge that has enabled it step by step, through the prevention of infection to bring nearly all parts of the human frame within the reach of reparative efforts, that this homage was rendered.

And the end of the work is not yet. It matters not what further advances in surgery the future may see, what still greater triumphs may be in store for surgeons yet unknown, all will be due in the last resort to the prescience and wisdom of Joseph Lister who discovered and gave to the world the great First Principles which have robbed surgery forever of its terrors.

The personality of the anesthetist as exhibited especially to female patients, is a factor of the greatest importance not only in its bearing on each surgeon's success but also on the comfort of each woman.

In the majority of cases, wherein the operation calls for the administration of an anesthetic by an assistant, the woman is usually prepared for and reconciled to the operative procedure itself—especially after being assured by her attending physician, in whom her faith is naturally established, that she "won't feel anything"—but what causes her constant uneasiness and gradually works her up to a state of great fear and apprehension, beforehand and even at the time of immediate operation, is the taking of the anesthetic.

How often the attending surgeon is questioned concerning his assistant—"you are sure he knows how much to give me"—and then, when the anesthetic is begun, "oh, if I were only asleep now"—all showing the more or less lack of confidence in the assistant, brought about by an exaggerated state of nervous tension and fear of the man she knows nothing of—except through the assurance of her. own physician.

The patient is not to be blamed in the least. It is no pleasant procedure for her to stretch herself out at the mercy and judgment of the physicians, and the mysterious drug which she realizes will totally rob her of her faculties. She trusts the operator, but she is afraid of the anesthetist; and why not? In most cases he is a total stranger to her, meeting her for the first time just before placing the inhaling apparatus over her face. She knows nothing definite concerning the man's ability, but must rely entirely upon her attending physician's recommendation and confidence.

For the moment the anesthetist is the all-important person to the patient; the surgeon is occupied with his own part of the work, and the woman is entirely in the hands of the assistant whose duty it is to place her under the influence of the anesthetic—and his position is necessarily a delicate and trying one. He must work often without the confidence of the patient which makes matters far worse for all concerned. What saves him however, is the drug, which sooner or later, renders the woman oblivious to his presence.

A woman is naturally endowed with an abundant sense of delicacy toward all things—personalities and mannerisms always affect her most readily—and in her highly nervous condition at this time, her temperament is markedly exaggerated, her likes and dislikes, whims and ideas more pronounced, and she is "all on edge." She has momentarily forgotten the operation in her great fear of "going to sleep"; the anesthetist is the one she sees and hears and she cannot help but respond in one way or another to even the most minute details in his management of her.

If he speaks in a rough, harsh, domineering manner, and handles her in a too pronounced business-like way, trying to hurry things along for the usually impatient operator, she naturally rebels. If he jams the inhaling apparatus down over her face and gives her a preliminary suffocating inhalation of the anesthetic, she responds with violent coughing and gagging, which at once arouses her very worst fears and convinces her that she is most surely about to die.

It might be well if the anesthetist, upon seeing a woman patient for the first time, especially in her own home, would pay more attention to the effect of his attitude, manner and bearing upon the patient. He can accomplish much upon "first impression"—especially with the afflicted female. His first endeavor should be to inspire confidence.

Perhaps a word about his personal appearance may not be amiss. He should be neat in dress and personally clean; a slovenly and careless appearing person often upsets a woman at once—for she is fastidious.

The odor of stale tobacco, beer, or any indication of alcoholic indulgence upon the breath or clothing, is at all times offensive to a woman, and because of his necessarily close contact with her, at the time of operation, may on the instant completely ruin the anesthetist's chances of gaining and holding her confidence.

A quiet tone in speaking, a gentle way of giving the necessary orders and directions, a little diplomacy in framing and asking delicate questions, combined with a certain air of decision, self-confidence and gentle firmness, will work wonders for the physician and patient.

During preliminary preparations, it is not essential to regale the woman with funny stories in an effort to make her laugh. A few remarks upon general topics are indicated to relieve her mind but attempts at super-nonchalance are frequently overdone—the patient becomes suspicious and mistrusting.

Selection of the anesthetic, method of administration, and the general technique of the procedure, do not come under this heading—that is another story, and it is taken for granted that the anesthetist is thoroughly competent. The vast importance of an experienced or expert anesthetist cannot be overestimated.

To sum up, everything without being fussy, should be done to impress the woman that she is receiving the very closest attention; that her welfare and comfort are the factors under consideration. And an important point to be borne in mind is, to let her take her time—within reason of course. Never hurry a woman, and especially during administration of an anesthetic. From start to finish, a gentle, refined, positive and professional manner of approaching the female patient, bearing in mind that one is dealing with an extremely delicate and sensitive human organism, will go far toward assuring rapid and effectual results from the anesthetist's efforts, and leave behind him, in the woman's mind, the impression of his being a competent physician and a gentleman.

Scientific research in the United States receives too little recognition. As a matter of fact we seldom give our scientists the commendation that their contributions actually merit, and it is not an infrequent occurrence that the work of American surgeons and investigators is more highly appreciated by those on the other side of the water than it is by their own countrymen. Take for instance the remarkable studies of Sajous on the internal secretions. Although the writer was more conversant with Sajous' contributions to the subject than the average American physician, it was not until he went to some of the medical centers of Europe that he began to grasp the far reaching, epoch making importance of the discoveries and researches of this truly great American scientist. As long ago as 1901-02, our European confreres saw that Sajous had tapped a vein of richest truths concerning matters previously shrouded in obscurity and was uncovering a wealth of

data and information that promised a new era of progress in the study of metabolism. Ten years have slipped by, and Sajous' two volumes are a monument to some of the greatest studies in human physiology and pathology. His name is known and his work is known—and admired—by those who ever stop to think of what he has done while pursuing a busy life as practitioner of medicine and editor. But what has his country done for him? What recognition, what gratitude and appreciation have been accorded him? Had he had the good fortune to have been born in England or Europe he would have been knighted, made a member of the Legion of Honor, or given a government grant that would have enabled him to devote himself to research work the rest of life.

So with Finlay and Agramonte of Cuba who showed the relationship of mosquitoes to yellow fever and thus made possible the practical obliteration of this disease. In this connection it is interesting to learn that these two scientists have been suggested for the Nobel prize in medicine. That they richly deserve it every American physician will agree, for few contributions to preventive medicine are more glorious and deserving of substantial recognition than theirs.

So with Gorgas, Flexner, Noguchi, some of our great surgeons like Halstead, Howard Kelly, Maurice Richardson, the Mayos, Murphy, Bryant, McBurney, Coley, Wyeth and many others.

So with some of those who have devoted their lives to medical journalism and whose work as great medical editors stands forth like that of Shrady, Hamilton, Foster and Stedman. Why do our colleges fail to honor these men and emphasize their unselfish, faithful work for humanity?

Are we unable to appreciate our own? Are we so indifferent that we will go on keeping from telling them while it could encourage them, that we are proud and grateful for their efforts? Are we not missing opportunities to foster and promote scientific research?

The American Medicine Gold Medal. Few American medical journals belong so completely to the medical profession. It may not be known but in the early history of the publication over 7,500 physicians bought stock in the enterprise and became financially interested in its future. While the present management made up of physicians exclusively, had nothing to do with this and feel that much criticism could be justly expressed at the way promises were given investors, we have felt that the situation entailed distinct obligations to the medical profession, and have consequently made service to American practitioners of medicine our principal aim. Proud of medical science as it exists in America to-day our one great ideal is to aid its progress and assist every physician to go forward. We realize how puny our aid and assistance must be. But believing that everything helps and knowing that sometimes the humblest efforts are able to set greater forces to work, the editors of AMERICAN MEDICINE have established the AMERICAN MEDICINE Gold Medal for Conspicuous Contributions to the Progress of Medical Science. It is to be donated each year to the American surgeon, physician or investigator who in the opinion of three trustees to be announced in our May issue, has made the most noteworthy contribution to medical science. The announcement of the first recipient will be made at the forthcoming meeting of the American Medical Editors' Associa-

tion and annually thereafter. Further details and design of the medal will appear next month. Readers of AMERICAN MEDICINE are urged to send in their nominations for this Gold Medal, for it is the support of the subscribers that has made this project possible. As AMERICAN MEDICINE grows, every dollar of profit is going to be turned back to the profession, for the welfare of the whole. This present announcement is only the beginning of what this publication proposes to do for the earnest workers in the field of medicine and surgery.

Will you kindly express your ideas as to whom in the whole country is today most deserving of recognition?

———

The prevention of conception is a matter which seems in a fair way to involve the medical profession in more or less controversy with theologians and statesmen. Sociologists and economists are apparently very largely of the opinion that the steady reduction of the birth rate has been beneficial, and that the dreadful distress found in lower races and lower layers of civilized societies, is at least partly due to unrestrained reproduction of the species. On the other hand, certain theologians are quite convinced that we have not nearly finished the divine task inherited from the sons of Noah who were charged to be fruitful and multiply and replenish the earth. Consequently the sacrament of matrimony is considered divinely appointed for the sole purpose of reproduction, and to many minds, both lay and clerical, there is an air of unholiness in even a discussion of the matter of limiting offspring. By extremists, any attempt to prevent conception, even by voluntary continence, is considered a heinous sin. Under such circumstances, it is evidently out of the question to discuss whether the descendants of Noah have not so fully complied with the Divine law as to have overdone it and have now through sheer lust brought into the world a mass of people unable to make a fair living. Statesmen as a rule, seem to side with the theologians and have passed prohibitive laws with severe penalties for sending any such information through the mails.

The public's opinion as to race suicide seems wholly at variance with its practices. If a married woman does not have a child within a year of the weaning of the last born, or much sooner as a rule, it is proof that something has been done to prevent pregnancy. It is very rare to find a family in which the maximum number of children have been born, so we must conclude that prevention of conception is well nigh universal among thinking people. Physicians know that there is no woman who considers herself divinely appointed to bear children to her maximum limit. It is therefore strange that there should be such a public opinion against limitation of offspring, for it is one of the things every woman knows is sheer hypocrisy. Physicians even go a step further and state that unrestrained child bearing is so harmful to the woman that it not only kills her and deprives the first few born of a mother's care, but that the later children are often too feeble to raise. Large families therefore tend to race suicide in comparison to the small families in which each child is vigorous and properly brought up. We personally know of one family where the husband openly stated that woman's sphere was solely that of a breeder to the maximum, in which the strain caused such bad offspring that one became a murderer and suicide, and though one case must not make a law it shows that big families of apparently healthy people are not necessarily good or safe.

The relation of large families to public health is what brings the medical profession into this theological matter. When a woman finds that a pregnancy is liable to kill both herself and baby she never hesitates to ask relief of her physician. There has never been the slightest hesitation on the part of Protestant physicians when consulting over such a case. The pregnancy is ended at once and the act is sanctioned by civil law, though it may be condemned by ecclesiastic law of some churches. Here at least religion and medicine sometimes conflict. Yet when it comes to the advice as to how to prevent future pregnancies without danger to health of husband or wife, medicine and civil law are at variance to some extent. Now that learned economists are asserting that public welfare demands prevention and lawgivers practice it, why should it any longer be considered criminal to advise it? There can be no harm in discussing what every woman knows and every man too. Indeed there must be an ethical course to pursue, which is also legal and it is high time to decide upon it. The subject is at last entering the stage of discussion in current medical literature, and we hope it will continue to be discussed in the calm method of every other public health measure. In England the largest families are found in the three unproductive classes which depend upon the public for support, —nobility, clergy and the submerged tenth. The real people, the self-supporting productive middle classes who furnish the funds,—are beginning to object quite loudly and so must we. Many a man has too much difficulty in feeding his own three, to give much to the clergyman's six.

ORIGINAL ARTICLES.

ADDRESS.
AUDITORY VERTIGO AND TINNITUS AURIUM.[1]

BY

ALBERT A. GRAY, M. D.,
Glasgow, Scotland.

In all branches of medical science there are certain manifestations of disease which may be termed "bugbears," whether they be considered from the point of view of the patient, the family physician or the specialist. To the patient the symptoms cause much suffering, to the family medical attendant they are the source of recurring worry, to the specialist they are at once a worry and a humiliation. The only persons who view their existence with satisfaction are the unqualified medical mountebanks and quacks who infest every country, because of the laxity of the laws regulating the practice of medicine. These gentlemen are cunning enough to know that in a great number of such cases, neither they themselves nor the most experienced specialist nor the regular practitioner can do much to help the sufferers, and consequently they see the opportunity of reaping a golden harvest.

That branch of medicine which has to do with diseases of the ear has, perhaps, to bear rather more than its share of these bugbears, and with your kind permission, I intend to speak for a few moments concerning two of them, auditory vertigo and tinnitus—subjective sound sensations.

Of these vertigo may be considered first, not because it is any less serious to the sufferer, indeed it is rather the reverse, but

[1] An address delivered by invitation at a meeting of the Eastern Medical Society, Nov., 1911.

because of the two it is, on the whole, more amenable to treatment than the subjective sensations of sound.

Now, in the first place, we must arrive at a diagnosis. When a patient comes complaining of attacks of giddiness, how are we to ascertain where the seat of the disturbance is? In respect to mere probability, it may be said at once that the great majority of cases of vertigo are due to disturbance in the labyrinth or its nerve connections, and it is a common mistake to forget this axiom. Very frequently cases come for consultation in which the vertigo has been attributed to a bilious attack or gastric catarrh, or to being run down in general health. And in one respect the diagnosis may be said to be correct, for these conditions not uncommonly precipitate an attack of the vertigo. But when the ear comes to be examined carefully, it will be found in many such cases, that the labyrinth is in an unstable physiological condition, and that the true cause of the symptom is to be found in that organ.

The diagnosis of labyrinthine vertigo is usually very simple if there is any associated symptom which leads the patient to refer to his ear. Thus, if the sufferer remarks that he had noticed he had suddenly become more or less dull of hearing after the attack, or that he was aware of noises in the ear after it, then the suspicions of the medical attendant are aroused at once and the ear examined.

But there are not a few cases in which these symptoms are so slight, and bulk so little in the mind of the patient as compared with the alarming vertigo and the nausea and vomiting which is apt to accompany it, that he may either never have noticed them, or may not think it worth while mentioning them to the physician.

These are the cases in which an error in diagnosis is apt to occur. As an example of this I may mention a case already reported by myself, but which will perhaps bear repetition. The patient had suffered from several severe attacks of giddiness and vomiting for several months, and these had been diagnosed as bilious attacks. Not feeling any improvement after treatment, he changed his medical attendant and the second medical adviser made the diagnosis of auditory vertigo; and for confirmation, sent the patient on to me. On examination it was clear that the second diagnosis was correct. The hearing power was slightly diminished on the right side, and the other labyrinthine symptoms functions were in a state of hyper-excitability. On questioning the patient, he said that he had had slight, but continuous noises in the right ear, but had never thought of associating these with the attacks. The exciting cause was found to be mental overwork, associated with considerable periods of fasting. With the removal of the causes, the attacks gradually diminished in frequency and severity, and ultimately ceased altogether. The hearing in the right ear, however, was not recovered, and got steadily worse as time passed, until it became very marked.

The case illustrates the importance of always examining the ear in cases of vertigo whether the patient complains of deafness and tinnitus or not. It is also to be noted that, while the labyrinth recovered so far as other symptoms were concerned, the hearing became steadily worse. In my own experience this is almost invariably the course of events. A few exceptions are found in cases in which the cause of the trouble is syphilitic and in which the patient is very rapidly brought under the full influence of mercury and iodide of potassium immediately after the first attack.

But the routine examination of the ear in cases of vertigo may bring to light more serious conditions than those in the case just described. I have found, for example, on more than one occasion, that the symptoms were due to the gradual erosion of the walls of the labyrinth by a chronic suppurative process in the middle ear, which the patient had not referred to because he had no idea that there could be any connection between the ear and the giddiness. In such cases the vertigo, distressing as it may be, is really a blessing, as it brings to light a state of affairs that, unknown to the patient, is a very grave danger to his life. In such cases the line of treatment is obvious. The suppurative process must be attended to without delay. If local treatment fails to remove the symptoms and cure the suppuration rapidly, the case must be subjected to the radical mastoid operation. It may even be necessary, if the cavity of the labyrinth itself is found to be the seat of suppurative disease, to open it freely.

Another, and comparatively frequent cause, of auditory vertigo is the syphilitic poison. In these cases the syphilitic infection may either have been acquired, or transmitted from the parent, but I am inclined to think that the former are distinctly more common. Of all the causes of auditory vertigo, with the exception of those due to suppurative middle ear disease, syphilis is the one in which a mistake in diagnosis may have the most disastrous results. And the reason is this, if the case be recognized immediately after the first attack, rapid mercurialization or the use of salvarsan, associated with absolute rest in bed may in some instances bring about a restoration of the hearing which is always more or less affected. If, however, the days are allowed to pass, before anti-syphilitic treatment is adopted, there will be no restoration of the hearing, though the giddiness and other labyrinthine symptoms will disappear. Unfortunately there is no sign, so far as aural symptoms are concerned, which will enable the physician to differentiate the syphilitic from the non-syphilitic cases. The diagnosis must be made on the evidence of other signs of syphilis in the body, and on the result of the Wassermann test.

But after eliminating such well-defined causes as suppurative middle ear disease and constitutional syphilis, there remain a considerable number of cases in which the syphilitic poison is absent, and there is no middle ear affection at all. The classification of such cases is a matter of difficulty, and indeed the aurist must frequently be content with an incomplete diagnosis. But in a considerable number I have found evidence that, in addition to the labyrinthine affection, there is present a state of instability of the vasomotor system of the body generally, and this in its turn may be due to disturbances in the alimentary canal or to a condition of exhaustion of the nervous system due usually to mental overwork and worry. In respect to this latter class, I may remark that I happen to have been consulted by a relatively large number of men of our own profession on account of auditory vertigo. This may merely be a coincidence, but on the other hand, it may be associated with the worry and close mental concentration that the practice of medicine demands from those, at any rate, who do their work faithfully.

Finally, there are some cases of auditory vertigo to which no cause can be definitely assigned. The patient suffers from attacks of vertigo associated with vomiting or nausea, when he is in other respects in apparently perfect health.

Before passing on to speak of prognosis and treatment, I must say a few words in regard to one of the methods employed in diagnosis about which much has been said in recent years. I refer to the so-called "nystagmus tests." These tests which were devised by von Stein and Barany, have for their object the ascertaining, by objective means of the stability of the functions of the vestibule and semicircular canals. In the "rotation test" nystagmus is brought about by rotating the patient a fixed number of times on a chair constructed for the purpose. In the caloric tests the nystagmus is produced by syringing hot and cold water into the external meatus. In the great majority of individuals, nystagmus is elicited by these means. The nystagmus is in different directions according to the direction of the rotation of the patient in the one case, and to the temperature of the water employed for syringing, in the other. Limits of time forbid me entering into a detailed account of the different types of nystagmus so produced. The important matter to remember is that if the nystagmus is increased beyond the normal limits, the vestibular functions are in a state of hyper-excitability, and if it is abolished or diminished below the normal, these functions are in a state of diminished sensitiveness. For my own part, I must frankly admit that I think a little too much has been made of the importance of these tests. The limits of the normal nystagmus reflexes are so very variable that it is, in many cases, difficult to say that these are exceeded. Still, in those cases in which the reflex departs very markedly from the normal, the nystagmus tests are of undoubted service in diagnosis.

Leaving this very brief and I fear incomplete reference to diagnosis, a few words must be said on the prognosis.

The general statement may first be made that the prognosis will depend upon the answer to the question, Is there any discoverable and definite exciting cause? and if so, to what extent can this be removed? Thus, is the patient obviously much overworked or worried? Is there any suppuration or other disease in the middle ear? Is there any severe digestive disturbance? Or, is the patient subject to constipation? If any such cause is present and is removable, then the prognosis is relatively good. At the same time, even in these cases, the vertiginous attacks may not cease at once, but they will gradually tend to get less severe and less frequent as the exciting cause becomes less active.

In respect to the cases in which the syphilitic poison is the exciting agent, I venture to be rather more definite in regard to prognosis. In these cases, the first attack is usually the last, unless, of course, the opposite ear is subsequently affected, in which case the second attack will almost certainly be the last. In this respect, therefore, the syphilitic cases are markedly different from many of the others in which the attacks are repeated at intervals varying from a few days' duration to several months, or even more.

With regard to the remaining cases in which no definite exciting cause is discoverable, the prognosis is much more difficult, and in many cases it is impossible to give an opinion. One of the most important factors in my own experience is the age of the patient. In young people the outlook is far more hopeful than in those who are passing into the later registers of life. In fact in these latter, it is well to let them know that there is considerable probability of their never getting permanently free of their trouble.

The physician has but little direct local control over the vestibular functions of the labyrinth, and so far as he is concerned the treatment consists of the removal of the exciting cause of the attacks. In this matter he must exercise the utmost systematic care in finding out every possible physiological disturbance in the body. These disturbances will be most commonly found in the alimentary tract or in the nervous system. Overeating and, what I have found, curiously enough to be a factor even more common, prolonged periods of fasting, must be avoided. Constipation is another serious disturbing element and in respect to this I would like to say a word or two more emphatically. For the purpose of relieving chronic constipation in cases such as these, it is wise to avoid, if possible, all the ordinary laxatives. Of course, during the attack of giddiness, if it be of long duration, a saline purge is desirable, but for regular administration, by far the best corrective, is the pure petroleum or parolein. It may be given in doses of from a teaspoonful to a tablespoonful three times daily. But even at the best, such treatment very frequently fails, and we are driven to other more drastic measures.

Of all forms of treatment for such cases, I have found that prolonged rest, bodily and mental, associated with change of air and scene is by far the best. A long sea voyage is the ideal for those who are able to stand the sea. It is remarkable how frequently this line of treatment is successful, and I have not the least doubt that its efficiency is in large part due to the mental, rather than the physical rest which it necessitates. The effect of the mind upon the vasomotor system is particularly close, and when the stability of the latter is brought into a normal condition, the vertiginous attacks diminish in frequency and severity and ultimately disappear.

Finally, a few words in regard to surgical treatment. With the exception of those due to suppurative middle ear disease operative procedures are very rarely justifiable. Only when the attacks are so frequent and severe as to interfere seriously with the activities of life, is it permissible to destroy the semicircular canals and vestibule. This is the very last resource; and before it is undertaken, the patient should be made clearly to understand that the risk is not small. There is neither the time nor necessity at present to describe the operation. Tinnitus, or the subjective sensations of sound in the ear, is a much more difficult problem in all respects than auditory vertigo. It is more common and the proportion of cases in which relief can be obtained is much smaller. It is moreover, practically always associated with deafness and usually with deafness very considerable in degree.

There is no doubt that tinnitus is the result of different causes in different cases. Thus, eustachian catarrh or even suppurative middle ear disease may be associated with it, but in these circumstances the noises almost invariably cause little trouble to the patient. In uncomplicated affections of the sound-perceiving apparatus, whether this be situated in the membranous cochlea or in the associated nerve structures, it is a curious fact that tinnitus is not usually a predominant symptom. The very severe cases of tinnitus are undoubtedly those in which the patient is suffering from otosclerosis with fixation of the stapes, and in which it is quite possible, though not by any means proved, that the nerve structures in the cochlea are coincidently affected. Furthermore, in these circumstances the sensation of the sound is frequently referred to as being in the head rather than in the ear. In very many cases the noise is heard by the patient in both ears, and even in those subjects in which the symptom is unilateral at the beginning, it is almost always destined to become bilateral sooner or later.

While the worst cases of tinnitus are always associated with deafness, there are not a few of the milder cases in which the hearing is normal. These form an important class not because the symptom is in itself very distressing, but because it is sometimes indicative of actual or threatened constitutional disease, which is sometimes very grave. Thus, it has fallen to my lot to see patients who come on account of tinnitus without deafness, in whom the symptom was, in reality, the first warning of such conditions as arteriosclerosis, diabetes, valvular heart mischief, anemia and aneurism. It is of the utmost importance to make a very careful examination of the heart, the arteries, the blood, urine, etc., in all cases in which tinnitus is present without deafness.

Prognosis.—As with all other symptoms, the prognosis depends upon the cause, and the extent to which it is removable. If eustachian or serous middle ear catarrh is present, the cure of these troubles will bring about the cessation of the subjective noises. Similarly, in cases of chlorosis or simple anemia, the same result will be obtained when the general condition is rectified.. Even in cases of arteriosclerosis I have seen improvement occur, not of course, because of any diminution in the thickening of the arteries, but because, under the judicious treatment of the physician, the high arterial tension was lowered to a certain and appreciable extent.

But in the really severe cases of tinnitus which are associated with otosclerosis it must be frankly admitted that the prognosis is not good, and the treatment is highly unsatisfactory. Further, it is an unfortunate fact that the more severe the subjective sounds are, the less can they be influenced by treatment. Local applications I have never found to be of any permanent value, though a course of blisters over the mastoid process may have some temporary benefit and the same may be said of pneumo-massage. The inflation of the middle ear, either by the catheter or the air-douche produces no improvement and may damage the hearing. With regard to the general constitutional treatment, I may venture to say that as far as this consists in improving the general condition of the patient, it is highly desirable. But, in so far as it consists in prescribing nerve sedatives, such as the bromides, I am inclined to think that in the end more harm is done than good. Iodide of potassium is frequently prescribed, and in those in whom the administration of the drug is not followed by objectionable symptoms, such as skin eruptions and nasal catarrh, the benefit obtained may justify the prescription.

Of greater importance than these is the abstinence from such substances as alcohol, tobacco, tea, coffee, etc. And in this, as in many other circumstances, the regulation of the bowels is of supreme importance. I may here again state that for this purpose, I have found petroleum in doses of from a teaspoonful to a tablespoonful, the most valuable.

The question of surgical interference, when all other means have failed, again presents itself. In the case of tinnitus, even more emphatically than in vertigo, it must be said that the circumstances which can justify such procedure must be rare indeed. For myself, I have never yet felt justified in operating. The operation, which consists of destruction of the cochlea, has been carried out several times, and it is a significant fact that it has not always brought relief.

Moreover, since the very severe cases are almost invariably bilateral, it follows that with the rarest exceptions, both cochleae would require destruction, with consequent complete loss of hearing of all sounds. In view of these circumstances, it may be said that the physician who can encourage his patient to bear his trouble, has achieved a much greater success than the surgeon who has destroyed the cochlea. For even in the worst cases the tinnitus may, in the course of time, abate or become more bearable, while the patient still has some useful hearing left. In such circumstances the sufferer may well repeat to himself the old Arab proverb, "Bless the disease, if it bring thee acquaintance with a wise physician."

––––

After operating on the perineum, it is bad practice to apply a perineal pad, for by so doing discharges are transferred from the anus and the wound is apt to become infected. You will have better results when no dressing is used.

––––

The rectum should be thoroughly dilated after all operations on the perineum, so that the bowels can be easily moved and gas allowed to escape.

THE THERAPEUTICS OF THE URIC ACID DIATHESIS.

BY

O. L. MULOT, M. D.,

Brooklyn, N. Y.

Woe be unto the physician who becomes interested in uric acid. The more he studies the literature concerning it, the more thoroughly will he find himself lost in a maze of contradictions and cant. Questions will suggest themselves to him and when he goes to the text-books for the answer he will find only disappointment. Such has been my case and no doubt that of many others and I only state this as an explanation why the following studies were undertaken.

In making quantitative analysis for uric acid in urines from cases of undoubted uric acid diathesis, I obtained results far in excess of what the text-books stated and this suggested the question of solubility. This is variously stated as from 1 part in 14,000, 16,000 or 18,000 parts of cold water and from 1 part in 1,400 to 1,600 parts of boiling water; these facts may have a chemical interest but they are absolutely valueless to the clinician, for patients pass urine at neither of these temperatures. Ogden, in his treatise on urine examinations, states that Riedel says that uric acid is more soluble in a solution of urea, but as Ogden failed to state where Riedel's assertion was published, I can say nothing as to the details of that work. I thought that it would prove more time saving for me to determine for myself, the solubility of uric acid in a urea solution at body temperature. Having prepared some uric acid from snake excrement, which in itself constitutes a valuable experience, in a study of this kind, a 1% solution of urea was prepared, and to it added a definite amount of uric acid, but in excess of any possible solubility; this was warmed and while still warm, run through a filter. This filtrate was then treated and assayed according to the Folin method with a result of 1 part in 1,150 parts of a 1% solution of urea at about body temperature. As a check upon the accuracy of our assay, the amount of undissolved uric acid on the filter paper was next determined. The sum of the two, equalled the original amount added to the urea solution, and proved that technique and method were correct.

This proportion of solubility corresponds to the amount of uric acid that is found in many cases of uric acid diathesis; cases that pass a urine that may be regarded as a saturated solution of uric acid at body temperature and from which uric acid crystalizes out on cooling. In one of my cases, in 1,250 cc. urine, there was 1.85 grammes of uric acid, which corresponds very closely to the figures obtained in testing the solubility; whether or not the phosphates still further help the solubility I cannot say as this phase of the question was not taken up.

Before taking up a recital of my next experiments it may be well to mention a change, not exactly in the method but rather in the technique of Folin's procedure, which I devised and found more accurate. In order to more fully understand this modification of technique, it will be necessary to describe Folin's method in the original. I will quote from Ogden's work: "Take 100 cc. of the urine, saturate with ammonium sulphate crystals, (it requires about 10 grammes) let this stand at least two (2) hours, filter and then wash the ammonium urate precipitate with a 10% ammonium sulphate solution until it is free from chlorine. Then dissolve the entire urate of ammonium precipitate in hot distilled water, add to this solution 15 cc. of concentrated sulphuric acid and triturate, while hot, with a twentieth normal permanganate of potassium solution. The latter should be added slowly toward the end of the reaction, which is marked by the first approach of a pink color, which should be permanent for an appreciable interval. Each cc. of the permanganate solution is equal to 0.00375 grammes of uric acid. The number of cc. of the permanganate used, multiplied by the above stated coefficient, plus a correction of one milligramme for each 15 cc. of liquid present will give the amount of uric acid in 100 cc. of urine used and with the 24 hrs. quantity known, the total can be easily calculated."

This is Folin's method and in practice. it will be found that the end reaction is uncertain and indefinite as there indicated, for it allows too much room for the individual experimenter's interpretation of what constitutes a pink color or what he understands as "an appreciable interval." To eliminate this, it suggested itself, to bring the filtrate plus the sulphuric acid up to a definite amount, say 50 or 100 cc., putting this into the burette and triturating this into 1 cc. of the permanganate solution, to a decolorization which would be a much clearer, more definite and more easily determined end reaction. In actual practice this proved so and it is the procedure that was followed in all the experiments and tests here recorded. Furthermore it eliminated the necessity of the addition of one milligramme for each 15 cc. of liquid, for our very first experiments proved that it would account for all of a definite known quantity of uric acid.

I wish to say right here that the quantitative estimation of uric acid sounds much more formidable than it proves in actual work.

From these primitive and simple experiments, several plans of attacking the uric acid diathesis, suggest themselves, The first would be to administer some substance that would heighten the solubility of uric acid; another to increase the quantity of urine and then to combine the two, which if we succeeded in keeping the urine always at the point of saturation might suffice to keep the system from storing uric acid. Whether any of the old remedies were capable of realizing the former has been the subject of much discussion and the preponderance of evidence is in the negative, on the other hand, just increasing the quantity of urine has not always sufficed to keep down the symtomatology of the substance; but I will leave the discussion of that phase of the question for later consideration and let us return to our experiments.

The first substance that interested me, was one discovered by Schmoll, 1904, and to which he gave the name of thyminic acid, not to be confounded with thymol which is sometimes called thymic acid. After I have described its behavior toward uric acid in the test tube and in actual clinical tests I will give its origin and history. To 30 cc. of 1% urea solution, 0.1 gramme of uric acid was added and then 0.2 grammes of thyminic acid; the whole was warmed and while still warm, filtered. An assay of the filtrate and the residue on the filter only yielded 29% of the original amount of the uric acid with which I started. This means that 71% had entirely disappeared or been converted into something else. As it was some three or four years since I had read up on this substance, the result was somewhat disconcerting; but when I referred to the notes that I had made at that time, I found that the substance was believed to change 1½ times its own weight of uric acid into a solution from which it was unprecipitable. Later on I performed the experiment over again with different proportions, but not having an incubator could not get an action of more than 1¼ times its own weight; that is, that 0.1 gramme of thyminic acid converted 0.125 grammes of uric acid into a shape that would not show in the assay.

Before I take up the action of thyminic acid in clinical tests I wish to say that I applied the same laboratory tests to piperazine; a mixture of uric acid, 0.2 grammes.

Uric acid .... 0.2 grammes.
Urea .... 0.2 "
Piperazine .... 1.0 "
Aqua .... 30.0 "

This was warmed for ½ hour, filtered, then assayed; the filtrate held in solution 0.037125 grammes; the residue on the paper showed 0.13875 grammes, a total of 1.75875 showing a loss of 0.24125 grammes. I will show the difference between the two substances in solution. I do not want it thought that I advance this as an argument against piperazine; simply because it does not act like the other substance in the test tube, proves nothing, but I will leave the discussion of that for later.

I will now take up the result on the urine of thyminic acid administration; Mr. H., aged 56 years, amount of 24 hours' urine was 1024 cc. (32 ounces) and assayed 1.8 grammes (28 grains). Five days after taking 12 grains of thyminic acid each day his urine for 24 hours amounted to 1820 cc. and the total amount of uric acid was 0.45 grammes (not quite 7 grains). During the time that he was taking thyminic acid, his 24 hours' urine was several times assayed but never did the uric acid go above 8 grains for the 24 hours and sometimes it was lower than the first figures quoted. Beside the uric acid figures, the increased quantity of urine is significant; there was no albuminuria whatever in this case. He

came to me complaining of a cough at night and some slight emphysema; with disappearance of his uric acid, his cough also disappeared. I do not mean to infer that this or any case of emphysema is due to uric acid.

I shall recite other cases, but prefer to take up the consideration of the theory which underlies thyminic acid medication. Schmoll found this substance first in the thymus gland and hence gave it the name of thyminic acid; later it was found to be a constituent of all nuclear gland tissue and therefore is also sometimes called nucleotin —a phosphoric acid derivative. Minkowski gives for it the chemical formula $C_{30} H_{46} N_4 O_{15}$; Kossel's formula differs materially from this, it is $C_{16} H_{25} N_3 P_2 O_{12}$. The preparation which I used is a synthetic one. There is much that speaks for the correctness of Schmoll's discovery and his theories about the relation of this substance to the uric acid metabolism. If this substance is found in all nuclear tissue, gland tissue, then the liver, the largest nuclear tissue gland in the body, must be the largest thyminic acid producer and this corresponds with the most recent clinical conception of uric acid, held by the physiologists.

All attempts, experimentally, to reproduce any or all of the symptom complex, which the clinician has believed to be due to uric acid, have failed. This is a forceful argument for the existence in the body of a substance such as Schmoll believes himself to have discovered. Many have held the belief that uric acid diathesis was purely of dietetic origin, but such a belief is irrational; for, if that were so, all living upon a similar diet would suffer from it. This is far from being the case; often one member only, of a whole family is afflicted, yet practically all participated in the same diet. There must be some integral fault in the particular economy, owing to which, it fails to properly metabolize the uric acid. The theories as to the etiology of uric acid are numerous and varied, but none of these theories will stand critical examination. If Schmoll is right, and I believe he is, that it is the lack of thyminic acid in the body that causes a failure of the uric acid to be held in its proper physiological state, it still does not explain what this lack of thyminic acid is due to, and that unknown "what" is the etiology of uric acid diathesis.

The failure to reproduce experimentally the phenomena of the uric acid diathesis, has led to scepticism as to whether any pathological significance is to be attached to uric acid *per se*. Not until the experimentalist finds some means to prevent the bodies of his subject animals from secreting this anti-uric acid substance, will he be able to contribute one iota to the question of uric acid possibilities. Until then the study of the picture will belong entirely to the clinician; but the clinician will not be able to draw it, until he insists upon actual assays of uric acid in the urine examinations and refuses to accept a thumb-rule estimate, based upon a ratio between urea and uric acid. Such an estimate may be correct when things are normal, but does not hold good in pathological states; only an actual assay can tell us this.

Sir W. Roberts, in his article on gout, in Albutt's System, Vol. III, speaks at some length upon the chemistry of the combinations between uric acid and sodium, says that uric acid normally exists as a quadriurate and that the sodium combines with this to form a bi-urate which is the form in which it is deposited in the joints and bone ends. But all this preceded Schmoll's discovery. Further he speaks of the solubility of this bi-urate and the danger of a free sodium administration; he says that pure water is the best solvent for this bi-urate. The older physicians used potassium salts and I once witnessed the results of an intensive potassium iodide treatment upon such deposits. From that case, I feel justified in sounding a warning against an attempt to accomplish this absorption, lest with its absorption, we create a condition worse than the one we aim to relieve, for in the case in mind the patient lost the power to hold anything between the fingers. Uric acid does not always manifest itself by a "brick dust deposit" in the urine, indeed maybe that is only a stage; and certainly gout is not the only role that uric acid has in its repertoire.

It never was the intent, nor is it within the scope of this article to write a full description of all the clinical features, which may, directly or indirectly be due to uric acid. I do not believe that at the present time these are even known in their entirety. I have spoken of its marked presence in a case of emphysema, but I do not wish to be understood as believing that this is a constant in every case of emphysema. Uric acid is *not* to be considered as the sole cause of all the ills to which human flesh is heir. There are, however, some things of clinical value in the recognition in uric acid diathesis; there is for instance a peculiarity in the urinary history, namely that the patients have times when their urine does not bother them; I mean by that, that they can hold their urine for a long time without discomfort; then comes a time for them when they must void their urine very frequently and the necessity as well as the desire to empty the bladder is most imperious and distressing; if for any reason this is impossible, the urine involuntarily escapes. My experience has taught me to look for this bit of history. With such a history, a search for acne-like pustules and scars on the back and the nates, should be made. Urine rich in uric acid is usually scanty in quantity, even in spite of the necessity of frequent micturition. Uric acid seems to me to be a powerful cardio-vascular irritant, and Haig has shown its effect upon the nervous system by its relation to some headaches.

In the case of a lawyer, who, by a scalp specialist had been told that he had too much uric acid in his system, came to me and I prescribed thyminic acid without first determining quantitatively his daily amount of uric acid. Later he told me that since using the thyminic acid, a little eczematous patch under his left knee had entirely cleared up, but three months after stopping its use, it returned, and on resuming the medication it again disappeared. Bulkley in a recent article, the date and publication, I unfortunately am unable to recall, shows the value of a non-nitrogenous diet upon certain skin affections. This opens the question whether the good effects of such a diet as Bulkley advises are not as attributable to the unloading of the excess of uric acid as well as to lack of urea forming elements. Heretofore we have had no effective means of ridding the system of uric acid, except by diet. A rigid diet would not be long carried out by patients, but with thyminic acid we are able to very well control it without resort to diet. It must be remembered that no curative powers are claimed for this substance, because it will not stimulate the economy to put forth more thyminic acid, but if we supply it steadily to the system we can certainly do much to prevent the accumulation and deleterious effects of uric

acid. Fenner in the *London Lancet* has shown that in a number of cases, the unloading of the system of its uric acid was also accompanied by a marked decrease and in some cases an entire disappearance of sugar from the urine where this had been present. Clinically the presence of uric acid and sugar has long been recognized, but were by most considered to be a frequent coincidence or a complication. From Fenner's careful studies and reports we must accept a much more close relationship between these two conditions in which a much more important role falls to the part of uric acid and one that in part seems to strengthen and justify the French conception of a dual role of the liver in the production of clinical types of glycosuria.

In closing this article, I wish to say that I realize fully, that I have contributed nothing to the chapter of uric acid diathesis from a diagnostic or pathological point; nor do I flatter myself that I have added anything new to the treatment. Neither of these things were in my mind when I started these studies; I had seen the claims for thyminic acid and in other articles again saw them most emphatically denied; to know for myself which of these conflicting statements were right; that was the mainspring of my experiments and justice is the excuse for this report.

BIBLIOGRAPHY.

Minkowski. *Die Gicht.*
Hess & Schmoll. *Arch. fur experimentelle pathologie und pharmacologie,* 1896.
Kossel. *Centralblatt fur die Wissenchaften,* 1893.
Kossel & Neumann. *Zeitschrift fur Physiologische Chemie,* 1893.
Schmoll. *Archives general de medicine,* 1904.
Richardiere & Sicard. *Goutte,* 1910.
Fenner. *London Lancet,* 1905, Vol. II.
Fenner. *London Lancet,* 1908, Vol. II.

After operations on the perineum the bowels should be kept free to prevent straining of the parts operated on.

THE FIRST WOMAN PRACTITIONER OF MIDWIFERY AND THE CARE OF INFANTS IN ATHENS, 300 B. C.

BY

GILBERT TOTTEN McMASTER, M. D.,
New Haven, Conn.

The late Theophilus Parvin, while lecturing to his students at the Jefferson Medical College, once said, "Sometime, you will hear of a new discovery in medicine. The propounder, of that *new idea*, will become famous. Some day, while looking over books of the forgotten past, you will find that this *new* idea, is not *new*, that it was known to the Ancients; they performed it in a queer manner, perhaps, but it was the same. For example, today we hear much of massage. Upon some of the stones of ancient Egypt, and Arabia, Dr. Schliemann tells me, we find illustrations of this procedure. Gentlemen, *there is nothing new under the sun."*

Dr. Parvin's assertion is better appreciated when we study past methods in medicine, crude though they may appear from their admixture with religious fads.

The Greeks certainly placed medical and surgical knowledge on a scientific basis. They were a nation of real culture, even though they were rude and unpolished in their forms of expression. But in the care of newly born infants they were much like us of today; like us in the little things, and that is what counts after all. They were strikingly like us, in enforcing the laws governing the practice of midwifery, in Athens, 300 B. C. The old Athenian M. D.'s were jealous of their rights, just as we are today, for jealousy, I am sorry to admit, has never been a stranger to those of the "Physic Art." As the story goes, there was a law in Athens forbidding women, or slaves from practicing midwifery. Men only had this right.

Modesty, then as now, was common to women, regardless of the assertion of the great Pope some 1700 odd years later. These women of Athens objected strongly to being exposed *"To the hands of men."*

The first midwife in Athens was one Agnodice, a woman who was evidently backed by her sex—*"the Sex"*—for when she got into trouble her Athenian sisters stood by her.

Agnodice disguised herself as a man, and repaired to Herophilus, a famous physician and anatomist of Athens, 300 B. C., and began the study of midwifery. She became proficient in her chosen profession, and then disclosed herself to her sex.

Women have always talked among themselves. *Eustathius* out of *Euripides* says in these immortal lines

"ἔνδον γυναικῶν καὶ παρ' οἰκέταις λόγος."

"Women should keep within doors, and then talk."

And they did talk—and settled the fate of some doctors, then as now. The result was that women about to be confined, would have none but *Agnodice*. The demand for her was excessive; greatly to the discomfiture of her brother physicians, to whom her sex was not yet known.

Her inroads upon their financial rewards were keenly felt. Then the Athenian physicians suddenly evinced the customary professional amiability and good will, and a violent devotion to ethical standards, by vehemently denouncing Agnodice, *"As one that does corrupt men's wives."*

To controvert this far from complimentary accusation by her loving medical brethren, Agnodice revealed her sex to her tormentors. The Medical Faculty of

Athens indulged in protests in highly flavored Greek, when this heinous crime became known. They persecuted the girl to the limit of human tolerance. They appealed to the law courts, for the law regulating the "practice of midwifery" had been violated.

as they stood before the lawyers were in reality pleading for their own lives, when demanding clemency for their learned sister. But their veils, as *Euripides* proves, were not so heavy as to hide their beauty:

"ἐγὼ δὲ λεπτῶν ὄμμα διὰ χαλυμμάτων·"
"ἔχουσ᾽,ἀδελφὸν τ᾽ουκἀνειλόμγν χεροτν·"

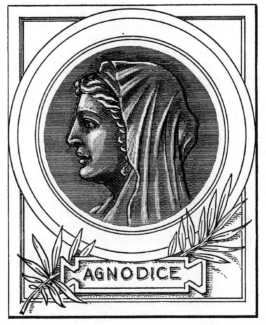

AGNODICE

Agnodice fell into the clutches of the law. Her ruin was imminent. Doubtless she already felt, in anticipation its penalties, when to the chagrin of the "most learned and reverent doctors," the matrons of Athens, waited upon the courts "en masse," fearlessly telling the jurists that *"they were not husbands but enemies, who were going to condemn the person to whom they owed their lives."* These veiled Athenian women

Iphigenia (Euripides Iphg.) Taur. V 372. "Seeing my brother through my thinnest of veils."

In this instance, it must have vastly enhanced female beauty. The Athenian lawyers, whose profession has never been proof against the charms of a pretty woman, repealed the law debarring women from practicing midwifery, and were chivalrous enough to rule that "three of *the sex* should practice this art in Athens." (*Archaeologia Graeca.* John Potter, D. D., London, 1764, Vol. II, pages 324-325).

Right here, about 300 B. C. is an instance of a medical practice act, laws governing a license, a state board, and all that sort of thing, with the foreshadowing of the Woman's Medical College.

I believe this to be the first time history mentions a female following any branch of medical practice.

It is evident that there was a united body of medical men at Athens at that period, who were pioneers in organized opposition to illegal practices. There were no doubt exams. and statutes governing the practice of medicine, where "fools asked questions, for wise men to answer," as Francis Bacon has wisely said.

The efforts of the Ancients for a painless delivery were absurd and clouded in mysticism, but a few of their superstitions may be of interest for psychologic study.

For example, *Elithera* and *Lucina,* among the Greeks, were supposed to care for women in the pains of child bed. Lucina, is believed to be light, hence the lines of *Ovid.* "—— Tu nobis lucem, Lucina, dedisti." "Lucina, you first brought us into Light."

Then Juno was supposed to have a hand in the game, as indicated by the lines, "Juno Lucina, ser opem"—"Juno Lucina, help assist the Labor."

Cicero declared that the Moon, or Luna, as the Romans called it, had a firm power over generation, at certain Zodiacal signs. (*Cicero de Nat Deor lib II*).

The Greeks and Romans alike believed that if a painless delivery took place, it was a positive sign as to the virtue of the woman, and a special dispensation of the Gods. Then it was quite the thing for the woman, when confinement was at hand to be in the vicinity of a palm tree or hold in her hand palm branches, which eased her pain, so it was thought. For example, when Latona was brought to bed with Apollo, Theognis bespeaks the God as follows:

—Σὲ δεὰ τεχε ωότνια Ληὶà Φοίνιχος δαδινῆζ Χερσὶν ἐφαψαμένη·

"When handling *palm* trees Latona brought you forth."

And even Horace (the greatest wit and poet of them all) in Liber III Od, XXII, says:

"Montium custos nemorumque virgo,
Quae laborantes utero puellas
Ter vocata audis, adimisque letho,
Diva triformis."

"Goddess, to whom belongs this hill, this brake
Where frighted deer their covert make,
Triple Diana, who dost hear,
And *help child-bearing women* after the *third* prayer."

When the child was born, common reason prevailed. No sooner had the infant made his entrance into "this vale of tears" than they washed it in water. (Warm, some say). For example, when Callimachus referring to Jupiter's birth:

"Ενθα σ' επεὶ μήτηρ μεγαλων ἀπθήχαῖο χόλπων,

"Αυζίχα διϛ́ήτο ζοον ὕδαῖοϱ, ὧ χε τοχοιο
"Δυμαῖα χϋίλὼσαῖιο, τεὸν δ' ενί χρῶτα λοέσσαι·

"As soon as you were born, and saw the light,
Your Mother's grateful burden, and delight,
She sought for some clear *brook* to *purify*
The *body of so dear a progeny.*" (*Hymno in Iovem, VI 4*).

But those of Lacedaemon, as Plutarch tells us in his life of Lycurgus, used not water but wine when the newly born saw light, "in order to estimate the temper, and complexion of the bodies of the newly born." If these Spartans had the idea that the child might be feeble or "have convulsions, or faint upon being bathed," this was usually most unfortunate for the child. While those of vigorous and powerful constitution, would "gain firmness and possess a temper like unto steel so hard would it be to overcome them."

Next came the division of the navel. This operation called ὀμφαλητομία whence arose the saying *"Thy navel is not cut."* The full import of this speech is not at first apparent, but this much: *"You are an infant scarce separate from one's mother,"* and later in bluff King Hal's time, *"Thou art yet tied to thy mother's apron strings, thou varlet."*

But just how this cord was severed, whether torn or cut by a sharp instrument, is yet open to argument. At all events it was done by the nurse, as the records show. After this operation, the child was wrapped by the nurse in "swaddling bands," lest its lower extremities, not being able to hold its weight, might become crooked.

The Spartans, however, used no such aid, but were of such experience that they brought up their young without such coddling and had straight strong children. The course followed by the Spartans Plutarch gives us fully in his life of Lycurgus as follows:

"Their management of children differed likewise from all the rest of the Grecians, in several ways, for they used them to any sort of meat, and sometimes to bear the want of it, not to be afraid in the dark, or to be alone, nor to be forward, peevish, and crying, as they generally are in other countries through the impatient care and fondness of those who look after them. Upon this account Spartan nurses were frequently hired by people of other countries; and it is reported, that she who suckled *Alcibiades* was a Spartan."

After this the religious ceremonies fill each hour and day, for strange as it may seem to us, these barbarians were more attentive to their gods, than are we of today to ours.

The last measure of note is the purification of the mother, which took place upon the fortieth day after confinement. This is so steeped in myth and symbolism as to hide the real medical facts, but looking backward one must agree that *"There is nothing new under the sun."*

SYMPOSIUM ON INFLUENZA IN CHILDREN.

INFLUENZA IN INFANTS AND YOUNG CHILDREN.[1]

BY

HERMAN SCHWARZ, M. D.,
Adj. Pediatrist, Mt. Sinai Hospital.

In giving a practical talk on influenza in infants, I must necessarily try to impart to you just what I mean by this term. For if I am to refer only to those cases of influenza in which the influenza bacilli are found, I am afraid that the discourse will be even shorter than it is. For it is a well known fact that since the large epidemic in 1889, true influenza bacilli are being found less and less often in the cases which we ordinarily speak of as influenza. Paul Krause suggests that those cases in which the bacilli are found should be called influenza, and those in which they are not found be called grippe; and Holt recom-

[1] Read as part of the Symposium on Influenza in Children at the March meeting of the Eastern Medical Society.

mends somewhat similarly that only those cases 'in which the influenza bacilli are found in large numbers should be classed as influenza. Anyone who has tried to search for and to grow the influenza bacilli knows how difficult it is and can hardly make this classification one of practical use. Furthermore, it is a well known fact that in healthy individuals, influenza bacilli are very often ' found, especially during the winter months. In addition 'they act as distinct saprophytes in the exanthemata.

In a large series of cases of respiratory infections in children reported by Holt, he found 19% of the normal individuals examined to have the influenza bacilli. In 76 cases of pneumonia, 37 cases showed influenza bacilli. In 20 cases of bronchitis, 3 showed influenza bacilli. In 29 cases of tuberculosis, 4 showed influenza bacilli. The germs seemed to grow better in combination with the streptococcus and staphylococcus. Curiously enough Jehle found the germ in the heart blood postmortem in only 3 out of 20 cases of pulmonary influenza; whereas in the exanthemata, the germ was very regularly found in the blood. Holt has shown that the germ is less likely to be found in the nose and throat than in the bronchi and the pneumonic areas, and it is therefore important to get bronchial secretion and not nasal-pharyngeal for examination. As will be discussed later, they occur in the bronchi ectatic cavities which are relatively frequent after influenza pneumonia. To sum up, therefore, our general conception of influenza, or grippe, in infants as seen in New York, we might term it an acute inflammatory disease of the respiratory system, less frequently, of the nervous system, and least or probably not at all of the gastro-enteric system.

In proceeding to the discussion of the symptoms and characteristics of infantile grippe, I can only give you some general impressions which I have gathered in seeing these infants during the winter. Contrary to the other diseases of infancy and childhood, influenza does not spare the young infant, nor does it draw much distinction between the bottle or the breast-fed. It seems to me in our climate to depend upon the character and the type of the infant in the first place, and ' secondly to the construction of the nasal-pharyngeal passages. There is no question that the exudative type of infant as described by Czerny, with its head and facial eczema, fat and chubby body, has less immunity against this disease than the normal infant. The deformities of the nasal-pharyngeal space, including adenoids and tonsils, and a superabundance of lymphoid tissue in the pharynx also tend to predispose to the disease. In addition to the deformities in the pharynx and nasal-pharynx we must not forget the deformities in the nose itself in these young infants and not let them be subjected to 3, 4 and even 6 adenoid operations, in order to prevent them from having colds. One must wait until the nose is fully developed and has stopped growing and go after the nasal obstruction which is often present. This grippe, then, in infants, manifests itself most commonly in an infection of the nasal-pharynx, most often due to the pneumococcus, streptococcus and staphylococcus; less often to the influenza bacilli.

The Coryza.—It is important to know that there are two distinct forms of acute rhinitis in infants; one of which is highly contagious, the other, not, and it is impossible to differentiate them. In a goodly proportion of the cases there is no coryza nor even a pharyngitis. Whenever the latter is present, however, the redness seems to be limited to the pillars and the posterior pharynx, so that looking into the child's mouth the buccal mucous membrane and roof of the mouth is usually pale, and the back of the throat profusely red. The presence of the rhinitis or pharyngitis alone will often give rise to a temperature in infants, which we commonly call grippe. However, in many instances, these symptoms pass over in a few days without marked fever, unless we have one of the characteristic complications, namely, the involvement of the ear, bronchi or lungs. The temperature curves in the uncomplicated cases of grippe, are extremely varied; last usually from two to three days, but may continue for a week or more. During the past winter I have seen a number of these cases with and without rhinitis and pharyngitis, with temperatures ranging from 103 to 105. There were two classes— one in which the curve was distinctly remittent, 99 or 100 in the morning, 104, 105, in the evening; in others, a perfectly constant temperature for five or six days, ranging around 104. These cases can only be called grippe at the end of the disease, and when everything else has been excluded, ears, lungs, and urine. And this brings me to the important point in the symptomatology of these cases, namely a careful examination of every part of the body, especially the ears. The leucocyte count does not help one out for it varies considerably, being low, 6 to 8 thousand in some, or 10 to 14 thousand in others. The polynuclears, however, are increased and eosinophiles are usually present. Blood culture is of very little avail. It is important therefore to know that during the winter time, we get a class of cases which may run a temperature for a number of days, with absolutely no physical signs or at the most, a slight coryza and pharyngitis.

The Ear.—One of the most frequent complications of grippe in these infants is the involvement of the ear. Influenza bacilli have been repeatedly found in the ear but much less frequently than the other bacteria. In 57 cases of otitis, of which 50 had influenza bacilli in the throat, Holt only found four cases where they were present in the ears. The infant's ear is more prone to involvement on account of its anatomical peculiarities. I can just touch lightly upon this as, no doubt, Dr. Oppenheimer will tell you much more. You must know that in infants the tympanic cavity is really not a cavity, but filled with folds of mucous membranes and septa. Therefore, the drainage is poor. The tube is short and wide, and the muscles are weak. Furthermore, the horizontal position in which the children are constantly kept, the obstructions in the nasal pharynx due to adenoids, especially in the fossa of Rosenmuller, all tend to cause obstruction and infection. In breast-fed babies, improper nursing occluding the anterior nares may cause a blocking of the tubes. Whether the infection may occur through the blood and not by way of the tube, is still an open question. The symptoms that direct one's attention to the ear, are with the exception of fever, often nil. Up to the fourth month, infants rarely point to the ear as the seat of pain. Restlessness, and inability to take the bottle or the breast, are often the only subjective signs. Pain is absent in very many cases. They do suffer perhaps on account of the pain that may be induced by swallowing, yet I wish to emphasize the fact that it is surprising how many of these children get their otitis, which can only be

208   **AMERICAN MEDICINE**
Complete Series, Vol. XVIII. }   ORIGINAL ARTICLES   {   APRIL, 1912.
New Series, Vol. VII., No. 4.

found out by looking at the ear. And this brings me to the forcible assertion that in order to examine any infant with temperature properly, one must have his head mirror and his ear speculum with him. One need have no elaborate apparatus, an ordinary head mirror, a convenient gas jet, and a decent applicator, is all that is necessary. It is often easier to clean the canal by moistening the applicator with warm water and cleaning the canal through the ear speculum. In looking at the drum in very young infants, one must remember that it is so placed that it is almost continuous with the posterior canal wall. The ordinary otoscopic picture I shall not go into, such as redness and bulging, except to mention that bullae on the drum membrane are very characteristic of influenza otitis, that when perforation occurs, granulations may often form at the point of perforations and discharge may continue for quite some time. The course of these cases is usually a few days of temperature, then a dicharging ear, and recovery in from two to three weeks. However, in many cases, perforation does not occur quickly because the drum membrane is thicker and relatively more resistant than in the adult, and inasmuch as the middle ear is not a cavity, it takes longer for an empyema to form, bulging and perforation to take place.

Let me add here, that in contra-distinction to older children and adults the temperature may keep up even after free discharge has taken place. Yes, it may keep up for weeks, without any true operative mastoiditis being present. I say this here because it is not fair to assume operative mastoid simply because one has profuse suppuration and temperature. How to judge whether a case is going on to perforation or not, is beyond me. Leucocytes do not count, temperature is, of course, some guide, yet I have seen perforation take place after the temperature has entirely disappeared. Distinct bulging and persistent temperature would be the indication.

The Lungs.—Pulmonary complications will be so well discussed by Dr. Northrup, that I will touch upon but two forms which very often follow influenza in infants.

First, the occurrence of chronic recurrent bronchitis with marked *dyspnea and fine crepitant rales.* Second, the subacute and chronic broncho-pneumonia with or without the formation of interstitial pneumonia. Here the disease is markedly protracted, remissions and intermissions of temperature and persistence of physical signs. These children often have attacks of bronchitis every 4 to 6 weeks throughout the year.

Gastroenteritis.—Whether gastroenteritic grippe occurs, I really cannot say, for I would not know how to recognize it. Vomiting at the onset of the attack has been a rather frequent symptom this winter. As far as the kidney and bladder are concerned infections are rather rare. Holt, Poltauf and Kretz have found nephritis and influenza bacilli in the kidney and in a case of my own, granular casts were present for a number of days. These disappeared and for the past five months the child's urine has been comparatively normal. Cystitis, I have never seen occur.

Treatment.—The rhinitis had better be left alone—for irrigations of the nose in these infants is very dangerous and often brings on an olitis. The use of urotropine has not been very satisfactory. Phenacetin and caffein preparations make the patient more comfortable.

INFLUENZAL MENINGITIS.[1]

BY

GODFREY ROGER PISEK, M. D.,
New York City.

Professor of Children's Diseases, Univ. of Vermont; Adj. Prof. Children's Diseases, Post-Graduate Hospital; Asst. Visiting Physician, Willard-Parker Hospital; Visiting Pediatrician to Red Cross Hospital.

While influenzal infection of the central nervous system is not common, it must be conceded that many more cases do occur than are recognized. In fact it is only in comparatively recent years, since the more common use of lumbar puncture, that this fact has become known.

Even the pathologist will fail to stamp some of the cases as due to Pfeiffer's bacillus if his attention has not been drawn to the possibility; since his media must be specially prepared and be of the blood-agar type to produce the most characteristic growth.

We can understand why a positive diagnosis was not made more often in the days preceding lumbar puncture, if it is remembered that the organism very readily loses its viability after death of the patient, so that even on necropsy the etiological factor may be destroyed. There is no question that the toxin of the influenza bacillus has an especial affinity for the nervous system, and if there is a general bacteremia present resulting from a virulent type of organism, the delicately organized nervous system of the child suffers profoundly.

If we are to profit by a discussion of this subject we must be aware of the fact that influenzal meningitis is a disease almost invariably fatal. Up to the present writing

[1] Being part of a Symposium on Influenza in Children, before the Eastern Medical Society, March, 1912.

there have been only 5 recoveries among the 58 reported, which can be regarded as absolutely authentic cases of influenzal meningitis.

Tuberculous meningitis alone can claim a higher mortality record. In the tuberculous variety our hands thus far have been tied and we see no rays of promise for the immediate future. Not so with influenzal meningitis. Here the organism lends itself more readily to sero-culture and judging from the results obtained recently by Wollstein in monkeys, we are hopeful that this high mortality may be cut down.

This infection may well be studied in children, for this variety of meningitis occurs like all other forms, more frequently in early life than in adults. Of the 58 cases reported only 5 were in adults.

Besides causing a sero-purulent meningitis with its usual dire results, clinical studies lead us to the belief that the organism under discussion may also cause less virulent infections which result in a non-purulent type of encephalitis. The minute hemorrhages which follow are not sufficient to cause marked cortical irritation, but may account for some of the children who frequent our clinics suffering from sclerotic changes of the brain, hydrocephalus, or even imbecility.

That a primary inflammation of the meninges ever occurs is questionable. The presence of the organism in the cerebrospinal system with symptoms pointing to the involvement of the respiratory system, the nasopharynx or the accessory sinuses of the middle ear, stamp the disease as metastatic in character.

Furthermore, in the clinical manifestations of influenzal meningitis we have no exact means of distinguishing it from a cerebrospinal or pneumococcic meningitis.

The diagnosis is more apt to be made in the presence of an epidemic, or if it follows closely in the wake of an influenzal type of inflammation in the cavities contiguous to the brain.

The symptoms do, however, exhibit a number of characteristics and some departures from the above forms of meningitides that are worthy of consideration here. In any case we are justified in considering a diagnosis of influenza if the severe constitutional symptoms are out of proportion to the temperature curve.

Meningismus, a condition due to cerebral irritation, is not uncommon in early life and must be distinguished from a true meningitis with parenchymatous involvement of the meninges. It is the toxemia which causes the intense headache and somnolence which are found in meningismus. The younger the infant the more severe are the symptoms.

In tuberculous meningitis the sensory symptoms predominate, and it is usually only late in the disease that motor manifestations occur. The contrary is true in infections with Weichselbaum's bacillus causing cerebrospinal meningitis; here the motor tract gives evidence of early involvement resulting in convulsive seizures, early rigidity of the neck and opisthotonos. In other words pressure is not exerted equally over the different parts of the cortex and localizing symptoms are induced.

In the type under consideration there is a rather sudden transition from the symptoms of cerebral congestion to those resulting from intraventricular and subarachnoid pressure. The headache suddenly becomes more intense and there is pain on pressure over the eyes and the supraorbital region. The restlessness which is present is produced by irritation of the sensory centers and later the pressure becoming excessive, these centers are depressed or altogether abolished. Convulsions may occur only at the outset or they may be intermittent. Retraction and rigidity of the head, with a mild grade of opisthotonos are usually recorded. Examination of other organs at this time may disclose the fact that there is also present an influenzal pneumonia, a mild peritoneal irritation, or that there is involvement of the head sinuses due to the Pfeiffer's bacillus. If there is an accompanying albuminuria the diagnosis is still more suggestive, as it occurs in 6-10% of all cases. The high remittent type of temperature that occurs when the meninges are involved is due to the absorptions of septic products from the coverings of the brain.

Other data suggestive of the influenzal type of meningitis are those referable to the heart and peritoneum. At first the toxin causes tachycardia or arrythmia, later the increased cerebral pressure destroys the irritability of the pneumogastric nerve and a continuously high pulse rate results. The general nutrition suffers severely and emaciation is steady and progressive. Delirium, stupor, or profound coma develop. Convulsions of a severe type (particularly in infants and younger children) are apt to occur at or near the beginning of the disease. The loss of flesh and strength is rapid and marked. Photophobia and irregularity of the pupils with loss of pupillary light reflex and nystagmus are quite regularly present. Neuroretinitis is found on ophthalmoscopic examination of the fundus in some cases. The respirations vary with the stage of the disease; they are increased when the fever is high, sighing and shallow when stupor begins and are irregular when coma develops. The respirations, as in other forms of meningeal inflammation may become Cheyne-Stokes in type from pressure upon the medulla due to the contained cerebral fluid.

The reflexes will help to establish the diagnosis, but must be interpreted with caution. The tâche-cerebrale is always obtained, but is only a minor confirmatory sign. The Babinski reflex, or extension of the great toe on irritating the plantar surface of the foot, is confirmatory, but valueless in children under two years of age, although negatively it may be of assistance. Kernig's sign, which is obtained in nearly all meningeal cases at some stage or other, is also present in all forms of cerebral irritation.

Macewen's sign, or the hollow note elicited by percussion over the parietal bone, is obtained only in cases in which fluid has accumulated in excessive quantity in the ventricles. The rigidity of the neck with dilatation of the pupils when attempts are made to flex the neck is also a helpful and confirmatory sign of meningitis.

The Brudzinski sign, or the synchronous flexion of the legs and arms when the chin is forcibly depressed to the fixed thorax and the contra-lateral sign in which we obtain involuntary flexion of the opposite extremity when one member is flexed, are confirmatory signs of value resulting from irritation of the cerebrum and posterior columns of the cord.

While the phenomena just enumerated may assist in drawing the attention of the observer to the form of meningitis present, the only absolute method of making an exact diagnosis is by examination of the cerebrospinal fluid.

Lumbar puncture not only establishes the specific etiologic factor but gives relief from intracranial pressure and assists in forming the prognosis. The procedure is not difficult and if performed with aseptic precautions and a due regard to the anatomy, is productive of no harm.

In influenzal meningitis the fluid is quite uniformly cloudy, with a well marked straw colored sediment. In those instances in which a clear fluid has been reported the presumption must be that not enough fluid was abstracted to have drained the subdural spaces. The fluid abounds in polymorphonuclear leukocytes while the bacilli are found to be both intra- and extra-cellular, and do not differ morphologically from those obtained from other structures of the patient.

Aside from making the diagnosis the practical feature is the treatment. Heretofore we have treated this type of meningitis as we would a pneumococcic, or in fact any meningeal inflammation with signs of intra-cranial pressure—namely by supportive measures and repeated lumbar punctures. The rapidity of the course in this type hardly allows us to await results with medication directed toward the invading organism, so that such a drug as hexamethylenamin (urotropin), for example, is of little avail.

Fortunately this disease has been studied at the Rockefeller Institute and Wollstein in her recent valuable contribution to this subject has shown the curative possibilities of an immunized serum made from a virulent influenza organism which is said to possess high opsonic value. As a result of a series of experiments with monkeys, she calls attention to the need of making the diagnosis by puncture promptly, and the necessity of resorting to the serum treatment immediately after the diagnosis is confirmed. To quote her own words: "In view of the severe conditions surrounding influenzal meningitis in human beings it would seem desirable to apply the serum to the treatment of the spontaneous disease."

The mode of use is that recommended for Flexner's serum. The results obtained in animals have been so encouraging that we should feel ready to employ this means when opportunity presents in an attempt to restore the life of a patient with influenzal meningitis that experience tells us is otherwise doomed.

36 East 62nd St.

COMPLICATION OF INFLUENZA AFFECTING THE EAR, NOSE AND THROAT OF CHILDREN.[1]

BY

SEYMOUR OPPENHEIMER, M. D.,

Associate Otologist, Mt. Sinai Hospital; Consulting Laryngologist and Otologist, Gouverneur Hospital, Philanthropin Hospital, Har Moriah Hospital, Monmouth Memorial Hospital, etc.

Undoubtedly influenza affects children much more frequently than is generally supposed and that this is so, can be readily appreciated when it is realized that Pfeiffer's bacillus gains its entrance into the system through some portion of the respiratory mucosa and while the affection largely affects adolescents, yet small children present pathologic changes in the ear, nose or throat in many instances. In the infant, it does not commonly involve this portion of the economy, but is most frequently observed in the school child, especially those between the fifth and fourteenth years.

On account of the marked tendency to involve the mucous membranes, this affec-

tion presents a serious aspect in many children and not only do acute changes occur, but secondary catarrhal affections become prominent at a later period, when the primary cause of the affection has passed away. It is characteristic of influenza, that it may affect any portion of the mucosa from the larynx to the middle ear, or the nasal accessory sinuses independently, so that a primary otitis may occur, or one may less frequently find the child complaining of a faucitis which reveals itself as part of the general infection. The microorganisms of the disease seem to possess a peculiar faculty of involving the various anatomical recesses of the upper respiratory tract and it has impressed me, that the serious morbid changes occur in those cavities where the lining is of marked tenuity and illy supplied with vascular channels, as the maxillary antrum, the frontal sinus (if the child is of sufficient age for this cavity to be developed) and the middle ear cavity.

Irrespective of the type of influenza present, some inflammation of the nasopharyngeal tissues is found in nearly every instance, as more or less hyperemia of the mucosa, but as a rule, the inflammatory changes are not equally distributed over all the surface. As far as a typical clinical picture of influenza is concerned, such is practically impossible when it affects the upper air passages, as any portion may be involved as a coryza or faucitis, which usually lasts for four or five days, and then subsides, but it will be found that in addition, some of the general symptoms of the disease are complained of; the catarrhal inflammation is of greater severity than usual "cold in the head"; it is more prolonged and the accessory sinuses are much more apt to become involved. It may also be pointed out in this connection, that

[1] Presented as part of a Symposium on Influenza in Children at a meeting of the Eastern Medical Society, March 8, 1912.

chronic alterations of the mucous membrane with more or less thickening and purulent changes, are apt to remain and prove most intractable to treatment, but differing from that observed in adults, in the absence of the hemorrhagic type in the child, which in my experience, is most unusual.

In a well marked case, there is acute nasal catarrh often extending to the nasopharynx, with the mucosa presenting a dusky red hue. Often the inflammation seems most intense in the vault of the pharynx and it is in this type that aural complications are most apt to occur, while at other times, the inflammation will assume the character of a purulent rhinitis and then the accessory sinuses become involved in a much larger number of instances than is generally appreciated. The nasopharyngeal lymphoid tissue becomes swollen and the inflammation remains persistent and severe, causing considerable distress to the child and undoubtedly in many instances, being the basal factor in the future development of "adenoids."

The pharynx and tonsils are also involved, but not as frequently as in the adult, except in older children where the pharyngitis may be severe. Rather characteristic, is that the dysphagia and pain are out of all proportion to the objective signs and the patient will complain bitterly of the distress, when the pharynx shows but a moderate degree of inflammation. Tonsillar and peritonsillar abscess occur infrequently, but when present, the inflammation greatly adds to the danger of aural complications and one also finds excessive swelling of the cervical glands which as a rule does not occur during an ordinary inflammatory attack. Should the tonsils be involved primarily, abscess not infrequently takes place, but it

differs in no way from that produced from other causes. In children, however, who have had previous tonsillitis, there frequently occurs a lighting up of the old process and either during the attack of the general infection, or immediately following, a rather violent tonsillitis not infrequently occurs.

One would expect that from this location, the next structure to be involved would be the larynx and while such occurs frequently in the adult, it is uncommon in the child and the presence of localized hemorrhages, edema or paralyses are rare. There may be, however, a severe catarrhal laryngitis, but an independent laryngitis without other symptoms, does not occur as a result of influenza in the child. When the larynx is involved there is hoarseness, or intermittent aphonia and in almost every instance there is also a trachitis, with its accompanying spasmodic cough. Examination of the larynx in the older child, shows a diffuse inflammation and rather characteristic is the desquamation of the superficial epithelium over irregular areas of the vocal cords or in their immediate vicinity. It responds most slowly to treatment and the intermittent aphonia may remain for a number of weeks after all signs of the original infection have disappeared.

Most important is the relation of influenza to pathologic changes in the accessory nasal sinuses, as in the child such a relationship is not fully appreciated and many cases are unrecognized during the acute stage and go on to chronic changes with the original cause apparently unknown. Within recent years the prevalence of influenza has caused a great increase in the number of sinusitis patients seen by the specialist and in a not inconsiderable number, the primary cause can be traced to an attack of influenza during childhood. As a rule the inflammation is not the direct result of infection by the specific organism of this affection, but a latent sinusitis occurs from secondary invasion by streptococci or staphylococci and I especially wish to emphasize that in children the results of an influenza sinusitis do not necessarily show themselves as a direct sinusitis, but may appear as a nasopharyngeal catarrh, indicative of the subacute sinus changes.

In acute sinusitis there is usually a preceding purulent rhinitis and this may involve any of the sinuses depending upon their development in the child affected. Usually this shows itself by the rhinitis not improving in a few days and then pain develops over the particular sinus involved, with a continuation of the nasal discharge. Should the affection run the usual course, within a few days the symptoms subside, but not uncommonly there remains some inflammation of the sinus involved, which continues for an indefinite time. Most frequently the antrum, or frontal sinus is involved, but the other cavities are also implicated depending upon the age of the child. It should be remembered in this connection, that the maxillary sinus exists in the newly born, but does not reach its full size until about the fourteenth year. The frontal sinus usually becomes differentiated from the seventh to the twelfth year; the ethmoidal cells exist at birth; while the sphenoidal cavity is usually found about the sixth year, so that sinusitis can be present in the child at a very early age, dependent upon the particular sinus affected. Most frequently the antrum is involved and rarely the cavity of the sphenoid, the symptoms differing in no way, however, from sinusitis produced by other causes.

Frontal sinusitis is apt to appear early in the course of the general disease and produces symptoms of great distress; the frontal headache so frequent in influenza, being the result of involvement of this sinus. Of necessity, there is some ethmoid inflammation in practically every instance of influenzal rhinitis and headache is complained of at the root of the nose, or over the vertex, while there is an augmented purulent discharge and the ethmoiditis is apt to resist treatment and continue as a chronic suppuration.

Finally, a few words as to the aural aspect of this affection; hemorrhagic otitis seen in adults, is not characteristic in children and the pathological changes which occur in the auditory apparatus, are the result of either a primary infection by way of the blood channels, or more frequently the invasion spreads from the nasopharynx and the secondary infection produces the suppuration so frequently seen in influenza. Usually the infection is secondary streptococcal with suppuration of the middle ear and rapid perforation of the membrana tympani. The otitis media has characteristics that differentiate it from aural suppuration, the result of other infections and most prominent is the intensity of the pain which frequently remains unabated even after the membrana tympani has been incised, or perforation has taken place. The onset is rapid and the constitutional disturbance marked, while in a few hours the drum membrane shows exaggerated hyperemia and even bulging from the accumulation of fluid behind it. Following this there is a profuse purulent discharge which has a remarkable tendency to become chronic despite active treatment and it is associated with impairment of hearing of greater severity than is usually found with other forms of suppurative otitis media.

At the same time in the majority of patients, the prognosis is good and despite these severe symptoms, recovery takes place rather quickly, although some deafness may remain for a considerable time. These cases are frequent and on account of the wide prevalence of influenza at times, there is a great increase not only during an epidemic period, but also following it, and the incident of aural diseases is also augmented by the lighting up of chronic cases, which had previously been quiescent.

A much more serious aspect, however, occurs in a rather large group of cases, in which the mastoid tenderness which is present but which disappears on the subsidence of the acute symptoms, increases in intensity with an augmentation of the purulent middle ear inflammation and within a few days the mastoid structures become involved, with rapid osseous destruction. If the cells are well developed, the septa are broken down and the entire mastoid area becomes converted into a large abscess cavity, which if not promptly operated perforates usually through the cortex with the formation of a subperiosteal purulent collection.

Most serious intracranial complications may of course ensue, but it must always be borne in mind in studying these cases in the child, that at times in the presence of a severe attack of influenza with high temperature and complicating suppurating otitis media, various symptoms resembling meningitis, or venous thrombosis may be present, which are not the result of the aural inflammation, but of the underlying general infection.

45 East Sixtieth St.

PULMONARY ABSCESS ASSOCIATED WITH INFLUENZA.[1]

BY

W. P. NORTHRUP, M. D.,
New York City.

The pulmonary complications of influenza in children are well illustrated by the following case history.

F. F.—14 months old was brought to the hospital on the third day of illness. It was not seemingly very sick and was brought in thus early because the child had been in hospital before and the mother had no prejudices. For our study this was fortunate.

The illness may be divided into three periods of which the short time elapsing before entrance may constitute the first.

First period—three days—the mother describes an ordinary cold. "Nose ran," hoarse cough, restless at night, vomited several times, "seemed sick," no chills, bowels regular.

Second period—eleven days, case under observation. Our first observation was that the child seemed "sick," that the depression was out of proportion to the physical findings, the temperature was not so high, but the child was "dopey." The mucous membrane of the nose and throat was congested, dusky, just the sort to lead one to suspect ear complication. True to the indication the ear drum was red and bulging, discharging a thin pus after incision. There were significant signs over the middle third of the left lung in the axillary line. Briefly stated these signs suggested a solid unaereated mass about the size of a golf ball, a "dead unaired mass." The position was next to the pleura, its inner margin of shadow not quite touching the heart shadow, when viewing it squarely in front. The words used in description intimate how definitely the mass was circumscribed and how defined it was. The half-dozen Roentgen radiograms accompanying the presentation of the case history are referred to in the description here

[1]Read as part of a Symposium before the Eastern Medical Society, March 8, 1912.

given. Each radiogram shows the advance of the process as described. The physical signs were marked dulness, pleural friction, rales and lack of all breathing sounds, evidencing a dead mass. The temperature of these eleven days fluctuated in wide excursions touching 106 F. twice.

We believed the dead mass to be an abscess and accordingly tried to reach it with a large aspirating needle. With a radiogram taken from each of two directions we could not extract any pus. So convinced of the presence of pus were we that we punctured from front and side and back, over and over, until it seemed useless and unjustifiable to repeat. Not a drop of pus could be obtained. Cultures were taken from needle points, from the throat swabs and from ear pus. Streptococci and staphylococci and pneumococci were obtained but no influenza bacilli. The conviction prevailed that nothing but the latter would satisfy the conditions. During the second period the shadow enlarged somewhat, still globular.

Third period—4 days—the 15th day of illness. Here began a change in the picture. Now the chart was that of a straight pneumonia and the radiogram showed pneumonic consolidation of the upper lobe, spreading also into the lower. The temperature ranged high and regular, the respiration-pulse ratio was approximating one to three, there were rales, bronchial breathing, etc. There was every reason to believe that pneumonia was present. After holding pretty regularly about 103 F. the temperature suddenly fell to normal and crisis, so far as the chart was concerned, was seemingly present. The general condition of the child was not favorably affected by the change, however, and steady failure was apparent.

The remainder of the story is short. The child went into collapse and on the 24th day of illness died.

After death puncture was again resorted to in the hope of finding pus. None was extracted.

The three periods of sickness might have appended a fourth and important chapter —the post-mortem record. The first shadow of a globular mass proved to be a globular mass of necrotic tissue within which were two small abscesses about the size of a bean each. The necrotic mass was beginning to liquefy but the process had not advanced far. It apparently required a secondary infection to liquefy it as in tuberculous coagulation necrosis. To our great satisfaction, from the cavities of the two small abscesses were isolated the bacillus of influenza.

At last the whole picture fits together and as sometimes happens the autopsy findings fit the clinical findings.

SOME REMARKS ON THE TREATMENT OF CANCEROUS GROWTHS WITH SELENIUM COMPOUNDS.[1]

BY

F. VON OEFELE, M. D.,

New York City.

I claim the priority of the treatment of cancer by selenium, for there are several short communications in the scientific press written by me before Wassermann announced his treatment of mice. There are also many physicians in this city, to whom I have spoken in the last 2 or 3 years regarding the possibility of treating cancer by selenium and who are well aware of my studies in this direction. But the most important point for my claim is, that I can give step by step the results as well as the dates of the researches that led me to become convinced of the possibility to treat cancer with selenium. I will tell you these conclusions and I hope they will be conclusive enough to convince you that I have been a pioneer in the treatment of cancerous growths by selenium. I also hope that from the discussion you will re-

---

[1] Read at a meeting of the Yorkville Med. Society, Feb. 19, 1912.

ceive an idea of its possibilities and that in the near future you will be able to treat your hopeless cases of cancer and obtain results by selenium, to the extent of palliation at least, without waiting to hear whether the experiments on mice are completed or not.

To understand this treatment we must start at the chemistry of albuminous matter. It is known that one part of the albuminous matter of the food is digested in an acid medium by the pepsin of the stomach and the other part is digested in an alkaline or neutral medium by the trypsin of the pancreas. For purposes of discussion I will divide all the albumins into these two kinds, calling the first the albumin group and the second the nuclein group. Our living bodies are known to contain these two groups of albuminous matter. In the plasma of the cells there is more of the albumin group, and in the nucleus of the cells there is more of the nuclein group. The albumin group contains more sulphur and the nuclein group more phosphorus. But most of the albuminous group contains a little phosphorus, and most of the nuclein group a little sulphur, while there are many links that connect each group with the other. The phosphorus is never lost in the analysis; therefore for a long time we have known a great deal regarding phosphorus metabolism. The sulphur however is mostly lost in the determination of the inorganic constituents. In the text books, therefore, we see very little regarding sulphur metabolism. The exact determination of sulphur in the feces 10 years ago received my special attention. From that I went to the study of the sulphur end-metabolism in the urine. After extensive work I made the statement that in various diseases the sulphur metabolism

is materially changed which change can be estimated by the urinary findings. In other words, from the quantitative determination of sulphur compounds in the urine we can diagnose different diseases. Especially was it noticed in my work that the amount of sulphuric acid in the urine was very strongly decreased in cases of carcinoma. In very malignant cases the sulphuric acid was more diminished than in the cases growing more slowly. The neutral sulphur was increased but not as much as the sulphuric acid was decreased. This special statement of the neutral sulphur I had never published, but Salomo of Vienna found the same and published it. Therefore, for this part I can claim no priority. But this is only a very small part of the whole statement. It may be good that Salomo did find it, thereby corroborating my results. From these studies it was evident that in the treatment of cancer it was necessary to improve the oxidation of sulphur. At this time I met Dr. F. Klein who had been doing some chemical work with selenium but he was not a physician and therefore did no medical work. He got me re-interested in selenium and I proposed it as the best agent which could raise the sulphur oxidation in the body without disturbing the metabolism. Selenium belongs to the same chemical family as sulphur and tellur. But it is always in the middle member of the family that the physiological power is the highest, as I stated in one of my papers on selenium.

Selenium unites in all chemical combinations, in which sulphur combines, organically or inorganically. But selenium easily takes oxygen for its first degrees of oxidation and gives it off to sulphur for the sulphur's higher oxidation. This is the essential property which makes selenium capable of improving the sulphur oxidation and changing the sulphur metabolism of a dangerous carcinoma into the metabolism of a less dangerous carcinoma. It has not been absolutely proven that this conclusion is true, but if it be true, and the amount of necessary selenium be no higher than the older homeopathic physicians have repeatedly used in their own bodies experimentally, it certainly did not seem dangerous to administer it to human beings in even smaller amounts than the homeopaths have used for 80 years. In these experiments on human cancer cases, we were successful as you can learn from the special communications of the physicians who worked with me. Dr. Eugene Kessler, who is present, is one of these gentlemen.

It seemed to me that it was absolutely unnecessary and inconclusive to attack these problems by animal experimentation. Cancer of rats and mice is never as malignant as it is in human beings. Carcinoma of mice can after 3 to 4 weeks of growing retrogress and disappear, which has rarely if ever been heard of in human cancer cases. Cancers in mice and rats may become so large that they reach the same size as the animal itself without destroying its life. This also is never possible in human cases. Therefore, I think it was more reasonable to go directly to humans, as was done in this city, instead of making inconclusive animal experiments.

But before this selenium treatment there were many other cancer remedies and some of these appeared to be very successful in a theoretical way. But none of them had reached the point of being a practical success. Many of these are chemical compounds which produce a high degree of oxidation in the tumor. Others were aniline derivatives. Twenty years ago in many cases I used aniline; it did not cure the cancer but it retarded its growing. From this old experience I realized the possible value of aniline, and therefore recommended the combination of aniline and selenium. Although this combination was only used occasionally, it is very evident that it comes very near to the eosin-selenium combination of Wassermann. I do not know the theories that led Wassermann to combine eosin and selenium. It is a fact that selenium improves the sulphur oxidation, particularly if used in a combination with aniline derivatives or other matter. The all important question is which selenium compound should be used? There are 100 to 1,000 different selenium compounds that have possible value in the treatment of cancer. But I believe that the best, from logical standpoints, is a compound of selenium, which comes nearest to one of the regular constituents of the body. The body contains thio-cyanate in the saliva and urine, and artificially a seleno-cyanate can be made corresponding to this thio-cyanate which can be used not only with minimum of danger but which will pass through all body liquids unchanged and improve in the cancer tumor the sulphur oxidation. I will gladly give directions for making this preparation to the profession or druggists, Or if any physician prefers another selenium preparation, I will furnish directions for its compounding, if it is possible to do so. The eosin-selenium preparation suggested by Wassermann is not very difficult to make. It is only a question of time and money.

In conclusion, let me express the hope that not only the researches I have just described but those of all other earnest workers may contribute to that result we all so long to see achieved, the ultimate conquest of cancer.

THE DIAGNOSTIC VALUE OF INTRADERMAL INJECTION OF GONOCOCCUS VACCINE.

BY

JULIUS LONDON, M. D.,

Assistant Genito-Urinary Surgeon to Mt. Sinai Hospital, New York City.

Bruck in the *Deutsch Medecin Woch.*, 1909, describes a reaction for gonorrhea obtained by vaccination of patient with

negative, but in the same patients the same vaccine *injected into the skin* showed a beautiful result similar to the Stich reaction obtained by Hamburger and by Dr. George Manheimer of this city in tuberculin diagnosis.

In this preliminary report I desire to call attention to the diagnostic value of this method of intradermal injection of a few drops of gonococcus vaccine—50,000,000 to 100,000,000 per cc. in saline solution. In positive cases an area of erythema develops from one to three inches in diameter, in the center of which there is a small red papule, a little deeper in color

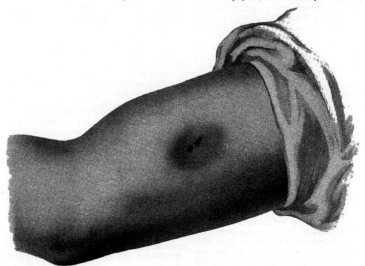

gonococcus vaccine according to the technique of von Pirquet.

Irons of this country has called attention also to this type of reaction.

In testing out a number of cases for this reaction by vaccination of gonococcus vaccine in saline solution my results were

than the surrounding areola. This central papule is really composed of two parts, one at the site of needle puncture and the other at the periphery of injection. Normal-saline solution may be used as control, but is not necessary as I have used a few drops of a solution containing 500,000,000 per cc. without any reaction in negative cases. Oftentimes the entire area of reaction is slightly elevated. Adjacent lymph nodes are not enlarged.

In negative cases there is no reaction or yellowish discoloration at site of injection. The reaction appears in from twelve to twenty-four hours and quickly fades in twenty-four to forty-eight hours, the central papule being the last to disappear.

763 E. 156th St.

THE ANNOTATOR.

Industrial Insurance in the Care of the Injured in Germany.[1]— Jaeger states that $1,500,000,000 have been paid to sick, injured and disabled workmen in Germany during the past 21 years.

The laws upon this subject originated in Germany in 1883 and similar compulsory insurance legislation has since then been enacted in England, France and most of the countries of Europe.

Industrial insurance legislation affects sickness, accidents, invalidism and old age.

Its principal merits are (1) It includes fundamentally everybody needing insurance, thus differing from other insurance companies.

(2) It furnishes for the workman the most comprehensive provision offering not only support by money, but free medical aid, free medicines, and free boarding in institutions.

(3) It offers the workingman the surest and cheapest system.

(4) The means and powers of the nation concentrated in the workingman's insurance have made it possible to solve other problems of civilization such as the systematic advancement of popular hygiene and the art of healing in connection with accidents, war against tuberculosis, housing of workmen, etc. These are very gratifying facts and show effectively that civilization is progressing in the most important matter of improvement of the welfare of those who have long been neglected. Let us hope

that the protective insurance physicians, on a large scale, will be the next step.

The Neglected Cold.[1]— Huber thinks that physicians and laymen alike are prone to minimize the significance of colds.

It is when we realize what their sequels, potential or actual, may be that they assume tremendous importance.

The two dominant sequels are pneumonia and tuberculosis.

It is not mere cold weather which invites one or both of these enemies, but alternating cold and warm, with the dust and germ laden atmosphere.

There are many things to be avoided in order also to avoid "catching cold," the superheated house with its deficiency of pure air and its excessive volume of CO_2, the germs in the clothing (hence the need of clean and well-brushed clothing), etc.

The actual cause of colds is, of course, bacteria, of more than one variety.

Some individuals are immune to such bacterial influence and hence to colds.

Apparent causes or coadjutants are mouth breathing, errors of diet, bad teeth, occupational influences, etc.

Prophylaxis is therefore all important in forestalling this most important disorder.

The timeliness of such warnings is perfectly apparent. There is no physical disturbance which the average individual is more inclined to slight and neglect than a cold, and too often it results as this writer has indicated.

Moral Problems of College Life.[2]— Seneca Egbert regards the three sins to which college students are most susceptible as gambling, drinking and licentiousness.

He thinks the first two of these are less prevalent than they once were, and that the third is the gravest from many points of view.

He therefore believes it is imperative that young men should have authoritative information as to the physical risks of venereal disease, their nature and their results.

[1] Chas. H. Jaeger, M. D., Am. Jour. of Surgery, March, 1912.

[1] John B. Huber, M. D., N. Y. Med. Jour., March 9, 1912.
[2] Seneca Egbert, M. D., N. Y. Med. Jour., March 9, 1912.

He emphasizes the important fact that sexual continence is not incompatible with good health, on the part of young men.

He also lays stress upon the fact that the teacher should appeal to the ethical and moral sense of the student in matters of this kind, on his own behalf, on behalf of his possible future family, and on behalf of the women with whom he might associate. Abundant physical exercise is advised as perhaps the best means of diverting the exuberant energies of youth.

This is a matter of the greatest significance and physicians will readily realize the responsibility which rests upon them as the teachers and guides of the youth who are under their care to a greater or lesser extent.

To no one will a young man more readily listen than to a wise and sympathetic physician in regard to the all important sex problems.

What a Father Would Tell His Son.[1]—
Wile notes the fact that nothing in regard to sex hygiene has heretofore been taught in the schools and he believes it devolves upon the father to instruct his growing son in regard to those matters which have so important a bearing upon his subsequent life. His own experience should fit him to be a guide for his son and he should encourage him in seeking knowledge which will inform him as to the care of his sexual organs and the care of his health in general. Stories about life in plants and animals will often prove very suggestive.

The hygiene of sleeping should be carefully attended to, courtesy to the entire female sex encouraged, and vigorous and fatiguing exercise recommended.

Teaching the evils of masturbation must not be shirked, and the physiological meaning of night emissions must be explained. The dangers of venereal disease must be pointed out and also the fact that except in very unusual instances sexual continence is not incompatible with good physical health. The education of children in sex hygiene should be supervised by parents from infancy to maturity.

[1] Ira T. Wile, M. D., *N. Y. Med. Jour.*, March 9, 1912.

The foregoing assumes of course, that the father is competent to give his son this useful advice. As a matter of fact, we know that in many, perhaps the majority of cases, he is not. It would seem to us that perhaps for another generation this most desirable advice could best be given by the teacher or the family physician.

What a Mother Should Tell Her Child.[1]
—Mary Sutton Macy answers this query by saying the truth, though not necessarily the whole truth. When the baby of three or four years of age asks the mother where he came from, let her take him into her confidence and show by the analysis of plant life, of seed and flower, how life in human beings also is propagated. If the mother does not know the answer to such questions she should find out as promptly as possible. When the age of eight or nine is reached the confidences of the hour of bedtime may be increased by simple information in anatomy and physiology.

Children should be warned against evil companions and the misleading stories which are so often told by them and encouraged to come to the mother for the answer to the sex questions which come crowding upon them.

When puberty arrives the girl should be plainly informed as to the meaning and importance of menstruation and the boy should be cautioned against the vices and sins by which he will be tempted.

The truth should be taught directly and the fact should ever be remembered that a child asks questions because he thinks, and he is entitled to information especially from those who are responsible for his existence.

Any comment would be the same as for the article which precedes this one that a greater degree of intelligence and a greater power of expression is assumed for mothers than most of them possess.

By all means let us insist that this important information be given but by one who not only can answer the questions of the child but can meet his objections if the answers seem unsatisfactory.

[1] Mary S. Macy, M. D., *N. Y. Med. Jour.*, March 9, 1912.

Chloretone as a Preventive of Post-Anesthetic Vomiting.[1]

—Biekle states that he never operates under a general anesthetic without first administering chloretone when possible. He gives fifteen grains in a capsule, one and a half hours before the operation.

Its advantages are said to be:

1. It lessens the patient's dread of the table.
2. The anesthetic is taken more quietly.
3. Less anesthetic is required.
4. The patient comes out of the anesthetic quietly. There is no tossing or restlessness, the quiet and absence of vomiting give physiological rest, healing by first intention being thus facilitated. Ligatures are thus less likely to slip and bandages remain undisturbed.
5. It minimizes shock to a remarkable degree.
6. Nourishment can be taken freely as soon as the patient becomes fully conscious.
7. In operating in private houses less nursing will be required and the nurse can clean up the scene of the operation while the patient is calmly resting.

The drug may cause slight dizziness prior to the operation but this is the only drawback which has been observed.

If ether has been administered there may be some ejection of mucus directly after the operation but there will be no subsequent vomiting.

Sanitary Conditions in Bakeries.[2]

—An editorial article on this subject informs us that of the 4,000 bakeries in New York City, the majority are in cellars or basements in which the sanitary conditions, especially as to ventilation and light, are woefully defective. The walls, floors and ceilings of many of them were found in a filthy condition, food was stored under most unsanitary surroundings, dirty clothing was often in contact with the food or the cooking utensils, and the latter were often in a condition which excited disgust. The bakers themselves, in many instances, were as unclean as was their environment. Such things are a menace to health and demand

action on the part of the municipal authorities.

In the factory bakeries the sanitary conditions were said to be good.

The following suggestions were made:

1. All bakeries should be licensed by the Board of Health.
2. No rooms should be licensed as bakeries which are less than nine feet high and none whose floors are more than four and a half feet below the level of the sidewalk.
3. A specific sanitary standard should be observed in all bakeries.
4. Bakeries should be inspected before and after a license has been obtained.
5. The Board of Health should have power to close and seal any bakery which does not conform to its orders, after forty-eight hours' notice.

The question naturally occurs why has the Board of Health allowed such a perilous condition of affairs to arise. Its powers are ample, it has inspectors who are supposed to be aware of such conditions, and the matter becomes exceptionally important because most of these insanitary bakeries supply the food for the poor who must take the cheapest they can get. We hope the time will soon come when all baker's food will be prepared in well-regulated factories, such as are now giving the most satisfactory results.

The Use of Saccharin in Food Prohibited.[1]

—An editorial states that the secretaries of agriculture and of commerce and labor have prohibited the use of saccharin in food after April 1, 1912.

Their decision is based upon the fact that saccharin is merely a sweetener and when thus used displaces the sugar of an equivalent sweetening power.

Since sugar has a food value and saccharin has none, foods sweetened with saccharin are adulterated under the food law as their food value is lessened.

The decision also notes that the use of saccharin in foods used by those who must abstain from sugar on account of disease need not be discontinued because it then falls within the class of drugs, the decision being restricted to foodstuffs.

[1] L. W. Biekle, M. D., *Therapeutic Gazette*, March 15, 1912.
[2] Editorial, *N. Y. Med. Jour.*, March 9, 1912.

[1] Editorial, *N. Y. Med. Jour.*, March 16, 1912.

Hence any food product containing saccharin may still be sold provided the label shows clearly that the substance is intended for persons who are prohibited by disease from using sugar.

It seems to us, if the decision is correctly stated, that there will be precious little difficulty in evading its provisions. It appears to be admitted that saccharin is not harmful but merely that it does not add to the food value of that which it sweetens, and if it does no harm it is straining a point to consider it as an adulterant, that is in a bad sense.

Besides what is to hinder anybody from buying and using as much as he chooses of the preparation which is labeled as intended for those who cannot use sugar? Isn't this slightly ridiculous?

Report of Progress in Sanitary and Moral Prophylaxis.[1]— Prince A. Morrow gives the following as some of the most apparent and significant evidences of progress in this field.

1. The change in the spirit and practice of the medical profession in sharing its knowledge with the public, the break with the policy of silence and concealment. The venereal infectious diseases may now be discussed before audiences of men and women with the same publicity as other infectious diseases dangerous to public health.

2. The change in the attitude of the public toward the sex problem. There is now open mindedness on the part of the public in marked contrast to the apathy or even hostility formerly prevalent. The question is even discussed in social circles with frankness, candor and competence.

3. The revolution in pedagogic and social sentiment on the question of sex teaching in schools, colleges and homes. Instruction in the laws of hygiene and sex is of supreme importance and it is most gratifying that conventional prejudice against such instruction is being overcome.

The importance of the work of this society cannot be over-estimated. It is singular that a question so important as the propagation of species and the organs whose health is essential to such propagation should for so long a time have been refused consideration by society in general. With free discussion and the diffusion of information on these matters the result cannot fail to be beneficial to the community.

Quinine in the Preventive Treatment of Migraine and Anaphylaxis.[1]—Herzfeld states that typical attacks of migraine have their origin in the gastro-intestinal tract and are due to autointoxication caused by the absorption of certain albuminoids. His statement has been questioned but it now seems to be conceded that the absorption of certain albuminoids gives rise to the condition now known as anaphylaxis, to which class the syndrome known as migraine or hemicrania is referred.

Having found in his own experience that during an attack of gastro-intestinal trouble certain foods which ordinarily caused no disturbance would then undoubtedly cause migraine he began to experiment with himself to endeavor to abort such attacks.

He was able to determine that when the stage of severe pain had been reached no abortive treatment was possible, the best he could do being to use palliative means.

But during the first stage of the trouble and even during the stage of scotoma, the gastro-intestinal trouble co-existing, quinine was specific if given early and in sufficient quantity.

Seven grains was the dosage which proved curative with him.

In urticaria, in serum exanthemata and in hay fever he also found quinine distinctly serviceable.

The Death-Dealing Influence of High Cost of Food Supplies.[2]— An editorial article calls attention to the influence upon the resisting power to disease of those who must adjust their diet to their limited earnings. It is shown that increase in wages has not kept pace with increased cost of foods. The evil results must fall heaviest upon the

[1] Prince A. Morrow, M. D., N. Y. Med. Jour., March 23, 1912.

[1] Herzfeld, M. D., Therapeutic Gazette, March 15, 1912.
[2] Editorial, N. Y. Med. Jour., March 23, 1912.

224   AMERICAN MEDICINE }
Complete Series, Vol. XVIII. }   THE ANNOTATOR   { APRIL, 1912.
New Series, Vol. VII., No. 4.

masses of the people, upon those who on account of their sanitary surroundings are most exposed to the evil conditions which make the body an easy prey to infection.

The poor resisting power of the countless millions who subsist upon rice is adverted to and the enormous rate of their suffering from infectious disease. Though such a diet supplies heat producing elements upon which muscular activity depends, it fails to supply albumin and nucleins which form the basis for our defensive or immunizing allies in the blood. Deficiency of food equally predisposes the body to infection, epidemics follow famine, abundant diet is an indispensable element in the treatment of tuberculosis and other wasting infections.

The albuminous foods are those which are now especially high in price and the result must be not only loss in efficiency but a decided increase in the infectious diseases. This is a situation which is not without alarming features. It is not the high-priced artisans, the plumbers, bricklayers, carpenters, machinists and many others, for whom the present scale of wages leaves a large margin of safety, but those in the humbler occupations who seldom have a chance to save anything if they would, for whom we should feel deep concern and for whom there should be help in the form of control of those organizations which monopolize the supplies of the necessaries of life. The food question was perhaps the most potent factor in bringing on the French revolution.

The Social Worker as a Factor in Solving the Dispensary Problem.[1]— Brown remarks that the dispensary evil is familiar enough to physicians in general, and he thinks the social service may be of assistance in remedying it. No physician who is in the least thoughtful or observant can have failed to realize the tremendous influence of free dispensary service upon the lay public, the profession and the resources of hospitals.

The average lay mind considers it good business to obtain for nothing any kind of service rather than pay for it. Many seem

[1] S. H. Brown, M. D., N. Y. Med. Jour., March 30, 1912.

to think they are conferring a favor on physicians by consulting them in a dispensary.

Again much of the dispensary work of the class just mentioned it must be admitted, would not be done at all, if it were necessary to pay for it. There may be an injury in such a service, in using time which is taken from the service of the really worthy poor. On the other hand, if poor patients happen to be very dirty or if their ailments are uninteresting, they may receive scant courtesy at the hands of dispensary doctors.

If however, the poor are clean and polite they usually receive all the consideration which could be desired and sometimes more than they deserve, especially if it is suspected that they have some kind of influence with the management of the dispensary. The suspicion that dispensary physicians are often guilty of toadying to this class of patients seems to have some foundation in fact.

The social service which is attached to many of the hospitals is composed of trained workers, both paid and voluntary, whose business it is to investigate the surroundings of those who seek free medical aid.

In many cases, perhaps in the majority, the need of assistance is found to be urgent. It is suggested that all applicants for aid, emergency cases being excepted of course, should first receive such investigation. This will enable all hospitals and dispensaries to weed out the *beats* and help the worthy. The visits of the social service worker at the homes of *beats* and impostors are not usually relished but they have been found very effective in stopping their impositions.

Notification of Venereal Diseases.[1]— To the ordinary mind venereal prophylaxis includes State regulation of prostitution, a measure which has been hastily condemned by moralists, and has met with so much opposition that one often fears that venereal disease will be allowed to spread without impediment, to the inconceivable detriment of the public health. It is an old rule in medicine that when we cannot

[1] Med. Press and Circular, April 3, 1912.

treat the cause of a disease we can always treat the symptoms. In the case of venereal disease, the cause is apparently at present beyond our power of control, but we may with profit limit its manifestations. To this end the early diagnosis and efficient treatment of all cases of venereal disease are essential, and just as important is the prevention of contagion. To carry out these aims with any prospect of success, notification is a necessary measure, and the Board of Health of New York City has taken action in a manner which should receive the careful attention of sanitarians in this country. It has been decided that those in charge of public institutions, such as hospitals, dispensaries, charitable and industrial institutions, including those which are supported in full or in part by voluntary contributions, shall report promptly to the Department of Health the name, sex, age, nationality, race, marital state and address of every patient under observation suffering from venereal disease. In addition, all physicians are requested to furnish similar information concerning private patients under their care, except that the name and address of the patient need not be reported. The Board of Health will undertake to make the necessary bacteriological examinations and tests for diagnosis, and to distribute curative sera, but only on condition that the data required for the registration of the case be furnished by the physician treating the patient. This is a step in the right direction, but we fear that it is in advance of what public opinion in this country will sanction.

The Pulmotor—A New Apparatus for Resuscitating the Drowned and Asphyxiated.—So much interest has been aroused by the press accounts of this new apparatus for performing artificial respiration and forcing a supply of oxygen into the lungs that we are glad to publish the following description from the *American Jour. of Clin. Med.* (April, 1912).

The pulmotor which the Commonwealth Edison Company has so far sent out is about the size of a large suit-case. In the lower portion of the case is an iron cylinder, 3½ by 21 inches, containing oxygen at a pressure of about 2800 pounds when completely filled. This life-sustaining gas also furnishes the energy which is required to induce breathing, in the following manner:

The oxygen from the tank flows through a reducing valve, which at the outlet side maintains a pressure of about seventy-five pounds, and from there to the controlling valve. Initially the passage to the lungs is open through this controlling valve. The latter connects with rubber tubes leading to a metallic face-cap with a rubber rim which closely fits the patient's face. This face-cap on one side is provided with a rubber bag, which permits a pair of forceps to protrude, by means of which the patient's tongue is held from obstructing the pharynx. The oxygen then has free access to the lungs.

When the pressure in the lungs has reached a certain value (about normal), a bellows interconnected with the lung cavity through the rubber tubes actuates the controlling valve. The pressure of the oxygen is now directed so as to create a suction over the connections which lead to the lungs, thereby causing exhalation of the gases previously forced into the lungs. When a certain vacuum is reached in the lungs and bellows, the outer atmosphere acts on the latter, which in turn operates the controlling valve and again admits the oxygen to the lungs. The frequency of these reversals depends upon the size of the lung cavity, a larger space requiring greater time, while with smaller lung cavities the operation is correspondingly more frequent.

This process is continued until the patient shows signs of natural respiration. The pulmotor action is then discontinued and the patient is allowed to breathe the pure oxygen through another small face-cap connected by a hose directly with the oxygen-tank.

Several patients can be treated at once. An extra tank of oxygen is carried in nearly all calls. This enables the operator to treat two persons at the same time, using the pulmotor on one and giving the other person oxygen from the oxygen bag. The majority of calls have been for more than one person—in several cases for four persons. In the latter cases it was possible to treat them all at practically the same time by having the patients close together and transferring the pulmotor and oxygen-tube from one to the other.

Ancient Egyptians and Modern Medicine.— As retribution follows crime, says a writer in the *Med. Press and Circular,* so with steps no less halting, science pursues disease. To cure the first colic, medicine was born, and surgery to treat the first cut. Considering then the age of these kindred blessings, we sometimes wonder that so many diseases are still beyond our power in regard both to cure and prevention. Professor Elliot Smith's researches into the relics of ancient Egyptian civilization have shown that many of the ailments from which we suffer today claimed their victims six thousand years ago. Rheumatoid arthritis was prevalent in predynastic times, as evidenced by the specimens discovered in the Nile valley. Urinary calculi were also found, and one on analysis proved to be composed of a central body of urates and a shell of phosphates, indicating that cystitis and ammoniacal decomposition of the urine, set up by calculi, are no new things. Gouty deposits in the shape of "chalk stones" occurred in several cases investigated. Though the symptomatology and treatment of appendicitis have been placed on a sound basis comparatively recently, the existence of the condition itself, six thousand years ago, was evidenced by the discovery of fibrous adhesions round the appendix. Little or no trace of syphilis, tuberculosis and rickets was found. The conclusion of the whole matter is the old truism that under the sun is no new thing, and perhaps even our science is but remembrance.

Origin of the Word "Ache."—An English writer, Basil Hargrave, in his book of "Popular Phrases and Names," gives the origin of the word "ache," now pronounced as one syllable, which, in the time of Shakespeare and much later, was pronounced as a word of two syllables, so that in "Tempest," where Prospero threatens Caliban, the true reading was:

Till all thy bones with a-ches make thee roar
That beasts shall tremble at the din.

The word ache comes from the Anglo-Saxon "acan" or "acian," the "c" pronounced "k." Jonathan Swift makes "old a-ches throb" and Isaac Disraeli in "Curiosities of Literature" says that what the poet and linguist wished to preserve was lost by the modern printer who, unaware of the old pronunciation, made "aches" one syllable and then to complete the meter crowded the word "will" into the line, making it "aches will throb." Butler in Hudibras used the old form:

Can by their pains and a-ches find
All turns and changes of the wind.

Latter Day Therapy.— A well-known physician on the Brooklyn Heights tells with some amusement of a time when a misunderstood word of his gave a patient an unpleasant time of it. A man, evidently used to a good deal of outdoor work, came to him, obviously tired and nervous and aching all over.

"Do you walk much," said the doctor.

"I sure do, Doc," was the reply.

"The trouble is you are all jarred to pieces on the pavements. Your nervous system is on the blink. Do you know rubber heels? Try some and see how you feel."

A few weeks later the man came in looking actually ill.

"Didn't you try my remedy?" said the doctor.

"That's just what I did, Doc," answered the man, "but I could hardly swallow it, and it made me right sick."

"Swallow what?" yelled the doctor.

"Why that rubber you said would heal me."

And across the street the barn robin chortled to the sun.

ETIOLOGY AND DIAGNOSIS.

The Epidemic of Septic Sore Throat.[1]—In a most comprehensive editorial article, Dr. Ruhräh discusses the prevalent serious epidemic throat disease. He notes that there have been reported from time to time epidemics occurring in European cities which have been characterized by sore throats of peculiar virulence. Sometimes these sore throats have been believed to be due to the influenza bacillus and at other times they have been traced to the milk supply. The first experience of this kind appeared in Boston last spring, and this epidemic was studied by Richardson and others, who found that the great majority of cases occurred in the users of the milk from one certain dairy. More recently the disease has been reported in Chicago by Davis and Rosenow, and there is also a recent report by Müller and Seligmann of an epidemic which occurred in Berlin. For the past few months the disease has also been prevalent in Baltimore, Maryland, and it has been so entirely different from anything which has been met with in previous years that a few words of description may not be out of place. In the Boston epidemic most of the cases oc-

[1]John Ruhräh, M. D., *New York Med. Journal*, Mar. 23, 1912.

curred in adults, and children were almost exempt; in the Baltimore experience the greatest proportion of cases occurred in children and even young infants, and while there was a considerable number of cases among adults, the disease, as a rule, was not as severe in them as in the younger patients.

The cause of the disease is a streptococcus, which may be demonstrated in exudates or in smears from the throat, or from the organs *post mortem.* In the smears it occurs usually as a diplococcus, or as a streptococcus in short chains. In cultures it appears as a streptococcus. The disease is apparently transmitted in two ways—by the milk supply and by direct contact, and it occurs in small household epidemics, usually all, or nearly all the occupants suffering more or less with the disease, while there will be one or two very severe cases. The onset of the disease is rather sudden, often with high fever and with sore throat, sometimes the picture of follicular tonsillitis, sometimes with a tonsillar exudate rather closely resembling diphtheria, and sometimes with a diffuse dusky redness of the entire mucous membrane. After a few days the disease usually remits, which is followed in a day or two by a recurrence of all the symptoms and a marked swelling of the cervical lymph nodes, so that the name of bubonic sore throat has been suggested. The fever lasts from a week to three weeks or longer, and there is usually considerable prostration. There is a marked tendency to complications of various kinds—formation of abscesses, erysipelas, otitis media, meningitis, peritonitis, and gastritis being the most frequent. Sometimes the joints are swollen and painful, and the patients old enough to talk complain of headache and soreness of all the muscles. Another curious manifestation is edema of the eyelids, accompanied by a very slight conjunctivitis; this edema is frequently unilateral. There is also frequent marked involvement of the nose and the accessory sinuses. In some instances the disease comes on very suddenly, with very high temperature, 105° and 106° F., or even more, and marked prostration, in these cases there is usually some disturbance of the bowel, occasionally symptoms suggesting peritonitis. These cases are often fatal, death taking place from failure of the respiration or the circulation, due to the intense toxemia. In other cases there is merely the picture of a continued fever, with slight angina, the fever lasting in some instances four weeks. In these cases the temperature is characterized by marked remissions. The disease may be differentiated from typhoid by the Widal reaction, and the spleen is not enlarged, or only slightly so; the liver may be slightly enlarged. The blood shows leucocytosis, involving chiefly the multinuclears.

The treatment of the disease is rather unsatisfactory; patients should be isolated, and as a preventive the milk should be boiled. The treatment is along general lines, and the most successful measures are those which tend to support the strength of the patient and keep up the nutrition. Fresh air in the sick room

and careful nursing are also important. As a rule, severe purges should not be used. Surgical interference is often necessary for involvement of the ear, or for abscesses, or for the peritonitis, but in most of the peritonitis cases toxemia is so great and the patient's condition so alarming that laparotomy offers but little hope of relief. The lymph nodes should not be incised unless there is definite pus formation, as, notwithstanding the fact that they reach an enormous size, they practically always subside without suppuration. Cold applications may be made locally, or such sedatives as lead water properly diluted, or belladonna ointment may be used.

The Diagnosis of Cerebral Hemorrhage.[1]—In the diagnosis of cerebral hemorrhage when the patient is in a comatose or semi-comatose condition, the first step is to decide whether the condition is the result of a cerebral lesion, such as hemorrhage, embolism, or thrombosis, or is due to a toxemic state, such as is found in uremic or diabetic coma, alcohol or opium poisoning.

The history of the case sometimes gives us a clue as to the condition we have to deal with, but very often it does not, and in many cases, especially in hospital practice, we must make our diagnosis by careful examination of the patient. Examination of the urine very often puts us on the right track, as, for instance, in diabetic or uremic coma, but it should be remembered that the presence of albumin in the urine of a comatose patient does not necessarily mean uremic coma, for cerebral hemorrhage occurs more frequently in Bright's disease than in any other condition. Moreover, albumin in the urine may be the result of a cerebral hemorrhage. In a case recently admitted to hospital I made a diagnosis of uremic coma, because the patient suffered from coma attended with bilateral convulsions, and his urine contained 1 per cent. of albumin, but at the autopsy his kidneys appeared normal, and examination of the brain revealed an extensive hemorrhage into the left lateral ventricle and blood clot also in the third and fourth ventricles.

Undoubtedly the most valuable evidences of a cerebral lesion are the presence of unilateral signs, such as rigidity or flaccidity of one side, conjugate deviation, inequality of pupils, the presence of Babinski's sign, or absence of the plantar reflex on one side.

It is a remarkable fact that Babinski's sign may be found as early as six hours after the onset of the apoplexy, and in two cases I found it present four hours after the onset of the attack.

In most cases of cerebral hemorrhage some of these unilateral signs are present, as the lesion is usually in the region of the internal capsule, and therefore the motor tract on one side only is involved, but in cases of ventricular hemorrhage the blood finds its way from the

[1]By F. X. Callaghan, M. B., B. Ch., Dublin, *Med. Press and Circular,* Mar. 13, 1912.

lateral into the third, and finally into the fourth ventricle, and therefore signs of bilateral paralysis or irritation are found. Consequently some other means of diagnosis should be used, and I think lumbar puncture the most trustworthy, as the presence of blood in the cerebrospinal fluid would settle the diagnosis.

As regards the differentiation between hemorrhage, embolism, and thrombosis, to discriminate between thrombosis and hemorrhage is the main difficulty, for in embolism the nature of the lesion is nearly always suggested by the presence of mitral valve disease, and, moreover, to make an early and definite diagnosis between hemorrhage and thrombosis is of the greatest practical importance, since the treatment of the two conditions is very different.

Many authorities lay stress on the following points as being characteristic of thrombosis:—

I.—Premonitory symptoms—e. g., headache, numbness, and twitching in the limbs about to be paralysed.

II.—Development of paralysis without loss of consciousness.

III.—Incompleteness of the hemiplegia.

IV.—Condition of heart and blood pressure.

These points are certainly of importance, and in some cases I have made what was apparently a correct diagnosis of thrombosis by consideration of these points, but, even in my small experience of cerebral hemorrhage, I have seen cases in which premonitory symptoms were present, and cases in which the hemiplegia developed without loss of consciousness. I have also seen a case which, from the success of the treatment adopted, I presume to have been one of thrombosis, in which the hemiplegia was complete, and in which the vigorous heart and blood pressure of 140 suggested hemorrhage.

Therefore, to differentiate hemorrhage and thrombosis, some more certain means is desirable, and I believe such a means is at our disposal in lumbar puncture.

In cases of thrombosis, as the blood remains inside the blood vessels, it does not find its way into the cerebro-spinal fluid, whereas in hemorrhage the effused blood passes into the cerebro-spinal fluid, and can be detected by lumbar puncture. It is, of course, necessary in such cases to discard the first few cubic centimeters of fluid, as blood present might be due to local injury caused by the needle.

In cases of ventricular hemorrhage, it is easy to understand why the cerebro-spinal fluid obtained by lumbar puncture should contain blood, because the blood passes from the lateral to the third, and then to the fourth ventricle, and through the foramina of Magendie and Luschka into the cisternae at the base of the brain, and so to the spinal meningeal space; but in cases of hemorrhage into the substance of the brain, it is not so clear why blood should be detected in the cerebro-spinal fluid obtained from the lumbar region. Purves Stewart, however, mentions lumbar puncture as a means of differentiating hemorrhage from thrombosis, and in one case of partial hemiplegia following an injury to the head, the cerebro-spinal fluid I obtained on lumbar puncture contained hemoglobin, the fluid, indeed being straw colored, and the color persisted after centrifugalisation.

The Various Tubercular Reactions and Their Comparative Value.[1]—According to Benker, the tuberculin reaction manifests itself differently according to the dose, the site of application, the clinical stage of the disease and also the individual susceptibility towards the tubercular endotoxins and exotoxins.

The phenomena of the reactions are at times local, that is, manifested by an inflammatory process at the point of application; and again general, of which at times a characteristic fever reaction is the only demonstrable effect of the systemic action. Other signs of the general reaction are malaise, lassitude, pain in the back and legs. At times a focal reaction takes place, consisting of severe inflammatory changes in the neighborhood of tubercular foci, producing even necrosis.

All the reactions manifest themselves to the eye or ear of the observer, or upon palpation, according to their location and intensity.

General and focal reactions occur only, as a rule, when a sufficient quantity of tuberculin is introduced subcutaneously and absorbed into the general circulation.

The five most important methods of application are:

1. Cutaneous method, after Morro (inunction of tuberculins in the unbroken skin).

2. Cutaneous method after Von Pirquet. (Inunction of tuberculin after superficial scarification of the skin as in vaccination.)

3. Intracutaneous or intradermal method after Mantoux and Roux. (Injection of 1-100 M. grm. of tuberculin into the skin of the leg.)

4. Subcutaneous method, after Koch. (Injection of tuberculin under the skin for absorption into the circulation.)

5. Application of tuberculin to the mucous membranes (of which the conjunctival method of Wolff-Eisner and Calmette is the most important).

6. Installation of a definite quantity of tuberculin into the conjunctival sac. Of the many tuberculins advocated for these tests the tuberculin O. T. (typhus humanis) has stood the test of time and is the best.

The cutaneous methods, after Morro and Von Pirquet reveal both active and inactive tuberculosis, except during the first year of life.

The subcutaneous method tends to produce general and focal reactions and is therefore dangerous to the patient.

The conjunctival method does not reveal all the early and active cases with one per cent. tuberculin solutions, as advocated by Wolff-Eisner; stronger solutions prove dangerous to the eye.

[1] O. H. Benker, M. D., Interstate Med. Jour., February, 1912.

The safest method to test quantitatively the tuberculin sensibility is the intradermal method with definite quantities of tuberculin.

The author has added to the intradermal method a control test of 1-10 c. c. of a ½ per cent. solution of carbolic acid, three extra dilutions of tuberculin O. T. representing 1-10 mgrm., 1-1000 mgrm., and 1-10,000 mgrm., and changed the site of application from the leg to the arm.

The technique is as follows: The place of inoculation over the biceps muscle is cleaned with alcohol; then with a sterile platinum needle and glass syringe, the eye pointing upwards, inject 1-10 c.c. of the following five solutions: Phenol, ½ of 1 per cent.; O. T., 1-10,000 mgrm., O. T., 1-1,000 mgrm., O. T., 1-100 mgrm., O. T., 1-10 mgrm., at a distance of 5 cm. from each other, and allowing the solutions ·slowly to infiltrate the skin, producing a small papule.

A positive reaction takes place as a rule several hours after the inoculation to 1-10 mgrm. and 1-100 mgrm., and often also to 1-1,000 and even to 1-10,000 mgrm., showing greater intensity to the stronger solutions. After twelve to twenty-four hours the infiltration becomes visible and palpable, and the inflammatory reaction increases accordingly. At the end of forty-eight hours it has reached its greatest intensity. We see now a central tubercle encircled with· a zone of redness, shading off gradually into the healthy tissues. This zone of redness varies from 1 to 2 cm. The reaction fades away, as a rule after two days, but occasionally persists for several weeks. The control shows a slight erythema, which becomes imperceptible after a few hours. The following are his concluding statements:

1. That we can demonstrate by the intradermal test, in doses from 1-10,000 to 1-100 mgrm., nearly all doubtful and early cases of active tuberculosis.

2. If after a 1-10 mgrm. injection no reaction occurs, we can exclude tuberculosis.

3. From reactions to doses between 1-100 and 1-10 mgrm. we can only conclude that latent tuberculosis is present.

TREATMENT.

Chronic Rheumatism.[1]—The pathogenesis of nodular rheumatism is still very obscure and yields no indications upon which to base a truly rational treatment, applicable to every case. The slow but progressive course of the disease entails the successive use of the most varied remedies. The changes involved in metabolism have been studied as completely as possible, and reveal an important failure in nutrition. Minute attention has been directed to searching for the least sign of tubercle, which Oppenheim considers responsible for the great majority of cases of chronic rheumatism. Finally, a more or less important part of the etiology· of polyarthritis deformans can be attributed to thyroid insufficiency, calling for examination of the gland and a careful hunting out of any symptoms of hypothyroidism. These provide the essentials for guidance in the lines upon which treatment is to be based.

General Treatment.—Diet should not be restricted systematically as in the case of gouty rheumatism. On the contrary, the necessity for generous feeding must be insisted upon on account of the failing condition in which most cases are found. The possibility of renal complications in later stages of the disease must· be taken into account, and may render it necessary to order a diet more or less strictly limited ·to milk and vegetables. In winter cod-liver oil should be given in as large a quantity as the patient can tolerate.

If, as is frequently the case, the urine is found to be hypo-acid, or rather shows a high coefficient of demineralization, it is useful to give phosphoric acid.

R Acidi Phosphorici Diluti, 3ij.
Sodii Phosphatis Acidi, 3iv.
Aquæ destillatæ, ad 3vj.
Misce. Fiat mistura.
Sig. "One tablespoonful to be taken in half a tumblerful of water before the two chief meals."

If there is any reason to suspect a thyroid origin of the rheumatism, the phosphoric treatment should be replaced by thyroid opotherapy. Small doses must be given—one or two cachets containing ½ grain of dried thyroid body. These must be taken for some considerable time with occasional breaks. Improvement is noticed after months of treatment, although these improvements are far from being the rule, as the treatment very often proves useless. To prevent the wasting and debility produced by thyroidin, treatment by arsenic—to be dealt with later—must be added.

· When the rheumatism is of definitely tubercular nature, specific treatment by tuberculin must be tried. Some excellent results obtained in this way have been recently published.

In the absence of the above three special indications, or concurrently with them, the general internal treatment of chronic rheumatism consists chiefly of the use of arsenic and iodine. Arsenic can be given either in the form of injections of cacodylate of sodium or in solution:—

R Sodii Arsenatis, gr. ss.
Aquæ destillatæ, 3x.
"One tablespoonful before the two chief meals."

Or 5 or 6 drops of Fowler's solution may take the place of this. This treatment is kept up for three weeks, then left off for three weeks and begun again. During the interval, the tincture of iodine should be given. It is of much better effect in these cases than preparations of iodine. At first 5 drops should be given in a glass of water three times a day at meals, increasing the dose by one drop a day for a week, keeping at the maximum for the next week, and returning by degrees in the third. If this proves intolerable for the

[1] _Le Progrès Médicale._

stomach hypodermic injections must be used.

  ℞ Iodi,   gr. xv.
      Potassii Iodidi,   gr. xxx.
      Aquæ destillatæ,   ℥iij.

An injection of 1 to 2 c. c. (mxv.-xxx.) is to be given deeply every day for a month. After a fortnight's interval the injections are given again.

Hypodermic injections of thiosinamine should be given for periods of a fortnight to three weeks to obtain its known resolvent action upon cicatricial and fibrous tissues.

  ℞ Thiosinamini,   gr. xxx.
      Phenazoni,   gr. xlv.
      Aquæ destillatæ,   ℥x.

1 c. c. (mxv.) is to be given by deep hypodermic injection every day. It must never be forgotten that this drug is strictly contra-indicated in the case of a patient suspected of tuberculosis.

The general treatment is completed by a series of remedies of a physical nature. Among these are specially to be commended the actual cautery dotted along the spine, repeated every 10 or 15 days, and very hot baths, taken every other day for 20 minutes while the temperature is gradually raised up to 107° F. or even to 113° F. Various drugs have been added to the baths, the most effective seems to be the turpentine bath, made by adding to the bath four ounces each of soft soap emulsion and turpentine.

Local Treatment.—This varies with the degree of pain present. When the pain is very severe it is a question of a subacute outbreak the treatment of which will be discussed later. When, however, the pain is moderate, local treatment is specially directed to overcoming the stiffness, the tendency to ankylosis of the joints and the resulting muscular atrophy. With this object use can be made of the following:—

1. Application of continuous currents of rather high intensity—50 to 60 milliamperes for 10 minutes through the affected joint. To be preferred to this is electrical ionotherapy by Leduc's method. The drug used may be sodium salicylate in two per cent. solution, or potassium iodide in three per cent. solution. The negative electrode soaked in one of these solutions is applied to the affected part; the other electrode is placed indifferently at some distance from the joint. The intensity of the current should be from 30 to 50 milliamperes. It should be applied for from 30 to 40 minutes three times a week.

2. Massage of the affected joints and of the neighboring muscles. This may be preceded most usefully either by a hot-air bath, the temperature of which should reach at least to 70-80° C., or by, what is better for the small joints of the hand and foot, a bath of hot sand. For the latter, the sand is heated in an oven, poured into a bucket and cooled to 50° or 55° C. The foot or hand is plunged into the bucket for from 20 to 25 minutes, night and morning. After the bath, massage is done for some minutes with the hand covered with the following ointment:—

  ℞ Unguenti Fioraventi,
      Tincturæ Nucis Vomicæ,   ana ℨi.
      Adipis Lanæ,
      Paraffini Mollis,   ana ℥ss.
      Misce. Fiat unguentum.

3. Passive and active movements of the affected joints are a most useful addition to the massage. The most complicated maneuvres of mechanical treatment are from this point of view not of such value as the movements of normal life performed by the patient in spite of the difficulty and pain set up. Thus for nodular rheumatism localized in the hands and wrists, it is essential that the patient uses his hands to feed himself, clothe himself, and attend to his usual occupations, difficult and painful as the movements may be. It is the only way to prevent ankylosis and positive impotence.

4. As an accessory local treatment may include the use of Bier's bandage, applied some distance from the affected joints and kept in place for from 4 to 10 hours a day, according to the way it is borne. Again, radio-active mud may be used enveloping the joint, but the results obtained by it in nodular rheumatism do not appear so brilliant as those in other forms of rheumatism, such as, for example, gonorrheal arthritis. Finally, local counter-irritation, frequently repeated, by actual cautery or tincture of iodine.

Treatment of Painful Subacute Attacks.—As soon as a subacute attack happens in the course of chronic rheumatism the treatment must be radically altered.

1. Locally the massage and movements must be stopped, absolute rest of the joints being necessary. They should be wrapped round with methyl salicylate, pure or mixed in a liniment or ointment:—

  ℞ Mentholis,   gr. xv.
      Guaiacolis,   ℨi.
      Methyl Salicylatis,   ℨi.
      Ol. Camphorat,   ad. ℥iv.
      Misce. Fiat linimentum.

Or

  ℞ Acidi Salicylici,   ℨi.
      Olei Terebinthini,   ℨi.
      Adipis Lanæ,   ℨi.
      Adipis,   ℨi.
      Misce. Fiat unguentum.

"To be applied frequently to the affected joints."

Or dermatol in an ointment for its analgesic effect.

  ℞ Bismuthi Subgallatis,   ℥ss.
      Paraffin. Moll.,   ad. ℥ijs.

This is spread over the affected part, which is then hermetically covered with absorbent wool and renewed twice a day.

2. Internally, all thyroid, iodine, or arsenical treatment must be stopped and large doses of aspirin given:—

  ℞ Acidi Aceto-Salicylici,   gr. vijss.
      Fiat pulvis.

"To be taken in a cachet four times a day before meals."

Colchicum appears to have a very marked sedative effect upon the pain.

℞ Tincturæ Colchici Seminum, ℥iv.
Tincturæ Aconiti, ℥i.

Twenty drops to be taken three times a day. After the third day a progressive reduction in the dose is to be made.

When the pain will yield neither to the action of aspirin nor to that of colchicum, one tablespoonful of the following must be given at night:—

℞ Chloralis Hydratis,
Potassii Bromidi,
Syrupi Codeinæ, ana ℥i.
℥i.
Aquæ, ad. ℥iij.
Misce.

Thermal Treatment.—Generally speaking, this sort of treatment does very little good in nodular rheumatism. It is possible to recommend the mud from Dax and from St. Amand, and the waters of Bourbon l'Archambault, Bourbon-Lancy, and Bourbonne. Patients should avoid damp and cold climates. They should be sent to dry localities, bathed in sunshine and sheltered from winds.

Treatment of Erysipelas of the Face.[1]—Castaigne and Fernet, reviewing the various remedies recommended for the treatment of erysipelas of the face, point out the method which yielded them the best results. Ichthyol proved to be the most useful of all, applied in a mixture with equal parts of traumaticine. This was swabbed over the affected part three or four times a day, and the application was continued for forty-eight hours after all local symptoms had died out. Ichthyol may be used in many other ways, often to greater advantage. It may be applied pure, diluted with half its volume of boiled water, freely bathing the parts every day or twice a day. As it dries it forms a thick scab, thus rendering the use of successive dressings unnecessary. When all active symptoms have subsided it may be applied in an ointment. In the case of severe inflammation with oozing and suppuration it is better, for the first twenty-four or forty-eight hours, to apply dressings moistened with a 1 in 10, or 1 in 20 solution, applying the pure ichthyol at a later stage. In an ointment it is not so active, and should be only used in cases with little inflammation.

℞ Ichthyolis .... ℥ss.
Zinci Oxidi .... ℥ij.
Adipis Lanæ .... ℥ij.
Paraffini Mollis ....ad ℥i.
Misce. Fiat unguentum.

This is an excellent application when inflammation has disappeared. It should be used while redness persists, or the following cream may be substituted:

℞ Amyli .... ℥j.
Zinci Oxidi .... ℥ij.
Adipis Lanæ,

[1] *Jour de Med. et de Chir. pratiques.*

Paraffini Mollis ....ana ℥ij.
Liquorisi Hydrogeni Peroxidi. ℥ss.
Misce. Fiat cremor.

ss

Should any telangiectasis persist the following ointment will be found more effective:

℞ Solutionis Adrenalini Chloridi
(1/1000) ....℥ss.
Zinci Oxidi ....℥ij.
Adipis Lanæ ....℥ij.
Paraffini Mollis ....ad ℥i.
Misce. Fiat unguentum.

GENERAL TOPICS.

The Red Cross Exhibition.—The American Red Cross desires again to invite attention to the exhibition in connection with the Ninth International Red Cross Conference, which will be held in Washington, D. C., from May 7 to 17, 1912.

The exhibition will be divided into two sections, which will be styled Marie Feodorovna and General. The former is a prize competition, with prizes aggregating 18,000 rubles, or approximately $9,000, divided into nine prizes, one of 6,000 rubles, approximately $3,000; two of 3,000 rubles each, and six of 1,000 rubles each.

The subjects of this competition are as follows:

1. A scheme for the removal of wounded from the battlefield with the minimum number of stretcher bearers.
2. Portable (surgeons') washstands, for use in the field.
3. The best method of packing dressings for use at first aid and dressing stations.
4. Wheeled stretchers.
5. Transport of stretchers on mule back.
6. Easily folding portable stretchers.
7. Transport of the wounded between warships and hospital ships, and the coast.
8. The best method of heating railway cars by a system independent of steam from the locomotive.
9. The best model of portable Roentgen apparatus, permitting utilization of X-rays on the battlefield and at first aid stations.

The maximum prize will be awarded to the best exhibit, irrespective of the subject, and so on.

The General Exhibit is again divided into two parts; the first will be an exhibition by the various Red Cross Associations of the world. The second will be devoted to exhibits by individuals or business houses of any articles having to do with the amelioration of the sufferings of sick and wounded in war, which are not covered by the Marie Feodorovna Prize Competition for the year. While the American Red Cross will be glad to have any articles pertaining to medical and surgical practice in the field, it is especially anxious to secure a full exhibit relating to preventive measures in campaign. Such articles will be classified as follows:

1. Apparatus for furnishing good water in the field.
2. Field apparatus for the disposal of wastes.
3. Shelter such as portable huts, tents and the like, for hospital purposes.
4. Transport apparatus (to prevent the suffering of sick and wounded) exclusive of such apparatus as specified for the Marie Feodorovna Prize Competition.

As with the Marie Feodorovna Prize Competition, for this country only articles having the approval of the Central Committee of the American Red Cross will be accepted.

Diplomas will be awarded for exhibits in this section of the exhibition as approved and recommended by the Jury.

Further information may be obtained from the Chairman, Exhibition Committee, American Red Cross, Washington, D. C.

It is perhaps to apparatus having to do with prevention of disease in armies that the energies of Americans have been specially directed since the Spanish-American War. Therefore, the last mentioned section of the Exhibition should make an appeal to them.

Amputation of Penis.[1]—Lydston and Steere report a case of complete amputation of the penis by a jealous wife. They state that the psychology of cases of genital injury by criminal assault varies: The causes are as follows: (1) Simple jealousy. Women sometimes injure not only the offending male, but also the female rival, making the genitals the object of assault. The male often makes the genital organs the objective point of assault upon a rival. The dominant idea is in most cases simply revenge. (2) The desire to deprive a rival of what seems to the jealous person the chief point of interest to the rival. (3) A desire to punish the one at whose hands the assailant has suffered injury. (4) Both women and men have been known to commit sex mutilation on persons in whom they no longer had an interest. (5) The desire to protect oneself from future encroachments on one's sexual rights. (6) Insane impulse. (7) Reversionary instinct, resulting in sadism. Apropos of this point the attack of the female spider and of the female *Mantis religiosa* upon the male after copulation are illustrations.

The Role of Germs in Disease.—Disease is not a germ, nor is a germ a disease, says Butler in *Am. Jour. of Clin. Med.* The specific germ is only one factor in an equation of many factors. Hence, the requirements of the case will not be met by tilting at a single factor—

[1] G. F. Lydston, M. D., and H. F. Steere, M. D., *New York Med. Jour.*, Feb. 3, 1912.

this is too narrow a conception of the nature of the task before us.

Disease is a commotion manifesting itself by a group of symptoms, and treatment means the recognition of each of these as parts of the disorder to be combated. For instance: in fever, the headache, the thirst, the dry skin, the enfeebled digestion, the constipation, the weakened action of the heart. Each and all of the conditions enumerated call for consideration; each is or may be a source of discomfort and an essential part of the whole disease; taking this word at its literal meaning, and by as much as we remove one or other, by so much we lessen the disease itself.

SOCIETY PROCEEDINGS.

THE EASTERN MEDICAL SOCIETY OF THE CITY OF NEW YORK.

The regular stated meeting was held Friday, April 12th, 1912, the President, Dr. S. J. Kopetzky, in the chair.

The Executive Session was devoted to the transaction of routine business, election of members, etc.

The Scientific Session took up the following:

I. **Presentation of Specimens.**
   MONSTROSITIES.
   (a) *Anencephalus.* By Dr. Nathan Ratnoff.
   (b) *Teratococus.* By Dr. Meyer Rabinovitz.
   (c) *Cranio-Thoracopagus.* By Dr. Isadore Seff.

II. **Presentation of Cases.**
   Two Cases of Cesarean Section. Dr. S. W. Bandler.

III. **Symposium in Obstetrics and Gynecology.**
   Papers,—
   (a) *Dystocia, Due to Faulty Presentation and Faulty Position.* Dr. Simon Marx.
   (b) *Repair of Injuries to the Pelvic Outlet.* Dr. Brooks H. Wells.
   (c) *The Treatment of Abortion in the Presence of Fever.* Dr. Herman J. Boldt.
   (d) *Immediate Operation for Tubal Pregnancy.* Dr. Louis J. Ladinski.

The discussion of the Symposium was by Drs. Le Roy Brun, John G. Polak, George L. Brodhead, S. W. Bandler, F. A. Dorman, I. L. Hill, A. Sturmdorf, and M. Rabinovitz.

The discussion of the questions brought out in the Symposium was of great interest from a clinical standpoint and was listened to with the closest attention by a large audience.

The Symposium, the description of the cases presented, and the description of the monstrosities reported, will appear in the May issue of AMERICAN MEDICINE.

233

American Medicine

H. EDWIN LEWIS, M. D., *Managing Editor.*
PUBLISHED MONTHLY BY THE AMERICAN-MEDICAL PUBLISHING COMPANY.
Copyrighted by the American Medical Publishing Co., 1912.

New Series, Vol. VII., No. 5. Complete Series, Vol. XVIII., No. 5.	MAY, 1912.	$1.00 YEARLY In advance.

The question of disinfection deserves a great deal more consideration than it has ever received. Ever since the studies of Pasteur, Koch, Lister and others placed the germ theory on a sound basis, the practical importance of disinfection in the prophylaxis of disease has been recognized. Countless disinfecting agents and innumerable methods have been employed with a confidence in their efficiency that has been little short of fatuous. For instance, certain substances have long been looked upon as germicidal, notably the phenol derivatives, the chlorine preparations, some of the rapid oxidizing agents, various coal tar products and quite a few other synthetic preparations, and a manufacturer has only had to effect some combination of these, coin some fanciful name indicating that the product was more or less bactericidal, extol its antiseptic virtues to the skies—and lo, the public—and we regret to say many physicians, health officers and sanitarians—have used it without question. A great many of our so-called disinfectants have this identical history. Thoughtlessly these preparations have been employed before a single step has been taken to check up the claims made concerning their germicidal power. As a matter of fact the disinfectant value of many of the most popular products is an unknown quantity to many of those who have been using them most extensively, and the menace of this condition must be evident. Without the facts that can only be obtained from definite and exact tests to establish the actual bactericidal power of a disinfectant, every person who uses it is working in the dark. The security derived from employing non-standardized disinfectants is, therefore, all too often a false security. The dangers presented by placing dependence—when disinfection means so much—on measures that—for all we may know—possess no greater disinfecting power than "saline solution," hardly need emphasizing. The resulting sense of safety is all too apt to create a confidence that is not only far from justified but extremely apt to lead to disaster. What explanation can be made to the innocent sufferers from such methods? What excuse can be offered to those who, secure in their belief that disinfection has been done properly, relax the precautions they would otherwise employ, and straightway become infected? Is there not every reason for criticizing and condemning every party to such a wrong?

The use of indeterminate disinfectants is little less than criminal. In other words employing disinfectants the exact disinfecting or germicidal power of which has not been definitely determined is an outrage against those whose health and lives are liable to be jeopardized by the false sense of safety created. Indeed, the culpability of using uncertain and doubtful disinfecting agents is to-day more pronounced than ever, since very substantial progress has been made, not only in evolving tests for the definite determination of disinfecting power, but also in establishing well defined standards. We refer especially to the work of two English scientists, Drs. Rideal and Walker. Their investigations have been epoch-making since they have placed the whole subject of disinfection on a practical scientific basis. The test which these investigators have developed—known as the Rideal-Walker test—has revolutionized the whole question of antiseptics and disinfectants, and the gain to humanity is incalculable. Over a year ago we took up the problem of the standardization of disinfectants editorially, and pointed out the great importance of the question. At that time we were not as familiar with the splendid studies of Rideal and Walker as we are now, but we saw the urgent need of research in this direction. The economic side of the question was recognized and the great loss in dollars and cents from the use of inefficient or useless disinfectants was especially emphasized. This phase of the matter is bound to receive greater attention, since the economic problem is of prime importance in hospitals, public institutions, municipal buildings and wherever it is necessary to secure maximum efficiency at minimum cost. The article in this issue by J. T. Ainslie Walker, F. R. S. M., F. C. S. is a notable one and we are especially honored in being able to present this valuable paper by one of the two men who have done so much to place modern disinfection on a sound and practical footing.

The **Rideal-Walker test** in brief consists of comparing the strengths of disin-

fectants which kill the typhoid bacillus in a definite time, under carefully standardized conditions, with the strength of pure carbolic necessary to perform the same work under the same conditions. For example, if a 1 in 2,000 solution of disinfectant X will kill a certain strain of typhoid bacillus in ten minutes, and a 1 in 100 solution of carbolic acid will kill the same organism in the same time (and *at* the same time) the carbolic acid co-efficient of X is

$$\frac{2000}{100} = 20.$$

Similarly when dealing with a disinfectant of lower bactericidal power than carbolic acid, if a 1 in 70 solution is required to perform the same task as a 1 in 100 solution of carbolic acid, the co-efficient is

$$\frac{70}{100} = 0.7.$$

By the use of this test it is possible to determine the germicidal efficiency of any preparation, under any given conditions of working, and thus convert disinfection from a speculative and frequently useless process to a reliable and scientific method of preventing the spread of infection.

The Rideal-Walker method has been officially adopted by all Government Departments in Great Britain, by numerous Colonial Governments and by the majority of municipal and other public bodies throughout Great Britain and her colonies. In this country it has been adopted by various city health departments, and by at least one State, that of Maryland, a copy of whose regulation is as follows:

"All disinfectants manufactured or sold in this State must bear a label showing the carbolic acid coefficient, or relative germicidal strength of such disinfectants as compared with pure carbolic acid.
In determining the relative germicidal value of disinfectants the application of the Rideal-Walker Test to the typhoid bacillus in a 24

hour bouillon culture may be made, and such results will be accepted until further notice.

The statement of the coefficient should be made as follows:

Carbolic acid coefficient 0.3, or 1.2, etc., etc.

This statement may appear on the principal label or on a supplemental label or sticker."

One feature of the test, which probably more than any other was instrumental in securing for it such wide official favor in Great Britain, is the fact that it enables the purchaser, without specifying any one disinfectant, proprietary or otherwise, to select the most economical and the most efficient.

The sentiment is rapidly growing—especially among the principal health officers of the country—that the manufacture and sale of disinfectants should be controlled by Federal or State legislation, on lines similar to that already enacted by the State of Maryland. It has been pointed out, however, that the well-known delays and difficulties attendant upon the passage of legislation affecting interests opposing progress in matters pertaining to disinfection may be avoided by the simple adoption of the following specification in all proposal forms calling for supplies of disinfectants:

"Any disinfectant fluid may be tendered, provided that its guaranteed bactericidal efficiency is expressed in terms of absolute phenol as determined by the Rideal-Walker method, when working with vigorous cultures of B. typhosus, and that it is homogeneous, miscible with water in all proportions, does not separate out on standing, and flows freely from the cask at all times. The coefficient must be given in the blank space left for the purpose in the Schedule."

The above, taken from the City of Westminster form, is suggested as probably the best worded specimen of a clause, which with very few exceptions, is to be found in all British proposal forms. By the adoption of this or a similar clause, large users of disinfectants can readily ensure the selection of the cheapest and most efficient disinfectant available.

The acceptance of the Rideal-Walker method as a reliable index to bactericidal efficiency was followed by the application of disinfection in circumstances previously regarded as outside the scope of this work. The most striking illustration of this point is perhaps the daily disinfection of schoolroom floors, a process which, during the past few years, has been adopted by hundreds of British educational authorities. The routine disinfection of public conveyances (railways and street cars) of places of public resort (theatres and halls) of factories, workshops and offices, are further instances. It may safely be assumed that without the conviction that they were obtaining some valuable return for their outlay, those responsible for this work would never voluntarily have carried it out as they did, and it is equally certain that prior to the introduction of the Rideal-Walker method, no means of obtaining such assurance was available.

The manufacture of high testing disinfectants, capable of bearing high dilutions without loss of efficiency is bound sooner or later to have an important bearing on many schemes of public disinfection. Already since there are disinfectants available which are highly efficient in dilutions of even one to 500 of water—and it is possible to obtain solutions that will destroy all organisms of infectious disease with two or three minutes' contact, and at a negligible cost of less than a cent per gallon—the practice of disinfecting public places is extending rapidly. Naturally in these high dilutions the objectionable smell, inseparable from the application of disinfectants of low dilution, and all too often low efficiency, is absent. The importance of this is illustrated by the fact that with such a preparation it is possible to sterilize the floor of a Pullman car or public theatre without any inconvenience to passengers or occupants. But most important of all, there is no longer any excuse for using disinfectants on the simple claim of the manufacturer that his product has high disinfecting power. Let us insist that the label tell the carbolic co-efficiency of every disinfectant under regulations and penalties of the Pure Food and Drug Law.

The institutional baby is receiving a commendable amount of study by various associations, with a view of determining if some means can not be found of lessening the present deplorable mortality. In prehistoric times it was fully recognized that a motherless baby could not be nourished; so it was allowed to die at once and in some races it was strangled with a wisp of its mother's hair and buried with her. Advancing culture made these practices too horrible, and regular institutions were created to care for the motherless, but we suddenly realized a few decades ago that it was no use, for they all died anyhow, generally long before they were a year old. So we reluctantly concluded that such a delicate pink bit of humanity really required the undivided care of one person, and that the family will always be the basis of society, all our Utopian socialists to the contrary notwithstanding. Then came all kinds of plans to end the dreadful mortality of babies deprived of a mother's care, and we were congratulating ourselves that the scandalous death rate was a thing of a horrid past—like a nightmare—but it seems that here and there conditions are as bad as ever; that is, many die before two years of age and under the best of care a third or more may die in the first year. Institutions

with good "records," have been detected omitting mention of sick infants sent to hospital or returned to the friends to die. Even "boarding out," to get family care of a woman who is carefully trained and daily visited, has not as good results as we had hoped. There is a fatal defect somewhere.

The feeding of motherless babies seems to be the fault, for in spite of all the wonderful advances by which we are able to raise so many children deprived of mother's milk, we fail far too often even when the child gets every other essential from loving parents. Such children nearly all died before the advent of scientific modification of cow's milk, and it is a great thing to save any, but to do so requires almost hourly watching for signs of indigestion so as to make instant changes—impossibilities except when the devoted mother is the watcher, and of course out of the question in an institution. Then there is the dreadful mortality in the lower orders even when the baby is breast fed, for its real struggle for existence begins after it is weaned and hordes of them perish before they acquire the digestive powers normal for the child of five. We have done a world of good by insisting upon every mother nursing her infant, as we have proved that every month of breast-food adds enormously to the chances of survival, but the present scandalous mortality follows weaning. These difficulties will prevent perfect success in raising the foundling, until our physiologists and chemists are able to make a perfect imitation of breast-milk—and that is still some distance away.

The defectiveness of the motherless is another point to be considered. There are hosts of perfectly normal people who as infants had been deprived of their mothers by accident, but it must be confessed that the class of babies usually thrown on society for their lives, come from the defectives and inefficients. Though the latest work in heredity proves that the characters acquired in the slums are not transmitted, it must be acknowledged that the baby will inherit the low organization which caused the parents to drift there, and even if we do raise it and start it as a self-supporting man, the chances are that unless given some aid all his life, he will drift into the slums like his father when the struggle for existence proves in turn too great for him. It is this essential basic defect which will always prevent the raising of as many foundlings as in the well-to-do families. Nevertheless we have no patience with those who assert that the death of foundlings is a "merciful dispensation of Divine Providence." If mercy were needed Providence would have shown it in the prevention of the birth, not in killing them. No! public welfare demands that every baby be saved on the general principle of making life safe to all. Then again, should only one in a million of illegitimate foundlings be as great as Alexander Hamilton or Abraham Lincoln, it would pay to save the million to find the one. So we commend the present movement, particularly of making the mother nurse her child whether it is legitimate or not; if this is impossible then wet nursing for the few in which it is possible, and for each baby the individual care of one woman who is trained and watched. Let the institutions be merely for collection and distribution as they are wholly impossible as homes and as such should be forbidden by law. Babies must be put where they can be fed right, cleaned right and watched right, and loved right; and then, to prevent too much coddling, as judiciously neglected as a well-fed puppy.

Dr. O'Loughlin, Senior Surgeon of the White Star Line who went down to his death on the ill-fated Titanic was a man whom his American and British colleagues are proud to remember, not alone for the nobility of his last hours but equally for the manner of his living. That he was a brave man with all the courage that we like to think our heroes possess has been attested to by many survivors who tell of his cool, collected demeanor in that last terrible hour before the Titanic sunk. Apparently Dr. O'Loughlin knew no fear, for he paid no attention to his own danger but went from one group to another, soothing the frightened, encouraging the weak and striving in every way to prevent panic and hysteria. As the last life-boat left the vessel, although he must have known that the end was near, he was seen standing in a companionway with the same smile on his face that had endeared him to countless travelers who knew and loved him.

And so after all the years he had spent at sea, he met the death he had often been heard to describe as the one above all others he desired. To him the ocean was a passion, for he loved it all his life. From almost the day of his graduation he had lived in touch with its many moods, and he never cared to leave it. It was kismet that he should have thus closed his career, for he never thought of settling down on the land.

Kind, gentle and thoughtful, Dr. O'Loughlin had all the gallantry and chivalry of the true Irish gentlemen. Although rather weakly in his early years, as soon as he completed his medical course at the

238   AMERICAN MEDICINE }
Complete Series, Vol. XVIII. }   EDITORIAL COMMENT   { MAY, 1912.
{ New Series, Vol. VII., No. 5.

Royal College of Surgeons at Dublin he promptly went to sea as a ship surgeon and rapidly gained health and vigor. A remarkably well read man and by instincts a scholar, Dr. O'Loughlin exemplified all the best traditions of the cultured physician. With the thousands of people he came in contact with every year, it is not surprising that he became an exceedingly capable

steerage or the millionaire in the "Royal Suite," it was just a suffering human being. This was enough to command his gentlest manner and most painstaking attention and skill.

Truly it is a privilege to pay a tribute to such a colleague, a man who had found his niche and had filled it so well. The memorial on another page represents AMERI-

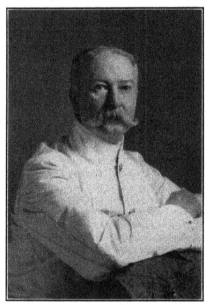

DR. W. F. N. O'LOUGHLIN.
Senior Surgeon White Star Line, Died April 15, 1912, on Duty.

physician and surgeon. He early learned the necessity of self-reliance and this combined with a fine medical education made him one of the most efficient medical men in the transatlantic service. Many an American traveler could tell of his skill and it never made any difference whether the call came from the poor immigrant in the

CAN MEDICINE's token to a physician whose life and death have added new lustre to the noble profession of medicine. It is not offered as a concession to sentiment, nor yet as a mere tribute to a doctor who lived and died well. But when a man goes through life making the most of himself as Dr. O'Loughlin did, honoring and respecting

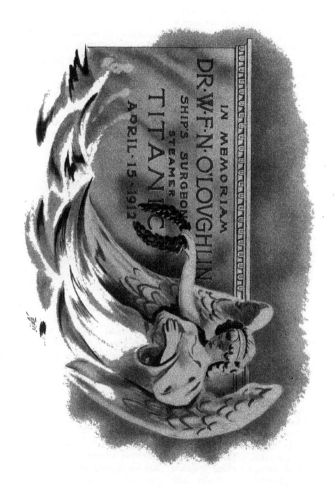

A Brave Man, a Real Gentleman—a True Physician!

his calling by proving capable and efficient, and then meets the Last Summons true to his work and manhood, all of his colleagues receive a certain strength and inspiration from his memory. And so this memorial dedicated as it is to a true physician, will represent to a certain extent the hope that we all have, that our lives may not be in vain, that our work may bear good fruit, and that our end may have some of the same nobility and unselfishness that so evidently characterized that of Dr. O'Loughlin.

The whole matter rests in the hands of these Trustees. No suggestion or advice will be offered them, or will the slightest pressure be brought to bear on their deliberations. All that American Medicine desires is that the Gold Medal be given each year to the American physician who has made the most notable contribution to medical science during the preceding twelve months. If the Trustees make the award to a clinician, a laboratory worker, an author, a surgeon, a sanitarian, or just to a great and good practitioner it makes

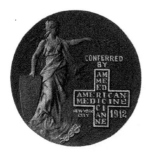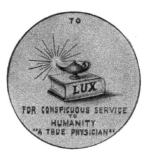

Rough Design of American Medicine Gold Medal. To be Awarded Annually by a Special Board of Trustees.

The Trustees of the American Medicine Gold Medal Award have been appointed by the Directors as follows: Dr. William J. Robinson, Editor of the *Critic and Guide,* Dr. Claude L. Wheeler, Editor *New York Medical Journal,* and Dr. H. Edwin Lewis, Editor of *American Medicine.* These gentlemen have consented to undertake the difficult task of selecting the American physician whose work during the past year can properly be considered the most serviceable to humanity. Their essential familiarity with current medical literature and extensive acquaintance with American medical men make it certain that no man's work will fail of careful consideration.

no difference. We know that the most deserving man in the opinion of the Trustees will be the one to receive this year's —and each succeeding year's—medal.

The one great purpose of the American Medicine Gold Medal Award is to emphasize to the world the work and achievements of some American medical man each year. As we stated last month we pay too little attention to what our American scientists are doing. Researches, discoveries and inventions by American physicians receive practically no recognition and as a consequence the great public have little or no conception of the real progress medical science is making. We thoroughly realize that the simple gold medal conferred by American Medicine constitutes little recompense for the work of the physician who may receive it. The medal itself aside from its intrinsic beauty is nothing. But when awarded by a board of honorable men—and representing a decision that the recipient's work is the most notable of the year—it can hardly fail to carry an honor and distinction that any American physician should be proud to receive.

In this connection, we wish to correct the idea some may have formed that this Gold Medal Award is competitive. This is not its purpose. The Medal represents an honor to be conferred, not one to be sought or to be competed for. Beyond all doubt, the physician who receives it will not know he is to be honored until he receives formal notice of the Award. Thus it will carry infinitely more significance and serve its purpose much more closely as a real testimonial to its recipient's worthiness. Competitive prizes and awards have their place and far be it from us to discredit them in the slightest. But the American Medicine Gold Medal as the years come and go will be an honor and distinction for work undertaken and achievements accomplished without thought of reward, rather than a trophy or prize.

American medical science—in the laboratory or at the bedside—compares favorably with that of any other country or nation. The American people have been indifferent and remiss in recognizing this; and simple as American Medicine's Gold Medal may be, with the help and cooperation of the physicians who are Trustees of the Award, it is to be hoped that it will do something to counteract this indifference.

The Study of Senility. We will never be able to treat the aged understandingly until we understand the senile organism. If we were to study senility as the pediatrist studies childhood we would realize that the degenerations that accompany the process of aging are as natural, normal and physiological at that period of life as are the regenerations that characterize the imperfect development of childhood. The senile degenerations are not diseases or complications of diseases any more than is a pulse rate of 100 in the child tachycardia, or its inability to digest certain foods, indigestion. Diseases in old age are not pathological conditions complicated by degenerations, but pathological conditions in organs and tissues that are in the process of degeneration. If we accept this view we will get a new conception of disease in senility. The usual text-book descriptions of senile rheumatism well emphasize the many errors in diagnosis and treatment of the ailments of the aged that are due to ignorance of the anatomical and physiological changes in senility. A thorough knowledge of these changes would clear up many puzzling features in senile cases and the causes of failure in their treatment. A recent number of the *Archives of Diagnosis* contained a paper on Sources of Error in Diagnosis in Senile Cases by Dr. J. L. Nascher, a pioneer in this work, in which the writer pointed out the following sources of error. (1) Mistaking the normal anatomical and physiological manifestations of senility for disease conditions which they resemble. (2) The manifestations of senility so pronounced as to mask the symptoms of a grave disease. (3) Ill defined symptoms and atypical diseases. (4) The unreliability of symptom complexes in old age. Not without reason did Seidel say in his

242   AMERICAN MEDICINE }
Complete Series, Vol. XVIII. }   EDITORIAL COMMENT   { MAY, 1912.
{ New Series, Vol. VII., No. 5.

article on diseases of old age, "the normal mortality of advanced life is considerably increased as a consequence of the hitherto neglected study of the anatomical and physiological peculiarities of the senile organism." No better practical argument for a more thorough study of geriatrics—a name, by the way, coined by Dr. Nascher to cover the study of the aged—need be advanced than the wide discrepancies between the diagnosis and clinical history of senile cases and the post-mortem findings. The inability of the pathologist to distinguish between senile contracted kidney and the kidney of interstitial nephritis will account for the frequent reports of interstitial nephritis which gave no evidence during life. Similar mistakes are made in connection with changes in other tissues, and it only requires intelligent study and investigation to make them much less common.

The sterilization of habitual criminals to prevent the birth of more criminals is being advocated more and more as it seems so scientific to most of the unscientific. For some time we have been trying to find out something as to the ancestry of our young criminals, to discover how many of them really are children of criminals, and much to our surprise there is scarcely anything known on the subject beyond the well established fact that the vast majority of convicts come from non-criminal families. The old jail-bird is not a family man as a rule and even if he has a wife, he has few children or none at all. We are slowly coming to the conclusion that there is actually no basis—in fact or theory—for the assertion that we will reduce the number of future criminals by sterilizing existing ones. The 1909 report of Elmira reformatory shows that of 18,801 young prisoners, nearly 80 percent were in good health on admission, over 15 percent being somewhat impaired and less than 5 percent sick or feeble. In their mentality nearly 5 percent are excellent, nearly 75 percent good, 16 percent fair and only 5 percent deficient. This shows that as a class they are normal. We also know that they are victims of a bad environment, having been given no chance to become money makers. That is, only 40 percent had a common school education, and less than 5 percent a high school or more, while 41 percent could simply read and write, and over 14 percent were illiterate. That is why they were nearly all common laborers, servants, cheap clerks and idlers. Only 17 percent were in mechanical work, showing how few had been apprenticed. It goes without saying, that the cause is parental neglect, and as a fact nearly all were allowed to form bad associations. The lack of education in the parents was practically the same as in the children, but it did not cause the parents to go wrong and cannot be the sole cause of the criminality of the children who would have been as good as the parents if not neglected. Many an illiterate man is highly moral. A hint as to one cause of the parental neglect, is the fact that in over 28 percent there was a clear history of ancestral drunkenness and doubtful in over 18—over half being temperate. Why these temperate respectable working people should have produced 52 percent of our criminals remains to be explained by our sociologists. By these paradoxical figures we would prevent more criminality by sterilizing the temperate, and letting the drunkards go.

The occupations of the parents of criminals and the insane have not been made the subject of much inquiry but should be investigated at once to find out who are producing these victims of environment. Our state lunacy commission in its 1910 report states that in only about a half of the cases can a family history of insanity, alcoholism or neurosis be obtained, so it is highly essential to find out why the other half broke down. They too must have been neglected or overcared for as is the rule in the neurotic histories. The parent's occupation might help to explain the matter. In the case of the criminal it is far more important to know the occupation and habits of the parents, now that we know they are not criminal. Ferriani (U. S. Consular Report by Britain) has shown that 80 percent of young Italian criminals are manufactured by a bad environment, more than half coming from wretched homes, and two-fifths having criminal parents—the very opposite of such American statistics as have been published, as far as known to us—but even these are so normal that they lead moral lives if so taught and nearly all can be reformed. That is, a criminal is a normal person in the vast majority of cases, and as he will have normal children it is ridiculous to sterilize him. We may find that professional men have more offspring in prison than habitual criminals have, but if so we would not like to advocate the sterilization of doctors, lawyers and clergymen. The whole matter is so full of absurdities, and there is such an absence of fact as a basis for the preventive propositions, that we beg our criminologists to give us the facts as to the parental occupations.

The propagation of paupers by England's poor-laws is the astonishing revelation made in the report of a committee appointed to consider the eugenic aspect of poor-law reform (*Eugenics Review*, Nov. 1910). It seems that charity has been carried to such absurd lengths, that the marriage of paupers has been favored, the women cared for in parturition and the children supported. It is shown by actual evidence that quite a high percentage of these present day social parasites are children of families pauperized for several generations. They are all hopelessly incompetent to make a living, generally through mental deficiency. There is an increasing demand that they be prevented from propagating their kind as burdens for the British Empire of 1930 or 1940. While charity must be organized to reform the victims of environment, such as young criminals, it does seem that the professional or salaried charity workers are out of their sphere in aiding the reproduction of those unable to support themselves—not to mention a wife and swarm of infants. We have been so impressed with the revelations of this poor-law investigation, that we would suggest an inquiry into the effects of our own charity organization society by disinterested auditors. We commend to everyone these simple ideas—if any person is compelled to ask help to keep alive, are not his offspring liable to be equally incompetent later? If so, what is to be done with him? Shall we put him on his feet to beget more like him, or segregate him so he cannot? If the English statistics are true, every dollar spent at 105 E. 22nd St., in 1911, makes it necessary to spend four more in 1931. Think of all this, and find out whither we are being carried by the money of rich sentimentalists.

———

Scandals in the American Red Cross Society must cease. Now comes the awful revelation that its noble founder, Clara Barton, was driven out of it by calumnious charges, through the machinations of its present head, Miss Mabel Boardman, who desired the position for social advancement. It is charged that the persecution embittered Miss Barton's later life, and that she died heart broken and an object of charity after she had spent her life and fortune for her people. Republics are always ungrateful, but are we Americans human? Or are we merely the brutalized off-scourings of Europe who always demand that people sacrifice themselves for them and give nothing in return? What is far worse, it is now charged that the Red Cross Society took no notice of her death whatever—an indifference bordering on brutality. We have repeatedly said that the society could be made a means of great good in times of local disaster when the people are so prostrated that they cannot help themselves. It now looks as though it will always fail of its purpose until it is freed of all self-seekers, social climbers, shirks, and salary grabbers who cannot make a living at productive employments. Already the scandals at home and embezzlements abroad have hampered its legitimate work to the point of paralysis from lack of funds, and it should not be thus. Incidentally we would like to know why a certain major of the medical corps of the Army, is not doing his legitimate duty with the Army—duty for which he draws a large salary—but is attached to this society which by the President's proclamation will not be allowed to serve anywhere near a battlefield? The longer anyone stays away from the Army, the more of its needs will he forget. If the gentleman in question can be spared from the Army now, we ought to economize by reducing the number of majors in its medical corps and let the Red Cross pay his salary—particularly if he is more valuable in the rear of a battle than at the front.

Misinterpretation of vital statistics is our besetting medical sin, and we ought to reform. The commonest error is to consider a place healthy if its death rate is small, whereas the main causative factor in a small death rate is a small birth rate. One of the axioms of sociology is that the bigger the birth rate the bigger the death rate. For instance, suppose a place of unchanging population is so healthy that every baby born there is reared and then lives a healthy active vigorous life and dies at 70. If the population is fixed, 1,000 say, then an old person dies for every baby born, and if 15 are born, there must be a death rate of 15, which is not as good as that of London. On the other hand suppose a place to be so unwholesome that few people are able to have babies and few of those survive. Here too, if the population is neither increasing nor decreasing, there is a death for every birth, but if there are only 10 births the death rate will also be only 10, though few people reach maturity and none old age. The main criterion, then, is the average age at death, and until we know that, the death rate gives us little knowledge of the wholesomeness of a place. The city has recently been defended as a good residence place, because its death rate is small, yet the babies are slaughtered, the average age at death is low, few of the survivors reach a green old age, the death rate in middle life is inordinately large and city families tend to die out. It is not yet the normal life for all, though in time by ordinary natural selection it doubtless will be. Some types are already better off in the city but until all are so, there must be a constant stream from the country for natural selection to work on.

May, 1912.
New Series, Vol. VII., No. 5. }   ORIGINAL ARTICLES   { AMERICAN MEDICINE
Complete Series, Vol. XVIII.   245

ORIGINAL ARTICLES.

DIPHTHERIA EPIDEMICS AND THE PUBLIC SCHOOL.

BY

A. W. COLCORD, M. D.,
Clairton, Pa.

During the year of 1911, twenty-two (22) cases of diphtheria occurred in Clairton Borough. Twenty of these were in the months of October and November, eighteen (18) of which were among the pupils of the public schools.

Clairton is a borough of 3,300 people, situated twenty miles from Pittsburgh, in the Monongahela valley and connected with Pittsburgh by the Pennsylvania railroad, which runs trains nearly every hour during the day and evening. These trains also pass through a number of other towns in the valley, such as Homestead, Duquense, McKeesport, Elizabeth, Monongahela, Donora, Charleroi, Brownsville and Uniontown. During the same months there were numerous cases of diphtheria in each of these towns. In some of them the schools were closed down for sometime and various methods for fighting the epidemic were used, according to the ideas of the local boards of health.

A large number of people travel daily, by train, from Clairton to Pittsburgh, McKeesport and other towns in the valley, using the railroad and street car service and, of course, mingling intimately with the people of Pittsburgh and the smaller nearby cities and towns. From this it will be seen how a diphtheria epidemic can easily spread from town to town and how difficult it must be to stop it when once started.

When the first few cases of our epidemic appeared, we used the usual methods prescribed by the State Board of Health. Each case was promptly reported by the attending physician to the health officer, who in turn reported it to the State Board of Health, placarded the home, placed it under quarantine and kept the usual watch over the premises. All children from the infected home were excluded from school for the legal period—21 days. Every infected room in the home was disinfected at the end of the quarantine period and, if a case developed while at school or a child came to school from an infected home before a diagnosis was made, the school was promptly dismissed and the school room disinfected. In addition to this our physicians worked with the local board of health and health officer to see that proper precautions were taken regarding care of the sick, exclusion of other persons, destruction of infected articles, etc.

Still in spite of these, what seemed to us vigorous measures, carried out as well as such things are usually done, the epidemic increased in violence and case after case developed in the schools. This was especially true of one room where four cases developed, one at a time at intervals of a few days, though the room was disinfected after each outbreak and every other means was taken to suppress it. At this point the School Board, Board of Health and all local physicians held a joint meeting to discuss ways and means of coping with the situation, which seemed to us alarming. The writer, then the president of the local Board of Health and a member of the school board advanced the idea that there were probably children then attending our public schools with the bacillus in their throats or noses—"diphtheria carriers." The doctors present suggested that we should not close the schools, but let the pupils attend regularly and that we start a thorough inspection of throats in all rooms of both school buildings; also that cultures be taken from every suspected case and sent at once to the City Laboratory of Pittsburgh for examination. This suggestion met with the approval of those present and the doctors offered their serv-

Pittsburgh City Laboratory for examination.

On our first examination of throats in the room where the four cases had developed two cultures were reported "positive." Upon investigation these two cases proved to have come from families where the children had had "bad colds," with sore throats or running noses or both, but where no physician had been employed. Both families were, at once, quarantined and the

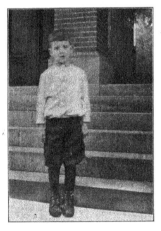

Paul Frazer, one of the "carriers."

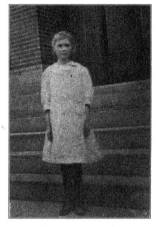

Mary Jane Flemming, one of the "carriers."

ices in the examination of pupils. The rooms where cases had developed were examined daily for a time, then twice weekly. Other rooms were examined two or three times weekly. Wooden spatulas were used for tongue depressors once only and destroyed. Sterile tubes with cotton swabs on wire handles were obtained from the Pittsburg Board of Health and from every suspicious throat a culture was taken. These were collected daily and sent to the

cases showing positive cultures each given 3,000 units of antitoxin.

From the time of the removal and isolation of these two carriers no more cases developed in this room. After two or three more scattered cases in other rooms the epidemic stopped and no more cases have developed. The inspection of throats was continued, at intervals, for two weeks after the last case developed. After the finding of the two carriers (there were at that time six cases from the one building) the whole building was fumigated and all books from this room were burned.

For a portion of the time two physicians were paid for making examinations and toward the last, during the severest of the Pittsburgh epidemic, the laboratory there was crowded with their own work, compelling us to hire it done at the laboratory of the Allegheny General Hospital. Each physician was asked to take a culture from every suspicious throat in his

1. Wrong Material.—The old dry sulphur fumigation, no matter how much was used, was practically worthless, as proved by the series of experiments at the Johns Hopkins Hospital some years ago.

It need hardly be mentioned to the medical reader that the most of the various methods formerly used to disinfect, by the laity or even many physicians, were useless, such as sprinkling carbolic acid water on the floor, burning a little sulphur on the stove, etc.

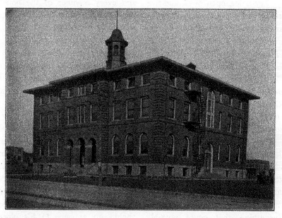

Third Street School Building. In one room of this building the "carriers" were found.

private practice and hand the tube to the local board of health for examination. All this expense was borne by the borough.

For the disinfection of school rooms, during the epidemic, 38 gallons of formalin and 154 pounds of permanganate of potassium were used. In our disinfection of both school house and private dwellings we add 50% to the amount recommended by the State Board of Health.

Much of the disinfecting that has come under the writer's notice has been poorly done. Some of the causes of failure are:

2. Insufficient Quantity of Material.— Many of the lamps and other apparatus for generating formaldehyde gas provide no adequate method for estimating the strength of the gas employed and are no doubt worthless. The best method I have seen is the formalin-permanganate method —using formalin solution one pint and potassium permanganate, eight ounces for each 1,000 cubic feet of air space. This is placed in a container having a capacity of, at least, ten times the quantity of disinfectant. The container is placed inside of a tub of water to prevent the generated heat from burning the floor. Newspapers may be spread around the tub to prevent soiling carpet.

The Philadelphia Board of Health uses formalin (20% solution) three pints to 1,000 cubic feet sprayed over floor. This is said to have produced negative cultures in 100% of all tests. Of course, the same method of sealing room must be used as in other methods.

3. Failure to Hermetically Seal Room. —All cracks, key-holes, open flues, and fire places should be sealed with gummed paper or paper and paste. There should be no fire in the room.

4. Gas Not Left Long Enough in the Room.—The room should be left sealed at least six hours.

5. Failure to Open Up Furniture, Drawers, Clothing, Bedding, Etc., so gas can reach them.

6. Failure to Disinfect Every Infected Room.—A room which has been entered by the patient, nurse or anyone coming in contact with the patient or with infected clothing, etc., should be regarded as infected, and fumigated.

7. Failure to Disinfect Every Infected Article.—Everything that could possibly have been infected should be either burned, boiled, soaked in a disinfecting solution or placed in a room and exposed to the gas. The disinfecting solution may be either formalin—one ounce to gallon, 5% carbolic acid—or 1-1000 bichloride and is convenient to use on all flannels or articles that cannot be boiled; also on all infected laundry that must be sent out from the house. The articles should soak two hours.

8. Failure to Disinfect the Person of the Patient When Removed from Quarantine.—The disinfecting bath is best given by the nurse in the sick room. For this 1-4,000 bichloride is recommended by the Pennsylvania State Board of Health, paying especial attention to hair and scalp. This is followed by soap and water bath, the patient is wrapped in sterile sheet and taken to a disinfected room, where sterile clothing awaits him.

In our work we have used only the soap and water bath for body, but used 1-2,000 cyanide solution for hair, face and hands. The same should be done with the nurse and every member of the household who has come in contact with the patient or occupied an infected room.

9. Dogs and Cats Allowed to Enter Sick Room and Then Allowed to Play with Other Children or Enter Other People's Houses.—These should be killed or scrubbed with a disinfecting solution of 1-2,000 bichloride.

10. A Careless Physician or Nurse.— The physician on entering a house containing a case of diphtheria, should put on a contagious disease gown coming to his feet. On leaving he should wash his hands, face and hair in 1-2,000 cyanide solution. Should a physician be called to a case and find it diphtheria, having no gown on, he should go at once to his office, without entering another home, store, street car, etc., and change his clothes, disinfecting hair, face and hands. Such an infected suit may easily be disinfected, as follows: Fold suit in ordinary wash-boiler, cover partly with heavy paper or oiled cloth, over this a thick pad of absorbent cotton. Pour on this four ounces of formalin solution, put on lid and seal edges with adhesive plaster, leave 12 hours, take out and air one-half day. The writer keeps a wash boiler in his office for this special purpose and has used this method for several years.

The bag carried into the sick room of a diphtheria patient is sterilized in the same way. The gown, when a case is discharged, may be sterilized in this way or boiled.

All toys and books handled by the patient should be burned as should all soiled cloths. The Pennsylvania Health Department recommends that the mattress also be burned. Our local board of health has not done this in most cases, but as we use one and one-half times the required amount of disinfectant (formalin 24-oz., permanganate 12 oz., to 1000 cubic feet) and care-

should have been normal several days and, if possible, two negative cultures should be taken. It is not, of course, necessary to keep the patient in quarantine for such sequelae as paralysis, weak heart, etc.

In my opinion disinfecting done less thoroughly than that outlined above is not disinfection. I am aware that there are other methods equally good, but the point I would emphasize is that "a chain is no stronger than its weakest link." There must be left no loophole for germs to escape and spread disease.

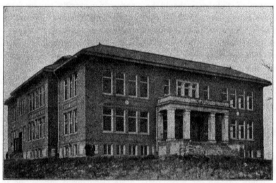

Shaw Avenue Building where a few cases occurred.

fully expose mattress, we believe it to be well disinfected.

When disinfecting a house the health officer should pay special attention to privy vaults, closets, etc., using methods commonly recommended. All dishes, spoons, etc., used by patient should, of course, be boiled before using again.

11. Discharging Patient from Quarantine Too Soon.—Not only should all membrane have left the throat, but all ulcers should be healed, the swelling and redness gone and discharges from the nose, throat and ears stopped. The temperature

It has been our custom to allow the wage-earner of the family to go to his work, provided:

1. He is conscientious, honorable and intelligent enough to follow exactly our instructions.

2. His work must be in the open air or well ventilated mill where only men are employed.

3. He must not work on food material, clothing or anything that would carry infection to others.

4. He must not, on his way to and from work, enter any store, public building, private house or public conveyance.

5. He must not enter the sick room unless, before again going to his work, he changes his clothing and disinfects hands, hair and face.

6. He must at the expiration of the quarantine period subject himself to the same personal disinfection as other members of the household.

We have allowed adult members of the household to be released from quarantine before the expiration of period on thorough personal disinfection.

Milk, cream, butter, etc., sold by a family having a case of diphtheria should be kept in a separate building and cared for by a person not living in the same house with the patient, nor entering it.

The control of a diphtheria epidemic depends not on one man, nor even on the local board of health alone, but upon "team work," good, earnest harmonious work by the Board of Health, Health Officer, Truant Officer, Local Physician, Principal and Teachers, School Board and the general public.

The Board of Health should be composed of some of the best men in the community and should contain, at least, two physicians. They should be fearless and earnest and should keep themselves well posted on what is latest and best in public hygiene.

It is best to have a health officer who can devote his whole time to the work. He should visit all parts of the town, daily, and work with the truant officer in ferreting out mild cases that have no physician. He should carefully guard all quarantined houses and kindly, but firmly, suppress any attempt to break over the rules. He should be taught the principles and details of good disinfection and should be

earnest enough to carry them out thoroughly.

The truant officer can do much in a diphtheria epidemic to aid the Health Officer and the Board of Health. He should report all unattended cases of sickness, at once, to the Health Officer.

Much depends on the local physicians. They must lay aside all petty jealousies and "get together." They should, during the epidemic:

1. Conscientiously report all cases.

2. In undoubted cases of diphtheria give antitoxin promptly and in large doses.

3. Give immunizing doses to other children in the family.

4. Take a culture of every suspicious case of sore throat, croup or rhinitis and keep such a case under a "provisional quarantine" until culture is heard from.

5. Aid board of health in maintaining a quarantine, instructing the family and nurse in the details of sick room disinfection and generally help to create the right atmosphere in the community favoring proper quarantine regulations. A doctor who "knocks" the Board of Health, the State Department, quarantine and disinfection, or who tries to favor his own families in these matters can do much harm.

6. Do all in their power to aid in school examinations, if necessary, without charge. State inspection as carried out in Pennsylvania is good, in a general way, but it cannot take the place of examination by local physicians, at a time like this.

7. Be extremely careful about their own personal disinfection when visiting a case of diphtheria. In these matters the physician should not be asked to bear the expense of such precaution. The Clairton Board of Health has furnished the physi-

cians with contagious disease gowns, disinfects suits of clothes for them when requested, pays for examining all cultures, including messenger service, and the state furnishes antitoxin both for treatment and immunization whenever the family is unable to buy it.

In our epidemic although there were a number of malignant cases there was but one death. In only two instances did more than one member of a family contract the disease. This shows how thoroughly our physicians use antitoxin, both for curative and immunizing purposes.

The teachers in the public school should enter heartily into the work and should watch the pupils closely, not only for sore throats, but also for hoarseness, rhinitis, nausea, fever, malaise, swollen glands, running ears, etc. Such should be promptly reported to the principal, who should call the examining physician. If suspicious cases, they should then be kept under observation at home, a culture taken and the child not returned to school until the culture is reported "negative." In our late epidemic, teachers were pleased with our attitude regarding the closing of schools and were glad to do all that they could to aid in the work. The same may be said of our school board, who gladly met with the board of health and conceded everything needed for the work.

In the writer's opinion, every school should have a regularly appointed school physician, who should examine all pupils, once or twice yearly, and in addition, should be ready to be called to the school building when a principal or teacher thinks it necessary for advice on any question of health. In this way a contagious disease as diphtheria may be early detected and measures taken, at once, to prevent an epidemic. If a teacher simply sends a sick child home, the parents may neglect to call a physician and an epidemic may be started and well under way before it is brought to the notice of the proper officers.

Not only should all persons from an infected home stay away from the public schools for the regulation period, but away from all private, parochial and Sunday schools and churches, theatres, nickelodeons and all public gatherings. The Board of Health may do much by using tact to keep ministers, influential citizens and the general public in full sympathy with the work of quarantine, disinfection and the general means of protection against contagious disease. It is only when this "atmosphere" is right that the best work can be done. In this respect the Clairton Board of Health has been extremely fortunate. The Borough Council, who hold the purse strings, have given us all the money required to carry out the necessary measures and have aided us in every way possible.

No attempt has been made to give full directions for disinfection, fumigation and general prophylaxis in diphtheria. The work of the Clairton Board of Health has been mainly in accordance with the instructions printed in three excellent circulars, distributed by the State Board of Health[1], which give the work more in detail and are, no doubt, similar to those issued by the health boards of the various states. The writer has only tried to emphasize what seem to him some of the most important features and to call attention to some things too frequently neglected.

---

[1] Rules to be Observed in the Care and Management of Cases of Diptheria—(Form No. 3).
Quarantine, Isolation and Disinfection—(Form No. 17), and Direction for Room Disinfection—(Form No. 16).—Pennsylvania Department of Health.

The most important thing after all is that the Board of Health and local physicians *believe* that diphtheria is a contagious disease; that it is caused by a living germ; that the germ can be carried and can be communicated to others by the patient himself or by clothing, toys, books, cats, dogs, or by the hair and hands of other people not having the disease; that this germ can be killed and rendered harmless by being exposed to heat or certain chemicals; that quarantine and isolation are effectual measures in preventing the spread of the disease and that antitoxin given at the right time and in proper quantities will cure or prevent diphtheria. The physician or Board of Health member who doubts these things is a dangerous member of the community. It is the duty of every physician, every member of a Board of Health, every teacher or minister to help to educate the public up to believe these things.

SOME POINTS IN OUR EPIDEMIC.

1. Schools were not closed, but children were daily assembled and kept under observation.

2. Systematic and frequent examinations of all throats in the public schools.

3. Cultures taken of all suspicious throats in schools or in private practice of local physicians and examined at the expense of Board of Health.

4. Finding of "diphtheria carriers" and the quarantine and giving of antitoxin to the same.

5. Both cases of "carriers" occurred in families where several children had been sick and no physician had been in attendance. These mild cases are a great source of danger.

6. No case occurred in room after the finding and isolation of the "carriers." Whole epidemic was soon stopped.

7. Nasal diphtheria is frequent—often mild—more contagious. During an epidemic, suspect a running nose, especially if reddened at opening of anterior nares.

8. An efficient health officer who devotes his whole time to the work.

9. The cooperation of all the local physicians.

10. Harmonious "team work" by board of health, school board, teachers and general public.

11. Disinfection that disinfects.

INEFFICIENT DISINFECTANTS.

BY

J. T. AINSLIE WALKER, F. R. S. M., F. C. S.,
New York City.

It is a curious and somewhat disquieting fact that while the last quarter of a century or so has witnessed enormous strides in the advance of bacteriological science, and, as a natural result, in that of disinfection, certain methods which have long since been proved to be of very restricted germicidal value still have a considerable —though a rapidly diminishing—body of adherents. One does not willingly accept responsibility for the suggestion that apathy, or inability, or disinclination to keep abreast of the times are responsible for this unsatisfactory state of affairs, but at the same time it is difficult on any other grounds to explain why the primitive methods of the pioneer workers should still find a place in any modern system of preventive medicine.

Sulphurous Acid. —Of these obsolete processes, fumigation with sulphurous acid gas (sulphur dioxide) by reason of its seniority no less than by that of the extent to which it is still employed, is entitled to pride of place.

Aerial disinfection or fumigation by the production of sulphur dioxide, either from burning sulphur or from a solution of sulphurous acid, is still used in many places, in spite of the fact that it has been repeatedly condemned by International Congresses and scientific experimenters generally. It is really a survival of the ancient fancy that infection was actually airborne. The aerial convection hypothesis has been in turn applied and discarded in the case of almost all infectious diseases. It survives today only in the case of smallpox, and although the school of epidemiologists which holds this view in regard to smallpox is influential, the aerial convection even of this disease, would probably be denied by a numerical majority among health officers. In the absence of such a hypothesis, it is obvious that to use the atmosphere of a room as a vehicle for conveying a disinfectant to the solid surfaces around and within it is a much less certain and more inconvenient method than the process of spraying or washing with a liquid. This objection is the stronger when account is taken of the difficulty of obtaining a completely sealed room, the consequent probability that the assumed disinfectant atmosphere will be diluted, and the great uncertainty of the extent to which uniform diffusion of the disinfectant will be obtained.

In his classic report of 1881, Koch said of sulphur dioxide, that with or without water, dry or damp, it was entirely useless for the disinfection of spores and quite unreliable for the disinfection of sporeless organisms in the presence of any superficial protection. He further demonstrated that in practice the unequal diffusion of the gas and its loss through various causes render its disinfecting effect much worse

even than in the laboratory experiments on which his opinion was based, and he strongly recommended that its use should be entirely abandoned.

A year or two later Cassedebat reported in similar terms. He exposed the organisms of typhoid, dysentery, cholera, and diphtheria to the action of the gas, both in the dry and the moist condition, and found that even when the maximum concentration possible in practice was used the results were wholly unreliable. Klein, Houston and Gordon, in a report to the London County Council published in 1902, showed that sulphur dioxide was useless for the disinfection of tubercular sputum on such common materials as wood, cloth, linen and paper. "It is therefore necessary to remember," they point out, "that as regard highly resisting microbes, some stronger measures than formalin or sulphurous acid gas have to be employed for disinfection of wood or cloth materials." Sternberg characterized the use of sulphur dioxide as a farce; Dr. Alvah H. Doty in his "Prevention of Infectious Diseases," says, "sulphur dioxide at best can only be employed for superficial disinfection and should never be depended upon to penetrate," and the *British Medical Journal* of November 3, 1894, refers to it in the following terms: "Our obstinate adherence to the old-fashioned sulphurous acid disinfection, which, while entailing the absolute maximum of inconvenience has been shown over and over again to be unreliable in laboratory use and simply ridiculous in practice, is even more difficult to understand. On the ground even of economy there is no comparison between this obsolete process and a disinfectant spray; and while cases of renewed house infection are familiar to almost every medical officer in this country, we have Dr. Dujardin-Beaumetz's authority for saying that where the disinfectant spray has been introduced they are practically unknown in France."

The conditions which must be fulfilled before sulphur dioxide can exercise its germicidal effect are most exacting. "The fireplace, window, and door were carefully and accurately sealed up with pasted paper and the room was left closed up for exactly 24 hours," we read, in the report of Klein, Houston and Gordon. The improbability of a room being so accurately sealed up as to render it air-tight and the impracticability of keeping a room so sealed for as long a space as 24 hours need not be emphasized. Then too, occur the questions of moisture of the atmosphere and of complete combustion of the sulphur—both essential factors. The difficulties presented by the former may be gathered from the fact that even experts differ as to the degree of moisture necessary to secure disinfection. Dr. Doty says, "Various estimates have been made as to the amount of moisture which is necessary for this purpose; theoretically, it is held that the volatilization of one pint of water at the time of the combustion of four pounds of sulphur is the amount required to secure the germicidal effect of the latter. The author's investigation does not confirm this statement, as experiments show that many times this amount of moisture cannot be depended upon to secure the required result."

It is manifest, then, that the conditions under which sulphurous disinfection is carried out are at best irksome. And, moreover, allow these conditions to be modified in the slightest degree, as must necessarily obtain at certain times in prac-

tice, even in the hands of the most careful operator, (such as failure completely to seal the room or completely to burn the sulphur, the presence of a damp lime washed ceiling which will absorb much gas and so remove it from the sphere of action) and ample justification will be found for the sweeping condemnation by the authorities quoted above.

Formaldehyde. —Expert opinion differs widely as to the bactericidal value of formaldehyde. The marked discrepancies in the results obtained over a long period of years by experienced observers have tended to raise doubts as to its general efficiency. These discrepancies indicate that disinfection by formaldehyde is subject to adverse influences beyond the control even of the best qualified workers, and certain therefore to interfere with the results obtained in actual practice.

It seems probable that under certain conditions formaldehyde may be used with advantage, but in the writer's opinion these conditions are strictly limited to naked organisms on exposed surfaces. For disinfection in circumstances which demand penetration, as is generally the case in practice, few workers probably would care to rely solely on formaldehyde. This opinion gains strength from Klein's report to the London County Council on his experiments carried out on behalf of that body in 1902. "In cases where wood flooring, unpainted or unvarnished articles of furniture or similar absorbing materials and cloth fabrics are to be subjected to disinfection on account of their being possibly polluted with tubercular sputum," he says, "disinfection with formalin (40% formaldehyde) will not suffice." From this it is clear that however efficient disinfection with formaldehyde vapor may be in the case of, say, scarlet fever, it cannot be relied upon in that of pulmonary tuberculosis and this fact alone constitutes a serious disability to its use as a disinfectant for general application.

Of formaldehyde in its liquid form (formalin) nothing more need be said than that its carbolic acid coefficient is 0.3. In other words it has only one-third the bactericidal efficiency of carbolic acid.

Carbolic Acid.—A common specification of carbolic acid is that it "must contain not less than 95 per cent of carbolic acid and be free from tar oils and sulphuretted hydrogen." The acid referred to in this specification was originally present in the form of phenol, a saturated solution of which may contain, say 5 per cent. Latterly however, more profitable uses have been found for phenol, of which there is little if any in the commercial "carbolic acid" of today. The specification quoted demands practically that the phenol be replaced by cresylic acid, an ordinary sample of which containing upwards of 98 per cent tar acids and in all respects up to the most exacting of specifications, requires 200 times its volume of water to dissolve it even with difficulty. If, for instance, 1 cc. of such substance is mixed with 200 cc. of water, it is only after prolonged shaking that it will dissolve. Wolf Defries in his "Standard Chemical Disinfectants" says: "The disinfectant value of commercial 'carbolic acid' cannot be estimated by methods of chemical assay, and the widespread impression, which appears in many forms of contract adopted by users, that the presence of a given percentage of carbolic, cresylic, or other tar acids establishes in itself a definite bactericidal efficiency is wholly unfounded."

These facts should be sufficient to demonstrate the fallacy of employing carbolic acid as a disinfectant for general use. A further objection, the cogency of which will be realized when one recalls the fatalities which occur from time to time through the handling of this dangerous preparation by unskilled persons, is its high toxicity.

"Chloride of Lime."—With any disinfecting process it must be remembered that reaction between the disinfectant and organic matters which may harbor infectious organisms requires the disinfection to be repeated until the whole of the organic matter has been removed. Disinfectants which require such repeated reactions are therefore of little or no value for practical work.

Notwithstanding that one of their chief characteristics renders them totally unsuitable for this purpose, the hypochlorites, of which chloride of lime is the commonest form, are largely used as disinfectants. When brought into direct contact with certain organisms, chloride of lime undoubtedly exercises marked germicidal effect. This however is immediately neutralized when organic matter is present, which in actual practice is invariably the case. Dr. Doty says: "When it is deemed advisable to employ lime as a disinfectant, it should be used largely in excess of the material treated, particularly if chloride of lime is selected, for in the presence of organic matter this preparation is decomposed and practically rendered inert."

A striking example of this characteristic is that of Klein's well-known experiment described in *"Public Health"* of October, 1906. Working with chloros, a liquid preparation containing ten per cent of available chlorine, (the active principle of chloride of lime) and *B. typhosus* in a watery distribution free from organic matter, he obtained the high carbolic acid coefficient of 21.0; but on mixing with the chloros an equal amount of organic matter (urine) allowing the mixture to stand for an hour, and then adding the typhoid bacillus, that coefficient fell as low as 0.8. This result has been confirmed by Rideal, Sommerville, Moore and others; while Gruber has shown that for the efficient disinfection of cattle wagons, treatment with a solution of chlorinated lime had to be preceded by a thorough cleansing with water under pressure, and preferably at a high temperature, and that the chlorinated lime solution had then to be applied six or seven times. To apply the solution once, or even twice, gave no satisfactory result.

It is of the utmost importance that all chlorine compounds should be carefully tested in relation with organic matter of such kind as presents in practical everyday disinfection; and apart from a plain statement of the germicidal work that it is capable of performing in the presence of such organic matter, no reliance should be placed on the amount of "available chlorine" contained in a solution.

Perchloride of Mercury.—The last of the disinfectants to be considered in this connection is mercuric chloride, more generally designated perchloride of mercury, bichloride of mercury or corrosive sublimate. Against this substance the charge of bactericidal inefficiency does not apply, for under favorable conditions its carbolic acid coefficient may be very high. But, like chloride of lime, it has one fatal disability and that is its well known incompatibility with soap, serum, etc. Another objection to its use is its extreme toxicity, for though with careful handling this objection need not prove insuperable, it will probably be admitted that, other things being equal, a non-toxic disinfectant is always preferable to a toxic, and there are modern preparations which possess germicidal efficiency equal to that of perchloride without the objectionable attributes of the latter. As regards its incompatibility with soap and serum, this is so marked as to prohibit its use under many common conditions of working; its corrosive action precludes its use on metal work and it is demonstrable that, working with one of the modern preparations referred to above, disinfectant results equal to those obtained with perchloride may be effected at half the cost. It was for this reason that the Government of India abandoned the use of perchloride.

The foregoing particulars of the unsatisfactory characteristics of the disinfectants touched upon should be sufficient to show the undesirability of their use in general practice. In the absence of efficient substitutes, there might be some reason for utilizing to the fullest extent the limited capabilities of these obsolete processes; but this argument is no longer tenable, for modern research has placed at our disposal methods of determining with great accuracy which, in any given circumstances, are the most reliable of the many disinfectants available. That reforms take root slowly is as true of scientific as of most other subjects, and while disinfection has already attained a recognized position in prophylactic medicine, it is to be regretted that in certain quarters there has been displayed a marked disinclination to take advantage of the new conditions which have arisen out of scientific investigation of the action and use of modern germicides. For this reason the common assertion that "thorough disinfection was carried out" is too often suggestive of that blessed word Mesopotamia. To slightly modify Koch's well-known dictum, disinfection can only be considered effectual when the specific cause of infection is absolutely destroyed in the infected article.

THE SPHYGMOMANOMETER—ITS PLACE IN DIAGNOSIS; WITH REMARKS ON THE SIGNIFICANCE OF BLOOD PRESSURE.[1]

BY

HUGH E. ROGERS, M. D.,
Brooklyn, N. Y.

The sphygmomanometer is an instrument devised to determine blood pressure.

History.— There is nothing particularly new in the determining of the blood pressure by means of instruments. As far back as 1828 there are records which show the adoption of the manometer by the Frenchman, Poiseulle of Paris, and by Ludwig of Germany. Poiseulle introduced the U-shaped mercurial manometer. These records are not very accurate.

In the year 1856, K. Vieroldt recognized the value of a knowledge of the blood pressure. His method was very crude and consisted of placing weights over the radial artery until the pulse was obliterated.

In 1876, Marcy also devised a method for determining the arterial tension.

It was not until the year 1887 that any definite instrument was devised—not only to determine but to record the blood pressure.

This was the discovery of V. Basch of Vienna, who devised the first instrument for determining and recording the blood pressure. But even this instrument recorded only the maximum or the systolic pressure and the records show that it was not very accurate.

About this time, or a few years later, Riva-Rocci, an Italian of Turin, devised a more efficient and reliable instrument of the mercurial type. This was the first real advance in the perfecting of the sphygmomanometer.

This has acted as a model for most of the mercurial sphygmomanometers of the present time, including the very latest, those of Janeway and Stanton. These are nothing more or less than modifications of the Riva-Rocci. The Stanton being even more simple than the Janeway; the Janeway using the old style U-shaped tube. The Riva-Rocci sphygmomanometer is still in use.

A brief description of a Riva-Rocci will suffice for comparison.

All of these instruments were of the mercurial type. They were cumbersome, large and bulky, adapted only for hospital or office use. Their size and mechanism precluded their use by the general practitioner. Not being portable, the physician is unable to carry them from patient to patient, and make his records as he goes along.

They are fragile, are made of glass and easily broken.

Their mechanism depending on the metallic mercury, presents the greatest disadvantage. Because of the strong affinity for moisture of the mercury, in mercurial manometers, moisture is bound to accumulate and because of this oxidation of the mercury is sure to take place, making the instrument more or less unreliable. This moisture itself increases the capillary attraction, causing errors in the reading. Because of the inertia, or slowness, or even absence of the contractility of the mercury, it is not possible to correctly determine the diastolic pressure.

It has remained for one of our own generation, Dr. Oscar H. Rogers, a medical director of the New York Life Insurance Co., to devise and help bring to perfection an instrument, which I consider to be one of the

[1]Read before the Brooklyn Medical Society, December 15th, 1911.

real advances in scientific medicine of the century—the portable sphygmomanometer. An invention which takes its place with the clinical thermometer and the urinometer— just as necessary and as infallible as either (assuming these instruments to be correct) and the time is not far distant when every doctor will not only carry his thermometer in his pocket, but will also carry his sphygmomanometer. Just as he records the temperature of every patient, so will he take the readings of the blood pressure.

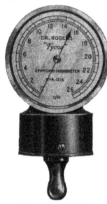

This new instrument is known as "Dr. Rogers' Tycos Sphygmomanometer."

By comparison with the older mercurial types you can readily see what a wonderful little instrument it is.

Its parts consist (as in fact, do the older types) of (*a*) The manometer; (*b*) The armlet; (*c*) The inflating bulb.

Compare the manometer of the Dr. Rogers Tycos with that of a Janeway or a Stanton or a Riva-Rocci, and you will appreciate what a wonderful piece of mechanism it is; the latter being of the mercurial type, are dependent for their operation on the contained mercury.

In the Dr. Rogers Tycos this is absolutely eliminated. No mercury whatever is used—the operation being dependent on the expansion of the diaphragm chambers contained in a small cylinder.

The pressure is exerted within the chambers and the resistance to the diaphragm chambers measured accurately on the dial.

This diaphragm is extremely sensitive and I would like to say incidentally that a large sum has been spent on the development of the temper and resistance of the metal which is used in its construction. What this metal is I do not know. As a result of the expansion of this very simple diaphragm we are able to obtain, not only the systolic or maximum pressure but also the diastolic or minimum. The determination of the diastolic in the mercurial instruments being quite unsatisfactory, by reason of the slowness of contractility of the mercury itself—the recovery of the mercury requiring approximately, one and one-half seconds, whereas there are one and one-quarter impulses of the heart a second—making them unreliable.

The determination of the diastolic pressure is very important. Not so much in life insurance work, as is the systolic, as in the treatment of disease—so as to determine whether or not the treatment of a given disease is increasing the force of the muscular mechanism of the arteries or reducing the blood impulses or both.

If you are familiar with the workings of an aneroid barometer you can readily appreciate the workings of Dr. Rogers' Tycos The aneroid barometers are made so small that you can put them in your vest pocket, and so delicate and sensitive is the mechanism that if you should take a trip up into the mountains, the atmospheric pressure will so work upon the diaphragm, that your ascent will be recorded, foot by foot, on the dial, as high as you go, without taking it out of your pocket.

In Dr. Rogers' Tycos the principle is almost identical—the pressure, instead of being atmospheric, being exerted by means of the inflating bulb and the armlet, the armlet containing a collapsible rubber bag. This rubber bag is connected with the manometer by means of a rubber tube—while a second tube connects the rubber bag with the inflating bulb. The use of the two tubes thus fully equalizing the pressure, so that no excessive exertion is put on the diaphragm, causing a complete circulation of the air by reason of a free inflow and outflow.

This rubber bag is 5 by 9½ inches, is sewed in a soft flexible sleeve of good quality and strength, the whole being forty inches long—tapering from five inches at the extreme end to about two inches at the rounded end.

Aside from its elegance and sightliness, a comparison with a Janeway or a Stanton armlet, will convince you that for comfort to the patient—utility—convenience and facility for the operator, it is far ahead of them all.

Modus Operandi:—(a) Application: In the standing posture the sleeve containing the rubber bag is placed around the left arm above the elbow over the brachial artery; in the recumbent posture, it is wrapped around the left leg over the femoral artery and never on the arm. The reason for the left side being obvious.

(b) To determine the systolic pressure: Palpate the pulse of the radial with the fingers of the left hand; then exert the pressure with the inflating bulb, held in the right hand; observe the amount of pressure required to collapse the arteries so that the pulse is lost at the radial. The point at which the pulse is obliterated is the systolic pressure.

The best way to try conclusions is to advance the pressure beyond point where pulse is obliterated, open the leak valve slowly and carefully, permitting air to escape, until you reach point at which the pulse returns. This is the systolic pressure.

(c) To determine the diastolic pressure: Observe the systolic pressure; that is, the point at which the pulse returns; turn off back valve and secure reading; the hand on the dial will then oscillate, due to the arterial impulse, between the point at which the pulse first appears, the systolic pressure and the point at which the artery regains its normal fullness and volume. The point at which the greatest oscillations occur is the diastolic pressure. The value of obtaining the diastolic pressure is so that the pulse pressure may be known.

(d) To determine the pulse pressure: Take the systolic—then take the diastolic and subtract, namely,

$$\begin{array}{ll} \text{Systolic} & 130 \\ \text{Diastolic} & 104 \\ \hline \text{Pulse} & 26 \end{array}$$

General Considerations.—What is meant by the blood pressure? By blood pressure is meant the amount of blood pressure which must be excited on outside of an artery in order to equalize that in the vessel.

In so far as the circulation of the blood is concerned there are three varieties of blood pressure: (a) The arterial; (b) The venous; (c) The capillary.

Of these, we have only to deal with the arterial. Not only because the arteries are more accessible and palpable, but because, by the very nature of things, the arteries not only receive the direct ventricular impulse, but by reason of their construction, they are more elastic and resistant. They do not act as mere conducting tubes, as do the veins and capillaries. Because of their elasticity and resistance, acting under the influence of the vaso-dilator and vaso-constrictor nerves, in overcoming the systolic impulse, what would be an intermittent becomes a continuous flow which is peristaltic in its nature. This constitutes what is known as the pulse wave.

In fact, the function of the arteries, besides acting as high pressure receptacles for the blood, by reason of their contained muscular fibres and consequent tonus, is to assist the heart in its efforts to propel the blood through its various arteries and exert a powerful influence on the current of the blood in general.

The veins and capillaries are merely conducting tubes. This is not so with the arteries. The function of the arteries is to assist the heart in its propulsion of the blood. In other words, the ventricular impulse and the arterial impulse are synchronous, that being accomplished by the elasticity and resistance of the arterial walls. "The disappearance of the pulse wave in normal arterial circulation is due to the elasticity of the arterial walls and resistance to the flow." (*Janeway*).

This elasticity and resistance constitute what is known as the peripheral resistance. It is the peripheral resistance which enables us to determine and record the amount of arterial tension or the arterial blood pressure.

Janeway. says: that the blood pressure at a given moment depends on (*a*) the energy of the heart; (*b*) the peripheral resistance; (*c*) the elasticity of the arterial walls; (*d*) the volume of the circulating blood.

The peripheral resistance is the main objective point. This is brought about by the elasticity of the arterial walls and consequent resistance to the flow of blood through the calibre of the artery. The greater the ventricular impulse, the greater the peripheral resistance, a purely reflex condition. Increase the ventricular impulse and by increasing the volume of output of the blood you cause a rise in the blood pressure.

Lessen the volume of the circulating blood and you will lessen the systolic impulse—lessen the peripheral resistance and you have a fall in the blood pressure.

So you see, in normal cases, the rise or fall of the blood pressure depends on the peripheral resistance remaining unchanged. That is to say, the arterial walls, by reason of their elasticity and resistance respond to the stimulation of the vaso-constrictor and vaso-motor nerves, a purely normal reflex action.

There are no two cases exactly alike, even in the normal. They must necessarily vary. If this be so in the normal, it is readily seen that great alterations can take place in the presence of disease.

There are two kinds of blood pressure. (*a*) Hypertension or high blood pressure; (*b*) Hypotension or low blood pressure.

Hypertension is either systolic or what is known as the maximum or diastolic or the minimum. It is divided into two classes:

(*a*) The functional or physiological.

(*b*) The essential or permanent.

The functional or physiological occurs in cases where there is no organic lesion of any kind. Any condition which calls for increased heart action, brought about by excitation of the vaso-motor nervous system, such as:

Muscular exertion, as in exercise.

Mental excitement.

Various functional nervous conditions.

Pain of any kind; even colic; labor pains.

Certain toxic poisons.

Various drugs, particularly digitalis.

Acute cerebral congestion.

Anemia.

In cases such as these the peripheral resistance remains unchanged. That is, by reason of the stimulation of the vaso-motor nerves—the vaso-dilators and vaso-constrictors—the elasticity of and resistance of the arterial walls meet the demands of the ventricular impulse and overcome it, constituting what is called compensation.

If, however, this stimulation is carried to the point beyond, this compensation breaks, goes over the borderland of the functional and organic and the pathological exists.

This point in functional hypertension bordering on the essential may be designated by the term abnormal.

"Abnormal high pressure cannot exist permanently." With undue excitement of the vaso-motor nerves there is an increased demand on the peripheral resistance. This increase in resistance must be met and overcome by the *vis a tergo* or the left ventricle. In normal cases it is met and overcome and as soon as the undue excitement dies down the blood goes on the even tenor of its way.

But, if this increase of peripheral resistance tends to become abnormal, the *vis a tergo* or the left ventricle must also meet this increase and overcome it. The left ventricle being a muscle, by reason of the extra stress that is put upon it, meets this demand by hypertrophy. This is functional hypertrophy and is just the condition that we meet in athletic heart.

However, when this increased demand goes a point beyond the abnormal, the compensation ruptures, it takes us into the realms of the pathological and we get the essential or permanent hypertension.

The essential or permanent hypertension includes cases which are associated with an organic lesion in some part of the body. Either in the arteries themselves as in arteriosclerosis or in organs directly connected with the circulation, as in the cardio-vascular lesions of diseases of the kidney or in any organ in which there is an interference with the circulation of the blood. "Increase the tension of the arterial walls and you decrease arterial distensibility." (*Janeway*[1]).

Arteriosclerosis.

Chronic Bright's disease, particularly what is known as chronic interstitial nephritis. Cardiac hypertrophy; angiosclerosis, not associated with the arteries; degenerative diseases of the blood vessels and the kidneys or toxemia causing same as a result of high arterial tension.

Gout: autotoxemia leading to actual atheroma. Dissipation; diabetes, in elderly and gouty people. Chronic emphysema, angina pectoris. Acute traumatic conditions of the brain, such as, acute compression, fracture of the base of the skull and apoplexy. The highest blood pressure ever recorded is on record as having occurred in these last three conditions.

In chronic interstitial nephritis, the small granular kidney—the contracted kidney, essentially a disease of the kidney, the arteries and the heart combined, we have a typical picture of permanent hypertension—registering higher than in any other organic condition—having registered as high as 200-240 m. m.

In aortic insufficiency we get a high systolic pressure; a high tension pulse accompanied by a low pressure between beats indicating strong cardiac action, but no increase of peripheral resistance.

In aortic diseases deficient circulation is due to insufficient supply of blood in the arteries; in mitral disease to increased pressure in the veins.

"Permanent hypertension cannot be maintained without hypertrophy of the left ventricle." (*Janeway*).

The coincidence of hypertrophy of the heart and alterations in the kidney were recognized by Bright as early as 1836.

It may be put down as a general proposition that abnormal hypertension cannot exist permanently—that when it passes the borderline the condition becomes pathological. By the abnormal is meant, that point in functional hypertension which borders on the essential or permanent.

For example, a normal man in a quiescent state has what we might call a normal hypertension; let him exercise and the high pressure is increased. This is known as the functional. If exercise is continuous the blood pressure sometimes falls to normal, constituting what is called "second wind." Let him overdo it by too much exercise and the abnormal takes place; the *vis a tergo* or the left ventricle and peripheral resistance are put upon the stretch and if necessary the left ventricle hypertrophies to meet the demand and compensation takes place. Carry it a point beyond and compensation ruptures and the essential or permanent hypertension exists.

Hypotension is simply the opposite of hypertension. It is brought about by a disturbance of the cardio-vascular nervous system which causes a loss of energy in the heart muscle itself as is seen in various forms of heart disease; the wasting diseases such as advanced tuberculosis or carcinoma of the stomach. From loss of tone in the circulatory apparatus; from dis-

eases resulting from deterioration of the blood, such as advanced syphilis, diabetes, pernicious anemia and various cachectic diseases; from certain drugs causing vasodilatation such as the nitrates, especially amyl nitrite, chloroform in which hypotension occurs early and must be carefully watched. From various infections and toxemias.

Typhoid fever: from profuse hemorrhage; collapse or shock. The process of dissolution is attended by a fall of blood pressure. In brief, hypotension is caused by any loss of cardiac energy, decrease in the peripheral resistance and lessening of the volume output of the circulating blood.

In hypotension the blood accumulates in the veins, causing a venosity, the arterial blood current slows up, there is little or no resistance in the arterial walls to the circulatory path of the blood—due to loss of tone either in a particular organ or to part of the vaso-motor system or the vaso-motor system in general.

The whole subject may be summed up in a few words—that the principle of arterial tension or blood pressure is dependent on the fact that the arteries are the high pressure receptacles for the blood and that it is not subject to the laws of gravitation but to the general law of hydrostatics.

The normal pressure for adult males is about 120 m. m., for females 10 m. m. less, in life insurance work we accept between 130 to 140 m. m.

Conclusions.—It is a good diagnostician who can recognize a disease in its incipiency. The recognition of disease in its first stage, makes possible the employment of prophylactic and curative measures which would otherwise not have been thought of, and early and prompt treatment may accomplish a great deal towards an early cure.

The expert diagnostician, more than on anything else, depends on the sense of touch, as in palpation, for his ability to recognize a disease and make a diagnosis.

The reliance that every doctor places on the palpation of the pulse is well known. And the value of a correct knowledge and interpretation of the pulse wave will not be doubted by anyone. Certain it is that some even without a very fine development of the tactile sense, can recognize and diagnose certain conditions by just feeling the pulse. While in others, the sense of touch is so finely developed that it is possible for them to make fine distinctions, which others otherwise cannot or do not take the time to make.

But the sense of touch has its limitations, especially where conditions of the circulatory system are concerned particularly in obscure cases, and it is in these cases that even the expert diagnostician, relying on the sensitivenes of his touch, fails. And where the tactile sense fails, as far as diagnosis is concerned, the sphygmomanometer steps in. As an aid to diagnosis in obscure conditions, a knowledge of the existing blood pressure is incalculable.

Dr. Henry Elsner[4] of Syracuse, says: "That one of the most important functions of the expert diagnostician is the correct interpretation of the blood pressure."

No better criterion can be found, than that all the large life insurance companies recognize the value of known systolic pressure as a determining factor in placing a risk.

Here it is a purely speculative business proposition as to just how long an applicant will live. An applicant presents himself for examination. He may be healthy or unhealthy. If he is healthy, well and good. If he is unhealthy and knows it and his general appearance is healthy as is often the case, he will evade and even lie. He tells us nothing, we must find out for ourselves. We must rely absolutely on the objective symptoms, just what we hear, see and feel. If there is any doubt as to the diagnosis of applicant's condition after the application of the sphygmomanometer, if a persistent hyper or hypotension exists it will enable the examiner to complete his diagnosis and get a good line on applicant's general condition.

If this be so in life insurance work which deals for the most part, only with the objective, the value of the instrument to the general practitioner, who not only deals with the objective but also with the subjective symptoms of diseases, as elicited from patients themselves, can be readily appreciated.

I quote Dr. Oscar H. Rogers[5] who has made a life study of the subject, who says: "I look upon blood pressure observations as so important a feature of clinical examination that I am sure the time is not far distant when every physician will have to provide himself with an apparatus for the purpose of making such observations just as he provides himself with a clinical thermometer or an equipment for making an examination of the urine."

REFERENCES.

1. Janeway, *Clinical Study of Blood Pressure*, 1904.
2. Bishop, *Heart Disease and Blood Pressure*.
3. Graham: White and Ritchie, *Physical Diagnosis*.
4. Henry Elsner, Syracuse, N. Y., "*Blood Pressure Study*."
5. Oscar H. Rogers, New York City.

102 Lewis Ave., Brooklyn, N. Y.

AN ATTEMPT TO COPE WITH THE ECONOMIC PROBLEM WITHIN THE PRACTICE OF MEDICINE.[1]

BY

OSCAR ROTTER, M. D.,
New York City.

From a careful investigation and study of medical economics, I am convinced not only that a great majority in our profession feel the existence and pressure of certain economic problems very keenly but that a more equitable material welfare to which we are justly entitled in return for our professional work can never be attained except by cooperation for mutual protection. That the day of purely individual self-help against the many unfavorable conditions under which we are compelled to practice our profession is over, is proven by the fact that physicians all over the United States have found it necessary of late years to organize themselves into fraternities or societies to improve their economic condition and social relations instead of adhering to their previous mode of regardless competition in the struggle for a fair livelihood. Competitive rivalry among them in the pre-cooperative period has often been of a nature which should be looked upon as below the dignity of self-respecting professional men and proved after all only suicidal to the majority.

So much for a general introduction. The rest of my address I shall deliver under three chapters. In the first chapter I shall speak of a message, in the second of a mission and in the third of personal and practical suggestions for the abolition of some of the most important evils that are a well known cause of the equally well known

[1] Read before the Medical Alliance, January 25, 1912.

progressive decrease in our professional income.

The Message.—First as to the message I have to bring to you. It is the news that the Yorkville Medical Society of which I consider myself at this moment a representative, has taken the progressive step to make the economic problem a permanent topic for discussion and practical action. At its regular meeting of October 16th, 1911, after a thorough general discussion of a paper read by me on "The Economic Problem as it Affects the Medical Profession" the following motion was made and carried unanimously:

Moved:

To establish a permanent Committee on Economic Research of the Yorkville Medical Society.

The Yorkville Medical Society through this committee is to work out a systematic program of dealing with medical economic problems and to invite the cooperation of all other medical societies of Greater New York.

In order to adapt the work of this committee to the real needs of the physician in private practice it is required that only such members be designated as are not in charge of hospital or dispensary work.

A committee of seven members was appointed forthwith with the instruction to begin and keep up work as outlined and laid down in the resolution.

The Mission.—Now as to the mission with which I have come to you. It is the first time since the creation of the committee on economic research within the Yorkville Medical Society that I as a member and at this moment the representative of this committee have had an opportunity to invite the cooperation of another medical society, to ask it to join us in the spirit of the resolution stated and to take part in the active work for carrying out its purpose. I therefore, herewith invite and solicit the cooperation of the Medical Alliance in this good and timely cause.

We cannot and should not expect any practical material benefits from this movement before we have succeeded in interesting actively all other local medical societies. The work at this stage is mainly educational and informal. We must try to establish a federation between the existing local medical societies for mutual economic protection. With an economic committee in every local medical society, it would be easy to arrange periodical joint conferences between these committees or delegates from them to discuss medico-economic questions, and formulate a program of action. In short our immediate aim must be to create a practical machinery of cooperation.

Practical Suggestions.—Now as to practical personal suggestions. Under this heading I shall refer to a number of evils which have a ruinous effect on the private practice of medicine. They are due partly to certain modern economic forces over which we have no control, and partly to our own reckless carelessness and thoughtlessness in taking care of our material interests in the struggle for existence. We must learn a lesson from the captains of industry as well as from laborers in other fields of endeavor. They both know that they have to combine, to cooperate, to unite their forces in the fight for a just and equitable share in the social wealth created by the work and toil of all. Only we physicians are naive enough to expect that all should be well with us because we feel and know that the work we do is necessary, useful, humane and because it often even requires great sacrifices of our

personal comfort. We should know however, that hard work and toil is as a rule underpaid unless they who do it know enough and are strong enough to compel a fair and just compensation. At the present age this is possible only by organization, cooperation, and efforts at mutual protection.

What are the evils with which we can economically struggle only through cooperation?

There is first the *abuse* of Dispensary charity by a host of people who could and would pay a physician in private practice for medical services if they were not supplied with them without question at many of the institutions created and supported for the benefit of the really poor. We certainly cannot blame the state for this condition of affairs. It has done all that can be expected from it in the interests not only of the deserving poor, but also of the private physician who has to live by his professional work and who has spent many years of study and the cash capital necessary to fit himself for his responsible work in compliance with the very severe and rigid terms required by the state before he is permitted to practice his profession and earn a livelihood thereby.

Here is the law of the state enacted for the purpose of preventing the *abuse* of Dispensary charity:

Section 25, Chapter 368, Laws of 1899.

Any person who obtains medical or surgical treatment on false representations from any dispensary licensed under the provision of this act, shall be guilty of a misdemeanor and on conviction thereof shall be punished by a fine of not less than $10 and not more than $250.

(Imprisonment until fine be paid may be imposed. Code Crim. Pro., No. 718).

So the law exists but it is not in actual operation. The fault is with the system of inquiry into the financial circumstances of persons applying for free treatment at the dispensaries. As a matter of fact, inquiry at the dispensary desks is only nominal. The attending physicians have no time to make inquiries or if they do they render themselves liable to censure by the hospital administrations, for hospitals and dispensaries are ever trying to out rival each other in the number of patients treated. A very simple and practical method of control and enforcement of the dispensary law would be that applicants would be required to bring a certificate of recommendation either from the Department of Charity or better yet from any physician in the neighborhood of the patient's residence, such physician's certificate of recommendation to be furnished free of charge. This would stop at once any attempt at misrepresentations. Free medical services to persons able to pay is an injustice to the community, to societies who furnish the means for the support of charitable institutions, to the dispensary physicians who do professional work without compensation, to physicians in private practice who have to earn their livelihood through their professional work, and last but not least, to the needy and deserving poor who would receive better because more individualized attention and treatment by dispensary physicians not so overcrowded with work as they are at present. Fully 40% of dispensary patients are actually in similar financial circumstances to the majority of patients who make up the circle of practice of the general practician and not a few have an income greater than many a physician himself! This form of graft practiced on charitable institutions maintained by public or private funds, and on the medical profession in private or dispensary practice, is certainly an evil that must be abolished sometime and somehow. There is simply no excuse for its existence.

Another evil seriously affecting the economic welfare of the physician is growing up more and more through the activity of the New York Board of Health. It no longer confines itself to its legitimate and original sphere of enforcing the laws of public sanitation and hygiene, or of assisting the physician in the diagnosis of certain diseases by laboratory tests, etc. It has become in more than one way a privileged competitor of the physician in private practice. It has practically, if not legally, taken from him nearly all cases of vaccination. It not only opens up dispensary after dispensary but even sends out physicians and nurses to the bedside of patients without taking any more trouble to limit the bestowal of such public medical charity to the really poor than do the hospitals or dispensaries. Against such an unwarrantable encroachment, the medical profession should enter an earnest and vigorous protest.

As regards the evil of lodge or contract practice, it is up to us physicians to start a movement through our societies and the medical press to agree among ourselves either to refuse to engage in it or only on such terms in regard to remuneration as may be formulated by a conference of the economic committees of medical societies and ratified by the membership of each society.

Next, what should we do to meet successfully the evil of competition with the various unqualified practitioners, who, though unable to diagnose a disease, nevertheless are engaged in the treatment of patients by some freak non-medical or non-surgical method? I refer to all those "would-be-doctors" who practice under various names such as hydropaths, naturopaths, Christian Science healers, dietists, fasters, masseurs under the cloak of osteopaths, etc., etc. Inasmuch as each of these methods has a certain but limited value and place in the auxiliary therapy of disease we should pay more attention to them, study their mode of action and application and use them ourselves in our practice whenever scientifically indicated. Patients know that only the physician is a "doctor" in the real and full sense of the word, but as long as they believe in the efficacy of these non-medical or non-surgical remedial agents, looking upon them as a "panacea," they will patronize those who make a routine practice of them while they would probably prefer to get these modes of treatment administered by a regular physician if he were willing and able to make them a part of his daily work. Sooner or later our medical colleges must supply their students with knowledge regarding them. We have in all our medical societies men who are scientific specialists, in hydrotherapy, dietetics, electrotherapy, mechanotherapy, etc. There is a good opportunity for them to teach their brother physicians the general principles and art of these methods of therapy through lectures and demonstrations, thus fitting them to recognize the indications for such special therapy as well as to refer patients in need of it to such scientific specialists in our own profession if they are not qualified to employ them actually themselves—just as we refer our patients when necessary to a surgeon, an oculist or a nose and throat specialist.

The evil of counter-prescribing by pharmacists can I think easily be done away with. The interests of the pharmacist and the physician are in many respects identical, as for instance, in regard to the abuse of dispensary charity. More than this, the pharmacist very naturally prefers to be on good terms with the physician. Every pharmacist as a man, especially as a business man, appreciates the reputation of being an honest and capable dispenser of medicines prescribed by the physician. Whatever grievances exist here and there can easily be adjusted by amicable cooperation between the medical and pharmaceutical societies and their respective press. There has already been held a joint meeting of the Yorkville Medical Society and the New York County Pharmaceutical Society for the discussion of this subject. Thus much practical work is already under way in this sphere.

One more evil I shall refer to which deserves attention. There exists as yet no uniform basis of reciprocity or mutual recognition of state licenses or medical college diplomas conferring the right to practice medicine between the different states. Eleven states do not reciprocate at all. New York only reciprocates with seven other states. In the absence of reciprocity with any state or with certain other states, a physician, no matter from what college he has graduated or how long he has been in actual practice, is required to pass a written examination before a State Board of Medical Examiners which is virtually a repetition of his college examination for his degree! It is needless to mention that no physician, no matter how good a practician he may be, is able to pass such an examination without a thorough and systematic review and preparation in the theoretical details of all branches of medicine which often require months of study. The examiners of medical state boards would probably fail themselves to answer satisfactorily their own examination papers without such previous preparation if they were candidates for license to practice medicine before a board of medical examiners of another state! As long as there exists no general reciprocity in regard to diplomas or licenses between all the states—which would be the most reasonable and fairest attitude—a *clinical* examination in the presence of actual patients *only* should be required of physicians. Their college diplomas should be accepted as a sufficient proof of a systematic theoretical knowledge of the science of medicine. Many a physician struggling hard to get along in an over populated state might do well and become prosperous in one of the younger states of our vast country. As regards Greater New York there is no doubt that more physicians would go away than physicians from other states would come here to try their fortune. The high cost of living in New York City would more than equalize matters in regard to such eventual new competitors.

A few words more and I am at the end of my remarks. I think there is no doubt in the mind of the majority of New York City physicians that they have many justified grievances as regards the unfavorable economic conditions and circumstances under which they have to make a livelihood to-day through the practice of their profession. And let it not be forgotten, an economic improvement for the physician means also an improvement in the medical services rendered to the average patient. A man depressed by financial care and worry in the struggle for existence is not the best man to bring relief and help to the suffering sick. It is liable to rob him of his energy and love for his responsible work. And yet the majority of patients require the services of the physician often in the middle of the night, not of the surgeon or specialist! Nor is this all. To keep abreast with the modern advancement of the science and art of medicine it requires ever more cash investment for modern equipment for efficient practical work, such as books, professional periodical literature, periodical post-graduate courses, instruments, apparatus or other office outfit than almost any other business or profession. Without some surplus in the financial income over the necessary expenses for our daily life such extra professional expenditures are impossible. This tends to lower the scientific and professional status of the average physician, the average patient being again the greatest loser. And last but not least, just as civilization in a country is measured by the culture and material condition of the majority of the people, so the respect that a profession commands, depends on the professional quality and material welfare of the majority of its members!

Physicians therefore, should strive for a degree of material welfare proportionate to their professional work and to their social status in the community for their own benefit as well as for the best interests of their patients.

In washing the vagina and external genitals, cotton or gauze should be used, rather than a brush. A brush is apt to abrade the parts.—*Waldo.*

A soft rubber or metal catheter is preferable to a glass one. "I have known of two instances," says Waldo, "where the end of a glass catheter was broken off and remained in the bladder. In sterilizing a glass catheter by boiling it may be so injured as to favor the occurrence of such an accident."

THE PLACE OF ANTITOXIN AND IN-
TUBATION IN THE TREATMENT
OF DIPHTHERIA.[1]

EDWIN RAPALJE BEDFORD, M. D.,
Attending Physician to the Cumberland St. Hospital; and Inspector of the Health Department, Brooklyn, N. Y.

Ten years ago the automobile was not so generally used by physicians as it is today. A number who used them were disap-. pointed with the results obtained and went back to the use of the horse and carriage or street cars to take them on their daily rounds. Some of these physicians have not returned to the use of the automobile, but others who have observed the improved mechanism, and how much can be accomplished in a short period of time, have ventured again to try the motor car, and the majority of them (i. e., those who use the right product) are getting quicker and more satisfactory results than when they employed other methods of travelling. Some of the disappointment at first was due to using a one cylinder engine when a four cylinder one was required. If there is a bad piece of road or a steep grade to climb, the one cylinder car will be a failure, but a more powerful car will carry you safely through; however, even then the increased momentum is generally required before you reach the worst place in the road if you are going to progress successfully. What the auto is to the physician as a means of conveyance in the making of his calls, so is antitoxin as a method in the treatment of diphtheria.

When the serum first appeared, some who tried it were enthusiastic, others

[1]Read before the annual meeting of the Homeopathic Society of the State of New York, February 13th, 1912.

were disappointed with their results and went back to their former methods of treatment. Some were and are still afraid of this "auto." Let us consider the cause of their disappointment. Many times the fault lay, as it did with the motor car, in not using a sufficiently powerful dose which the occasion demanded. A small dose of antitoxin given in a severe diphtheritic infection will result in a failure; whereas, if a powerful enough dose is given the result is usually quick and gratifying. As it is necessary to speed the motor engine before you reach the steepest incline of the hill in order to get the best results, so if you would pull your case of diphtheria safely through, get the antitoxin in before the vitality is so low that recuperation under any method of treatment is impossible.

It seems unnecesary at the present time to advocate the use of diphtheria antitoxin, yet there appear to be some who still fail to see the advantage of it, just as there are still a few who are reluctant to trust to the auto which is doing such good work for the majority of us.

Many have hesitated to use antitoxin for fear of ill effects upon the heart and kidneys, and also for fear of paralysis following its use.

Let us deal with the facts and see if these fears are well grounded. Previous to the use of antitoxin, diphtheria was a much dreaded disease, necessitating a long period of confinement to bed, with great fear of attempting to get up, because of a possible fatal collapse, due to a diseased weakened heart. Again, nephritis was a frequent complication prolonging the confinement to bed; while post-diphtheritic paralysis was far from uncommon and many times only partially recovered from. What has become of these complications since the use of antitoxin has become general? Some cases are not confined to bed at all, and many for a few days only. In fact, cases have recovered so quickly after an injection of serum that it has been impossible to convince the patient of a correct diagnosis, although the latter has been confirmed by the microscope as well as by clinical evidence.

Albuminuria, when seen at all by the writer appears to be only transient as a rule; and other symptoms of nephritis are very rare. Paralysis is seldom seen except that which I believe is largely due to the pressure from the amount of fluid injected, and which usually passes away in from thirty-six to forty-eight hours after the injection. Where paralysis has occurred later, I believe that it is due rather to the disease than to the treatment and probably would have been prevented if a larger dose of the serum had been used. Many times it is very difficult to keep the patient in the house for ten days after the first injection.

When a case can be seen within the first or second day, as occasionally happens when secondary cases develop in the same family, the writer has found 1,000 to 2,000 units to be a sufficient curative dose, but usually 3,000 to 5,000 units will be required; and if the case is exceptionally severe, or the disease has existed for five days or more 5,000 to 9,000 units should be injected.

In laryngeal cases, 8,000 to 10,000 units should be the initial dose, and unless the case is a mild one, this dose should be repeated within twenty-four hours. It is seldom necessary to again repeat the dose, although I have frequently done so without observing any ill effects afterward.

This leads us to the subject of intubation, which is simply an emergency operation for the relief of the patient, that has

saved many lives while the antitoxin is getting in its work. Intubation is not required so frequently as formerly, as the timely use of antitoxin has prevented the extension of the membrane to the larynx. When it is required, it can be done with few assistants by wrapping the patient in a sheet or blanket, securely, placing him upon his back upon a table. One assistant to steady the head is often all that can be obtained among the poorer families where this ordeal is most often required, for it is these people who are apt to neglect the illness until the larynx is involved.

The writer has more than once performed intubation in very young children without the aid of any assistant.

The mortality of intubated cases probably averages from 20 to 33% according to the length of time that stenosis has been present before the tube was inserted. The mortality where the larynx is not involved probably varies from 8 to 12% according to the number of days that the disease has existed before the injection was given.

Antitoxin is used for the purpose of immunizing in doses of 500 to 1,000 units and although it is difficult to prove whether any drug is a prophylactic yet the writer has seen very few secondary cases develop in probably over three thousand children that have been immunized. Those that did develop were generally mild cases, or did not develop until after two weeks, i. e., after the period of the protection had expired. During the past year in over 600 persons immunized *no* secondary cases have developed.

During the past eight years the writer has given on an average of 150 to 200 curative injections a year, and has performed about forty to sixty intubations each year. During one period of seven months fifty intubations were performed.

Of course, laryngeal cases are more prevalent during the winter months, and during January, 1912, I performed seven intubations. Often when the weather turns cold after a mild day, we will have two or three intubations within twenty-four hours.

In closing I wish to affirm my strong belief in the homeopathic law of cure. Dr. Laidlaw, I believe, is authority for the statement to the effect that antitoxin does not act homeopathically but as an antidote. I believe that he is right for the more severe the infection, the larger will be the dose required.

I have seen the indicated remedy do wonders in various potencies, but I have not seen it or any other method of treatment save the lives in the severe cases of diphtheria that antitoxin has. Therefore, I would prefer to practice medicine in the Borough of Brooklyn without the assistance of an automobile than to treat diphtheria without the aid of antitoxin.

352 Hancock St.

MY EXPERIENCE IN THE WRECK OF THE TITANIC.

BY

HENRY W. FRAUENTHAL, M. D.,
New York City.

Recalling the Titanic as I saw it from the tender just before going on board at Cherbourg, it is almost impossible to conceive that this magnificent vessel of 880 feet could have sunk. Up to the time of the accident, the trip had been ideal.

On Sunday night, I retired at about ten o'clock, and my wife and I were sleeping soundly, when at about twelve o'clock, I was awakened by my brother pounding on my cabin door, and insisting upon my getting up. Thinking that I had overslept and was late, I asked what was the matter, and he said that something had happened to the boat. On going to the door, he informed me that he had overheard the captain informing Colonel Astor that something serious had occurred to the boat, and advised that everyone put on life preservers, and they were lowering the lifeboats. When I went on the boat deck, there were a few people there, but no confusion, and I saw them lowering the boats. There seemed difficulty in filling the boats. I returned for my wife to my cabin, No. 88, Deck C, and in passing Mr. Widener, who was in No. 80, Deck C, I informed him that I had learned the boat was in danger, but he said that it was ridiculous. This answer probably describes the mental state of nearly everyone on the boat, thinking that it was impossible for anything serious to happen to this paragon of modern ship architecture. I returned to my cabin, and insisted on my wife putting a life preserver on. We went on deck, and got in the boat which was in charge of Third Officer Pittman. In this boat, there were an equal number of men and women, thirty-four in all. The boat on the port side, which was lowered at the same time as ours, was sent off by order of Captain Smith *with only twenty-two passengers*, because at that time *there were no more who were willing to trust themselves to the life boats.*

In the process of being lowered, several times we thought we would be thrown into the water. When nearing the water, it was discovered that the plug in the bottom of the boat had not been safely inserted, and this was attended to. Had this been overlooked, this lifeboat would have sunk as one of the others did, in which the plug was not inserted. After rowing a short

distance, I inquired of Third Officer Pittman what had occurred to the boat, being
under the impression that the trouble was
with the machinery and we were likely to
be blown up. *I learned then for the first
time, that we had struck an iceberg.* I
asked when we would return to the Titanic,
and he said within half an hour, as he
thought there was no danger to the vessel
and only as we observed one row of port-
hole lights after another disappearing below the water line, did we begin to realize

scraped like a ferry-boat going into the
slip. Pittman was awakened by a sailor,
and said he went down to see what had
occurred and met some of the stokers
coming out of the hold, saying that water
was rushing in and driving them out. He
then went on deck and aided in loading
the other boats. He was ordered to take
charge of the lifeboat in which I left the
vessel, which I think was No. 5.

There was no moon, but the stars in the
sky were numerous and it made the sur-

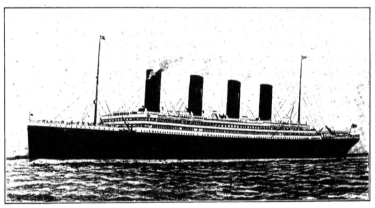

"STEAMER TITANIC."

Largest and most luxurious in the world. Launched at Belfast, Ireland, May,
1911. Length, 882 ft. 6 inches. Displacement, 66,000 tons. On her maiden trip
struck a mammoth iceberg on Sunday, April 14th, at 10.25 P. M., 41° 46 minutes,
north latitude; 50° 14 minutes, west longitude. Sunk at 2.20 A. M., April 15,
1912, with a loss of over 1,500 lives.

how serious the accident was. One of the
sailors in our boat was on watch at the
time the accident occurred and said that
the iceberg was above the upper deck and
through concussion several tons of ice were
thrown on the upper deck. Pittman, the
3rd officer, who like myself, was asleep,
was not awakened by the accident. Those
who were awake at the time, said there was
no concussion, but it seemed as if the boat

roundings appear as light as it would with
a quarter moon. We rowed about a mile
from the Titanic, believing that if she went
down, it would be a protection against the
suction of the vessel. In the boat *I*
was in, and *in all the other lifeboats* which
I inspected as they were hoisted in the Carpathia, there was *no compass, no lantern,
no water, and no food!* The only light in
any of the small boats was a lantern taken

off by Fifth Officer Lowe and his reason for taking it was, as he said, that he had been in two shipwrecks previously and realized its need. It was by the means of this light that the Carpathia was able to sight us, as they saw the light at a distance of ten miles. After daybreak, it would have been difficult for the Carpathia to have detected us in the ice field we were in. The ocean surface during the whole night was as smooth as glass, nor was there any wind. The air was intensely cold, and nearly everyone suffered from the low temperature.

We watched the boat and timed her as she sank, which was about 2.20 a. m., according to the officer's watch. The time of

about six o'clock, being on the water just about 5½ hours. Some of the smaller boats did not arrive until nearly nine o'clock, after which we circled around for about three hours, hoping to pick up some of the shipwrecked. During the night we could see the large iceberg which we struck and several smaller ones, and I cannot see how so large a mass of ice could not have been seen in ample time by the lookout. At about 8 a. m., two big vessels arrived on the scene and they were left on the ground to see if they could pick up any of the survivors. When day broke, we saw about two miles away what seemed to be land, but which was a field of ice and which I since learned was 200 miles long. So had we

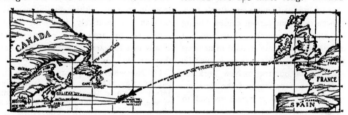

Chart showing place where Titanic struck iceberg, and sank at 2.20 A. M., April 15, 1912.

the accident was about 10.45 p. m., *showing that the boat remained afloat for only about three and a half hours.*

One of the boats rowed up to us, which had but twenty-seven passengers in it and three men from our boat were transferred to this lifeboat.

When the vessel went down and for some time after, the cries of those who were on life preservers and floats were indescribable and no one who heard these cries, will ever forget them.

The Carpathia was in sight at about 4.30 a. m., when all the small boats rowed towards her. We were taken on board at

missed the large iceberg, going at the rate of 21 or 22 knots an hour, we would have driven into the field of ice just ahead of us.

The passengers from the small boats were taken into the Carpathia by means of a pilot's ladder. For safety, the women had a looped rope under their arms, and when they lost their footing on the rope ladder, they were drawn on board the boat. Many did lose their footing on account of the nervous state they were in and the cold which made them stiff; and in being hauled on board, received many bruises.

One cannot speak in too high praise of the arrangements for our reception on board the Carpathia. As each one got to the deck, they were given a large *hot* drink, of either hot water or hot tea, or hot diluted brandy. If this did not warm them up, they were covered with blankets, and additional drinks were given. By this means, a reaction was brought about, and in place of being blue, they became pink and moist, and out of the 705 survivors, no case of bronchitis or pneumonia occurred to my knowledge, and the vessel came into port with a clean bill of health. Although all the papers were filled with the account of the large number of ill on board, it was not a fact. A certain number suffered from the exposure and from injuries and were taken to St. Vincent's Hospital. A number of sprained ankles and Pott's fractures occurred from various causes. Owing to the fact that a number of women lost their husbands, a certain amount of nervous hysteria prevailed. This was intensified by the fact that on our trip to New York for four days, we were most of the time enveloped in fogs and everyone seemed to dread the recurrence of an accident.

About $6,000 was collected on the Carpathia from the survivors to meet the immediate needs of the Titanic passengers, of which $4,000 was afterwards given to the crew on the Carpathia, in recognition of their services.

The large death list was due to the fact that *the majority of the people did not know the nature and extent of the damage done to the boat*, and *a great number knew that the Carpathia had been in communication, and that she was coming to the rescue.* The fear of going into the small boats on account of the danger in case of a high sea, deterred many from entering. *There was a general feeling that the boat could not possibly sink before* *some of the larger boats near by would come to the rescue.* This was particularly true, as some of the people refused to depart shortly before the boat went down, thinking it safer than venturing in a small boat.

REPORT OF A CASE OF ACHONDRO-PLASIA.

BY

LOUIS CURTIS AGER, M. D.,
Brooklyn, N. Y.

Among the dystrophic conditions of infancy and childhood achondroplasia, or chondrodystrophy fetalis, so named by Kaufmann in his very thorough study of the condition, published in 1892, is one of the most interesting. Although this condition is seen comparatively frequently in the clinics of our large cities, cases are sufficiently rare to warrant the recording of any that are seen for the first time.

On November 26th, 1911, the following patient was referred to me from New Jersey. Female, six years and two months of age. The first living child; two induced miscarriages previously. The father was normal, of American parentage, and gave absolutely no indication of specific disease. Mother neurotic, poor nutrition, history of gastric ulcer since marriage, but no indication of specific trouble.

Child was born in normal labor and was apparently normal at the time of birth. Whooping cough at two years, measles at three years of age. The digestive tract has always been normal. Child was nursed through the second summer. The parents noticed the small size of the child as soon as it began to walk, but no especial attention was given to the matter for several years.

A physical examination was as follows: General nutrition apparently good, although the muscles are somewhat flabby. The reflexes apparently diminished and mentality seems to be normal in this case, which is exceptional in this disease. In the neck the lymphnodes are slightly palpable, probably due to bad teeth, elsewhere they are negative. The thorax slightly funnel shaped; the lungs normal; heart normal, and abdomen markedly protuberant. The feet are entirely normal in contour. The epiphyses are very large but symmetrical. The child is 36½ inches in height and weighs 37½ pounds, whereas a child of this age should be forty-four inches in height and weigh about forty-five pounds. Compared with her actual height, her weight is normal. The head is of the typical shape found in these circumstances, the bulging forehead and compressed at the root of the nose. The lateral diameter is 6½ inches, antero-posterior 7½ inches, arm is 5½ inches, length of forearm 5½ inches. There is no spinal curvature in this case and all the extremities are symmetrical in their development. The head is also symmetrical.

According to Kaufmann, there are three types of this condition, the most frequent is the combination of hypo- and hyper-plasia which results not only in dwarfism but in marked deformities of both the spine and extremities. At the present time this patient shows no deformities, and is, therefore, of a pure hypoplasia type. It is, of course, possible that the various deformities, bowlegs, scoliosis, lordosis, may develop later in life.

There is one point in the clinical history which is of some significance. The child suffers from abnormal thirst and very frequent urination particularly at night. This suggests polyuria, although I have not been able to get full quantity of urine for twenty-four hours.

As the pituitary gland is generally believed to have some control over the mechanism of growth, as well as an influence over the flow of urine, we have here a further indication of the relation of the pituitary to this type of dystrophy. It would be of extreme interest to treat some of these patients seen very early in life with pituitary extract with the possibility of stimulating growth of the long bones.

137 Clinton St.

SOME COMMONPLACE REMARKS ON THE TREATMENT OF MEASLES AND SCARLET FEVER.

BY

J. L. MARBOURG, M. D.,
Seattle, Washington.

After twenty-three years' experience, with no fatalities, in the treatment of scarlet fever, it is my earnest opinion that it is not absolutely necessary to quarantine in this disease or lose a single case.

The treatment of measles and scarlet fever that I have followed is based largely on the idea of destroying the germ, in the skin. I use an oil, which consists of a ½ of 1% solution of beta-naphthol in linseed oil, the combination being effected by heat. Olive oil or any other oil would probably do as well. This is applied thoroughly after a warm sponge bath, plain or medicated with lysol or creolin. For use as a systemic internal antiseptic, I give six to eight grains of calcium sulphide to an adult, preferably in tablet form; children in proportion. For the fever I use phenacetin, advise a nutritious diet in conjunction with some digestive ferment, such as essence of pepsine or liquid rennet, containing fluid extract of cactus; guard the kidneys with a solution of lithium salicylate; regulate the bowels with castor oil in port wine; allow no fruit or fruit acids; and for throat complications, invariably use a gargle as in diphtheria. In all cases of scarlet fever, the nurse is advised to put a few drops of formaldehyde in a shallow dish, placed under the bed, and insist on the use of formaldehyde in all utensils used for the excretions.

In my early practice, I was called to see some very virulent cases of scarlet fever; one of six children died before the parents thought of getting a doctor; another was dying when I arrived at the house; but the remaining four under the treatment I have outlined quickly recovered.

In 1908 I was called to some interesting cases of scarlet fever, in Youngstown, Wash. Bessie J—age seven, was taken with a severe form of scarlet fever on April 23rd. She had throat complications, high fever and delirium; simple treatment as above was instituted; three days later, called again, found her out of danger, and did not call again until after desquamation.

Sept. 4th, her sister, Mary, was taken with the same disease and same complications, only if anything more severe; placed her on simple treatment; called next day, and then not again until it was time to raise the quarantine. Sept. 19th, their brother James, who had not been quarantined, but who was attending school every day (the school afterward was closed because of the disease) was taken down with scarlet fever, with symptoms equally as severe as his sisters'. The second call on this case was made Sept. 24th, and then once again, to release him from quarantine. These cases were especially interesting because of the fact of the imperfect sanitary conditions, the house having no sewer connections and being built on swampy ground. The mother who nursed these children was not well herself, having a history of tuberculosis. I could not be certain that my instructions were carried out, but had them 'phone me when things did not go right. The results from the line of treatment I have described were all that could be desired, with the result that the children were in better health after, than before acquiring scarlet fever.

PERMANENT MOUNTS OF MICRO-SCOPIC PREPARATIONS.

BY

G. R. WILLIAMS, M. D.,

Paris, Illinois.

An important question often presents itself to the physician. It is usually advisable after a diagnostic microscopic examination to file the preparation for reference. In such cases we may well select a method which will answer both purposes —that is, give us the most information in regard to the disease process and yet serve well as a permanent mount.

During the past few years, our laboratory has been compelled to investigate thoroughly this question. Now and then, perhaps months after the preliminary examination, someone questions the findings and if a good microscopic preparation is at hand, a hasty reference will verify the correctness of the initial report.

Vermes. This diagnosis rarely passes unquestioned. It must be remembered that teniae may be kept alive several days in warm water to which a little egg white has been added. When ready to fix, they may be killed in a 1% eucaine hydrochloride solution, fixed in 10% formalin, gently washed and then immersed in aqueous alum-carmine. Flatten gently between two slides held together by a rubber band. Decolorize in 75% alcohol and then transfer to 95% alcohol, absolute alcohol and eventually to carbol-xylol. Now quickly remove one slide and while the preparation is still wet, add balsam and a large square or oval cover glass.

Round worms may be killed in the same manner but must be sectioned. These sections are treated in the same manner as described below.

Arthropods. If these are to be mounted entire, two principles must be held in mind:

1. All fixing and staining reagents must penetrate deeply.

2. Any stain which destroys or fails to preserve calcareous tissues, is to be avoided. Therefore alum carminè cannot be used. Kill in 1% eucaine solution, fix in concentrated picro-sulphuric acid, wash out in successive warm 70% alcohols; stain in Mayer's alcoholic cochineal—old formula; dehydrate with successive alcohols —70%, 90% and absolute; clear in carbolxylol and finally mount in xylol balsam.

In this connection, I desire to describe a more simple method which we have tried for two years with certain of these parasites, notably the phthirius pubis. These lice were placed under a small bell jar with chloroform and were quickly killed. Immediately they were placed on a slide and covered with warm balsam. The preparation was completed with a cover glass. These specimens were not stained but are well preserved, being easily seen when the diaphragm is contracted.

Urinary Sediments. Here is a stumbling block. We have, as yet, been unable to devise or learn of any one method constantly suitable to the preservation of all urinary sediments—inorganic, organic or mixed.

For inorganic sediments, centrifugalize, decant and add filtered distilled water. Shake well and again centrifugalize, going through this process twice. Repeat the technique the fourth and fifth times, substituting absolute alcohol for the filtered distilled water. This finishes the washing. Obtain the sediment by means of a pipette and place on a slide. When the alcohol

evaporates, the crystals are left well distributed. Drying may be hastened by slightly warming, taking care not to expose preparation to the free flame. If these crystals are urates, uric acid, calcium carbonate, cystin, tyrosin, indigo or bilirubin, a drop of balsam and a cover glass may be added. But when we are dealing with oxalates or phosphates, glycerin jelly is substituted and a shellac ring painted around it. Before this dries, a cover glass should be pressed into place and another ring of shellac run around the edge of this to keep out all air. Cholesterin or the other thin crystalline plates may be mounted in a dry cell without the glycerin. If the sediment is known to be cholesterin, it may be well to omit the alcohol washes. In one urine, a case of intestinal carcinomata, we were able to demonstrate the presence of cholesterin plates, but there were not enough of these to justify the preparation of a permanent mount. Our experience with a large number of pathological urines during the past few years, would lead us to believe that cholesterin is a rare urinary sediment. When mounting triple phosphate crystals, a little ammonia should be added to the glycerin jelly.

If the cellular elements alone are to be studied, a dried droplet of the sediment, stained with Wright's blood formula and mounted in xylol-balsam will give satisfactory results.

When dealing with urinary casts, the sediment should be washed with filtered distilled water in the manner described above. Instead of proceeding with absolute alcohol, however, the following formula is substituted: Add to a mixture of equal parts of glycerin, water and 95% alcohol, about one-fourth percent perosmic acid. After two washings in this solution, carry out a third in which the perosmic acid has been omitted from the formula. After a thorough and final centrifugalization, transfer the sediment to the slide and mount before drying, in a shellac cell, as described above.

Of late, we have made several beautiful preparations of organic sediments by the following simple method. Spread and dry in air; fix in flame taking care not to let the glass become hot enough to melt or destroy the casts; add a few drops of an aqueous solution of bismarck brown and after one minute, wash thoroughly. Dry between blotters and mount in balsam. We are unable to tell at this time how well these sediments may be preserved by this method, but an examination of preparations made four months ago, is exceedingly promising.

Treponema Pallidum. In our hands, the Giemsa's Azur-eosin stain has given poor results, apparently owing to a tendency to fade. By the use of a powerful mantle flame, some of these organisms may still be identified after many months. For this purpose, the new kerosene mantle burners are to be recommended above the gas light. The intensity of the white blaze of the former varies but little and the candle power is twice that of the Welsbach. For the purposes of differential diagnosis, we regard the Giemsa stain as a valuable asset, owing to its property of differentiating the mouth spirochetes. Those smears and sections treated with the Goldhorn and Levaditi formulas, keep much better.

But as permanent mounts, our India ink preparations have given us the best results. The method for this preparation was described in a communication by us, two years ago—*Archives of Diagnosis* of January, 1910. We have one preparation in particular, filed in November, 1909. This was taken from a typical mucus patch on the tonsil and, in addition to cellular elements, bacilli and spirochetes, still shows many treponema well preserved, often without the loss of the characteristic windings. This would tend to show the fixing and preserving as well as the differential properties of the ink. The suspension of the treponema, was concentrated according to a method described in the original communication, and a droplet of this and a like amount of the ink mixed on a slide and permitted to dry. Finally a drop of balsam and a cover glass were added. It would seem that this simple method is to be especially recommended and is gaining favor with practitioners.

Molds. Although molds are easily stained, desiccation results in extensive structural alterations. For this reason we have adopted the following technic suggested by Novy and have several excellent preparations, some of which were filed several years ago.

1. Tease out the specimen in some weak alcohol, to which has been added a couple of drops of ammonia.

2. Pour off excess alcohol.

3. Add enough glycerin to cover the preparation and mix thoroughly.

4. Transfer a drop of this mixture to a slide.

5. Around the edge of the preparation, place a ring of cement or asphalt.

6. Apply a round cover glass. This completes the technic.

Bacteria. After considerable experimentation in this field, we have concluded that any of the following simple solutions stain satisfactorily: fuchsin, gentian violet and methylene blue. Such preparations must however, be protected from the light.

Contrary to most statements, I feel that methylene blue gives the best results. When exposed to the rays of the sun, it quickly fades, but when the preparation is filed in a tightly covered slide box, its beauty is preserved for years. Some fading invariably takes place, so that it is well to overstain. For this purpose, we do not use the Loeffler's alkaline solution, but a concentrated alcoholic stain which has been diluted with distilled water until it is barely transparent, and filtered. Fuchsin has proven a valuable stain, and vesuvin, which is being tried at present, bids fair for a permanent post in our laboratory. Somewhat less useful is gentian violet, a dye which works quickly but readily fades. However it will stain all microorganisms of the plant family and must be used occasionally, especially in the Gram's method.

Mounts should be made in xylol balsam rather than chloroform balsam as the latter shows a tendency to be colored by the coal tar dyes. The balsam should be clear and colorless—not yellow and not acid. We prefer the paper filtered balsams.

A preparation of bacteria suitable for reference filing, seldom demands more than a simple stain. A notable exception is the tubercle bacillus. These preparations should be kept from the light because of the susceptibility of the counterstain rather than the colored tubercle bacilli. Capsule stains are preserved with difficulty. Now and then a Gram's stain may be preserved for years with success.

Tissues. Hemotoxylin and eosin have proven best in routine work. When dealing with nervous tissues, we have been obliged to use special methods to bring out histological structures but in many instances, we have been able to preserve our specimens for future reference. Alum-

carmine stains quickly and does not readily fade. It must be remembered that it does not preserve calcareous structures. Sections stained in carmine cannot usually be mounted in glycerin for permanent record. Acetic-acid-carmine preparations cannot be preserved which is rather unfortunate, since preliminary fixation is not necessary. Legal's picro-alum-carmine gives beautiful permanent mounts. With other carmine stains, our experience has been limited. Thionin may be used with advantage in staining frozen sections but fails as a permanent stain.

Blood, Pus and Exudates. Our experience has been limited almost entirely to Wright's formula which has never failed us, either for diagnostic or filing purposes. Those few Romanowsky stains which we have attempted, have proven much less useful—in one instance giving excellent results and in the next, failing miserably and without apparent reason. I must concede that excellent permanent preparations may be obtained now and then by the Romanowsky method.

109 E. Court St.

THE ANNOTATOR.

Asexualization of the Unfit.[1]— J. M. Taylor thinks there are in every community a certain number of individuals who are defective in the genital sphere, and the community is bound to suffer by their licentious acts. Every community also contains individuals who are defective in mind and morals and must also suffer from their acts. Having freedom of action such individuals are a perpetual menace particularly to the young and unsuspicious of both sexes. In addition to the foregoing there are the degenerates who are lower than the beasts. Concerning these three classes it has been shown:

[1] *St. Louis Medical Review*, March, 1912.

(1) Many of them are capable of some improvement especially after asexualization.

(2) Whenever they are brought in contact with individuals of the opposite sex they have no power to control the sexual impulse.

(3) Their offspring are almost invariably as bad as or worse than themselves.

Should we deny these degenerates the privilege of asexualization? It has often been shown that glimmerings of the light impelled such individuals to recognize the benefits of this procedure and to ask that it be performed. A legislator or governor who blocks the course of such a reformatory procedure assumes a grave responsibility, and must be held accountable for his acts in this direction.

There is no doubt about the existence of these dangerous elements nor of the mischief which they cause. There is doubt in the minds of many as to the wisdom of the proposed procedure. Admitting at the start that we believe the measure to be desirable and that it will come in time, we must not balk at the difficulty in obtaining an impartial tribunal to decide when it should be done and upon whom. Legislatures and governors will not take such a momentous step until there is a mighty wave of public opinion behind them insisting that such a step be taken. It is rational, it is not inhumane and the public should be educated up to the point of demanding it.

There is such a law in Indiana, recently passed. Let us watch its effect with careful scrutiny.

means semi-invalidism, recovery from which is generally slow.

The treatment of such ulcers has usually resulted in wastefulness of materials and in neglect of the patients especially if they are treated at a dispensary. The advice to such patients that they should not work and should keep off their feet is not of a very practical nature. The results of treatment of a series of such cases at the Massachusetts General Hospital during a period of five years were not flattering, being better in the young, the intelligent and the careful, than in the badly nourished, the careless and those who live amid unsanitary surroundings.

Operative procedures in this series gave rather better results than prolonged treatment. The writer thinks that the social service department of our large hospitals and dispensaries should take pains to reach this class of patients and place them under conditions which will enable them to do their work comfortably and well, and he suggests a special clinic for the treatment of varicose ulcers and flat foot with which the former condition is almost habitually associated.

This condition may be classified among the occupational diseases to which more and more attention is very properly being given. One who has not seen cases of this nature can scarcely realize the handicap under which such sufferers labor. The suggestion as to a clinic, which has been made is a good one and is in line with all proper efforts to improve the social and physical conditions in the community.

Varicose Ulcers.[1]—I. S. Wile states that in the fight for the preservation of health certain unfavorable conditions may be present, no matter what improvements may be made in the hygiene of occupation, of factories or of the personal mode of living.

One of these conditions interfering with usefulness in industrial work is varicose veins, which are usually caused by constant standing in one's occupation, the condition being sometimes aggravated by tight garters or constricting garments. If the varicose vein becomes ulcerated it usually

Increased Use of Hospitals and Dispensaries.[1]—I. S. Wile quotes from published reports that the number of hospitals in the Saturday and Sunday Association of New York has increased 114 per cent during the past 25 years, while the number of patients has increased 600 per cent. The number of free patients has increased 523 per cent and the free hospital days 230 per cent.

The municipal hospitals care for many of the sick and injured poor but their limited capacity throws a heavy burden on

---

[1]*American Journal of Surgery*, April, 1912.

[1]*American Journal of Surgery*, April, 1912.

the voluntary hospitals, and the allowance which the latter receive for the care of the city poor is less than half the cost. In view of the volunteer medical aid which the city receives, the writer thinks the financial assistance from municipality to the volunteer hospitals should at least equal the cost per capita in the city hospitals. The distribution of voluntary funds to hospitals should be in direct proportion to the benefit which is derived from them. A clearing house of hospital information which has been established will enable donors to designate the channel in which they desire their gifts to be directed. It is also desirable that hospital methods be unified that the standards of all may be raised. This might mean improvement in caring for patients of the middle class, assuming that the interests of the rich and the poor have already been attended to. Those who have been in practice in and about the city during the last quarter of a century cannot be unmindful of the great changes which have taken place in hospital methods and management during that period. Not only do the poor in far greater numbers than formerly, avail themselves of hospital advantages, but the rich as well. Though a physician who is not a member of a hospital staff can usually find hospital accommodations where he can treat and retain control of his patients the expense, especially in cases of prolonged illness, is usually prohibitive. We are told of families which have been utterly impoverished by such a prolonged drain. It is a question whether the elaboration of hospitals and nursing systems has not gone too far, so that to many individuals of good intentions but small financial ability the alternatives seem to be an intolerable burden of expense or the acceptance of charity. Neither of these conditions is ideal and we must look and hope for a more rational system of procedure in the near future.

The School and the Doctor.[1]—G. Straubenmuller observes that the universal war cry is "death to disease and dirt." This means that school teachers and men of

[1] *N. Y. Medical Journal,* April 20, 1912.

science must cooperate and the war on misery should begin with the child.

The writer urges a scientific study not only of the obvious dangers to the physical welfare of school children, but of the less obvious ones, together with remedies for their removal. Since the state makes education compulsory it should provide hygienic surroundings and hygienic instruction for the child. The work of medical school inspection is only in its initial stage. Apparently its object is to prevent the spread of contagious diseases and to correct physical abnormities, thus permitting mental advancement, but it should also go much further.

School hygiene should be prophylactic, constructive and remedial and this will include many things not now included in medical inspection. Aside from inspection the duties of the school physician must be advisory and preventive; he should be the medical counsel for youth looking after their hygienic interests. The knowledge of specialists is frequently of importance especially in determining the more obscure questions as to physical and mental status. Medicine and pedagogy must work together in order that the product may be a strong and virile body of citizens.

The proposed broadening of the work of the school inspector, by the foregoing article, by an official in New York City school department, is a very timely suggestion. At present the school inspectors may be divided into three classes; those who are interested in the physical condition of the scholars, those who are more or less interested in the hygiene of the school buildings, and those who are chiefly interested in drawing their wages, and the latter is by far the largest class at present. This work should be placed upon a more scientific basis. The perfunctory examination of school children as now performed in so many cases is farcical and a waste of money. It is certainly desirable that the teacher and the school physician should work and plan together for great ends for the children, not merely to detect contagious disease but to forecast the child's future development.

282   AMERICAN MEDICINE
Complete Series, Vol. XVIII. }   THE ANNOTATOR   { MAY, 1912.
New Series, Vol. VII., No. 5.

Some of the Abuses of Surgery.[1]—H. B. Delatour refers to the efforts of the profession to keep bad men from its ranks and to obtain wise and just legislation. These efforts had not always been successful.

The tendencies of the profession in many communities were towards commercialism. Examples of this were seen in the occasional receiving by physicians of commissions from pharmacists and instrument makers. If there were an anti-tipping law it was thought that such conduct would be actionable. It was thought, further, that the family physician when meeting a consultant should charge more than his ordinary fee. The division of operating fees was believed to be bad from almost every point of view as the physician would be likely to select an operator who would pay him the largest percentage irrespective of the operator's ability.

Some physicians were inclined to minimize the value of surgical operations by incorrectly stating the financial condition of their patient or by referring the patient to a hospital where the work would be done for nothing. Men who were inexperienced too often attempted operations which they were not competent to perform. The family doctor too often attempted to do operations which were supposed to be simple and did them imperfectly or even with fatal result, which might have been avoided had the work been done by an experienced operator. Such abuses tended to bring surgery into disrepute.

There is no doubt of the justness of some of this writer's criticisms. It should be beneath the dignity of a physician to accept a commission or a portion of a surgical fee, or any other form of bribe or graft which is really such, but if the average physician's income (as stated by one of those who discussed this paper) is only $12.00 per week, less than an unskilled mechanic's, not more than a street sweeper's, the temptation will often be .great and ethics will crack if they do not break. The work which is done by so many inexperienced operators certainly should be criticized with severity, men who are lacking in judgment, lacking in elementary knowledge, lacking in technical skill; there are many of them as the author says, who are

on the staff of hospitals where they have been placed without any regard for their unfitness or their possibilities for mischief. With regard to incomplete operations one need not have had very extensive experience to know that some operations must necessarily be incomplete, especially in the surgery of malignant disease, and the wise surgeon is the one who knows when it is best to stop.

The Duty of the Physician Toward the Antivivisection Movement.[1]—Drs. J. D. Bryant and J. S. Nacher, the committee of the State Society on Experimental Medicine warn the profession against the campaign of the Antivivisection Society which seeks the abolition of experimental work upon animals on the ground that it is cruel and unnecessary. This society distributes circulars containing false statements and false implications concerning animal experimentation, while its agent Mr. W. R. Bradshaw lectures to granges and other societies throughout the state, representing laboratory procedures which do not accord with the facts.

He intimates that animals are tortured to death to satisfy a craving for cruelty.

He denies that bacteria cause infectious diseases and that diphtheria antitoxin has any value.

At the close of each lecture he presents a resolution proving the legislation proposed by the New York Antivivisection Society.

The committee states that its work is to oppose such activities but it has been compelled for many years to be constantly on the alert. It desires the active cooperation of all physicians especially in places where the lectures referred to may be given. They also should urge upon members of the legislature the unwisdom of all antivivisection legislation thus far proposed.

The committee, finally, will be glad to furnish literature, free of cost, showing the methods and the value of animal experimentation.

In the face of the beneficent results derived from experiments upon animals in the last half century, in the face of the utter inability of the bigoted opponents of

---

[1] *N. Y. Medical Journal*, April 27, 1912.

[1] *New York State Journal of Medicine*, April, 1912.

such work to bring forward adequate evidence of the cruelty of workers in this field—which would be detestable enough if it were true, it does seem strange that this misguided cult can continue to get a hearing among intelligent people, and still more that any senator or member of assembly can be found who will be simple enough to assist them in their desire for obstructive legislation. It seems that the only safety from such mistaken enthusiastics is in the constant activity of the above-mentioned committee of the State Society.

_____

The Medical Situation in Europe.[1]— M. A. Austin states that in England the proportion of physicians to the population is 1 to 1,400, and in the United States 1 to 500. The great number of benefit societies in England together with the new Lloyd George Benefit Bill have so cheapened medical service that there are now only about half a million of the population in England who need pay more than 1.50 each per year for such service. It is believed that this means ruin to a large number of physicians.

In the United States the condition is not quite so bad though the increase in cost of living and in extravagant habits are making deep inroads into the possibilities of getting a decent living. The author proposes the following suggestions with regard to possible contracts between physician and client for a period of not less than a year, fees being paid quarterly in advance and computed on a basis of the following factors: (1) Financial responsibility. (2) Income of the family. (3) Number in the family. (4) Children under 14. (5) Children over 14. (6) Occupation. (7) Sanitary condition. (8) Family history as to tuberculosis, rheumatism, cancer, heart and kidney disease. (9) Habits as to alcohol, tobacco and drugs.

Combinations of several physicians are suggested for cooperation in obstetrical, surgical and special work. It is thought that the peculiar advantages of the specialist in obtaining large fees are passing, inasmuch as the preparation of the average

[1] _American Journal of Clinical Medicine_, April, 1912.

physician is gradually qualifying him to treat most of the conditions which are likely to come under his observation. These propositions are rather startling, but no thoughtful man will deny that the situation must be faced.

Organization and combination which are gradually involving all departments of human industry cannot be expected in the long run, to make an exception of the work of the doctor. The requirement is to act calmly, wisely, and with a view to the best interests of all concerned.

The question of self preservation is the dominant one but it must not be allowed to overshadow the altruistic aspect of the situation from which the true physician can never be dissociated.

_____

Sex Mutilations in Social Therapeutics.[1] —G. F. Lydston has made many useful contributions of a sociological nature and this, his latest one, is by no means of least importance. It will certainly be regarded as advanced thought on this line and we are not yet prepared to accept it _in toto_.

The following is a brief summary of his article:

Consumptives, epileptics, insane, incurable inebriates and criminals should not be allowed to marry unless they will consent to sterilization. This would prevent many social ills including the birth of degenerate offspring. The State should stand in a parental relation to the children of the poor and to orphans and should see that all children are physically, mentally and morally trained. Every school should be a military school or a gymnasium in modified form and manual training should replace some of our modern school methods. Criminals, insane, epileptics, prostitutes and confirmed inebriates should be regarded as _culls_ until they have established their right to be considered cured and worthy of replacement in society. If incurable, they should be placed beyond the possibility of contaminating the social body. Society should protect itself against loss through ill advised matrimony. The loss includes the expense of hospitals, insane asylums, prisons, workhouses and ponderous legal machinery.

[1] _N. Y. Medical Journal_, April 6, 1912.

284   AMERICAN MEDICINE
Complete Series, Vol. XVIII.   THE ANNOTATOR   MAY, 1912.
New Series, Vol. VII., No. 5.

The Physician as a Business Man.[1]— Sigmund Epstein thinks the observation and study of the healing art tend to make men narrow, and such men lack the wisdom gained by experience in the world. Medical men will always be indispensable, however, in connection with disease and injury, in public sanitation, in matters of dietetics, whatever be their shortcomings as business managers.

The present highly organized condition of business should indicate that a similar plan of procedure would be advantageous for the doctors. Instead of cooperation, with a few notable exceptions, the tendency among doctors is too often to belittle and under-rate one another. The church, the school, the press, and the drama all advertise and take pains to bring their wares before the public. The tendency, at least in some countries, is for the doctor to advertise in a mild kind of way also. The doctor and the public are beginning to approach each other in many ways. They are more and more becoming identified with the daily press and in many other lines of work quite distinct from the practice of the healing art. A bright business outlook is predicted for medical institutions and ideals in America.

There is much food for reflection in the author's suggestions. Many more doctors than formerly have the commercial and gainful disposition and we doubt whether there is anything like the laxity in business methods among doctors which used to be so prevalent. Of course there is still much room for improvement in those methods. Doctors must first agree among themselves and be loyal to one another, which so many of them are not. If they were loyal to each other they could at once demand that their business relations with the public be on exactly the same footing as those of anybody else who serves the public—the butcher, the grocer, the plumber for example.

Habit Formation.[2]— W. H. Baldwin says there are two factors in the formation of a habit, the psychological and physi-

[1]*New York Medical Journal*, April, 1912.
[2]*Medical Council*, April, 1912.

ological, the former presenting itself first.

When a habit-forming drug is used frequently or continuously a physiological process takes place and the habit becomes fixed, absence of the drug causing organic craving and discomfort, no matter how decided the change in the mentality. Nature endeavors to eliminate foreign substances and if unable she throws out protective processes or counteracting substances. If the avenues of elimination are closed and secretion is checked recourse is had to the protective forces of the ductless glands, an antitoxin being formed whose action is opposed to that of the drug which has been taken.

Absolutely necessary to a cure is an honest desire to be cured, and a willingness to sacrifice comfort in the effort. The prospect of cure will be improved if the victim is in a well regulated sanitarium in which the moral atmosphere is positive and the bodily complications can be met as they arise. The time element is important, months may be necessary before the sub-conscious mind will cease to respond to outside stimuli. The sanitariums in question are usually very expensive and quite out of reach of many who need them. It is a little like asking a patient to take his medicine out of a gold spoon when the condition of his finances would compel him to take it from the bottle—if he took it at all.

The Physician Himself.[1]— I. W. Voorhees thinks the profession is at last waking up to the problems of internal relations and those which concern the public welfare. We are now in a state of unrest which is aiming at organization for defense against our enemies as well as offense against great combinations of commercial interests, which would use the profession of self aggrandizement.

Attention is particularly called to the recent symposium of the Manhattan Medical Society upon the subject noted in the title of this paper. In the six papers which were read there was little reference to self-interest, all of them being concerned with matters which are vital to the profession

[1]*Med. Review of Reviews*, April, 1912.

as a whole. Some of those who participated in the discussion however, showed that they were still bound by old prejudices and errors. In spite of these and similar lucubrations it is evident that the profession is undergoing a rapid evolution of feeling on the subjects which lie nearest to its own interests and those of the public and that effective organization is needed against the powers of darkness. This should indicate conservation in place of wasting of strength. The calumnious utterances of the profession and its internal dissensions are probably amusing to the layman. More than that they destroy his confidence in our steadfastness and integrity. This endangers our well-being and is bad business policy as well as bad ethics.

There is a world of truth in this author's remarks. We see the effect upon the public of the recriminations of those who are in high position as they go about the country berating and accusing each other, lowering their dignity and making many statements which they will sometime regret and desire to recall. Such also has been medical history, to a large, to a too large extent, individually and collectively. Now let us stop pulling down and build up—for a while, and note the result.

Sanitation at Panama.[1]—W. C. Gorgas states that from 1520 when the route across the isthmus was first established until 1904 when the United States took charge it has been universally regarded as the most unhealthy spot in the world. Yellow fever, malarial fever and dysentery were endemic, and those who crossed the isthmus or tarried there did so at the imminent peril of their lives.

The mortality from 1850 to 1855 when the railroad was being built was so great that the work stopped, from time to time, because the workmen were all sick or all dead. Negroes from Africa and Chinamen all shared the same fate. The mortality from 1881 to 1889 when the French were working on the canal was excessive though their hospitals were good and their care of the sick excellent. Their loss by death during this period was 22,189. The United States during a period of equal

duration out of an average force of 33,000 has lost less than 4,000.

At first the mortality was 40 per 1,000, now it is 7.50 per thousand thanks to the discoveries in tropical medicine and improved methods of sanitation. Sanitation expenses on the isthmus are about $365,-000 per annum for a population of 150,000.

The cleaning up of Panama is one of the glories of American medicine and will cover the name of Gorgas with undying fame.

Without such work by the doctors the canal could not have been built.

How many of the people at large reflect upon this?

Federal Public Health Bills.[1]—An editorial comments upon the two bills relating to Federal Health activities which are now before the United States Senate. The Owen bill provides for an independent public health service with a director who shall not be a member of the cabinet. All appointments in this service shall be made without discrimination, in favor of or against any school of medicine or healing.

This new department is also to include the Public Health and Marine Hospital service, a portion of the Bureau of Chemistry in the Department of Agriculture and the Division of Vital Statistics in the Census Bureau. It also provides for a bureau of child conservation and divisions of sanitary engineering, of publications and of personnel and accounts.

No provision is made for recruiting the Marine Hospital service and the medical service as at present organized is apparently to be discontinued with the death or resignation of those who are now in office. The heads of the other five bureaus included in the proposed plan will probably be laymen or at any rate not physicians. No provision is made that the director of the department be a physician. It is well known that the Marine Hospital Service at present comprises a large number of physicians well adapted by long training for useful public health work together with a number of highly trained scientists in the hygienic laboratory. The provision against discrimination as to any particular school of medicine apparently means that the various sects of medicine and healing will demand recognition as they have demanded and received it from most of the states and from the Canal Zone.

What is now offered is thought little less than insulting to the medical profession of this country. The Smoot bill enlarges the health activities of the Federal Government but does not incorporate a portion of the Bureau of Chemistry of the Department of Agriculture. It provides for an assistant secretary in the Treasury Department who shall devote all his time to public health work. The Public Health and Marine Hospital Service is to be the predominating bureau and include the division of vital statistics. Of the two bills the Smoot bill should therefore be the more acceptable to the medical profession. Of all interests which affect the public vitally those which have to do with the profession of medicine seem to have the hardest time in obtaining recognition in organized form from the Federal Government.

Is not the health of the people of as great importance as say the animal bureau of the Department of Agriculture? And why has the vital matter of quarantine been left out of both bills, a matter which concerns the country at large, and not any one state in particular? We would suggest that the author of the Smoot bill call for consultation with a sufficient number of broad minded physicians, from all sections of the country if need be, and so amend his bill that it becomes a law that it may accomplish the greatest amount of usefulness quite apart from any consideration of dignity or politics medical or otherwise.

ETIOLOGY AND DIAGNOSIS.

Differential Diagnosis of Lymphatic Infection and Tenosynovitis of the Hand.—Kanavel calls attention (*Infections of the Hand. Lea & Febiger, Publishers, Phila.*) to the fact that one may mistake a lymphatic infection for a tenosynovitis. Here, however, the red lines of lymphatic involvement running up the arm without the localized tenderness over the tendon sheaths, the slight pain on moving the fingers, the generalized edema of arm and hand in contradistinction to the localized swelling found in the early stage of tenosynovitis aid us in the diagnosis. Again, we may be in doubt as to whether we are dealing with a tenosynovitis of the ulnar or radial bursa or a rheumatism of the wrist. Kanavel has seen several such cases. In one case it was difficult to determine whether the patient was suffering from a gonorrheal rheumatism of the proximal interphalangeal joint of a finger or a gonorrheal tenosynovitis with secondary involvement of that joint. The latter assumption was later found to be the condition present. In those cases where there is a lack of traumatic history, and the apparently spontaneous development of an inflammation, especially at the wrist, the diagnosis may be most difficult in spite of the ease with which a theoretical differential diagnosis is made. Here again, however, the localized tenderness over the sheath and pain on extension of the finger are of the greatest importance; moreover, these cases are always virulent and extend rapidly, so that if it be a tenosynovitis the hand grows rapidly worse. In a rheumatism there is as much pain on the dorsal as on the Volar surface; the swelling involves the wrist more than the hand, fingers, or forearm; and other joints may be involved. The presence of a gonorrhea does not aid us materially, since either condition may follow. Subcutaneous infections are seldom difficult to differentiate. One case of gonorrheal tenosynovitis of the tendon sheaths of the dorsum of the wrist came under my notice in which the diagnosis of rheumatism had been made. Here the absence of any tenderness or swelling on the flexor surface combined with swelling and tenderness localized to the sheaths confirmed the diagnosis.

The Diagnosis of Gastric Ulcer.—Speaking of ulcer of the stomach, Martin (*Surgical Diagnosis, Lea & Febiger, Publishers, Phila.*) says that the diagnosis of gastric ulcer is based upon hemorrhage, which may be occult, slight, profuse, or very exceptionally promptly fatal; pain, often localized, markedly aggravated by taking food, and relieved by vomiting or stomach lavage or orthoform (Murdoch); tenderness, also frequently well localized, hyperperistalsis, and excess of hydrochloric acid in the gastric content.

When the ulcer is situated near the pylorus, and either by its hyperemia, induration, or cicatricial contracture causes spasmodic contraction or pronounced mechanical narrowing of this orifice, there will be added to the symptoms just noted those of pyloric obstruction characterized by retention of food, hyperperistalsis, dilatation, absence of hydrochloric acid, and lactic fermentation.

As symptoms of corroborative, but not diagnostic value, anemia, emaciation, constipation, and the occasional association with pulmonary tuberculosis may be mentioned.

Referred pain and cutaneous hyperalgesia are at times well marked, the seats of preference being over the ensiform cartilage or to one side of it, and at a point in line with the scapular angle at the level of the ninth dorsal spine (Head).

The one symptom upon which most reliance can be placed is hemorrhage. This, if profuse and vomited, in the absence of adequate traumatism, blood dyscrasia, or vascular back pressure, can be regarded as almost pathognomonic of ulceration. Constantly recurring slight hemorrhage shown by the presence of occult blood in the vomited matter or that drawn from the stomach by lavage, is considered equally diagnostic in the absence of either renal or hepatic disease.

Abdominal arteriosclerosis may cause acute attacks of pain, suggesting perforation, or may be characterized by recurring paroxysms closely simulating those of ulcer or carcinoma. Berger reports cases suffering from postprandial pain, emaciation, and bleeding, in which an autopsy failed to demonstrate the erosions from which the bleeding came.

Though in typical cases the symptoms of gastric ulcer are sufficiently characteristic to make the diagnosis well-nigh certain even in the absence of exploration, the frequency with which the first symptoms, barring slight digestive disturbance, are those of acute perforative peritonitis, proves that ulcer may exist without offering any symptoms upon which even a probable diagnosis can be based.

From the surgical point of view the diagnosis is important because of the complications of hemorrhage, pyloric obstruction, diffuse perforative peritonitis, localized peritonitis with gradual extension of inflammation, perigastric adhesions, or pus formation. These conditions, developing in the absence of a preceding history of gastric ulcer, can be distinguished as to their etiology only on the basis of probability and exclusion.

The distinction between a chronic indurated gastric ulcer and gastric carcinoma may be impossible both clinically and at operation. The subsequent course of these cases shows that even careful microscopic examination may leave the examiner in error. Hence, when radical surgical procedure is possible, this in doubtful cases should take the form applicable to cancer.

TREATMENT.

The Treatment of Acute Infectious Gastritis. —Aaron states (*Diseases of the Stomach, Lea & Febiger, Publishers, Phila.*) that the treatment of these severe forms of acute gastric catarrh is based upon the same principles as that of the milder forms. The stomach must be emptied and cleansed as quickly and thoroughly as possible by means of lavage. When the disease is due to infection it is well to wash out the stomach with antiseptic solutions: for example, salicylic acid 1 to 2 parts in 1,000 of water, or dilute boric acid solution (3 to 1,000 to 5 to 1,000). Emetics should not be employed if it is possible to empty the stomach in any other way. Food should be interdicted

for a number of days in the case of robust patients, to give the stomach needed rest. Thirst and persistent vomiting are to be met by small doses of cold mineral waters, carbonated waters either with or without fruit juices, cracked ice, or cold tea. The general condition of the patient, his pulse and temperature, must be constantly under observation. Wine, brandy, cognac, champagne, Tokay wine and strong coffee are to be administered to the aged and weak as indicated.

Since in these severe acute cases the hydrochloric acid is diminished, dilute hydrochloric acid should be given three times a day in doses of 0.75 to 1 gm. (10 to 15 minims), well diluted with water. This will serve the additional purpose of allaying the thirst. Resorcinol may be given for nausea and bad-smelling eructations. Persistent vomiting is combated by the use of menthol, or by Potio Riveri (citric acid 2 gm., bicarbonate of soda 3 gm., water 100 cc.), to which may be added cocaine, 0.065 gm. (1 grain); this is given in teaspoonful doses as occasion requires. To reduce fever, 0.3 gm. (5 grains) of quinine or phenacetine may be given; or recourse may be had to the tepid or cold bath. Calomel, 0.015 gm. (¼ grain) three times a day, will often exert a good influence on the course of the disease.

When the infection has passed to the intestine, calomel should be given, to be followed if necessary by resorcinol with salicylate of bismuth; the following formula has been recommended:

	Gm. or cc.
℞-Bismuthi salicylatis	3.0 gr. xlv
Resorcinolis	2.0 gr. xxx
Glycerini 15.0	℥ss
Aquae 200.0	℥vij

Misce.

Sig. One tablespoonful every three hours.

The Induction of Labor.[1]—Induction of labor is suitable treatment, says McDonald, in contracted pelves of moderate degree, provided the size of the baby be estimated by measurements of the uterine fundus and fetal head and by the relation of the fetal head to the pelvis.

Labor may then be induced at the most suitable moment, so as to get the largest sized baby that will pass the pelvic strait and avoid unnecessary prematurity. It is essential that mothers be examined at least four weeks before the expected labor in order to estimate the proper time for induction.

The lowest limit of pelvic contraction, suitable for treatment by induction of labor, is 8 cm. true conjugate, as this will allow the birth of a 2,500 gramme (five and three-quarter pounds) baby, with an average 8 cm. biparietal diameter. This weight of baby avoids the dangers of unnecessary prematurity and has a mortality but little more than the average. Better results are obtained with pelves larger than this, but this is the lowest limit.

[1]Ellice McDonald, M. D., *N. Y. Med. Jour.,* March 16, 1912.

288   AMERICAN MEDICINE
Complete Series, Vol. XVIII. }   TREATMENT   { MAY, 1912.
New Series, Vol. VII., No. 5.

If the child is measured in all cases by the methods of the author, the dangers of prolonged pregnancy and overweight babies will be avoided, because they will be recognized and may be treated.

·Caesarean section has a mortality in 3,000 cases of seven per cent. and should be reserved for cases with pelvic contraction through which it is not advisable to have a baby pass (below 8 cm.), or to cases in which the child has already grown too large to pass through the moderately contracted pelvis. In these cases it may be done as a primary operation and the mortality reduced.

The Rational Treatment of Furuncles.[1]— Given a furuncle late in the first stage, what is the most rational method of treatment? It would seem to be, says Skillern, to establish an outlet, not for the beneficent serum and leucocytes, but for the products of liquefaction necrosis which are formed by nature according to her best judgment, *secundum artem*. With the scalpel scratch off the little central vesicle; this causes no pain. A drop of seropus follows and the ulcerating hair-follicle and sebaceous gland are exposed. Apply a Bier cup and suck out as much as possible of the exhausted serum and blood. In the wake of the latter from near-by tissues comes fresh blood, with fresh serum and fresh, vigorous leucocytes. It is these that are going to cure the furuncle, and not the surgeon's knife. The knife inflicts unnecessary trauma and gives the tissues two lesions to deal with instead of one. Often the vesicle does not even have to be scratched, in which case the cuticle is thin enough to be readily ruptured by the cup alone. Apply a dressing of plain sterile gauze wrung short of saturation from a solution of normal saline with sodium citrate. An important consideration in this method of treatment is that of drainage. If a gauze drain is inserted, it plays the rôle of a cork in a bottle. If left alone and allowed to dry, the lymph coagulates, thus plugging the furuncle.

In keeping with modern pathologic conceptions, what is desired is free bathing of the bacteria with fresh serum from the blood, with its highly antitrophic power. Sodium citrate, one-per-cent. solution, precipitates the calcium salts in the lymph and insures a comparatively free outlet of the serum. By osmosis, the sodium chloride sets up a flow of lymph through the walls of the furuncle, the citrate maintaining the fluidity of the serum. Thus there is brought about a continuous flow of lymph of high antitrophic power from the congested blood-vessels through the wall of the furuncle and out through the wound. A bit of rubber dam may in addition be inserted if there is much tension on the outlet. The citrate is required for only about three days, and during its use the surrounding skin should·be

[1]A. D. Skillern, M. D., *Jour. A. M. A.*, Sept. 16, 1911.

protected from pustulation by an ointment. The patient may make up his own solution for home use by adding a teaspoonful of sodium citrate and two and one-half teaspoonfuls of table salt to a glass of hot boiled water. Over this aseptic drain-poultice apply a piece of waxed paper or oiled silk, then a compress of non-absorbent cotton or wool and a cotton bandage. If the patient is going to lay up, leave the dressing open, instructing him to renew the drain-poultice frequently. The solution prevents the vesicle crusting over and the gauze absorbs the products of disintegration as nature dispenses them. Sodium citrate should also be administered internally, 15 grains three times daily after meals, both for its alkaline action on the blood, and for its diuretic action on the kidneys. The cupping and dressing may be repeated and renewed frequently (every four hours) until the slough is loose, when this may be readily removed by a pair of small dressing forceps. After this, no matter how the resolving furuncle is treated, resolution proceeds rapidly and uninterruptedly, and the resulting scar is always the smallest obtainable in proportion to the size of the furuncle. In most cases it is invisible.

In some cases the granulations, instead of being firm, red, and rapidly growing, are flabby, bluish, and sluggish. The trouble here it is believed is due to relaxation of the tissues and mobility of the part. These conditions may be overcome by strapping the edges of the wound with adhesive strips, which compress the granulations and immobilize the skin. Then the granulations are dried, mopped with tincture of iodine, and dusted with Bier's powdered nitrate of silver. Exuberant granulations should be snipped off with scissors; for, as Colles long ago pointed out in his lectures, the silver stick does not "burn down" granulations, as it is commonly supposed, but stimulates them. To promote epithelial regeneration— which, in this method, has a very limited area to cover—8-per-cent. scarlet-red ointment or amido-azotoluol may be employed.

The author objects to flaxseed poultices on the ground that, while they may soothe the patient, yet they devitalize the edge of the furuncle, prolong the period of resolution, and leave a legacy of an unsightly depressed scar. He objects strongly to the bichloride of mercury on the ground that it is a corrosive poison, that it devitalizes the vigorous leucocytes and disintegrates the beneficent serum; that it destroys feeble bacteria in the depths of the wound, and that on tender skin it causes pustules to spring up anew. He asserts that he is unalterably opposed to incision for the reasons given above. If incise you will, then excise the furuncle entirely; otherwise withhold the knife.

How is autointoxication of the adjacent hair-follicles to be prevented? By shaving the area of skin wide of the furuncle and disinfecting it with 70-per-cent. alcohol or tincture of iodine with benzine, a dilution of liquid formaldehyde or of aluminum acetate. Local disinfection should be repeated at each dressing, benzine being an excellent medium to thoroughly cleanse the skin of wound discharges, effete products, and remnants of adhesive plaster.

Of course, if a patient presents himself for the first time with a furuncle well advanced in the second stage, where there is marked softening and fluctuation, in fact, merely a subcuticular abscess, a small incision through the thinned skin is indicated on the surgical principle of *ubi pus ibi evacuo*. This principle is in no way applicable to a furuncle in the first stage, because there is no pus to be evacuated. The writer strongly objects to squeezing a furuncle in any stage. Squeezing is unsurgical in that it causes acute suffering quite needlessly, traumatizes the furuncle, breaking the barrier of protecting leucocytes, and provokes hemorrhage, which interferes with drainage. Make the drain, aided by the Bier cup, remove the pus. It is less painful and at least equally efficient. To hasten the subsidence of the enlarged lymph-nodes and of the acute hyperplasia about the furuncle, thiosinamine may be given by mouth in 1½-grain doses three times daily after meals.

The Treatment of Acne.[1]—Brocq advises that local treatment must vary with the class of case being dealt with. In juveniles and in many other cases strong massage, a regular kneading, will give unexpected results. When the skin is delicate and irritable it is well to order, for washing the face, boiled water as hot as possible to which has been added a few drops of Eau de Cologne or of borate of soda. After washing, a swab of absorbent wool, moistened in camphorated spirits, should be passed over the face. At bedtime a little of the following ointment should be applied:

R Zinci Oxidi .... ʒiss.
Acidi Salicylici .... gr. v.
Adipis Lanæ .... ʒi.
Paraffini Mollis .... ʒij.
Misce. Fiat unguentum.

With this by degrees is incorporated a little precipitated sulphur, beginning with 8 grs. and going up, if it is borne, to 30 grains.

In medium cases all the affected points are to be soaped at bedtime with hot water and ichthyol soap. Afterwards the following ointment is to be applied:

R Camphoræ,
Resorcini ....aa gr. viij.
Sulphuris Præcipitati......gr. xlv.
Cretæ Præparatæ ....ʒiss.
Saponis Mollis ....gr. x.
Paraffini Mollis ....ad ʒss.
Misce. Fiat unguentum.

This must be kept on all night and washed off with soap in the morning. It may be replaced by this lotion:

---

[1] *Jour. de Medecine et de Chirurgia pratiques.*

R Sulphuris Præcipitati ....ʒvj.
Glycerini ....ʒss.
Spiritus Camphoræ ....ʒij.
Aquæ Rosæ,
Aquæ Destillatæ ....aa ʒvij.
Misce. Fiat lotio.

This must be well shaken up before use and applied with a fine brush.

In obstinate cases with many comedones and pustules the former must be removed as much as possible and each pustule opened with the point of a "flamed" scarificator. The points are then dried and touched with a drop of spirits of camphor or of *Eau d' Alibour* diluted with half its volume of boiled water. If any abscess is present it should be opened with the galvanic cautery. At night the affected parts must be vigorously soaped with sulphur soap or soft soap, then moistened with spirits of camphor, and finally the following ointment applied:

R B-Naphthol,
Camphoræ,
Resorcini ....aa ʒi.
Sulphuris Præcipitati ....ʒij.
Cretæ Præparatæ ....ʒiss.
Saponis Mollis ....ʒss.
Paraffini Mollis ....ʒij.
Misce. Fiat unguentum.

This must be removed before going to bed by means of pure vaseline, and the following paste applied:

R Zinci Oxidi,
Adipis Lanæ,
Amyli,
Paraffini Mollis............aa ʒiss.
Misce. Fiat pasta.

The following morning after washing well with soap and dabbing over the face with spirits of camphor, a thin layer of the following should be applied:

R Zinci Oxidi,
Pulveris Lycopodii..........aa ʒi.
Paraffini Mollis ....ʒij.
Misce. Fiat unguentum.

This may be powdered over with oxide of zinc or colored starch powder.

HYGIENE AND DIETETICS.

What and How to Eat.—It is a very old saying, says Dr. J. N. Hurty in a recent article, that "most persons dig their graves with their teeth." "He is writing fool on his tombstone" was the remark of a well-known physiologist when a young man at the next table in a cafe ordered a cocktail, a two dollar beefsteak with the usual trimmings of Worcestershire sauce and rich, highly spiced viands. "The young man's eliminative organs will be equal to the task of throwing off the excess foods and the poisons which proceed from his high living, for some years," said the physiologist, "but when he arrives at about forty-five or fifty, when he should be in the bloom of useful life, he will find himself stung. Before his joint pains, rheumatism, bilious attacks, eczema, and bad kidneys come to him, he will say: 'Oh what's the use of living if one can't enjoy himself and have a good time when young?' When the troubles predicted arrive he will say: 'What a fool I was not to have lived rationally and enjoyed a painless, useful and happy old age.'" Truly, "youth is the time to praise the Lord." The foundations for the regrets of old age are all laid in youth. To praise the Lord after middle life does not avail much. To preserve and strengthen our inheritance of strength and comeliness, we must first of all pass up wine and flesh. Nothing new in this, for Daniel was fully cognizant of it and had the will and force of character to put his knowledge into practical use. See first chapter of Daniel.

To live rationally, live simply. The most that is in life is only to be obtained by living rationally. When you leave the stuffy, foul air of the theatre after the play, how good and how refreshing is the outdoor air! Now, after the foul air assault on your body, don't visit the cafe and then continue the assault. True, you enjoy the rich and unnecessary food, but your kidneys don't. They don't say anything at the time, but just keep on pounding of them, and then after a few years you can enjoy the pains their protest brings and finally join the caravan of the 100,000 who annually go to their graves in the United States with kidney trouble. You will be about fifty years old at this time, and in the course of nature, had you eaten wisely, breathed wisely, and attended to the functions of your body wisely, you would have before you another fifty years of pleasurable, useful life, and then the instinct of death would come to you and at last you would—

> Approach thy grave
> Like one who wraps the drapery of
> his couch
> About him and lies down to pleasant
> dreams.

Eat only plain foods, eschew spices, alcohol and all stimulants, avoid immoderation as to quantity and chew thoroughly. This will be rational eating, and in a lifetime your sum total of pleasure will be maximum.

The Role of Garden Vegetables in the Dissemination of Typhoid Fever.[1]—Whatever the medium by which the typhoid fever germs may be spread, says an editorial· writer in the *Medical Record*, the question of their viability outside the human body is of primary importance. This problem has been worked out by many investigators so far as the usual media of water, milk, and soil are concerned, but until comparatively recently very little attention has been paid to the role of raw foodstuffs, such as

[1]Editorial *Med. Record*, Mar. 23, 1912.

fruit and vegetables, in conveying infection which they may have acquired during cultivation.

In order to increase our knowledge on this phase of the subject, R. H. Creel (*Pub. Health Reports*, Feb. 9, 1912), carried out a series of experiments in raising radishes and lettuce on soil which was infected with the *Bacillus typhosus*. This infection was accomplished subsequent to the seeding, but prior to the appearance of the plants. As a result of this work he found that plants would take up with them on their leaves and stems the microorganisms which they encountered as they pushed their way through the infected soil. Furthermore, it was found that *Bacillus typhosus* could be recovered from the leaves and stems of plants that were to all appearances entirely free from adhering particles of dirt. In order to determine how far natural rainfall might be expected to free the vegetables from the organism, a leaf of lettuce from an infected bed was repeatedly washed with sterile water, and then the leaf, in an almost macerated condition, was rubbed on an Endo plate culture. This experiment yielded positive results, · and seems to warrant the conclusion that ordinary cleansing by rainfall, or under the kitchen faucet, will not free the infected plants from the germs. Furthermore, under conditions most unfavorable to the growth of *Bacillus typhosus*, the infection lasted at least thirty-one days, which is a period sufficiently long for the maturity of quick-growing varieties of lettuce and radishes.

In view of the results of his experiments, and considering the fact that other observers have proven that the life of *Bacillus typhosus* in soil may be prolonged to sixty or even seventy days, Creel considers that the fertilization of garden soil by human excreta assumes a twofold importance. First, the vegetables, such as lettuce, radishes, and celery, may directly convey the infection, and second, the soil may serve as a reservoir for bacteria. Drainage from such germ-soaked areas may carry the microorganisms to streams of water, and thus keep up the infection much longer than if the water were directly infected.

In view of the already well-known dangers incidental to the exposure of night-soil in such situations as to render it easily accessible to the house fly, it would seem that these experiments serve to add another strong argument against the use of human excreta as a garden fertilizer.

SOCIETY PROCEEDINGS.

THE EASTERN MEDICAL SOCIETY OF THE CITY OF NEW YORK.

Stated Meeting, May 10, 1912.

The regular monthly meeting of the Eastern Medical Society was held Friday evening, 8 P. M., April 12, 1912, at the Cafe Boulevard. President S. J. Kopetzky in the chair. During the Executive Session routine business was transacted, with the usual election of new members, etc.

During the Scientific Session the following program was rendered:

I. Presentation of Cases.

Ligature of Internal Iliac Arteries in Pelvic Cancer. (Six Cases.) By Dr. Irving S. Haynes.

II. Symposium.

Reports of Research work on the Cancer Problem in Medicine.

(a) *The Present State of the Cancer Problem.* By Dr. W. B. McCullum.

(b) *Modern Methods of Diagnosis.* By Dr. M. J. Sittenfield.

(c) *Specific Therapy of Cancer.* By Dr. I. Levin.

(d) *The Surgical Aspect of Cancer.* By Dr. W. L. Rodman of Philadelphia, Pa., (by invitation).

III. Discussion by

Dr. Henry C. Coe, Dr. Charles H. Peck, Dr. Harlow Brooks.

After the meeting a collation was served, to which members and guests were invited.

Resolutions on the Death of Dr. Lipschutz.

Whereas, Death has suddenly snatched from our midst our co-worker, Dr. J. M. Lipschutz,

Resolved, That we, the Medical Board of the Bronx Hospital and Dispensary, hereby express our deep regret at the loss of an earnest, energetic and promising young physician, and

Resolved, That a copy of these resolutions be sent to his family and to the *New York Medical Journal, Medical Record, American Medicine* and *The Critic and Guide.*

William J. Robinson, President.
M. Aronson, M. D.
Alex. Goldman, M. D.
H. Schumer, M. D.
Martin Rehling, M. D., Secretary.
Committee.

GENERAL TOPICS.

A Splendid Issue.—Following are the special contributions for the Greater New York Number of the *American Journal of Surgery,* June, 1912: "Sources and Treatment of Bleeding from the Genital Tract of Women," H. J. Boldt, M. D., New York; "Prognosis in Surgery of the Prostate in the Aged," Howard Lilienthal, M. D., New York; "The Columns and Crypts of Morgagni; Their Influence in Rectal Diseases," James P. Tuttle, M. D., New York; "The Suprapubic Two-Step Operation for the Removal of the Hypertrophied Prostate," Drs. L. S. and P. M. Pilcher, New York; "A New Technic for Extirpation of the Penis," Edward L. Keyes, Jr., M. D., New

York; "The Operative Treatment of Cardiospasm," Willy Meyer, M. D., New York; "The Female Perineum from a General Surgeon's Standpoint," Robert T. Morris, M. D., New York; "Some Peculiarities of Deep-lying Abdominal Inflammation," C. N. Dowd, M. D., New York; "Removal of Foreign Bodies from the Eye," Chas. H. May, M. D., New York; "Breast: Consideration of Border-Line Tumors," John F. Erdman, M. D., New York; "The Illustration and Discussion of the Temporal Bone, with Reference to the Parts Involved in Surgery," W. Meddaugh Dunning, M. D., New York; "Clinical Observations in Puerperal Infections," John Osborne Polak, M. D., New York; "When Shall We Operate on Simple Fractures of Long Bones?" J. P. Warbasse, M. D., New York; "Unusual Fracture Cases and Commentaries and some of the more Usual Forms," Walter M. Brickner, M. D., New York.

Smallpox in Michigan.—During the first three months of 1912 there were reported 283 cases of smallpox in Michigan. The vaccination history of these cases is as follows:

2 cases vaccinated		"50 or 60 years ago."
3 " "		"14 years ago."
1 " "		"years ago."
1 " "		"at the time of exposure."
1 " "		"12 years ago."
1 " "		"infancy and again 10 years ago."
1 " "		"about 10 years ago."
1 " "		"some 20 years ago."
1 " "		"one week after exposure."
10 " "		"about 3 years ago" (some doubt).
1 " "		"some years previous."
2 " "		"in childhood."
2 " "		"when very young."
1 " "		"30 years ago."
2 " "		"6 years ago."
1 " "		"2 years ago."
1 " "		"4 years ago."
1 " "		"5 years ago."
5 " "		"doubtful if ever."
245 "		"NEVER VACCINATED."

Total, 283 cases.

It costs Michigan $150,000 a year to take care of indigent smallpox patients and to protect the unvaccinated.

Pasteurization Not Recommended.—At the Chicago meeting of the American Association for the Prevention of Infant Mortality, says *Life and Health*, Dr. George W. Goler, of Rochester, said that most Pasteurization is done for the purpose, not of preventing disease, but of keeping the milk from souring. He believes that people should be taught to Pasteurize their milk at home, and asserts that the New York law requiring Pasteurization was a political measure intended to delay the passage of a law requiring the tuberculin test. The law requiring Pasteurization, according to Dr. Goler, will help the man who produces dirty milk to go on in his dirty old way.

A New Bandage for the Eye.[1]—The bandage devised by Layson can readily be made from a piece of 2½ or 3 inch gauze roller bandage. Cut a strip sufficiently long to tie around the patient's head and split this at each end, leaving about 6 or 7 inches unsplit. Two tails are thus made on each end of strip. The two which are to be applied on the side of the closed eye should be slightly longer than on the side of the eye which is to be left open. To apply the bandage, place the unsplit part over affected eye and pass the two longer tails one above and one below the ear. Carry the other end of the bandage over the forehead above the unaffected eye to a point above the temple. At this point have the upper tail to cross over the lower one and then pass back under the occipital protuberance to be tied securely with the lower tail of the opposite side. The two remaining tails are then tied at a point well above the occipital protuberance. The cross prevents the bandage slipping up too far on the side of the eye left open.

A New Medical Society.—A number of medical men of upper Manhattan and the Bronx have just organized a new medical society under the name Northern Medical Society of the City of New York. The following officers have been elected: President, Dr. William J. Robinson; First Vice-President, Dr. A. L. Goldwater; Second Vice-President, Dr. Alex. Goldman; Recording Secretary, Dr. De Witt Stetten; Corresponding Secretary, Dr. H. Schumer; Treasurer, Dr. M. Aronson. Meetings will be held monthly. Only members of the medical profession in good standing are eligible to membership.

A Special Gynecological Number.—The May issue of the *International Journal of Surgery* is devoted to a very remarkable symposium on gynecological subjects. The material in this issue is of great practical value and the following titles indicate the scope and importance of the articles presented:

The Appendix from a Gynecological Viewpoint, by H. C. Coe, M. D., New York.

Some Observations on the Vaginal Removal of Submucous Fibroids, by Samuel W. Bandler, M. D., New York.

Circumcision in Girls, by Robert T. Morris, M. D., New York.

The Single Stitch Perineorrhaphy, by Ralph Waldo, M. D., New York.

Sterility: Lesser Semen Defects and Minor Lesions of the Female Generative Tract as

[1]By Z. C. Layson, M. D., Hinton, W. Va.,

Causative Factors, by W. H. Cary, M. D., Brooklyn, N. Y.

A Modification in the Repair of the Pelvic Outlet, by John C. MacEvitt, M. D., Brooklyn; N. Y.

The Silver Stem Pessary for Amenorrhea and Dysmenorrhea, Sterility, etc., by J. H. Carstens, M. D., Detroit, Mich.

A Common Abuse in the Practice of Gynecology, by H. A. Wade, M. D., New York.

Uterine Displacements and Their Treatment, by C. L. Bradford, M. D., Pittsburg, Pa.

Indication for Caesarean Section, by J. Bertram Dowd, M. D., Brooklyn, N. Y.

A New Self-Retaining Female Catheter, by James Allmond Day, M. D., Jacksonville, Ill.

In addition to these splendid papers, many of which are beautifully illustrated, there are a number of notable editorial articles, as follows:

Yeast in External Infections, by G. K. Dickinson, M. D.

The Diagnosis of Ectopic Pregnancy, by Ellice McDonald, M. D.

The Relation of Arrest of Development to Gynecology and Obstetrics, by Charles P. Noble, M. D., and a Plea for Improving the Prevailing Character of Expert Testimony, by Emery Marvel, M. D.

There are also the usual departments on Surgical Gleanings, Book Notices, etc.

All in all, this May number is one of the best ever issued by the *International Journal of Surgery* and well indicates the service this high class journal is rendering its many readers.

Reform in Naming Remedies.—In an address to manufacturers the Council on Pharmacy and Chemistry shows that it is possible to provide medicines with names descriptive of their composition and that the interests of both the manufacturer and the consumer, the physician and his patient, can be sufficiently safeguarded if to the descriptive name of an article there be appended a distinctive word, syllable, initial or sign that shall identify its manufacturer. The feasibility of coining proprietary names that shall indicate the important constituents of a remedy is shown by illustrations taken from "N. N. R." The objectionableness of names which suggest the use of a remedy to the public is discussed and it is also pointed out that names suggestive to physicians are objectionable because there is a tendency that physicians will base their use of the remedy on the name without giving due consideration to the condition and symptoms of the patient. Since therapeutically suggestive titles have been applied to proprietary medicines without any intention of appealing to the public and since it is difficult to change a name once established the Council has decided to make no objection to such titles if they are already in use provided they are not liable to lead to the use of a remedy by the public. (*Jour. A. M. A.*, March 30, 1912, p. 953.)

American Medicine

H. EDWIN LEWIS, M. D., *Managing Editor.*

PUBLISHED MONTHLY BY THE AMERICAN-MEDICAL PUBLISHING COMPANY.

Copyrighted by the American Medical Publishing Co., 1912.

New Series, Vol. VII., No. 6.
Complete Series, Vol. XVIII., No. 6.

JUNE, 1912.

$1.00. YEARLY in advance.

The American Medicine Gold Medal for 1912 was awarded to Dr. William Crawford Gorgas, Colonel in the Medical Corps of the United States Army, member of the Isthmian Canal Commission and chief sanitary officer of the Panama Canal Zone. The Trustees of the Award unanimously selected Dr. Gorgas as the American physician who in their opinion, has performed the most conspicuous and noteworthy service for humanity in the domain of medicine during the past year. The American Medicine Gold Medal has therefore been conferred upon this eminent physician who through his splendid labors in Havana and more recently in Panama has shown to the civilized world what hygiene and sanitation can do for mankind when intelligently employed. Probably no better idea can be gained of the work Dr. Gorgas has been doing than to quote the following from an article of his in a recent issue of the *Jour. of the American Medical Association:*

"The health conditions at Panama when the United States took charge, in 1904, were very bad. For four hundred years this isthmus had been considered the most unhealthy spot in the world and the mortality records will sustain this opinion. The official pilot chart, in 1903, says:

"'The Panama Canal District is one of the hottest, wettest and most feverish regions in existence. Intermittent and malignant fevers are prevalent, and there is an epidemic of yellow fever at times. The death rate under normal circumstances is large.'

From the best information which I can get, and which I consider accurate, I believe the French lost 22,189 laborers by death from 1881 to 1889. This would give a rate of something over 240 per thousand per year. I think it due to the French to say that we could not have done a bit better than they, if we had known no more of the cause of these tropical diseases than they did.

The great discoveries in tropical medicine made during the time between the coming of the French to the Isthmus and the coming of ourselves, however, namely, that certain species of mosquito transmit both yellow fever and malarial fevers, have enabled us to protect ourselves against these and other tropical diseases.

The French, with an average force of not more than 10,200 men, lost in nine years 22,189 men; we, with an average force of 33,000 men, in nearly the same length of time have lost less than 4,000. The death rate among the French employees was something more than 240 per 1,000; our maximum rate in the early days was 40 per 1,000; our rate at present is 7.50 per 1,000. Malaria, from a maximum of 821 per 1,000 taken sick—i. e., that out of every 1,000 of our employees in the course of the year we have 821 taken sick with malaria—we have reduced at present to 187 per 1,000. But most important of all, yellow fever has been entirely banished. We have not had a single case since May, 1906, now a lapse of almost six years. The general death rate has been reduced from a maximum of 49.94 per 1,000 to a rate, for the year 1910, of 21.18 per 1,000. Such a rate compares favorably with that of many parts of the United States.

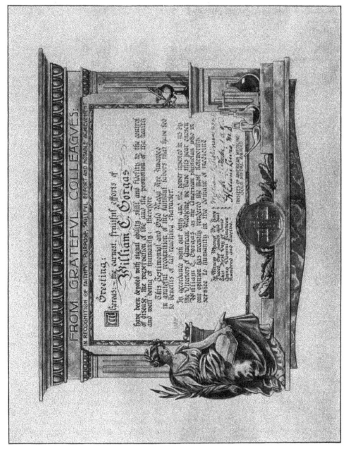

Certificate of Award of the American Medicine Gold Medal for 1912.

While the great work in tropical sanitation, of Laveran, Ross, Reed, Finlay, Carter and many others, have enabled the sanitary department on the Isthmus to take a vital part in the work of building the canal, this is not the greatest good that we hope, and expect, will flow from this conspicuous object-lesson. We hope that our success at Panama will induce other tropical countries to try the same measures; and that thereby gradually all the tropics will be redeemed and made a suitable habitation for the white man."

a slight degree, to emphasize the splendid achievements of the earnest, resourceful and efficient physicians of America.

In closing we cannot do better than to quote the inspiring words of Dr. W. H. Welch of Johns Hopkins University in presenting Dr. Gorgas for the honorary degree of doctor of laws at the commencement exercises at that institution:

"In behalf of the Academic Council I have the honor to present for the honorary

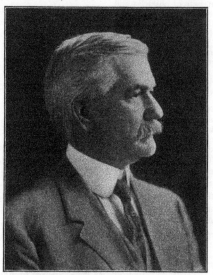

Photo by Harris and Ewing, Washington, D. C.

William C. Gorgas, M. D., LL. D.

Truly it is work of this kind that makes us proud indeed of our profession. The American Medicine Gold Medal is a very slight and humble means for conveying the respect, esteem and genuine admiration we hold for this great American physician and sanitarian, but we earnestly hope that its award to Colonel Gorgas for 1912—as well as its award every year hereafter to other worthy medical men—may serve, if only to

degree of Doctor of Laws, Dr. William Crawford Gorgas, Colonel in the Medical Corps of the United States Army, member of the Isthmian Canal Commission and chief sanitary officer of the Isthmian Canal Zone, formerly president of the American Medical Association, physician and sanitarian of the highest eminence, who by his conquests of pestilential diseases has rendered signal service to his profession, to his country and to the world. With high administrative capacity and with full command of the resources of sanitary science Colonel Gorgas has given to the world the most complete and impressive demonstration in medical history of the accuracy and the life-saving power of our knowledge concerning the causation and mode of spread of certain dreaded epidemic and endemic diseases. He it was who, by application of the discoveries of Major Reed and his colleagues of the Army Yellow Fever Commission, was mainly instrumental in freeing Cuba of yellow fever, and he it is who, in spite of obstacles and embarrassments, has made the construction of the Isthmian Canal possible without serious loss of life or incapacity from disease—a triumph of preventive medicine not surpassed in importance and significance by the achievements of the engineer. In the conquest of science over disease, in the saving of untold thousands of human lives and human treasure, in the protection of our shores from the once ever-threatening scourge of yellow fever, in the reclamation to civilization of tropical lands—in results such as these are to be found the monuments of our laureate, his victories of peace, to which this university now pays tribute by such honor as it can bestow."

We believe the medical profession as a whole, and the readers of AMERICAN MEDICINE in particular will universally commend this first award of the American Medicine Gold Medal.

The Meeting of the American Medical Association held at Atlantic City June 4, 5, 6 and 7, was fully up to the standards of former meetings—in every respect except attendance. The registration—3,600—was ahead of that of the 1910 session, to be sure, but when one considers the accessibility of Atlantic City, its closeness to the great medical centers of New York, Philadelphia, Baltimore and New England, the splendid program arranged, the coincidental meetings of other societies, and the many social attractions announced, it is certainly surprising that so few doctors availed themselves of the opportunities offered.

There can be no question but that the A. M. A. meeting is the main event each year in medical affairs. The program of each meeting is an epitome of the annual progress that has been made in every branch of medicine. The discussions in each section bring out the work that is being done in medicine and surgery all over the country and to a certain extent the section meetings serve as clearing-houses for striking a balance in medical opinions. No physician can attend the various section meetings and take active part therein without receiving substantial benefit. There is a stimulation obtained from rubbing elbows with men working along similar lines that is always beneficial. More than this, a man invariably gains new strength and courage by detaching himself from his own sphere of activity and coming in personal touch with the aims and efforts of other men, thus learning first hand of their ideas and methods. It is safe to say that no man with red blood in his arteries and veins ever fails to profit immeasurably from attending these splendid meetings of the leading medical organization of the United States. We do not hesitate therefore in openly stating that it is a matter for genuine regret that only about 2½ per cent of the physicians of America—or approximately 10 per cent of the whole membership of the Association—attended the 1912 convention of the American Medical Association. To belong to an association and not go to its meetings seriously reflects on the interest that is felt in its affairs. Membership in any organization is ordinarily supposed to entail certain obligations, not the least of which is to attend and take an active part in its deliberations and work. We are old fashioned enough to believe that members of the A. M. A. are not fulfilling their duty to the Association, their fellows or to themselves when they stay away from these meetings. It is unfair to those who each year prepare an interesting and profitable program, and arrange attractive social events for the pleasure and enjoyment of the members and their guests. In other words it discounts the efforts of those who labor to make each meeting a success, and consequently places a handicap on every detail of the Association work. We do not intend to scold or set ourselves up as critics of the members of the Association. Our interests are no other than those of the average member. But knowing how essential enthusiasm and interest are to the future—as well as to the present—success of every organization, we cannot help but feel that the indifference and lack of interest indicated by an attendance so out of proportion to the membership calls for more than passing notice. Surely there must be some explanation for the fact that the number of physicians registered as in attendance *was only a trifle over one-half the total membership in the three adjacent states of New Jersey, New York and Pennsylvania!* But when it is considered that the program was excellent, well advertised and many of the leaders of the profession were expected to be present, the basic reason for the dereliction of nearly 90 per cent of the active members belonging to the Association, is not easy to ascertain.

Small attendance is not the only disturbing feature. For several years we have been discussing these matters pertaining to the Association, and while we know that anything we may say will be interpreted in certain quarters as vicious criticism, and an attack on the A. M. A.

we feel that we, in common with all other earnest members of this great medical organization, owe it to our sincere desire to see the Association grow and extend its influence on the medical affairs of the country, to consider openly and fairly these great questions of attendance and membership. The American Medical Association from a small, inconsequential organization has become a powerful society, national in its scope and influence, and a potent force in the solution of the medical problems of the day. Every physician should look upon membership in the Association not only as a privilege and an honor, but as one of his obligations as an American physician. The American medical profession should be a factor in shaping and directing the affairs of the nation. The great problems of the conservation of life, the social progress of the American people and the public health are so closely associated with each other that no physician who is alive to the larger duties of his calling can conscientiously limit his activities to the simple treatment of disease. Not only sanitation, hygiene and the fundamental questions of the prevention of disease fall within the field of the modern physician, but if he aims to fulfill his whole duty as a member of the most humane and unselfish of professions he must extend his consideration and influence to the problems connected with the mental, moral and social welfare of the race. As an individual each physician's efforts will necessarily be circumscribed by the limitations of his field of active endeavor. To make his influence felt he must unite with his fellows, and the American physician who wishes to see the medical profession become a strong powerful factor in the progress of the American people should ally himself with the American Medical Association. In union there is strength and if the medical men of the United States ever reach the point where they have the influence and power that their work and motives warrant, it must come through organization. The American Medical Association offers the opportunity. It is for the physicians of the country to decide what they will do with it. Will they unite with this splendid institution, which already includes a large proportion of the foremost medical men of the United States, and shoulder to shoulder march on to achievements and triumphs that will assure not only new honor and recognition for the noblest calling that mankind can follow, but also place the physical, moral and social conditions of the people of America where they should be? Or will they refuse to affiliate with the Association and allow a golden opportunity for constructive work to go by? The hour is pregnant with possibilities far beyond the comprehension of the most enthusiastic. Can the physicians of the United States prove indifferent to the situation and its needs?

There is no standing still for the American Medical Association, any more than there is for any organization with work to do. The membership situation of the Association certainly justifies genuine alarm on the part of those who have its future interests at heart. Both the outgoing president, Dr. Murphy and the incoming president, Dr. Jacobi, recognized the menace of the situation and handled the subject without gloves. Dr. Murphy said in his address to the House of Delegates, June 3: "The activities in organization have been decreasing from year to year until now they have about reached a standstill. The number of members May 1, 1911,

was 33,960; 299 members have died; 1,301 members have resigned; 500 members have been dropped as non-eligible, and 1,987 have been dropped for non-payment of dues, and 64 reported not found, making a total of 3,151 names to be deducted from the membership list. There have been added 3,474 to the membership roll, of which 2,253 were transferred from the subscription list. The membership of the American Medical Association May 1, 1912, is 34,283. There have resigned from the Association in the past four years 4,899; there have been dropped for the non-payment of dues 2,726, making a total of 7,635 members taken out of the Association. Why? This means an annual loss to the Association in dues alone of $38,175 and a still greater loss in prestige and education. No business house would permit such a loss of patronage without the closest scrutiny and the most careful analysis. Again, we have in the United States practically 102,000 medical men, with only 34,000 of these in the American Medical Association. Some states are thoroughly organized having as high as 66 per cent. of the physicians in the state as members of the American Medical Association, as North Dakota; while others have as low as 22 per cent.— Tennessee. It appears to me it is the obligation of this Association to determine why the state of North Dakota has not 80 or 85 per cent. and the state of Tennessee an equally high percentage. Are we doing a sufficient amount of work for the every-day practitioner to keep him interested? Are we giving him sufficient for the $5 which he pays for his membership and the *Journal?* Or, what in addition must we do to keep alive the interest in the Association and to obtain his support and membership? All these questions should be worked out by a body of men who have special ability and facilities to determine the cause and remedy the evil effects of this diminution in membership. It will be said that we have taken in more than we can assimilate. That is not a rational explanation. It will be said that we have taken in a large number of members who were undesirable. That I do not believe is true. The fact, as it appears to me, is that we have a colossal number of desirable members of the profession outside of the organization who are not reaping the benefits in the way of education and stimulation to higher work which they should receive from this Association."

Dr. Jacobi in his inaugural address likewise said:

"In order to be powerful and influential, you must not only be wise but numerous. In last year's official report you were told that it was not prudent to increase our number. In fact, you are 35,000, and the largest medical association of the world. But please remember that yours is also the largest country of the world. There are 100,000 medical men besides us, with the same rights to enter and the same duties to perform. We have been told that reasons of finance are among those which should restrict our number. I appeal to you and to those 100,000 outside. A big bank account appeals to our treasury, but glittering gold never saved a country nor a soul. If you have money, it is yours to spend as you have made it. See to it that your House of Delegates spends it in increasing, and consolidating, and strengthening your Association. Our colleagues in the vast country want to be invited; then they will come in. They must learn what we are, and where their interests are— and the interests of the public—from better sources than the hordes of irregular manufacturers and the "freedomers" whose bitter attacks convey what knowledge many millions are permitted to have of the American Medical Association. Let the people understand the meaning of the American Medical Association and its doctors through *our* doings, and not through the scurrilous lies of our and the people's enemies. My hope is for an annual increase of thousands of members. Multiply and be fertile. *Stand still awhile, and you invite decline.* (Italics ours).

It is by vast numbers only that our profession will ever attain its legitimate influence in politics and in society, and such beneficent power as Socrates, Descartes, Kant and Gladstone claimed for it."

The Secretary in his report on membership gave the following:

"The membership of the American Medical Association on May 1, 1911, was 33,-960. During the past year, 299 members have died, 1,301 have resigned, 500 have been dropped as not eligible, 987 have been dropped for non-payment of dues and 64 have been removed from the rolls on account of being reported 'not found,' making a total of 3,151 names to be deducted from the membership list. There have been added 3,474 names to the membership roll, of which 2,353 were transferred from the subscription list. The membership of the American Medical Association on May 1, 1912, was 34,283, a net increase for the year of 323."

In other words, but for the transfer of names from the subscription list to the membership list *there would have been an actual loss of 2,030 members!* The net increase of 323 referred to in the Secretary's report—eliminating the fact that it was made possible by the transfer of 2,353 names from the subscription list—is a pitifully small gain when it is remembered that on May 1, 1911 there were at least 70,000 physicians not affiliated with the Association who were eligible to membership. Looked at from every angle this condition is not a healthy one. Something is to blame not only for the fact that 90 per cent of the members fail to attend the annual meeting—even when it is held in the most desirable place in the country—but also that over two-thirds of the eligible physicians of the United States cannot be induced to become members of the Association.

What is the reason for this state of affairs? Here again we realize we are treading on dangerous ground, for whatever we may say, or however kindly and earnestly we may say it, there will be those who will see some ulterior motive or malicious purpose in our statements. But, knowing that a considerable proportion of our readers are members of the Association and men who have confidence and respect enough in our words and work to credit us with honorable intent, we are willing to risk the criticism of the mental myopes and trust to common sense and judgment to establish the kindliness and sincerity of our motives as well as the truth and soundness of our remarks. We believe that no little part of the condition confronting those who have been trying so hard to build up and increase the membership of the Association can be attributed to the lamentable indifference of the average physician. Wrapped up in the problems and controlled by the circumstances that constitute his daily routine he may have little time or wherewithal, even if he has the inclination, to take up the duties of membership. Many times it is nothing but procrastination that keeps a physician from taking the steps leading to membership. Countless other things, small and inconsequential in themselves, may serve to determine the matter for the individual physician—the psychologic moment has failed to arrive, or the proposition has not appeared under conditions sufficiently moving to lead him to do the things essential to affiliation. We have got to admit that little—sometimes ridiculously little—things determine our action in joining a movement or an organization and this will account for a goodly number of those who continue to remain non-members.

But there is another factor that year after year we have been referring to as the prime influence in keeping down both the attendance and the membership, and that is the present system of organization. With no other feeling than sincere regret and an honest belief that the Association is hopelessly handicapped by the disfranchising of the individual member, we do not hesitate to say that our national organization will never grow to its full stature until provision is made for two things—*1st*, opportunity for the expression of the opinions of the members present at each annual meeting, and *2nd*, the exercise of the veto by the president. It is all very well to refer to the need of having the business sessions divorced from the scientific. No one can quarrel with the institution of some method like the House of Delegates which will enable the transaction of the business and executive details of the Association with facility and despatch. But it would be an easy matter to set aside one day for open discussion of the policies and work of the Association and afford the members present an opportunity to vote on the ratification or rejection of the acts of their delegates and officers. So also the election of officers should be in open meeting. That the presidents and other officers have been beyond criticism thus far, does not mean that the time may not come under present conditions when men will be given office who will fall far short of representing the members. As for giving the president more power, we feel that the dignity of the office requires it. At present, the president is little more than an honorary officer. He can do nothing but advise and recommend. This ought not to be. The men who have graced the office in recent years have been big men, men who have stood for the best in medicine. Can it be doubted that their influence would have been infinitely greater if they had had the power to institute needed reforms and insure that they were carried out? The president of the American Medical Association should be invested with a power that would make him a force not only in the Association but in national affairs. As long as the office is so distinctively honorary—when it should be executive, the results each year will continue to be as they have been. It is generally known throughout the rank and file of the medical profession that the individual member of the Association has no voice in the direction or management of its affairs. The only place where he can register his vote—except in a section meeting on section business—is in the county medical society. But every county society member has a like privilege whether he is affiliated with the national body, or not. About the only thing that membership carries at $5.00 per year is a subscription to the *Journal* and the right to wear the Association button. This statement is not intended to raise the question of values. As a matter of fact the *Journal of the A. M. A.* is well worth the membership fee, for it would be the rankest prejudice to deny the literary and scientific excellence of this splendid publication. But the thought we wish to convey is that membership in the A. M. A. is mighty barren of any rights or privileges. Since it is asking a great deal of intelligent men to join an organization that denies them any influence as individuals and offers no opportunity for expressing any opinion whatsoever concerning its affairs, the disbursements of its funds or the election of its officers, it is perhaps not so surprising after all that as Dr. Murphy said, "the activities in organization * * * * have about reached a standstill."

In behalf of an organization that has done a most excellent work, that has accomplished great and substantial good for humanity, and that has untold possibilities for the uplift of the profession and the future welfare of the people we earnestly plead for a reorganization that will recognize the individual member and give him an active voice in the affairs of the Association. Intelligent physicians will never long continue as nonentities in any organization, and if the A. M. A. is to grow and achieve the ends its present adherents earnestly desire and hope to see, those in power must read aright the conditions before them. *Progress is not only possible but sure if the organization is only put on a true democratic basis. But if the present oligarchical system is maintained, decline is certain and inevitable.* It remains to be seen if the men who have done so much to bring the Association to where it now is are big enough to meet the crisis that confronts them. If they prove so, there are no limits to which the Association can extend its usefulness as a great all-powerful American institution.

———

Scientific efficiency is receiving some pretty hard knocks of late; but, according to a wise editorial in the *N. Y. Times,* the objectionable features are not part of a truly scientific system, in that they tend to strain and exhaust the "speeded" workman, and in that condition his output is less and inferior. Fortunately the employer in his self-interest looks after that side of the matter in the case of wage-workers, while the piece-workers learn their safe gait by experience, as a rule. There is a story that the Bank of England discovered that clerical blunders involving serious losses were generally made after 3 P. M., so that, as a matter of economy, clerks were forbidden to work after that hour. The fagged brain or muscle is unreliable and it is injured if goaded to further exertion. The true scientific management stops labor just before exhaustion reaches the stage of unreliability, or undue slowness. Yet there is a danger which neither employer nor employed considers—the danger of a daily or weekly exhaustion just beyond the powers of repair by recreation and rest. This deficit increases until disability results—a matter which does not concern the employer whose employees are constantly changing, but it is of vital importance in life positions where experience is the real thing paid for. In the latter case, the employer takes measures to preserve the worker's ability, but in the former the tendency is to squeeze the man's energy dry and then hire someone else—a matter the laborers are trying to prevent.

The really scientific management will try to prevent loss of efficiency due to the confinement of workers too long at one operation in a minute division of labor. Yet here a similar conflict of interests exists—the more minute the subdivision of labor the easier to replace the disabled whose welfare is of no consequence to the money-maker. In some lines in the steel business ten years is the limit of endurance; and yet there is no difficulty in filling the vacancies. There is a growing suspicion that if the sole purpose of scientific management is to increase the output where labor is plenty, there may be no limit to the destruction of individual efficiency. In ancient times slaves were deliberately underfed in mines and field, as it was cheaper to buy a fresh lot every year to replace the last purchased, who were so soon killed by starvation and overwork. If scientific management does not consider the worker's future, it will merely be a modern form of the same thing. This is the basic reason for the recent opposition to the spurious scientific management which speeds the worker to get the tem-

porary energy he can sell for the wages, and it is a wholesome opposition as the ultimate welfare of society is not its wealth, but its citizens, whose disability must be delayed. In time the really scientific methods will come as a pure matter of evolution. It might be said in passing, that scientific management is not new, but as old as man himself. The whole course of civilization is a succession of new ways of getting more product out of an hour's or day's labor. The most efficient ways succeeded and the inventors became prosperous. Every factory owner of a century ago was keen to take up suggestions to increase his product without increasing the number of laborers, and the successful ones survived times of stress. The enthusiasm for our last inventions of new methods is misplaced as the question of strain is now introduced and public health is involved.

A better plan is to devise economies where time or material is wasted.

———

Feminine dress is receiving a great deal of attention in the public press just at present and there seems to be a growing sentiment that certain reforms are urgently needed if the truest ideals of modest womanhood are to be preserved. The subject falls well within the scope of a scientific medical journal since there can be no question but that human apparel—of the female particularly—reflects to a marked degree the manners and morals of people as well as of periods. Clothing and dress have always exerted a potent influence on the problems of every day life. Primarily evolved by the urge of physical necessity—the need of protection from cold, wet, or the heat of the summer sun—gradually mankind and womankind found

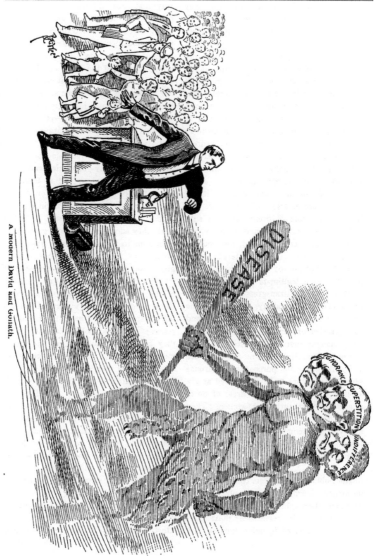

A modern David and Goliath.

that dress afforded opportunities for many things besides the mere attainment of physical comfort. Other emotions and desires soon made themselves felt and so human clothing has long been representative not only of the physical needs, but also of the moral and mental views of every race. It is the truth of this that makes certain tendencies in the dress of the American girl and woman matters of serious moment to the thoughtful analyst of human manners and customs. To the human female, dress has ever had its value as a means of attracting masculine attention and stimulating masculine interest and desire. As a detail or factor in sexual attraction it has served a more or less useful purpose. As long as this role of dress has been subordinate to good taste and modesty, no criticism has been warranted, nor could a word of condemnation be uttered. But alas, the features of female dress which have served a legitimate purpose as long as they have not transgressed the bounds of decency and modesty, have for some time been tending to an accentuation and exaggeration of certain details of the female anatomy that are disgusting to every decent instinct. Styles and modes which are designed for no other purpose than to arouse sexual passion are to be condemned as absolutely out of place in the dress of pure-minded, modest girls and women. They are a pitfall and a menace to the innocent and virtuous female, and as such are intolerable for our daughters, sisters and womankind in general.

The hobble skirt and its congeners have no artistic charm. One has only to stand on a main thoroughfare in any large city to recognize the evils presented by these monstrosities of modern feminine apparel. The way that hips, thighs, breasts and other portions of the anatomy are exposed and exaggerated is a sad commentary on the morals and mental processes of the future mothers of the race. The more the situation is studied the more bewildered one is apt to become. Surely, it cannot be that our girls and young women are losing their moral sense or lowering their standards of virtue? No, it is not this—yet. At present, the disgusting and depraved methods and styles of dress that are so deserving of criticism are attributable solely to a desire that so many young girls and women have of being modern and up-to-date, to be just a little more daring or "risque" than their associates, and to win the reputation of being stylish dressers. Thoughtlessly they adopt extremes and give no consideration to the spectacles or freaks they become, or the concession they make to good taste and conscientious scruples. This is the explanation for the great majority of the girls and young women who dress themselves in the most vulgar manner with utter disregard of all modesty or maidenly reserve. They do not realize the dangers they are surely fostering, or the terrible menace that they are bringing closer and closer to their daily lives.

The great evils of present-day styles of feminine dress are, therefore, the wrong impression they give of good pure girls, the invitation they let innocent women offer to insult and attack, and finally their indisputable tendency to lower or destroy ideals of womanly modesty and self respect—which, after all, are just about the best armor that virtue and chastity ever had, or ever will have.

What an illustration of the irony of fate it will be if modern woman in her frenzied effort to win favor in the eyes of the male sex, adopts the latest and most brazen styles only to find that she has sacrificed the qualities of modesty and reticence that alone can make her attractive to the men worth while!

———

Typhoid fever in rural Virginia has been the subject of considerable study by Freeman and Lumsden (*Amer. Jour. of Public Health*, Ap. 1912). The conditions found raise considerable doubt as to whether we are yet civilized, for it must be impressed on everyone that what is in Virginia is in every other rural district to more or less degree. It is a disease of the country which is imported into our cities, largely by foods, and we must bestir ourselves to prevent the transfer. There is no question, of course, that a sudden outbreak, particularly in winter, is generally due to the transference of the bacillus by "clean" water. But in summer time, when light can kill the bacilli, water pollution is a minor factor. Moreover the filthier the water, the sooner do saprophytes kill the organisms. Water filtration checks the disease only when there is a short distance between the sick and the well. That is, the sewer outlet is near the water intake. Where there is a long period for the bacilli to be damaged or killed, filtration has little effect as Washingtonians now realize to their sorrow.

The source of typhoid infection is now very evident—a nearby case, and nearby means time rather than distance. Actual contact is the main way of getting the disease, but nearly all the rest of the cases get it mediately. Any medium which will keep the bacilli alive must be suspected. This is as near to "fomites" as we can come. If a "carrier" farmer in northern

New York is so filthy in his personal habits that he really washes his hands in the milk he squeezes from a cow, he is practically in close contact with everyone who drinks the milk. If the milk is cooled at once and kept cold, the danger is minimized, but this is impossible in hot weather when the bacilli multiply in warm milk. Hence it is a disease of warm weather. Freeman and Lumsden show that the morbidity curve is parallel to the temperature curve. So we have another weapon with which to cudgel the dairyman. The selling of warm milk should be made a crime. The house-fly is also an agent of the devil in this disease; but really, like the devil himself, he is not as black as he was once painted. Let there be no let-up on fly extermination, but if we are so clean that the fly can find no bacilli to collect and then smear on our food, we need not bother about him. We had better starve him to death. Attention to his medium of exchange may lessen our proper efforts to isolate the carriers, disinfect their discharges and protect our foods. It is the distributer we are now after, the walking typhoid and convalescent carrier.

Commercialism must be ignored in future crusades. One of the blackest spots on the honor of the Norfolk, Virginia, profession was the way they denied rural typhoid at the time of the Jamestown Exposition. The city was perfectly willing that visitors should come there for the money which could be squeezed out of them, but such denials for a temporary advantage, work the other way. The navy now wants to shun Hampton Roads in the typhoid season. It would have been infinitely better to have been clean, and compel the farmers to be clean. San Francisco suffered dreadfully for denying the existence of plague, but it will never be so foolish again. People fear a concealed danger, but not an open one. The great Exposition of 1915 will be a grand success if sanitation is made a great feature and everything is made public. It has the world's best wishes, and will be worthy of our faith.

Cardiac hypertrophy at high altitudes has long been known. It seems to be due to the increased respiration needed in rarefied air, and even horsemen have taken advantage of the phenomenon to train racers in high altitudes, so that they can win at lower races by reason of greater power of the heart and respiratory muscles, and possibly also of a mild emphysema permitting of more air contact with the blood. Watkins-Pitchford (*Transvaal Med. Jour.,* Dec. 1910) now shows that even in school children of S. Africa more than half had this condition, and in some it led to dilatation. Only one-third had normal hearts. Severe exertion like cross-country running was not possible on account of exhaustion. By residence in S. African table-lands, the viscosity of the blood was unduly increased, temperature raised, pulse and respiration increased in volume and rate, metabolism of carbon increased and of proteids decreased, body weight unduly increased, arterial tension increased, and the blood changes already mentioned—a doleful record showing the utter impossibility of permanent colonization by Europeans. To us in the American lowlands it shows the dangers of sending certain cases to the highlands. To advise a consumptive of weak heart to go to such places is theoretically wrong, and as a matter of fact the results in Quito are known to be

bad. Certain British medical journals have made a tremendous blunder in advising the tropical highlands for consumptives with weak hearts. There is some evidence that if the heart can stand the strain and undergo slight hypertrophy, it increases the blood supply in the lungs and this may be the main factor in the remarkable cures at moderate elevations, which are also in part due to the increased erythrocytosis due to elevation.

The ash bath does not refer to a new therapeutic measure nor does it suggest medicinal value; quite to the contrary, it is a most, disgusting and pernicious nuisance to which the people of New York City, and perhaps elsewhere, are daily subjected. We refer to the careless removal of ashes from the ash cans and streets.

The ash receptacles are emptied into wagons usually in such manner that great clouds of dust and finely divided particles of refuse, borne by the wind and gentle zephyrs so active at the particular moment, blow upon the passer-by as well as into every open window and doorway in the vicinity.

How often have we walked along the street to suddenly find ourselves lost in a storm of ash dust? And yet, we seem to like it—perhaps giving vent to a few forcible expressions of passing anger, and with attendant casual brushing of our clothing and wiping of the face.

We are of course always exposed to dust and its contaminating ingredients, but to be completely snowed under a cloud of ash dust is positively revolting from an esthetic point of view, and decidedly injurious to our physical well being. Aside from the mechanical irritation to eyes, ears, nose, throat and in fact the entire respiratory tract, there undoubtedly exists a potent etiological factor of disease, in the special germ and general pathological bacteria contained in the dust.

This careless removal of ashes, dirt and refuse in large communities is disagreeable, uncleanly and positively unhealthy. A more careful handling of the ash cans, and perhaps the employment of covered wagons, might offer possible solutions to the problem—at any rate, it is entirely unnecessary and out of accord with civilization and high taxes for the "common people"—meaning all who walk or even ride—to be subjected to repeated bathing in ash dust.

Some effects of bright light on the eyes have been investigated by Dr. J. Herbert Parsons of London, Eng., (*Jour. Amer. Med. Ass'n.*, Dec. 10, 1910), and we are constrained to say that American ophthalmologists have sadly neglected this field though they have a profusion of cases in our more sunny climates. It is amazing that they should actually surrender the leadership to one practicing in a foggy, smoky, cloudy city where the inhabitants do not know what sunshine really is. Parsons apparently shows that the ultraviolet rays are the dangerous ones, and that for ordinary amounts of light, they as well as the infra-red are completely absorbed by the cornea, aqueous and lens. Few reach the vitreous and none the retina. Where they are too strong to be thus stopped, as in glass blowers and metal workers, they cause cataract. Incidentally he shows that people vary greatly in their perceptions of the colors at each end of the spectrum, some of us being blind to what causes red or violet sensations to

others. Red-blindness therefore amounts to a normal protective variation as red rays are very irritating and it must be much more common than supposed. Perhaps those cases so injuriously affected by red light have too great a range of light perception, and we have a hint as to why redfree illumination is becoming so popular with printers and other night workers. Babies appear to absorb more of the short rays than adults, and and the lower animals show great variations probably because of their differing habitats. Parsons quotes numerous other European investigators who have described the pathologic changes in the lens and capsule after excessive light exposure. Unfortunately he does not make a distinction between the hyperesthesia or irritation (day-blindness) of moderate exposure and the hypoesthesia (night blindness) or exhaustion of longer and greater exposures.

The absorptive power of spectacle glasses is now about to be put on a scientific basis, for the manufacture of almost any kind is an accomplished fact. All this is of much importance in America, where the whole white population comes from lands of lesser light and have not evolved the protection of the races of light climates. Gould has described at least a dozen or more very effective contrivances for shading the eyes, pigment, etc., which shows how important it is. So we must supplement nature when we drift away from our ancestral home. As the wave lengths in the yellow band give the greatest visual effect, it is found by experience that glass which transmits this band and cuts off the two ends of the spectrum, prevents many of the troubles due to excessive tropical light. Green is also very comfortable as it was in our natural habitat when forest dwellers and we are adjusted to it, but it obscures vision so much that it can be used only for therapeutic purposes. The effects of the other wave lengths and the effect of their exclusion, is a vast unexplored field which Americans are preeminently situated for studying. Are we to remain purely "practical" men and supinely wait for our European brethren to work out the facts for us? Why don't some of the research laboratories take it up, and give it as enthusiastic attention as the serums and vaccines? There is some evidence that blue is really very injurious and unless we are protected from undue sky glare there is a chain of pathologic symptoms, from the lids and conjunctiva all the way back to the optic disc and nerve. So let us get at the facts at once that we may lessen the stream of patients flocking to our eye clinics. Surely our southern ophthalmologists find different kinds of cases than the northern, and the very blond population should have vastly different needs than the very brunet.

Our Correspondence department is designed for those who have some special communication to make to our readers, or who wish to discuss *pro* or *con* any of our editorials or articles. AMERICAN MEDICINE is committed to the utmost freedom of thought and every physician and gentleman who addresses us in good faith without malice or discourtesy will be given a hearing and the space his communication merits. We realize that a great many will differ from the opinions we express editorially. We lay claim to no infallibility of observation, judgment or opinion. Mistakes will often be made. Our first aim is to discuss subjects earnestly, honestly, and with independence. We strive to take a liberal, fair and sententious view of the topics we take up. The views expressed represent our convictions at the time they appear. We are always open to argument, and if we are wrong or any man can convince us that his views are more nearly correct than our own, we will gladly change. Obstinacy, stubbornness and dogmatism have no place in the work of the honest editor. At the same time we do not propose to be vacillating, with one opinion today and another on the same question tomorrow. We intend to be as nearly right as possible every time.

So we ask our readers in reading our editorials to credit us with honesty and clean intent. Criticise us, correct us and amplify our work all you can. AMERICAN MEDICINE will meet every kindly, courteous and friendly criticism half way every time.

Consider the letters in this current issue. Our correspondents take issue with us, but since they are courteous and fair in their remarks we gladly publish their letters. No man has a monopoly of truth and we are always willing to give those who honesty differ with us ample space to express their views.

IN MEMORIAM.

W. F. N. O'LOUGHLIN, M. D.
Surgeon of the Titanic.

While nations weep, and muffled bells are rung
  For loved ones lost and men of shining mark,
  Why should the surgeon of the fated bark,
The noble man of healing go unsung?
He to the sick, the aged and the young,
  Was friend and mercy's minister. But hark!
  His deeds of love, though hidden in the dark,
Are theme, perchance, of some celestial tongue.

He stood and smiled, as in his manly prime
  He bade farewell to all that earth possest:
And none can say with what a faith sublime,
  In that last hour of glory's mighty test,
  He laid his head on ocean's icy breast,
And pass'd beyond the mysteries of Time.

Morrisville, Pa.   RICHARD OSBORNE.

ORIGINAL ARTICLES.

THE REPAIR OF INJURIES TO THE PELVIC OUTLET.[1]

BY

BROOKS H. WELLS, M. D.,
Professor of Gynecology at the New York
Polyclinic, New York City.

In the short time at my disposal I propose to leave out, as far as may be, theory, statistics and literature and to deal only with the practical aspect of the question, how shall we best repair the late effects of injuries to the structures of the pelvic outlet resulting from childbirth?

These conditions for our purpose may be broadly classed as:

1. Cystocele.
2. Relaxed pelvic floor, or perineal laceration.
3. Prolapse of the uterus.

The several operations now used by competent gynecological surgeons for the relief of these conditions have been evolved from the experience, the successes and the failures of many good men through many years, and to apply them with the best results one must have had surgical training and experience along these special lines.

In spite of elaborate theories, continued discussion and innumerable modifications none of the operative methods now most successfully used really restores the parts anatomically to their antepartum or normal condition, but they do substitute for a condition producing many distressing symptoms, one of comfort and normal functioning.

Thus, in cystocele, the bladder is deliberately placed at a level higher than normal; in relaxed pelvic floor, the anterior or

[1]Read before the Eastern Medical Society, April 12th, 1912.

proximal borders of the levator muscles, structures never normally in contact, may be sewed together; in prolapse, the fundus of the uterus is often deliberately placed under the bladder and between it and the anterior vaginal wall.

Cystocele.—To relieve this condition the modern operation separates the bladder widely from the anterior vaginal wall and from the anterior surface of the uterus and reattaches it or allows it to readjust itself at a higher level.

The patient is placed in the lithotomy position. The anterior vaginal wall over the cystocele is picked up on either side of the median line and with slender bladed, blunt pointed, dissecting scissors an anteroposterior cut is made through vaginal mucosa and the thin fascia underlying it. The points of the scissors are then pushed carefully up in the median line under the fascia to the urethra and down to the cervix, opened and withdrawn. The median incision is then completed from cervix to urethra and the bladder completely separated from its vaginal and uterine attachments with gauze, sometimes aided by a few snips of the scissors at its cervical attachment. The vaginal wall is resected so that the edges of the incision come together without tension and without redundancy and the incision is closed with interrupted sutures placed so that the first three or four include in their bite uterine tissue and hold the vaginal wall against the cervical portion of the uterus, thus holding up the bladder so that it becomes reattached at a higher level.

In very marked cystocele with retroversion, after freeing the bladder, the peritoneum may be divided transversely at the vesico-uterine reflexion and, after having shortened the round ligaments or done other necessary work, the base of the bladder is picked up in the middle line, as advised by Goffe, at a point which, when carried to the edge of peritoneum on the middle of the anterior face of the uterus, will take up the slack in the base of the bladder. A suture is passed through these points. Two other points are then selected one on either side at the edge of the peritoneal reflexion from the broad ligament and corresponding points at the base of the bladder and sutures are passed so that when tied all the slack in the base of the bladder is taken up smoothly. The vaginal walls are then resected and sutured as already described.

Either of these operations gives satisfactory and very permanent relief.

Perineum.—Irrespective of the shape or method of denudation, or of the material or manner of placing the sutures, or of the name by which the procedure is known, all operations for the restoration of the relaxed pelvic floor which give clinical satisfaction bring together, more or less completely, certain lateral pelvic structures, namely: the fascia or proximal edges of the levators and the tissues external to them. This indication is not new. It is accomplished by the Emmet operation when properly done.

Hadra, in a paper published in the *American Journal of Obstetrics* for April, 1884, spoke clearly of the importance of the levator ani and especially of the fact that its anterior portion must be torn or relaxed to allow the symptoms that we now speak of as due to relaxed pelvic floor and said that to most satisfactorily cure the condition it would be necessary to seek the levator muscles and sew them together.

Reynolds Wilson, in 1898,[1] in a paper which I have always admired for its sim-

[1] *American Journal of Obstetrics*, Vol. xxxvii, page 20.

plicity and clearness of diction, describes the pelvic floor and the indications to be met in its repair so lucidly that I am tempted to quote him somewhat freely.

"The muscles of the pelvic floor are divided into two layers; the deeper layer, made up of the levator ani muscle, which descends in the shape of a cone from the sides of the pelvis to the point of attachment of the more superficial layer in the center of the perineum; and the superficial layer, made up of, first, the transverse muscles of the perineum, which stretch from the tuberosities of the ischium and are inserted in the center of the perineum, and, secondly, of the muscles which surround the vaginal outlet. These muscles are attached to the various fascial layers as follows, naming them from within outward: First, the recto-vesical layer of the pelvic fascia, which is deflected from the sides of the pelvis over the *pelvic* surface of the levator ani muscle. Second, the perineal layer of the obturator-coccygeus fascia, which is reflected from the sides of the pelvis over the *perineal* surface of the levator ani muscle. Third, the anterior and posterior aponeuroses of the perineal septum, which include the deep transverse perineal muscle. Fourth, the two layers of the superficial perineal fascia, including the superficial transverse and the bulbo-cavernosus muscles.

"We may divide the pelvic and perineal fasciae into two sets of layers corresponding to the deep and superficial muscular layers. The deeper fascial layers are united to the more superficial layers in the perineal raphe. The superficial layers stretching forward from a line connecting the tuberosities of the ischia to the pubic rami, shut off the outlet to the pelvis, save at the vulvar opening.

"In an extensive laceration of the perineum the muscles which are respectively held between these layers of fascia become separated both as to the insertion of their fibers in the center of the perineum and as to the attachment of the deep and superficial layers at the same point. As a consequence the more superficial muscles are free to retract in the direction of their proximal attachment—namely, away from the center of the perineum—and the levator ani, which constitutes the deeper layer, is drawn, at the point of laceration of its fibers, outward laterally by the action of the more superficial muscles. It is in this way that the deep furrow, or sulcus, on either side of the bulging rectocele is formed.

"Such being the lesion, we may select a variety of explanations of the effectiveness of operation in such cases. If we follow Emmet we will believe that by denuding an elliptical area on either side, corresponding with the curve of the posterior commissure of the vagina and within the introitus, and introducing sutures in an antero-posterior direction, we are able to reunite the deeper fascial layer of the perineum to its attachment at the vulvar outlet. If we follow those who assert that restoration of the perineum and support of the posterior vaginal wall is only accomplished by bringing the divided fibers of the levator ani muscle together, we will look for our result in re-establishing the function of this muscle and thus drawing the posterior wall of the vagina upward and replacing the rectum in its normal position. It is then a question, not of restoring the fascial attachments, but of enabling the muscle to become again an 'elevating' muscle.

"The objects, therefore, to be attained in the operation are: First, the union of the fibers of the levator ani muscle with their proper perineal attachment; second, the restoration of the fascial covering of this muscle; third, the union of the two layers of fascia, the pelvic and perineal, at their points of mutual attachment—namely, in the center of the perineum; the restoration of the action of the transverse muscles of the perineum, which have hitherto drawn upon the severed fibers of the levator ani muscle in a lateral direction, flattening the calibre of the vagina and causing it to gape. Thus with the upward and forward action of both sets of muscles—that is, of the levator and of the superficial muscles—restored, we have a restoration of the tone of the pelvic floor together with a closure of the vaginal outlet."

It would seem that the situation as here presented could not be more clear and simple and yet the question, how best to accomplish all this has caused much discussion and promises to remain in the field of controversy for our successors yet unborn to wrangle over.

At the Polyclinic I have always taught the necessity of approximating the levator edges and of restoring the central attachments of the transverse perineal muscles and fascial layers and have obtained clinically and anatomically very satisfactory results in the restoration of the lifting function without drawing the levators from their sheaths. During the last four years, however, the edges of the levators have been definitely exposed and sewed directly together.

The patient is placed in the dorsal position with flexed legs held by stirrups. A symmetrical incision is made with scissors, beginning in the center of the perineal com-

312   AMERICAN MEDICINE }
Complete Series, Vol. XVIII. }   ORIGINAL ARTICLES | JUNE, 1912.
New Series, Vol. VII., No. 6.

missure at the muco-cutaneous junction and extending in a curved direction upwards and inwards below the orifice of the vulvo-vaginal gland to beyond the remains of the hymen. The mucous flap thus outlined is dissected free with snips of the scissors through whatever scar tissue is present and is then freed as may be necessary by blunt dissection with gauze. In general this freeing is carried up about an inch in the center and on the sides as high as the levators, scissors being used as in the separation of the bladder in the cystocele operation. The levator edges can then be pulled forward and sutured in the middle line with two or three sutures of number one or two ten-day chromic gut. The levators should be handled gently and it is not desirable to free them from their sheaths extensively, as advocated by Strumdorf, for the reason that we wish to include, as far as may be, the fascial edges. Another layer of buried stitches in front of the levators brings together the remaining layers of fascia and the insertions of the transverse perinei.

When the levator edges are brought together the rectocele disappears and with it much of the apparent redundancy of the vaginal flap, so that very little trimming is needed to make it fit. It is fastened in place with No. 1 plain catgut which is continued as a subcuticular stitch to bring the edges of the initial incision together. Finally the sphincter is stretched as this, with the subcuticular suture of the skin, does away with much post-operative discomfort.

Instead of using buried sutures, the operation may be done with the Holden figure of eight silkworm gut stitch or even with deeply placed circular sutures. Personally I prefer the buried sutures.

Prolapse.—In prolapse two methods of operation have been found to give most satisfactory results; the method by interposition of the fundus of the uterus between bladder and anterior vaginal wall, which is the method of choice; and the method by vaginal hysterectomy with suture of the broad ligaments.

In the "interposition" or Watkins' operation the cervix, if much hypertrophied or diseased, is amputated, the bladder is then separated from the anterior vaginal wall and from the uterus, the vesico-uterine peritoneal fold is opened, the fundus of the uterus turned forward and brought out under the bladder, where it is held by a couple of catgut sutures, and the vaginal walls closed over it as in the operation for cystocele. This places the uterus in extreme anteversion and at the same time very radically gets rid of the cystocele and the falling of the anterior vaginal wall. Then the relaxed pelvic floor is repaired as already described and the operation is completed.

This method has given me very uniformly satisfactory results in forty-eight cases and I employ it, except in instances where the sub-pubic segment of the vagina, that is, the urethra and the adjacent tissues, is prolapsed, or where the uterus is so diseased as to make its removal advisable aside from the fact of its prolapse. In the presence of these indications vaginal hysterectomy is done and the stumps of the broad ligaments, as so strongly advocated by Goffe, are stitched together to make a shelf across the pelvis and over this shelf the bladder is placed and held by two or three sutures, very much as in the operation for cystocele. The perineum is repaired in the usual way.

523 Madison Avenue.

DYSTOCIA DUE TO FAULTY POSITION AND PRESENTATION.[1]

BY

S. MARX, M. D.,
New York City.

In a large measure mal-positions and mal-presentations are provocative of difficult labor. Therefore it behooves the accoucheur in all cases of dystocia to make a careful finger—if necessary, a hand—examination where a labor is unduly prolonged and severe. This must of necessity clear the atmosphere and where the presenting part is neither obstetrically faulty nor the position of that presentation wrong, there can only be one factor to consider, namely, a pelvis that is either relatively or absolutely contracted. While dystocias due to this latter condition are of the supremest importance, and the difficulty to overcome them forms one of the most serious problems in midwifery, the subject must be omitted since it is germane to the article.

Obstetrically considered mal-positions are more frequent than mal-presentations, the latter seldom occurring alone, but nearly always accompanied by concomitant disturbing factors and probably caused by them—witness the frequency of breech presentations, and placenta previa in the presence of contracted pelvis. And I wish to go on record by stating that repeated mal-presentations in successive labors are nearly always associated with deformities in and anomalies of the pelvis. It is necessary to have clearly in mind what is position and what is presentation.

By presentation we mean the part of the fetal ovum that first presents itself to the examining finger. By position, the relation which the presenting part bears to fixed obstetric, anatomic points in the pelvis; and again it must be remembered that while a presentation may be normal, its position may be absolutely abnormal; as witness an occipital advance but in which the occiput lies posteriorly. I mention the posterior occiputs advisedly, for in an overwhelming majority of cases a posterior occiput is the cause of dystocia in all obstetric head presentations, a posteriorly placed occiput is the cause of primary dystocia in surely over 90% of the cases. Primarily they are so frequent that the writer (at least in primiparous women) looks upon them as nothing unusual. With all mal-positions as well as presentations well defined and pronounced symptoms arising early become only too evident even to the casual observer. A part presenting almost beyond the reach of the examining finger and of necessity above the brim, is a condition which should always make the accoucheur suspicious of trouble for no normal presenting or positioned fetal part behaves in this fashion, with one exception, i. e., in the presence of a contracted pelvis and associated with it. Again slow engagement and nagging inefficient pains form more corroborative evidence; and last and of great importance the early rupture of the membranes with the escape of the waters make a triad of symptoms, which make strongly presumptive the diagnosis of a mal-presentation as well as position, even before a vaginal examination is undertaken.

Diagnosis.—External examination forms an important link in our diagnosis, again mapping out the outline of the fetal ovoid and the auscultation of the fetal heart, both are never to be omitted. A rule I have always found good and true is one in reference to the fetal heart. The

[1]Read before the Eastern Medical Society, April 12, 1912.

further away from the median line that the fetal heart can be heard with the greatest intensity, the greater is the probability of a mal-position. Again the same tentative diagnosis can be made, the higher the fetal heart is heard at or above the umbilicus.

Yet even though all signs are strongly presumptive of a mal-placed or mal-positioned head, the clinching evidence is obtained by a thorough vaginal examination by finger or hand even if it necessitates a complete narcosis. The exact relation of the head to the pelvis is of the supremest importance and upon its exact knowledge depends our rational and scientific management of the case. Many men can make out presentations, few, I know can diagnose positions. It is a sad commentary on our obstetric teaching that such a statement is truly and honestly made after twenty-five years of obstetric experience. To make the grievous error of dilating a fetal anus mistaking it for a one finger dilated os uteri was one of the most flagrant mistakes I have ever encountered. To continue along in this vein of thought would make this rather sketchy article as ludicrous . as it would be sad. ·Still it would reflect seriously on me as well as all teachers of this most important branch of medicine. Even though vicious positions be present and their presence diagnosed timely, the proper and early treatment is so satisfactory that rarely a case ought terminate any other way than favorable, simple and successful. Abnormal presentations can in many cases be overcome if time be given them to undergo normal restitution. In obstetrics patience is truly a virtue. This is the one secret of success. Two forms of treatment must always be considered in abnormal postures

of the anatomic head, and I refer especially as included in these positions, posterior occiputs and mento posteriors. Mento anterior positions I consider as belonging to the class of normal cases. In the first of these forms of treatment it is to remember strictly the mechanism of the normal cases and exaggerate by all means within our control such mechanism. Hyperflexion in occiput cases or hyperextension in face cases, performed either by direct pressure with hand or finger; and the 2" form purely orthopedic is the postural treatment—in short place the woman on that side corresponding to the position of the presenting part—chin or occiput to the right, patient on the right side and the reverse in left-sided cases. These two methods with a reasonable degree of patience will give wonderful results. In transverse cases immediate version to the breech and in breech cases, a waiting policy till the os is dilated and then no forcible traction on the legs but guide the body by moderate traction, and institute powerful pressure from above to maintain a firmly flexed head for safe delivery. Note again the exaggeration of the normal mechanism. More *vis a tergo* less *vis a fronte*. If our temporizing means fail when are we to interfere? I can only repeat the following words which surely ring true: "When and how to operate during labor are gifts possessed· by few obstetricians even among . the best of us. Far better is the accoucheur who knows *when* to operate *not how* to operate. The best operator is he who possesses the faculty of knowing both how and when to operate. Were I asked at this moment to select an obstetric attendant for my own· family I should ask that man who possesses the reasoning power of placing the indication over and opposed to one with requisite operative skill minus that peculiar erudite sense that makes him a master of the situation. Erudition is not born; it is made by sound preliminary training and profound experience. Generally speaking it can be stated as an unalterable truism that no labor should be interfered with except (1) there be present symptoms of a beginning maternal exhaustion as shown by rise in temperature and pulse rate, and on the presence of a contraction ring, all indicating the futility of the labor.

(2) Fetal exhaustion as evidenced by marked excursions of the fetal heart's action, the presence and continuance of an umbilical souffle and the discharge of meconium. Should one or all of these manifestations arise the labor must be terminated to save fetus or mother. But how far can we go in the attempt to deliver a suffering fetus through a genital canal illy prepared for such rapid work? Os dilated or dilatable membranes recently ruptured, makes the operation one of relative simplicity for a safe delivery of mother and child. Version when head above the brim, forceps when presenting head engaged. But when conditions are otherwise, how are we to act? Placing the life of the mother and the child on one plane and where a non cutting operation cannot be done, a Dührrsens by splitting the lower uterine zone or a vaginal Caesarean section in the cases where the cervix has not yet merged would seem to be the measures at our command. To attempt to deliver the fetus rapidly no matter what the indications, simply defeats our own ends and to this adds risks to the mother. To cope successfully with such an emergency in a woman whose os is hardly dilated, are we justified in subjecting her to the risk of a serious operation in order to attempt to deliver her of a living child? Can we operate quickly enough or deliver

sufficiently rapid to succeed without producing dangerous lesions? I think not. Where the canal can be easily dilated for rapid work it ought to be done. Under all other conditions I speak strenuously in favor of a waiting policy. This may be indirectly a plea for the use of craniotomy instruments. Be it as it may I feel that the furor for operating during labor has swung the pendulum too far. Where the child is in dire distress or where one feels that any prolonged operative interference will nullify that life in the attempt at delivery, or in all cases where the fetus is dead, we possess a useful and yet conservative field in the destructive operations on the unborn child. These are the indications for craniotomy and such allied operations. No indication for delivery should be determined by the clock, nor should the convenience of the physician nor pressure of practice ever be a determining factor for active interference. Neither should the insistence of sympathetic surroundings be the sole cause for consequential interference in what may only be an apparent dystocia. He who interferes only in the presence of definite indications will show himself the master mind of obstetrics. In any and all other cases he will regret at leisure—even though forced to act by environal circumstances and surroundngs.

Major operations in mal-positions and mal-presentations are rarely called for and can be dismissed in a line. I can readily imagine a case of dystocia from the above causes, which might cause a relative contraction of the pelvis. The head high up, waters long escaped with the concomitant spastic uterine contraction making version a dangerous operation and the fetus in good condition—calling for a Caesarean section, from the standpoint of scientific midwifery—but how very seldom is the privilege and sanction given us by the family to do this operation? Pubiotomy I ignore and wave to one side because of the uncertainty of the end results, especially in the primipara in whom there can be no question these complications are most likely to occur. The mortality may be low, but what about morbidity and future results, the unknown complications, and the fetal death rate, in an operation that is essentially a child's life saving operation?

We have therefore left only manual interference, version and forceps. A preliminary version might be done early but this savors too much of meddlesome midwifery for in the vast numbers of cases normal restitution occurs sooner or later. Version done late is likely to be dangerous, for we must remember that one of the earliest symptoms is the discharge of the amniotic fluid and if the labor be at all prolonged tetany of the uterus occurs and a forced version done under these conditions may cause a uterine rupture. But if these conditions do not obtain a deliberate internal version and breech delivery by the mechanism hinted earlier in the paper, should give good results. Manual interference, whether the face or vertex presents is from a personal standpoint immaterial. Both are readily managed, for I· look even upon a face as requiring little attention, except as advising forced extension and postural treatment. Any complex manipulations are not in order. To convert to a posterior occiput a normal chin anterior case is irrational since it is well known that the former positions give us more trying conditions when they fail to rotate than normal face cases. Where post chin cases fail to rotate—and this is very seldom, I have repeatedly, by full hand introduction, flexed the head and obtained a normal anterior

occiput. Repeated attempts have been made by the writer to correct post occiputs by rotation of the entire body and the head. But in most instances failure has been the result or at best temporary success only.

And finally the head engaged or in rare cases where version in contraindicated and yet the head is above the brim, forceps and their use finish the discussion in this subject. The keynote of this article before the attempt at forceps delivery, must ever be remembered. Indications must be present, then go ahead. What form or variety of instruments is used depends upon the forceps one is used to. The success depends not upon what forceps is used but upon the man behind it. Follow nature as much as possible, rotate with or without nature's efforts and attempts. If rotation occurs under your unconscious influence, well and good. Failure simply means that nature's efforts at rotation are futile, then the manual dexterity of the accoucheur substitutes artificial rotatory means and for this purpose the axis traction instruments are simply perfect in their marked mechanical skill.

947 Madison Ave.

THE TREATMENT OF ABORTION IN THE PRESENCE OF FEVER.[1]

BY

HERMAN J. BOLDT, M. D.,
New York City.

Different kinds of bacteria are recognized as causative in the production of temperature during the puerperium. Owing to the fact that anaerobic bacteria have been found in the blood, and that in many fatal cases, anaerobic streptococci were found, it would seem that we would do well to regard every

[1] Read at a meeting of the Eastern Medical Society, Apr. 12, 1912.

instance of fever during the puerperium as a genuine infection.

The treatment of this class of patients has become a subject of much discussion. Winter of Koenigsberg, has questioned whether it would not be better policy, in cases in which fever is present, caused by a piece of retained placenta, to make use of the expectant plan of treatment, and wait for a spontaneous expulsion of the foreign substance, for such it must be regarded under such circumstances. Frequently after the removal of a part of a retained placenta, an elevation of temperature already being present, the patient has subsequently died of a fatal infection. Is this brought about by the original retained piece of placenta or the traumatism caused by its removal? The answer is entirely speculative.

Because of Fromme's bacteriological investigations, it has been advised by some authors, that in the presence of virulent hemolytic streptococci in the uterine cavity, not to enter it for the purpose of removing retained parts, but to limit such intervention to cases where only decomposition products were present. Most observers agree that if other micro-organisms, except gonococci and liquifying staphylococci, are present, to the exclusion of streptococci, one should undertake active intervention. Of course imperative indications as profuse hemorrhages contraindicate a "let alone policy," despite the presence of dreaded micro-organisms.

Another class of clinicians consider that other clinical symptoms as chills or an increase of micro-organisms in the blood are an indication for active therapy.

Another author denies the possibility of sapremia or putrid intoxication and believes that every elevation of temperature indicates a genuine infection. He advises that the uterus should be emptied and cleaned out immediately.

A number of years ago I reported two patients from my postgraduate hospital service, who had micro-organisms circulating in the blood, one having staphylococci and the other streptococci. No active treatment was undertaken for either, and both made an uninterrupted recovery. The temperature was not higher than 103 degrees F. at any time, so the mere fact that micro-organisms are in the blood does not necessarily give an unfavorable prognosis. Although the presence of micro-organisms in the blood need not lead to an unfavorable prognosis in all cases, yet we must realize that true bacteremia is a *very* serious condition, and that the mixed infections. are particularly dangerous.

The most important result of the bacteriological studies, combined with clinical observation, is, that we cannot, from the bacteriological examination of the blood, give an invariably correct prognosis. But we can make some important deductions as to the treatment of patients with fever which is caused by an incomplete abortion. Placental remnants undergoing changes by saprophytic or virulent bacteria making their habitat there, are in intimate relation with the maternal circulation and some organisms may find an entrance into the blood. We are not likely to believe that when bacteria are circulating in the blood and were caused to disappear as the result of emptying the uterus, that the condition was a genuine septic infection. Yet even if we take it for granted that we have only a saprophytic infection, it cannot be denied that in some cases at least, a more serious condition may result therefrom so that staphylococci, bacillus aerogenes capsulatus, and other forms may be mingled with virulent types of micro-organisms, and therefore we should at the earliest possible moment, change the incomplete abortion to a complete abortion.

Taking a careful review of the scientific work in the bacteriological studies and considering the frequent positive bacteriological findings, one is drawn to the conclusion that in all cases of incomplete abortion, no matter what the bacteriological findings may seem, the uterus should be divested as soon as possible of its placental remnants. This should be done without inflicting traumatism. If we cannot enter the uterine cavity with the finger because of smallness of the canal, the cervix should be most carefully dilated and the remnants removed manually. A curetting should *never* be done.

REPORT OF TWO CASES OF CAE-SAREAN SECTION.[1]

BY

SAMUEL W. BANDLER, M. D.,
New York City.

I wish to report these two cases of Caesarean section, one a primigravida, the other pregnant for the third time. In each case the possibility of a Caesarean section was held in mind for some time before labor. In both the placenta was encountered in making the uterine incision.

The first patient showed measurements somewhat below the normal. At no time during the latter months of pregnancy could the vertex be readily made out per vaginam. During the last two weeks there was no attempt at fixation of the head in the pelvic brim, a thing which in the primigravida is always significant. This patient went into labor, and after a labor of

eighteen hours there was absolutely no progress toward fixation, much less toward moulding. The question of Caesarean section was broached and readily acceded to inasmuch as I had mentioned the probability of this procedure to the husband two weeks before. I removed her to the Post Graduate Hospital on December 20th, 1911, promising to give her an additional test for several hours. She was given a further test of labor for several hours and was then in a very exhausted condition, but the fetal heart was well heard. Abdominal Caesarean section was performed and she was delivered of 9½ pound boy. In this case the placenta was encountered in making the incision through the anterior uterine wall.

The second patient had had two children. One is living which weighed only five pounds when born. The second child weighed over ten pounds and was extracted by forceps with great laceration of the perineum, and was born dead.

The patient was seen by me for the first time during the middle months of her third pregnancy. She was very stout, had a large amount of liquor amnii, and it was not easy to make out the size of the fetus, as at no time during the last few weeks of pregnancy did the head present to the examining finger. Because of the previous favorable experience with the small child the patient was allowed to go to term instead of having labor induced some weeks before the expected time. The patient went into labor at full term and after a little manipulation the vertex presented at the pelvic brim. She was given the test of labor for a period of twenty-four hours. Examination showed a very large head, absolutely no moulding. Patient had the choice between abdominal Caesarean section, or vaginal extraction with death to the fetus as the probable outcome.

[1]Read at a meeting of the Eastern Medical Society, April 12, 1912.

She chose the former. I operated upon her on the 11th of February, at the Post Graduate Hospital, and delivered her of an 11 pound baby. In this case too the incision through the uterus encountered the placenta.

In sewing the uterus I made use of a suture which is useful in keeping the subsequent field of uterine sewing clear of blood from the uterine cavity. This suture is passed from side to side in a longitudinal direction, very much like a subcuticular suture but close to the endometrium. It serves to shut off the uterine cavity from the area which we are uniting, and it allows us to pass the sutures which unite the two edges of the uterine incision down to this suture and thus assures that we are close to the mucosa but not through it. At the same time the field of operation is not obscured by blood.

134 W. 87th St.

FOUR INTERESTING OBSTETRICAL CASES.

BY

A. J. RONGY, M. D.,
New York City.

Adjunct Gynecologist, Lebanon Hospital; Attending Surgeon, Jewish Maternity Hospital; Consulting Gynecologist, Rockaway Beach Hospital.

I believe the cases here reported well illustrate the rapid progress the practice of obstetrics has made in recent years. The indications and contraindications for the various obstetrical operations made necessary by pelvic deformity are being studied and classified so carefully that it will be only a short time before the obstetrician will have a definite course to pursue in a given case of dystocia.

CASE I. *Vaginal Caesarean for Eclampsia.* Mrs. B., patient of Dr. Max Bressler, 18 years old, para I in last month of pregnancy. In the second month patient began to vomit and suffered from general symptoms accompanying the first three months of pregnancy. In the fourth month the legs became edematous and evidently showed signs of nephritis. At the beginning of the 9th month of pregnancy patient began to suffer from headaches, dizziness and disturbances of vision; she vomited a few times and passed a scanty amount of urine. A few days later she was suddenly seized with convulsions of a rather severe type lasting one to two minutes.

At this juncture I was asked to see the patient, found her in complete coma. She was constantly kept under chloroform to prevent another on-coming convulsion. I hurriedly transferred her to the Jewish Maternity Hospital and ordinary anti-eclamptic remedies like fluidext. veratrum viride, etc., were immediately administered. Vaginal examination proved the cervix thick, elongated, not taken up by presenting part. It was evident that manual dilatation would be impossible in this case. Notwithstanding the treatment, patient began to have convulsions again, lasting for a few minutes at a time and became thoroughly cyanosed.

At this stage the patient's condition was such that rapid delivery was the only course to resort to in order to save her life so that vaginal Caesarean section and high forceps extraction was decided upon, and a live baby weighing 6 lbs. was extracted. Baby lived for six hours. Patient had one convulsion after operation was finished.

Her convalescence was very stormy as she developed a double lobar pneumonia on the third day which lasted fully two weeks. She finally commenced to improve and was discharged from the hospital at the end of four weeks.

Vaginal Caesarean section particularly in the last month of pregnancy is a difficult operation and it should be undertaken by obstetricians of fair gynecological training. The more pregnancy is advanced the more difficult is the operation if forceps is to be used in extracting the child. In order to have sufficient room the uterus should be divided both anteriorly and posteriorly for unforeseen lacerations in the uterine wall

320   AMERICAN MEDICINE }
Complete Series, Vol. XVIII. }   ORIGINAL ARTICLES   { JUNE, 1912.
New Series. Vol. VII., No. 6.

may take place if delivery is attempted through an anterior opening only. Vaginal Caesarean section has an advantage over forcible dilatation even if such a procedure were possible in some of these cases, because we are dealing with a regular cut surgical wound which can be treated in a surgical manner while in the other methods of delivery the lacerations and injury to the cervix and uterus are so irregular that repair is almost impossible, if not futile.

Rubin Patterson, in his last analysis of over 500 vaginal Caesarean sections for eclampsia proved conclusively that the maternal as well as foetal mortality is less by this method than by the combined other methods. The shock from the operation itself is practically little and does not interfere with proper convalescence. It has an advantage over the abdominal section that the peritoneal cavity is not entered and also the shock that usually accompanies abdominal operations is absent.

Vaginal Caesarean for eclampsia should be performed in those cases only where the cervix is rigid, elongated and manual dilatation is apparently impossible. I think this condition mostly found in primiparas is better treated by this method than by any of the other methods, including the non-surgical, non-scientific, and greatly injurious method of Bossi. I think the method advocated by Bossi of forcible dilatation of· cervix by a four-pronged steel instrument is never justifiable, and should not be performed. I also believe that a cervix that is long and rigid cannot possibly be forcibly dilated by either hand or instrument so that the foetal head can be safely delivered through it; that in cases in which forcible dilatation is used and followed by immediate delivery that a great deal of irreparable injury to the soft parts is done and the patient is left in a poorer physical state than if vaginal Caesarean would have been performed.·

CASE II. *Pubiotomy.* Mrs. A. S., patient of Dr. I. Ritter, age 34, para I. Patient began to have labor pains on Jan. 3. Pains were rather irregular and weak. During the 4th membranes ruptured. On the same day about 8 p. m. pains became stronger and came more often. Breech presenting and cervix was fully dilated. Jan. 5, during the entire day, notwithstanding strong pains she had had there

was very little progress. Patient began to show signs of exhaustion towards evening, pulse rose to 120-130, temperature 101.

I was asked to see patient about 8 p. m. of the same evening and on examination I found breech presenting, child rather large, pelvis contracted, of the justo minor type. Diagonal conjugate measured 10 plus. It was evident from external examination that the child was large and out of proportion to the pelvis. Foetal heart sounds were good. The chances of delivering a living child under these conditions was apparently improbable. In the interest of the child pubiotomy was suggested as a method of procedure and with but little additional risk to the mother. The attending physician and the family concurring, the patient was removed to the Jewish Maternity Hospital. The patient was prepared for delivery and a Gigli saw introduced as a prophylactic measure, and the legs of the child brought down. It was very evident from the appearance of the lower extremities that the child was large and well developed and that extraction through a contracted pelvis was impossible. The foetal heart sounds still being good, pubic section was performed and a living child weighing 9 lbs. 10½ oz. was delivered.

The separation of the cut ends of the bones was almost two inches giving just sufficient space to deliver the head. The child was born asphyxiated but was finally resuscitated at the end of ½ hour.

Pubiotomy has a definite field in modern obstetrics. It should never compete with abdominal Caesarean section. Cases in which pubiotomy is indicated, Caesarean section is contraindicated and vice versa. It is an operation of emergency and should be performed in those cases which have been misjudged or neglected, when the child is still viable. The operation adds but little risk to the mother and it certainly saves a great number of children. I think the method of Döderlein is the one best to follow and that the hemorrhage accompanying this method can be very readily controlled by pressure. Convalescence is not very much prolonged if no complication sets in. I usually allow them to leave the bed on the 15th day and discharge them from the hospital at the end of three weeks.

One of the greatest dangers in this operation is injury to the bladder but if the ordinary precautions are taken I believe this danger will be minimized. In this case the birth of a live child would have been impossible as the diameters of the head (bi-parietal 10) were out of proportion to the pelvis, in addition to which both arms were extended.

CASE III. *Central Placenta Previa.* "Mrs. N., patient of Dr. J. Chasis, 28 years old, para III, last pregnancy eleven years ago. All previous labors instrumental. Patient's condition during present pregnancy normal. She began to bleed profusely three days before being seen by me. Internal examination revealed a moderately contracted pelvis with central placenta previa presenting. Os rigid and cervical canal intact. As a result of these findings patient was taken to hospital. Abdominal Caesarean section performed, live full term child extracted. Post-operative T. 99.8, P. 126, R. 28. Immediately afterwards, patient began vomiting a brownish fluid, 1-2 drams at a time and this most distressing feature continued with slight periods of intermission for four days. There was slight abdominal distention and some pain; urine scanty with some traces of albumen but no casts. At this time P., T., R. were 140, 99.6, 32, respectively. For relief of vomiting a lavage with one quart sat. sol. Mag. sulphate followed by one pint sterile water was given. Patient became markedly worse, respiration rose to 58, pulse to 140, with restlessness and cyanosis. Administrations of morphine, nitroglycerine and digitalis quieted the patient. Patient began to show uremic signs; vomiting became fecaloid, there was distention, constipation and suppression of urine, only vi ounces being passed in next 24 hours. Temperature reaction was slight, 99.2-100.2; P. 120-148, R. 30-50.

A few of the therapeutic measures tried were hypodermoclysis, hot packs, salines per rectum, poultices to kidneys, cardiac stimulants, etc. Notwithstanding all therapeutic measures, kidneys refused to act, patient only passing vi.5i in the next 24 hours, finally dying of cardiac failure, 4 days after the laparotomy."

I believe that abdominal Caesarean section is indicated in a small per cent on centrally implanted placentae previae, where the cervix is rigid and not taken up and where the hemorrhage is active. These patients will lose less blood by this operation than by the older methods of treatment and it was particularly indicated in this case as she had given a history of difficult instrumental deliveries and the parts were quite rigid on account of eleven years interval between this and the last pregnancy. We had no opportunity of studying her kidneys as her operation was urgent, but I believe that this was the proper procedure in this case notwithstanding the probable slight affection of the kidneys that would have shown had her urine been thoroughly examined beforehand. I can recollect a number of cases of centrally implanted placenta previa which have terminated fatally from acute anemia that would have been saved if Caesarean section had been performed before active hemorrhage took place.

One of the great advantages of preventing secondary post partum hemorrhage, usually a great danger in these cases, is that the uterus can be tightly packed from above so that additional loss of blood will not take place. Once hemorrhage in placenta previa cases is stopped in time so that the patient does not become acutely anemic, the risk of undergoing abdominal Caesarean section will add very little to enhance recovery.

CASE IV. *High Forceps.* Mrs. R. S., patient of Dr. N. Schechter, 26 years old, Russian, married 4½ years ago, para III, first pregnancy normal, child small (mother's statement). Second labor instrumental, child surviving only a few hours.

Patient went into labor on Jan. 1, having weak irregular pains. Pains became stronger on Jan. 2, membranes ruptured and cervix was 2 fingers dilated. At one a. m. Jan. 2, cervix was fully dilated, pains regular and strong, coming at intervals of 5-7 minutes. Notwithstanding these pains patient made very little progress during the entire night, head attempting to engage but could not pass obstruction in the form of an exotosis situated between the first and second sacral vertebra. Patient began to show signs of exhaustion and her attending physician thought that immediate delivery was imminent.

I was called to see her about 10.30 a. m. Jan. 2, and on examination found cervix fully dilated, uterus rather thin, waters drained off, head attempting to engage above the bony obstruction. Patient having no living children, anxiety for a living child was great. It was evident that the delivery of a living child through this pelvis with a head unmoulded, was not likely. The surroundings of the patient to attempt any important operation were not ideal and therefore I advised her removal to the Jewish Maternity Hospital where she was admitted about 12 m. same day.

The general condition of the patient being poor and the long history of labor eliminated any surgical interference and a conservative plan of treatment was decided upon. She was given a hypo of ¼ gr. morphine and her pains ceased, giving her time to rest and doze off for the next few hours. Her pains commenced again in the evening and became quite strong and regular forcing the head into the inlet of the pelvis. Once engagement of the head took place we thought it better to wait and see whether the bi-parietal diameter could not pass by the obstruction and on examination at 10 p. m. we found the head wedged right into the inlet, somewhat moulded, apparently making it possible to deliver by high forceps. Patient was prepared for delivery and after a rather difficult extraction a living child was delivered.

I believe that the high forceps operation should be eliminated from the category of modern obstetrical procedures; formerly when this operation was resorted to, it was the only alternative the obstetrician had as a life saving measure to the mother but with modern surgical technique, and asepsis and antisepsis developed it should not any more occupy the prominent place it has heretofore in our obstetrical work. It fails to meet with the three essential elements that should govern the practice of obstetrics to-day. It produces the greatest amount of morbidity of the mother. Probably no operation causes more septic infections than this. It causes the greatest number of children to be still born, the infant mortality of high forceps delivery in the hands of the experienced is nearly 50%. It is non-surgical because an attempt is made to drag through by sheer force a fetal head that is out of proportion to the cavity through which it is to pass. Plastic operations on the vaginal vault are brought about by the indiscriminate use of the high forceps operation and in many instances the repair of these lacerations and injuries is almost impossible. In this case high forceps was used as the only conservative operation as far as the mother was concerned because her general health being so poor it was dangerous to undertake any other method of procedure.

ALTITUDES.

BY

E. S. GOODHUE, A. M., M. D.,
The Doctorage, Hawaii.

Fortunately for us, our charts and maps of a smooth, round earth, are to be taken as figuratively true only. As an actual fact, we have mountains and valleys, plains and plateaus, sea-level and the rising slopes which pass upwards into regions of rarified air. These inequalities of surface prevent climatic alignment along regular sections of the earth's surface, disturb geographic homogeneity, and force isothermal lines outside of mere parallels of latitude.

The mountains of a torrid zone endow their slopes with the coolness of more northerly climates, and, despite their location, are crowned with perpetual ice and snow.

Climatic isotrophy then, must be determined by other methods than a mere graduation of the earth's surface into regular mathematical zones. In other words, altitude comes in, that is, height or elevation above sea-level. And yet climate—that intangible and variable entity which is dependent upon so many phenomena—does not readily yield its attributes to one factor, but is modified in turn by various other influences.

The weight of air above upon a given space (barometric pressure), bears its relation to height, and we are at no trouble to determine the matter, but temperature while affected by altitude and latitude, is greatly modified by humidity and the movements of air. All, in turn, are modified by the proximity of high mountains and large bodies of water; by the local influences exerted by forested areas; by extensive treeless plains, sandy deserts or barren lava beds. The climate of a place then, is the result of the action and interaction of these various influences which, in the long run, are permanent and regular, provided the topographical conditions over which they act remain unchanged. The arrival of a glacial age, of course, would alter all the laws of ordinary modification, or the sinking of a continent under the sea!

There are certain definite effects of mere altitude, and the general influences of elevation upon the body are definite, modified by locality, as well as temperament and idiosyncrasy. Even in similar latitudes, where the elevation *is*, makes all the difference, whether in Colorado or different section of Colorado; in New Mexico, inland California or up in the Adirondacks. And in the tropics your high point in altitude must be greater than it is in the temperate zone to claim geographical characteristics. For instance, from the 46th to the 50th degree of latitude, an elevation of 8,000 feet and over is almost unbearable for long continued residence. The St. Bernard monks who live in arctic isolation with curtailed lives, are an example. While in Bogota nearly under the equator, at 9,000 feet, the climate is even salubrious; at La Paz, Bolivia, equally so, and in Arequipa, Peru, at an elevation of 8,000 feet, there is a temperature range of from 50 to 60 degrees only. The air being relatively dry, body heat is quickly reduced and health maintained.

"With the air at 50 or 60 degrees, there need be little perspiration unless there is free exercise. It is fortunate that the highest relative humidity of dry countries occurs at the time of lowest temperature, so that there is no discomfort from heat. When the air temperature is near that of the human body, or above it, the relative humidity is so low that temperatures of 5 or 10 degrees above the body heat are hardly noticed, so rapid is evaporation from the skin. Hence it is true that the perceptible temperature of the air may be very different from that shown by the thermometer."[1]

Pure air and sunlight are no doubt important factors in the restoration and maintenance of health. In defining an ideal climate Dr. Wheaton says:

"It would appear to be one possessing the greatest possible amount of sunshine; a mild climate; a pure, dry atmosphere; light winds, and porous soil, with elevation sufficient to increase the respiratory act in depth and vigor. But Dr. Bridge does not entirely agree: "Altitude," he says in his excellent book on tuberculosis, "has long been held to be beneficial in pulmonary tuberculosis, and probably with good reason. An elevation of three to five thousand feet above sea-level often starts a process of better nutrition in patients who come from lower levels. The change sometimes begins an improvement that goes on to recovery. The reason for the benefit is a matter of some speculation. A favorite theory long held was that the more rapid and deeper breathing required by the rarified air expanded lung vesicles and so helped to cure the disease. But I believe this theory is untenable, because it is no benefit to the dis-

[1]Tuberculosis, by Norman Bridge, M. D.

eased lung tissue, but the contrary, to have it expanded extremely.

It is well established now that as one journeys from a lower to a higher altitude the red corpuscles of the blood increase in number, there being perhaps a slight reduction in their diameter. In the time required to travel quickly to the top of a high mountain the number increases by some thousands for each cubic millimeter of blood. But not all the increase shown by the usual examinations of the blood is real; some of it is due to a rapid flow of the red corpuscles from the deeper vessels to the surface of the body. Such rapid changes in the blood elements are a hint of further changes as vital in the other physiologic conditions, that can explain any benefit to the sick far better than a suppositious influence on the mechanics of the lungs, due to rarified air."

Dennison of Colorado found that with increasing elevation there was a diminution of dust, smoke, and moisture in the air, and consequently greater purity. He concludes that as diathermancy increased with altitude, purity, dryness, coldness and rarifaction were concomitants.

Dr. Remondino who has made valuable contributions to our meteorological knowledge, thinks that "a low elevation with a dry soil" is to be preferred as a health location to more elevated regions. Now while an elevation of 3,000 to 10,000 feet may be beneficial in many cases of disease, it is not in all; it is disastrous in some, although all the other conditions of life may be favorable, and, excepting those patients who do better at sea-level and in a relatively humid area (and quite a number most certainly do), it seems to be agreed by our best climatologists that a "medium climate" and a moderate elevation is, on the whole, the safest place for persons sensitive to meteorologic influences.

"Regions at or about sea-level, some above and some below it, are as dry as any habitable place on earth. At the same time we have along our southern Atlantic and Pacific coasts many places where a mild sea climate can be found in perfection. There is a medium climate, less dry than the arid lands, but more so than the sea coast, with elevations approaching two thousand feet, that is grateful to a large proportion of pulmonary patients; it is beneficial to many of them as well."[1]

Dr. Carrington whose experience and judgment are worth considering, thinks that in New Mexico at least, the best results are secured at an elevation of 3,000 to 6,000 feet, but the majority of physicians who have made a study of the subject, believe in moderate elevations.

Dr. Bowditch recommends that sanatoria be placed "anywhere from 250 to 1,500 feet," and Dr. King believes that "sanatoria situated in high altitudes, that is, from 5,000 to 10,000 feet are far more limited in the scope of usefulness than is the case with those at more moderate elevations." His choice is 1,000 feet above tide-water, while the special committee appointed by the governor of New Hampshire as to a site for a state sanatorium, decided that an elevation of 500 feet was their preference.

In his account of the effects of extreme altitudes (12,000 to 14,000 feet) upon residents in Bolivia, Dr. Foster says that obese persons of limited lung capacity, suffer greatly from shortness of breath. Generally, respiration and pulse-rate are not increased, although the latter is perhaps more

[1] Tuberculosis, by Norman Bridge, M. D.

forcible. "The great amount of electricity present places the nervous system under a constant strain. Ten hours sleep at night are a necessity—a few suffer from insomnia. There is also a tendency to a loss of weight."

On the leeward side of Hawaii at sea-level, the climate is rather warm, especially in some locations, although the relative humidity is low, as at Lahaina, on Maui, Kailua, on Hawaii, and Waimea, on Kauai.

But at an elevation of 850 to 2,000 feet, especially on the Island of Hawaii where the great central mass of mountain slopes gradually to the sea, the leeward sides have a grateful as well as a salubrious climate. Here in this forested belt is the place for homes, and here nature has provided a natural sanatorium for many forms of disease. I doubt if there is a better climate in the world—a more comfortable climate, or one more conducive to the maintenance of a normal standard of health in the young and in the aged; yet is there not a worse place in the world for invalids who seek health, because we are absolutely without means of caring for them.

I should that on the Kona side of Hawaii an elevation of 900 feet is best for all classes of disease. As specified elsewhere, some locations even in this belt are preferable to others, according to topography.

On the windward sides, at sea-level, it is cooler owing to the constant trades, but, as a rule, it is humid and may often be sultry at night, and this humidity extends some distance up the mountainside.

Here are copious showers, and too great an annual rainfall for comfort. Between these places the climate partakes of both sections. At an elevation of 4,000 feet on the leeward sides, may be found a delightful bracing climate during summer, a little cold, even frosty in winter, and up as high as 8,000 feet, the weather in summer is delightful. Were these altitudes more accessible, I am sure they would furnish us with our most healthful and pleasant resorts.

ABYSSINIAN SUPERSTITION IN GYNECOLOGY.

BY

FELIX VON OEFELE, M. D.,
New York City.

Many times the practising physician meets with failure in his treatment of disease. This is so the world over. The sick may call their physician with every confidence; the physician may make an accurate diagnosis and inaugurate the best known and most appropriate treatment; but all too often the physician will observe that his patient fails to follow his instructions. The reason for this is usually found in the fact that the instruction or directions of the physician in some way run counter to some personal or general superstition of the patient, which superstition rules stronger than the reason. Therefore, it is very important for the practising physician to know and recognize the various superstitions that are common to the sick room. Dr. Glogau recently in the "gesellig-wissenschaftlichen Verein" considered the subject in a general way and sufficient for laymen. For medical men it is quite impossible to cover superstition of the laity in one writing. Therefore, I will consider only one chapter of this great subject and that will be Abyssinian Superstitions Relative to Abortion.

This chapter will show you also that medical superstition is pretty much the same not only throughout all countries of the world but also throughout all the thousands of years of history. Abyssinia was in the olden time close to the civilization of Egypt, Arabia and Babylonia. During the past two thousand years it has been far from the centre of civilization, in fact isolated in darkest Africa. The first evidences of Abyssinian superstition were found in certain small collections of native products and drawings, which came

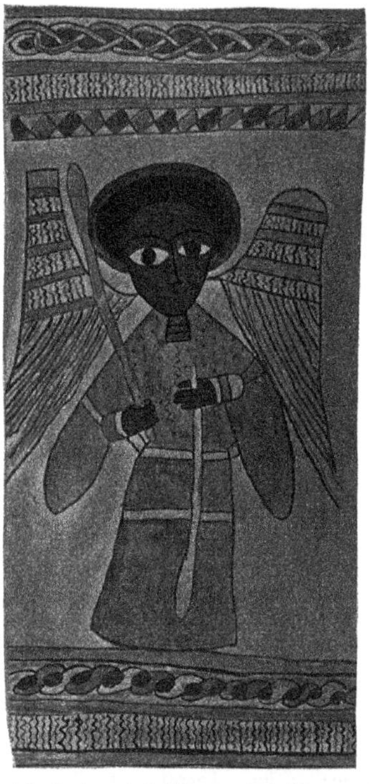

his material. A new and larger collection of native drawings and designs showing Abyssinian medical superstition is now in the Princeton University at Princeton, N. J., the illustrations herewith having been kindly loaned to me therefrom.

Professor W. H. Worrell of Hartford, Conn., has made a special study of this collection and I had the pleasure of meet-

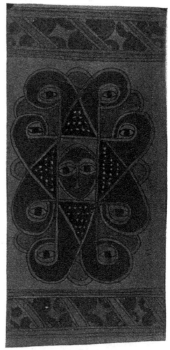

Fig. 1—Archangel fighting against demons of certain diseases—Original in the Princeton University.

Fig. 2—The twelve houses of the horoscope of astrology arranged as a cross and 2, 3, 5, 6, 8, 9, 11 and 12th house with an eye— Princeton University.

from Abyssinia to Russia, and were described in various publications by Turajeff, a Russian friend of mine. I received all his articles and have been in correspondence with him, therefore, I am familiar with

ing him this spring at an Orientalistic gathering at Columbia University. He sent me a number of painted drawings, copies of Abyssinian amulets. These amulets present to anyone with an astrological knowledge abundant proof of their astrological origin. The accompanying pictures particularly show that these amulets are mostly used against abortion. The basis of the charms is found in old Babylonian mythology concerning the demon "Labartu," the main idea throughout being that which happens in the heavens to the planets, happens in a similar manner on the earth to every human or living being.

Abyssinian charms or amulets—as Worrell describes—are made of from one to three strips of parchment or leather, which vary greatly in thickness and quality, sewn together with thongs of the same material, the whole forming a strip from 20 inches to 6 feet in length and from 2 inches to 10 inches in width. Many specimens of the Princeton collection have lost the beginning or end. The scroll thus formed originally was rolled tightly together and bound with cord or inserted in a telescoping capsule, sewn tightly in leather. Capsules and leather covered rolls are often strung together, to the number of five or six, and ornamented with beads.

Upon this material the Abyssinian *dabtara* writes the legends, spells, words of power, secret signs or other devices which are to make the charm effective. The appearance of such scrolls is unique. At the top is usually a picture of the Archangel Michael or Gabriel (Fig. 1) with sword in hand accompanied by smaller angelic figures or faces. Schematic horoscopes of spider-like forms, often with eyes (Figs. 2 and 3) or the twelve houses of the horoscope appear as a cross (Fig. 4) with sun and moon on either side, sometimes the fish, the serpent, the lion (or dog?) and the whole in indescribably fantastic figures combined with geometric designs in endless yet characteristic array. Only very rarely is there an illustration

bearing upon the accompanying text, as in the pictures noted in three instances of the saint Susneyos, the protector against abortion, who is seen mounted and attacking the demoness Werzelya, the original cause of abortion. The name of the possessor of the scroll appears many times throughout the roll. The space for the insertion of the name is left blank by the maker, the name being afterward filled in for the purchaser, and subsequently changed as many times as need be, as the roll passes from hand to hand, which is very often the case.

The substance of the spells is written in a script generally very much debased and in some instances assuming a character attributable only to a desire for the bizarre and mysterious, mixed with magical signs, (Fig. 5) suggesting on the one hand Abyssinian or Arabic letters, on the other, the signs which are found in Coptic and late Greek magical texts. The language is a more or less successful attempt at Gehez, the ancient, ecclesiastical and literary language of Abyssinia, commonly known as Ethiopic. The Amharic speaking scribe is everywhere evident; and in some instances the writer passes completely into the latter language.

Abyssinian charms are worn about the neck, or merely kept in the house of the possessor. It would seem from the texts that the presence of the roll is in itself sufficient for complete protection—a fetishtic idea which is common. There is also frequent mention of the immunity that comes to the one who reads the book.

The text of the scrolls, besides the figures, etc., above described, contains both simple spells and words of power, the whole being accompanied by legends explaining how they originated, were first used and came to have their efficacy. The

latter device is well known in magic literature from earliest Babylonian times onward. Prof. Worrell has gone into these
facts in detail.

The legend of Susneyos and Werzelya is
the most common against abortion. The
origin of this is as follows: The sun stands

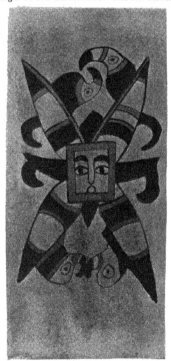

Fig. 3—Corruption of the horoscope cross above
—Princeton University.

in the center of the astrology. The sun in an
eclipse, the sun in the night or the sun
in the winter was for the superstitious people a dead or stolen sun, and the sun after
an eclipse or in the morning or in the spring,
was in one way the son of the previous
dead sun or the resurrected sun, or on the

other hand, the resurrected new born son
of the sun. That is the basis of the dis-
membered child in the astral myths according to Stucken. A superstitious
pregnant woman in uncivilized or unhealthy countries is liable to many accidents that may occasion an abortion. Naturally she wants to save her unborn child
from abortion as the sun is saved from
the dead. The people believe that some

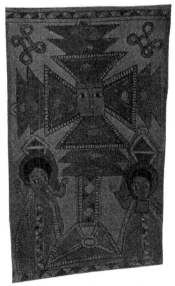

Fig. 4—More christianized corruption of the
horoscope cross—Princeton University.

short traditional incantations save the sun
every night and every winter. Every superstitious woman believes therefore that
the story of the resurrected sun, including
the original powerful incantations, will
protect and preserve her unborn child.

This story is the legend of Susneyos and
Werzelya. The general index of the
original legend is as follows: A man *A*
has impregnated his wife *B* (his sister?)

with an embryo C. In the absence of the father A there comes a wicked woman D and steals the embryo from the womb of the woman B. A comes back and finds B crying. Then A takes his horse and spear and pursues D in the desert. A has a liaison with an old woman sitting on a fence. This takes the place of the three ancient obstacles of the pursuer, the sitting woman replacing a transformation of D and the fence replacing a comb. Later on the pursuer finds D with some male companions (the planets Saturn and Mars) in a sexual orgy sacrificing the embryo C. Now comes a christian contamination in the Abyssinian form of the story. There is only a prayer of A to Christ left and the promise of Christ that A will overpower D. In the following fight between A and D, A spears D in the side and D must give out the stolen child C. Also A forces D to tell all her different names, because a knowledge of these names gives him, and also the special amulet, power over D and she is also forced herself to recite an incantation of the seven archangels (instead of "the seven planets of incantation of the seven old Babylonia) which keeps D and other influences away from every pregnant woman. D must swear in the future to stay away from every worshipper of A.

It is very interesting that the same story as found in many of the Princeton amulets was retained in Abyssinia in its ancient form until this century. It is especially noteworthy because Prof. W. Max Müller of the University of Pennsylvania has found other ancient traditions of Babylonian medicine in Dârfûr in Central-Africa. We find the same idea of overpowering D by A in old Babylonia and in the gospel, among the Moslems, the Koptes, the medieval Greeks, among modern Slavonic people and elsewhere in the world. The name of A in the Abyssinian texts is Susneyos and the name of D Werzelya. In other languages she has different names; in old Babylonia, Labartu, in medieval Greek, Gyloo. B has the Greek name Meletia. Instead of A we find sometimes

two brothers corresponding to the Dioscurs. In other stories instead of D often the tempter of the sister B is killed by the two brothers. The name Werzelya, in Coptic Berzelia, may be an old translation of the wife of the god Moloch to Greek as Basileia, but again changed in a Semitic meaning to Bersilia, meaning "the iron wife," in the same way as the name Berzelius, the well known chemist, means "the iron man." The text attributes to Werzelya from her name, iron hands killing the children. Susneyos may also in Semitic signify lily-man. In a parallel story of the gospel the woman B has the name Susanna, meaning lily-wife; the prophet Daniel there corresponds to A and two wicked men correspond to D.

To American physicians it cannot fail to be interesting in connection with the rich collection of amulets at Princeton that phases of this superstition are very frequently encountered in gynecological practice among Slavonic immigrants. But the persistent worshipping of Bersilia has more interest for the United States in another direction. The hoo doo cult of the American negro is only a derivative of an old Bersilia cult. The hoo doo cult of Louisiana and still of New York is Vaux doux-cult in Hayti and vicinity. There is reason to believe that in old Babylonia, there was a cult of the goddess Labartu. But we know more of the parallel cult of Moloch and Astarte in Phoenicia. In oldest Palestine there were frequent killings as a sacrifice to these gods. As a sacrifice to Astarte the girls had to sacrifice their virginity in the temple. Consequently the later Jewish priest must always wed a virgin, because his wife obviously should not be a worshipper of Astarte. Then there was in old Palestine a sacrifice of the first born son to these gods. As a consequence, we observe in the oldest part of the gospel the first born

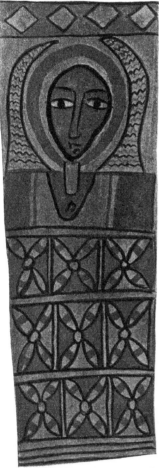

FIG. 5—An old Egyptian mummy as an Abyssinian protective picture—Princeton University.

everytime disappearing, as did Ishmael and Esau. So also Abel disappeared, the older

brother of Solomon from his mother Bathseba and very many others. We hear also, that Isaac should be sacrificed. We hear also in the gospel that Solomon and other Jewish kings made sacrifices of children to these gods. Also in Egypt the God of the Jews killed all of the first born sons of the Egyptians in Moses' time. In the later Jewish religion the freedom of the first born son is bought by two doves; and that is the end of the ritual killing of children in the prehistoric time in the Jewish religion.

But the other Palestine people, as for instance the Phoenicians, kept up the sacrifice of children, and it went over to Carthage and for a short time—as Pliny tells —to Rome. But it went from Carthage more to the South to Dahomey, where the French government even up to to-day has been unable to stop it. From there it went a long time ago to Hayti, where to this very day every year about 80,000 children are ritually sacrificed and eaten up by the worshippers of Vaux doux-cult. The main points of this hoodoo cult are the incarnation of a wicked god, an enemy of the Christian God often in the form of a snake; the use of stone amulets, the sacrifice of young pork, of young goats, of chickens (instead of doves as in Phoenician times) and of children, eating the flesh and drinking the blood of these sacrifices, and finally communistic sexual excesses. The cult music is produced from drums and triangles. Between four male priests, a priestess, the Mamaloi (instead of Mama Roi; means mother-king, or the highest woman of an oriental state) as a human representative of Werzelya has to kill the children. Only a few weeks ago we read in the newspapers of a negro girl of Louisiana, a recognized priestess of hoodoo, who had killed 17 other negroes. The American neurologist or better, psychologist in studying such cases, will find that they are traceable back to the Werzelya superstition.

From the foregoing it will be evident that all or nearly all of the superstitions of the civilized world are interwoven one with the other, and all of them are frequently encountered in scientific medicine, especially in connection with diseases of the genital tract of the female. Medical superstition is rife in every country; it is surprisingly prevalent in New York city. One can prove this from the astrological fakirs at the watering places. Unfortunately a sick woman will rarely if ever tell her physician of the superstitions that trouble her. Therefore, it is necessary for the practical physician to have a broad knowledge of different kinds of superstition, their sources or derivations and all about them in order to accomplish all that is possible in the mental as well as the medicinal treatment of disease. For this reason I am convinced that a knowledge of Abyssinian superstition is of value from a practical as well as from an anthropological point of view.

The illustrations herewith of specimens of drawings by Abyssinian natives are reproduced through the courtesy of Prof. W. H. Worrell of Hartford.

VISUAL MEMORY.

BY

AARON BRAV, M. D.,
Philadelphia.

Visual memory belongs to the domain of psychology and like all other psychic processes depends upon a physical stimulation or excitation that has made its impress upon a psychic centre.

Visual Memory.—Under this term we understand that phenomenon in the domain of psychology which enables us to recall to our consciousness whenever we so desire, objects we have seen and reproduce them in the form of a mental image. This is purely a psychic phenomenon and does not depend upon the visual acuity. The acuity of vision may be below normal, may even be so reduced as to prevent us from obtaining an absolute pure image of an object sighted, yet the visual memory may be perfect. Even after the visual acuity has entirely been destroyed the psychic element known as visual memory may still be present. The man who by accident has become blind is still able to recall to his mind's eye images that he has observed long before he became blind. On the other hand we may find a normal visual apparatus whose physiologic function is harmonious, giving rise to perfect vision, in which the psychic phenomenon of visual memory may be either deranged or entirely destroyed so that objects are plainly seen but are not recognized.

Function of Visual Memory.—The function of our visual memory is:

(1) To store up images seen to enable us to recognize them when we see them again.

(2) To enable us to analyze and differentiate objects that have a close resemblance to one another.

(3) To reproduce mentally in our consciousness images seen before.

(4) To reproduce physically images seen before and improve them if necessary by the aid of the imagination.

(5) To stimulate the imaginative powers.

Recognition.—By this term we understand that psychic process that enables us to know certain things that once formed a part of our consciousness and reproduce them in a conscious form through the aid of the visual memory. It is obvious that the sense of vision is an important factor in the development in this psychic process. When an object is seen the excitation produced in the optic nerve fibres is trans-formed into a sensory sensation so that the object comes within the domain of consciousness. The excitation produces permanent changes in the ganglionic cells which becomes so intense especially after repeated excitation by the same object, that if years afterward we encounter the same object although perhaps long forgotten 'we are still, even without any effort, able to recall the object to our mind. Recognition differs however from visual memory in so far that in recognition we have again a physical excitation by the object which we recognize as one we have seen before, the stimulus or excitation traveling over the same path where the previous excitation left permanent changes and like a phonographic record reproduces the previous impression, while in visual memory we recall objects, although we also recognize them, not by means of physical excitation for the object in reality is not present but by a subjective sensation in which the mind alone acts as the excitant. The principle however is the same.   A permanent impression on the path leading from the visual tract to the visual psychic centre and from there to the visual memory centre. Recognition means the power of identifying objects that at present set up the same excitation in the visual tract, that a similar object produced some time ago. It is reasonable however to state with a degree of certainty that the same mental process is produced in mental imagery but here we do not have the object in physical form to stimulate the visual tract and the

psychic path, but the thought of the object, or the object in an idea, stimulating primarily psychically the visual tract and then is transformed into a sensory sensation. The cycle essential for visual perception however is practically the same. The point I wish to make is this, that no mental image can be produced without first stimulating the visual apparatus either by means of physical or through psychical forces or objects. The congenital blind therefore cannot mentally form an image in his consciousness as there has never been any permanent change or path formed by a previous physical stimulation of an object.   Physical stimulation of the optic nerve is therefore essential in mental imagery.

Conditions Influencing Visual Memory. —It is the experience of every observer that certain objects seen before cannot be either recognized or identified while others can be recalled with ease and vividness and it is necessary to explain this rather curious phenomenon. The following conditions influencing visual memory may offer a solution to the problem.

Visual Attention. —When in the regular walk of life we see numerous objects every minute, the various physical stimulations rapidly succeed one another without making any special impression; under such circumstances the confused impression arising from the images superseding one another quickly fade away leaving no imprint upon the visual and psychic part. The visual wave if it could be measured would be found to travel on an equal level without rise or fall, visual memory under such circumstances is either imperfect or entirely impossible. When however in the routine act of vision one object is attended by visual attention there is at once a rise in the wave of visual sensation making a marked impress on the visual path by producing a permanent change; such objects that are attended by this visual attention can easily be recognized years later either in physical form or in mental imagery. Permanent changes therefore in the visual tract are in direct ratio to the interest any object seen evokes in our consciousness. Thus an object of vital interest to us in which we are largely concerned which we have carefully observed for any length of time, and which have made an impression upon us, can be brought to our consciousness with the aid of our will.

Objects seen frequently also can be recalled to our consciousness for the same reason, although not accompanied by visual attention for they have through repeated stimulation left an impress upon the visual path.

Visual memory may be cultivated by means of attention or concentration of mind at the time when the object is first seen.

The Relation of the Motor Apparatus in Visual Memory. —This subject seems to have escaped both the ophthalmologist as well as the psychologist. But the question is a fair one, what about the accommodation and convergence? Do the internal and external ocular muscles perform any physiologic function in the psychic process of mental imagery?

We all agree of course that every psychic process must have some physical stimulus either in the present or past for its basis. We have further endeavored to show that visual memory is merely a reproduction of a former psychic concept that had as its primary basis a physical excitation. We also tried to explain that every image formed or rather perceived as

a mental image of visual memory must go through the same visual arc, namely excitation in the retina and optic tract to the psychic centre, with the only difference that while in physical vision or objective vision the stimulus comes from without, in the process of visual memory the excitation comes from within reflexly, stimulating the optic nerve and tract even as in ordinary vision. That being the case the optic nerve being stimulated the question arises, are the muscles also stimulated to activity in this form of subjective vision, even as they are and must be active in objective vision in order to produce a clear image? To this question if my observation be correct my answer will be in the affirmative. To this conclusion I came after the following experiment which we all observe while looking at some object from far and near. By looking at an object especially of a large size from a distance of several meters, then bring some object to about 15 centimeters from the eye, we at once feel a change of effort in our eye which is attributable to the action of both the internal and external ocular muscles. Now the same experiment can be tried with eyes closed. When we close our eyes and bring to our consciousness a visual image of say a large building standing at a considerable distance and then suddenly change this mental picture by thinking of a small object say a pencil about 10 centimeters distant we at once feel a sensation of effort of muscular contraction. The eyes actually fix the object near and are in a state of convergence. This proves that the stimulation reflexly excites the periphery of the visual apparatus and has to pass through the same visual arc, as is the case in objective vision. We can appreciate this more markedly if we with eyes closed try to read by means of our visual memory or image some lines from a book when we find that our eyes will make the same movement for fixation as if we were objectively engaged in reading a book.

Disturbance of Visual Memory.—As in the visual function there is a reduction in the acuity of vision when the various media that enter into the visual act are diseased so in mental imagery there is a diminution in the power to recognize objects or recall them mentally when the cortical visual memory centre is disturbed or the path leading up to this centre. This may entirely be absent. This has of course been experimentally established. In presenting this paper it is not my intention to intrude upon the domain of neurology but report this little observation relative to the subject of the motor and sensory apparatus of the eye in mental imagery or visual memory.

917 Spruce St.

THE DISPENSARY PATIENT.[1]

BY

LUCETTA MORDEN, M. D.

Brooklyn, N. Y.

I chose this subject because of its interest to druggists, physicians and dentists. Perhaps not so much to the last at the present time as it promises to be in the future.

We all realize the necessity and value of the dispensary, particularly in large cities. They, like hospitals, should be located where they are most needed—in congested districts, where medical attention needs

---

[1]Read before the American Medico-Pharmaceutical League.

to be obtained quickly and without expenditure of car fare.

Dispensaries are supported by the city, by voluntary contributions, and by receipts from sale of drugs and tickets.

In every one there is posted in a conspicuous place a notice of the law stating who are entitled to treatment and the punishment for violation. Are there offenders? Are they punished? I think you will agree with me that the answer to the first question is "yes," and to the latter, "no," in most instances at any rate. I have never heard of an offender being prosecuted.

Just a glance at the different motives prompting patients to go to the dispensaries:

1st. Poverty—The only reason why they should go.

2nd. Recommendation of others—"I go there, why don't you come too?"

3rd. There are better physicians or specialists there. Their opinion and advice is preferred.

4th. Matter of convenience—"It is only a few steps away so I also go."

5th. Ignorance—"I did not know that dispensary doctors have offices or make house calls."

6th. "Drug bill is higher than doctor's bill, therefore, I go to the dispensary." I know of a case of a bookkeeper who goes to the dispensary regularly for pepsin.

7th. Grafters—"The city pays for everything, why should I go to a private doctor?" Those with large bank accounts have said, "why pay out money when you can get it for nothing or next to nothing?" Recently a tenant met her landlady, a large property owner, at a city dispensary where even medicine is free!

So much for the abuse of the dispensary. There are three things which I wish to emphasize particularly concerning its proper use.

1st. The establishment of more evening clinics.

2nd. Dividing the city into districts for dispensary classes, as the Board of Health has divided it for supervision of tuberculosis.

3rd. Investigation of patients.

At the present time, very few dispensaries are open at night. To do the most good for the greatest number this should not be the case. Now men and women, married and single who are obliged to go to work, are the sufferers, i. e., the wage earners—those who should be in the best possible physical condition. Why should they neglect themselves? Because being absent from work means deduction in week's wages, or if repeated, loss of position. The result is, they stick to their work while their physical condition becomes worse and worse until they are obliged to stop work, and they and their family become a public charge. I think we agree that the best directed philanthropy is dealing with the curable rather than the incurable—that is, *before too late.* It seems to me that the employees of all factories, laundries, department stores, etc., should have compulsory systematic examinations by physician and dentist and made to follow out treatment advised. This would be beneficial not only to the individual but also to their families, their fellow employees and to the public generally. Is is right to allow a patient to work in a cigar factory with advanced tuberculosis? Should we not have evening classes where she can go—is made to go if necessary—when she has the first symptom? Mothers often find it difficult to leave little ones at home under proper care

while they go to the dispensary for treatment during the day. Evening classes are especially desirable for diseases needing long treatment while the patient is still able to or is obliged to work in the meantime.

Districting the city is another important matter upon which I wish to speak a few minutes. It would be of material advantage to the patient, doctor, nurse or social worker.

Advantages to the patient:

1. He would attend more regularly.

2. No time or money lost in transportation.

3. He would not be taking medicine from several doctors at the same time.

4. Ultimate result more satisfactory.

To the doctor:

1. An opportunity would be afforded him to pursue a definite line of treatment.

2. He would see the results of his labor.

3. He would not be taking a history, examining and advising a patient who had gone through the same program in another dispensary or several of them a few days before.

4. He would do better work, knowing that his responsibility is greater.

To the nurse or social worker:

1. More than one nurse from different parts of the city should not be visiting the same family.

2. She would learn more about the family and advise more judiciously.

3. Know if others in family needed medical attention.

4. She would be looked upon as a friend —not an intruder.

Cases have been known where as many as half a dozen, if not more, cards from various dispensaries have fallen out of a patient's pocket. There are patients who are attending more than one dispensary and being treated by a private doctor at the same time. Finally, there are patients who wander from dispensary to dispensary because one bottle of medicine or a day's time will not cure a disease requiring weeks, months or years to cure or that is possibly incurable.

Districting will do a great deal to remedy the above. It could be reduced to a perfect system eventually. Great good by so doing has been accomplished in the tuberculosis campaign, but even here there is room for improvement. A patient will be directed to go to a certain dispensary in his district. He goes once—concludes he doesn't like it and then wanders off to another or several, thus losing time as far as his own physical health is concerned and needlessly putting the physician to great trouble—increasing his work and thus preventing him from giving the necessary time to other patients to whom it is due. In intervals such a patient is quite likely to get in the hands of the "sure cure" advertiser who treats with X-ray or inhalations.

Home conditions and financial standing of dispensary patients should be investigated. As far as I know, there are no dispensaries where this is carried on. The clerk who gives tickets may question—if the patient is well dressed or adorned with jewelry, etc. Nine times out of ten, the patient is wise enough to reply, "No, I cannot afford to pay a private doctor." Some dispensaries, I believe, refer a few to a charitable organization for investigation. The dispensary is one of the most abused privileges today. Men, women and children, are all guilty of violating the law. As a rule, it is not the established physician or the noted specialist who suffers, because their clientele come from a different class, but it is the young physician whose charges are modest and who could easily be paid by

these violators. This also holds good in operative work. And it is the patient who could not pay $25.00 to have her child's adenoids removed, but who could pay $5.00 or $10.00 who is the most frequent transgressor.

In annual dispensary reports in which appeals are made, the average contributor is attracted by the number of patients treated. This factor decided the amount of the donation, hence all dispensaries seek large attendance to make a good showing at the end of the year. I think this is one reason why practically none are refused treatment and why investigations are not made. I understand that physicians are not supposed to refer any patient to another dispensary if that particular ailment is treated there.

Managers of hospitals and dispensaries feel under obligation to contributors, and the latter expect the best care gratis to all their employees, or those in whom they are especially interested, regardless of their position or financial standing. Among them we find ministers, bookkeepers, stenographers, chauffeurs, all of whom are able and should patronize private physicians.

145 Milton St.

_____

APPENDICITIS AND THE BEST TIME TO OPERATE.

BY

BEVERLEY ROBINSON, M. D.,
New York City.

It is refreshing indeed, to a man who has followed the doings of physicians and surgeons for many a year, to have the truth told about an important disease, which occurs daily. The man who tells the tale is Sir G. T. Beatson, *Lancet*, May 11, 1912; the disease is appendicitis.

According to Beatson it is judicious in only very rare instances relatively, to interfere surgically, during the acute stage

June, 1912.
New Series, Vol. VII., No. 6. }   CORRESPONDENCE   { AMERICAN MEDICINE
Complete Series, Vol. XVIII.   337

of the disease. By so doing, life is jeopardized *not* infrequently owing to peritoneal inflammation, brought about by transport of poisonous bacteria. If we wait until the acute symptoms have completely disappeared; pain, fever, increased white blood count—indeed, until the interval period, there is, as is well known, little, or no danger to life.

Acting after this manner in over 370 operations, Beatson had a *mortality* of but 3.3 per cent as compared with the statistics of several other English surgeons, who had pursued a different plan—i. e, the one of immediate operative interference in all cases of acute appendicitis, which was very low indeed.

Further Beatson believes in the careful, sane medical management of cases of acute appendicitis—and is of opinion that small, or moderate doses of Dover's powder—bismuth and gray powder, are often desirable. Feeling as I do—and have long maintained, that *appendicitis* should not be regarded as a surgical disease, more than, or even as much as it is a medical affection, I am greatly pleased to have my views in part endorsed by an eminent authority in surgery.

Further, I am very hopeful if Beatson's ideas prevail and especially in the United States, we shall have a diminution in operations and dread of them. Again, if one be performed, it will be done by a thoroughly competent man of high character, after due consideration of all the facts involved, and after proper preparations have been made, without hurry, nervous excitement, and often hasty removal from home to hospital and consequent increased shock, or risk of extension of peritonitis.

It remains to be proven that first, or second attacks, should be followed by others unless operated, and whether such attacks are graver, or less so, if they occur—I am convinced they would not occur if people would merely be careful as to a few simple rules of health and they would not be really dangerous to life in a very large proportion of cases if they were properly treated medically—by rest, liquid diet, warm local applications and enemeta. In some instances local blood letting with leeches in the beginning and afterwards the use of salicin by the mouth is of undoubted and great value.

CORRESPONDENCE.

ETHICAL OR UNETHICAL—WHO SHALL DECIDE?

BY

I. L. VAN ZANDT, M. D.,
Fort Worth, Texas.

To the Editor AMERICAN MEDICINE:

In connection with your January editorials in which you fairly and without prejudice discuss the work of the Council on Pharmacy and Chemistry of the American Medical Association, permit me to record my own experience, which has been more or less peculiar.

In '99 after I had been using beechwood creosote in the treatment of pneumonia for almost six years, on seeing that Cassoute and Cardier of France had been using the carbonate of creosote, (trade name Creosotal). I began using the same, as a substitute.

Early in 1901 I sent a paper to the *Medical Record,* advocating the use of Creosotal. The paper was promptly returned by the then editor Dr. Geo. F. Shrady, because it "advocated a proprietary article."

He, however, later accepted the paper on condition of a change in wording from Creosotal to carbonate of creosote. This was after I had written him a letter showing what I thought of the inconsistency of his position.

In 1904, after having already published in 1902 a statistical paper on "Creosote in Pneumonia," he rejected another paper recommending Creosotal on the same grounds urged in first rejection. The Council on Pharmacy and Chemistry have accepted Creosotal.

In 1899 I became acquainted with and began using Collargolum in the form of a 15 per cent ointment called Unguentum Crede, which like Creosotal, was patented in Germany and manufactured I believe by von Heyden. Since Oct., 1904 I have been using the same in other forms, by mouth and rectum, and often find it more effective than any other remedy in infections.

But now the "Council," steps in and denies it admission to New and Non-Official Remedies. That is, two-thirds of a special committee do, Dr. Solis Cohen making a minority report in its favor.

I am a member of our county society, (was its first president), and of the State association, and have always striven to be ethical and honest. The editor of one of our great journals said I was using an unethical remedy, and the Council on Pharmacy and Chemistry now says I am using another.

Dr. Shrady, were he living and editor of the *Medical Record*, would probably now publish my article referring to Creosotal but reject one mentioning Collargolum.

What am I to do? Throw aside a remedy that has served me most satisfactorily and which, I think from my experience is more effective in certain conditions than any other known agent? No, I long since concluded, and so told Dr. Shrady, that I would rather my patients would get well unethically than die ethically. I will still continue to use it and proclaim its virtues abroad, hoping that the Council will see the error of its way and let down the bars, so that the severely ethical can use it without doing violence to their consciences.

The thoughtless way in which some physicians accept the dictum of the Council —allowing pharmacists and chemists to think for them—reminds me of a question put to me in my early professional life, about the year '69, viz.: "Doctor, is there somewhere gathered together a lot of smart men, who study out what to do for different kinds of sickness and then write it out for the rest of you to follow?"

I. L. VAN ZANDT.

THE FARMING CLASSES—ARE THEY DETERIORATING?

BY

WM. M. GREGORY, M. D.,

Berea, O.

To the Editor AMERICAN MEDICINE:

In reading the April number of AMERICAN MEDICINE just now, I came across an editorial article, entitled "The Deterioration of the Farming Class," which contains such astonishing misstatements that I felt moved to contradict them. I am a practising physician 54 years of age, and I live in a town of 3,000 people which is a suburb of a city of 600,000. Some of my patients are village people, some are country people, and some are city people. I am the 20th practising physician in our family and we have nearly all been country, or village doctors. I was raised in the country and have lived in the country or in small towns all my life except the years spent in medical college. I wish to state that the mental, moral, and educational standing of our country people has been raised several hundred per cent in the last few years. The writer of the editorial says: "Let us look into it a little to see if the charge is true, that we are evolving a peasantry too stupid for our form of government." Bless the man! Doesn't he know that we have no peasantry in the United States unless he wishes to call the colored people in the south by that ugly and opprobrious name? Doesn't the writer know that the great bulk of our farming class is made up of descendants of the New England pioneers? Has the writer any knowledge of the number of Farmers' Institutes that are held in this country every winter? Does he know who furnishes the papers for these institutes? Has the writer ever attended one single meeting of a national, state, or subordinate Grange? Does the writer know anything of the Boxwell law whereby states like Ohio have provided "That any child that has finished the required grammar school or graded course in a country school 'shall have free tuition at any high school in the state?'" The writer also speaks of "The dulling monotony of isolation." Who is isolated? Not the farmers that I know anything of. The practically universal use of the telephone, the daily paper delivered at the door by the R. F. D. man, and the countless electric car lines that traverse the country in every direction, prevent anything like isolation. Speaking of free high school tuition, we in this little town usually have about 40 boys and girls from the surrounding townships attending our high school, many of them driving in four or five miles every school day in the year. I wonder if the writer ever saw a *centralized school?* We have many of them in Ohio, and as the name indicates the system provides for a large *central* school containing all the various grades and departments and to which *all* the children of the township are conveyed every day by public conveyances. The writer's contention as to the public health of the country is quite mistaken in its reversion of actual conditions. I have lived all my medical life on the border line between city and country and before coming here I was a dispensary physician in the city of Cleveland. The country has the best health, next comes the small towns, and the large cities have the most sickness per thousand. The city infects the country or the small town every time. I have been health officer and have observed that in the four small epidemics of smallpox and diphtheria that we have sustained the contagion was conveyed to us from Cleveland every time. It could not very well be otherwise in a city with an enormous foreign population, and where a great number of mild cases of smallpox, diphtheria and scarlet fever, are never seen by any physician, and never quarantined. Our farmers almost universally are scientific, up-to-date men, cultivating the soil according to modern methods, and using modern implements for their work, and having modern conveniences in their homes. If any class of skilled labor is making more money than they are at the present time I would like to know who they are. As to the bunko man and his gold brick friend, the time has long gone by when they could do anything in the country. Their happy hunting ground is right in the heart of our largest cities. Reason. The city man is sure of his ability to take care of himself. The country man, since he has been reading the daily papers for a few years, absolutely *will not* have anything to do with any proposition offered by a stranger. I do not make this assertion from my own observation, but on the authority of the police and detectives in our largest cities. New York city alone gives more and better picking to the confidence man than all the country districts in the United States. As to public morality in the country the writer should remember that many things will pass in a large city that would cause a man to be shunned by all decent society in the country, for in the country "everybody knows all about every body else's business" and in the city it is quite possible to lead a double life.

Respectfully,
WM. M. GREGORY.

ACHONDROPLASIA.

BY

A. ROSE, M. D.,

New York City.

To the Editor AMERICAN MEDICINE:

In the May number of your esteemed journal Dr. Louis Curtis Ager has published a very valuable report of a case of achondroplastia. The more I appreciate his publication the more I regret the term achondroplasia. It is not Dr. Ager with whom I find fault but with Kaufmann, who has introduced the ungrammatical term and therefore I hope Dr. Ager will pardon me for my criticism. The compound under consideration does not come directly from the words achondros and plasis but from the compound adjective achondroplastos from which the noun achondroplastia is derived; consequently the word achrondroplasia should be replaced by achondroplastia. In this way and only in this way all the similar compound terms must be spelled, namely neoplastia, autoplastia, pseudoplastia, zooplastia, cheiroplastia, neuroplastia, organoplastia, osteoplastia, heteroplastia, hyperplastia, polyplastia, etc. And I am confident every one who wishes to write elegantly will appreciate this correction.

A. ROSE.

173 Lexington Ave.

THE RELATIVE EFFICIENCY OF NEGROES AND WHITE MEN IN VARIOUS OCCUPATIONS.

BY

REV. HORACE BUMSTEAD, D. D.,

Boston, Mass.,

Former President Atlanta University.

To the Editor AMERICAN MEDICINE:

In your editorial comment in the March issue, you assert the impossibility of negroes competing with white men in many of the callings created by civilization. You claim that even as mechanics they are less efficient, owing to a lack of intelligence and inability to perceive phenomena. You therefore deplore the fact that, as you say, schools for negroes set before their students an unattainable ideal and only increase their bitterness when failure comes. May I ask, as one who has had more than thirty years' experience in the education of negroes and study of their race, the privilege of presenting some facts with which your view is hardly consistent?

As a teacher, I would remark at the outset that ability to compete with white men is not the sole justification for holding up the highest ideals in schools for negroes. It should be borne in mind to how large a degree negroes are today a segregated race, finding an increasing market for their talents among their own people. if not among the whites. Consequently the more they compete with one another, with the highest ideals and unlimited educational opportunity before them, the more will they develop and diversify their capacities and promote the efficiency of their people. Even if they cannot now reach the white man's highest standard in all callings, they can in many callings surpass the lower standards with which thousands of white men everywhere are content, and can find profitable employment among both races where lower standards prevail. To limit the educational opportunities of negroes, as you propose, would check the development of much valuable talent and result in great economic waste.

But your depreciation of the ability of negroes in mechanical work is certainly very surprising. It is a well known fact that negroes monopolized nearly all the mechanic arts in the south while slavery lasted. Their high grade work in southern mansions and churches is even today pointed out with pride by old time southerners. Much of this fine work, of a kind now produced by machinery, was then wrought by hand with great skill and by tools now fallen into disuse. And today the great industrial schools at Hampton and Tuskegee can furnish plenty of evidence of the highest skill among the descendants of these slaves, now studying within their walls.

You say, however, that in your criticism you are referring to the real negro—not the more intelligent half-castes; and, presumably, you would meet the evidence presented by attributing the successes of these slaves and students to their white blood. This plea, if true, let me remark in passing, is a sufficient answer to your contention that schools for negroes should limit their efforts to education within the limits of a supposed racial inferiority—since a very large proportion of the students within these schools have more or less white blood in their veins and are therefore, to that extent not being confronted with an unattainable ideal.

But how about the pure negro? If he is to be found anywhere in the world, it must be in Africa. What is the testimony as to his mechanical skill in his native land? Let me cite a single authority: Professor Franz Boas of Columbia University, in an address a few years ago, referring to the excellence of native African work, spoke of the sceptres of African kings, carved in hardwood and representing artistic forms; the dainty basketry of the Congo and the grass mats with their beautiful patterns; the symmetrical lance heads almost a yard long, and axes inlaid with copper and decorated with filigree; the bronze castings of the West Coast which, (though perhaps due to Portuguese influence and even in that case showing the educative capacity of the natives) have so far excelled in technique any European work that they are even now almost inimitable. Evidences of this native African skill are abundant in the museums of London, Paris and Berlin.

In conclusion, permit me to express my surprise that you should seem to have based your discouraging view of negro capacity on Professor Woodworth's article in *Science*, though perhaps this was not our intention. I find nothing in that article to justify your view. Professor Woodworth has, indeed, controverted the alleged *superior* perceptions of lower races but, at the same time, he seems to me to be, throughout his article, in entire accord with his colleague in Columbia University, already quoted, Doctor Franz Boas, professor of anthropology, who in his recent book, "The Mind of Primitive Man," contends for the essential equality of original endowment in all races and their capacity for even rapid advance under the influence of improved environment. Dr. Boas remarks in his final chapter: "We do not know of any demand made on the human body or mind in modern life that anatomical or ethnological evidence would prove to be beyond the powers of the negro."

HORACE BUMSTEAD,
Brookline, Mass.

THE ANNOTATOR.

The Opportunities for Professional Work Afforded to Medical Officers of the U. S. Public Health and Marine Hospital Service.[1]

—Rupert Blue (Surgeon-general) states that this service offers opportunities to physicians for a career along numerous lines.

It cares primarily for sailors of the merchant marine in twenty-one government hospitals and one hundred and fifteen relief stations. Furthermore it tests the vision of master and pilots, examines surfmen of the Life Saving Service, and examines physicians for the Revenue Cutter Service, who have an extensive tour of duty including Alaska.

It operates forty-three quarantine stations in the United States besides others in all our colonies and in numerous foreign ports.

It examines all alien immigrants who come to our shores, excluding the unfit and placing the sick in government hospitals.

It co-operates with state and local authorities in preventing the spread of disease and in managing epidemics.

It has several laboratories for collating and disseminating facts relating to disease and their prevention.

It affords opportunities for special students at certain hospitals, as for pellagra at Savannah, Ga., and for the animal parasites of man at Wilmington, Del.

Its Hygienic Laboratory has active working divisions in pathology and bacteriology; zoology, pharmacology and chemistry.

Officers who enter the service must specialize on hygiene and sanitation; thus some give themselves to the study of one disease, others to questions of quarantine and immigration. The first detail of an officer is usually a short one, the second is usually to a quarantine or immigration sta-

tion or to a revenue cutter. The Hygienic Laboratory follows with its important and fascinating fields of work.

Examination for promotion comes in four years. One must serve in any climate or port where sent, the opportunities for advancement being good, indeed the author thinks no public medical service in the world offers greater facilities for advancement in public health work.

Sanitarians are trained in this service for expert work, as they are not trained in our colleges and a wide field of usefulness becomes available for those who have obtained such training.

The service as a whole is believed to be fully as attractive as any which at present engages the attention of physicians.

We believe that Surgeon-General Blue's exposition of this important public service, about which the average physician knows nothing, will prove of great value.

Particularly should it be attractive to those who are beginning their life work, and who can here find opportunities for usefulness and very good compensation which would be denied them in many portions of the country where the field has been occupied, threshed, and everything of value garnered by the multitude which has crowded in before them.

Influenza-Pneumonia.[1]

—An editorial on this subject thinks the danger from influenza consists in the surprises which it prepares for its victims. In its early stages the patient often thinks his complaint a trivial one. Then come complications and secondary infection and the physician has a problem of grave importance to grapple with.

The pneumonia of influenza has a 50% mortality or more.

There is still difference of opinion as to whether the bacillus of Pfeiffer alone causes influenza pneumonia or whether it is aided by the bacillus of Frankel which causes lobar pneumonia. The fatal result in so many cases is favored by the fact that the vital forces during the preliminary influenza have been greatly weakened by the influenza bacillus and its toxins. Influenza pneumonia does not begin with a rigor, sel-

---

[1] Medical Review of Reviews, April, 1912.

[1] St. Louis Medical Review, March, 1912.

dom has a crisis, has little pain or inflammation and seldom has rusty sputum or hepatization. Most of the physical signs are obscure. Very marked however is the depression of the vital forces, and the contagiousness. Hence those who are its victims should remain at home as well for their own good as for that of others. No antitoxines to this disease have as yet been discovered.

Treatment should be stimulating and strengthening, including digitalis, strychnia and quinine and a suitably nutritious diet is indispensable. The widespread prevalence of this disease (influenza) its insidious nature, and the complications which are often so distressing bid every practitioner watch each case with the utmost care and be prepared for almost any kind of an explosion. The great difficulty often consists in persuading a patient with grippe that anything of importance is really the matter with him, and inducing him to put up with the restraint which prudence should always impose upon him.

Report of the Committee on Hospital Dispensary Abuse.[1]—H. S. Anders as chairman makes the report to the Philadelphia County Medical Society. The investigation included a definition of hospital and dispensary abuse and a letter with queries to department heads in various hospital dispensaries. The following are the queries.

1. Was any effort made in your department to eliminate patients who were able to pay a physician?

2. Did you direct your assistant to inquire from patients as to their ability to pay for medical service?

3. If this question was answered affirmatively did you refer the patient to his physician, if not what did you do?

4. Would the dispensary abuse have been diminished if applicants had established their inability to pay for services in a medical registrar's office, as a preliminary?

In answer to the above questions some replies were affirmative, some were nega-

[1]N. Y. *Medical Journal*, April 20.

tive, and others non-committal. The following recommendations were offered:

1. Every dispensary physician should sincerely and steadily strive to abolish dispensary abuse.

2. A social service department should be established in each dispensary to ascertain the ability of patients to pay for medical services and the cases should be followed up with thoroughness to obtain accuracy of information.

We do not perceive anything startlingly new or unusual either in the questions or the recommendations of this investigation. The abuse is and long has been a real one, to correct which spasmodic attempts have been made from time to time somewhat after the fashion of the investigation which is here referred to. Those who maintain and derive advantage from the clinics can hardly be expected to manifest any very great enthusiasm in efforts which are designed to diminish their work and directly or indirectly their opportunities for benefit and income.

The Vivisection Report.[1]— An editorial informs us that this report of the Royal Commission has been in preparation for four years during which conclusive work has been done on spotted fever, infantile paralysis, sleeping sickness, typhoid fever, hydrophobia and diphtheria.

The report is unanimous and the commission gives the following excellent advice to the public: "We desire to state that the harrowing descriptions and illustrations of operations inflicted on animals which are freely circulated by post, advertisement or otherwise, are in many cases calculated to mislead the public, so far as they suggest that the animals in question were not under an anesthetic.

To represent that animals subjected to experiment in this country, are wantonly tortured would in our opinion be absolutely false."

The commission reports upon the great results, the many diseases overcome, which have followed directly upon animal experimentation.

[1]N. Y. *State Journal of Medicine*, April, 1912.

Animals themselves have been enormous gainers in the animal diseases which have been subdued.

They state that they were satisfied that anesthetics were generally used in experimental work, and that the animals suffered no pain in most cases. Their ethical conclusion is that "experiments upon animals adequately safeguarded by law faithfully administered are morally justifiable and should not be prohibited by legislation."

This report is an extremely satisfying conclusion of a most exhaustive investigation, with the English public very, largely against experiments upon animals in any form.

So trying has the matter been for years in Great Britain that students were able to obtain the necessary practical information connected with investigation of disease by means of animal experimentation only by visiting the laboratories of France, Germany, and other countries where a freer spirit of tolerance for investigation prevailed.

Post-Operative Secondary Hemorrhage.[1]— An editorial warns us that secondary hemorrhage may follow any operation and that we should be on the lookout for it quite as much as for sepsis. Heart failure, shock, emboli, etc., are explanations which are alleged for many fatal cases which doubtless proceed from hemorrhage, especially when the patient has been too long under the anesthetic, arteries have been tied hastily, and the operator has lacked experience and judgment.

It is believed that hemorrhage in many cases, results from operating during shock. Perhaps the operation could not be postponed or it may have been done too hastily, and when reaction came increase of blood pressure came with it.

Unwise stimulation after operation also causes the accident in question, the blood pressure being unduly increased by alcohol or strychnia. The symptoms of secondary hemorrhage are well-known; when they are observed the wound should at once be reopened, moderate narcosis being produced by chloroform. Hot water and adrenalin are recommended as the best astringents when astringents only are required.

[1]*Medical Council*, April, 1912.

Next in importance to the ligature for arresting secondary hemorrhage is placed the Mikulicz tampon, which is to be kept in position forty-eight hours and then gradually withdrawn after loosening its attachments with peroxide of hydrogen at 110° F.

The accident in question is an unpleasant one, often a grave one, but it is our experience and observation that it is not nearly so frequent as in days gone by.

Not only hastily applied ligatures and the want of ligatures but the want of ligature material—catgut which has untied or broken or dissolved, is too often responsible for secondary hemorrhage. So too is the reprehensible method of operating by the watch, which very few surgeons can do successfully—for the patient. Those who boast of operations performed in a few minutes or seconds seldom care to speak of their patients who have died from secondary hemorrhage.

The Mikulicz tampon certainly does give valuable pressure at times but its removal is usually difficult in forty-eight hours or even longer and its use has been abandoned by many surgeons.

Post-Operative Drowning.[1]— Greenbaum and Greenbaum observing that infusion is practised in most cases of surgical collapse whether the latter be due to loss of blood or lowered blood pressure remark that while the immediate results may be, brilliant the final one may be tragic.

Post-infusional death from pulmonary edema suggests that this result might sometimes be avoided.

Ether being the anesthetic usually employed in the fatal cases the authors advise caution in the rapidity with which it is given, and also as to the constitution of the intravenous injection material, its temperature, and the quantity injected.

In many of the reported cases disease of the kidneys and lungs pre-existed.

Intravenous saline infusions should be used only to replace fluid which has been lost by the body, fall in blood pressure due to other causes does not demand infusion.

Infusion should be performed with as great care as the operation for which it is used.

[1]*Therapeutic Gazette*, April 15, 1912.

If it is anticipated that infusion will be required ether should not be used as the anesthetic.

It should not be used when renal insufficiency is present.

Rectal infusion is less dangerous while subcutaneous infusion holds an intermediate place.

We are glad to see this timely warning. Too often intravenous infusion is used when rectal injection would answer the same purpose. The dangers of the operation, especially to the lungs and kidneys, are too apt to be ignored especially by the inexperienced, the rash, and the injudicious.

It is doubtful whether, on the whole, this procedure has done more good than harm. At the same time in the hands of one who is wise and cautious it has often done magnificent service.

A Federal Commission of Industrial Relations.[1]— E. T. Devine notes the recommendation by President Taft of such a commission to inquire as to the relations between employers and employees in the hope of avoiding industrial conflicts or of adjusting them fairly and quickly when they have occurred. Physicians as public spirited citizens have an active interest in this commission, though the suggestion originated with social workers and economists on the ground of public interest. The inquiry to be made is to consider the following questions:

How are rates of wages, hours and conditions of work determined in the principal industries? What are the grievances of workmen and the methods for considering them with their employers?

What obstacles do the managers of industries have to contend with and what are the methods for overcoming them?

Are there grave dangers to the nation from underpay, overwork, human exploitation among the inarticulate workers who may not even be conscious of grievances?

What have been the relations and trade agreements between trades unions and employers associations? What voluntary schemes have been tried for adjusting differences between employers and employed, and how have they worked?

What machinery have other countries devised for raising industrial standards or settling industrial difficulties, and how would they be applicable here?

How would the Eudmann act apply in the several states for other than railroad troubles?

What is the trend of statute law in the various states regulating contract work, also the trend of court decisions on the relations between employers and employed?

What are the powers, activities, and resources of bureaus and departments of labor and what do they need to produce the maximum of usefulness?

The Prevention of Blindness.[1]—An editorial notes that one-half the births in New York State are attended by midwives, also that one-quarter of the inmates of schools for the blind derived their blindness from ophthalmia neonatorum. It is further noted that the practice of midwives is practically limited to the poor in large cities, that those who employ a midwife are usually too poor to employ a nurse and doctor and that the midwife will usually lend a hand about the house, assisting in the care of the children, in the cooking, etc.

This means that in the homes of the poor the midwife is likely to continue an element of importance and it is a notification to the profession to see to it that midwives be educated to keep clean, to do as little harm as possible and to recognize and report ophthalmia neonatorum.

Failure to report such cases should be followed by fine and imprisonment or by revocation of their license. Such a plan in Boston has been followed by admirable results.

But the medical profession should go further than this. It should unite with the clergy in demanding laws which would forbid those who have venereal disease to marry and endanger those who are innocent. This would be going to the root of the matter and more effectively than Crede instillations, it would abolish much of the blindness by abolishing ophthalmia neonatorum.

---

[1] *Medical Review of Reviews*, April, 1912.

[1] *N. Y. State Journal of Medicine*, May.

The Economics of Food.[1]—A. L. Benedict thinks that food seldom receives the attention, economically, from the average individual which it deserves. This remark also applies to institutions which seldom go further than the estimation of a fair minimum per meal per capita.

The true nutritive value of food stuffs in families is seldom appreciated, their economics is limited to a knowledge of price at which one can afford to purchase them, their freshness, palatability, etc. Almost the entire trade in food considers nothing but price and unit of measure. It is as important to consider the possible economics in food supply as the cost and hygienic requirements of housing.

The cost of food can be greatly reduced if one knows what substances to select, moreover dietetic economics may be readily acquired for it concerns only proteids, carbohydrates and fats for the average individual. Such an individual requires 2,500 calories or heat units per day, proteids yielding 4.9 calories per gram, carbohydrate 4.1, fat 4.9. One of the most economical foods in calories is sugar, it should include from one-sixth to one-third of a day's ration and would cost about seven cents. One-sixth of the ration should consist of fat, either butter or lard or both, at a cost not exceeding eighteen cents per day. Cereals in the form of breakfast foods are so light and bulky that life could not be sustained by them alone. Fresh vegetables are not so nutritious as is supposed, and much of them is wasted. Potatoes, peas, beans and corn are the richest in proteid as well as carbohydrate. Fresh fruits contain nourishment in sugar, a large orange representing about one hundred calories. Three and a half quarts of milk would be necessary for a day's ration but this would give too much fat and too little carbohydrate to be economical physiologically. An egg represents one hundred calories, about one-tenth of the fat or proteid of a pound of lean met. Eggs at one cent a piece would correspond economically with meat at ten cents per pound. The caloric value of the meat proteid ration should be two hundred per day.

From the economic standpoint of price and calorie the cheapest ration would consist of sugar, breadstuffs and lard or similar fat. The meat, fresh vegetables and fruit will increase the cost of the first mentioned substances three-fold. It could easily amount to fifteen cents per day and might be double or treble that amount.

A Study of Industrial Diseases.[1]—An editorial states that there are distinct groups of diseases, injuries and causes of death in the 35,000,000 industrial workers in this country. Dust affects the lungs of miners and many varieties of factory workers, while workers in coal, petroleum, coke, acids, dyes, gasoline, and aniline colors suffer from inhaled gas and vapors.

Workers in metals and their salts suffer with metal poisoning and vapors affect those who are in chemical industries. Intense heat causes skin diseases and intense light, eye diseases. Each industry has its own injuries, mining being about the most dangerous. As to mortality, agriculture is the most favorable occupation for all ages, the various industries less so, and transportation and commerce still less.

The stone and earth industry shows the most favorable average mortality figures, then come in succession the metal trades, the machine industry and the chemical industry.

The mortality in the textile trades is not high except in the clothing and cleaning trades. The building trades have a low mortality up to the age of 30 and the foodstuffs to the age of 40.

The Germans have done most to safeguard workmen, insurance of operatives against illness and injury being obligatory.

The reporting of occupational diseases by physicians is compulsory in six states, California, Connecticut, Illinois, Michigan, New York and Wisconsin.

Occupational neuroses are classified by Dana as (1) pains and symptomatic cramps (2) neuritis and atrophy (3) aeroparesthesias (4) true occupational or professional cramps. Germany teaches its workmen sanitation, hygiene of the house and general hygiene, and furnishes institutions where the diseased body can be treated by mechanical devices adapted to each portion of it. Commissions are con-

---

[1] *Interstate Medical Journal*, April.

[1] *Medical Times*, May.

sidering employers' liability and workmen's compensation in Colorado, Connecticut, Delaware, Iowa, Massachusetts, Michigan, North Dakota, Pennsylvania, Texas and West Virginia. The United States Steel Corporation, the International Harvester Corporation and the Brewers' Association have consummated plans for compensating death or injury among their employees. The subject of industrial diseases and accidents is in its infancy in this country, but eventually we will take our place with other enlightened nations in the conservation of the life and health of our toilers.

It is well that we are awakening to a sense of duty and obligation to those who toil and it is not very creditable to the humanity of our rich and over-rich employers that we should be behind all other civilized nations in adequately protecting those through whom it becomes possible for the fortunes of the rich to be rolled up.

Vaccine Therapy.[1] — An editorial states that the value of bacterial vaccines in the treatment of infectious disease is now established, and that a working knowledge of their indications and methods of employment is a necessary part of modern therapeutics.

The extermination of an infection depends upon the ability of the body tissues to produce a sufficient quantity of antitoxines. It frequently happens that the tissues are unequal to this task, then the injection of bacterial vaccines outside the immedate area of inflammation brings more tissues into activity in the production of antitoxines, the latter are carried by the blood current to the seat of infection and recovery may be the result. Bacterial vaccines differ from alums in that they stimulate the production of antitoxines within the patient. If the patient cannot produce sufficient antitoxines they must be supplied by injecting serum.

Serums give the best results in acute general infections while bacterial vaccines are most effective in localized infections. While autogenous vaccines are theoretically the best, good results are often attainable with stock vaccines, especially in infections from gonococci and staphylococci.

Before beginning vaccine treatment it is best to determine the identity of the infecting germs, but this does not preclude the use of a well selected stock vaccine, thus boils, carbuncles and septic wounds can be successfully treated with a staphylococcus vaccine though the particular organism in the infection may not have been determined.

Reaction from vaccine administration shows that a proper vaccine has been selected and this is often a matter of diagnostic importance especially in obscure cases. The size and frequency of dosage are best determined by the degree of reaction but the response from an initial dose cannot be determined in advance. If the reaction from the initial injection is profound the second injection should be a smaller one.

If there is no improvement after the initial dose, the subsequent doses should be increased until the inadequacy of bacterial therapy in this particular case has been determined. The interval between injections should be from three to five days though in acute conditions a shorter interval may be required. This mode of treatment is not unerring and may be regarded as auxiliary to other measures.

The method of bacterial therapy is revolutionary. It is as yet only in its infancy. It will be the privilege of the younger generation of physicians to watch its development and its progress and upon them will devolve the task in large measure of furnishing the clinical evidence that this system is the correct and rational one for the treatment of infectious disease.

ETIOLOGY AND DIAGNOSIS.

A New Diagnostic Reflex Sign in Typhoid Fever.[1]—The sign is obtained as follows: The arm of the patient is bared to the shoulder. Arch the thumb and middle finger in a horseshoe and place over the biceps so that the arch is filled: press firmly and continuously and briskly raise the hand till the thumb and finger come together with a slight concussion. The result, if the sign is present, is the forma-

[1] *Medical Council*, May.

[1] C. B. Burke, M. D., *N. Y. Med. Jour.*, Dec. 16, 1911.

tion of an oval ridge of contraction on that portion of the biceps traversed, without any complete contraction of the muscle. The ridge thus formed disappears slowly. If the sign is absent there is no typhoid fever present: all cases which gave a Widal, or in the blood of which the typhoid ba. illus was present, gave the sign. The intensity and persistence of the sign vary with the virulence of the infection and the stage of the disease. The author considers that the sign is probably due to peripheral nerve irritation from toxin. He has obtained it in, amongst other conditions, a number of cases of pulmonary tuberculosis, all well advanced. We look upon the sign as a new and useful way of eliciting myoidema, and its presence in advanced tuberculosis confirms this, as in this disease myoidema obtained by direct percussion of the thoracic muscles has been long recognized as a useful sign.

The Diagnostic Importance of Hemoptysis.[1] —Dr. Bartlett draws the following conclusions from his study of hemoptysis.

(1) Bleeding from the upper air passages must be ruled out by careful inspection and history.

(2) Hemoptysis may occur in certain constitutional or blood diseases as merely another manifestation of the general tendency to bleed.

(3) Hemoptysis frequently occurs in broken compensation in heart disease.

(4) Ninety per cent. of all hemoptyses are tuberculous. As a rule definite signs and symptoms are present. Not uncommonly, however, they are in abeyance for months or even years.

(5) Hemoptysis may occur in any ulcerating or eroding pulmonary disease. It should, therefore, be expected in abscess, gangrene, bronchiectasis or pulmonary cirrhosis.

(6) Hemoptysis in pneumonia, bronchitis, asthma or following trauma should lead to the suspicion of an underlying tuberculous process.

(7) It is very doubtful if vicarious menstruation or hysteria can produce hemoptysis in normal lungs.

(8) Hemoptysis occurring without warning in young and healthy adults, and passing off without the development of further signs or symptoms of tuberculosis is probably of tuberculous origin and should be so treated.

(9) Broncho-pulmonary hemorrhage without definite symptoms or signs of cardiac or ulcerative pulmonary disease is due in nearly every instance to tuberculous infection, which is merely another way of saying that hemoptysis should be considered as due to pulmonary tuberculosis unless proved to be due to some other cause.

Differential Diagnosis of Lymphatic Infection and Tenosynovitis of the Hand.—Kanavel calls attention (*Infections of the Hand*, Lea &

Febiger, Publishers, Phila.) to the fact that one may mistake a lymphatic infection for a tenosynovitis. Here, however, the red lines of lymphatic involvement running up the arm without the localized tenderness over the tendon sheaths, the slight pain on moving the fingers, the generalized edema of arm and hand in contradistinction to the localized swelling found in the early stage of tenosynovitis aid us in the diagnosis. Again, we may be in doubt as to whether we are dealing with a tenosynovitis of the ulnar or radial bursa or a rheumatism of the wrist. Kanavel has seen several such cases. In one case it was difficult to determine whether the patient was suffering from a gonorrheal rheumatism of the proximal interphalangeal joint of a finger or a gonorrheal tenosynovitis with secondary involvement of that joint. The latter assumption was later found to be the condition present. In those cases where there is a lack of traumatic history, and the apparently spontaneous development of an inflammation, especially at the wrist, the diagnosis may be most difficult in spite of the ease with which a theoretical differential diagnosis is made. Here again, however, the localized tenderness over the sheath and pain on extension of the finger are of the greatest importance; moreover, these cases are always virulent and extend rapidly, so that if it be a tenosynovitis the hand grows rapidly worse. In a rheumatism there is as much pain on the dorsal as on the volar surface; the swelling involves the wrist more than the hand, fingers, or forearm; and other joints may be involved. The presence of a gonorrhea does not aid us materially, since either condition may follow. Subcutaneous infections are seldom difficult to differentiate. One case of gonorrheal tenosynovitis of the tendon sheaths of the dorsum of the wrist came under my notice in which the diagnosis of rheumatism had been made. Here the absence of any tenderness or swelling on the flexor surface combined with swelling and tenderness localized to the sheaths confirmed the diagnosis.

Diagnosis of Duodenal Ulcer.[1]—As a general rule it may be stated, says Herschel, that the symptoms of duodenal ulcer are those which were formerly at first called acid dyspepsia and more recently hyperchlorhydria. The writer thinks, however, that we are not justified in the assertion recently made by Moynihan, of Leeds, in a monograph upon duodenal ulcer that "*persistent* hyperchlorhydria * * * is the medical term for the surgical condition duodenal ulcer." We undoubtedly find symptoms, which in practice cannot be distinguished from those of duodenal ulcer, in chronic gall-stone disease, and in chronic appendicitis; and there are most certainly both a condition of hyperchlorhydria due to prolifera-

[1] W. B. Bartlett, M. D., *Boston Med. and Surg. Jour.*, Dec. 26, 1911.

[1] Geo. Herschel, M. D., *Interstate Med. Jour.*, March, 1912.

tive gastritis and also one which is a purely nervous condition. Nevertheless, the fact remains, and this is as far as the writer thinks we are justified in going, that there is a group of different affections comprising those enumerated above which are characterized by the symptom-complex to which stomach specialists for the last ten years have given the name of hyperchlorhydria, and that of these duodenal ulcer is by far the commonest.

Vital Resistance of Patients.[1]—With the great strides made in the technique of surgery in the last two decades there has developed an unfortunate tendency among many surgeons to look upon the surgical condition they are called upon to treat as something quite apart from the individual to be treated. Such surgeons examine the region of the appendix in a case of appendicitis, for instance, but do not look over the lungs or heart of the individual before advising immediate operation; still others are always ready to urge operation for a simple inguinal hernia, for a varicocele, for a chronic gastric ulcer, without considering whether the operation may not be a much graver source of danger than the morbid condition itself. However, there has recently developed the opposite tendency, which strives to counteract the unbounded enthusiasm of the technician for an immediate surgical interference, a tendency to study the patient as well as his disease, to consider the factors of safety present in the individual under consideration, and to take all possible means of increasing the chance of recovery from the operation itself as well as from the disease.

In a paper by Dr. Joseph C. Bloodgood, which embodies this tendency to a striking degree, in the May number of *Annals of Surgery*, the author insists upon the necessity of estimating the vital resistance of each patient, with the exception of those, of course, in whom no choice can be made because of the urgency of symptoms. He thinks that in the preoperative interval physical rest must be obtained, the function of the kidneys ascertained, blood pressure recorded, and food and stimulants modified in kind and quantity to suit the individual's needs. Of equal importance is mental tranquillity and this must be obtained by natural allusions to the operation as simply as of the general therapeutic procedure; in some cases the knowledge of its urgency should even be kept from such patients as may be thought to become too much frightened by the coming ordeal. Rest, then, physical and mental, fresh air, restricted diet, moderate catharsis, increased water, restriction or complete elimination of alcohol and tobacco are the preoperative measures that conserve or increase the vital resistance of the operation.

During operation, anesthesia is the main item. Bloodgood speaks against trusting anesthesia to anybody but a physician; he thinks

that the anesthetist should be a senior, not a junior, member of the resident staff and should be skilful in the latest anesthetic technique. In the author's experience nitrous oxide and oxygen anesthesia is the best for all purposes, while the additional use of a local anesthetic to "block" the nerves adds a great deal to the prevention of postoperative shock. Blood pressure estimations during the operation tell the condition of the patient and approach of danger better and earlier than the pulse and respiration, and a rapid and marked drop in pressure is to Bloodgood a sign that saline infusion is immediately needed. Such infusion, too, should be administered to a patient *before* he leaves the operating room if collapse in the early hours after operation is apprehended. In postoperative treatment, Bloodgood advocates salt solution by the continuous method of Murphy in all cases, so that the kidney functions may be started early; morphine in small doses to allay restlessness and pain; careful watch and early treatment of any complications, such as dilatation of the stomach, excessive distention of the abdomen, acidosis, etc. Recovery from the operation and the condition operated for should be followed by watching the patient for the development of any nervous complications, and in this the family physician and the surgeon should cooperate.

Bloodgood's paper, cursorily sketched above, is a welcome one, for it is evidence of progress in the attitude of the surgeon toward the patient, of progress that cannot but reflect further credit upon the well deserving art of surgery as practised in America.

The Etiology of Lupus Erythematosus.[1]—From an exhaustive study and review of the disease and its literature, Freshwater draws the following conclusions:

(1) Characteristic examples of the two main varieties of the disease differ in so many respects that it is difficult to conceive that they have a common cause.

(2) In view of our imperfect knowledge concerning the etiological factors in skin diseases, we are not in a position to state that all eruptions apparently alike must be due to a single cause.

(3) There is not sufficient evidence, clinical, histological, or bacteriological, to show that lupus erythematosus is always a tuberculous lesion.

(4) The supervention of the disease on local injury to the tissues, as in the case of frostbite, sunburn, etc., strongly suggests that a purely local cause is at times responsible for its occurrence.

(5) A large number of cases suffer from some anomaly of the circulation, so that the skin may be unable to bear an increased strain such as might be produced by a toxin circulating in the blood.

---

[1] Editorial, *Medical Record*, June 1, 1912.

[1] W. Freshwater, M. D., *British Jour. of Dermatology*, February.

JUNE, 1912.
New Series, Vol. VII., No. 6. }   TREATMENT   { AMERICAN MEDICINE
Complete Series, Vol. XVIII.   349

(6) That the exact nature of the toxin or toxins is uncertain.

(7) The primary involvement of the blood-vessels, together with the symmetrical distribution of the eruption in the majority of cases, favors the supposition that the causative agent acts through the blood-stream.

TREATMENT.

Nocturnal Enuresis.[1]—Ruhräh points out that nocturnal incontinence of urine in children is one of the common and one of the most troublesome conditions which the physician is called upon to treat. The physician, after one or two therapeutic ventures, dismisses the case with the suggestion that the adenoids should be removed, or if it is a boy, that he be circumcised, and then if these suggestions are carried out, and a cure does not result, the family of the child become resigned to what they regard as inevitable. If we exclude those cases in which there is evidence of mental deficiency and those caused by congenital malformations, we have a group of cases which were formerly regarded as "essential" or idiopathic enuresis. As our knowledge of the subject has increased, the idiopathic cases have gradually diminished in number, and Bazy aptly remarked that essential enuresis means essential ignorance. Many children with enuresis suffer from an overirritable nervous system, and this may account for small lesions causing the urine to be passed through reflex irritability. In other cases the lesion is marked, and would affect the nervous system of the normal child. Bed-wetting may result from mere laziness, and in other instances a child may sleep so soundly that the warning of the distended bladder is unheeded. Another cause is abnormal muscle tone, and Merklen considers enuresis an element of weak motor inhibition. Among the more interesting of the newer suggestions as to treatment are the results of Williams in treating these cases by the use of desiccated thyroid. His cases had subnormal temperature and evidence of thyroid insufficiency, and he obtained wonderfully satisfactory results in all except one case, and in this case the child did not have a subnormal temperature. Williams gave one-half grain of the dried thyroid twice daily to children between two and six years of age and this may be increased for older children. The increase in dosage should be made slowly as directly opposite effects are occasionally induced by overdosage. Ruhräh has used this method and in a small proportion of cases in which there were more or less marked signs of thyroid insufficiency, the results were quite remarkable. These were children with adenoids and enlarged tonsils, or in some cases, children in whom the adenoids or tonsils had been recently removed.

In his cases the effect was obtained promptly or not at all. In every case in which a favorable result was obtained, a marked difference was noticed after the administration of one or two doses of the drug, and in all cases within a week. Another remarkable observation coinciding with that of Williams' is that the undersized children gained weight rapidly. When there is no other indication for treatment he has found the use of atropin to give better results in a greater number of cases than any other one thing, and to be of any service it must be given in full doses. In nocturnal cases a dose at five o'clock and at bedtime is all that is required. In cases occurring both during the day and night the drug is advised every three hours. He usually prescribed one grain of atropin sulphate in two ounces of water, each drop containing about 1-1000 grain, and usually as many drops will be required as the child is years old. The proper method of dosage, however, is to start with one or two drops, increasing each dose one drop at a time until flushing of the face and neck occurs some twenty minutes after taking the drug. The dose should then be diminished one drop, and this amount continued until the child has ceased urinating at night and for at least two weeks later, when the drug may be dropped gradually, diminishing a drop at a time until one drop is reached when it may be stopped.

Simplified Technic in Prostatectomy.[1]—By following a few simple suggestions, most of the difficult features of prostatectomy can be eliminated, says Ochsner, and all of the advantages without any of the disadvantages of both suprapubic· and perineal operation are be attained.

1. Introduce a grooved Van Buren sound into the urethra down to, but not through, the prostatic portion.

2. The straight portion of the sound should extend up over the pubis. An assistant holds this firmly and pushes the curved end against the perineum.

3. An oblique skin incision is made from a point half-way between the scrotum and the anus to a point half-way between the anus and the patient's left tuber ischii.

4. An incision is made through the upper end of this incision through the urethra exposing the grooved sound.

5. The end of a probe-pointed long, narrow bladed, lithotomy knife is placed in the groove of the sound.

6. The sound and the knife are then carried together into the bladder, care being taken to have the sound pulled forward, hugging the pubic bone, after the fashion of the old perineal lithotomy operation, splitting the membranous and prostatic portion of the urethra quite into the bladder.

[1] John Ruhräh, M. D., *Amer. Jour. of Med. Sciences,* February, 1912.

[1] A. J. Ochsner, M. D., *Med. Council,* June, 1912.

7. Be careful not to injure the rectum.

8. Approach the prostate from above precisely as in case of suprapubic prostatectomy by passing the finger into the bladder through this incision.

9. In case this is not ·ssible because of adhesions, remove the gland with the Ferguson gnawing forceps.

10. Search the bladder for stones with the sound and finger.

11. Catch the capsule with fine-toothed clamp forceps.

12. Introduce a drainage tube.

13. Tampon the capsule around this tube with gauze while holding it in place with the clamp forceps.

14. Leave the gauze and drainage tube in place for two days, then remove these permanently.

15. Administer from two to five drops of aromatic sulphuric acid in half a pint of distilled water every hour to prevent formation of earthy phosphates.

16. Let the patient sit up on the third day.

17. Give daily hot tub baths after the first week.

The Treatment of Duodenal Ulcer.[1]—While there is no question that ulcer of the duodenum is a surgical condition, that operative interference is the only radical cure, that there is danger from prolonged ulceration causing adhesions to or inflammation in adjacent organs, that an ulcer in healing may cause narrowing of the duodenal canal and perhaps more or less obstruction, and that an unhealed ulcer may be the irritating cause of a future localization of carcinoma, still, many patients will not submit to operation, and instances of cure and healed ulcers are frequently seen on autopsy and apparently often clinically occur. Consequently, there is plenty of justification for the medicinal cure or medical management of duodenal ulcer.

Prerequisites of such treatment are:

1. The teeth, gums, mouth, tonsils and pharynx, if in bad condition, must all be properly treated and put into as nearly perfect order as possible.

2. A test breakfast, a test of the duodenal regurgitated fluid and a test of the feces must be made to determine, if possible, exactly the amount of disturbance in the digestive tract that is present.

3. The urine must be carefully examined to determine any liver, pancreatic and kidney disturbance.

4. The blood must be studied to determine the seriousness of the condition and the latent or reserve strength of the patient.

All of the above having been accomplished, the physician is ready to carry out the treatment. The treatment consists of:

[1] Special Therapeutic Article, *Jour. A. M. A.*, June 22, 1912.

1. The administration of a cathartic the night before the patient begins his treatment, such as the following:

℞

	Gm.		
Hydrargyri chloridi mitis ..	15		gr. iiss
Pulveris rhei	25	or	gr. iv
Sodi bicarbonatis..........	50		gr. x

M. et fac chartulam 1.

Sig.: Take at bedtime with a cup of malted milk or other bland nutriment.

2. Absolute rest in bed for three weeks.

3. Early in the morning of the first day the patient should receive 10 gm. (2½ drams) of Rochelle salt, given in a glass of hot water. This, with the cathartic of the night before, will cause as near as possible surgical cleanliness of the intestine; and, as elsewhere, an ulcer must be kept as clean as possible.

4. Dry heat should be applied to the abdomen more or less constantly for ten days, best with an electric pad.

5. There should be no food for forty-eight hours.

6. A glass of hot water with a quarter of a teaspoonful of salt and a quarter of a teaspoonful of sodium bicarbonate should be given every four hours for four times. There should be no more water given for ten or twelve hours, except in sips as needed for thirst. The object of this is to clean off the mucus thoroughly from the inflamed duodenum, and then to give the stomach and upper intestine an absolute rest.

7. After forty-eight hours, viz.; on the third day, very small quantities of nourishment should be given. The food must not excite the stomach to the production of much hydrochloric acid, as it is better to prevent its production or secretion rather than to administer olive oil, butter or atropin to stop it. This means that no meat or meat-juices or meat extracts or broths should be given, although some clinicians seem to find meat chopped fine and prepared in various ways a most valuable food, even in the early stage of the treatment of this disease. The nourishment should be in small amount so as not to cause distention of the stomach and thus to interfere with the cure of any dilatation that may previously have been present. As soon as possible, of course, the food must contain sufficient calories to prevent further loss of weight, even if not much is gained for the first ten days. A very good nutriment for this period, viz., beginning on the third day, is a predigested and alkalized milk, i. e., 2 ounces of peptonized hot milk with an ounce of Vichy, drunk slowly, and given every three hours during the third day of treatment. On the fourth day 3 ounces of peptonized milk and 1 ounce of Vichy should be given hot every three hours.

8. Two and one-half hours after every other administration of peptonized milk, viz., every six hours, and one-half hour before the next feeding, a glass of hot water should be given to wash the stomach and duodenum; or, if hot

water is objected to, a clear, clean, fresh clam broth may be given.

9. On the fourth day the bowels should be moved by an enema, and this should then be daily repeated until later in the treatment.

10. On the fifth day 5 ounces of peptonized milk and one ounce of Vichy should be given every six hours, alternating every six hours with 5 ounces of a thin, strained oatmeal gruel given hot, and followed by 2 ounces of warm Vichy; in other words, one or other of these feedings every three hours.

11. As the patient needs iron, and he is receiving no meat, a 3-grain tablet of saccharated oxid of iron should be given twice a day with the nourishment for a period beginning with the fourth day of the treatment. The tablet should be powdered before taking.

12. On the sixth day the cereal (oatmeal gruel, salted) should be continued and a raw egg on cracked ice with a trace of lemon juice should take the place of one milk feeding. The other feedings of milk on this day should be not peptonized but given with Vichy as before.

13. Hot water at least twice a day should be given one-half hour before a nourishment.

14. After ten days there should be a gradual increase in the food; first two raw eggs; then they may be cooked; shredded wheat biscuit, malted milk, junket and gelatin flavored with lemon or orange (no alcohol, tea, coffee, and only exceptionally tobacco, should be allowed) may be given. Later, finely chopped fresh chicken, roasted oysters in season, fresh steamed soft clams, chopped little necks served in broth, mutton, chicken and beef broths may be gradually added to the now increasing diet. Still later, chopped beef made into a pate and broiled may be given once a day, and the frequency of the feedings changed to five times a day, then to four times. Water may now be taken cool but not cold, but not much liquid should be given or allowed with any one meal, so as to prevent still longer the stomach becoming distended.

15. The daily enema for the bowels should be given for ten days, which, with the four days before such treatment was used, means up to two weeks from the beginning of the treatment. Nothing else should be given to cause bowel movements unless they are very unsatisfactory. If such is the case, a sufficient amount of effervescing sodium phosphate may be given each morning, in hot water, but it should not be taken until it has nearly finished effervescing—not while it is storming.

16. After two weeks the enema should be stopped and sodium phosphate in the morning should be relied on to cause a movement of the bowels.

17. The patient having been in bed for three weeks, convalescence to last a week should be inaugurated. This means a gradual getting up as from typhoid.

18. The patient having recovered from his illness and its treatment, should take one month's rest, i. e., at the end of the four weeks, at some country, mountain, or sea shore resort, depending on the time of year. Or, if this is impossible, a month's rest at home, with plenty of out-door rest, should still be insisted on. At the end of this time, viz., eight weeks, there should be a gradual resumption of his occupation, the patient being careful for a long time not to take into his stomach anything irritant, too cold, too salty, or any harsh, rough food, or anything that is acrid or may become acrid, as grape-fruit, strawberries, or anything that is too acid, as vinegar, pickles, etc. He should also be careful about getting chilled.

19. A laxative tablet will probably be needed for some time. A very satisfactory one is as follows:

℞	Gm.	
Sulphate of strychnin....	0015	gr. 1/40
Aloin.....................	02	gr. 1/3
Powdered ipecac.........	03	gr. 1/2
Extract of belladonna.....	006	gr. 1/10

This should be taken after supper and not on an empty stomach. If it acts in the night when given at this time, it may be given at bedtime, but not on an empty stomach. The patient should have a cup of malted milk with a cracker or two broken into it before the tablet is taken.

The Treatment of Gonorrhea by the General Practitioner.[1]

—Treatment at its best is unsatisfactory for the reason that, says Stapleton, the patient is not aware of the difficulty of curing the disease. As a rule they are very careless in following advice.

My opinion is that where we are able to put the gonorrhea patient to bed and then treat him we have better and quicker results.

First.—I tell him that absolute cleanliness is necessary—warning him as to danger of infecting his eyes and mouth. Have him wear a suspensory.

Second.—Have him discontinue all forms of alcohol—no intercourse or any form of amusement such as dancing—reading which is sexual in character—cut down amount of meats—have him eat plenty of vegetables and drink copiously of water between meals—when not working to rest as much as possible.

Make a microscopical examination of pus to determine presence of gonorrhea germ as routine practice. Easily and quickly done.

Examine urine to determine acidity.

If urine too acid I have patient add soda bicarbonate gr. v to glass of water when drinking.

In the beginning I never use an injection, but place the patient upon the old reliable Lafayette mixture which as you know contains oil of sandal-wood, potassium hydrate—sweet spirits of nitre—mucilage of acaci and syrup making an emulsion. This is given in teaspoonful doses after eating and at bedtime.

In an ordinary mild case the medicine gives almost immediate results. I continue on this

---

[1] W. J. Stapleton, M. D., *Med. Era.*

352   AMERICAN MEDICINE }
Complete Series, Vol. XVIII. }   HYGIENE AND DIETETICS   { JUNE, 1912.
{ New Series, Vol. VII., No. 6.

until the discharge is considerably lessened—in fact until there is only a drop or two to be found. Then I .change to a mild alkaline mixture internally and use an injection containing zinc sulphocarbolate, boric acid, hydrastine muriate, and morphine sulphate. This is in brief the ordinary treatment of the office patient.

I have never had any success with the so-called abortive treatment. The ideal method would be to have our patients who expose themselves use the method employed by the Germans and in the United States Army with such excellent results, i. e., the use of a 33 per cent. calomel paste as a preventive of syphilis and gonorrhea. The paste is injected into the urethra immediately after intercourse.

HYGIENE AND DIETETICS.

Diet in Cardiovascular Diseases.[1]—Evidently animal tissues to a considerable extent should be restricted, says Cornwall, and in some cases they should be altogether excluded. It is my practice in the great majority of cases to allow a small amount of meat, fish, or poultry from one to four times a week; in a smaller number of cases, for a time at least, no animal tissue at all is allowed; these last are the cases which show marked symptoms of putrefaction toxemia. It is not usually difficult to get cardiovascular patients to reduce their animal food to a very small amount after they have experienced the beneficial effects of such abstinence.

The broths made from animal tissues seem to have no reasonable place in the dietary of cardiovascular disease; they are little more than solutions of the nitrogenous extractives (artificial urine); their only claim to consideration is found in their ability to excite the secretion of gastric juice and that merit is not sufficient to counterbalance their positive disadvantages.

With animal tissues occupying a very small place in the dietary of cardiovascular disease, we have to rely for protein chiefly on milk and the cereal foods. Milk supplies easily digested, nonputrefiable protein in considerable amount, and also a fair quantity of easily digested fat and nonfermentable carbohydrate, and it is free from the purins. A quart of milk contains nearly as much protein as a half pound of beef, and considerably surpasses the latter in calorific value. The objections to its digestibility which obtain in many cases can be overcome very easily by dilution with cereal gruels, alkaline waters both still and carbonated, or even plain water, or by fermentation outside the body with the lactic acid bacillus. Milk thus modified is not only very digestible, but is an important factor in making the diet antiputrefactive, which is one of the indications in cardiovascular disease.

The cereals, including bread, contain a con-

[1] E. E. Cornwall, M. D., N. Y. Med. Jour., June 22, 1912.

siderable amount of protein, a large amount of carbohydrate, and a very little fat, and are almost entirely free from the purins. The deficiency of fat can be supplied by the addition of butter, which makes them more palatable. The moist cooked cereals should never be served with cane sugar to patients with cardiovascular disease. Seven ounces of cooked cereal, which is a large saucerful, contains more protein than a lamb chop and possesses nearly twice the fuel value. Two ounces of bread without butter contain more protein than one ounce of sirloin steak, and possess a fuel value more than twice as great. Cereals, beside being an important source of easily digested protein and carbohydrate, supply sugar in the lower part of the digestive tract where, by being converted into lactic acid, it helps to keep down intestinal putrefaction.

All the green vegetables which are easily digested are generally acceptable in the dietary of cardiovascular disease, unless special contraindications exist. They supply necessary salts, add variety to the diet, and are laxative.

Most fresh fruits which are easily digested, and which do not contain so much sugar as to be unduly fermentable, are valuable adjuncts to this dietary for nearly the same reasons as the green vegetables.

The roots, particularly potatoes and carrots, are ordinarily allowable.

Butter and olive oil are digestible and agreeable fats. A little fat bacon is occasionally useful for variety, and adds only a very small amount of putrefiable protein to the diet; but this small amount sometimes has to be considered.

The soups made with milk and green vegetables (the vegetables purées) also add variety to the diet and possess considerable food value in the milk they contain.

Cheese, particularly cream cheese, can be allowed in many cases, and is a valuable source of nonputrefiable protein.

Cane sugar should be excluded largely or completely from this diet, but any craving for sweets can be satisfied by honey, which is acceptable to most people, though some have an idiosyncrasy which makes it impossible for them to take it without disturbance. Milk sugar is perhaps the least objectionable of the common sugars, but its lack of a pronounced sweet taste prevents it from being popular. It is not often necessary to consider the sugars by themselves in the dietary of cardiovascular disease, for the starch of the cereals, to say nothing of the milk sugar in the milk supplies sufficient carbohydrates.

In prescribing a diet for cardiovascular disease, it is not sufficient to prescribe the articles and the quantities; it is also necessary to state how the food should be taken. It may be possible to arrange the food in three daily meals, but it often happens that a larger number of smaller meals best suit the conditions present. In any case the evening meal should be the lightest, and the patient's stomach should be empty when he goes to sleep.

American Medicine

H. EDWIN LEWIS, M. D., *Managing Editor.*

PUBLISHED MONTHLY BY THE AMERICAN-MEDICAL PUBLISHING COMPANY.

Copyrighted by the American Medical Publishing Co., 1912.

New Series, Vol. VII., No. 7.
Complete Series, Vol. XVIII., No. 7.

JULY, 1912.

$1.00 YEARLY in advance.

The political situation can hardly fail to interest every progressive physician, not only because of the many questions which essentially concern him as a good conscientious citizen, but more especially because certain matters of great professional importance are at stake as never before. We refer particularly to the organization of the national public health agencies under one head. To the great chagrin of a great many physicians the Republican convention at Chicago completely ignored the subject and the platform adopted did not make a single reference to this great question which means so much to the American people. To those who followed events at the Chicago convention, it was hardly surprising that the people's interests were of secondary or negligible importance, for elements were in control that could be depended upon to satisfy their own purposes first and ignore everything that did not promise some selfish advantage or gain. Furthermore since Mr. Taft's supporters were able to dominate the whole situation— an achievement which apparently entailed methods and manners that offer little grounds for pride or satisfaction—any strong positive stand on public health matters was not to be expected. Mr. Taft's whole attitude on questions pertaining to public health has been one of indifference, ignorance and neglect. The treatment ac-corded Dr. Wiley may well be cited, for if the President had estimated the administration of the Pure Food and Drug Law at its full importance, the Department of Agriculture would have been cleaned up when the true situation was revealed, and men of unquestionable integrity placed in charge. Dr. Wiley may have had his faults—we have not been one of his blind supporters, although we recognized his ability and earnestness—but to let a man who had been so largely responsible for the real progress made in pure food and drug matters withdraw from the service of the people, and retain at the helm those who were generally considered to be playing politics was an evidence of indifference on the part of President Taft that the medical profession will not soon forget. Neither will the rank and file of the profession overlook President Taft's ukase giving Christian Science practitioners special privileges in the Canal Zone. In fact, the medical men of the country should recognize without delay that the great questions pertaining to the public health which they have for so many years been striving unselfishly to place on an effective basis, have nothing to expect from President Taft or any administration of which he is the head. The future can usually be pretty accurately predicated on the past, and President Taft's past relations to the national public health agencies offer little promise that he will awaken to their importance or do anything to promote their efficiency.

Our political preferences have been asked by so many correspondents that we are going to take this opportunity of stating our position. There was a time when medical men were supposed to keep aloof from politics, to remain neutral—affecting a sort of political hermaphrodism—and be "all things to all men." But this role soon became intolerable to intelligent physicians, since their education, training and mental attainments qualified them to be positive factors in their various communities. Hence it is that for several years medical men have been taking a definite stand on all questions concerning the public welfare and few will deny that the people have gained thereby. By the same token, we believe that a wide awake, earnestly conducted medical journal should not hesitate to come out into the open and take a clear cut position on the great civic and political questions of the day. Medical men are interested in everything that has the slightest influence on human progress and well being, and what is more important than clean honest government, municipal, state and national? This is our excuse for taking up the subject, reinforced by our further belief that the medical profession and all of its instrumentalities should actively support every movement or policy that aims to advance public health efficiency.

The question confronting us as earnest physicians and good citizens is which party offers greatest promise of advancing the policies that the medical profession has been earnestly fighting for, for so many years? Which candidate, through inclina-

tion, interest or qualification can be depended upon, not only to recognize the real fundamental importance of the present day public health movement, but to advance it and its various details most intelligently and forcefully?

It is true that the Democratic platform has an unequivocal plank advocating all that the medical men of the country have been so long contending for. The nominee of the Democratic party is a cultured gentleman of scholarly ability and· high mental attainments. But he is an unknown quantity in some respects and owes his nomination so definitely to certain interests that are known to be strongly antagonistic to genuine progress in pure food and public health laws that grave fears may well be entertained as to any material advance in this direction if Governor Wilson is elected. We are not disposed to refer to certain other conditions which may lead many to doubt the advisability of turning the country over to another party committed to drastic tariff revision and diametrical change of many existing conditions that have brought the country to its present state of prosperity. No, it is pretty good judgment to cling to known forces that have demonstrated their qualifications and fitness to lead.

On this basis, we feel that the medical profession should support Colonel Roosevelt, our honored ex-president. He more than any other leader in public life has done more to recognize the honest unselfish work of the medical profession. It was during his administration that the present Pure Food and Drug Act came into being, and his attitude has always been one of consistent cooperation with every practical movement for the advancement of the public health. Of the three candidates,

Colonel Roosevelt has expressed himself most strongly in favor of proper organization of the various public health agencies under one head in a department which will make them of prime importance in their work. It is immaterial whether we have a Health Department with a Cabinet officer or not. The important point is to have all the public health agencies under one head, with an organization that will insure the greatest efficiency in promoting the health and physical welfare of the American people. Colonel Roosevelt is a known quantity on these as well as the other problems confronting our nation. No other man before the public embodies more of what we can term the American spirit. Honesty, courage, broad intelligence and a sober sense of civic integrity so typify this great American citizen that it is not to be wondered at that he has the following he has. To a certain number, the "third term misconception" alone stands in the way of supporting Colonel Roosevelt. In all frankness we feel that to withhold support on such grounds from a man who has proven himself so useful to his country, would be a grave mistake, and we doubt if in the end such a view will prevail against his candidacy. Summed up, therefore, Colonel Roosevelt is the one man among the candidates who will be able, not only by reason of his personal qualifications, but through his vast experience, to meet the needs of the hour not only with greatest surety of maintaining the country's present prosperity, but with greatest certainty of advancing the future welfare and prestige of the American people.

In concluding these remarks we want it distinctly understood that we are not electioneering. Many of our readers may entertain views entirely different from those expressed. We have every respect for them if they are only sincere and born of conviction. Each man, after all is said and done, must decide for himself who he will support and vote for. To us, Colonel Roosevelt represents an ideal and the means of its practical attainment. We trust him because we love him and we love him because we know him. To us he stands as typical of our idea of a true American citizen, a cultured gentlemen who loves his country and is willing to sacrifice his own comfort and personal desires for the duty he sees before him. We are not disposed to deny that he has faults or that he never makes mistakes, but his faults are human faults—those that every honest man can account for and understand. If fate places Theodore Roosevelt in the presidential chair when March 4th comes around again, we shall feel that the American people not only have much to look forward to, but that the medical profession has better prospects than ever before of seeing the public health interests of the nation placed on a sound substantial basis that will insure a new era in the prevention of disease and the reduction of human mortality. We have tried to state our position fairly and squarely without affront to any one. We claim no monopoly of judgment and those who think differently may have better reasons for their views. But the virile and intensely human character of the man Roosevelt has always appealed to us and we are glad to place ourselves under his leadership. We confidently believe the earnest work of the medical profession stands better chance of fruition under his leadership than any other.

———

Popular sanitary errors are mentioned by Prof. E. O. Jordan, University of Chicago, in an article devoted to the most profitable lines of present day research (*Science*, June 2, 1911). We urge physicians to read this article, as the lesson for us is the fact that these false ideas of laymen are old medical theories which once accounted for all known facts but were more or less promptly discarded when new facts were discovered which could not be thus explained. Even educated physicians hold to false ideas long after the error is abundantly proved, but the laity are far more conservative than we are. We have great difficulty in convincing them that a new theory accounts for newly discovered facts, but when they are convinced they hold to it with prim determination in spite of later discoveries. Thus the remarkable reduction of deaths following the campaign of cleanliness inaugurated nearly a century ago, gave rise to the natural conclusion that filth causes diseases, and that typhoid could originate *de novo*. We dropped those ideas when we found the real causes of infections and how transferred to us. Yet, as Jordan says, the laity still hold to the old theory and when disease breaks out, here or there, they insist upon spending money upon more or less futile measures and let the real dangers continue. Garbage disposal is of course a vital matter, especially now that the sentence of extermination has been served on the rat, but it has not the popularly believed transcendent importance in the ordinary infections not carried by rats. Similarly it was well to wage a war against sewer gas when we found contact diseases in hot stuffy rooms, but we do not seem able to convince people that sewer-air of itself is not particularly harmful in the ordinary amounts encountered. So they spend untold amounts on a plumbing inspection, quite well in its way but there

would be far less diphtheria if the plumbing were neglected and the money spent upon isolating and disinfecting the carriers.

Sanitation must be aimed at the causes of disease, for we are wasting too much money on non-essentials. Jordan's warning is most timely and should be heeded at once. The evidence is now conclusive that we contract infections from living carriers as a rule, and not from dead materials, except the infected foods of course. The regulations as to disinterment of corpses are ridiculously archaic and cause unnecessary expense to the relatives, while the only good accomplished is increased business of undertakers. A cholera corpse is absolutely sterile in less than three weeks after burial, as far as Koch's bacillus is concerned. Similarly there is need of great simplification of plumbing arrangements. Our disinfecting rules are almost criminal, for we have wasted money to kill the dead germs, of diphtheria say, on the walls—if any are there at all—and allowed the little patient to return to school weeks before the bacilli have disappeared from its throat. Here and there, a few advanced sanitarians are working on right lines, but the laity still hold to the false ideas, and demand "fumigation." We have long thought that we are too lax in the management of notification, but now we see a few laymen are taking the matter up with a view of keeping track of every infection until we know the convalescent is no longer a carrier. So it is not too much to hope that the new era is already inaugurated. Future sanitary research must be devoted exclusively to the way the living agent gets from one person to another; then practical means of isolation and disinfection of the persons will suggest themselves. In time we will not need an artificial immunity against anything—not even smallpox, though it will be a long time of course.

Overpopulation and cost of living are occupying the serious attention of Japanese statesmen who have apparently rediscovered the facts which worried Malthus over a century ago. Darwin proved that overproduction was normal and necessary if there is to be progress or evolution by selecting the fittest. There must be unemployed workmen for the factories to call on, to fill the vacancies which constantly occur and the same reasoning can be followed into all walks of life; but Malthus did not know this and was much concerned over the future when the usual checks to population—war, disease, etc.—would diminish so that there would be more people than food and the struggle for existence be terrible. As we have repeatedly shown, the process is the exact opposite and the stress of living is lessening in the world at large through a lessened birth rate and increased food production. There are now dense comfortable happy European populations fed from America—a condition beyond the wildest dreams of Malthusians, and moreover the improvement occurs without resort to any of their suggestions. A Japanese governmental commission is not aware of these natural phenomena, and has gone to the trouble of calculating that by the present rate of increase of population and food, there will be, in thirty years or so, some twenty or thirty millions of Japanese without food. They have not shown how so many people can grow up without food—but that's a mere detail. The evident purpose is to show the alleged necessity for expansion of territory to grow more food like the United States, or expansion of trade so as to import food like all of N. W. Europe. Will they fight for territory and trade to raise the surplus babies, or let occasional famines keep a proper balance?

The Chinese prefer famine and plagues to war if we can believe a writer in the *Journal of the Amer. Med. Ass'n.* (May 27, 1911), for he states that the belief is universal that they are real blessings in reducing overpopulation so as to make it easy to obtain food where formerly the struggle for mere subsistence was dreadful. Their hatred of war is well known, and they never migrate for a home but merely to make money so that they can return to live in comfort. With oriental fatalism they prefer plagues and famines—that is, the survivors do after the damage is done to others. A reduction of the birth rate is almost blasphemy in a land of ancestor worship, and the Japanese consider it a sacred duty to produce soldiers for the Mikado, so both peoples wax; but are they to grow strong without food? Will the advocates of peace be able to prevent them fighting for any food in sight? Starving men do not arbitrate, when they can take with none to hinder. At the present time there is a rice shortage which threatens famine in the whole Orient, and the world seems destined to witness the death of all the increases since the last famine.

The food question in Europe is just as critical as in Asia. France has checked the birth rate so as to have more food, and as an actual fact the per capita meat consumption doubled in the last half of the last century. Nevertheless, in spite of an enormous increase of wealth and ability to import food, there are now bread riots in France on the part of those unable to buy the importations, and also in Spain and Belgium. Germany on the other hand has always been industriously multiplying and sending out hordes to replenish the earth or steal it for the food unattainable at home. When they couldn't go in military formation to France, Italy, Spain or Russia they migrated individually, chiefly to America in recent centuries for the meat famine at home made them covet our beef and corn. But so many others have been coming here for the same purpose, that there is not enough to go round now and we hear all kinds of complaints of the poor man's inability to buy meat—as though it were some new human phenomenon. Germany knows that the exodus of her citizens will end when it will be as difficult to get meat here as there—and then comes the deluge for which she is apparently preparing like the Japanese. "Land or food" is the cry now, as with the Goths and Franks from the same place. No wonder the Moroccan question will not down and may lead to war in spite of ourselves. What has been the benefit of that enormous birth rate which the German medical profession has been praising? What is the use of immigration here, when every newcomer only hastens the meat famine? Cannot our dietetists realize that in a short time the poorest paid of our population can not afford meat more than once a week or month or not at all? What will the human harvest be?

Foreign famines increase our cost of living, so that the present crisis in Europe and the Orient is bound to have far reaching consequences on our public welfare. In spite of the fact that in the world as a whole, civilization has been making it possible for increasing millions to live in more and more comfort, there still is food shortage, and an inequality of distribution with more or less famine in spots and an exodus to food areas. The victory will go to the strongest battalions fighting for subsistence—and the source of the trouble is, now as ever, the German birth rate. As for American public health, let us suppress those illogical men who complain of the high cost of food from relative scarcity due to the greater demand for it, and who at the same time advocate more births and more immigration to increase that demand and high price. Every arrival on Ellis Island from famine areas shoves up the price of beef another notch. The dietetic lesson is the fact that a meat diet belongs to a primitive hunting stage of evolution, or the settlement of a new country inhabited by savages, and that with an increasing density of population we cannot afford grazing areas, so that meat becomes less and less available until it disappears entirely from the diet of the poor. We are destined to be largely vegetarians like orientals even if we must evolve a new type of man to digest the stuff.

———

Sanitary chemistry has grown so greatly in the last two decades, as to warrant more men specializing on it. We are producing a good crop of sanitary engineers, to be sure, but neither by training nor opportunity are they able to make the chemical researches for the data upon which all sanitation ultimately depends. At present, all sanitarians depend upon a great variety of chemists who are pri-

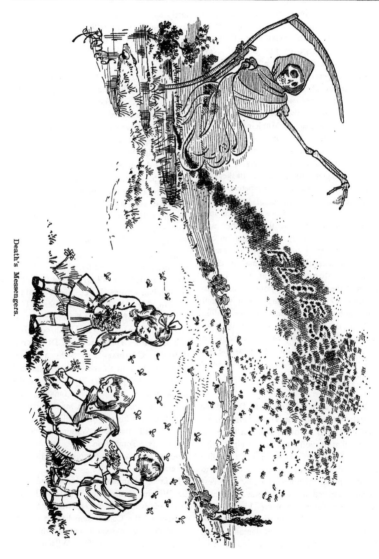

Death's Messengers.

marily engaged in something else which has a bearing upon sanitation only secondarily. Prof. Chas. Baskerville, Prof. of Chemistry, College of the City of New York, organized in 1910 a series of lectures by experts on the application of the principles of chemistry to the city, and these lectures are now published in an abridged form by the McGraw-Hill Book Co., under the title of Municipal Chemistry. It is remarkable how many chemical specialties are contributing more or less to public health and particularly to the solution of urgent city problems. Baskerville is correct in stating that a competent chemist must now be a member of every public works commission, and we can go a step further and assert that this member will often find it necessary to specialize on one problem. There is enough work in sewage alone, to take the entire time of many chemists. Moreover it is an urgent matter, and the time is long gone by for commissions to go blundering ahead without the slightest idea of what they are dealing with or the chemical changes it will undergo. Baskerville is to be thanked for calling attention to the indispensable social use of chemistry, and his advice must be heeded.

The long awaited Report of the British Royal Commission on Vivisection was issued on March 1, 1912. It is not to be expected that it will have any weight with the declared antivivisectionist, for, like most fanatics, he has subjected himself to the domination of a fixed idea by a process of auto-suggestion; and anyone conversant with psychologic problems knows how nearly impossible it is to disperse such obsessions by any reasoning or demonstration, however convincing such may be to ordi-

narily sane individuals. It may, however, carry some weight with intelligent people misinformed as to the actual state of affairs, to relate briefly what the report represents.

In consequence of the antivivisectionist agitation and the charges freely bandied about in England, that the Antivivisection Act of 1876 failed to check the alleged brutalities of animal experiments; that the officials appointed to administer the act did so unfairly, being partial to the experimenters; that in defiance of the law animals were experimented on without anesthetics and were allowed to linger in torture afterwards, etc., a Royal Commission was appointed by the British government on September 17, 1906, to inquire into the charges made and into the subject of vivisection generally. The Commission was composed of Lord Selby, Colonel Lockwood, Sir William Church, Bart., M. D., Sir William Collins, M. D., Sir John Macfadyean, Mr. MacKenzie Chalmers (Under Secretary of State for the home office), Mr. Abel Ram, K. C., Dr. Holbrook Gaskell, Mr. James Tomkinson, and Dr. George Wilson. Of these Lord Selby and Mr. Ram may be said to represent the judicial aspects of the question; Mr. Chalmers the official aspect; Sir John Macfadyean, veterinary science (he is also a medical man); Sir William Church, Sir William Collins, Dr. Gaskell and Dr. Wilson, medicine; while Mr. Tomkinson may perhaps be taken as representing the open mind of the general public.

In favor of animal experimentation were Sir William Church and Dr. Gaskell, the latter of whom, however, was the only member of the Commission having expert knowledge as an experimenter; while Sir William Collins and Dr. Wilson, with

Colonel Lockwood, may be taken as leaning in various degrees towards the antivivisectionist interest.

The instructions to the Commission were: "To inquire into and report upon the practice of subjecting live animals to experiments, whether by vivisection or otherwise; and also to inquire into the law relating to the practice and its administration, and to report whether any, and if so what, changes are desirable." For the purpose of carrying out their instructions the Commissioners held upwards of 70 meetings and examined a large number of witnesses, including representatives of the Universities and Medical Colleges, the Royal Society and other learned societies, delegates from antivivisection societies, prominent experimenters (physiologists and medical scientists), ministers of religion and others. The evidence taken before this Commission was published (verbatim and in extenso by question and answer) in 1907. The present report reviews this evidence and states the conclusions therefrom, and is signed by all the surviving members of the Commission (Lord Selby and Mr. Tomkinson having died in the course of the inquiry), including the three members more or less sympathetically inclined towards the antivivisectionist cause.

With the second part of the Commission's inquiry, inasmuch as it is of purely local interest to Great Britain, we shall have nothing to do. It is, however, gratifying to learn that the Commission expressed itself as "of opinion that, on the whole, the working of the act has been performed with a desire faithfully to carry out the objects which the framers had in view." It is further stated: "So far as we can judge we believe the holders of li-

censes and certificates (to perform animal experiments), with rare exceptions, have endeavored with loyalty and good faith to conform to the provisions of the law."

But the Commission did not confine itself to a consideration of the administration of the English Act; it investigated also the following questions relative to the entire subject of experiments on animals: (1) How far, if at all, such experiments have materially aided the cure of disease and the advancement of physiological knowledge upon which the cure of disease is based; (2) the possibility of producing in animals operated on complete immunity from pain; (3) whether under any circumstances even if the beneficial results claimed can be established, such experiments are morally justifiable.

We cannot follow the Commissioners though their detailed examination of these points. We can only cite their conclusions thereon, using their own words, and at the same time emphasizing the fact that the signature of every surviving member of the Commission of those whose previous bias was against such experiments, as well as those who were from the outset in favor of them or who had an open mind thereon was appended to the statements quoted; and although three of the members also signed separate memoranda containing reservations, they only affected certain points of detail or had regard to the advisability of particular procedure in the working of the Act.

Regarding the results of such experiments on the cure of disease and the increase of physiological knowledge on which the cure of disease depends, the Commissioners say that, after a full consideration of all the evidence pro and con, they are led to think:

"(1) That certain results claimed from time to time to have been proved by experiments upon living animals and alleged to have been beneficial in preventing or curing disease, have, on further investigation and experience, been found to be fallacious or useless.

(2) That notwithstanding such failures valuable knowledge has been acquired in regard to physiological processes and the causation of disease, and that useful methods for the prevention, cure, and treatment of certain diseases have resulted from experimental investigations upon living animals.

(3) That, as far as we can judge, it is highly improbable that without experiments made on animals mankind would at the present time have been in possession of such knowledge.

(4) That in so far as disease has been successfully prevented or its mortality reduced, suffering has been diminished in man and in lower animals.

(5) That there is ground for believing that similar methods of investigation if pursued in the future will be attended with similar results."

With regard to the possibility of inducing anesthesia in animals under experimentation, they state:

"After careful consideration of the whole question of anesthetics as applied to experimental investigations on living animals, we are led to the conclusion that by the use of one or other or of a combination of several well known anesthetics complete insensibility to pain can be secured."

Finally, as to the moral aspect of the question, it is stated that:

"After full consideration we are led to the conclusion that experiments upon animals, adequately safeguarded by law, faithfully administered, are morally justifiable and should not be prohibited by legislation."

In view of the fact that these conclusions were unanimously arrived at by a commission consisting for the major part of men either holding opinions at the outset more or less antagonistic to animal experimentation or having no prepossessions whatever on the subject, and after a careful consideration of the opinions, not only of eminent scientists but of prominent antivivisectionists and of well known moralists mostly of pronounced antivivisection views, it would seem difficult to think, as Lord Cromer, the president of the Research Defense Society, recently stated in a letter to the *Times* "that any impartial person will be able to read this illuminating report without coming to the conclusion that, broadly speaking, the supporters of vivisection have proved their case."

The "back to the farm" movement has a few medical aspects which it would be well to consider. It seems that the world over, agriculture requires an amount of painful, exhausting, deadening, monotonous labor out of all proportion to the wages. It is the oldest of the arts and was exclusively in the hands of the women for many thousands of years when conditions were so unsettled that a man could not be burdened with any work interfering with his duty to fight for his family. It was the first step in the ever increasing struggle to raise more food for the surplus who could not find enough in the wild. It was therefore a most unnatural life for primitive man who was built for fighting and hunting, and we can well imagine that as the hunting grounds disappeared and all men had to settle down to food raising or die, there was frightful destruction of life from physical unfitness to the calling. The women were strong, the men active. Ever since then, any man who could use his wits for obtaining his food in easier ways has been leaving the farm. Even yet the women do hard farm labor in many places. There has been a constant selection going on in those who drift to the city and the survivors are by that token unfit to return to the country. These types fit for city life are constantly increasing in number and proportion, for every labor saving farm invention releases laborers for the city factories. Instead of advising these people to go back to the farm, where they are not needed and could not do the work even if there was any to do, we must make the cities fit to live in. Back to the farm is medical nonsense for these city types who can't live anywhere else. In some places in Europe, the opportunities of industry or trade have actually drained the farms of brains, and the country laborers are as remarkable for stupidity as those of ancient Greece. In America we are beginning to witness the same selection, and as a result the standards of honesty, honor and civic pride are very high in the city as well as the intellectual level. Adams County, Ohio, vote-sellers are not exceptions by a long shot, and we have ceased to boast of the "honest farmer." It is therefore quite evident that as the least efficient are just able to keep body and soul together and often not that, farming is not remunerative for that reason alone. Brainy men can make money at it, but prefer easier work in the city.

City environment for the sick is a new idea which has been developed by the new medical anthropology. Beddoe's investigations in England have long made us familiar with the idea that certain types have greater morbidity to certain diseases. Shrubsall's work on Physical Characteristics and Morbid Proclivities (*St. Bartholomew's Hosp. Reports,* 1903) has pointed out the races that are most liable to tonsillitis, rheumatism, heart dis-

ease and osteo-arthritis. Numerous observers have shown that the tall blond Baltic man so eminently fitted to live long and healthy in the cold, black cloudy Scandinavian uplands is really unfit for any other life. He survives in northern Scotland, the Alps and in our Alleghanies, but dies out in the lowlands particularly where it is sunny or hot, the city is deadly to him and confinement in factories is worst of all. On the other hand certain short brunets thrive in the city factories and even in the sweat shops which would kill a Norwegian in twelve months. Dr. J. S. Mackintosh has also taken up this matter (*Brit. Med. Jour.,* Oct. 8, 1910) and shows that the roving open-air-loving blond cannot submit to confinement, particularly in rest-cures. He notes that Sir Wm. Bennett (*The Practitioner,* June, 1910) has found that certain cases of tuberculosis do best at their native places, others at the coast and most marvellous of all Mackintosh says that some do best in a London hospital. We have often called attention in these columns to the fact, now emphasized by Mackintosh, that the physical type of the patient must be considered in selecting a place for any invalid, particularly the tuberculous. The seashore may be good for some and bad for others, a big blond might get well at once in the Adirondacks where the little brunet Sicilian would shiver into his grave. Some may go back to the farm, and others must stay in the city where their type belongs. We have magnificent opportunities for observing the effects of our climates on all the various types of the world, but somehow we must depend on European observers. While they are noting marked morbidity differences, say between blonds and brunets, American physicians are denying the far greater differences in America. New Orleans climate has killed off the. blonds among the French, and yet no one even noticed the slaughter as it progressed. A similar process is going on in our sunny northwest, but there are few who are able to see it.

***

Reform in feminine dress must receive the attention of every thoughtful person. It is inconceivable that modest, pure minded women will be willing to adopt styles that admit of conclusions concerning their morals so contrary to their real intentions. But the extremes to which many young and imprudent females have gone in the effort to be up to date and *chic* are dangerous in the extreme, not alone because of the constant invitation to improper advances from the wolves in men's clothing who are ever seeking their prey, but also because of the effect on the sexually perverted and the possibility of inducing sexual crimes by degenerates. It is all well enough for the superior-minded purists to say that "to the pure all things are pure," and that the so-called evils of feminine dress are born in the minds of the lascivious and lustful. Some of this may be true. Nearly every man of normal appetites has a bit of Adam in him. Happily most men are dominated by innate decency and the respect they feel for womankind. Our daughters, sisters and wives have little to fear from most men, no matter how they dress. But every medical man of large practice and experience knows only too well the fires of perversion kindled by the present dress of young, voluptuous females. Freud's studies showing the sexual origin of countless nervous and mental affections emphasize the foregoing and leave no doubt that immodest dress is responsible for many a young girl's downfall and ruin.

Our remarks on this subject last month evidently struck a responsive chord in the minds of many people, for the communications commending our criticism of questionable styles of dress were unusually numerous. It would seem that here is an opportunity for accomplishing a much needed reform. Good women—and thank God, most women *are* good—will refuse to wear extreme and immodest apparel when they realize what construction is placed on their bravado or imprudence by mankind in general. No good girl can afford to allow even the slightest suspicion to attach itself to her character. Therefore she cannot choose her dress with too great care, for a single indiscretion or bit of daring may create an impression in the mind of some one that can never be removed. We are quite willing that a few may question the propriety of a scientific journal entering the province of woman's fashions. We and every other experienced physician know that the *risque* styles of the present day have a psychologic bearing on a good many susceptible mentalities, and as the modern physician is beginning to realize the importance of prophylaxis as well as treatment in ministering to diseased minds as well as diseased bodies, we doubt if we are very far afield, after all. Our only hope is that thinking men and women will awaken to the great importance of the subject and do their part in spreading the gospel of dressing modestly and decently. Let a certain class of femininity go to the extremes of immodesty and indecency, if they will, but not those who know the real significance of modesty and chastity.

The necessity for cooling hospital wards is at last receiving the attention its importance demands. We have called attention to the fact that though we deliberately expose the tuberculous and pneumonic to cold air to cure them in winter, yet when summer comes along we allow the heat to kill them when it is a very simple practicable matter to make the room as cold as we wish. Indeed the cooling of office buildings, clubs and hotels has long passed the experimental stage and yet we have atrociously neglected the use of the system to save the babies slaughtered by every hot wave. We also know that dysenteric adults have great difficulty in getting well if the thermometer is over 82° and may die if it is over 95° and yet they recover marvellously in cold air, indeed even cool air is beneficial and in the tropics anything below 78° or better 75°. The whole matter is being studied experimentally with infected animals in a cool room at the Liverpool School of Tropical Medicine by Prof. Ronald Ross and Mr. J. G. Thomson who have made a preliminary report (*British Medical Journal*, Mar. 25, 1911) as to the effect in trypanosomiasis. There seems no doubt that cold air prevents the development of some parasites, delays incubation and prolongs life, and hopes are raised that it may be beneficial if not wholly curative in human cases. In one case reported there was decided improvement. The authors review the scant literature on the subject, mentioning the benefit in malaria and tuberculosis.

———

The dangers of all the short ether waves have been repeatedly demonstrated, and it is now the routine technique to protect X-ray operators by opaque screens. Those who have not done so, are about all killed off by this time. We have then, not been at all surprised to hear of Madame Curie's illness, nor that the cause is the ether waves from the radium she has worked with so many years. We now learn that actinic eczemas, visual disturbances and neurasthenia are beginning to disable wireless operators who are more or less immersed in the same short waves. These conditions have long been recognized as some of the results of excessive exposure to the electric light and to the ultra-violet and shorter visual rays of the sun on skins insufficiently pigmented, and it is gratifying to see the profession turning against the dreadful sun baths once so popular. An ignorant tropical savage would not let his children expose themselves that way. We are quite sure our school teachers will not tolerate overlighting much longer.

The unwholesome stimulation of dazzling school rooms is being so widely recognized as causing nervousness and other damage, that the trend is all the other way and school rooms are now being lighted only to the degree needed for good vision without the strain of too much shade or too much glare. Electric stimulations will do as much nervous harm as overlighting and must be strongly condemned. The negro classes may like strongly lighted hot rooms and thrive in them, but the northern types would be killed therein. The degree of light and heat must be a compromise not specially harmful to the little dark Italian or little blond swede.

———

The maximum age for ship commanders is again brought up by the dreadful Titanic disaster. There is no question that somebody made a blunder and in the absence of exact information one naturally thinks of the person whose final decision counts—

366   AMERICAN MEDICINE
Complete Series, Vol. XVIII. | EDITORIAL COMMENT   {   JULY, 1912.
New Series, Vol. VII., No. 7.

the captain. This brings up the question to which AMERICAN MEDICINE has referred time and time again—why is it that so many disasters occur to ships commanded by men who have had splendid records for seamanship, alertness and good judgment for forty years or more? Everyone knows that the natural changes in the brain sooner or later cause a senile dementia which utterly prevents good judgment. The question is, at what age do these changes prevent that active mentality needed to meet new situations. Some ship companies have decided that no captain should be over sixty, and then elderly experienced men are given shore duty or pensioned. The navy, through sad experience, apparently does not wish to trust ships to men over 55, preferably less than 50. The Titanic disaster seems to indicate that 55 is the extreme limit for such responsibilities as a gigantic liner. There was a new situation—a new ship to make a speed record, the report of the position of gigantic icebergs whose proximity might have been known without wireless by the changes in the temperature of the air and water and yet the lookouts had no glasses, their warnings were apparently ignored, and the ship plunged along at 21 knots an hour. Would a younger man have been more alive to the new danger and stayed on the bridge every minute? Was the older man really warped in judgment by a long life of success?

There is a cock-sureness of long experience as well as of inexperience. Let it be investigated. Grandfathers are invaluable in council, but out of place as the actual managers. When should a man hand over the reins to his sons? Is there such a thing as the delusion of success or mania of never being wrong? There has long been proved to be an "officialism" which mentally afflicts those long in office and leads them to believe themselves infallible and subordi-

nates always wrong if of a different opinion. But the real reason is the fact that memory is so fickle towards the end of the sixth decade of life, that few men can remember all the little things they did to bring the success which made them famous. This is apparently contradicted by the large number of ship captains over 65 or 70, but it is proved by the appalling number of "accidents" falling to those who have never made a blunder "for 40 years." It fully explains why so many landsmen do some foolish thing after 60 to destroy much of what they did before. It is a fact that the man on the bridge of a modern floating palace, must be in the fullest vigor of his mental powers before it is possible for the natural and inevitable senile changes to have caused any deterioration.

The puzzle of black-water fever seems to be solved by the valuable study of Deeks and James on the Canal Zone and published by the Sanitary Department. They show that the disease is never found except where there is a non-immune population in a malarial region, the estivo-autumnal cases being numerous. Moreover in every case there is more or less proof of a long period of malarial attacks which were not properly and promptly treated with quinine. It seems to be a profound change in the blood and blood vessels from a long continued toxemia. Any depressing influence or an acute malarial paroxysm, or even quinine may evoke the symptom, but that neither malaria alone nor quinine alone is capable of causing it. The problem of prevention is merely that of curing malaria. The appearance of the disease in persons in whom a history of malaria was difficult to elicit, had given rise to a widespread theory that it was a special disease with an unknown specific cause found only where malaria is possible. This can now be definitely abandoned.

ORIGINAL ARTICLES.

THE HARMFUL EFFECTS OF SMALL AMOUNTS OF HEAT AND LIGHT.

BY

CHAS. E. WOODRUFF, M. D.,

U. S. Army Med. Dept., San Francisco, Cal.

Psychologists assure us that after forty years of age, it becomes increasingly difficult to change our habits of thought, and that our mental inertia becomes so great after 60 that we actually resent changes. Only the unstable young are plastic and as a fact we rarely get far away from the form in which the environment moulded us in childhood. Moreover the young are the most observant and nearly every great revolutionary idea has been conceived by a young man, generally less than 30, often in his teens. The work power which goes with stability can not reach its maximum until after we lose plasticity and, saddest of all, when we acquire a vast store of knowledge and experiences we rapidly lose the power of using them. Men can do good work as long as they live, but the quantity and quality of the yearly output progressively diminishes even though the culmination such as a history or a philosophy is not reached until very late in life. Some positions, requiring stability, conservatism and knowledge, should not be open to candidates much less than 60 years old. It thus happens that while the experienced leaders are generally balance wheels preventing the majority from running after false gods, they hold to false ideas themselves with a persistence truly harmful. This has led Osler to assert that where progress is rapid, men ought to retire at 60 to prevent undue obstruction.

He was misunderstood and greatly criticized, but as a matter of fact our greatest soldier, General U. S. Grant, placed the age younger still, and has often said that the history of the world, particularly our disgraceful failures in the war of 1812, shows that no general officer in war should be over fifty—this in spite of apparent exceptions like von Moltke whose plans are now known to have been dreadfully defective but who was lucky in not having a young Napoleon opposing him.

There is then no mystery about the persistence of ideas for long periods after they have been proved to be false. It seems impossible to eradicate the belief in the absurd story that wheat has been grown from seed found with mummies several thousand years old. The history of medicine is one long painful series of persecutions of those who have discovered new things. We were once convinced that consumptives were so delicate that they should be carefully housed in warm rooms and protected from drafts. It was quite logical, then, that we should have been horrified at Bodington's apparently murderous cruelty in putting them outdoors. In the supposed interests of humanity we drove him out of practice.

When an idea becomes crystallized in a text-book, the difficulty of eliminating it seems increased many fold, for it is copied from one authority to another as an accepted axiom not needing proof or confirmation. Jordan mentions (*Science*, June 2, 1911) many ways in which money is being squandered on fruitless public health measures, due to the impossibility of eradicating sanitary hypotheses inherited from the days before the real causes of infection and their methods of transfer were known.

There is no evidence whatever that sunlight is beneficial in tuberculosis, nor that the ideal climate should have a maximum of sunshine; moreover, a careful investigation carried on for several years has shown that the evidence is all the other way; nevertheless the baseless assertions are still repeated from book to book and have recently been approved at medical meetings. The error is an inheritance from the days of Bodington's persecution. So convinced were we that consumptives needed warm air, that we would not believe it was the cold air which cured them, and we insisted that it was due to the light. So we began the construction of the dreadful hot sunparlors to let in the harmful light and keep out the saving cold.

Luckily there are signs of a reaction in professional opinion, following upon the enormous number of experiments as to the effects of light and heat, and the revelation that in excess both are very deadly. The literature is so voluminous and progressively increasing, that it is not possible to keep up with it in reviews. The articles on radium alone are legion. The slowness of the reversal of opinion as to the effects of all radiant frequencies is in part due to the conservatism of the leaders, as previously explained. An editorial in the *Journal of the American Medical Association* (May 20, 1911) says: "The theory of Woodruff, that the deterioration of the white man in the tropics is due more to the actinic rays of the sun than to exposure to excessive heat, has found many adherents." It is presumed that the remark refers to the present writer as he is the only one of that name among the many who are investigating the subject. As he has never written a word as to the relative damage of the long and short waves in the

sun's rays, and as he has always believed the heat more harmful than light and as he knows of no one who believes otherwise, the editorial is triply erroneous. When the very best men in the profession, its leaders in fact—the editorial writers of our national association—can be so wholly wrong, as in Bodington's day, it is quite evident that the mass are uninformed. It is with a view of calling attention to the damage of heat that this article is written.

The effects of long and short rays are really phenomena of different orders and not comparable at all. It seems accepted now, that the infra-red rays cause vibrations of molecules (temperature) while the short light rays (blue to violet) and the ultraviolet cause movements within the molecule, stimulating or disrupting it. The midrays can do both and in addition cause the sensation of light, but there is more or less actinic effect in all frequencies. The heating and actinic effect are as different as the action of a corrosive poison and chloroform.

The new view point is that the short rays really are harmful—a complete revolution in thought from the time when we considered light as always beneficial in all amounts and never harmful. The original observations of von Schmaedel as to the necessity of skin pigment to exclude the harm, were at first completely ignored like the observations of that other German, Mendel, who has revolutionized our ideas of inheritance. Calling attention to the harm of light has been misinterpreted as trying to prove it the only cause of injury of misplaced migrants, whereas it is only one among thousands, many of which are more powerful.

It was presumed of course that every one knew of the effects of excessive heat, for H. C. Wood at the University of Pennsylvania proved by animal experimentation a half century ago that the typical sunstroke with coma and high fever was due to the dark infra-red rays, and should be called thermic fever. We even see it in negroes exposed to dark high heat—higher than that of the blood—for in such conditions the black skin keeps out most of the light and yet absorbs more heat than white skins. Negroes cannot stand as high a heat as white men, though the contrary is generally believed. When the external temperature is lower than 98° F. they are at a great advantage, for they radiate more. So great indeed is the damage to white men, by this inability to radiate heat in air temperatures above 80° F., that it is found practically impossible to cure certain cases in that range though they promptly recover in cool or cold air. It is now considered more necessary in certain affections to cool hospital wards in summer than to heat them in winter. All the sick babies slaughtered by a hot wave could be saved by putting them in a cool room but unfortunately we use the cooling machinery only to keep their poor little bodies from decay after the heat has killed them. The dead room should be the living room.

In passing it might be said that the condition known as "heat exhaustion" with the opposite symptoms to "thermic fever" is quite generally believed to be due to excessive light for it never appears except when the light is excessive, though it may be complicated with "thermic fever" in an infinite variety of forms. In India, thermic fever is strictly related to heat as to season, climate, time of day and degree of infra-red rays. "Heat cramps" so common and fatal in hot rooms are due solely to excessive perspiration for they are in-

stantly cured by intravenous injections of salt water, and are worse in negroes of course.

We have long known that the vast majority of living forms are not injured by reducing their temperature. Many fish can be frozen a short time yet will live after thawing, and simpler organisms can be reduced to absolute zero for awhile. On the other hand, death always results if the temperature is raised only a few degrees above that at which the species functions best. Some pathogenic bacteria will die at 104°, and trout at 70°. It seems that cold merely stops activity but heat disrupts by too much activity, and the same may be said of the short rays. Consequently we find that nature, besides being very careful to guard all protoplasm from too much light, is more particular still to prevent any rise of temperature. Complicated mechanisms are provided to aid the escape of heat in hot surroundings.

The benefit of cold air and the damage done by moderate heat are the two great modern ideas now being substantiated by experiments all over the world. E. O. Jordan says, (*Science*, June 2, 1911) "if the work of Beu (*Zeitschr. f. Hyg.* 1893, 14, p. 64), Heymann, Paul, Erclentz, Flügge (id. 1905, 49, p. 363), Leonard Hill and others means anything it demonstrates that the whole effect from 'bad air' and crowded rooms is due to heat and moisture and not to carbon dioxid or to any poisonous excretions in expired air." "Crowd poisoning" can be eliminated by electric fans without fresh air. Yet so obsessed are we with the old ideas, we cannot appreciate the proofs of the harm of small degrees of heat—over 75 or 80°. Quite a number of tropical practitioners have noticed that the higher the air temperature

370   AMERICAN MEDICINE
Complete Series, Vol. XVIII.   ORIGINAL ARTICLES   JULY, 1912.
New Series, Vol. VII., No. 7.

rises above 80°, the more difficult or impossible it is to cure certain cases, and that above 90° they die like the city babies in a hot wave, but that a storm which lowers the temperature below 80° will cure cases apparently moribund. A trip away from the tropics will save cases otherwise doomed. So it is now suggested to cool all hospital wards in climates where the air temperature is over 80°.

Our phthisiographers in particular have not yet grasped the full significance of their cures in the open air; for it is assumed to be due to almost everything else except the main cause—relief from the damage of small degrees of heat in confined rooms. When Trudeau found that animals infected with tuberculosis recovered outdoors while the controls in the laboratory died, it was assumed, of course, that the light did it in spite of the cold air, although everyone knows that the amount of sunshine in the cloudy Adirondacks is not worth quarreling over. Recent experiments in France have shown that they recovered by reason of the cold air in spite of the light.

In the *N. Y. Med. Rec.*, July 9, 1910, it is reported that Lannelongue and Achard have performed the following experiment: "They took several parcels of guinea pigs of the same age and as far as possible the same weight and the same day inoculated them in the peritoneal cavity with the same amount of the same culture of tubercle bacilli. Then these different parcels of animals were placed in different hygienic climatic conditions; the country, the seashore, the coast of La Mancha, high altitudes, the South, the North; the last lot was kept in the laboratory in a dark room, but with a window constantly open. The guinea pigs of each lot received daily the same food; whenever a pig died he was

sent to the laboratory of Lannelongue for an autopsy. Those that resisted to the last were those in the laboratory."

Ross and Thomson of the Liverpool School of Tropical Medicine have carried the experiments further (*Brit. Med. Jour.*, Mar. 25, 1911) by confining animals in cold rooms, and find that they are livelier and better, and that those infected with trypanosomes have delayed incubation, longer life, fewer parasites and greater phagocytosis. They mention the fact of phthisis being benefitted by cold air, and also the experiments of Crane (*St. Louis Medical Review*, July 7, 1906) that cold prevents or cures tetanus, while heat brings it out. There is much evidence that both malaria and yellow fever are checked by cold air —that is, the infected have far better chances of recovery but die in hot air. Pneumonia is cured in the cold, but is very fatal in the tropics. On the other hand, Sir Wm. Bennett (*Practitioner*, June, 1910) shows that while most consumptives do best by return to their birthplaces, some do best in the hospital even in London with its fogs—providing of course the rooms are cool. That is, it is now proved that the only thing outdoors in greater amount than in properly ventilated cold rooms, is the light, and therefore it must be the harmful factor in these cases which do not get well in the sunshine, and it explains the better health of those animals kept in the cool laboratory.

It might be well to inquire as to how much the heat of work rooms is responsible for the high sick rates of barbers, printers, tailors and other indoor workers.

In the modern rest cure it has been found necessary to darken the room to prevent the stimulation of the light, a fact which G. R. Rowe mentioned in 1817 in his work on Hypochondriasis. Most significant of all, it is now frequently stated—though no statistics have been given in proof—that blonds do not stand the rest cure as well as brunets and it is well to inquire if they have not been kept in glary rooms. The statement of Clarence Wheaton of Chicago, that "sunshine promotes repose of mind" is the opposite of the reports from all light climates, where the physicians are often compelled to send cases away on account of this mental irritation and subsequent exhaustion. Newcomers in Los Angeles, Cal., are recognized by their activity due to this stimulation—facts long known in the tropics.

In fact, every new observation published tends in the same direction of proving the damage done by moderate amounts of both long and short rays in sunshine. Experimenters are now trying to differentiate between the two. The most amazing fact brought out is the damage done by small amounts we formerly considered beneficial. Moreover we are finding that the animals we once thought to be the most resistant to both light and heat are in fact very susceptible, and survive merely because they hide from the danger, as their range is exceedingly limited. We have long known that white ants are killed by a few minutes' exposure to a diffused light without any increase in temperature, and die after a few seconds' exposure to the direct rays of the sun but here heat is also a factor. We have also known of the rapidity with which a cold light, such as that of Schott's uviol lamp, will kill the insects attracted to it. We now find that tropical fleas which we know are protected fairly well from light and which we formerly considered as inured to heat also, are easily killed by heat. In the search for simple means of

disinfecting flea ridden clothing in Indian plague epidemics, Lieut.-Col. Bannerman found that exposure to the sun for three hours was sufficient, but Capt. Cunningham ("The Destruction of Fleas by Exposure to the Sun," Calcutta, 1911) now finds that ten minutes is sufficient in the direct rays, while 45 minutes are needed for the fleas on the under surface where the short rays do not penetrate, and that a temperature of 120° F. must be obtained. Lieut. W. L. Hart of the medical corps, exposed to the direct rays at Cebu, P. I., some young rats found in a dark room, and in twenty minutes all were dead. Castellani and Chalmers thus killed rabbits with shaved heads in about an hour at Colombo, Ceylon, but those under red glass survived. They were inclined to believe the more effective rays were in the visible violet, but the result was thermic fever, with its characteristic congestion of the cerebral meninges.

Hans Aron of the University of the Philippines, has made many experiments in this line (The Phil. Jour. of Science, Ap. 1911) and the general trend of them all was to the effect that death was due to thermic fever and the pathology was the same, as far as known, as in the experiments of H. C. Wood. Death was often prevented by keeping the animals cool, in the draft of an electric fan. Without this aid, monkeys would die in less than two hours, and it was due to body heat for if the body were protected and only the head exposed death was prevented. Post mortems showed hemorrhages into the heart muscle and cerebral meninges. No wonder Ruhemunn found that cerebro-spinal meningitis was worse in the sunlight (Klin. Woch. 1906) and Huddlestone found that two children convalescent from pneumonia had "sunstrokes" from sun-exposure outdoors. (*N. Y. Med. Rec.*, Feb. 9, 1907). These facts should be seriously considered by those who like Knopf of New York expose the naked bodies of consumptives to the direct rays of the sun. Their body temperature may rise several degrees, as proved by White of Colorado. This is more important in the case of white men, as a brown or black skin, though it absorbs more of these direct rays, radiates more to the surrounding cooler air in accordance with the laws of heat. Aron found that with equal sun exposures tropical natives had cooler skins than white men. R. W. Felkin reported in the *Archives of Röentgen Ray,* 1905, that in North Africa, Europeans have an axillary temperature of 99.5, Arabs 99.1 and Negroes 97.8, and that for every degree of increase of air temperature white men have an increase of .005° body temperature from the difficulty of radiating heat. When the brown or black men are in a temperature higher than tropical air generally is, they cannot radiate heat and the results are the reverse.

Aron's results with monkeys were in accordance with recent clinical experience in zoological gardens. These animals live in cool air and in the shade of trees. At night the air in tropical mountains is often quite cold, and as this is their natural habitat we now find that those kept outdoors all winter keep in perfect condition but those in the hot monkey house die of tuberculosis. The inconsistencies of heliotherapists are illustrated by one living in Chicago who says that the ideal climate possesses "the greatest possible amount of sunshine, light winds and dry atmosphere and porous soil with elevation sufficient to increase the respiratory act in depth and

vigor," and yet in another communication states that professional opinion is almost universal that arid regions are not suitable though they mostly have all the alleged ideal conditions. He even states that there is no ideal climate. Now we find Sir William Bennett obtaining fine results in climates the exact opposite of this "ideal" —little sunshine, high winds, wet atmosphere, non-porous soil and low level!

In fact every bit of the new evidence supports von Schmaedel's original theory that skin pigment is to keep out the light rays. The least pigmented animals must hide from the light or live in dark climates. Wherever the air temperature is above 80° and less than 98°, this pigment is also a great advantage in keeping cool by radiation as explained in "The Effects of Tropical Light on White Men," so that the color becomes intensified; but such black animals cannot live in very cold climates without radiating too much heat nor expose themselves to the direct sun's rays without absorbing so much as to die of thermic fever. It thus happens that if any animal must go out in the sunshine, it must have a second or outer garment of light shade to reflect the heat. The Arab or negro puts on white for this purpose and so do many breeds of horses and other animals, but the majority use yellow, like plains animals. White is also used to conserve heat in cold countries as it radiates less as in the case of Coreans. These generalizations are all confirmed by the experiments with orange-red underclothing, though they are quite generally interpreted otherwise. (An Experiment with Orange-red Underwear, Dr. Jas. D. Phalen, *Phil. Jour. of Sc.,* Dec., 1910). As the writer had nothing to do with the initiation or conduct of the experiments, he has no knowledge of the reasons for them. They were certainly not designed to test a hypothesis that light is more harmful than heat, as stated by the *Journal of the Amer. Med. Ass'n.*, for as far as known no one has ever expressed such an idea. Nor is it known why this particular color was used. Nature never selects it. In the process of dyeing, the material thickened up and the garments were warmer than those used by the majority of people in cold climates, and the wearers suffered the same as though they wore furs, and when exposed to direct rays, the color of course absorbed heat like Aron's monkeys. If a white man exposed to strong sunlight elects to dress in thin white garments like the Arab horse or Chinese pony, then the undergarment should be opaque, preferably black like the skin of these horses; but if he dresses in yellow like the lion, then the undergarment will not be necessary at all provided the outer one is sufficiently opaque. The details reported have little scientific value in determining the relative efficiency of different kinds of clothing as a protection against heat and light. According to the *Arch. of Röent. Ray*, Jan., 1911, Prof. E. C. C. Baly, F. R. S., London Univ. College, proved that red-lined cloth does stop the ultra-violet rays and prevent the skin injuries they are known to cause, and people in the tropics who have used it, say the same thing.

The matter will be taken up more widely now as it has been found to have great economic importance. Dr. Robert Wallace, Prof. of Agriculture in the University of Edinburgh, has been observing the colors of tropical domestic animals for twenty-five years, his first article appearing in the *Proceedings of the Edinburgh Royal Society* in 1887. He finds pigmented skins universal and the absence of pigment prevents the acclimatization of northern stock in southern latitudes. I have unexpectedly encountered much data showing that certain colors of horses are at a disadvantage in hot climates. The articles have been published elsewhere,[1] but it might be said that all known facts confirm the generalization that animals must be protected from both the long and short rays of the sun.

The hair of the head is undoubtedly to shade the subjacent cerebral cells as the tissues are very transparent. It has very little effect in heat retention and the necessity of keeping the head cool is obvious. But Aron finds, as to be expected, that when exposed to sun's rays, the air in black hair is very hot. Such men then are like black animals which must seek the shade. Schmidt (*Arch. für Hygiene*, 1908) showed that the cerebral cortex becomes overheated by the transmitted heat as well as that radiated, and he advocates opaque clothing. We now see why it is that black-haired tropical people are so careful to wear big hats or other elaborate protection, why negroes and Arabs don white to reflect heat, why Coreans don it to conserve heat in cold climates, and why black is so popular for indoors or evenings in the tropics as it radiates better.

Liebe (*Zeitschrift für Physikalische Diätatische Therapie*, July, 1907) reported the stimulating effects of light baths, and mentioned that Hovorka often found them to cause headache, palpitation, insomnia, and even hemorrhages. Burton-Fanning reports in his work on tuberculosis the same things in cases exposed to light, and so does Carling of New York. (*N. Y. Med. Jour.*, Aug. 29, 1908), while many physi-

[1] *U. S. Cavalry Journal*, Sept., 1911, and May, 1912.

cians have noticed the tendency to pulmonary hemorrhage during sun exposure. When we realize that the temperature in a light bath is often 120° we can well see from Aron's work how dangerous they are from cerebral congestion due to this heat. Indeed Grawitz of Berlin was compelled to warn against sun baths, particularly in children whom he often found to be seriously affected. (*Deutsch Medizin. Woch.,* Aug. 19, 1909, No. 33). In view of the fact that all animals instinctively hide from the sun's rays unless highly protected, it is extremely difficult to account for the mania for heliotherapy, particularly as there is no evidence of any benefit. It is no doubt true that direct rays cure local superficial tuberculosis but experiments in Finsen's Copenhagen Institute showed that the rays do not kill the bacteria at all, and that the water in the cooling apparatus absorbs ultra-violet as well as infra-red rays. Numerous other observers have shown that the results are due to the serum poured out in reaction as after any other irritant, or in passive congestion. Similarly numerous writers have shown the curative value of exposing infected ulcers to direct rays, but here too it is shown to be due to a reaction from irritation and not due to disinfection. Of course the heat may disinfect as in the case of the fleas, but one can hardly say whether hot applications (air of 125° for a half hour) to gonorrheal arthritis cure by reason of the germicidal effects as we once thought or to the congestion resulting from the irritation. The appearance of carcinoma on the site of lupus cured by Finsen, (*Lancet,* Mar. 7, 1903, quoted by Watkins-Pitchford), the same as the ordinary x-ray cancer, shows how serious the irritation really is. In certain infections the skin lesions appear only on surfaces exposed to light (pellagra) or are worse there (smallpox). When the whole body is exposed to light or heat, the irritation must be very severe.

While the physicians of dark northern Europe and some in America (*N. Y. Med. Jour.,* Sept. 12, 1908) are beginning to warn against sun baths, the system is still in use on the sunnier continent, but the reports are very significant of the damage, and also show false premises. For instance, Malgat of Nice (*Annal. de la Societe de Medecine Physique de Anvers,* 1905) for years used light baths to the naked body on the theory that the light rays penetrated deeply, but we now know that they are largely stopped at the surface and always irritate. We know of course that the mid-rays (light) are stopped in proportion to the density of the pigment, and Sambon (*Jour. of Tropical Medicine,* Feb. 15, 1907) proved that it also excluded the ultra-violet in like proportion, confirming the results at the Finsen Institute. Indeed so efficacious is the pigment, that Stein and Hesse (*Arch. of Röentgen Ray,* Aug., 1907) have found that it required 45 minutes for utra-violet of the uviol lamp to cause an evanescent redness on a brunet skin, while 10 minutes' application to the delicate skin of a young girl raised a blister. In one dark skin a daily exposure of an hour for a whole week had no effect. Similarly, brunets resist x-ray burns. A negro, then, may enjoy a sun bath in a northern climate which is fatal to a white man from the light alone or the heat alone, for the latter absorbs both but cannot radiate the heat; but the tropical negro not only hides in huts in mid-day to escape overheating, but must also huddle up indoors at night when the temperature is below 75 or 70° as he chills so easily by radiation.

All these facts are confirmed by the results of treating tuberculosis in the Swiss Alps by Rollier's method of sun exposure. (*Bost. Med. and Surg. Journal*, Oct. 27, 1910). He apparently hasn't the slightest conception of the value of cold air, and imputes all the benefit to the light, though he says that there is little or no improvement until the skin gets heavily tanned and keeps out the light! Blonds who won't tan, won't improve—so great is the light damage, 'for we know that blonds are more benefitted by cold than brunets. Moreover the best results are obtained in winter when the light is the least intense. American physicians have noted similar phenomena, (*N. Y. Med. Jour.*, Sept. 13, 1908) particularly as to the greater morbidity and mortality of misplaced blonds, though we find that in proper cold and dark environments they are healthier than the brunets. In the Philippines the white tubercular are very largely blonds, and this is true in minor degree of central France and even in southern England but not in cold cloudy Scotland or Scandinavia or our own cloudy mountains. In view of these facts it almost insults one's intelligence to read in the London *Lancet* of Nov. 12, 1910, that another Swiss heliotherapist, Dr. Révillet actually sends Geneva tubercular children down to the sea-shore at Cannes, for sun-baths in the very season, October to June, when Rollier gets the most improvement higher up than Geneva. His results, 52 per cent of cures and 41 of improvements, are not nearly as good as in places where the little ones are not given sun-baths, for he does not accept cases with open lesions, and he has to hustle them off home as soon as the hot light season begins—the season in which we can get excellent results in cold shady mountain forests.

It might be well to remark here that Jacobi in an article on the difficulty of early diagnosis in tuberculosis (*Archives of Diagnosis*, Ap., 1911) mentions the possibility of frequent errors of omission and commission. Perhaps most cases are overlooked, if we can believe the post-mortem findings as to alleged healed lesions in such a large percentage of mankind, some say as high as 90 per cent. We may recognize only the progressives who do not recover spontaneously, for now Welch of Baltimore is reported as saying that a very large proportion of slum children become infected. On the other hand, one of the whispered scandals of the profession is the large percentage of cures of alleged incipients in certain institutions who were not tuberculous at all. In collecting statistics some years ago, I was compelled to reject the report of a private sanatorium because of the ridiculously large percentage of cures and arrests of even the incurables.

It has long been known that racial characters are evolved to make one fit to survive a certain environment, but the data collected in the last five years show that each type is tied by a much shorter tether than we imagined. Of course we knew that migration to a widely different climate was always fatal, but it now appears that even shorter movements are followed by extinction. Blond French in New Orleans died long ago, but they are also largely gone from Canada and from the English New Englanders. The low death rate of the English in India and Americans in Panama and the Philippines is due to the fact that the expert practitioners know what cases cannot recover, and ship them out. As a matter of fact, scarcely a week goes by that we do not hear of the death or suicide or return home broken in health of one of the "old timers" in the Philippines—men who have been there more than 10 or 12 years, and who have been held up as proof that God was foolish to go to all the trouble of making racial differences.

I have made an attempt to find out the effect of two years' service on a cavalry regiment. Reports were received from five troops containing 323 men. There were but two deaths from disease, both men with blue eyes, fair skin but dark brown hair. Six were sent home with illnesses not curable in the tropics; five of these had blue eyes, fair or ruddy complexion and the usual brown hair of our lighter types, one being light brown, and one was a light brunet with brown eyes, dark skin but brown (not black) hair. The only man who committed a serious crime (murder) had a fair skin, blue eyes and light brown hair. Of the six who had been overcome by the heat, five had blue eyes, and one brown but as he had brown hair and ruddy skin he was not a brunet. One troop reported 32 as having been overcome with the heat, evidently misunderstanding the question—as no organization ever has that many prostrations, and they had the usual percentages of blonds and brunets. Three troops said that no one had improved in health, one reported two who were of medium complexion, and one reported twelve with the usual percentage of types. That is, a blond underfed recruit can improve in health even under adverse conditions, but from the large number in this one company where others had none, the figures cannot be accepted. Sixty reported that their health had deteriorated, and 169 that there had been no change in their health, but on the way home 79 of the regiment broke down and went into hospital, 60 with malaria, one of them being fatal. As they were a rather anemic thin looking lot, they were not as well as they thought. As a rule deterioration does not begin before a year, and in two years some really get to understand how to behave themselves. A bank clerk who works under a swinging punka is in a different environment and doesn't show the same deterioration in two years. I know one blond clerk who has been here 40 years. The figures as to soldiers nevertheless confirm what is now known of the harm done to white men by minor degrees of heat and light. It might be of interest to the *Boston Med. and Surg. Journal* to note that Twining as far back as 1829, states, in his work "Clinical Illustrations of Disease in Bengal," that sprue cases "were generally of light complexion, active habits and *sober*."

The statement of the *Journal of Amer. Med. Association* (June 10, 1911) that the idea of a general deterioration of the white race in the tropics will possibly become obsolete, is so viciously unscientific as to be positively murderous, and should receive the condemnation of the medical profession. Its statement also that it is my idea as well as others that the "white race" "is at its best only in a cool and cloudy climate," is absolutely false—only the least pigmented of the white race require such an environment, short, darker types thrive best in glary hot Italy.

This reluctance to acknowledge the facts in America or even find out the truth as to climatic adjustment is most amazing, for the British government is using them in selecting civil servants for tropical colonies, utterly ignoring the British Medical Journal's opinion that the idea of the harmfulness of light is "little short of ridiculous"—as ridiculous as Bodington's idea of the damage of heat. There is also an increasing number of articles describing the special diseases of misplaced types in the British Islands, but we have infinitely more material to work on. Life insurance statistics show greater morbidity and lessened life of overweights so healthy in N. W. Europe, and English have noted the same in India for generations, yet I have known a big blond naturalist to doubt Darwin's law of adaptation because he (the big blond) had not died after twelve years in the tropics. There is a remarkable physical decay of the Baltic type after one generation in our cold sunny northwest, carrying off such men as the late Governor Johnson of Minnesota—and it is almost criminal not to find out why.

Types the most displaced are of course the unfittest and furnish the largest percentage of "failures." Our negroes produce a dreadfully disproportionate amount of crime, pauperism and disease. Where the blonds are the most unfit they are disproportionately represented in the unfit. When this was first published some readers got the idea that I had said that all tall blonds ought to be in jail, myself included as I am one of them, and I received two very indignant letters from our northwest, one man threatening to tell Mr. Taft on me. For twenty-four years I have been urging the sanitary necessity of short hair for soldiers, but warned against removing all shade by shingling, particularly in the tropics. One officer got the idea that all blonds ought to wear long hair like vikings, and when taken to task blamed it on me—so I received a right sharp reprimand for "misdirected activity."

The proof of the disappearance of misplaced blonds and their unfitness for city or factory life, has been misinterpreted as meaning their disappearance from the earth, but they will last as long as the conditions which caused their evolution, and they seem to be permanent fixtures of N. W. Europe and every other cool cloudy climate in the world. What we must realize is the fact that though they can stand higher heat and cold for short periods than a negro, they are really tied to a very limited zone and are specially harmed in the temperatures for which the negro is eminently fitted, 80°-98° F. Negroes demand a room temperature over 80° and the Pullman porter can not understand the complaints of his passengers when the car is so comfortable to him.

These recent revelations of the damage done by minor degrees of heat and light, at last put us in possession of the key to solve the riddle of climatic treatment of the tuberculous. In an article on this subject read in Boston by Hinsdale and in the discussion of it (*Bost. Med. and Surg. Jour.* Ap. 27, 1911) the old baseless dogma was repeated that the ideal climate for all human beings had a maximum degree of sunshine, and though it was acknowledged that some cases did get well in the Adirondacks, it was stated that some did best at home even in the city. The trouble is that no one seemed able to tell which is which, and we are not informed how to decide whether to send a new case to the mountains or lowlands, hot or cold, seashore or inland, plains or forests, north or south. We Americans have the most material to study but here again the British are taking the initiative. The statements of Dettweiler and Knight that there is no specific climate, and that any case can be cured in any, are also being proved untrue.

Shrubsall was the first to take up the matter, (Physical Characteristics and Morbid Proclivities, St. Bartholomew's Hospital Reports, 1903) and showed that even in England there were marked differences in the types which have migrated there after evolution by a different environment. J. S. Mackintosh, M. R. C. S., has continued the investigation (*Brit. Med. Jour.* Oct. 8, 1910) and shows that the constant tendency is for a type to be restricted in habitat, through the death of immigrants from other environments. These two investigators find that certain diseases are more common in the blonds and others in the brunets in England, where both types are migrants very little out of adjustment to the climate. How much more marked should these differences be in America! From the proofs that the blond is a product of a free and open air life, while the city brunets are very largely the result of the opposite conditions, we have a biological reason for the fact mentioned by Mackintosh that sufferers from claustrophobia are largely blond and those from agorophobia brunet —anthropologic matters our neurologists might look into a bit. There is also abundant reason for believing that there is an ethnic basis for the observations of Sir Wm. Bennett (*Practitioner,* June, 1910) that even in England, some tuberculous cases must be sent to their birthplaces, others to the seashore, and others kept in the city hospital. Our phthisiotherapists are neglecting their duty by not telling us which is which. This much is certain, no black consumptive should be sent where the temperature is ever below

75° or over 95°, and no blond one where it ever goes above 80°. There is evidence that a slender short brunet cannot possibly digest enough carbohydrates to keep warm in a very cold climate, and will shiver himself to death where a bulky tuberculous patient is comfortable in his shirt sleeves, whether he is as dark as an Eskimo or blond as an Aryan. We now know why very sunny climates have fine results in certain brunets but worry the blue-eyed to death. We now know why the blond Irish would all go back to the old sod if they could get enough to eat, for there the thermometer is rarely over 70° and the sunlight never fierce enough to drive one indoors. Ireland must always remain the breeding ground for types who migrate to help rule the world under Anglo-Saxon flags. Why not send the tuberculous Irish back to Ireland to be cured, as Bennett suggests, instead of sending them to hot glary places to die? We also now see why incipients were formerly cured in the old style cold sailing ships, but become rapidly worse in the hot modern steam boats.

The damage done by heat now shows us why the more crowded the slums and fewer the windows, the greater the tuberculous record; and why the more expensive, less crowded, cooler upper stories with more windows, occupied by the better fed, have the best records in spite of more light. This is not a plea for treating the consumptive in darkness as a few readers have imagined, but a plea to keep them alive longer by protecting them from the damage of minor grades of both light and heat, as proved by the Paris experiments with tubercular test animals. It is also a plea for preventing the stimulation of neurasthenics at sunny seashore resorts, and for sending them to cool cloudy places high or low, north or south, at the seashore or inland. Ide's statement that the seashore is both sedative and stimulating at the same time (*Neurologisches Zentral blatt*, No. 14, 1906) cannot be taken seriously. And the suggestion of *The Journal of the American Medical Association*, that "the so-called tropical neurasthenia may prove to be avoidable," has no basis in fact—for its main causes, light and heat, are not avoidable without confinement intolerable to northern types and even the confinement causes it. (See King, *Jour. Am. Med. Ass'n.*, May 19, 1906—Watkins, *N. Y. Med. Jour.*, Dec. 30, 1905—Fales, *Am. Jour. Med. Sc.*, Ap., 1907—Van Allen, X-Ray Atmosphere, *Bost. M. & S. J.*, Mar. 9, 1905—Heustis, *Western Canada Med. Jour.*, Feb., 1907—House, *Med. Sentinel*, Mar., 1906—Stuart, *Mil. Surgeon*, Feb., 1907).

Wilfred Watkins-Pitchford, Government Pathologist, Pietermaritzburg, South Africa, has taken up the matter quite extensively, led to it by facts seeming to indicate that light was one of the predisposing causes of cancer, a conclusion as to skin cancers to which the late Dr. Hyde of Chicago, had independently arrived. (*Amer. Jour. Med. Sc.*, 1906). Watkins-Pitchford is now finding that the cool highlands of South Africa are not the elysium for white men, we have been so often told and that there are many diseased conditions which in time must eliminate these migrants (*Transvaal Med. Jour.*, Dec., 1910) as they are due to such unavoidable causes as barometric pressure as well as light. He completely disproves our Association Journal's statement (June 10) that "the idea of the general deterioration of the white race in warm countries will possibly

become as obsolete as those formerly held concerning many of the tropical diseases have become." Indeed L. W. Lyde, Professor of Economic Geography, Univ. of London (*Contemporary Review*, Feb. 1911) has been so impressed with the impossibility of avoiding the causes of deterioration of migrants, that he goes to the extreme of predicting the disappearance of the least pigmented types everywhere, leaving the earth to the brunets. His data have led him to believe that no white man can stand more than seven years in the tropics even by avoiding all avoidable harm, a conclusion in harmony with what we now know of the damage done by heat and light of low degree, as shown by the shortened life of "old timers." It is strange, by the way, that men in cold places will spend immense sums to secure a harmful heat in dwellings and assembly rooms, but not a cent in hot climates to cool these places, though everyone knows the harm and also knows the cheapness and ease of cooling the air by modern machinery.

E. H. Starling, Professor of Physics, Univ. of London, and Wm. Ridgeway, Professor of Zoology, Univ. of Cambridge, have both called attention to the fact that man's physique limits him to restricted environments, (*Science*, Sept. 24, 1909, and *Pop. Sc. Mo.*, 1908) though neither of them was aware of the damage done by light, a damage vastly overestimated by Lyde. Wm. Wallace, of Edinburgh University, is now applying the same laws, showing the utter impossibility of acclimatizing any domestic animal in a climate markedly different from that which evolved it. Breeders are under a permanent necessity of constantly importing brood animals to keep stock from inevitable deterioration.

A word ought to be said about the use of alcohol by white men in the tropics to prevent their inevitable deterioration. The original statement was met by the Editor of the *Boston Medical and Surgical Journal* in 1900 by the remark that the use of it had been proved deleterious "beyond the possibility of discussion," yet tropical experts are still discussing it, some for and some against. The Editor of the *Jour. of the Amer. Med. Assn.*, who most wisely takes the total abstinence end of such arguments, when there is any doubt, now cavalierly dismisses the matter by the assertion that as to moderate use, "the best authorities, however, give this notion little support," a rather rude shock to such accurate and able men as Brown, noted for his works on bowel infection in the tropics; and a statement, too, rather unbecoming one who has never lived in a hotter climate than that made famous by the insane antics of the pitiable paretic, the late Carrie Nation. It is also rather rude to those German physicians who reported benefit in their African Herero campaign (see synopsis in the *N. Y. Med. Jour.*, Ap. 9, 1909) to say they are not among the best tropical experts.

The lesson to be drawn by biologists in general from the new data as to heat, is that they must learn why it is that mammalian and avian protoplasm of nerve cells will not function except at a temperature within a degree or two of 99° F., and why such elaborate means are taken to keep up the temperature and prevent overheating. Chemists may also find out something as to the actual size of a protoplasmic molecule, by studying the size of the wave which most easily breaks it up. Therapists using thermic baths or applications must realize that they are dealing with a far more dangerous thing than we formerly realized. If sunlight will kill a naked tubercle bacillus in ten minutes and a monkey in ninety, tuberculous or not, it must also do harm to a man in thirty minutes, from both the long and short rays. The sun of Texas will kill an infected yellow fever mosquito in two hours, and a naked infected man in less time, while the man's chances for recovery are vastly enhanced by putting him in a shaded cold room and blanketing him to prevent too great a reduction of body heat. Even plants are all killed or will not function if the light is too intense for their defenses (Duggan, *Science,* Jan. 23, 1905) no matter what the heat may be, and we know that too much heat will kill them even if protected from excessive light.

The mental and nervous effects of meteorological changes have long been known, and Cattell of Columbia has shown that minor changes in barometric pressure make great changes in mental activity. Kullmer of Syracuse University shows that the most progressive countries have the greatest and most numerous changes of air pressure, and now Watkins-Pitchford shows that we must also revise our opinions of high altitudes. It is true that as far as temperature is concerned, 250 feet equal one degree of latitude, and that arctic species thrive in Alpine conditions, but when one gets above the cloud-line, he gets the light damage and as a fact the blonds thrive only below that line. But now we find that when we go above 2,500 feet, the lessened density of air causes a very great increase of red blood cells, greater viscosity, more arterial friction and compensatory hypertrophy of the heart, followed later by the inevitable dilatation. Some years ago I was greatly chagrined at the mortality of my pneumonic patients in our western plateau, but I now find that they save such cases arising in the Mexican plateau by merely sending them to lower levels and now at Ems, and also in France (Rooaz and Delmas) they treat chronic bronchitis, emphysema, sequelae of pneumonia, and whooping cough under a pressure of 5-19 to 8-19 of an additional atmosphere in a pneumatic room, and Watkins-Pitchford suggests continuous pressure for pneumonia in high altitudes where removal to lower level is impossible. We now have a hint as to the greater prevalence of pulmonary hemorrhage in consumptives sent much above 2,500 feet.

A low level race cannot acclimatize itself to a high altitude as we once thought. It is as impossible as for the wide-nosed negroids to narrow their nostrils to be able to live in cold climates, for the wide nose does not warm the air and is evolved to admit large volumes of rarer warm air. It is therefore to be expected that Bauman (*Transvaal Med. Jour*, July, 1908) should find only 34 per cent of Johannesburg school children with normal hearts. It shows that permanency of colonization is impossible and that as in all other British colonies and America, the civilization will be dependent on an everlasting immigration from the breeding grounds in northwest Europe. An enormous number of our "colonial" families, like the "Spanish" families of Cuba, and the "English" of Australia, owe their survival to new blood from the home land.

That is, very small differences of light, heat, moisture, pressure and perhaps winds and all other climatic factors have very much more marked effects than we once thought. They eliminate migrants chiefly by killing the infected who would recover if in an environment like the ancestral ones. So let us give the tubercular patient the best chance by the climate which is ideal for him, but bad for any other racial type. Every climate on earth cures the cases physically adjusted to it, even in the Philippines, where every white case promptly dies, but the results with Malays are good if properly fed. Will it take the profession as long to acknowledge these facts as it did to acknowledge Bodington's?

Those in authority must not receive the new data as to heat and light and pressure like our forefathers treated Sir Isaac Newton's work—"Authority scowled upon it, and taste was disgusted by it, and fashion was ashamed of it." It will not always be fashionable for medical theory to accuse nature of foolishness in the way she uses pigments, so let us acknowledge her laws at once in our therapy. Come, gentlemen, wake up. Compel the *Journal of the Amer. Med. Ass'n.* to cease its attacks on these public health measures.

SUNSTROKE.

BY

O. L. MULOT, M. D.,
Brooklyn, N. Y.

Prevention. In the prevention of insolation, clothing plays a very important part, quite as important as diet, drink, etc. In considering clothing, it is not simply a question of the weight of the material only, but we must consider the question of whether we are to wear clothing made from a good or from a bad conductor of heat; nor is this all, the question of color is also of some importance. It is well known to-day that sunstroke, not simple heat prostration, is in reality more due to the actinic rays in sunlight, than it is to the actual temperature. We have al-

382   AMERICAN MEDICINE }
Complete Series, Vol. XVIII. }   ORIGINAL ARTICLES   {   JULY, 1912.
New Series, Vol. VII., No. 7.

lowed the haberdasher and the tailor a little too much say as to what is cool and what we should wear and have ignored the findings and dictates of science. Personally, I believe that non-conducting fabrics are preferable for all seasons; the undergarments may be woven as thin and gauzy as the manufacturer can make them, but they should contain a goodly percentage of wool. Wool undergarments even when thoroughly wet with perspiration, never strike the skin as cold; whereas the cotton or linen garment when wet, gives a feeling of cold. Thus the body clothed in a cotton or linen undergarment, wet with perspiration, is exposed to repeated chillings extended over a longer or shorter period as the case may be, during which the body makes repeated futile attempts at reaction. Some may contend that this is beneficial; no more so than getting the feet wet and letting them get dry in the same shoes and stockings, a most common and effective cause of colds.

We must realize that in the summer we wear our clothing to protect our bodies against the surrounding heat, especially in the sunlight where the temperature is higher than that of the body, therefore a non-conductor will not conduct the outer heat to our body. The old darkey who wore an ulster in the summer, 'kase what'll keep out de col' 'll keep out de heat?' may be laughed at, but scientifically he was not so very wrong. We know that the body temperature remains the same; in the winter we need the non-conductor to prevent the radiation of our body heat and in the summer we need the non-conductor to stand between the greater surrounding temperature and our body and prevent this from being conducted to our body. Let our clothing be as wide meshed and as light in

weight as the weaver can make it, but let it be of wool. Most of our suffering in the summer is due to the humidity which prevents the evaporation of the perspiration; while woolen does not absorb moisture as readily as does the cotton or the linen, it however does not chill the skin when it is wet as do the others.

A word about color; the dark ones absorb the light while the lighter ones reflect it, but the point in color is, that it should be one that filters out the actinic rays. If we lived in our aboriginal conditions our skin would protect us from these actinic rays by taking on a good coat of tan, but running around bare headed with only a pair of bathing trunks about the loins, would be too sensational and we would be stopped long before the desired coat of tan had been developed and we must dismiss it as Utopian. Still it is this color of the skin which practically gives the negro his immunity from sunstroke. Khaki owes much of its popularity for troops in tropical climes to its peculiar color which is the very best actinic filter so far produced by the dyer. Of course there are objections to seeing everyone garbed in this monochrome and it would not be becoming to all, but this color could very well be used in linings or in the underclothing where the color would not be of such importance and could not be seen. In many southern countries this color is very largely used in the lining of hot weather hats.

Insolation. It may be well to review a little the clinical types and symptoms of insolation. There are two forms: the asphyxial and the hyperpyrexial. In the former which is also the rarer, the premonitions are often scanty; dizziness, chromotopsia, cessation of sweating, headache, shortness of breath and gastric disturbances; with these premonitory symptoms the patient may suddenly fall, have a few convulsions and die. The coma may or may not be complete. When the symptoms are less severe, there are cramps, nausea and vomiting with thoracic oppression and stertorous and labored breathing. The headache is intense, the skin hot and dry and may show petechial spots. Delirium is usually present and may be either wild or in the severer form low muttering; the temperature ranges from 102 to 106 F.

In the hyperpyrexial type the temperature has been observed to go to 110—even 115 F.—and death occurs through paralysis of the respiratory center. The prodromal symptoms of anorexia, progressive physical weakness, cramp-like abdominal pains, restlessness, vertigo, lack of sweating, headache and irritability of the bladder, all of which may be present for one, two or even three days before the patient is stricken down. We must not confound heat exhaustion for true insolation. In heat exhaustion while there is dizziness, the headache is slighter; there is a tendency to fainting with the nausea. In these cases the initial temperature is more often subnormal. In this latter condition the indications for treatment are to remove the patient to a cool place, spray with cool water, stimulate with ammonia or better still with inhalations of amyl nitrite. If the temperature still remains sub-normal in spite of such stimulation, a warm bath may be used to advantage. The subsequent weakness must be combatted with suitable stimulating tonics. This condition is mild in comparison to true sunstroke and patients usually get well without much ado.

In true sunstroke we are confronted with a most formidable condition against which we must act with firm, strenuous and even heroic measures, if we are to hope at all to save our patient. If we contrast the symptomatology of insolation with that of meningitis we will be struck with their similarity and this similarity gives a clue to treatment. Beside the old classic treatment of tubbing in water in which pieces of ice are floating, venesection, hypodermoclysis and stimulants, lumbar puncture is to be added. But before we discuss reasons and results of the last named therapeutic measure a word about the nature of the stimulants to be used may not be amiss; these should be of the arterio-capillary dilator type such as nitro-glycerin, amyl nitrite, belladonna or atropia. If these do not suffice to keep the heart up, strychnia and strophanthus should be used, but not digitalis. As soon as the patient is removed from the bath, and he should not be kept there when his temperature has been brought down to 102, lumbar puncture may be performed with advantage.

This operation is not advised solely upon the similarity between the symptoms of sunstroke and meningitis, but because Dopter[1], who has made a study of the cerebro-spinal fluid in sunstroke, has found that even in mild cases, the fluid is under hypertension and in the severer cases it is albuminous, blood stained with initial polyneucleosis. Later there is a persistent lymphocytosis. This is a clear proof that in insolation the meninges are involved and that there is an imperative indication for lumbar puncture and in actual practise its use has not been a disappointment. It lightens the coma, and lessens the headache and the somnolence. It should be used early and should be repeated until the cerebrospinal fluid

[1] Dopter. Soc. med. des Hop., Dec. 4, 1903.

has become entirely normal, macroscopically, microscopically and chemically. De-Massary & Lian[2] speak highly of the good results obtained. Dufour[3] speaks especially of the good of this operation in the relief and cure of the sequelae of sunstroke. The operation is so simple and so free from danger when done under aseptic conditions that there should not be the slightest hesitancy in employing it in any case of sunstroke.

SURGICAL OPERATIONS IN HOT WEATHER.

BY

ROBERT T. MORRIS, M. D.,
Professor in Surgery at the New York Post-Graduate Medical School.

Theoretically surgical operations are best borne during the cooler months of the year, when less of the patient's potential energy is required for resisting the influence of hot weather. Practically the law of compensation seems to come to our aid in giving during the summer months a greater amount of fresh air from the open windows. This sounds a bit superficial to one who is fond of statements more scientific in character, but hospital records would seem to indicate that the patient's chances of recovery from major surgical work are about as good at one time of the year as at another.

The idea that patients make better recovery during the cooler months has been fostered unconsciously perhaps by surgeons who look forward to their summer vacation, and time for experimental work and library work without interruption.

[2] DeMassary et Lian. Soc. med. des Hop., Paris, Feb. 15, 1907.
[3] Dufour. Revue Neurologique, March 30, 1909.

Perhaps patients will do better on the whole at the time of the year when the surgeon thinks they will do better, for we then have the potent influence of suggestion. I would not care to set sail on Friday on a sailing craft; not because I have any superstition in the matter, but because the sailors, feeling sure that something will happen, suggest accident so strongly that a real menace is introduced arbitrarily, and the sailors are not as alert in avoiding accident as they are when each one believes that the inwards are auspicious for the voyage.

On one occasion I had to return to my hospital work rather early in September because a number of doctors and members of doctors' families were awaiting operation. A number of these were operated upon during the first forty-eight hours, and we then had a blaze of torrid humid weather, with the temperature ranging about one hundred in the hospital rooms in the middle of the day, and with exhausting nights. There were a number of abdominal operations in the series, but all of the patents did remarkably well, in fact it seemed to me unusually well. The experience on that one occasion has done much to confirm my belief that operative cases may be conducted about as well during the heated season as during the more temperate days.

My personal feeling is that the argument against operative work in hot weather relates to the surgeon rather than to the patient. This, however, is a really serious matter, and not to be taken jocularly. The responsibilities of the surgeon are so great that ample time for rest should really be taken, on the ground stated by Daniel Webster that "a man could do a year's work in ten months—but not in twelve." Then again it is impossible for a surgeon to keep up to date when his mind is filled daily with the details of cases under his responsible guidance. Time must be taken for traveling about, and seeing other men at work, or for doing experimental work, or turning the switch for library contact.

On the ground of advantage to the patient as a corollary to advantage to the surgeon it is my belief that operations should not be done, for the most part, during the heated season.

THE SUMMER DISEASES OF THE NOSE, THROAT AND EAR.

BY

HAROLD HAYS, A. M., M. D.,

Assistant Surgeon in Otology at the New York Eye and Ear Infirmary.

New York City.

The climatic changes in a city like New York are accountable for variations in temperature and moisture on the mucous membranes, particularly those of the nose and throat. The humid atmosphere which occurs during our summer months is probably accountable for as much trouble as the sleety murky weather of winter. That the nose and throat specialist has less to do in the summer than in the winter is due to many causes, particularly the exitus of patients to summer colonies and the ability of patients to increase their resistance during the summer months by living in a more healthy atmosphere.

However, there are certain conditions, symptoms and diseases which are particularly prevalent during the summer and it is with these that we shall deal.

Among the throat conditions which one is called upon to treat frequently are pharyngitis, tonsillitis and laryngitis. Their treatment differs in no wise from the treatment accorded them during the winter, but their cause, aside from a true infection is usually different. Pharyngitis is mainly caused in men by too great an exposure, too much smoking and an increased violence in exercise which increases the congestion of the parts for which relief is sought by the drinking of ice water and other cold drinks. This brings about congestion and anemia of the throat which increases liability to irritation. As a rule one or two applications of a one per cent. solution of silver nitrate to the pharynx and naso-pharynx is all that is necessary to effect a cure provided the patient refrains from too active exercise, exposure and an unnecessary use of the throat. One of the simplest remedies to allay this irritation is equal parts of some of the simple antiseptic solutions and witch hazel with which the patient should gargle every few hours.

Tonsillitis, of course, is an infection and is almost as prevalent in the summer as in the winter. The patient is most liable to suffer longer during the summer months for the reason that he will not take as good care of himself with the result that complications such as rheumatism are often more frequent after summer tonsillitis than winter tonsillitis.

A patient with tonsillitis should be kept in bed, should be absolutely quiet and should follow a regime of treatment which should entirely eliminate the infectious process.

A few months ago I advocated the use of strong solutions of silver nitrate in the treatment of this condition, and I am still of the opinion that an application of 50 per cent. silver nitrate to the infected area will produce a cure quicker than anything else. Of course, such treatment must be associated with the usual treatment of infectious conditions, such as absolute rest, free catharsis, and the application of ice compresses to the neck. For both pharyngitis and tonsillitis it is wise to keep the throat as clean as possible by the use of some medicament which is not too irritating. I therefore, in these cases advise the use of a lozenge composed of one-eighth grain formaldehyde, one grain of boric acid, flavored either with oil of orange or oil of cinnamon. These lozenges are made for me by a well known pharmaceutical firm. I have proved by laboratory experiments in the test tube that such a lozenge will inhibit the growth of such rapidly growing bacteria as the colon bacillus and the staphylococcus aureus. I frequently prescribe these lozenges in infectious diseases of the nose and throat with excellent results. They are far superior to any gargle and the formaldehyde is eliminated from the system very quickly.

Laryngitis in the summer time is frequently due to excessive use of the voice, and to over-heating with subsequent overcooling of the body and may often be secondary to a pharyngitis.

Silver nitrate in very mild solutions directly applied to the larynx seems to accomplish wonders, particularly if this is accompanied by complete rest of the vocal cords. Base ball games with the usual erratic shouting of the fan is often accountable for the summer hoarseness which lasts until the world's series are over. Where the laryngitis shows a tendency to become chronic it is positively necessary that the patient use extreme care in order that his voice may subsequently be restored to normal.

The common cold has occupied a great deal of space in our literature within the past few years. Whether it is due to that often accused organism, the *micrococcus catarrhalis* or not, is a question yet to be decided. Old fashioned remedies for the cure of the common cold are still in vogue and the patient seldom sees a physician until the condition has resulted in some complication such as a sinus infection, a secondary pharyngitis or an acute ear condition. The prevention of the cold is of far more importance than its cure, and if one were to follow the advice given by various physicians he would at most times be acting in direct variance to his own wishes.

During the summer months too little clothing is a great deal better than too much and the over-heating of the body with a lack of elimination of the excreta from the skin is accountable for more colds than anything else. Abrupt variations in temperature cause a disturbance of the heat center and may result in such serious conditions as pneumonia and nephritis. A recent article in the *N. Y. Medical Journal* (March 16th, 1912) by our venerable associate, Abram Jacobi, is replete with timely suggestions for the avoidance of cold. "To put shoes and low socks and knee breeches on a three-year-old child, and leave the calves uncovered in October and April is not done by *women* but by *ladies* who should not have children."

"Some, indeed, have fewer than they might have, the undertaker takes some." Again this author says: "Animals when suddenly cooled exhibit an increased disposition to infectious diseases, that is why starved and underfed school children and people are more easily infected. * * * * * In man the peripheral parts of the body are cooled, the blood vessels of the skin contract, then those of the brain and lungs and the kidneys may become congested. * * * * * The contraction of the blood vessels in the skin causes also a paralysis of the controlling nerves in the skin with congestion, cold and finally gangrene * * * death * * * by obstruction of the circulation, mostly during sleep, hunger and alcoholism."

Wet feet during the summer months when the body will not feel uncomfortably cold as result of it, may often be accountable for a consequent congestion of the body. The patient takes little care and the result is a cold which may finally end in a severe pneumonia. As I said before, the best cure for a cold is prevention. During the summer months the clothing next to the skin should be light, loose, and porous, so that the perspiration is not kept clinging to the body but is allowed to evaporate quickly. If the pores of the skin are kept clean and well open, if the patient when overheated from exercise does not allow himself to cool off too quickly, and takes proper cognizance of the fact that the drinking of iced fluids creates a disorder of the heat mechanism, he will avoid nine-tenths of the causes which create colds. If patients during the summer were to consult their physicians and follow their advice at the beginning of a cold instead of at the end we would have fewer complications.

Rhinitis or coryza is a similar condition which is often considered so simple that no care is taken. It may be aptly termed a localized cold. So-called rhinitis or coryza tablets are accountable for more troubles in the way of complications than anything I know of, for they prevent the patient from consulting a physician when he should. What applied to the treatment of colds in general applies here. Prevention

is worth more than cure. Aside from the general treatment, local applications or treatment may be necessary such as the use of mild non-irritating sprays and the use of such solutions as dilute silver nitrate or argyrol. There are various snuffs on the market at present which seem to furnish considerable relief.

Sinusitis resulting from the subsequent coryza is a far more serious condition to deal with and often occurs during the summer months particularly in affections of the frontal sinus or antrum. After bathing the patient's nostrils are filled with water and in the act of blowing this water too vigorously out of the nose some of the fluid is forced into the sinus, or some infection above it reaches the sinus, or the mucous membrane of the sinus is merely congested as a result of the irritation. The treatment of such conditions is either operative, depending upon the severity of the infection and whether there is any channel open for drainage. Non-operative treatment such as the use of astringent and antiseptic sprays, suction massage, etc., will cure nine-tenths of the cases of sinusitis; but where the condition appears to grow worse instead of better under this treatment, operative interference is absolutely necessary.

Many cases of summer neuralgia of the eye or of the teeth are due to infection of the sinus and the use of analgesics is absolutely forbidden. I believe that the majority of so-called neuralgias occurring during the summer months are of sinus origin and the sooner they are looked after by the specialist the better.

Hay fever is an extremely common condition occurring during certain periods of the summer. This term may be used interchangeably with rose cold which usually makes its advent in the later spring. Numerous monographs have been written on this subject and it would be impossible to attempt to outline a cure in a paper such as this. Let me say, however, that aside from eliminating irritation points within the nose caused by bony excrescences that the use of the ultra violet ray every other day for a period of weeks prior to the expectancy of the trouble has caused more relief than anything I know of.

There are a great many patients who never realize the uncleanliness of their ears until the summer comes round, and if it were not for the advent of a suspicious pain that makes them fear that a mastoiditis is imminent they probably would not know it then.

Bathing, particularly sea bathing, which under ordinary conditions causes a cleansing of the body apprises many patients of the fact that their hearing is worth something. After an ordinary bath in the ocean water not only goes into the nose in volumes but also into the external auditory canal as well, and if the latter is the case the swelling of a small particle of cerumen up against the drum may cause a pain in the ear which is as great as if the middle ear was infected. The patient goes to the specialist with the complaint that the hearing is 'decidedly' diminished or lost, that there is a rumbling sensation in the ears and that for a short time at least there was considerable pain. On examination one sees that the canal is filled with wax and that the violent pressure of a drop of water has caused a swelling of this wax to such an extent that it presses upon the drum or makes it act as a complete plug to the entire canal. Washing the wax away

with a dilute solution of bicarbonate of soda causes marvelous results and the most grateful patients I have seen are those which come into my office in a despondent mood and in five minutes walk out of it feeling like a new being.

However, there are certain cases where the pain in the ear is due to the advent of some water or infection in the middle ear by way of the eustachian tube. The patient has increased the congestion of the mucous membrane of his nose by frequent blowing and this congestion has crept up the eustachian tube until it has affected the delicate mucosa of the ear. These cases are serious and it is oftentimes necessary to allow the inflammatory products such as serum or pus to escape by making an opening in the drum.

However, this should not be done until other measures have been tried which will attempt to open up the eustachian tube. I have often found that a solution composed of one drachm of adrenalin, an ounce of Dobell's solution and seven drachms of physiological salt solution used in the form of drops through the nose and nasopharynx will diminish the congestion around the tube sufficiently to open it up and allow the escape of the serum from the middle ear. Many a patient has been saved the necessity of a paracentesis by using this simple method. In those cases where it is absolutely necessary to open up the drum this should be done as quickly as possible, for if prompt measures are not taken the result may be a mastoiditis with its consequent prolonged recovery.

I have attempted to outline in this paper the more important conditions of the nose, throat and ear with treatment during the summer months. There is no disease of the nose and throat that cannot occur during the winter as well as the summer yet there are certain conditions which are more prevalent during the warm weather and which persist for a longer time because the patient takes less care of himself. If it were not that the majority of people increase their resistance to infections during the summer by leading a more wholesome existence either at the mountains or sea shore, I am sure that the ordinary infections would take greater hold upon more people.

11 W. 81st St.

CRUDE INVESTIGATIONS IN MEDICINE AND WHERE THEY LEAD.

BY

BEVERLEY ROBINSON, M. D.
New York City.

Almost every week, something new or startling appears in the medical papers, regarding research discovery. To the careful, thoughtful man, when called upon to express judgment, there can be but one answer, i. e., I do not yet know; I shall wait and see. Again and again the thing recurs and again and again the same reply is given. To the young man with time, opportunity, laudable ambition—there is a natural tendency to take hold of any novel idea that attracts and to see in it for a while, something revolutionary, something to help his own reputation and also be to the great advantage of many ill people. If the old practitioner is lukewarm, protests, is not convinced, waits for more and later facts, before believing, he is regarded as behind the times—*emeritus* perhaps—but all the same, clogging, or stopping the wheels of progress.

In like manner, if one clings firmly to the faith within him, based upon years of observation, and repeated trials in practice, in which a remedy has been found efficient and innocent, his testimony is often gainsaid, or bluntly questioned by the overzealous aspirant for fame, or fortune. Drugs, applications, methods, once thoroughly believed in, which have shown their value frequently with few failures, when used properly and under suitable conditions, are put aside with scarcely a thought, for this or that new finding, until finally they are lost sight of entirely, or if still made use of by a few older men, may almost be considered as fresh discoveries, when in reality, they are of ancient date and are revivified merely, by the trust of a number of physicians. It is easy to give examples: leeches for inflammatory lesions of acute type; blisters where changes are chronic; Warburg's tincture for malaria; foot baths for colds; opium internally for many distressing complaints; antimony for pneumonia, etc.

Again, the undue search for causes of disease handicaps many physicians in their usefulness. The cause may not be readily found, it may not be single, but many sided, or multiple; it may never be clearly discovered. Are not these sufficient reasons to try to relieve symptoms and conditions which are evidently present, as much as possible? Not infrequently, the scientist regards such conduct as recognition of ignorance, that is wrong-doing, with which he has no sympathy, and in which there should be no trust. Because the unworthy empiricist who has had neither instruction, nor real desire, to keep abreast with progress, may be a power for evil in the community, it is not true of the physician who apt to learn all he can from younger members of the profession, attaches due importance to things proven good, although not in common use at present. One difficulty with the ultra-scientist is that while he waits for demonstration of truth and meanwhile does little to relieve symptoms, the old practitioner who may be called, mitigates much of the distress with simples, or mixtures widely known and employed long ago. What they have done, they will again accomplish, when prescribed.

The body of man, despite physiology, does not essentially differ in function every few years, although it goes through certain well-known changes. These changes, moreover, are not other to-day, than they were when the present practitioners were unknown.

The foregoing and much that might be added, should be laid to heart and make us unwilling to adopt every fanciful scheme of treatment because enthusiasts, or seekers for notoriety, proclaim prevention, or cure of blighting, or painful disease. Witness many vaccines and serums already in daily use. It would seem merely because we have no trustworthy remedy that can throttle contagious, or infectious disorders of divers sorts. Therefore we must risk putting in one's ill body remedies still unknown and untried except by purveyors of such goods, and abandon useful and innocent remedies of long standing and also, judicious, wise conservatism. It is not unlike the quality of mind which makes the too bold surgeon risk life, or mutilation to a patient merely because medicine rightly employed cannot promise cure. Again, it is like the same man who does exploratory operations simply because medicine is not yet an exact science (nor

ever can be) and cannot always accurately tell what precise condition of organ exists, or what nature of growth is present, and its every relation and complication.

To my mind, one explanation of the wide extent of quackery is the fact of imperfect research work and unwarranted conclusions deduced therefrom. The practice advertised by these men is followed for a time by many honest practitioners who wish solely to help cure, or relieve, their patients, and later given up in sheer disgust because found worthless, or not nearly so useful as old-fashion remedies. Frequently indeed they do much harm physically as we know—not to speak of the loss of faith and hope, thus engendered. In a case lately seen by me for what was regarded as an infection with suppuration of the cellular tissue of the neck, vaccines were injected several times with no appreciably good effect upon the local condition. What they did obviously cause was a mild degree of acute nephritis. For a while there was a notable quantity of blood in the urine of renal origin, which disappeared soon when vaccines were no longer used. Also, there was partial paralysis of one foot and leg, caused, as I believe, by the vaccines. This condition also disappeared when the vaccines were abandoned.

No amount of research and science, even the best, can wholly compensate for wise empirical knowledge, so-called, of observing, all around practitioners of large experience. Nor except in few diseases is it clear that much has been attained practically, in this way for the cure of disease, acute, or chronic, during the past two or three decades. There are some great and shining illustrations of the contrary fortunately and with which we are all familiar and of which we are justly very proud. The *immense* and *most* remarkable work done by Gorgas and for which he has just received the gold medal from trustees of *American Medicine* is perhaps the latest example of what science may and can do—when supported, however, by executive talent of pre-eminent value also—and highest personal rectitude.

Antitoxin against diphtheria might also be cited; vaccination against typhoid fever seems to be another great conquest. Anti-tetanic serum another and so also, the serums for cerebro-spinal meningitis and for rabies. But we also know how many pitfalls and difficulties are in the way of absolute belief. As to Salvarsan, to-day, we are conscious that our fond, original hopes are not supported by facts collectively that have come to light and there are great and lamentable drawbacks to its extensive use. So it is with tuberculin in any one of its modifications, and while good observers employ it, even these use it with much care and frequent questioning. Other reliable observers do not use it at all and others only in rare instances. The fact is finally, the new experimental science has brought with it many problems of intense interest and possibly of great and lasting value, if solved correctly, but their importance to the race, indeed to humanity everywhere, must largely depend upon the influence of the broad, judicial mind which is now, more than ever, required to separate wheat from chaff—always in the best interests of fellow men and women.

To whom does the highest rôle pre-eminently belong? In my judgment to none so truly and beneficently, as to the mature, wise practitioner who stands at the very top, and who like Moses on Mount Pisgah gazes at the promised land beyond.

FORMALDEHYDE IN THE REMOVAL OF VERRUCA, CLAVUS, CALLOSITAS, NEVUS PIGMENTOSUS AND CORNU CUTANEUM.

BY

R. L. HAMMOND, M. D.,
Woodsboro, Md.

So far as the writer has been able to ascertain no one has recorded their experience with formaldehyde in the treatment of the above skin affections, and it occurred to him to do so, inasmuch as his experience with it has been very encouraging.

Warts which had become very large and painful have been effectively removed by this agent with much less pain than attends their removal by other escharotics: (nitric acid, sulphate of zinc, caustic potash, arsenous acid, corrosive sublimate, etc.)

The technique of the procedure is very simple.

Formaldehyde of 40% strength is invariably used, undiluted or unmixed with any other agent; a wooden tooth pick or a match stick is dipped in it and the adherent drop is applied to the surface of the wart, corn, callosity, or mole, every 3 or 6 hours for two or three days. The normal skin should not be touched by the agent, as an undesirable dermatitis is thereby occasioned, and the attending infiltration of tissue increases the liability of a scar being left.

If the patient desires the objectionable growth more quickly removed, the intervals of the applications should be proportionately lessened. The dimensions of the tissue to be removed will determine the quantity of the escharotic that needs to be applied; but only as much as is required to saturate and completely cover the surface, without over-flowing on the normal surrounding integument, should be used at each application.

After several days, in small excrescences, and in about a week in the larger ones, an application having been made three times daily, pain is experienced, devitalization of the tissue occurs, and the application of the agent having been discontinued, the growth will desiccate; and after exfoliation the under surface or dermal layer will be found to be free from the blemish; if it is not, another application or two will secure the desired result.

If an open sore is produced a good healing ointment—oxide zinc or simple cerate—is usually all that is needed.

In the case of small excrescences the applicator should be whittled to a fine point so that the drop may be as small as required.

In extensive callosities the remedy can be applied with a brush, three times daily for several days, or until the surface becomes sensitive, then the applications should be discontinued, and the parts allowed to dry, then by soaking the epidermis with warm water it can be rubbed off; and this process can be repeated until a cure is effected.

If any excrescences treated exhibit a tendency to return they can be prevented from doing so by a recourse to the treatment.

In a case of cornu cutaneum, the horny growth should be clipped away as near to the dermal or matrix attachment as possible, or as near as the patient will allow; the agent should then be applied as often and as thoroughly as it can be with comfort. These latter annoying deformities however had better be referred to the care of the surgeon, but if his good offices

through prejudice against the use of the knife are eschewed, a very satisfactory cure can often be effected by the physician if time and patience are invoked.

Summed up, therefore, if plenty of time be consumed in the removal of these annoying growths comparatively little pain will be experienced, and a satisfactory cure will be the usual reward.

Local Anesthetic Power.—Formaldehyde is a local anesthetic of great power, and after the surface has been saturated with it, sensation is almost completely destroyed; the part can be cut or handled as roughly as possible and no pain whatever will be experienced; its anesthetic effect however does not protect the part against its own irritating escharotic action and pain to a certain extent is experienced at each application.

A CASE OF OCCUPATIONAL "NEUROSIS," WRITER'S CRAMP, SUCCESSFULLY TREATED BY MODERN METHODS OF PSYCHOANALYSIS AND REEDUCATION.

BY

TOM A. WILLIAMS, MB., CM., (Edin.),
Corresponding Member Paris Neurological Society, etc.
Washington, D. C.

The true professional neurosis should be of psychic origin; otherwise there would be an incapacity of the affected limb in the accomplishment of other acts.

For instance, it is impossible that hypotonia, as supposed by Hartenberg,[1] should be the cause of true professional capacity, for in that case, other limbs should be affected, and all actions would suffer.

Neither can we accept Kouindjy's idea of an ataxia.[2] The good effects of reeducative discipline in his hands by no means proves the genesis of professional troubles to be of the same nature as those of tabes.

Indeed, the cramps and most of the professional weaknesses and tremblings are in reality tics of the muscles with which any particular act is performed and which derive their origin from the inception of the act or even as soon as the idea is conceived. Naturally, a muscle while in tic cannot make a different contraction in order to perform another movement. Hence the incapacity.

A striking example, even in a physiological sense, is the emotional contraction of the throat in certain people which hinders vocalization in painful situations. By a similar mechanism, the fear of not being able to perform a certain act so impresses the brain that the muscles which should relax contract involuntarily. They begin to tic, and the act is not accomplished.

By the understanding of this mechanism, I have been able to cure cases of writer's cramp; though the procedure is often difficult and fatiguing.

In the first place, psychoanalysis is necessary in order to find the cause of the anxiety which prevents the patient's performing the act necessary in his profession and which is always the root of his affection.

The analysis being made, one proceeds to the discipline after the manner employed by Brissaud and Meige[3] in the reeducation of the "ticquers." The principles and the methods are the same; but one must always be prepared for the patient's return to the idea of a physical disability being the cause of the affection.

It is only when the mechanism of their normal automatic movements is understood that one can hope for a cure. Relapses occur nearly always if the patient does not understand completely the source of his troubles.

In a forthcoming monograph, (loc. cit.) these opinions are demonstrated in detail. Several long cases are analysed to show the psychogenesis. There I consider also telegrapher's cramp.

I do not wish to infer that all cases of professional disability are psychic, and to show this, there are added several cases brought on by over-work, drink, tobacco, etc., without any psychic symptoms. But the distinction between the cases is easy; for the latter recommence their work after rest quite well, and it is only after a certain time that the cramp, the trembling or the fatigue returns. While the true professional case, i. e., of psychogenic type, is attacked the moment he takes his tool to begin his work; and he often adopts useless and often absurd fashions of holding his implement.

Case of Writer's Cramp Arising from Impatience of Routine Letter Writing.—Married woman, aged thirty-eight, referred by a physician relative on account of aching in the back and inablity to write much on account of pain in hand, arm and shoulder. It first occurred seventeen months before, after much writing in acknowledgment of Christmas gifts, etc. But much writing had always tired her because she held her pen too tight. There has been no special anxiety or ill health upon this occasion.

Family History.—Negative except that her sister was very timid, and that all the children were bashful from being held back; her own children are in good health.

Personal History.—As a girl she was delicate and anemic. There were no difficulties of menstruation, which began at sixteen, and created no psychological perturbation as she was intelligently enlightened. She used to go North in the spring time on account of the heat. She played quietly there, vigorous exercise being too tiring.

She read much and was less dependent upon companions than most girls. She was also fond of sewing and the piano, but did not excel in either. She was perfectly tranquil and happy, a little timid in company, but without fears or qualms. She was conscientious and particular and much distressed by any rare failure in school. She disliked leaving; her favorite study was mathematics. She liked drawing and painting and kept them up after leaving. Cooking was given up from the fatigue caused. Aged sixteen, walking tired her much in the front of the legs. A craving for chalk and other minerals led her to take them, only occasionally. She developed a fear of mice and rats. She remembers no erotic fancies or dreams. After leaving school her life was uneventful, she did not dance to excess. She was happily married at twenty-three, having children at twenty-four, twenty-six and thirty-one without serious trouble. There were no abortions. She had a severe attack of malaria at twenty-five. Child bearing ceased spontaneously. Menorrhagia occurred and an operation was undertaken which relieved her.

For the last few years she has had recurrent, severe headaches lasting days at the time and requiring powerful drugs to arrest them. They were not determined by emotion. Twice during these, after influenza, spots came before the eyes and the page she was reading for some hours, and there was numbness of the left limb and side of the tongue. Numbness has occurred on other occasions but never on the right side. There has been no constipation, dyspepsia, vomiting or nausea during the headaches. There are no prodromes, but sometimes the catamenia postpones them for a week. She is not sure if they are ever determined by emotion.

Physical Examination.—She looks healthy, equable, well nourished and is powerfully built. There is no disease of the alimentary, respiratory, circulatory, genitourinary or integumentary systems.

The Nervous System.—Motility is very strong and equal. There is no modification of the reflexes.

Sensibility to temperature, pin prick, touch, compasses, is not abnormal; but the diapason is felt less clearly and less long on the right hand, wrist, shoulder, elbow and external malleolus of the ankle. This is more marked on the radial side of the arm. Stroking is better felt and more ticklish on the left arm than on the right.

Sight.—She thinks she can see further to the left but there is no hemianopsia, dyscromatopsia or visual defect.

In writing, her position is faulty, the wrist and elbow being turned so that the back of the hand is outward, and she uses mainly the extensors of the wrist and fingers. The elbow is turned outwards very awkwardly, the whole arm and shoulder is held very stiff, and she clasps the pen, a short one, very tightly in the fingers. She sometimes drops the pen; and on some occasions her sewing may fall from the hand and certain kinds, more particularly hemming, she cannot do. For a time, too, she feared to lift heavy crockery, thinking she might drop it, because the thumb would quiver in certain positions.

Her writing has always been jerky, because she hates it; but pain has only occurred since Christmas, seventeen months ago. It varies with the amount of writing, and was worse during a pleasant visit when she was doing nothing in particular, when it had however, been severe before she left home. The cramp and other symptoms came on after a period of stress while her sister's children were in hospital with scarlet fever. Her sister was then staying with her, and she feared for her youngest child, who had not had the disease; for although the doctor believed that the children upon recovery were safe, she could not help dreading infection, because her nephews had contracted the disease. The constant prepossession of these fears increased the tension of mind with which she always accomplished the writing of the distasteful formalities incident to Christmas. She hastened her writing more and more, and in consequence became more and more cramped, so much so, that she became unable even to hold up a newspaper, so constant was the cramp of the muscles. From possessing the reputation of writing faster than any one she knew, she had to descend to ceasing writing entirely.

Treatment.—The pathogenesis of her inability was explained thoroughly and she was instructed to begin slow writing exercises in a large, round hand. For detailed method see my article in *Journal für Neurologie, (loc. cit.)*. Only a little was to be done at a time, four or five times a day. The following week there was much less pain, except when she had to use her arm much: two minutes was her limit of endurance, after which the muscles would tighten in spite of her.

Progress of the Case and Further Analysis.—At times there is pain in the shoulder even when lying down and during her sleep. To obviate this, she has to hold her head well back. This first occurred after running hard before breakfast on account of being alarmed. There is a creaking of the left shoulder joint when it is moved. There is no tenderness of the skin there, but sometimes the muscles are tender especially after she has had one of her headaches. For these I prescribed a mixture of alkaline sulphates and bicarbonates to be taken morning and night, four days before the catamenia and when headache threatened. She was instructed that the evening meal should consist mainly of carbohydrates and succulent food. My endeavors to see her during, or after, a severe headache did not succeed. But some days after a very severe headache I found a marked subjective hyperesthesia to the tuning fork over the right elbow, ankle and knee. There was also a contralateral flexion of the toe on stroking the sole; the neck was constrained and painful; and there was interlacement of the visual fields and the arteries of the fundus oculi appeared very small, ratio of the veins being 1-4. But there was no projection of the papilla or haziness of its margin.

One week later, no headache having occurred, the hyperesthesia to the tuning fork was less marked. The right knee reflex was perhaps less responsive than the left. The ophthalmic arteries were no longer small and there was dyschromatopsia only in the temporal fields.

The writing, however, was even worse.

She has never presented astereognosis, impairment of attitude sense, dysdiadocokinesis. Her neck still hurts on movement, but much less than before and no longer while in bed, even when extended. She was instructed to practice free calisthenic movements of the shoulder and arm.

Two months later she was much improved, only one headache having occurred; but she does not write much.

Since then the improvement has been uninterrupted. The writing is practically normal and she can conduct the correspondence demanded by her social position.

Compare in *N. Y. Med. Jour.*, 1911, October.

REFERENCES.

[1]*Rev. Neurolog.*, 1911, June.
[2]Nouv. Icon. Salpètr., 1905.
[3]Les Tics et leur Traitement, Paris, 1901.

1758 K St.

A TRUE SNAKE STORY.

BY

HOWARD CRUTCHER, M. D.,

Roswell, New Mexico.

An old newspaper friend once said to me, "We never turn down a good snake story."

Readers of AMERICAN MEDICINE may appreciate the following, which is as true as steel, every thread wool, and a yard wide:

A Mexican sheep herder was struck in the right tibial region by a large diamond back rattled (*Crotalus adamanteus*), which appears to be the only reptile of his class that ever inflicts a wound, according to general report. The man who would be wounded by a snake of inferior grade would probably lose caste in the community. The sheep herder was given prompt treatment by those near at hand and within a few days was able to return to his usual duties.

"But every year, on the seventh of May, about five o'clock in the afternoon, his leg swells up, gives him a lot of pain, and finally breaks open and discharges freely something like green corruption. During this time his body is covered with diamond patches, exactly like those of the snake that bit him."

· During a sojourn in the White Mountains of New Mexico I made it my business to interview this patient, and am able to confirm the story, with the exception that his wound healed perfectly within a few days and has never caused him the slightest trouble since.

From snakes to coyotes is but a step, so to speak, and probably the editor of ·this journal, who spends most of his time around the mouth of the Hudson River, may be so tinctured with the salt air of the East that he may be unable to appreciate the marvels of the mighty western plains. But, to my story:

A Mexican plainsman was bitten on the hand by a coyote. The wound healed kindly, but every year thereafter, on the anniversary of the injury, the hand "bloated up, broke open and run green matter for about two weeks." During this distressing time the victim of the accident took on the manners of a coyote, ate goat meat, howled like a wolf, and was the cause of much alarm to those about him. This man is said to be alive at this time and I hope some day to interview him and to report his side of the case for these columns. It must not be understood that I vouch for the truthfulness of the story, although it contains no more elements of improbability than many things that appear in print.

THE ANNOTATOR.

Anaphylaxis in its Relations to Clinical Medicine.[1]—B. White states that this subject is coming to assume great significance for the clinician, relating as well to preventive as to curative medicine. Its processes are concerned not alone with infectious diseases but with those of the digestive and respiratory tracts due to different causes.

It is equivalent to hypersensitiveness and is a changed reacting power of the body to protein, due to introduction of the same or closely related protein.

It is a digestion outside the gastro-intestinal canal which gives use to more or less intense symptoms of intoxication.

Fatal intoxication following intravenous· or intra-peritoneal injection of a protein substance into a guinea pig which on some previous occasion has been subjected to similar treatment is an illustration of anaphylaxis in its highest known power.

The theory by which the processes of anaphylaxis are explained is as follows: introduction of protein substances into the body by any other way than through the gastro-intestinal tract is responded to by the production of anti or immune bodies which have the nature of a proteolytic ferment. Hypersensitiveness will .not be demonstrable in less than eight days. If then the same protein be again injected into the body in the same manner as before it will be attacked by the ferment-like antibodies and digested into simple substances, some of which are very poisonous. In a very short time these poisonous products attack the body cells and cause acute intoxication. The sensitigation is produced by the protein molecule, the intoxication by derivatives of the protein. This induced hypersensitiveness may continue through life.

Eugenics and the Doctor.[1]—An editorial informs us that the physician is a biologist and not a sociologist, though he may desire to be one. Eugenics consists in mixing a paint of white sociology and red biology, just enough of the latter to give a tint, a homeopathic biology which is likely to fade. Eugenics must have a skeleton as well as a soul, and the physician must furnish the biological basis for this science. ·

Eugenics seems to be taking too much account of environment and too little of the man. Sex relationship should be placed upon a higher plane than a mere biological one. Too much stress is laid upon sex pathology. We should seek the normal, determine the elements which maintain the normal, and then apply the principles of

[1] N. Y. State Journal of Medicine, May.

[1] Medical Council, May.

preventive medicine to the elimination of sexual sins and the destruction of sensuality which is the pathological outgrowth of perverted physiological sexology. Sex hygiene will do much to prevent sensuality. The physician's duty is to attend to the work as a biologist and healer of the body, the sex propaganda and eugenics in most of their phases being left to others.

Occupational Hygiene in the Navy.[1]— Surgeon General C. F. Stokes and Passed Assistant Surgeon J. L. Neilson state that there are problems of hygiene and preventive medicine in the navy which result directly from the conditions and modes of life on board ships where everything must be subordinated to military efficiency.

The personnel of the ship live in cramped spaces amid complicated mechanical and electrical contrivances, exposed to sudden changes of weather and climate, while their duties are arduous and exacting. The problem is to keep this personnel at a high standard of physical condition. The diseases and injuries to which these men are subject are divisible into five groups.

1. Affections which depend upon possible predisposition.
2. Those which depend upon environment of recruits.
3. Those which depend upon ship life.
4. Those which depend upon exotic exposure.
5. Special hygienic problems.

(1) Flatfoot is the most important of the first group and is to be regulated by proper shoes, practice marches, and special exercises for the feet.

(2) This group includes especially general infective, skin and venereal and nonvenereal diseases of the genito-urinary tract. They necessitate careful instruction in personal habits and cleanliness. The dangers of venereal disease are taught and there is prophylactic inoculation for smallpox, typhoid and diphtheria. There are isolation rooms for contagious diseases on the ships and fumigation and steam, disinfection at stations, hospitals and hospital ships.

(3) This group includes drowning, eye strain, the effect of gun fire on the ears,

heat exhaustion and thermic fever. Swimming exercises are compulsory. Eye strain on board ship is a grave problem and the vision is almost sure to deteriorate as service progresses. No satisfactory device has as yet been found to obviate the shock of gun fire. Heat prostration comes chiefly to those who are in the fire-room force and is apt to be accompanied with painful cramps.

(4) This group includes malaria, dengue, and dysentery which are especially due to shore duty in the tropics.

(5) Tuberculosis in this group is frequent owing to poor ventilation and unrestrained contact with the infected sputum of expectoration. It is most common among those whose life is spent below decks.

The monotony of life in the tropics, nostalgia and nervous disorders are also common. Injury and loss of life from noxious gases in ship compartments also demand special study and suitable pulmotors will utimately be installed in ships, stations and hospitals.

Life on a man of war from a hygienic point of view abounds in conditions which are far from ideal.

The wonder is that with exposure to such dangers as are ever present in this most complicated of machines, the rank and file are able to retain for any length of time that degree of physical well being which is indispensable for the purposes for which war ships are constructed and maintained.

The Prevention.[1]—An editorial notes the opening of the new building of this institution at Farmingdale, N. J. It takes children from four to fourteen years of age from homes in which tuberculosis exists, and gives them fresh air constantly.

They sleep out of doors, eat in rooms with wide open windows, go to school under the trees or in a wide open class room and play in the fields and woods. Their average stay is four months and the treatment is free. During this period a trained social worker goes to the child's home and recommends such changes as will make it sanitary when the child returns.

[1] *Medical Times,* May.

[1] *N. Y. Medical Journal,* May 4.

The departments of health and charities and various relief agencies aid in the matter of the necessary changes. Aid has thus far been given to 350 children. The method should be applied to diseases other than tuberculosis while the plan of housing and caring for the children might be adopted with advantage in all the so-called fresh air homes.

It is refreshing, amid so much that is disturbing and distressing in social conditions at the present time, to note these various practical efforts for the relief of those poor who are always with us and always need a helping hand.

We should imagine the problem of changing the sanitary condition of many of the homes from which children have been taken to the preventorium so as to prevent a relapse into disease would be very difficult, often impossible.

Results of Anti-Typhoid Vaccination in the Army in 1911 and Its Suitability for Use in Civil Communities.[1]—Surgeon Major F. F. Russell reaches the following conclusions:

1. Antityphoid vaccination in healthy persons is a harmless procedure.

2. It confers almost absolute immunity against infection.

3. It is the principal cause of the immunity of our troops during the recent Texas maneuvers.

4. The duration of immunity has not yet been determined, but it is at least two and a half years and is probably longer.

5. Its administration causes an appreciable degree of personal discomfort only in exceptional cases.

6. It apparently protects against the chronic bacillus carrier and is at present the only known means by which an individual can be protected against typhoid under all conditions.

7. All individuals whose occupation or duty involves contact with the sick should be immunized.

8. The general vaccination of an entire community is feasible and could be done without interfering with general sanitary improvements. It should be urged wherever the typhoid rate is high.

[1] _Journal of the A. M. A.,_ May 4.

Bacterial Therapy.[1]—W. O. Wetmore says that bacterial therapy depends upon the power of dead bacteria in proper doses and menstruum of stimulating the production of antibodies when injected into the tissues, thus acting as a protective or curative agent. These resisting elements occur as the result of the presence of bacteria or their toxines, and recovery depends upon their elaboration. Immunity may be natural or artificial and the body is fairly protected from the entrance of pathogenic germs by the skin and mucous membrane.

Certain glandular products in the tissues inhibit or destroy bacteria and their toxines. Infection depends somewhat upon the number of invading organisms, the result of their reaction is inflammation.

Fixed cells proliferate, white cells migrate and endeavor to capture and destroy bacteria. If the invading organisms destroy the white cells the contained enzymes are liberated and the blood becomes surcharged with these resisting elements. If the germs and their toxines are walled off by the cell elements, the circulation in this area is disturbed, the tissues disintegrate and pus is formed. Fever is thought to exert a detrimental influence on microbic life.

Antibodies to counteract toxines may be agglutins, bacterins or opsonins, but if the toxines are too abundant and too deadly the antibodies are ineffectual and death will result. Nature tries to confine invading organisms to the point of entry and here the greatest number of receptors are produced to attack them.

Injections of solutions of dead bacteria not only stimulate the cell elements locally to make antibodies but the whole system begins to produce receptors against bacterial invasion, after a period of twelve to twenty-four hours. When an animal is treated to produce antitoxine it receives toxine produced by bacterial growth or bacteria themselves in increasing doses, until its blood becomes charged with antibodies. These may be separated from it and transferred to the blood of an individual suffering with the given disease, thus acting as a curative agent. When a bacterin is injected the individual makes his own antibodies.

[1] _N. Y. Medical Journal,_ May 4.

Several injections at proper intervals may be necessary, but the results are often more gratifying and the immunity more lasting than the serum treatment.

The use of bacterins is founded upon a more rational basis than most therapy and becomes valuable as it is used with confidence. It is the stimulating of natural processes and this should be the main guide in medication.

The Registration of Contagious Diseases.[1]

An editorial recalls the fact that the community is dependent upon doctors for cooperation in order to ascertain whether contagious diseases are present, how they may be eliminated and how the community may be protected from infection. State boards of health usually supply the necessary machinery for supervising the health of communities but they can be efficient only as they are backed up by all the municipalities and communities.

The various states also must cooperate for there is interstate disposal of sewage and interstate sources of milk and water and they should have common standards as to the public health and a common basis for regulating traffic in those commodities which have direct relation to the health.

The physician in most states practises under a state license, if he fails to report contagious disease he violates the obligation imposed upon him by his license and there should be a penalty for such omission. In some of the states this omission is punishable by cancellation of the license. Another point of importance is that there should be a common standard in all the states regarding that which is infectious, for failure to have such uniformity may bring about serious complications.

It is the duty of the medical profession to insist upon the promulgation of preventive legislation and the first step in such legislation would be a uniform notification act requiring physicians to report to the proper health authorities, local or state, all cases of disease which may be decided upon as contagious. The far reaching significance of such a law adequately carried out can hardly be overestimated.

[1] Medical Review of Reviews, May.

The Health of Alaska.[1]

A. C. Reed tells of the deficiencies of the government with regard to the hygienic condition of Alaska. It has a native population of 25,000 scattered in small communities many of which are quite inaccessible. A report as to the sanitary condition of this immense country was recently made to Congress by Dr. M. H. Foster after a careful tour of investigation. He noted a death rate of 85.4 per 1,000 which was mostly attributable to tuberculosis. The population has decreased fourteen per cent in ten years, the birth rate being high but the death rate higher. Four per cent of the natives suffer with tuberculosis owing chiefly to their filthy and unsanitary modes of living. Eye diseases are very common and there are many blind. Syphilis is also very prevalent. The death rate would be much higher were it not for the healthful out-of-door occupations of the natives, chiefly salmon fishing. The streams and the ocean receive the sewage, and the water supply is derived from wells and springs.

Clothing is often washed with urine because of the ammonia which it contains, and also because water is not in all places plentiful.

Infant mortality is high owing to the entire absence of cows' milk, and the poor opportunities in general for feeding. Tuberculosis of the bones and joints and other chronic diseases of infants are common. A sanitarium for pulmonary tuberculosis and a home for destitute blind and crippled is recommended, also a commissioner of public health for the country. It is also recommended that the medical work be extended in connection with the Alaskan school system.

Medical Examination and Treatment of Prostitutes.[2]

An editorial notes that the enactment providing for the examination and treatment of prostitutes has been held constitutional by the appellate division of the supreme court. This court holds that disease acquired in their mode of life requires medical assistance and not punishment and that their reform be attempted. Their detention is not so much a punish-

[1] Medical Review of Reviews, May.
[2] Medical Review of Reviews, May.

ment for crime as a means for their reformation and for the conservation of the public health.

The jurisdiction of the courts over them is therefore rather reformatory than penal. The editor doubts whether the lower courts would treat male prisoners on this theory or that the legislature would enact laws to be similarly construed in regard to male offenders. He asks why we do not arraign as a vagrant or disorderly person the male who is responsible for the transmission of gonorrhea to his children's eyes, subject him to examination, commit him for treatment until cured and otherwise treat him as a subject for penalization.

It is the policy of society to expend nearly all its reformatory and sanitary efforts upon the most unfortunate victims of its own viciousness. This victim happens to be of no social consequence, is a fallen woman, is a paw for officialism to treat as it wishes, is degenerate and has no sensibilities.

Why not treat her kindly not only when diseased, but when not diseased?

Some of the Peculiarities of Old Age.[1]

An editorial notes that medical essays on this subject now abound. The poets had their turn in idealizing this period of life among us, a generation ago, when the chief interest among the medical men was with the strong and lusty.

Nascheis' recent essay on this subject calls particularly for criticism for he directs attention to the loquacity, the egotism and the clinging to life which mark the approach of senility. He also finds in this period a tendency to moral deterioration, an indifference to surroundings and a carelessness as to one's person and habits. These things, as the editor very properly remarks, are by no means characteristic of approaching age, for they are the very qualities which stand out prominently in adolescence and young manhood. It is admitted that there are certain features of old age which appeal to the student of physiology who is in search of data but that there are others, which are so foreign to the subject that their mention excites ridicule.

[1] Interstate Medical Journal, May.

The mere reference to the peculiarities of some aged men and women is not likely to be productive of much good, but there is a great field of usefulness in the discussion of means by which this period of life may be made more attractive and more useful, especially in the homes of the poor where the aged are too apt to be the victims of neglect or something worse. To make old age something to look forward to without dread or apprehension, that is a subject which ought to call for some of the best thought of the day. Improvement in the social state in general must by no means overlook those who have done the severer part of life's work.

On the Presence of Bacteria in Fresh Eggs.[1]

— R. C. Rosenberger has stated that he believes fresh eggs are sterile. A clean fresh egg has no distinctive odor, and the white and yolk should not mix, even after vigorous shaking.

There are no acid or gas producing bacteria in fresh uncracked eggs. If an egg is cracked and its membrane broken, colon bacilli may enter, the same being true when dirty eggs are broken carelessly, by dirty hands. The colon bacilli may also gain access by the dust of the air. A clean egg will remain fresh for ten months in an ordinary refrigerator.

The white and yolk can be mixed in an egg which has been kept for six months, in a refrigerator, but it has no odor and could be eaten raw without unpleasant results. During this period it usually loses eleven grams, by weight, by evaporation, but it may still be wholesome.

Eggs which are called fresh in the shell or frozen, and which contain gas and acid forming bacteria together with countless colonies of other bacteria, in reality are not fresh. Their contamination may have been caused by dirty nests, hands or receptacles, or possibly by the air.

Perfectly fresh eggs may be bought in summer, placed in the refrigerator and kept for use the following winter with entire safety. Frozen or dried eggs should contain nothing which when injected into a guinea pig would cause its death. If death has taken place the bacteria can be determined

[1] New York Medical Journal, May 11.

by examining the heart blood. Injection of this blood into a second guinea pig will sometimes cause its death also.

3. Experiments to determine the pharmacological effects of extracts of the organ with adrenalin for example.

4. Efforts to demonstrate in the blood of patients or animals, substances having the properties of an extract derived from an organ, that is to demonstrate in the blood an internal secretion of that organ.

What is Internal Secretion?[1]— E. L. Opie remarks that twenty years ago we were quite ignorant of the function of the ductless glands. To-day we have little precise knowledge of the thymus but we have much experimental knowledge of the functional disturbances which follow disease or removal of the thyroid, the pituitary body, the adrenals and the parathyroid. Internal secretions were described by Brown Signard as hypothetical products formed by the parenchymatous cells of an organ and discharged into the blood vessels in contact with the cells of the part. The ductless organs with cells like those of the glands are now believed to have functions which are essential to normal metabolism and these affect other organs only by way of the blood stream. The functions of organs are brought into correlation (1) by the nervous system, (2) by substances formed by one tissue and carried by the blood stream to other tissues whose functions are modified thereby. The latter are called hormones, an example of which is secretion which is elaborated in the cells of the duodenum, under the influence of acid and when carried to the pancreas excites the secretion of pancreatic juice. No line can be drawn between such products and the so-called internal secretions. Knowledge of the functional activity of raw thyroid, parathyroids, adrenals, pituitary body and pancreas is based on the following experimental efforts.

1. Extirpation of the organ to determine the effect of its removal and to bring the resulting disturbances into harmony with those which obtain in connection with disease of the organ.

2. Extirpation followed by the injection of extracts of the same organ.

A Contra-Indication to the Administration of Antitoxin.[1]—The editor remarks that most physicians who have used antitoxin serum have observed more or less serious symptoms following its administration, especially when given to those by whom it had been used for a similar purpose, months or years previously. As it is desirable to determine in advance whether a second administration of the serum will cause dangerous anaphylactic phenomena, W. L. Moss and others devised a local cutaneous anaphylactic reaction which will indicate hypersensitiveness in rabbits to horse serum.

Moss's test which he tried in thirty cases consists in cleansing the inner side of the upper arm with alcohol, drying with. a sterile sponge and then injecting intradermally one one-hundredth of a cubic centimeter of normal undiluted horse serum preserved with a few drops of chloroform.

If there is a positive reaction an inflammatory zone, one to two centimeters in diameter will appear at the site of the injection within twenty-four hours and will last from one to three days, but without constitutional symptoms. If the results are negative nothing but the needle prick will be observed. In the thirty individuals who underwent this test, nine had never received antitoxin and gave negative reactions. The remaining twenty-one had received antitoxin from four months to ten years previously. Of this number ten gave positive and eleven negative reactions. In three of the ten positives the reaction came with explosive suddenness at the end of six, eight, and twenty-four hours. In each of them there appeared a very annoying urticarial wheal, one a half centimeter in diameter with a surrounding areola of inflammation five or six centimeters in diameter. The reaction subsided promptly but it is thought that in such cases there might be danger from further injection of antitoxic serum. It is suggested that in all cases in which delay is warrantable this

---

[1] *Interstate Medical Journal*, May.

[1] *American Journal Clinical Medicine*, May.

test be made twenty-four hours before using antitoxin.

If the reaction is positive and the indication for antitoxin slight the antitoxin may be withheld, but if the indication is pronounced the antitoxin should be given and the risk taken.

Utilizing Criminals.[1]— The editor remarks the difficulty presented nowadays as to the disposition of criminals. What we ought to do with a convicted murderer is a question which is still unanswered. One writer suggests that such criminals be utilized as subjects for experimentation. Life imprisonment puts the community to the expense of supporting them, and if they are allowed to labor their work competes with that of free and virtuous citizens with a consequent lessening in the market value of the latter.

It would seem to be desirable in putting laboratory work to the practical test to make use of a doomed criminal rather than to risk the lives of investigators. The first object of punishment, it is said, is its deterrent influence, hence the value of penalties is to be determined by their deterrent influence. Life imprisonment is not deterrent, murders have increased where this is the supreme penalty, and there is always the chance of a pardon.

For a lesser crime than murder castration would be an ideal penalty and it would be life long. The peril would be that it might result in insanity and the criminal would then be a public danger and a public charge. The utilization of a murderer for experimental purposes has something mysterious and appalling about it which would certainly rouse the antagonism of the sentimentalists. They would be likely to say we could kill the prisoner but we might not torture him. Of course, there would be little or no pain in the experimental work but the criminal and the public would think there would be and herein would arise the deterrent influence. It would also provoke abhorrence of the medical profession, and the possibility of the benefit to humanity would count but little in comparison with this feeling.

[1] *American Journal Clinical Medicine*, May.

Surgical Anesthesia.[1]— R. H. Ferguson summarizes as follows the lessons to be learned from a study of the influence of alcohol, ether and chloroform upon the resisting power of the body to disease.

1. Alcohol must not be given in the infectious diseases especially in pneumonia and sepsis.

2. For surgical anesthesia administer the smallest possible quantity of any anesthetic.

3. Alcohol must not be used as a stimulant during or after anesthesia if the opsonic power of the blood is of any importance.

4. The anesthesia should always be as short as possible.

5. Only ether or chloroform which is absolutely pure should be used.

6. Special precautions for asepsis and antisepsis must be taken in all operations which are of considerable duration. Slight infections may develop into serious conditions after anesthesia owing to impaired resistance.

7. Six ounces of olive oil should be injected high into the rectum in all septic cases and also in others in which resistance to infections will be required.

8. Time is important in restoring the opsonic index hence the oil injection must not be forgotten.

9. The oil must be injected slowly lest it may not be retained.

10. Pure limpid olive oil must be used in order that it may be absorbed quickly.

11. When uncertain about the value of the injection of oil, always use it to be on the safe side.

Puerperal Infection.

A large percentage of puerperal infections start as wound infections, and usually originate not far from the vaginal outlet.

Strictest antiseptic precautions at the time of delivery, and moistening the pad that comes in contact with the vulva with a solution of bichloride of mercury (1-5,000) for the first five days after delivery, will prevent sepsis. I always wear rubber gloves during delivery.

[1] *New York Medical Journal*, May 11.

ETIOLOGY AND DIAGNOSIS.

The Relation of Heat to Infant Mortality.[1]—

Drs. Leitmann and Lurdemann contribute an important article to the discussion of the causes of infantile mortality in relation to the heat of summer in Berlin and some other large towns such as New York and Munich. As *Public Health* (London) well says, the paper deserves some special notice, since the authors have been at great pains to tabulate the daily mortality of infants for several years, together with a daily thermometric record taken at 2 p. m., with a maximal temperature. Reasons are given for preferring the 2 p. m. temperature in endeavoring to find a correlation between it and the mortality.

On looking over these one cannot help being struck with the remarkable parallelism of the two curves, and it is difficult to avoid the conclusion at which the authors arrive, that there must be some very close connection between heat and mortality. The two main views are represented by two schools, in one of which—represented by Meivert—a direct effect is attributed to heat, and in the other an indirect effect through the heat causing decomposition of food, and as a consequence infection through the alimentary canal. The authors incline to the former view, and state that the parallelism is most striking in the early summer, and they are led to the conclusion that the heat must constitute an immediate source of danger to infants, and that it does not require decomposition of milk by heat, or the spread of infection to increase the mortality among infants. Their reasons for this view are as follows:

1. In almost every year one finds a striking parallelism on hot days between the temperature and the infantile mortality in early summer.

2. Only temperatures of over 23° C. are connected with a distinct rise of the mortality.

3. Years of abnormal conditions of temperature show a like abnormal behavior of the mortality.

4. The mortality of breast-fed children is increased.

5. Infants which live in underground rooms and frequently, owing to the high temperature outside, receive milk decomposed during transport, do not show increased mortality.

6. The mortality rises often so quickly with the temperature that an immediate injury to the children must have taken place. If death occurs one or two days after the beginning of the heat, it must be considered that (a) the illness began at the time of the greatest heat; (b) that the injurious agent is the heat of the dwelling, which follows after and remains longer than the temperature of the outer air.

7. On hot days of the early summer the children do not die mainly of gastro-intestinal

[1] Drs. H. Leifmann and A. Lurdemann, *Deutsche Vrerteljahresschrift fur offentliche Gesundhertspflege*, Vol. 43, parts 2 and 3.

complaints. Convulsions come first. These symptoms are similar to those that one finds in adults on over-heating, viz., heat convulsions.

8. The mortality follows a falling temperature remarkably quickly. This cannot be explained either by infection or decomposition of food.

The authors' conclusions are amply supported by the clinical data which they have collected.

The Diagnosis of Atypical Scarlet Fever.[1]—

Miller sums up his paper in the following manner:

1. The differentiation of unusual forms of scarlet fever will remain a stumbling-block to the practitioner, until we have discovered the cause of the disease, and are able to employ similar tests to those that we now apply to diphtheria, typhoid fever, syphilis, etc.

2. Not one of the individual symptoms can be depended upon to establish the diagnosis. The disease may occur without rash, desquamation, fever or strawberry tongue. The whole clinical picture must be carefully considered and the individual symptoms critically studied.

3. The most constant symptom is the angina; and its presence, associated with a scarlatinal eruption, however slight, however evanescent and however limited in its distribution, should be regarded as sufficient to establish the diagnosis—or, at least, to demand isolation and close observation.

4. Next to the throat the condition of the tongue is the most reliable symptom, some enlargement of the papillae of the tip and border being usually observable, although this symptom is much more frequently missing than is the angina, and may occur in other conditions.

5. Of all the exanthemata, scarlet fever is the most varied and uncertain in its symptoms; and of all the symptoms, the rash presents the greatest vagaries. Hence, no rash, especially in a child, is too trivial to be disregarded, whatever the general symptoms may be.

6. Scarlet fever with well-marked rash may occur without desquamation.

7. Rubella scarlatinosa is often diagnosed when scarlet fever presents itself as a pronounced erythema with mild constitutional symptoms. This error is a fruitful source of dissemination of the more serious affection. The diagnosis of rubella should be accepted only upon the strongest evidence.

8. The history of a previous attack of scarlet fever should not prevent us from treating with suspicion apparently anomalous cases of the disease.

9. Differential blood-counts have produced nothing of value in the diagnosis of scarlet fever.

[1] J. D. M. Miller, M. D., *Archives of Pediatrics*, April, 1912.

10. Surgical scarlet fever and scarlet fever following burns are scarlet fever in the wounded, and should be treated and regarded as ordinary cases of the disease.

11. Scarlet fever without eruption, and other anomalous forms of scarlet fever, are a fruitful source of dissemination of the disease.

12. Finally, all doubtful erythemata, and all cases in any way resembling scarlet fever, should be quarantined until the diagnosis is reasonably established.

A New Indican Test.[1]—Dr. Nalonek has tested the efficacy of Gürber's method in 100 cases. Gürber recommends osmic acid instead of chloride of lime or chloride of iron. An equal amount of concentrated hydrochloric acid is added to the urine, then two to three drops of a one per cent. solution of osmic acid. Depending upon the amount of indican present the urine will now turn violet, bluish-violet or a pure blue. If necessary, chloroform may be added like in the other tests. An excess of osmic acid does not matter, since this is not able to further alter the indican. Vatoned found that this test is very reliable.

The Weather and Acute Catarrhal Enteritis.—We have learned that it is not merely an elevated temperature which is productive of this disease, especially in children, says a writer in the Medical Council; it is unclean or contaminated milk and other articles of diet. But weather conditions very largely influence when there are sudden changes in temperature. An abrupt fall in temperature is greatly provocative of diarrhea. On the Pacific coast, where there is an equable summer temperature, and where sudden changes are infrequent, catarrhal enteritis is uncommon. We of the Atlantic seaboard must meet it from June to September.

Be exceedingly careful of the babies when sharp summer temperature changes occur. Protect the abdomen, and keep them warm when summer temperature suddenly falls, and reduce the diet when it rises.

THERAPEUTIC NOTES.

Lobelia in Asthma.—Dr. Vance, of Somerset, Ind., in a late issue of Ellingwood's Therapeutist, says: I recently surprised myself and my patient a great deal more, when on being called to a very severe case of asthma, with all the disagreeable symptoms exaggerated, I administered a hypodermic of 30 drops of lobelia. Almost immediately the patient had re-

[1]Med. Press and Circular, June 19, 1912.

lief. The benefit was marked right from the first. After half an hour I gave 15 drops more, and the patient laid down and slept as quietly and as naturally as ever in his life.

Heat Prostration.[1]—Ice or cold applications to the head are almost invariably indicated. If the face is flushed, the skin red and hot, the pulse bounding and the heart acting tumultuously, the entire body should be rubbed with ice or bathed with cold water. Cold drinks are indicated. If the surface of the body is cool, use warm applications, mustard to the feet and internally hot drinks, whiskey, ammonia, etc.

Remedy for Poison-Oak or Poison-Ivy.[2]—A hot solution of potassium permanganate made strong enough to be quite dark, rubbed in so as to reach the poison in the vesicles, is effectual. If the skin is broken, the solution should be quite dilute, and may be applied by means of a compress. The stain may be removed by applying a solution containing a mixture of oxalic acid and sodium hyposulphite, freshly made, say a tablespoonful each of oxalic acid and hyposulphite to a pint of water.

HYGIENE AND DIETETICS.

Cold Storage Regulations.—The Massachusetts Cold Storage Commission, after an exhaustive study of all the important phases of the question, have reached the following conclusions:

1. Cold storage warehouses should be subject to the supervision of the State Board of Health, and should be required to take out licenses and submit regular reports. The main object of the proposed inspection is to ensure the proper condition of goods upon entry into storage and their proper treatment during the storage period.

2. Food products deposited in cold storage should be marked either on the individual articles or on the containers with the dates of receipt into storage and of withdrawal from storage. The reason for this requirement is to afford a means of identifying cold storage commodities as such in the trade, and of conveying to purchasers information to which they are entitled with respect to the commercial history of the food products which they buy, including the length of time goods are held in storage. (Two members of the commission

[1]Med. Summary, July, 1912.
[2]Life and Health, Washington, D. C., May, 1912.

dissent from the recommendation with regard to the marking of the date of withdrawal.)

3. The time for which products may be held in cold storage should be limited to twelve months, with discretionary power vested in the State Board of Health to extend the time limit for particular consignment of goods, and also to fix a shorter time limit than twelve months for any article of food if such further restriction of the storage period should be found upon investigation to be desirable. .

4. The fraudulent sale of cold storage products as fresh goods should be prohibited. It is generally admitted that the purchaser has a right to know whether he is getting cold storage or fresh goods. A provision requiring that purchasers shall be informed upon this point is a legitimate and desirable measure for the protection of consumers against deception.

5. The return to cold storage of goods that have once been withdrawn and placed on the market for sale to consumers should be prohibited. Such goods are presumably not in fit condition for further storage. The prohibition of restorage is not needed to protect consumers against a practice that unquestionably leads to abuses.

The commission recommends that the regulations apply to fresh meat and meat products, fresh food, fish, poultry, eggs, butter and other commodities that the State Board of Health may see fit to add.

To summarize it may be said that the two most important conclusions of the commission are (1) that cold storage is not to any great extent a public health question and (2) that cold storage does not ordinarily increase but rather diminishes the cost of living. It is, however, rightly recognized that cold storage foods, like all other foods, come to some extent within the purview of the guardians of the public health.

We are of the belief that the wide distribution of this report should have a great effect in disillusioning the public of many fallacious beliefs concerning the cold storage of foodstuffs, and should lead to a better appreciation of one of the most important discoveries of man.

A Refrigerator Without Ice.—Medical men are often called upon to give advice concerning the preservation of food during the summer months, and as ice is many times out of the question for the poorer classes, the following from the *Fresh Air Magazine* is well worth remembering. The writer says:

If there is no refrigerator in the home, and ice can not be afforded, milk can be kept cool for twenty-four hours in a home-constructed "cooler," which will cost only twenty-five or thirty cents, and will last the entire season. To make such a cooler buy a butter tub with lid at the grocer's. It should cost ten cents. Purchase ten cents' worth of sawdust (or your butcher or grocer may be willing to give you the small amount required). Make a bag of denim or other material of a size that will fit the top of the tub closely, and fill this with sufficient sawdust to make a cushion about an inch thick. Sew up the open end of the pillow, so that no sawdust can leak out. Fill the tub with sawdust to within an inch of the top. As soon as the milk arrives in the morning, sink the bottle into the center of the sawdust, leaving some sawdust underneath, and the rim of the bottle above, so that it may be pulled forth easily. Place the sawdust cushion on top and shut the lid on tightly.

Sawdust is a non-conductor of heat, and will not allow the cold of the bottle to escape or the heat of the atmosphere to penetrate to it. However, whenever the milk is used, the bottle should be drawn forth, the amount desired poured out, and the bottle returned at once to the sawdust. Sawdust will not cool milk which has been allowed to get warm in the air.

When one or two cents' worth of ice can be afforded, a good little refrigerator can be constructed with the butter tub and a lard can. Place a thick layer of the sawdust on the bottom of the tub, then put in the lard can and pack sawdust all around it, as high up as the can lid. A little piece of ice, wrapped in newspaper and placed in the bottom of the can, will keep all day, if the can is covered with the sawdust cushion and the lid of the tub is kept tight. Butter and milk can be placed in the can with the ice, and kept good and cold.

Care of Ice-Chest.—In the late summer, says a writer in *Good Health*, housewives find themselves well stocked, sometimes overstocked, with fruit and vegetables. Prompted by the desire to keep everything from spoiling, their first thought is to cram the motley lot into the ice-chest along with butter, milk, cream and the dozen-and-one little left-overs that the frugal housekeeper utilizes in some appetizing way. What wonder that there are so many smelly, disorderly, positively dirty ice-chests!

If the celery be left loose, broken leaves will fall. Rings of cream and milk tell where dripping bottles have stood. Crumbs of butter dot the shelves. Fruit juices in tippy receptacles leave unsightly stains. Then there is the slime that oozes down from the storage part, clogging up the pipes and causing a bad smell. Too, there is the accumulation of bits of hay or straw or whatever is used at the ice-houses for packing. All these conditions necessitate frequent systematic cleanings.

Once a week is none too often to wash out the ice-chest, using always a clean cloth and clean suds, not the regular dish-cloth and water through which a lot of dirty dishes have been passed. After giving the whole interior a thorough washing, including the part wherein the ice is stored, the pipes and all the racks, rinse again and again with clear water, taking care to flush the pipes until the drip-pan shows not a trace of slime or refuse. Baking soda slightly moistened will remove all stains. One housewife who is classed among those "painfully particular," yet whose family is known to be in the best of health always, insists on having everything clean before it goes into the icechest. She wipes off the butter-jar and the cream and milk bottles; washes the eggs and puts them on a granite pie-plate; rinses well all the vegetables such as cucumbers, tomatoes, radishes, egg-plant and cabbages, while she prepares for serving and places in bags made for the purpose lettuce and celery. Fruit and melons, too, are subjected to a thorough scrubbing and rinsing before being chilled.

The Care of the Baby in the Summer.[1]—The *Medical Summary* advises the practitioner to enlighten the mother, if she needs it, on these simple yet all-important matters:

Less food is required in summer than in winter. More fluids are required in summer thar, in winter.

Teach her the value of giving the little one a drink frequently in warm weather. It is a good rule to always give water before feeding or nursing.

If the bowels are irritable, distilled water or water that has been boiled and cooled is to be preferred.

If the child is artificially fed, lime water should be used each time in the milk, and milk sugar should be used as a sweetening agent.

In severe gastro-intestinal troubles lavaging the bowels with soapsuds is a good procedure. This may be best accomplished by attaching a soft rubber catheter to a common syringe.

Too many young children are overdressed in warm weather. If not dressed suitably any treatment directed at the ailing child is in a measure defeated.

Teach the mother the futility of giving a young child medicine aside from small doses of calomel and castor oil.

THE DOCTOR'S AUTOMOBILE.

When the Gudgeon is Guilty.—Gudgeon pin knocks are almost always caused by natural wear, the only exception being those due to a lack of oil. The knocking is never heard when running light, and scarcely ever, except when pulling hard on top speed or on a hill. It can only be cured by renewing the pins, or the bushes, or both.—*Am. Med. Compend.*

Rain on the Glass.—Frequent source of trouble to drivers of cars with fixed wind screens is the collection of rain on the glass in small globules, which are very detrimental to the vision, and, in consequence, necessitate frequent stoppages for the purpose of cleaning the glass. An effective method of preventing this is to carry a bottle of kerosene and glycer-

[1] Editorial, *Medical Summary*, June, 1912.

ine, mixed in equal quantities, and, on the commencement of rain, to rub a few drops of this over the surface of the screen. The rain will then spread over the glass in a thin sheet, enabling the drive to be continued in comfort.—*Motor Print.*

The Regulation of the Spark.—The spark should be regulated in conjunction with the throttle position, says an automobile expert in *Leslie's Weekly*, and that for slow running of the motor with closed throttle should be retarded so that the ignition does not occur until the piston is on its downward stroke. An exceedingly late spark, however, or one that occurs after the piston has proceeded a quarter or a third of its way down, is harmful and has a tendency to overheat the motor. Naturally the gases are hottest at the time of the explosion, and they cool as they expand. If the ignition of the explosive charge occurs at the top of the stroke, but a small portion of the cylinder walls will be in contact with the hot gases. A late spark, however, causes the ignition to take place after a certain portion of the cylinder walls has been uncovered by the downward motion of the piston, and thus a large area of the motor is subject to a high degree of heat. Continued running under these conditions will cause the motor to overheat, even though it may be running slowly. Furthermore, inasmuch as a late spark causes the explosion to be retarded until the piston is well on its way downward, it is quite possible that the charge will still be burning at the bottom of the stroke and that "live" flame will be discharged through the exhaust valves. This will corrode the valves and their seats and will warp the stems.

MEDICAL HINTS.

If a cathartic is given to a woman the night before an operation on her perineum or cervix, says Waldo, she is very apt to have an evacuation from her bowels during its performance. It is better to give the cathartic forty-eight hours before the expected operation or an enema on the morning it is done.

According to Waldo all late operations for perineal laceration in order to be successful must contain the following elements: 1. They must extend well up the posterior vaginal wall. 2. The denudation must go through the entire thickness of the mucosa. 3. The stitches must be inserted into the tissues so as to catch the muscle.

American Medicine

H. EDWIN LEWIS, M. D., *Managing Editor.*

PUBLISHED MONTHLY BY THE AMERICAN-MEDICAL PUBLISHING COMPANY.

Copyrighted by the American Medical Publishing Co., 1912.

New Series, Vol. VII., No. 8.
Complete Series, Vol. XVIII., No. 8.

AUGUST, 1912.

$1.00 YEARLY in advance.

The dangers of too much and too little clothing are both known in a general way, yet it is surprising how few people really strike the happy mean. The *Boston Med. and Surg. Journal* of Mar. 7, 1912, calls attention to the frequency with which sick people are found overclothed, more or less constantly dripping with perspiration and very susceptible to "colds" due to sudden cooling of the overheated body. The most harm seems to be done by retaining the winter wear too long in the spring, and it is probably a fact that this season does cause more "colds" than cold weather. We have frequently mentioned the fact that over-heating by furnaces or clothing is generally the basis of colds, irrespective of season or temperature of the air, but that people who constantly live in cool or cold air often seem immune though apparently much underclothed. On the other hand the *Journal of Tropical Medicine*, Feb. 1, 1912, calls attention to the wretched health and physique of those few young Britishers who are habitually underclothed. There ought to be some way we can determine the proper amount of clothing and instruct our patients. We suggest as a subject for future discussion that physicians look to the state of the skin, whether habitually too moist or too dry. There seems to be no question that perspiration is for the purpose of carrying off surplus heat by in-visible evaporation, and that the production of visible moisture is an indication that evaporation is being prevented by too much clothing.

The skin should never be absolutely dry nor appreciably wet. Of course, a bank clerk must work in a warmer room than a butcher, and must have less clothing, but either would be overclothed were he to exercise violently and would be underclothed if he were to sit outdoors in a snow storm. The athlete when exercising is sufficiently clothed in "running pants" and likewise those who must work in warm rooms need astonishingly little clothing. Horsemen know that a heavy coat of hair keeps a stabled horse too hot and also is too hot for exercising. So the animal is clipped in winter and clothed only when at rest to prevent the "colds" due to cooling off a sweat-soaked coat. American physicians have called attention to the few colds among the scantily clad women living in our overheated houses, while the English think the women underclothed in their cooler houses and injured by it. There is no question then that it is solely a matter of the environment and those whose daily life submits them to rapid changes must have outer garments to don or doff as occasion demands. Even those who stay indoors or outdoors, must vary the amount

408   AMERICAN MEDICINE
Complete Series, Vol. XVIII.   EDITORIAL COMMENT   AUGUST, 1912.
New Series, Vol. VII., No. 8.

worn, to avoid visible perspiration which soaks the undergarments and causes chilling.

The use of wool next the skin seems to be disappearing and the use of vegetable fibers becoming more common. Cotton absorbs extra perspiration like a towel, and evaporates it to the outer layers much more quickly than wool which becomes sodden. The woolen garments then seem to keep the skin too wet and subject to "colds" from chilling, while the skin under cotton is dry. Wool seems to be designed by nature to keep outer dampness from reaching the skin, and no wool clothed animal has sweat glands. So the ideal cold weather clothing seems to be cotton underneath and woolen outer garments, but all varying in weight and number of layers sufficient to retain warmth but keep the skin dry. The man who dances in a hot ball room, wearing heavy woolens under his dress suit, is sure to be overheated and so drenched with perspiration that chilling is sure to occur on the way home when he is fatigued and specially susceptible to infections. There is some sense then in the fad for wearing cotton summer undergarments in such a tropical environment. The skin is dry, and a heavy ulster on the way home prevents chilling. There is also a great deal we can do in regulating the absurd clothing of business men.

Votes for women are beginning to assume the practical stage in politics. We might as well bow to the inevitable as there is no cause for worry. Whether it will do any good is another question, for there are men mean enough to say that bad women are just as numerous as bad men. There is no question of course that as a class women are unalterably opposed to immoralities which their more complacent husbands are inclined to ignore. But it is a mistake to assume that this opposition will take the course of prevention. The first thing the women legislators of Finland did, was to urge the legitimization of children born out of wedlock. Kings have that privilege so why not peasants? Women votes did not purify Colorado politics very markedly at first and they turned one State from "dry" to the "wet" column. The wives of the rich may vote for rich senators, the wives of rum sellers are likely to vote for liquor and the wives of the clergy—stay home. We may be unlocking a Pandora's box but we can not help it.

The qualifications for voters change with the progress of civilization. Time was when men voted with swords, and women were very glad they were not voters. The franchise was a pure matter of physical prowess to protect the tribe or nation against enemies, and no weakling had any voice in State affairs. Nations are too big for that sort of thing now. Only a very few of the huge mass can possibly get on the battle line, and for every man with a gun there must be another to bring him food and ammunition, and several others back home preparing the supplies and many more working for the funds. A physical weakling may be infinitely more useful in war than the man who pulls the trigger. The actual fighters are no longer the ones who decide when we shall fight. The money lenders have more weight, and those who pay the bills and supply the materials also have more of a deciding vote than the few who finally go out to do the dying. A national movement is now the resultant of all the nation's brains, and the muscles have ceased to have a deciding vote. In such questions many men are less competent than many women. Public opinion is composed of all opinions, and a male vote does not express it. Why not have the full opinion?

Will women prevent war? History seems to show that they have brought on' wars. If they fear an invasion with the resulting loss of home and honor, their vote is solidly for war; and they glorify the defenders. Nevertheless the placing of such decisions in the hands of those who cannot do the actual fighting will probably cure many a war fever. The wisdom of such a course cannot be decided off hand, and whether the world will be better or worse for placing its destiny under the joint control of women governed largely by altruistic emotion and men governed by brutal selfish calculation, no one can say. The only thing we are sure of is that there is a world wide movement for making a national election expressive of a real public opinion—the will of all its citizens—male and female, big and little, strong and weak. When every woman was the wife of a soldier, she was as powerful as he in national decisions, but now there is an enormous unmarried class who cannot express their will without the ballot and they must have it or we may go wrong in national affairs. At least, our action may be wrong in the minds of the many who do not vote. So let it come if it will. Perhaps it may result in disfranchising the mentally incompetent of both sexes—and if this were the only result we would promptly join the ranks of the suffragettes. The last three years have shown that the movement is a perfectly natural one and cannot be successfully resisted. The unreasoning extravagances of the advocates merely counterbalance the equally unreasoning opposition of the conservatives. The nation's soul goes marching on.

The psychology of the franchise must be considered by the anti-suffragettes. In former times all men were married and it is common knowledge that a man's opinions are unconsciously but profoundly modified by "suggestions" of his wife. It was possible for the men to express the real public opinion. There is no question then that bachelors can not form or express public opinion and as in many ways they act in defiance of public opinion, they may vote in defiance of it. They may be doing as much harm now, as unmarried women may subsequently do from harboring fixed ideas of an impractical nature. As matrimony is denied to a large and constantly increasing number of both sexes—some of our best citizens too—it seems that their opinions should be added when we wish to get the real will of the nation. The connubial state cannot possibly be taken into consideration in the right to vote, but as a matter of fact maids and widows are deprived of their right to modify the expressed will of the nation though they do much to form the real public opinion. Any sociologist who is learned in evolutionary laws could have predicted the present movement and the ultimate success of the suffragettes, but no one can predict the result. Women may have poorer reasoning powers than men, but they make up for it with very powerful intuitions and emotions which men lack. Emotions guide nations as much as reason—but whether for weal or woe depends on circumstances. Whatever happens the world will still rotate.

Where two or more causes are operative for the production of a certain result it is often difficult to impress on people and especially those whose personal interests or feelings are concerned—the necessity for abolishing that cause which perhaps alone is capable of abolition "Because," some people argue, "there are lots of other ways of disseminating the infection of tuberculosis besides spitting. What's the use of sifting that out and making it a punishable offence? Are we not told that whenever we speak or cough we are disseminating droplets and these are infective if we happen to be diseased? You cannot prevent people speaking or coughing." And in like manner, "What's the use of closing the schools because measles has broken out? The children are just as likely to get the infection from their playmates as in their own homes."

But are they? A carefully reasoned investigation by Dr. A. Banks Raffle, school medical officer of South Shields, England, in the *Lancet* for Feb. 3, 1912, which appears to depend on a concurrence of data as apt as though they had been the result of careful and deliberate experiments, tends to show clearly that they are not. An epidemic of measles broke out in the spring and summer of 1911 in 15 out of 21 infant schools in South Shields. The number of children exposed to infection in these fifteen schools was 4,470. Of these 2,190 were susceptible, never having had measles (a fact ascertained during the preceding three years of school inspection). During the period before the closing of the schools 618 became infected. In the 14 days following the closing, i. e., in the period during which the infection might have begun

at school, another 140 were infected. That is to say, during the period in which infection at school was a possible factor, 758 out of 2,180, or 34.77 of those susceptible, became infected, either at school or at home. That left 1,422 susceptible children clearly free from infection contracted at school at the time of closing the schools. Of these only 75, or 5.13 per cent contracted measles from all the other possible sources, the school room alone being excepted. It seems fair to assume, therefore, that of the 34.77 per cent who might have contracted their measles in school 29.64 did actually so contract it, as against only 5.13 per cent who possibly became infected from home sources.

The medical inspection of schools has passed beyond the stage at which it is necessary to adduce arguments in support of its desirability. Yet if such were wanted it seems that the present instance gives an indisputable proof of one of the benefits that may be looked for from it. The great practical value of the preceding record as to the amount of susceptible measles material in the schools is here clearly demonstrated and in like manner often in a few years a vast amount of valuable statistical data of various kinds, if the work of school inspection and medical history recording is conscientiously performed, will inevitably be accumulated. Let no fact, therefore, be held too trivial for consideration, but let everything that can conceivably have any bearing, even a remote one, on medical statistics be systematically recorded, even though the direction in which it may become ultimately of value be not at the time definitely apparent.

Our remarks last month on the presidential candidates were received in the very spirit in which they were offered, with only four exceptions. We carefully avoided any political discussion believing that other mediums are much better adapted and fitted than our own for that careful consideration of politico-economic questions that is essential in handling these problems at all satisfactorily. But since a goodly number of earnest physicians, men whose good will and respect we prize highly, seemed anxious to learn which candidate AMERICAN MEDICINE was most inclined to support, we openly stated our preference and the reasons therefor. Believing that most honest men respect an open, clean cut expression of opinion even though diametrically opposed to their own, we did not evade the issue and tried as fairly and squarely as possible to show the grounds for our honest convictions. We are free to say that the interests of the medical profession, the work and aims of its members, and the forces contributary thereto, are first and foremost to us. With every power or influence at our command we are striving to support the splendid objects and undertakings of the medical profession, to help in promoting the efficiency of the agencies that have been evolved from medical knowledge and research, and to secure due recognition for the unselfish, high minded motives that we know are back of the plans and objects the medical profession is so earnestly advocating in behalf of humanity. The respect, appreciation and genuine whole souled admiration which we entertain for every faithful physician and his work have ever dominated the pages of this journal and we have no apologies to make for our enthusiastic regard for our profession. We have had occasion to learn the true worth of the work of the American physician and it merits all the appreciation and commendation we in our humble capacity can possibly bestow.

Consequently it is not to be wondered at that the writer, like any other loyal physician seeking to arrive at a decision as to which national party or presidential candidate to support, with the work and objects of his profession naturally uppermost should give his allegiance to that party and that candidate offering greatest promise and prospects of furthering those things closest to his heart. Before committing ourself, or responding to those who had asked us to declare our views, we carefully studied the situation and ascertained as far as possible the exact position of the three foremost candidates on the great public health questions of the day. President Taft's ideas have been well indicated by certain events that have transpired during his administration. His attitude toward the Pure Food and Drug Law, and failure to recognize the pernicious conditions attached to its administration, show how little appreciation he has of the actual needs of the situation. Then again, if President Taft appraised the public health problem at its proper importance he would not have allowed the platform of his party to ignore it entirely. We have no desire to reflect on the President's ability, honesty or conscientious work. He has repeatedly shown himself to be an able, high minded, hard working official. But he has neither the respect for the medical profession nor interest in what it is trying to accomplish that promises any tangible cooperation in promoting the humane endeavors of an adequately organized public health service. President Taft's attitude has been one of comparative indifference, and in some re-

spects actual antagonism, so the profession must turn elsewhere for the aid and
assistance it has a right to expect from the
Chief Magistrate of the United States.

Governor Wilson, whom we gladly acknowledged to be a most able and conscientious man, has pleaded lack of familiarity with the questions of public health
administration, and while the Democratic
platform advocates proper organization
under one comprehensive head, we had no
alternative than to state that Governor
Wilson on his own statement was an unknown quantity, at any rate as far as these
vital matters are concerned. Certainly with
all the attention that has been devoted to
pure food and drug legislation and the
agitation that has been going on relative to
a national department or bureau of health
there is today little excuse for begging the
question. We have no doubt that Governor
Wilson has very definite ideas in regard to
these problems which are all that any intelligent, broad minded man might be expected to have. If, however, for reasons of
policy or diplomacy he refuses to express
them, the medical profession cannot be
blamed for turning to the man whose position is known and who has not hesitated
when asked, to state frankly and fearlessly that he is strongly in favor of raising
the efficiency of public agencies to the
highest, of organizing them under one
proper head, and of strengthening every
measure that will promote the health and
lower the mortality of the people. It was
during Colonel Roosevelt's administration
that the Pure Food and Drug Law became
effective. More than any other public man,
Mr. Roosevelt has shown that he recognized the noble, unselfish efforts of the
medical profession to advance the welfare
of the people. He has seen that medical

men were good citizens and has never
neglected an opportunity of showing how
deeply interested he was in the progress of
public medicine. In no uncertain language
the platform of the Progressive Party
comes out forcefully for what the medical
profession have been so long advocating.
Colonel Roosevelt's speech of acceptance
likewise takes high ground on these matters so near to every American physician
—Governor Wilson ignored them—and
it seems to us that if any one of the
candidates especially deserves the support
of the medical profession it is Theodore
Roosevelt.

**Every man, however, should decide for
himself** who he will support in this as well
as in all other political campaigns. As we
stated last month a good many may look on
these matters in a different light. The
strength of the American people is the right
of each man to think for himself. We lay
claim to no infallibility of discernment or
judgment. Others having different or
broader knowledge may think differently.
Is that any reason for us to question their
good faith or honesty? Should we villify
our brother who holds different views and
looks on these problems in some other way?
Have we any monopoly of common sense
or good judgment? Most certainly not and
we frankly state that we have no quarrel
with any honest physician who questions
our belief that Colonel Roosevelt will if
elected president, do more than any of the
other candidates to further the objects that
the medical profession has so long been
trying to bring to pass. We think we are
right, for we carefully canvassed the situation before expressing our views, but
we have no ill feeling or hatred for any
one who believes that we are wrong or

holds that our ideas are ill founded and illogical. We have intelligence enough and sufficient breadth of view, to know that a good many of our readers are much better informed politically than we are. It is not our desire to precipitate a political controversy. We trust, therefore, that our democratic and republican readers will understand that we are not trying to convert them or to offer the slightest criticism if their ideas of the situation are the reverse of our own. Hold fast to your opinions and ideas if you have reached them after due thought and study. Honest convictions on the side of any question deserve respect and it is one of the fine, noble things of our modern American life that men can hold diverse opinions on important questions of religion, politics, art and business, and yet be warm personal friends, with a wealth of respect for each other. This is uplifting and makes for progress.

In response to our comment on these matters last month, we received, as usual, a considerable number of letters, the most of which were highly gratifying. Many agreed with us, quite a number questioned the correctness of our conclusions—giving reasons for their difference of opinion,— *and only four were intolerant and abusive!* Not a bad result when one stops to think of the thousands who doubtless read our remarks. We were as pleased with those honestly taking issue with us, as we were with those agreeing in every particular, for the men who disagreed with us were earnest gentlemen who gave us credit for clean motives and were able to state their opinions courteously and honorably. Such men accomplish things in the world's work and we are grateful to have them write to us even though they hold radically different views, and tell us we are wrong.

But for the four intolerant "gentlemen" who cursed us and villified us for daring to have ideas disagreeing with their own, we have nothing but the deepest contempt. Without knowing it we committed the unpardonable sin of expressing opinions opposed to those they have somehow acquired—possibly by inheritance—and lo instantly "stop the journal!" Can one imagine greater depths of smallness and bigotry than to discontinue a monthly journal—costing one dollar per year—that has admittedly given good service otherwise, just because it happens to print something one does not like or believe? Does any one take any periodical and expect it to give no other material or present no other views than those with which the reader is in accord? Certainly not, and every intelligent person realizes that negative facts are often as helpful as are the positive.

We feel in all truth that we can well dispense with "the unhappy four" who are so convinced of their infallible judgment that they can see no honesty or good intent in ideas differing in any way from their own. Such men are an injury to any cause, the one they espouse most of all, for their intolerance engenders antagonisms, and instead of winning converts their coarse, ill mannered tactics disgust and repel those who would otherwise be open to the influence of reasonable argument. A hundred years ago it was men of their type who were the first to hang poor old innocent women for erstwhile witchcraft, just as earlier in the Christian era, it was their kind who were readiest to lift their raucous voices and cry "crucify him, crucify him!" They have always existed and they always will, but thank Heaven, they are growing less and less as the world grows better and kindlier.

We are glad to think that all but an insignificant few were of a mental calibre to understand that our remarks last month were simply in line with the great underlying purpose that dictates the policy of AMERICAN MEDICINE, first, last and always, to uphold the principles and honor of our profession, to safeguard its best interests and to advance its faithful efforts in behalf of the people. We believe that the man who best appreciates the true purposes of our profession and will aid us most to consummate them is Theodore Roosevelt. In saying this let us repeat that we cast no reflection on any other candidate. But the hour is at hand when medical men can make their voices heard and their influence felt as never before. If we can do so consistently and with no sacrifice of honest convictions and belief, let us give our support to the man who has shown himself most in sympathy with the American medical profession and the splendid efforts it has so long been expending for the American people; the man who up to the present time has most openly and positively committed himself to an effective organization of all public health agencies under one head, the strengthening of pure food laws and the promotion of everything capable of improving the public health and lowering human mortality; a man who has no monopoly of virtue or ability, but who well represents in his private as well as in his public life, the true spirit of Americanism, earnestness, courage, honor, and a hatred for injustice and wrong. In brief, Theodore Roosevelt is the man whom we can count on to stand with the medical profession in all its laudable undertakings, and this is why we hope to see him elected. If there are any who can see any heinous design in these words or

any other purpose than to exalt and advance the interests of the profession we are trying to serve, God pity their pin head intellect and myopic vision. As a matter of fact, we are not addressing our remarks to the bigoted and narrow minded, but to those who are big enough to grasp our honorable meaning and purpose, and whether agreeing or disagreeing with us to realize the desire that actuates us, the desire to promote to the best of our humble ability the culmination of the fundamental objects of American medicine, the better control and prevention of disease and the reduction of mortality.

House refrigeration is bound to receive more attention now that it has been shown to be possible and practical. For several years we have been pointing out the desirability of giving as much consideration to cooling our homes in summer as we do to heating them in winter. The great suffering occasioned by excessive heat in hospital wards is only too well known and if some of our new hotels and theatres can have systems devised for them which allow their temperature to be kept at comfortable degrees, surely equally effective methods should be provided for use in our hospital wards and sick rooms. It is one of the anomalous conditions of our social organism that the demands of luxury always receive a readier response than those of necessity. Thus our pleasure seekers will know the comforts of scientific refrigeration long before our sick and suffering, even though it needs little argument to prove that the benefits that would accrue to the latter would be far greater and infinitely more worthy of commendation. Several years ago we commenced to urge the artificial cooling of hospital wards and rooms during the hot months. We showed the feasibility of cooling systems and a goodly number of sanitary engineers and experts agreed with our views and gave the subject practical thought. Last year it was our privilege to publish a notable paper on the cooling of hospitals by Lt.-Col. Chas. E. Woodruff at that time stationed in the Philippines. This attracted a great deal of notice and was quoted extensively. .

A few other journals have also done pioneer work in pointing out the urgent need of some thought being directed to this important detail of hospital hygiene, notably the *American Journal of Surgery.* The latest editorial on the topic in this esteemed publication is so timely and comprehensive that it deserves widespread consideration. As the editor says, unquestionably unusual atmospheric heat does, at least occasionally, tip the scales against very ill patients balancing between life and death. And we need no statistics to satisfy ourselves that, at any rate, heat spells add enormously to the suffering of patients swathed in dressings and struggling against the effects of narcosis and a major operation.

In a small room an electric fan adds enormously to a patient's comfort on a hot day; but what is to be done for the sufferers in large wards? An adequate automatically regulable cold air supply is the most rational system, and it would seem only a matter of mechanical experimentation to evolve it. Air sucked over brine pipes can, by means of a pump or blower, be delivered through ventilators sufficiently cold to cool a large room. The chief cost would be that of installation. The operation in a building supplied with refrigerating pipes would not be expensive; nor would it be required except during periods of unaccustomed heat. Moreover, the installation in hospitals already constructed

might be provided for only a few wards or large rooms, to which patients most affected by the heat could be moved. In hospitals being erected or yet to be built it can hardly fail to excite criticism if a complete ward cooling system of some character is not included in the plans.

"But," continues the writer quoted, "in the absence of some adequate system of cooling by cold air or cold pipes, what can be done during torrid spells to reduce the discomfort of sufferers in hospital wards? This is the practical problem that immediately confronts us, and since in many of the older institutions the ventilation systems lack the efficiency of those more recently erected, its solution is often as difficult as it is necessary. The editorial we have referred to suggests that in rooms not too large a series of fans, not too near any patient, might be operated at one end; and, indeed, the air might be blown from them over large blocks of ice, as is sometimes done in theaters. If this is not expedient, the sickest patients should be removed to well-shaded small rooms, where they may have the benefit of wall, ceiling or window fans. Water curtains can be operated to reduce room temperatures, but they constitute a crude method. Light, frequently changed bedclothes, cool drinks, frequent sponge baths and protection from flies and mosquitoes are the nursing contributions towards the amelioration of the patients' discomfort. The surgeon can contribute as much—prophylactically, by postponing operations of election during unusual heat spells; actively, by minimizing the bulk of dressings and bandages. Caps, tapes and straps can often be substituted for bulky roller bandages about the head and neck, while abundant wound discharges may be managed with small dressings if frequently changed."

At any rate now that we are alive to the possibilities of reducing the discomforts and ill effects of excessive heat, to neglect every available means of relief is to shirk a very evident duty. We hope the whole subject will continue to receive the thought it manifestly deserves.

———

The diphtheria carrier seems to be receiving attention the world over, now that we have about made up our minds that we generally if not always get this disease from a living person and rarely if ever from houses or "fomites." The bacillus dies very soon in light, or heat and when dried, and as we frequently remark sanitarians no longer try to kill dead things. The last plan is to sterilize the throat and nose by dry hot air, because of the ability of a mucous membrane to stand a higher temperature than the bacillus can. Apparent success is following this treatment in Lyons, France, by a Doctor Rendu so we are told. If this is true, it may be another instance of success following wrong reasoning from true premises. Finsen thought he was curing lupus by killing the bacilli with light—as that is what he started out to do. Now we know the light is not strong enough to be deadly or it would kill the tissues too. It irritates both and the inflammatory serous reaction finishes the bacilli with an overdose of a germicide. We find that this is the probable way hot water irrigations cure gonorrhea, though originally given for the germicidal effect. Local dry heat may act the same way in diphtheria and as we think it also does in various kinds of arthritis—particularly gonorrheal. No matter how it works, it is well worth a trial, to see if it really does work.

The antagonism between staphylococci and diphtheria bacilli was discovered by Schiotz of Copenhagen and put to practical use in sterilizing chronic carriers. Major Henry Page of the Army confirmed these results. (*Arch. of Int. Med.*, Jan., 1911 and *N. Y. Med. Journal*, Dec. 23, 1911). Schiotz found that people with "staphylococcus sore throats" rarely if ever contracted diphtheria even by close contact. Moreover he found that a diphtheritic sore throat often ended up with a staphylococcus invasion. So he conceived the idea of planting the staphylococcus during convalescence to shorten the period the bacilli held on—a matter often of several months. He was successful and no ill results were seen. Though it is now over a year since the facts were made known in America there has been but one use made of this apparently invaluable weapon, so far as we have noticed. Catlin, Scott and Day of Rockford, Ill., report that they ended an epidemic of institutional diphtheria this way and saw no ill results whatever. (*Jour. Amer. Med. Ass'n.*, Oct. 28, 1911).

There has elsewhere been amazing neglect to take it up and prove it to be good or bad here. Is this to be another epoch-making discovery rejected by smug orthodoxy? The genius of research is heterodoxy and we hope our laboratories will not become too conservative. An occasional error from undue enthusiasm, though deplorable, is infinitely better than this neglect of conservatives.

———

The therapeutic uses of cold air and cold water are slowly becoming appreciated and there is a desirable increase of exact literature on the subject. Blackader of McGill University recently called attention to the effects of a dry cold climate (*N. Y. Med. Jour.*, Aug. 3, 1912). For many years Baruch of this city, like a prophet crying aloud in the wilderness, has been vainly urging the proper uses of cold baths, but has been strangely ignored. Baths both cold and hot have been used empirically for untold ages and even yet we do not fully understand how they accomplish their wonderful results—but there is no doubt of the results, nor of their certainty if we use water accurately as to duration, temperature and technique. It is an exact art which is now being placed on a solid scientific foundation. The main results are due to reflex action on the circulation, which is such a complicated matter that unless we are accurate in details we are liable to produce the opposite effect than intended. Blackader now states that cold air rapidly increases hemoglobin, and there are numerous observations that both heat and light diminish hemoglobin. There must also be physiologic differences due to the fact that cold air contains so much more oxygen per volume than hot. At any rate we know that patients breathing cold air get well when those breathing hot perish and we will not be long in finding out the reasons. But don't let us ignore heat in our rush for cold. Homely remedies may be possessed of more virtues than we have been accustomed to impute to grandma's poultices. They are comfortable anyhow, and that's a big point. They rarely do harm and that's a big point too.

The refusal to release Thaw has evidently given profound satisfaction to those elements of the nation whose opinions are worth considering. We have repeatedly · said that the time has long passed for condoning any murder unless it is clearly proved to be in self defense. The people are out of patience with our carnival of bloodshed and have determined to end it. The new unwritten law is that if the murder is without provocation the murderer must die. If there has been a provocation which would have been considered justification a century ago, and the act is in "hot blood" we make allowances for human weakness, but the criminal must be locked up until we are sure he will not do it again. Where there is mental weakness from disease or defect, then there does not now seem to be any two opinions—the man is liable to do it again and must be under control in jail or asylum the rest of his life as he is not able to resist slight provocations which to the normal are not considered provocations at all. The murderers of Rosenthal have mistaken the new public opinion. They must die even if it requires a modernized vigilance committee working within the law. This conspiracy of murder must be the last.

The scandal of expert testimony is again in the limelight, though it was hoped that it had been definitely buried. It is certainly discouraging to see our ablest alienists so divided that some will declare sane a man whom others declare a hopelessly incurable lunatic. Psychiatry is too great and exact a science to tolerate such differences of opinion any longer. Its experts must devise ways of getting together to discuss their cases to clear up disputed points before they go on the witness stand. At present the court has no other course than to give a certain weight to each side, and decide for itself without their aid. This course is too dangerous, as a layman might give undue weight to an opinion which is absurd from bias. So we must start all over again the old crusade to exclude partisan experts from the stand. None of the bills so far presented are perfect, but each is workable and better than the present scandal in states where none have been passed at all. Let Thaw hire all the experts he desires, but keep them off the stand and treat them as hired advisers. Then their opinions are as valuable as the attorney's—no more no less. The court must depend on its own impartial experts and no others.

* * *

The increase of suicides in the United States seems to be a fact. Mr. Frederick L. Hoffman, our greatest statistician, thinks the condition alarming according to a report he has recently made from the offices of the Prudential Life Insurance Company. There is absolutely no question that every suicide is mentally sick and the means of prevention must be studied by pathologists and sanitarians. The most fundamental sign of mental health is the desire to live and it stays with us as long as the brain works right, in spite of the most painful physical ailments. To a well man, life is always worth living and he struggles for existence no matter how few other joys it gives him. All this is so well known that it is difficult to understand why anyone does not recognize the desire to die as a sign of illness and immediately consult a psychiatrist. Well, many do ask help, but the majority skilfully conceal their trouble and even invent the most ingenious ways of "ending it all." In every case there is a reason which the sufferer considers adequate for the act, and it must be confessed that in a very small percentage the reason does appear adequate to normal minds, as when a leading man in a community is detected in crime. The life of an outcast is not worth living to such. Yet even here we are justified in suspecting that an acquired mental weakness is the basis of the loss of the normal inhibition to crime, he had all along life. Why, then, are so many men neurasthenic to such an extent?

Neurasthenia is becoming more prevalent here but not in Europe. The usual explanation is the rush and roar, the struggles and strains of modern life, but they are the same in Europe. Dr. J. Madison Taylor of Philadelphia, is convinced that it is largely climatic, from living in a southern climate to which we are physically unadjusted, (*N. Y. Med. Jour.*, July 6, 1912). Why not prove this by a study of the physical types of our suicides and neurasthenics? There are more suicides in the light months than in the dark and that ought to indicate that people originating in dark lands are the more numerous. We hope some one will gather the statistics as it may result in measures of prevention. There is not nearly enough of such work done in America. Europe is in the lead. Our pathologists seem to think that all types are equally subject to every disease, but the sole idea of the agriculturist is to obtain plants which are adjusted to an environment as he knows they differ in resistance. Let us begin with the suicides and extend it to every disease. There is a wealth of data in this new field, so let us get to work at once. Time is too precious to dally over it, as Hoffman says the conditions are alarming.

ORIGINAL ARTICLES.

SYPHILIS OF THE EAR, WITH ES-PECIAL REFERENCE TO THE USE OF 606.[1]

BY

IRVING WILSON VOORHEES, M. S., M. D.,

New York City.

Schaudinn's discovery of the spirocheta pallidum as the exciting cause of syphilis gave a new impulse to the study of this ancient disease. Wassermann's investigations, following shortly afterward, helped to confirm Schaudinn's work, and paved the way for more accurate methods of diagnosis in obscure syphilis.

It seems almost a travesty of justice that one hears so little about the greatness of Schaudinn's work in comparison with that of the famous Berlin serologist, but since the trend of modern scientific medicine is more toward the study of the blood and problems of immunity than toward the less difficult but not less important bacteriologic cause of disease the disparity may perhaps be thus explained. Certain it is that Schaudinn's discovery ranks very high in the scale of medical achievement.

Since syphilis is in the beginning a circumscribed local disease it is obvious that our first efforts should be directed toward early diagnosis and prompt destruction of the infected area, followed by an attempt to exclude the spirochetae from the blood stream and to effect an immediate and permanent cure. The old rule not to begin treatment until secondary symptoms became manifest can no longer be adhered to by up-to-date physicians.

Diagnosis of the causes of complications in syphilis must ever remain difficult since it is often quite impossible to say whether a given lesion is due to syphilis itself or to some remedial agent used by the physician in his effort to cure the patient. Perhaps a careful examination of the records of the past can do more toward clearing up this knotty problem than any amount of argument concerning the advantages or disadvantages of this or that remedy. There are, however, some facts which have been determined as a result of long years of experience in the study of syphilis, and one of these is that the syphilitic poison possesses a selective action on the nervous system. From the otologist's standpoint the cochlear and vestibular branches of the eighth nerve are especially prone to attack. Moreover, one may find a destructive periostitis with pressure and inflammation of the nerves, especially those of the internal auditory canal. The facial may be affected, causing a paralysis of the muscles of the face. A polyneuritis cerebralis syphilitica is not confined to the third stage or late in the course of syphilitic disease but may be an early manifestation.

Site of Manifestation.—Primary lesions of the external ear are not so infrequent. About 40 cases are on record and doubtless many have been unreported. Primary lesions of the eustachian tube and nasopharynx, especially in the fossa of Rosemuller, are quite common from passing a dirty catheter, but less so than before we knew the value of asepsis.

Secondary lesions of the auricle and external auditory meatus exist as an exan-

[1]The material for this article was derived from a study of cases and many conferences with physicians connected with the various departments of the Allgemeines Krankenhaus, Vienna, Austria.
Read before the Manhattan Medical Society, New York City, April 26, 1912.

420   AMERICAN MEDICINE · }
Complete Series, Vol. XVIII. }   ORIGINAL ARTICLES   { AUGUST, 1912.
{ New Series, Vol. VII., No. 8.

themata papilides, and ulcerations as part · of a general skin syphilis.

The pinna may be partially destroyed by the formation of deep ulcers and contractions of scar tissue. The most frequently observed specific lesions of the meatus are condylomata and ulcerations. Condylomata are usually concurrent with symptoms of general syphilis, skin syphilis, pharyngeal ulcers, and swelling of the glands.

Tertiary lesions in the ear are rare, although gummatous ulcers may occur. The most serious forms of syphilitic ear disease occur in the internal ear. The labyrinth may become involved, either early or later in the disease, but one seldom finds labyrinthine symptoms due to syphilis alone within twelve months after the initial lesion. The insidiousness of this condition has been well described by Jonathan Hutchinson as follows:

"We know of no form of ear disease, other than that due to syphilis in which without any obvious destruction of parts, complete permanent deafness in both ears can be brought about in the course of a few weeks. But this is not a rare occurrence in the subjects of inherited syphilis."

Syphilis of the labyrinth is more likely to occur in the tertiary stage. Labyrinthine syphilis may be of slow onset, of rapid onset, or may begin with apoplectiform suddenness. In the latter, exudation into the labyrinth is extremely rapid and is probably associated with hemorrhage.

Otosclerosis may possibly belong to the slow type of syphilitic degeneration bringing about immobility of the stages, formation of new bone in the middle and internal ear, and spongification of the labyrinthine capsule.

For a long time it was thought that there is a connection between otosclerosis and lues, but recent investigations go to show that there is little or no connection. Beck, of Vienna, has made Wassermann's test of all individuals in several families showing otosclerosis. The test was negative in the majority of cases, only two patients out of fifty having had lues. One must remember, however, that if a patient with otosclerosis contracts lues, the prognosis for hearing is bad.

Diagnosis of Aural Lues.— It is not possible to find the spirocheta pallidum in discharge from the middle ear, because the pyogenic bacteria probably kill the spirochetae, but it may be that our staining methods are at fault. Deafness and loss of vestibular reaction may be present even with quite normal membrana tympani, in fact this is the rule rather than the exception. However, if there is complete loss of both vestibular apparatuses the patient walks like a congenitally deaf-and-dumb person, that is on a broad base with the feet far apart.

Sudden deafness in a child during the night usually means hereditary syphilis. This is probably due to a primary neuritis and not to labyrinthitis as Gradenigo asserts.

Pemphigus bullae on the feet or fine vesicles behind the ear in a new-born child are always suggestive of syphilis.

If careful examination of the ear shows a lesion of the cochlear nerve with intact vestibular reaction, there must be some cause for this in the nerve itself or in its central connections. If one can exclude all other causes of nerve degeneration such as long exposure to loud noises, traumatic injuries of the head, all infectious diseases especially scarlet fever and typhoid, and the presbyacusis of old age, the cause is likely to be syphilis since in a study of 50 cases of nerve deafness, exclusive of the above causes, 30 per cent gave a positive Wassermann.

A patient with only a few skin symptoms in syphilis is likely to have nerve lues. Marked skin manifestations offer better prognosis and better results from treatment because the blood coming to the surface of the body contains many spirochetae, and, therefore, the use of inunctions in these causes is very helpful.

Multiple sclerosis is sometimes difficult to differentiate from nerve lues, but one should remember that the symptoms of multiple sclerosis are rather capricious while the symptoms of aural syphilis are fixed, definite and unchanging. For example, examination of a patient suffering from multiple sclerosis shows the following:

Deafness, with no reaction of the labyrinth at one examination changing to hearing with a reacting labyrinth at another examination.

The patient does not fall in the direction of the slow component.[1]

The patient may be nearly blind for some days and then see again very well. We must differentiate this defect in vision from hysterical eye disturbances.

On one examination there may be a partial paralysis of the abducens muscle, and at another examination no sign of abducens paralysis.

---

[1] A word of explanation is, perhaps, in order here. Nystagmus consists of a rhythmic associated movement of both eyes in a given plane. This movement is slow in one direction and rapid in the opposite direction—the slow component being of vestibular origin; the rapid component of cerebral origin. Patients showing nystagmus with disturbances of equilibrium due to labyrinthine disease always "fall away from the nystagmus": i. e., they fall opposite to the quick component, and in the direction of the slow component. Obviously any patient who falls contrary to this rule is not suffering primarily from vestibular nerve disease.

Let us now cite a few cases according to the respective groups under which they seem to fall: First, aural disturbances due to syphilis alone; second, aural disturbances due to syphilis or mercury; third, aural disturbances of mixed origin; fourth, aural disturbances due probably to the use of 606.

I. Aural disturbances due to syphilis.

Case I.—Man, 23. Large glands in right side of the neck. Diagnosis by the surgeon was tuberculosis. In the skin clinic the Wassermann reaction was found positive. The patient is suffering from an extra-genital primary chancre, due to infection by a razor in a barber-shop. He now shows a typical syphilitic rash, and an o. m. c. c. in the right ear. The eustachian tube is closed from secondary infection of the fauces. This man was recommended for an injection of 606 because his aural catarrh is due to syphilis, and was not a pre-existing condition.

Case II. Man, 50. Had lues four years ago—now has pain in the head and ears. He forgets easily, sometimes cannot find his house, and becomes so excited he could commit murder. Examination June 24, 1911. The pupils are unequal. The left is smaller. They react poorly to light, and accommodate slowly. The patient has paresthesia of the tongue. He is unable to speak a sentence quickly and accurately. The knee reflexes are both diminished. Chief complaint, pain in the head and ears. This is probably a beginning tabes, or a general paresis.

Wagner of Vienna and Fischer of Prague use tuberculin in these cases of old syphilis with beginning tabes, chiefly because of the continuing fever. Fischer inclines more to the use of nuclein, many other neurologists use Zittmann's decoction, but this causes bad diarrhea and an increased amount of urine, and is not so agreeable in action as pilocarpin. Some of these cases do well on baths at the various hot springs.

Case III.—Man, 32. In August, 1910, he had a primary lesion. He had a marked exanthem, papules in the pharynx and in the mouth, combined with suppuration in the middle ear. He was first treated by mercury, and then, some weeks later, one injection of 606 was given. Eight days later the middle ear was dry. The question is, whether the otitis media was due to lues. This seems probable because of the effect of treatment. In this connection one should remember the necessity of knowing the exact condition of the pharynx and naso-pharynx because of their influence upon the middle ear in lues. It is very important to examine the ears of every case of syphilis, inasmuch as syphilitic papules occur in the external auditory canal from irritation of the skin by middle ear discharge. For the diagnosis of ulcerations in the pharynx and naso-pharynx, where the drum is defective, Ernst Urbantschitsch uses alcohol. The head is inclined toward the shoulder, some alcohol is dropped in the external ear, and when the ulcers are present the alcohol causes burning in the region of the tube. Personally, I do not regard such evidence as at all conclusive.

Case IV.—Child, 13. Had keratitis punctata one year before the onset of her present deafness, for which gray oil was given, but this did not prevent loss of hearing, in both ears later. Examination shows degeneration of both the vestibular and cochlear nerves, therefore, there is little hope of recovery. This girl has had two injections of .4 and .3 gram of 606 with seemingly no effect.

Case V.—Child, 6. Sister of girl aged 13 above cited. The only symptom of syphilis which this child shows is notched teeth. It is, therefore, very important to prevent the oncoming of eye and ear symptoms in this case, and it is much better to give 606 now as a preventive. Hutchinson's triad is of great value in making the diagnosis of congenital syphilis and consists as is known of first, interstitial keratitis, second, the so-called, Hutchinson's teeth, which are peg-shaped, notched and poorly covered by enamel, third, deafness or hardness of hearing.

II. AURAL DISTURBANCES DUE TO SYPHILIS OR MERCURY.

Case VI.—Man, age 30. In August, 1909, he discovered his primary lesion. He has had numerous injections of mercury into the muscles. In December, 1909, he had marked dizziness for two days, followed by disturbances of equilibrium and noises. Examination showed no vestibular reaction in the left ear, but fairly good hearing. The vestibular reaction in the right ear is normal, but the hearing in this ear is bad. There is also partial paralysis of both abducens nerves. His condition remained unchanged after a long period of observation.

III. AURAL DISTURBANCES OF MIXED ORIGIN.

Case VII.—Man, 40. Initial lesion 7 months ago, then six weeks later a rash was seen covering the entire body. Admitted to the hospital and treated from March 7th to 28th, 1910, with injections of mercury into the muscles. This treatment improved the symptoms very much, but on March 30th an injection of 606 was given into the veins. A second injection was given one week later. Six weeks after this second injection the man found he was hard of hearing, and three weeks after this he noticed facial paralysis. It is to be remarked that before the injection of 606 he had normal hearing on both sides. Therefore, no otosclerosis could have been present. Examination showed: Right ear, conversation voice 1½ meters, whispered voice 10 centimeters. Schwabach a little shortened, Rinné minus with air conduction much shortened. Left ear: Conversation voice *ad concha*, whispered voice not heard, Weber to the left, Schwabach shortened, Rinné minus. The patient has normal drums on both sides. In reference to the shortened bone conduction, one may say that all patients with well-established lues have shorter bone conduction than normal. This man has no head noises, no dizziness, no nystagmus, no vomiting, therefore his affection cannot be in the endolymph; that is, it cannot be due to labyrinthitis. On May 23rd, he was given a third injection of 606, but his condition remained the same, no better and no worse. In such a case it seems advisable to go back to mercury.

Case VIII.—Woman, 35. This patient has had lues for 3½ years. In October, 1910 she was given 606. She had sensations of itching in both external ears (parasthesias). She complains of ringing in the ear, which may mean degeneration of the labyrinth or luetic catarrh of the middle ear. She sometimes hears well, sometimes badly, which leads one to suspect lues. She shows tenderness over the mastoid, which is probably due to luetic periostitis. Examination shows both drums fairly normal, but some redness over the promotory. The possibilities of diagnosis here are catarrh of the tube, catarrh of the middle ear, otosclerosis, and beginning inner ear trouble. Conversation voice on the right ½ meter, on the left 2 meters, whispered voice on the right 0, on the left 10 centimeters, Weber to the right, Rinné positive on the right and left, Schwabach shortened on both sides. There is no change in the hearing after inflation; therefore this cannot be a simple middle ear catarrh. It is probably a beginning otosclerosis with aggravation of symptoms by lues and 606, and it seems better not to repeat 606 but to use inunctions of mercury.

IV. AURAL DISTURBANCES DUE PROBABLY TO 606.

Case IX.—Man, 43. Had a primary lesion December, 1910. In January, 1911, rash over the entire body. The cochlear and vestibular apparatuses were normal. On February 1st, the patient received .4 gram neutral solution of salvarsan. Six weeks later he experienced noises in his ears after a bath. Examination showed marked deafness of the right ear coming on after severe noises, dizziness and vomiting. The patient was kept in bed until the violent symptoms had disappeared, and it was then noticed that he had facial paralysis on the right side, accompanied by slight ptosis. On the right side the cochlear apparatus, the vestibular apparatus, the facial nerve and the trigeminus were all affected. This was diagnosed as a case of polyneuritis cerebralis Menieriformis or Frankl-Hochwart's disease. After some time the vestibular and facial nerves on the right side showed improvement, but the cochlear affection as evidenced by the deafness still remains.

Case X.—Man, 38. Occupation, chauffeur. In February, 1910, a primary lesion occurred, coming on three weeks after intercourse. Administration of 606 was first tried by the mouth but was vomited. The patient was then given an injection of 606

into the buttocks. Six weeks later, early in the morning, he found himself suddenly hard of hearing on the right side. On the next day he had noises, vomiting, dizziness, and disturbances of equilibrium, in which he fell toward his left side, that is, away from the side of the lesion. Spontaneous nystagmus to the left, rotatory to the left and horizontal to the right. This is rather characteristic for labyrinthitis. The patient was very nauseated upon looking to the left. Examination of the right ear showed no caloric reaction upon the use of hot water, no turning nystagmus and no galvanic nystagmus. The patient's condition remained about the same until January 11, 1911, when he experienced a new attack of noises, this time in the left ear, vomiting and spontaneous nystagmus to the left. It was found that the left labyrinth was not irritable, and this was followed two weeks later by complete deafness on the left side, occurring five months after the administration of 606. Curiously enough, the Wassermann reaction was never positive. This case was referred to Professor Ehrlich, who advised another injection of 606, but no improvement has since occurred. The patient shows some aphasia and mild convulsions in one-half of his body. His ears were apparently normal before the administration of 606. It is interesting to note that on the right side the cochlear nerve was the first to go, and then the vestibular nerve. On the left side the vestibular nerve was first to go and then the cochlear. In addition the patient now has a probable encephalitis. Examination of the urine showed the presence of arsenic seven months after administration of 606. After the use of pilocarpin the arsenic in the urine began to disappear, and the patient heard a little on the left side, but the right side was evidently too old a process to improve. The patient now shows marked ataxia when he walks with closed eyes. After the loss of both vestibular apparatuses a patient may know to which side he is turned, but this patient has lost this sensation.

Case XI.—Man, 25. In January, 1911, he had a primary chancre. Before the Wassermann was reported positive he was given 0.4 gram, and two weeks later another 0.4 gram of 606. Seven weeks after the first injection there were noises and hardness of hearing in the right ear.

For thirteen years this patient has worked in a place where there was a great deal of noise. Examination of the ears before the injection of 606 showed normal hearing for all tests. This ear difficulty began after the first injection of 606. In contradistinction it is noteworthy that in 600 cases treated with mercury there was only one case of deafness occurring in less than one year after the beginning of the treatment.

Treatment of Lues.—In the treatment of aural lues the aurist must be guided by the same principles which govern the treatment elsewhere in the body, depending upon constitutional rather than upon local means.

Hereditary Lues.— The best results of 606 are seen in congenital lues, and although mercury may be used it is not altogether satisfactory. Inunction is probably the best form of mercury in cases of hereditary lues, but the patient may get better for a few days and then become as bad as ever. Hyd. Tannicum (Lustgarten) can be given internally or Ung. cinereum may be rubbed in, and if so, should be used strong. When the skin is gray and shiny, this is an indication that the mercury is being properly given. The salicylate of mercury in oil is probably the best form of mercury for administration by the injection method.

℞

    Hyd. Salicyl .... 2.0 grams
    Petrolatum liq. ....20. grams
    Sig. For injection.

It is best to inject ½ c.c. (0.5 c.c.) every fourth day into alternate quadrants of the buttocks.

One of the best drugs in hereditary lues is pilocarpin.

℞

    Pilocarp. mur. 0.01
    Aq. Destil. 10.00
    1% sol.
    Sig. Subcutaneous injection.

Old Lues.—Old cases of lues do well with pilocarpin. If a man has a negative Wassermann, but says that years ago he had lues, it is best to try this drug.

In a big strong man one may use this drug as a 2 per cent. solution, but this causes severe sweating and discomfort. The injection may be given every second day. It is best to begin with 3 or 4 parts of the solution in a graduated syringe, and cautiously increase this dosage up to 10 parts.

In old cases of lues, sodium iodide may be given in warm milk .5 gram to 1 gram in a day. If the hearing is not better stop— then, after two months, begin again with 3 grams per day, but the patient must be watched closely for severe headache and burning in the eyes. When these symptoms take place the treatment should be stopped for a few days.

Probably the best treatment in lues of the nerves is inunctions according to the old French rule, but in some cases these seem to have no effect.

If one finds albumen in the urine in a patient under treatment with mercury, one must not stop the treatment, but simply watch the patient carefully, attending to the general hygiene of the body, cleansing of the mouth, etc.

Ehrlich's 606 heralded by many persons both among physicians and laity as a never-failing cure for syphilis "at a single stroke" is still warmly discussed. There are men of wide experience, such as Wassermann of Berlin, who praise it very highly; while others of equally great experience, like Finger of Vienna, believe that it very often produces harmful results. Certain it is that very different effects may be obtained in different individuals. These differences may be due to varying resistance of the individual, strong persons being less affected than weak ones. According to Ehrlich, these differences may also be due to degeneration or thrombosis of blood vessels supplying the nerves, therefore, no 606 is carried to these nerves and the spirochetae are thus unaffected. Consequently we got recurrences of syphilitic manifestations.

We know that arsenic is a quick poison for the lower forms of animal life. It kills the spirochetae very quickly, but also has a toxic influence on the normal nervous system. The Jarisch-Herxheimer reaction on the skin is a common result after 606. It may be that this reaction occurs in the inner ear also, giving rise to labyrinthine disturbances. However, we cannot be sure of this.

Arsacetin causes a rapid disappearance of the symptoms of syphilis, but also causes degeneration of various cerebral nerves, especially the optic nerve. When white mice are injected with 606 they are converted into dancing mice. They have disturbances of equilibrium and no idea of straight line movement. By the end of the 30th day these mice cannot see well. Histological sections of the cranial nerves show degeneration affecting especially the optic and auditory trunks. Curiously enough, histological preparations of Japanese dancing mice show degeneration of the vestibular nerve which is evidently congenital.

A person with an absolutely normal ear is not likely to get ear symptoms after 606, but on the contrary, if there has existed a middle or inner ear disease for some time, it is certainly risky to use this powerful remedy. This holds especially true for nerve degeneration. Wittmaack has found that exposure of animals to loud noises for a long time, followed by histologic examination of the inner ear, showed degeneration of the nerve cells in Corti's organ; therefore, it is not very safe to give 606 to workers in loud noises.

It has been said by some writers that severe ear and eye symptoms after 606 occur chiefly in cases of recent lues. On the contrary the worst results I have seen have occurred in old lues; for example, a man in whom Beck had injected 606 into the muscles developed a large abscess at the site of injections seven months later. Nothing happened immediately after the injection, but sometime later the man became completely deaf in the left ear. His lues was thirty years old.

The following groups of the results of 606 used in the Vienna clinics have been arranged by Docent Dr. Hugo Frey:

Group I. Cases which one or two days after the injections developed vestibular troubles, consisting of dizziness, nystagmus, and loss of vestibular irritability. These are variously explained, either from pressure on the nerves and luetic recurrence, or a toxic reaction of the injection fluid upon the eighth nerve. The last explanation is probably the true one—bearing in mind our studies on the common mouse, which, after the injection of 606 becomes a dancing mouse, and shows characteristic changes in the vestibular nerve ganglia.

Group II. Cases of deafness only, with no vestibular symptoms, such as dizziness.

Group III. Cases of deafness and vestibular irritability (dizziness) Méniere's Syndrome.

Different results are obtained from different fluids and different methods of injection. In Vienna either acid solutions, alkaline solutions or emulsions or arsenic are used.

Professor Gustav Alexander made some observations of his experience in aural syphilis both before and after the use of 606· at a recent special meeting of the Vienna Medical Society.

Professor Finger asked Professor Alexander the following question: "You have examined my clinical material a long time before 606 was invented. Did you observe then cases with such symptoms as one now sees after injection of Ehrlich's fluid?"

Professor Alexander answered:

"My entire material comprised sixty-eight cases; if I exclude cases of ear disease of meta-luetic origin, that is to say, tabes and paralysis. In the course of six years I have seen altogether 112 cases of ear diseases in a recent stage of lues. Three of these cases manifested diseases of the external canal and of the middle ear, and are to be excluded. In the comparison of the cases observed by Professor Finger and Professor Urbantschitsch more or less severe eighth nerve affections are dealt with solely. My nine cases correspond to a period of six years; the three Finger cases to a period of six months. In one of the Finger cases the ear affection occurred in a lues six weeks old. In the remaining two cases about three months after the initial lesion. Among the cases under my observation I can find only one in which the disturbances of hearing developed after thirteen weeks. In all other cases the disturbances arose in a recent stage of lues, but not earlier than the fourth, fifth, or sixth month.

"Let us compare the severity of the affection itself. Four of my cases showed slight disturbances of the auditory nerve with slight dizziness or subjective noises; slightly diminished hearing and quick favorable course. Diseases of the severer type, as in the Finger cases I have observed only in five of my cases. Among them is one case after atoxyl treatment. The remaining four were treated with mercury by inunction or injection. It would seem that acute luetic neuritis of the eighth nerve has a selective action on the cochlear or vestibular branch of the nerve. Heretofore cases of labyrinthine syphilis with respect to syphilitic inflammation of the eighth nerve in the recent stage were almost unknown. Von Frankl-Hochwart reviews in his book forty cases of lues with the Méniere's symptom-complex, which is nothing less than a disease of the static labyrinth or of the vestibular nerve. Von Frankl-Hochwart's 40 cases represent inveterate latent lues. He has never observed a case of Méniere's symptom-complex in a recent stage of syphilis. Politzer reported symptoms of labyrinthine syphilis in one case of lues of seven days' duration. This observation occurred in 1878, and remains unique until now.

"One must conclude from all that has been said that the cases reported by Professor Finger so far as the eighth nerve was involved in recent lues, must be attributed to the use of arseno-benzol. One thing is certain, that in cases of recent lues where any disease of the eighth nerve already exists, the danger is that the disease will be made worse by the use of arseno-benzol. After what has occurred, it is recommended that in cases of acute lues greater care be taken. Especially if there is a previously existing disease of the eighth nerve; for in such a condition an injection of arseno-benzol may cause a· pejoration of the ear disease."

This much may at least be said whatever the personal bias of the reader, that Ehrlich's 606 improves some cases only, especially cases of recent infection. Old ear cases show little or no good result, and some cases of syphilis are not improved by anything, mercury, potassium iodide or 606.

But we are not so sure that some of our bad results have not been due to unwise use of mercury and that 606 should not alone stand condemned. For instance, Beck reports four children in the same family who were infected with extra-genital lues of the mouth from an older sister. Two were treated with mercury and two with 606. All four had recurrence of the disease. This seems to show that 606 is a quicker but not more permanent cure for lues than mercury. Beck thinks it may be possible that tabes, which is so much more frequent in males, is the result of mercurial treatment. Tabes is not common in females, because many women do not know that they have lues, the diagnosis is never made, and therefore they are not treated by mercury.

CONCLUSIONS.

1. Salvarsan (606) is of value in syphilis of the ear.

2. It is especially useful in recent aural lues.

3. Its use in old lues of the ear should be guarded, especially if degeneration of the cochlear or vestibular nerves be present.

4. It may be of use in congenital deaf-dumbness due to syphilis if injected while the child is still young.

5. If aural lues is suspected and 606 is under contemplation, the advice of an otologist familiar with "neuro-recidives" should be first obtained.

14 Central Park West.

VERTIGO.

BY

LESTER MEAD HUBBY, M. D,.

New York City.

Vertigo is the hallucinatory sensation of subjective or objective rotation. Orientation is the conscious placing of the body in a certain relation to a plane horizontal to the earth's surface, and is in large part automatic. Equilibration consists in the correct adjustment of the muscle tension of the body, so that the desired orientation and equipoise result. Imperfect orientation produces imperfect equilibration and vertigo.

The cerebellar cortex contains the sensory elements of orientation, while the motors centers are chiefly located in the intrinsic nuclei of the cerebellum and in the para-cerebellar nuclei. The sensory nerve paths of orientation are the vestibular, the ocular, and the nerves of pressure and tension sense from the muscles, joints and internal organs. Disorder of one of these paths or centers may produce vertigo, until the body learns to orient without their assistance. The vestibular tract is the most important, and its involvement results in greater and more prolonged vertigo than that of any of the others.

The vestibular nerve begins in the semi-circular canal ampulae and the maculae acusticae of the utricle and saccule passes by way of several collections of bipolar ganglion cells in the auditory nerve (Scarpa's ganglion) in the internal auditory meatus, and terminates in several nuclei in the medulla, of which Deiter's, Bechterew's, and one lying in the posterior portion of the floor of the fourth ventricle seem to be the most important.

The vestibular nuclei have many associatory nerve-connections with the cerebellum, (nucleus fastigii, etc.,) the motor nerves of the eyeball, the cerebral cortex, etc. That with the motor nuclei of the eyeball is especially close, which explains their over action with the production of nystagmus and vertigo on vestibular stimulation.

Vestibular vertigo never occurs without nystagmus, is always in the direction of the slow component of the nystagmus, is always rotary in the plane of the nystagmus, and the direction of the swaying is altered by changing the position of that plane. It can be artificially induced by rotation of the body, by pouring hot or cold water into the ear, or by galvanization of the ear. Sea, car and elevator vertigoes are combinations of vestibular and ocular types.

Vertigo may occur on irritation of the vestibular nerve tract or of any of its associatory nerve fibres in the brain. The latter is called irritative shock or diaschisis, and consists in this instance in the production of symptoms from the vestibular tract which is connected by associatory fibres with the original lesion elsewhere.

Disorders of the external auditory meatus and of the tympanum occasionally produce vertigo by alterations in the endolymphatic pressure in the static labyrinth. This alteration in pressure is brought about either directly through the stapes (more rarely the round window) and the perilymph, or indirectly by sympathetic variations in the vascularity of the static labyrinth.

Local causes for changes of pressure in the labyrinth such as exudations (Voltolini's disease, etc.), hemorrhages, (Meniere's disease), scleroses, exostoses, and growths, may cause vertigo, the more acute the change the more violent the symptoms.

In those due to hemorrhage, even death may supervene from shock to the bulbar vital centers.

Irritations such as pressure, trauma or inflammation of the vestibular nerve in any part of its course from the labyrinth to its centers in the medulla may cause vertigo. This partly explains its frequent occurrence in pontine affections.

The vertigo occurring immediately after paralysis of one vestibular nerve is vestibular in type and is due to over action of the vestibular nerve of the other side, and the tendency to fall is toward the affected side. Later when this nerve over action with its nystagmus subsides, there still remains some vertigo which is due to quite a different cause, and is not vestibular in character. The falling is not always in the same direction, the direction of the swaying is not altered by the position of the head, and there is no nystagmus. The explanation for this is that the body has to learn to orient without the assistance of the vestibular nerve, and to depend upon the ocular, muscular, arthrodial and other sensory nerves in its place. This vertigo gradually disappears until when attempting some unusual act, or acting in some unaccustomed position, is it apparent.

The cerebellum is the principal co-ordinating center of the brain. Its cortex is mainly sensory, receiving afferent nerve fibres from the proprio ceptors of the entire body, probably including the viscera. Its motor nuclei are probably in the cerebellum itself (for the head and neck) or in the nearby medulla and pons. It is apparent therefore that involvement of the cerebellum, medulla, or pons, may cause incoordination, ataxia and vertigo, depending on the number of nerve-paths affected. As these paths are concentrated in the three peduncles and the vermis, vertigo is a prominent symptom in their involvement.

On the other hand a lesion of the cerebellar cortex, if produced slowly enough not to upset the intra-cranial pressure-balance may exist without vertigo.

Cerebellar vertigo is generally rotary in type, and the body tends to fall in the direction of the lesion. Thus in lesions of the right half of the cerebellum, the body tends to fall to the right—when in the anterior part of the vermis, the falling is said to be forward, etc., etc.

Cerebellar vertigo is generally accompanied by nystagmus, but the latter is slower and lacks many of the characteristics of the vestibular type, unless the vestibular nerve tract is particularly involved. Many times the nystagmus is simply hyper-physiological. The tendency to fall is not affected by the direction of the nystagmus, and is generally toward the lesion. Moreover, cerebellar vertigo is not changed in direction by altering the position of the planes of the head.

Localized lesions of the cerebellum from depressed fractures, hemorrhages, effusions, scleroses, tumors, etc., may cause vertigo. This is particularly true of the flocculus. Whether this is due to the termination of a large number of vestibular nerve fibres in this part of the cerebellar cortex or to pressure on parts of the vestibular tract in the adjacent region (such as the middle cerebellar peduncles, etc.), remains to be proved.

Vertigo occurs in general disorders of the cerebellum such as congenital defective cerebellar development; hereditary cerebellar ataxia; at the moment of epileptic seizures (petit, grand mal, and focal); occasionally in the neurasthenic and the hysterical; in the cerebellar neurosis of essential vertigo (which consists in epileptiform vertiginous attacks); and in Gerlier's disease (kubisafari) a disease of unknown etiology, characterized by transient and recurring attacks of vertigo, ptosis, neck palsy, etc.

Ocular vertigo results when there is a sudden paralysis of one or more of the extrinsic muscles of the eye-ball with that production of diplopia. It is sometimes accompanied by nystagmus of a simple vibratory type. The vertigo ceases on covering the affected eye, or when it is not used, and the sensation of falling is in no particular direction. It gradually disappears as the false image becomes disregarded.

The vertigo occurring on looking at rapidly revolving objects, is ocular in type.

There is little if any swaying, and the sensation of falling, etc., is in no particular direction.

Severe involvement of the nerve tracts of muscle and arthrodial sense sometimes causes verginal attacks. This accounts for its occurrence occasionally in tabes.

Starr thinks that in some ataxics it is due to primary atrophy of the vestibular nerve.

The vertigoes of multiple scleroses have different explanations depending on the anatomical distributions of the plaques. When in the pons, medulla, cerebellum or the vestibular nerve tract, the type of vertigo will correspond to that of the part involved.

In caisson disease the vertigo may be of a mixed type, due to the synchronous ear, eye, and intra-cranial disorders.

The vertigo of migraine may have a different etiology in each instance, depending on the type of the disorder. Instances have been recorded showing a distinctively cerebellar syndrome.

Sudden or marked increase in the intra-cranial blood pressure produces vertigo by the venous congestion induced in the entire brain but especially in the equilibration centers, e. g., intra-cranial hemorrhage, exudations, abscesses, growths, depressed fractures, venous congestion from heavy lifting and stool straining, etc.

Vertigo likewise occurs in sudden or marked intra-cranial circulatory anemia, e. g., general circulatory weakness following severe exertions, shock, hemorrhages, etc., temporarily depriving the cerebellar centers of sufficient blood to functionate.

Blood that is abnormal—containing either toxins or abnormal amounts of normal constituents, may produce vertigo, either by causing changes in the intra-cranial circulation or by direct irritation of the equilibration nerve cells. Examples of this are—blood containing alcohol, caffeine, nicotine, opium, auto-toxins, bacterial and protozoal substances, gouty diabetic and uremic products, etc.

The vertigo occurring in over doses of quinine and possibly the salicylates may be. due either to congestion of the static labyrinth (Kirchner) or to irritation of the nerve cells in Scarpa's ganglion.

Psychical vertigoes are due to shock with its coincident sudden intra-cranial anemia. They coexist with some phobia, e. g., height dizziness from fear of falling, etc. Rarely is there any swaying in this form of dizziness.

Alcohol, ether, chloroform and other hydro-carbon narcotics produce vertigo through direct action on the cerebellar nerve cells. C. C. Stewart has observed diminution and fusion of the Nissl granules in the Purkinje cells after their use. Vestibular nerve irritation sometimes occurs in partial ether anesthesia as evidenced by vestibular nystagmus.

Then there are various so-called reflex vertigoes. In chronic gastritis and gastric dilatation of vagal centers, passing thence to the various centers of equilibrium, or to absorption of cerebellar irritants, remains to be proven.

The vertigo occurring in the laryngeal crisis of tabes or other attacks of laryngeal spasm, is due to increased intra-cranial pressure from the dyspnea, struggling and excitement.

The vertigo which occurs in inflammation of the antrum of Highmore, ethmoids or sphenoidal sinus is due to toxic absorption with the production of intra-cranial congestion, which when considerable is seen in the optic papilla.

Suddenly stooping forward, or bending the head backward increases this intra-cranial congestion, producing vertigo.

When sufficient orbital congestion and inflammation reach the extrinsic muscles of the eye so as to interfere with their action, diplopia and vertigo result.

In Conclusion:—

Diagnostically considered there are four types of vertigo.

1. Simple. In this there is no tendency to fall in one particular direction. There is no nystagmus.

2. Ocular. Same character as the simple, but sometimes there is a purely oscillatory nystagmus.

3. Cerebellar. There is a tendency to fall always in one particular direction even when the head is placed in different positions. Nystagmus may be present, but is liable to be slower than the vestibular type. Moreover it may be merely hyper-physiological, i. e., only brought out on turning

the eyes strongly in each direction seriatim.

4. Vestibular. The swaying is in the direction of the slow component of the nystagmus, and in the plane of the nystagmus. Nystagmus of a vestibular type is always present, though it may be necessary to turn the eyes strongly in one direction to bring it out. The direction of the falling is altered by changing the position of the planes of the head relative to the earth's surface.

27 W. 68th St.

SOME EXPERIENCES WITH BAC-TERINS IN THE TREATMENT OF AURAL VERTIGO.

BY

G. H. SHERMAN, M. D.,

Detroit, Mich.

In the April number of AMERICAN MEDICINE appears a very excellent article by Dr. Albert A. Gray, of Glasgow, entitled "Auditory Vertigo and Tinnitus Aurium." While it is admitted that the diagnosis of these conditions is usually a very difficult and intricate procedure, the successful treatment is even more difficult. It is quite possible, then, that a recital of some very encouraging results in the treatment of this condition with bacterial vaccines might be interesting to readers of AMERICAN MEDICINE.

Extensive research into the cause of vertigo has been conducted by investigators abroad and in this country during the last few years. That the cause of this disagreeable ailment has been traced to disturbances in the internal ear is indicated in an exhaustive article by Dr. George E. Davis which concludes:

"The internal ears are the special sense organs of equilibrium. With the internal ears we recognize (orientation) and maintain our relations to space (equilibration).

"The visual sense organs (the eyes), and the kinesthetic sense organs (the muscles, etc.), are accessory sense organs of equilibrium (the internal ears), through the mediation of the cerebellum.

"The two special sense organs of equilibrium (the internal ear on either side) are normally symmetrical in structure and function, and any factor whatever, whether it be physiologic, experimental or pathologic, which innervates, stimulates or irritates one of these twin organs in excess of the other (or on the other hand accomplishes the same thing through enervation, depression or destruction of one in excess of the other), in that measure tends to or creates proportionately a disturbance of equilibrium sufficiently marked or intense that we also get nystagmus and that unpleasant and complex phenomenon termed vertigo."

Dr. Edward Bradford Dench (*New York Medical Journal*, Jan. 6, 1912, p. 1) reports a number of cases of vertigo treated by operation and other methods, and among other things says:

"As the end organ of the complex mechanism controlling the equilibrium of the body is situated in the semicircular canals, all cases of vertigo must, in their broadest sense, be considered as aural vertigo, inasmuch as they represent an involvement either of the ear itself or of some portion of the auditory nerve trunk or of its central or cortical filaments."

"We may classify cases of this disease as follows:

"1. Cases due to a chronic non-suppurative inflammation of the middle ear.

"2. Cases due to a residual suppuration of the middle ear.

"3. Cases due to aural suppuration.

"4. Cases due to involvement of the auditory nerve trunk, as the result either of a specific inflammation involving the nerve trunk, or due to a degeneration of the end organ of the auditory nerve as the result of some middle ear inflammation or of some general diathetic condition.

"It should be borne in mind that when any portion of the auditory apparatus, either of the middle ear, the labyrinth or the nerve trunk, is in a pathological condition, any slight stimulus, particularly an increase in the blood pressure, may be sufficient to bring on an attack of vertigo."

I will briefly review his cases because they are specially instructive in showing the relation of inflammatory processes of the aural mechanism to the production of vertigo.

Case 1. Non-suppurative otitis media with tinnitus was successfully treated with a two per cent solution of pilocarpin introduced into the tympanic cavity through an Eustachian catheter.

Case 2. Another case of .chronic non-suppurative otitis media with progressive sclerotic changes within the middle ear and labyrinth was treated by opening the vestibule with a small knife and allowing a certain amount of the labyrinthic fluid to escape. This aggravated the vertigo for a time but the condition gradually subsided and finally recovered.

Case 3. One case of grippe was followed by acute otitis media with mastoid involvement which was operated upon six weeks after the initial attack. A month after the mastoid operation severe vertigo suddenly developed. The acute symptom subsided but a slight vertigo remained, and two months later a radical operation was performed relieving a fistula in the horizontal semicircular canal. Drainage was instituted and the patient made a complete recovery.

Case 4. This was a case of perilabyrinthitis with vertigo, and was almost entirely deaf. As no fistulous opening into the labyrinth was found, the radical opera-

tion was performed and primary grafting employed. The patient made a good recovery.

Case 5. .This case gave a syphilitic history. The patient complained of hardness of hearing with vertigo. He was given large doses of salicylate of mercury and began to improve at once under this treatment and completely recovered. In some special remarks on this case the author says: "In this case we had to deal undoubtedly with a syphilitic inflammation, either of the auditory nerve trunk itself or of the meninges in the immediate neighborhood of the internal auditory meatus." The complete recovery of the patient confirms the correctness of the diagnosis.

Case 6. This man showed involvement of the auditory nerve trunk with severe tinnitus and some vertigo. Operation of dividing the auditory nerve at its emergence from the base of the brain was performed, and the patient was absolutely relieved for a number of months. There was some slight return of the tinnitus, but the other conditions remained good.

These cases show that a large variety of inflammatory conditions in and around the internal ear may be responsible for the single symptom of vertigo. In cases 3 and 4 operations were performed for the purpose of establishing drainage, but unfortunately no report of bacterial findings was made to show the etiologic cause of the inflammatory condition.

The syphilitic case demonstrates that a specific causative organism—the spirochete —may be responsible for an inflammatory process that will subside under specific treatment, with a resultant disappearance of the vertigo.

Putnam (*Therapeutic Gazette*, Feb. 15, 1912, p. 119, review *Boston Medical & Surgical Journal*, Sept. 28, 1911) says:

"The functional efficiency of the apparatus of which these canals are an essential part may be impaired, even though the cochlea and auditory apparatus are in a normal state, so that tests for hearing are an insufficient guide in the determination of the labyrinthine condition in cases of aural vertigo."

It is now quite generally admitted that aural vertigo is associated with some inflammatory condition connected with the semicircular canal and that this inflammation may be acute, subacute or chronic. It is also found that when such inflammation exists, variations in blood pressure have a great influence on the vertiginous attacks, causing them more frequently when the blood pressure is high than when it is low. This would indicate that in cases of arteriosclerosis the attacks of vertigo are due primarily to an inflamed condition of the aural apparatus while ordinarily they are attributed to the sclerotic condition.

Cases of vertigo associated with suppurative and non-suppurative otitis media are commonly met with. Bacterial examinations of the pus in the early stages of this disease show that in a large majority of these cases the streptococcus is the primary infecting organism. After a rupture of the ear drum, outside contamination soon takes place and staphylococci are found. Later they often supplant the streptococcus. From clinical observations we find that the streptococcus is an organism that may cause an almost endless variety of inflammation and many kinds of tissue may be involved.

I have seen cases of chronic erysipelas where the inflammatory process was practically the same for months. Chronic rheumatic joints are good illustrations of persistent infective processes without pus formation. As streptococcus infections are of such common occurrence in middle ear infections, the inflammatory processes associated with vertigo can very readily be attributed to this organism.

In chronic non-suppurative otitis we have a subdued inflammation associated with inflammatory deposits and adhesions. This condition often extends into the bony structure around the semicircular canals without pus formation. This is quite similar to the condition in the bony structure of enlarged joints in chronic rheumatism. From our present knowledge of germs and their relation to inflammation the inference is conclusive that the inflammatory process in these cases of vertigo is due to an infecting organism. It seems entirely probable that the streptococcus is responsible for many of the conditions which produce vertigo. Streptococcus vaccine is the specific for streptococcus infections, and my experience, which now includes the successful treatment of 20 cases of aural vertigo with this vaccine, seems to conclusively show that this inference is well sustained.

A somewhat detailed report of several of these cases will be of particular interest, as the subject is barely mentioned in present-day medical literature.

Case 1. A man called at my office for treatment. He was tall, well developed, and appeared in good health, but complained of persistent attacks of vertigo. This condition was steadily growing worse, although he had been under the care of one of the best physicians in Detroit for four months. He was a foreman in a pattern-shop, and found it difficult to walk about to attend to his work. No well-defined reason for the vertigo could be found. There was no tinnitus and hearing was normal. The ear drums were also normal. On careful investigation I realized that by giving medicines probably nothing more could be accomplished than by the previous treatments. Shortly prior to that time I had treated a case of nasal catarrh with streptococcus vaccine in which a peculiar dizziness or "nervous dancing of objects" as the patient described it, was incidentally completely relieved. From this clue I decided to treat the case empirically

434   AMERICAN MEDICINE }
   Complete Series, Vol. XVIII. }   ORIGINAL ARTICLES   { AUGUST, 1912.
   { New Series, Vol. VII., No. 8.

with streptococcus vaccine, giving 30,000,-000 with each inoculation at seven-day intervals. After the second dose he was much improved. Treatment was continued for two months, and a complete cure was effected. It is now nearly five years since treatment was started, and the vertigo has not returned.

Case 2. A man working in a dynamo room of a large power plant would be seized with spells of vertigo sufficiently severe to cause him to fall to the floor. He had been treated by several physicians but was steadily growing worse. His hearing was good, but he complained of tinnitus in one ear. Four doses of streptococcus vaccine at intervals of one week effected a cure. A year later the vertigo returned. This time it required six doses to effect a cure. About fourteen months after the second attack, the vertigo returned again, when but two doses of streptococcus vaccine were required. It is now ten months since the last treatment, with no return of the vertigo.

Case 3. I was called to treat an old lady having vertigo with a vaso-motor disturbance, which caused the skin to become markedly flushed. The vertigo was persistent, whether walking or lying down, and was so severe that she could not walk across the room unaided. This condition existed for some months. I persuaded her to allow me to treat her with vaccines. When I called to give her the third dose she sat in the hall at the open door. Expressing my surprise at seeing her there I asked her how she got down stairs. She informed me that she walked down alone, and in my presence she walked up stairs to her room alone. The improvement in her vertigo was remarkable. She very much disliked hypodermic injections, but I managed to get her to take the third dose. I have since lost track of her and am unable to say how she is now.

Case 4. A young woman with previous good health had been under treatment by a physician for vertigo and other disturbances that went with it, for seven months. She had some neuralgic pain on the left side below the heart. The appetite was poor and she had lost twenty pounds in weight, weighing at the first visit to my office 108 pounds. She described the sensation as being similar to that of riding in a small boat on rough, rolling water. The vertigo improved steadily after using the streptococcus vaccine, and after taking ten doses she was entirely restored to health. Her last inoculation was given eighteen months ago, and the vertigo has not returned.

Case 5. A middle aged man employed as a wagon maker complained of vertigo of six weeks' standing with tinnitus in the right ear. The vertigo entirely subsided after the sixth inoculation of vaccine.

Case 6. A middle aged lady complained of tinnitus in the ear with vertigo and difficulty of hearing. This condition had existed for about three weeks. After three inoculations her vertigo disappeared and the hearing was materially improved.

Case 7. A man employed as chief electrician in a large power plant consulted me concerning a vertigo of five months' standing. He described his condition as "feeling about half drunk all the time." There was no apparent ailment that the condition could be ascribed to. Hearing was normal and the habits were good and regular. I gave him inoculations of streptococcus vaccine at seven-day intervals. He began to improve after the first inoculation, and was completely cured after five doses. It is now nearly three years since the last treatment, with no return of the vertigo.

Case 8. A middle aged man who had charge of the power plant in a large manufacturing plant, after a bad cold had some pain in his ears, with a fullness in the head. Hearing was somewhat impaired and vertigo was almost constant. This had been going on for four weeks. Streptococcus vaccine was employed, and four doses were given from five to seven days apart. Improvement was observed after the first inoculation, and he made a complete recovery. As one of the members of the family was sick with tuberculosis, I had occasion to see the man frequently, and he assured me that there was not the slightest return of the vertigo.

Case 9. An elderly lady complained of being almost deaf for about one week. She also was troubled with severe attacks of vertigo. Examination showed that hearing was almost entirely gone in the right ear and she could only hear loud conversation with the left. There was no pain or apparent inflammation in either ear. Streptococcus vaccine was given for the first dose, and a streptococcus-staphylococcus combined vaccine was given a week later. Two weeks after the first inoculation when the third dose of the combined vaccine was given the vertigo had left her but her hearing was not improved. I have lost track of her and do not know what the ultimate result was.

Case 10. A young woman of 29 had suffered with repeated attacks of vertigo for four months. Hearing was normal. There was some digestive disturbance and the question as to whether or not the vertigo was due to nausea was carefully considered. I found that it was not. In consideration of the digestive disturbances I gave her a combined colon bacillus and streptococcus vaccine. Six doses at weekly intervals effected an entire cure.

Case 11. This was a man 74 years old, with marked arteriosclerosis. Attacks of vertigo would come on at intervals several times a day with great severity. During these attacks he was obliged to sit down or take hold of some object, to keep from falling. His hearing was somewhat impaired, but he could hear a loud conversation quite well. His general health was run down and he had in a degree lost control of coordinating the legs while walking. Streptococcus-staphylococcus combined vaccine was given at from five to seven-day intervals. He had a single attack of vertigo after the first inoculation. I gave him altogether ten doses, with the idea of procuring the tonic effect of the vaccine. His general health improved some, but the treatment was discontinued. So far as I know the vertigo has not returned.

Case 12. An apparently well-preserved old lady complained of severe tinnitus, taking on the form of music and imaginary people talking to her. This annoyed her so that she could not secure proper sleep. Her hearing was fairly good. The vertigo was quite severe. I gave her seven doses of combined streptococcus-staphylococcus vaccine. Her vertigo soon left her after using the vaccine and the tinnitus

became some better, but is still troubling her.

Case 13. Man with vertigo of two years' standing. Tinnitus in both ears. Hearing normal. Three doses of streptococcus at weekly intervals relieved him of his vertigo, but the tinnitus was not markedly improved.

Case 14. A case of chronic non-suppurative otitis with tinnitus in both ears. Can only hear loud conversation and has been suffering with a vertigo which came on gradually for some time. The patient also had some bronchial trouble at the same time. I administered seven doses of streptococcus-staphylococcus-pneumococcus combined vaccine at about weekly intervals. The vertigo subsided soon after using the vaccine and the tinnitus and hearing improved. Two months after receiving the last dose she returned, complaining of some dizziness. I started the vaccine treatment again and the vertigo subsided after the first inoculation. The case is still under treatment.

Case 15. Chronic non-suppurative otitis in a man of sixty, with vertigo of seven years' standing. At first the vertigo was intermittent, but for the past year it has been almost constant. He reports that for some days the vertigo was so bad that he was obliged to sit in a chair all day. The hearing is such that conversation can be carried on with a moderately loud voice. The vertigo began to improve after the first inoculation of streptococcus vaccine, and after the third dose it had entirely left him. I have so far given eight doses, but treatment is still being continued with the hope of possibly improving the hearing a little more.

Case 16. Chronic non-suppurative otitis media with tinnitus and vertigo of four years' standing. During the week prior to the time he first consulted me the vertigo was especially bad. Some days he was obliged to stay at home. The hearing is fair, he can hear a watch tick two inches from the right ear and five inches from the left ear. I started treatment with streptococcus vaccine. Improvement was observed after the first dose and after the third inoculation there was no more vertigo. So far only five inoculations have been made. On account of a concomitant nasal catarrh the last two inoculations consisted of a combined streptococcus-pneumococcus-staphylococcus vaccine. He is encouraged and still under treatment.

Case 17. A case of chronic non-suppurative otitis media in a woman with vertigo of over a year's standing, and tinnitus in both ears. Cannot hear a watch tick next to the ear. Bone conduction poor. Has so far received three inoculations of combined streptococcus and staphylococcus vaccine. The vertigo has almost entirely left her, but the other conditions are about the same, and she is still under treatment.

Four other cases of vertigo were successfully treated, the details of which would not materially add to what has been said in my other cases.

Dr. Harold Payne Lawrence, of Pinconning, Mich., courteously reports the following case: "Mr. D., age 48, musician, consulted me in regard to a case of vertigo to which he had been subject for one and a half years. A number of internists had diagnosed his trouble as auto-intoxication, but the treatment was of no avail. I also diagnosed his trouble likewise, but failed to benefit him. He then told me that he suffered from a running ear several years ago, and that naturally drew my attention to the chronic affections of the middle ear. I then thought of a possible infection of the semicircular canals (for which I wish to give thanks to Dr. Emil Amberg of Detroit, who gave me several valuable hints on the subject). He was injected with the streptococcus vaccine, 60,000,000 every seven days for five weeks, and showed improvement. I was not thoroughly satisfied that the staphylococcus was not also present, so I used combined streptococcus and staphylococcus for six weeks. His trouble has entirely subsided, but he is still under treatment."

The successful treatment of vertigo with vaccine is one more illustration of the very wide scope and real therapeutic advantage of vaccine therapy. In these cases the inflammation is deep-seated, in such a position that local antiseptic treatment is practically impossible, and operative interference is always a serious procedure. By this simple process of immunizing the patient, the trouble may be reached in any part of the body, and if it should be supposed by some that the results referred to here are only temporary (in spite of the fact that years have passed in several of the cases). it is at least incontroversible that results have been secured even though the skeptic desires to call them "temporary"—the patients are pleased!

THE MODERN TREATMENT OF SYPHILIS.

BY

D. A. SINCLAIR, M. D,.

Adjunct Professor of Genito-Urinary Surgery, New York Polyclinic Medical School and Hospital; Adjunct Attending Genito-Urinary Surgeon Bellevue Hospital,

New York City.

During the past year the treatment of syphilis has undergone almost a complete change, due to the advent of salvarsan (606); and so true is this as far as my own practice is concerned, that to-day I have comparatively few syphilitics under the regular treatment of mercury and potassium iodide. Such a state of affairs is not hard to understand, when we consider the great therapeutic value of this new remedy. In my opinion this drug has established a firm and valuable place in our therapeutics in the treatment of syphilis. I have administered it to over 127 adult female and male patients and have had therefore, ample opportunity to observe its effects. This experience has led me to form opinions which, of course, may demand modification for further observation and time.

That salvarsan in the treatment of syphilis is the most powerful drug we have at the present time, needs no further testimony; the literature has and will teem with reports mostly favorable to its effects; my own experience however must add its meed of praise, to the end that the profession at large, by such additions may the sooner arrive at some definite conclusion, as to its final place in our therapeutic list. Up to the present time all of the patients who have received salvarsan at my hands, have not been put upon mercury or iodide of potash after its administration, because in the first place I do not think they are necessary, and secondly our powers of observation would be clouded, for we would then be unable to say in any given case so treated, which of the drugs were acting favorably and the result would be confusion and doubt.

What is salvarsan? What are the indications for its use? What is the dose? How given? If it should be repeated, when and how often? Does it cure syphilis? What are its benefits and what are its dangers? These in a general way are the questions which our patients may ask, and which we may ask ourselves. My belief is that we should be guarded and conservative in our promises so far as a complete cure after a single dose is concerned, for we have no positive knowledge as to the ultimate effects of this drug, nor will we have for many years to come.

Salvarsan or "606" is an arsenical compound called chemically "Dioxydiamido-arsenobenzol." It is indicated in primary, secondary and tertiary syphilis and their sequelae, especially in cases where mercury and iodide of potash are not well borne or where they fail to control the symptoms. It is said to be contra-indicated in locomotor ataxia and other parasyphilitic conditions of the central nervous system, optic atrophy, marked cachexia not due to syphilis, fetid bronchitis and marked derangement of the circulatory system. It is desirable and advisable to have a Wassermann test or one of its modifications before the administration of salvarsan; it is also desirable to have a urinary, ocular and general physical examination. This is the ideal method of procedure, which is, as a matter of fact, carried out only in exceptional cases, in which we are led to suspect something radically wrong likely to be a contra-indication. Such examinations are rarely practical in poor people who cannot afford consultations and who are averse to confiding their illness to more persons than absolutely necessary. When a patient has clinical evidence of syphilis a Wassermann examination is, it seems to me, a useless expense unless it be for the purposes of convincing a doubting individual, or for our own information and statistics. Then there are many of our old patients whom we know have syphilis for we have treated them in days gone by and remember how indifferently they followed our instructions, taking mercury or iodide of potash when they would have an outbreak and ceasing treatment when their symptoms disappeared, going on in this way for years, following what may be called a patched-up, haphazard form of treatment; again, there are patients referred by their family physician who supplies the same kind of clinical history, the doctor feeling morally certain in the light of experience that in the particular case referred his patient cannot be. free from syphilitic taint; these individuals I believe should have salvarsan whether or not they have had a blood examination. Lastly, we have to deal with a certain class of patients who have had syphilis and although they may not have had any symptoms for years, and in spite of their having taken a faithful course of mercury and iodide of potash during the first three years of their disease, and in spite of negative blood tests, they demand salvarsan and are bound to get it from some one—these patients I believe should receive it, unless there is some contra-indication as mentioned above. In regard to the Wassermann test or its modification by Noguchi, I consider it valuable but not absolutely reliable for I have had the blood of several patients who had syphilis examined by different pathologists with contradictory findings and I think the experience of other clinicians will bear me out in this statement. I rely first of all on clinical manifestations of the disease seen by myself or by some competent physician even if no signs are manifest at the time the question of giving salvarsan comes up; where there is any doubt, I resort to the Wassermann test; and when this is positive I do not hesitate to administer salvarsan; if it is negative I advise the patient of that fact and if he still insists and will not be satisfied until he has received the consoling assurance that such a procedure seems to give, I feel that it is not only justifiable, but necessary to treat him, for in my experience in medicine there are no more difficult patients to manage than conscience-stricken syphilophobes. As a therapeutic test salvarsan fills an important place in medicine.

Dose.— The average dose of salvarsan for an adult is 0.6 grammes, which amount is estimated to contain about 3 grains of organic arsenic in such a form that it does not injure the cells of the blood nor the healthy tissue if given in an alkaline or neutral medium, but attacks the *spirochete pallida*, the germ of syphilis, killing it in a short time. In selected cases I have given as much as 1.2 grammes without any deleterious effect and for aught I know even more than this may be administered. Up to the present time I have given 127 intravenous injections of salvarsan, all to adult male and female patients in varying doses as follows:

One of ....0.5 grammes
One hundred and twelve..0.6   "
One of ....0.75   "
One of 1.0
Twelve of ....1.2   "

The first infusion I gave was alkaline but in the cloudy state from the sodium hydroxide, not enough having been added to clear it up; no ill effects followed. I have given several neutral, clear infusions, and two acid infusions.

The patients treated by me with the usual data follow:

With clinical syphilis, positive Wassermann 26.

With clinical syphilis, negative Wassermann 3.

With clinical syphilis, no Wassermann 61.

Without clinical symptoms, positive Wasserman 17.

Without clinical symptoms, negative Wasserman 8.

Without clinical symptoms, no Wassermann 6.

Patients who received a second infusion 6.

I gave an intravenous infusion of 0.6 salvarsan in a case of myelogenous leukemia for Dr. H. L. Hunt at his request. The patient was cachectic and his spleen extended from his diaphragm to his pelvis filling half his abdomen laterally. He left the hospital in a few days none the worse for the treatment. I have been unable to learn his exact condition further than that Dr. Hunt informed me that he was at his home in Pennsylvania about a month later, but further news of him I have not.

I gave an intravenous infusion of 0.6 salvarsan for a patient of Dr. Packard who was suffering from epilepsy, whose Wassermann test was negative, but as the doctor thought he had improved under iodide of potassium, he was desirous of giving him the therapeutic test of salvarsan which while of no benefit did not have any untoward effect.

Administration.—The preparation of the patient before the infusion consists in cleansing the arms from the mid-humeral region to the wrists with green soap and water, followed by alcohol and ether; whoever does this preparation should be instructed not to overdo the scrubbing as the skin is delicate in this region and more harm than good is often done by over scrubbing. After cleansing the arms, a sterile bandage should be applied to keep them so. I prefer that no stronger bichloride solution be used than 1 to 10,000 for this purpose. Salvarsan should only be administered by the intravenous method, the technique of which is simple, observing the usual antiseptic and aseptic precautions ordinarily followed in all surgical operations.

The gravity apparatus is the one I use, and consists of a 300 cubic centimeter glass percolator; or glass funnel holding this amount answers the purpose admirably. To either of these is attached a rubber tube three feet long. The preparation of the salvarsan solution is as follows:

The ampule containing the salvarsan having been previously immersed in a strong antiseptic solution of bichloride of mercury 1 to 500 or carbolic acid 1 to 20 is filed at the neck and broken open; the contents are emptied into a glass graduate of a capacity of about 500 c.c.—very hot distilled water, or saline solution, freshly sterilized is added to it—about 100 c.c. this should be stirred with a glass rod until a perfect solution of the salvarsan takes place, which it quickly does if a very hot solution is used. After it is thoroughly dissolved we have a bright amber colored solution which when tested will be found to be sometimes neutral but more times acid. If it is neutral we may proceed with the infusion at once. If acid we add, drop by drop sodium hydroxide (15 per cent in strength); after we have added eight or ten drops the fluid becomes very turbid, but on the addition of about 15 more drops it becomes perfectly clear—as it was before the addition of the sodium hydroxide. If it is now tested it will be found to be alkaline. On close inspection, if the solution is found to contain any undissolved particles or foreign material, it should be filtered through filter paper or absorbent cotton or fine gauze until it is perfectly free from all extraneous matter. Into the glass percolator or funnel we pour filtered saline solution or distilled water at a temperature of 110 degrees F. in sufficient quantity to displace the air in the rubber tube, which is now clamped at the distal end. The salvarsan solution is now poured into the percolator or funnel and held by an assistant.

We should use every precaution to prevent any air being carried into the vein during the intravenous infusion. I have on several occasions, in my early cases unwittingly allowed a small bubble to be carried in with the fluid. No symptoms aside from a slight irritating cough which lasted but a minute resulted and indeed others have reported instances where quite a large volume of air entered causing a churning sensation within the heart when examined at the time, but otherwise no serious consequences ensued; nevertheless we should be cautious in this regard. The needle used for introduction into the vein should be of about number 16 gauge, sharp pointed, the angle of which should be at 35 degrees; it should have a smooth high polish as this facilitates its introduction. The patient being in the recumbent posture, his arm is held perfectly straight, resting on a high stool at the side of the table for support; a tourniquet of rubber tubing or a catheter is applied, encircling the arm four inches above the elbow and clamped in place with artery forceps. This cuts off the return circulation and brings the veins prominently into view. The most prominent vein is selected, and with a steady deliberate thrust of the needle an attempt is made to introduce it into the lumen of the vein. Occasionally we may be *unsuccessful* in the first attempt, the needle entering the skin, but between it and the vein, due to the loose connective tissue in which it lies and the facility with which blood vessels slip away from all instruments so invading the tissues of the body; the absence of a free flow of blood undeceives us when we think we have succeeded in entering truly the lumen of the vein. If then we fail to get the flow of blood, we should withdraw the needle until its point is approximately one-quarter of an inch under the tissues, when directing it against the wall of the vein, with a second thrust we endeavor to enter it. In this we are generally successful, a free flowing of blood insuring us of our premises. The position of the needle when in the vein should be such that the concavity of the pointed bevelled end should look opposite to the point of entrance. When this as accomplished, we quickly connect the coupling at the end of the rubber tube to the needle—the clamp at the distal end having been removed the saline solution or distilled water in the tube flowing meanwhile; at the same time the assistant removes the tourniquet, thus releasing the obstruction to the flow into the vein, as may be easily verified by watching the top of the fluid in the glass funnel or percolator. It is very important that the patient's arm be held perfectly quiet, and equally so that the hand of the operator holding the needle shall not be moved even to the slightest degree, otherwise the needle may become displaced. If, when the fluid is allowed to flow, we notice puffing up of the tissues, corresponding to, or about the point of the needle, it is a signal for desisting at once, as our needle undoubtedly has become displaced. Herein we see the advantage of having distilled water or saline solution in the rubber tube, because the leakage of either one into the tissues is harmless, whereas any leakage of salvarsan solution would cause more or less inconvenience, if not absolute pain amounting even to ankylosis of the joint, depending upon the amount of leakage. If then, the puffiness above referred to occurs, we should immediately clamp the rubber tube near the distal end and detach it from the needle. We may then try to re-adjust the needle in the vein with the help of tourniquet re-applied, but if we do not succeed in this second attempt, we should abandon the operation at once, so far as that particular vein is concerned and either try another vein in the same arm, or one in the other arm. If we fail after a second attempt, or if in our opinion the veins are too small, or that they are covered with much adipose tissue, which always makes an otherwise simple operation difficult, and this is especially noted in women whose veins are as a rule very much smaller than men's, we should at once proceed to the open method. For this purpose, we should always be provided beforehand with a complete infusion set which consists of the following instruments:

1 hypodermic needle and syringe; one-fifth percent cocaine solution; 1 scalpel; 2 pair thumb forceps; 1 pair of scissors; 1 grooved director; 6 artery clamps; 1 tube of No. 1 plain catgut; needle holder and needle; and a canula for intravenous infusion.

The tourniquet should be reapplied as above described and the vein selected, injecting the cocaine solution over its surface to the extent of about one inch. The skin and subcutaneous tissues are now incised and the edges of the wound picked up with thumb forceps and the vein isolated by blunt dissection. The grooved director is now pushed under the vein which brings it free into the wound directly under our eye; it is now easy to introduce the needle into the vein and complete our infusion, in this way sparing the vein, bleeding from which is controlled by stitching the wound in the skin and subcutaneous tissue and the application of a snug bandage. Again failing, two pieces of catgut are introduced underneath the vein, one at

the proximal, and one at the distal end of the exposed section of the vein. The distal end of the vein is now tied and an opening made near the middle of the exposed portion about half way through its diameter, or if the vein be large, then just enough of an opening is made to accommodate the entrance of the canula, which is introduced, having been previously adjusted to the rubber tube of the salvarsan container and the air in it displaced by a small amount of fluid. The catgut at the proximal end is now tied over the vein enclosing the canula with one knot only, the ends of the suture being left long; the fluid now will flow into the vein and when it has reached the point to where the container joins the rubber tube, the tube should be compressed with the fingers of the operator to arrest the flow, and saline solution or distilled water to the amount of a couple of ounces is poured in—the tube freed from compression and the solution allowed to flow again; this last addition of saline solution forces the salvarsan solution in the tube into the vein, with a small quantity of saline solution. When this has been accomplished the canula is withdrawn from the vein, and, at the same time, the assistant tightens the catgut ligature which enclosed the vein and canula and ties securely. It is well before closing the wound, to flush it out with hot saline solution, then, with a couple of stitches through the skin we close the incision putting a wet boric acid pad over it held in place by a snug bandage.

I generally keep patients resting for twenty-four hours in bed, but frequently in robust individuals I allow them to get up in twelve hours and occasionally in extraordinary cases, they have left for home immediately after the infusion and have suffered no harm thereby. If they insist on going home before twelve hours are over, it is better that they go at once, as whatever disagreeable symptoms are apt to follow the infusion, come on generally in about two hours.

These consist in the average case of more or less fullness in the head or headache, nausea and vomiting, with perhaps some mild abdominal discomfort and looseness of the bowels. Not infrequently they have slight chilly sensations or more rarely distinct chills. Some have complained of "peculiar sensations" as though the infused fluid were running up and down their spinal column and lower extremities. There is generally a slight fever, and almost always a sleepless night following the treatment. All of these symptoms subside within 24 hours, and frequently are entirely absent; occasionally I have seen them remain two or three days and in two cases the patients were sick for a week. In full blooded individuals while the fluid is passing into the circulation, a sudden redness and apparant bloating of the face and neck is observed, sometimes accompanied by a slight irritating cough, all of which symptoms subside in from five to ten minutes after the infusion—hence in such cases I use a smaller quantity of fluid, not more that 125 or 150 c. c. altogether.

Intramuscular injections of salvarsan 1 have no experience with as far as the giving is concerned, but have seen several patients who had been so treated elsewhere and who applied to the hospital for relief from bad local results following . this method. I refer mainly to the sloughing of the tissues at the site of the injection, which left large cavernous looking excavations, taking many months to heal, the destruction of tissue was so great. I personally believe that in nearly all, if not all, of the cases treated by intramuscular injections of salvarsan, that this necrosis of tissue takes place to a greater or less extent. Where it is not manifested externally as in the cases I have referred to, I believe that nevertheless it does occur, but that absorption takes place. I cannot understand how this could be otherwise, judging from my experience with the intravenous method in my early cases, where I accidentally got but a small amount of salvarsan into the tissues; in every one of these cases there was sloughing, and in one case a most intractable ulceration with partial ankylosis of the elbow joint remained for months. The material which I stripped from these cases consisted of what appeared to be salvarsan and broken down tissue, and they all took from several weeks to several months before resolution was completed. At this juncture we are reminded in a forceful manner, of the necessity of being very careful when giving the intravenous infusion, not to get salvarsan into the tissues, and hence the advantage of using the small amount of saline contained in the tube attached to the percolator before the salvarsan itself reaches the tissues. If we should perchance get any salvarsan into the tissues while giving the infusion, we should assiduously endeavor to strip it out as completely as possible.

I do not believe that one dose of salvarsan of 0.6 grammes cures syphilis. I have given many such doses within the last 14 or 15 months, and while I have seen but a few relapses, the majority of the patients so treated have remained up to the present time, as far as I am able to judge, free from the disease. That one intravenous infusion of 1.2 grammes of salvarsan may cure the disease I think possible, but believe that it should be repeated several times. I am aware that there is a great diversity of opinion as to the number of repetitions and the time of giving them. In the present state of my mind, I consider it advisable to give an initial dose ot 0.6 grammes and in selected cases, as high as 1.2 grammes, in either event, repeating it . within one or two weeks, this is to be reduplicated every three months for one year. We should have the blood examined every three months during the second and third year and if it is negative, and there is absence of clinical manifestations, we may consider our patient cured. This will be as far as we have ever been able to determine a cure in syphilis treated by the mercury and iodide of potash method, and beyond the moral certainty, accompanied by the repeated salvarsan treatments and negative blood examinations, and in the absence of clinical manifestations, nothing but time, and a very long time at that, will determine the ultimate effect of this very potent remedy in the treatment of syphilis. With reference to the suggestion of giving salvarsan and following it with mercury and iodide of potash, I have no opinion to offer other than it is an excellent one, but we would be no nearer judging whether our patient was cured or not than we would be by treating him with salvarsan alone, as above suggested; neither were we more convinced when we prescribed the regulation three years treatment with mercury and iodide of potash before the advent of salvarsan. We all have seen relapses in patients who took their mercury and iodide potash for three consecutive years faithfully, and from my own experience in this particular, I would, if I were the victim of

syphilis, rather rely on a thorough course of salvarsan than on mercury and potassium iodide, for I have seen such rapid and remarkable effects from a single dose administered intravenously, where the other drugs but indifferently showed improvement, that I am satisfied that a single dose of salvarsan is superior to months of treatment of mercury and iodide of potash.

The dangers in the use of salvarsan are, as far as my experience goes, limited to the local manifestations following leakage into the tissues during an intravenous infusion, and a more extensive inflammatory reaction seen in the cases above referred to following the intramuscular injection. I have seen a macular syphilide clear up in 24 hours, and a noticeable paling of a vicious tubercular syphilide in the same space of time. I have also seen the disappearance of a well defined macular syphilide accompanied by mucous patches of the lip completely disappear in four days and an initial lesion as large as a 5 cent piece reduced to the size of a match head in the same space of time. Most remarkable of all are the statements made by some of my patients who were suffering from nervous phenomena which they described as "pecular sensations" in their head and limbs, that they were much improved or altogether better within so short a time as twelve hours after the infusion. The psycological effect of the treatment might account for this in some instances, but as reported in the case of M. J. McC.—there must undoubtedly have been an actual pathological process underlying his sensations which, after the first infusion cleared up within 24 hours. Similar symptoms were likewise complained of in the case of J. J. D. and disappeared within 24 hours. The nervous phenomena coming on two or three months after an infusion of salvarsan manifested by headaches and the above mentioned "peculiar sensations" I have noted in a few of my cases, and in two of them these symptoms were present before any treatment whatever was given. I also have had one case of deafness accompanied by diplopia and paralysis of the external oblique muscle of the eye follow within 8 weeks an intravenous infusion, which cleared up completely after a second treatment. Many cases similar to these have been observed by clinicians all over the world, and the explanations offered vary. My personal opinion is, that these symptoms are due only to syphilis and not to salvarsan, because cases so affected have cleared up both under mercury and iodide of potash or a second treatment with salvarsan. Similar conditions arose too, before salvarsan was discovered, both in patients who were and were not under mercury and iodide of potash treatment. Did we then stop our drugs and blame the occurrance on them? Certainly not; but we rather increased the amount up to the tolerance of the individual. Why then should we not adopt the same line of thought in regard to salvarsan?

The conclusion that I have arrived at in explaining relapses of syphilis after salvarsan, is the same one that explains relapses after mercury and potassium iodide viz.: insufficient treatment. If a patient suffering from tertiary syphilis, for instance, should be treated with iodide of potash, we would not stop at a certain number of grains, but would increase the dose many times even as high as several hundred grains three times a day, or up to the tolerance of the particular case in hand, until the symptoms for which it was given were completely dissipated. Similarly in any other ailment, as kidney colic, severe abdominal pain, etc., where morphine was indicated, we would not stop at an eighth or a quarter of a grain, but would if necessary give one-half, three-quarters or even a grain; and so with all other drugs for no matter what symptom we were combatting, we would give the maximum dose compatible with safety. This principle of therapeutics I always follow and apply it in the giving of salvarsan; hence I believe those suffering from relapses of any kind, simply do so because they have had insufficient treatment. The fact that subsequent infusions have cleared up relapses is sufficient evidence, both as to the specific action of the drug and also to an inadequate dose having been originally administered. Therefore I believe the idea of Prof. Ehrlich of destroying all the spirilla at one blow should be carried out, and to this end, as large a dose of salvarsan as is compatible with safety should be given at once.

Case 1.—Mr. H., single, age 30. Chancre latter part of July, 1910. Secondary symptoms in September, 1910. I saw him for the first time October 31st, 1910, when he presented the following symptoms: deeply fissured tongue covered with mucous patches, and mucous patches on tonsils. Loss of flesh to a marked degree. Vigorous treatment with intramuscular injections of salicylate of mercury, and iodide of potash to the point of tolerance, with but partial success. This man was most conscientious and faithful to his treatment, but in spite of all, his lesions persisted. On Jan. 26th, 1911, I gave him my first intravenous infusion of 0.6 of salvarsan. I gave it alkaline, but in a turbid state due to insufficient sodium hydroxide being added to clear it up. He stood the treatment well and within four days the mucous patches were markedly changed for the better and disappeared entirely within a week. I saw him a month later and he looked and felt perfectly well and promised to return if the slightest symptom returned but up to the present time I have not heard from him.

Case 2.—Miss F. S., age 25. Contracted syphilis in February, 1910. Received ten injections of some mercurial preparation, was salivated, and after recovering from the latter, was put on internal medication consisting of pills and liquid medicine which she had been taking up to the time I saw her in February, 1911, one year after the onset of the disease. At that time she has a papulo-squamous syphilide of the nose, chin, arms and palm of the hand. I assisted her doctor in giving her an an infusion of 0.5 gm. in the right median basilic vein. There was considerable leakage of the salvarsan into the tissues, resulting in a very severe inflammation lasting for nearly three months, leaving an ankylosed elbow joint, which I subsequently forcibly broke up. The lesions quickly disappeared from the nose, chin, arms and the palm of the hand within I should say ten days. On June 10, 1911, her blood was negative to the Noguchi-Wassermann test and there were no clinical evidences of syphilis.

Case 3.—Mrs. U., age 29. Chancre on the posterior lip of the os uteri in December, 1902. Secondary maculo-papular syphilide January 31st, 1903. Treatment by the writer consisted of intramuscular injections of mercury salicylate in 1½ grain doses during the next succeeding three years, besides the internal administration of potassium iodide in ten grain doses three times a day during the third year. No symptoms appeared after the first six months' treatment until January, 1911. She then noticed swellings on the gluteal regions, upper part of the back, chest and head, which later broke down, leaving deep excavations into which one might easily place one's finger, and which gave vent to a foul smelling discharge. There were no m.m. symptoms. This young woman had been a heavy drinker of late years, but during the five or six years after her infection she was quite moderate in this respect. Here then is a case in which an approved course of treatment had been given and followed, remaining free for years of any syphilitic symptoms and yet presented a very severe tertiary relapse. On February 12th, 1911,

I gave her an intravenous infusion of salvarsan 0.6 gm. and repeated the infusion one week later. I saw this woman one month after the second treatment and was gratified to see that all the lesions had filled in and at that time had only a dry scab on them. Since that time I have not seen or heard from her.

Case 4.—(referred by Dr. J. T. Meehan). Mr. E. K. Initial lesion 1895. No treatment until the fall of the same year when he went to the Marine Hospital in New York complaining of a sore throat, which was treated there for a month before it got well; he took no medicine whatever until three years later, when being then at the Panama Canal he was taken sick with malarial fever. He was placed in the hospital and says he was given iodide of potash, at the same time noticing spots on his legs, penis and right arm, which the doctors there told him was syphilis. He took with more or less regularity the K. I. getting up as high as 75 grains a day, continuing it up to the time I saw him which was February 14th, 1911. At that time he was suffering from a large crustaceous rupial syphilide on the left arm, covering the lower two-thirds of the post-humeral region, the crust on which was half an inch thick. He was suffering considerable pain and his arm was practically out of commission. On February 14th I gave his 0.6 gm. salvarsan intravenously. The pain in his arm disappeared in 48 hours and the crust was completely gone in two weeks. August 23rd, 1911, six months later, I administered 0.6 gm. salvarsan intravenously, although the patient was in perfect health and his blood was negative; he had gained six pounds since his first treatment. Incidentally he told me that ever since his trip to Panama that his malarial fever never left him. He suffered from what he called a "dopy" feeling which left him after the first infusion.

Case 5.—Mrs. J. H. R., age 26. Referred to me April 1st, 1911. History: Syphilis beginning nine years ago. Had sore mouth, headaches and hair came out. Spots on body. Took mercury tablets for one year; when symptoms disappearing, she stopped treatment. Two years later, sores around the knees and calves of the legs appeared. She then took iodide of potash for six months—symptoms disappearing. No treatment thereafter until a year ago, when her nose became sore and she consulted her family physician, who operated on her nose and who also prescribed iodide of potash, which she took off and on ever since. The only symptom now, is that her nose clogs up and gets sore if she stops the iodide of potash. Examination showed a papulo-squamous syphilide of the right ala of nose. Noguchi-Wassermann test positive. Intravenous infusion of 0.6 gm. salvarsan. One week later soreness had completely disappeared from her nose and the lesion was barely visible. Patient felt very much better. Ten days after the infusion, patient was covered over the entire surface of her body with a measly eruption. This eruption came on very suddenly, and I think was due to the salvarsan. Catharsis was prescribed and the rash completely disappeared in a few days. On July 28th, I saw the patient and there was absolutely no sign of syphilis present.

Case 6.—Mr. F. Z., age 24. Single. Chancre. July, 1910, incubation of which he says was one month. Secondaries in July, appearing on chest. Treatment by mercurial injections of which he received five in all. Internal medication was taken faithfully until Feb. 8th, 1911, at which time he presented the following symptoms: Large deeply excavated mucous patches over the entire surface of the tongue; papulo-squamous-circinate syphilide the size of 25 cent pieces on neck at hair line; papulo-squamous syphilide of the right external ear, also at the bend of the elbow and covering the entire glans penis. Intravenous infusion of 0.6 gm. in 600 c.c. of hot saline solution. Noguchi-Wassermann test was positive before infusion was given. Within two weeks the patient was free from all the above mentioned lesions, only staining of the skin remaining.

Case 7.—Mr. J. D., age 26, married. On May 11th, 1911, I gave him an intravenous infusion of 1.2 gm. salvarsan. This man I was unable to get any history from, he throwing a mysterious air about the origin of his malady. Clinically he presented a very active and virulent form of syphilis. His entire body, from head to foot was covered with a large tubercular syphilide, and so large were they, that they actually were deforming to his face. Mucous patches present on tongue. He also complained of quite severe pain in his right leg over the tibia, which impaired its function. His wife, whom I examined was free from any signs of the disease, as was his infant child which was not his own, being adopted. He stood the large dose of salvarsan well, and the next day told me the pain in his leg had entirely disappeared and that he could use it freely: there was a noticeable paling of the tubercles on his face which was remarked by his wife and his physician, Dr. Palmer of the police department. I have not seen him since, but he wrote me a letter one month later expressing his gratitude and telling me his spots had disappeared but the stains still remained. The disappearance of the pain in his leg I wish especially to call attention to, as a similar condition was noted in the case I will next recite.

Case 8.—Mr. M. J. McC., age 30, single. Referred by Dr. M. C. O'Brien. Intravenous infusion of 0.6 gm. salvarsan July 5th, 1911. On examination the patient presented the following symptoms. Initial lesion on the mucous layer of foreskin, dorsal aspect; secondary maculo-papular syphilide covering the abdomen, back and legs. He complained of a "peculiar, annoying sensation" over his right temporal region and over his tibia in the right leg. The next day after the infusion he left the hospital saying that he was free from the sensations in his head and leg. His physician reported a marked blanching of the eruption was noticeable on the third day and an entire disappearance of the rash in one week with complete healing of the initial lesion in the same space of time. On August 30th, 1911, a little more than seven weeks after this treatment the patient came to my office (his physician being out of town) and presented the following symptoms: Deafness in his left ear; can only hear a watch tick two inches away; headache; itching of the skin of the right side of the face over the temporal region. I prescribed catharsis together with phenacetin and quinine. The next day he reported that his headache was better, but that his ear continued to buzz and that his head felt as though it was swelled up. I referred him to an aurist, who later told me that he thought his deafness was due to syphilis. This aurist, after watching him for several days sent him to an oculist on account of the development of some eye trouble. I had a consultation with the oculist, who referred the patient back to me, and he told me he believed his eye trouble was due to syphilis. The patient was at this time suffering from complete deafness in the left ear, paralysis of the external rectus muscle of the right eye, diplopia or double vision, fullness in the head, and walked with a wabbly gait with the aid of a cane. Indeed, this man was as sorry and as miserable a spectacle as I have ever seen from this disease, so early in its course. The question of what was best to do for this unfortunate was at issue. I inquired of both the aurist and the oculist if, in their opinion his condition might be due to salvarsan, but they expressed their inability to decide such a momentous question. They both had seen exactly the same train of symptoms in patients suffering from syphilis who had and who had not been under mercury and iodide of potash treatment before the advent of salvarsan.

The patient who is an intelligent man begged me to do with him as I pleased, he being willing to share the responsibility for any consequences which might follow my course of action, for I had explained the situation to him in a thorough manner, and had ventured my own opinion that his trouble was due to syphilis and not to salvarsan, as he had complained of threatening nervous symptoms before the first infusion and found almost immediate relief after its administration. Also that it was too long after the treatment for him to suffer from it, as in my opinion any untoward effect would have shown itself within a few days or a week. We decided to repeat the infusion and to give a sufficient amount compatible with safety. I accordingly sent him to the hospital and on September 8th, 1911, I gave him an intravenous infusion of 1.2 gm. of salvarsan. He remained in the hospital one week and was quite sick from the treatment, vomiting and in general very much upset for two days; his bowels moved five times within the first four hours; there was no abdominal pain. He said he had a feeling as though the fluid infused was running up and down his spinal column. He visited me on September 19th, eleven days after the infusion and was greatly improved; his headache and fullness in the head was gone, but there was still a slight soreness in the temporal region; external rectus muscle of the right eye appeared normal; sight was no longer double, but vision still a trifle hazy; could hear a watch tick 6 inches away from his left ear, appetite good, bowels regular; no dizziness when he walked. I next saw him on October 14th, 36 days after the infusion. He felt and looked well. The oculist had recently examined his eyes and pronounced them normal. His ear as far as he could himself judge was normal; hears excellently over the telephone which he could not do before the infusion. He still feels a "peculiar" sensation over the right temporal region, similar to what he felt before the beginning of the salvarsan treatment, but very slight and at times not at all. He was anxious to get more salvarsan treatment, but his physician thought it best to wait a while.

REFLEX PAIN IN OCULAR CONDITIONS.[1]

BY

SAMUEL HORTON BROWN, M. D.,
Philadelphia.

It is very difficult at times to differentiate in many cases between the so-called "reflex" and "direct" pains encountered in the body, and this doubtless is due to the vague conception entertained by all of us as to the vital force, or molecular energy, or what not, that transfers a stimulus to the centers and returns an impulse expressed as motion, sensation, special sense, etc. It is customary to regard pain experienced directly in or very near the disturbed structure as "direct" while that at a distance, provided some other association

[1]Read before the Mt. Sinai Hospital Clinical Society, May 21, 1912.

with another affected part is not proved, is regarded as "reflex" pain. This appears to simplify matters very much but if anatomic and physiologic knowledge is allowed to enter into consideration the so-called "reflex" pains will be found to be direct or at least "referred" in most cases. Clinically, the practice is to regard pains, the exact cause of which is in doubt as of the nature of "reflex" pains.

The relation between ophthalmology and these "reflex" pains is very important, since the eyes are in active use the entire working day. The finely balanced mechanism which fuses the two images seen by the eyes into one knows no rest from the time the subject arises in the morning until he goes to sleep at night. Not only is this delicately arranged mechanism constantly in action but there is also the function of accommodation as exercised by the ciliary muscle, constantly changing the focus of the eye for all kinds of ranges. It can be readily appreciated that even in the presence of perfect health these mechanisms are subjected to considerable strain and it is a great wonder that the centers governing them are not the subject of fatigue. But we seldom encounter any evidence of such condition when the eyes are normal as regards refraction and muscle-balance, and when the patient is not possessed of the so-called "neurotic temperament."

This brings into consideration the ocular troubles that may produce pain either direct or reflex. The great bulk of painful conditions that may be attributed to the eyes may be said to be due to eyestrain. These are so great in number and so various in character that practice advocates examining the eyes of patients so affected and prescribing glasses, no matter how weak the necessary correction may be. It is assumed that these patients are so responsive to the most ordinary stimuli, that therefore they should not be allowed to exercise the ocular functions the slightest beyond what is absolutely normal. This it may be readily seen is similar to the rest cure of S. Weir Mitchell for the treatment of neurasthenia and allied disorders, and, indeed, it is the principle enunciated by him in the early seventies when he definitely determined a relationship between headache and eyestrain. Previous to 1872, and for a long time afterward, glasses were prescribed only when vision was defective. S. Weir Mitchell showed that the formula necessary to produce these head pains were a disturbance of the refraction or muscle balance of the eyes, plus an overworked, fatigued physical condition or a frail delicate, worn-out nervous system. This is confirmed daily by observing robust healthy persons who are able to overcome quite considerable defects in their eyes without experiencing the slightest discomfort.

The subject of errors of refraction in reference to "reflex" and "direct" pain is one that has been greatly overworked for the purpose of essays but there are a few facts connected with the same that warrant repetition. To begin with, there are three principal optical defects, hyperopia, myopia, and astigmatism, which may exist singly or in several forms of combination. Simple hyperopia, unaccompanied by other optical defects, or accommodative or muscular trouble is never attended by the ordinary symptoms of eyestrain. It is the condition present at birth, and is also seen in steple-jacks and others similarly employed. Simple myopia, unaccompanied by astigmatism or muscular or accommodative disturbances is never associated with painful or distressing symptoms such as we are disposed to recognize as those of eyestrain. The bad effects of the prolonged close work of the myope with a simple defect are expended upon the eye itself, and while it may terminate in disease of the choroid, posterior staphyloma, or detachment of the retina, the condition will be painless. Astigmatism, simple, compound, or mixed, symmetrical or unsymmetrical, with or against the rule, is the pain producer. The ciliary muscle is called upon to contract unevenly to change the curvature of the lens to compensate for the curvature of the cornea. This it fails to do but the repeated efforts force it into a condition of spasm which is followed by congestion of all parts of the eye where there are blood-vessels. This causes more or less pain and tenderness within the globe itself.

The central nervous system seems to appreciate this deficiency of the ciliary muscle and attempts to make up this by increased activity in the extraocular muscles. Accommodation and convergence being closely allied, this is readily understood and often there is spasm of convergence. Various ocular phenomena may be observed during the evolution of this condition, but attention is usually first called to the condition by the complaint on the part of the patient of headache. According to the enthusiasm of the particular observer, from 50 to 90 percent of headaches come from this cause. Certain it is that a very large proportion of the cases of headache or rather pains in the head are due to this cause. They may be frontal or temporal, either side or both, but they are seldom occipital, parietal, or nuchal. Now if we recall that the fifth nerve is the sensory nerve of the eye, and that it is the sensory nerve of a large part of the face and front

of the head through the plexuses and ramifying nerves with which it is connected, we readily appreciate that these ocular head pains are being experienced over the distribution of the fifth nerve and in a sense are "direct" pains.

The close association of the mechanism of the pupil with the sympathetic system doubtless aids in the explanation of those cases of nausea, vomiting, and gastric pain that accompany eyestrain especially when the eyestrain occurs in the presence of unequal errors of refraction or imbalance of the extraocular muscles. In practice, the subjects of this condition are those who complain of an inability to look at moving pictures, or to gaze upon a parade, or to look at the crowds such as seen in a large store. Whether this is the reason why many men refrain from attendance upon church or reform political meetings is a question for discussion.

Turning from the painful possibilities incidental to ametropia, accommodative errors, and muscle-imbalance to the surgical condition of the eye in which plain, localized or disseminated, is observed we find many features of interest.

Here we must pause for a few moments while we refresh in our minds the orgin and distribution of the fifth cranial nerve. We find that (quoted from Morris's Anatomy) "the sensory root of the trigeminus may be traced through the Gasserian ganglion into the cerebellum and into the terminal nucleus of the pons. After leaving the semilunar (Gasserian) ganglion, in pursuing its course toward central structures, it gives off T-shaped fibers which divide into peripheral and central branches. The central branches divide into ascending and descending branches on entering the brain-stem and find their nuclei of termination in a dorsolateral column of gray substance which consists of the upward continuation of the gelatinous substance of Rolando of the spinal cord. Opposite the entrance of the nerve the column becomes somewhat thickened, constituting the sensory nucleus of the trigeminus, the part below being known as the nucleus of the spinal cord. The branches of the entering fibers bifurcate and terminate about the cells of these nuclei. The descending branches are longer and passing downward, form the spinal tract of the trigeminus, which may at times be traced as far as the second cervical segment of the spinal cord. The ascending branches are short and terminate, as a rule, in the sensory nuclei."

"The axones from the nucleus of termination are distributed to the nuclei of its motor portion of the same and opposite sides; to the nuclei of the motor cranial nerves, and to the thalamus of the same, and chiefly the opposite side. The sensory nuclei are connected with the somesthetic area of the cortex by the fibers of the medial lemniscus (fillet) and with the motor nuclei of the other cranial nerves by the medial lemniscus."

While the motor root of the fifth nerve is not directly connected with any ocular functions, it may be well to trace its origin in order to show the close association with the nuclei of other cranial nerves.

"The nucleus of origin of the motor root of the trigeminus is composed of two portions. The principal nucleus lies on the dorsomedial side of the sensory nucleus. It gives rise to the greater part of the motor root and its fibers are distributed to the muscles of mastication. Above the principal nucleus and along the line of the locus coeruleus extends the nucleus of the mesencephalic (descending) root. The cells of this nucleus are thinly scattered as high up as the posterior commissure of the cerebrum and the mesencephalic root arising from them gradually increases as it passes through the encephalon to the superior level of the pons, where it joins the fibers arising in the principal nucleus. The distribution of the fibers of the mesencephalic root is not clearly settled. The motor nuclei of the fifth nerve are connected with the lower part of the somesthetic area of the cerebral cortex of the opposite side by the geniculate bundle of pyramidal fibers, and they are associated with the sensory nuclei of other cranial nerves by the medial longitudinal fasciculus."

From the foregoing it will be readily appreciated how closely related are the central portions of this nerve with the central portions of other cranial nerves, sensory as well as motor, and it is scarcely conceivable, in view of this, that they do not have common functions at least.

So much for the detail of the central distribution of the nerve. As we all know, the peripheral distribution is through three large branches, the ophthalmic, the maxillary, and the mandibular. The ophthalmic is exclusively sensory, and before it divides into frontal, lachrymal and nasociliary (nasal) nerves, it receives communicating filaments from the cavernous plexus of the sympathetic and likewise communicates by three branches with the third, fourth, and sixth nerves. This affords a structural explanation of some of the peculiar associated extraocular muscle-palsies and other muscle phenomena, such as twitching of the lids, blepharospasm, etc. Later in its course, through the medium of its nasociliary (ganglion) branch it communicates with the third (oculo-motor) nerve and filaments from the cavernous plexus of the sympathetic. The long ciliary nerves are branches of the nasociliary (nasal) branch, while the short ciliary nerves are derived from the ciliary ganglion, which receives its sensory root from the nasociliary (nasal) nerve. Thus it will be seen that sensory impulses except those directly referable to the sense of sight are carried by the fifth nerve, most by the ophthalmic, a few by the maxillary branch. Ocular pain is made possible only through the fifth nerve. The other nerves arising from the fifth nerve are distributed to certain of the muscles of mastication and to the teeth. Through the superficial communication with the facial nerves, pain arising from diseased conditions of the face may be referred to the eye and vice versa.

Having assumed an important relationship between the fifth nerve and the eyes, especially as regards the production of referred pain, and having proved it, to our own satisfaction, at least, from an anatomical standpoint we turn to the clinical conditions that appear to confirm these findings. Beginning with the skin of the eyelids, the most common painful condition encountered is Herpes Zoster Ophthalmicus, or shingles along the distribution of the fifth nerve. This is a most painful condition and the pain is not only in the eye but diffused over the face and brow and temple. In this condition the disease originates, perhaps, in the nerve but in glaucoma in which the underlying disease is in the eye the pain has the same character and distribution. In cases in which the Gasserian ganglion is removed for obstinate trifacial neuralgia we may see the eye affected with all kinds of inflammatory and other disturbances without the slightest pain resulting.

Leprosy in which there are anesthetic areas on the face and brow due to cellular deposits about and within the nerves, is seldom if ever attended with symptoms that would call attention to the eyes. Objectively, the examiner will determine corneal ulcers and other affections but there will be few if any subjective signs.

While these may be regarded as direct conditions there are several well-recognized forms of reflex trouble the origin of which lies in the ocular structures. For instance, Markus (Ophthalmoscope, January 1907) reported a case in which there was tonic contraction of the right frontalis, resulting in a continuous elevation of the right eyebrow. This was not compensatory as is seen in ptosis. There was twitching of the left supercilii and the right pupil was slightly larger than the left. The patient was more or less hysteric and was also the subject of almost continuous leftsided headache.

Tonic cramp of the orbicularis (blepharospasm) due to the irritation of foreign bodies in and inflammation of the conjunctiva or cornea is by no means uncommon and owes its production to irritation of the terminal filaments of the fifth nerve. Not only does this reflex action find its expression in this tonic spasm, but pain, photophobia, lachrymation, and redness in the anterior ocular structures may be attributed to it. Conjunctivitis ordinarily is not attended with dilatation but occasionally when the swelling is great and attended with pain the pupil will dilate as the result of reflex influence. In the conditions known as snow-blindness, conjunctival asthenopia, retinal hyperesthesia, etc., the distress produced will be manifested over the nerve distribution.

Conjunctivitis has been attributed to teeth disorders by Förster, Kempton, and others in certain cases and relieved by the extraction of the offending teeth. While most of this apparent relation is speculative, and has decreased with the evolution of the knowledge concerning eyestrain, it is possible to point to a tangible connection between painful conditions of the trigeminus and many forms of corneal ulceration. Indolent ulcers, dendritic ulcers, ulceration associated with carious teeth, neuroparalytic ulcers, etc., are acknowledged to be dependent upon the disturbance of the trophic influence of the fifth nerve. While most of these examples illustrate an influence on the eyes from disturbances elsewhere along the course of the fifth nerve, we have an example of the reverse condition of affairs in the case reported by Stevens in 1877 in which a case of obstinate toothache was relieved by the correction of astigmatism by the wearing of the appropriate cylindrical lenses.

In connection with affections of the iris, it may be assumed that the pain is directly due to involvement of the fifth nerve, since it is the sensory nerve of that structure. The possibility of the fifth nerve being the intermediate factor in those cases of mumps attended with iritis is worth investigating. True iritis has been shown to have produced neuralgia directly referable to the teeth by Galezowsky and others. Cyclitis secondary to dental disease has been observed by Juler. The pain and distress in sympathetic ophthalmia is often referred over the distribution of the fifth nerve through the disturbance of the ciliary nerves.

Glaucoma is an example of pain referred to parts unaffected by the underlying disease and the symptoms may be attributed to the influence of the fifth nerve. The trophic disturbance is manifested by the anesthesia of the cornea, and by the changes in the optic nerve, but the predominating symptom the intense pain and neuralgia represents the sensory disturbance of the fifth nerve.

After reviewing the many painful conditions that are associated with ocular conditions we come to the conclusion that reflex pains may be the cause or the result of ocular conditions, and that this probability becomes increased the closer the association of the symptoms with the distribution of the fifth nerve.

1901 Mt. Vernon St.

BRONCHIAL ASTHMA IN CHILDREN.

BY

C. K. JOHNSON, M. D.,

Instructor in Pediatrics, University of Vermont, Burlington, Vt.

Bronchial asthma is a condition characterized by recurrent attacks of bronchial spasm, the intensity and duration of the spasm varying widely in different cases.

Kerley divides his cases into two classes:

1. Those cases in which the paroxysms are produced by direct irritation, as by the pollen of plants, or the odor of flowers or animals, these producing the condition known as "hay fever" with the accompanying bronchial spasm.

2. Cases presenting the "lithemic diathesis" i. e., a rheumatic or gouty condition.

He believes the majority belong to the second class. This disease is comparatively rare in early life. Salter reports 225 cases, 11 of which occurred during the first year and 60 occurred between the first and tenth year.

Enlarged bronchial glands may act mechanically as an exciting cause. Again, many cases are accompanied with bronchitis and this is often the immediate cause of bronchial spasm. Personally, I am inclined to endorse Kerley's view, that many cases of so-called recurrent bronchitis may be due to a lithemic diathesis and should be treated with this fact in view.

A. Sachs[1], noting that anaphylaxis in guinea pigs bears a striking relation to an asthmatic attack in man, advances the view that attacks of hay fever brought on by the odor of animals, rag weed, pollen may sometimes be due to an anaphylactic reaction. The symptoms of bronchial asthma do not differ greatly from the adult type except catarrhal symptoms are more common.

Diagnosis.—A word regarding the diagnosis of this condition.

In any given case it may be difficult to decide the class to which the patient belongs, as for instance adenoids may be present in the lithemic type as an accessory cause. If we bear in mind that few well marked cases of hay fever have been reported before the 10th year, this may be of assistance.

Blood. The blood will give us aid in diagnosis and in defining the line of treatment that should be followed.

Von Noorden[2] in 1892 reported a case in which while the eosinophiles were 5% when free from symptoms, after repeated attacks they were 33⅓%.

Billings[3] reported a case with 53% of eosinophiles.

In encountering this condition we should bear in mind other known causes than bronchial asthma. Eosinophilia is present in patients harboring parasites such as trichinae spiralis, in scarlet fever, in many skin diseases especially of the chronic type, such a psoriasis and the like, also in leukemia.

Hanna Hirschfeld[4] after examining the blood of children afflicted with the various forms of tuberculosis with the view of learning the relation of the white blood cells found that the cases with a favorable prognosis often showed a lymphocytosis and in some cases as eosinophilia.

Herrick[5] reports a case of bronchial asthma (adult) in which the eosinophiles reached 77% after repeated attacks.

Sputum. Muller in 1899 described an increase of eosinophile cells in the sputum of patients with bronchial asthma.

Treatment.—The treatment of bronchial asthma as laid down in text books is rather vague and indefinite. The following case is reported to outline a systematic and successful method of treatment.

Male 5 years. This boy's mother is said to have had attacks when small which in all probability were asthmatic. One uncle and two aunts have always had asthma and rheumatism. The father is in good health. This boy was apparently in good health until 22 months old when he had an attack of what was diagnosed as bronchitis. He apparently completely recovered from this but within a few months had a second attack during which he had much difficulty in breathing for several days. From this time until I saw him Nov. 1911, he had been having these attacks of bronchitis with bronchial spasms at intervals varying from two to eight weeks summer or winter. When first seen he was sitting propped up in a chair, breathing labored, a short harsh cough, slight cyanosis, temperature 100 3/10 F, pulse 130, respiration 38. Auscultation revealed noisy, labored breathing with sibilant and sonorous rales over whole chest. Calomel was given to clear the intestinal tract and sodium bromide and antipyrin for the spasm which nearly disappeared in 48 hours. He was now given aspirin 5 grains three times a day. Meats were restricted to twice a week, and sugar reduced to minimum. Twelve days later he had another attack of equal severity. At this time he was given adrenalin chloride 1-1000 solution 7 minims subcutaneously; this afforded marked relief and within a few minutes he said he breathed easier. The diet was continued as before, aspirin being given for ten days alternating with ten days of sodium bicarbonate 15 grains three times a day. The blood during the first attack showed the following:

Polynuclears 47.
Small lymphocytes 20.
Large lymphocytes 17.
Eosinophiles 16.

The eosinophiles during the second attack were 16 percent and in the interval 11 percent. The sputum was not examined. This treatment has been continued to date, June, 1912, with short intervals without drugs, no other paroxysms having occurred except one very slight attack which required no treatment.

Some text books advise the restriction of carbohydrates in this condition and recommend potassium iodide for long periods, this drug being considered especially efficacious in the lithemic type.

Herrick states that potassium iodide is most valuable in cases showing a marked eosinophilia.

Leman strongly recommends the iodides in all types of bronchial asthma.

Kerley treats the attacks with antipyrin and sodium bromide and in the intervals reduces the food in infants to ½ the amount suitable to the age, and gives one grain sodium bicarbonate to each ounce of milk food given. Proper bowel action is carefully maintained, since intestinal toxemia is considered an important causative factor. In older children he follows the same line of treatment as for rheumatism, chorea and recurrent bronchitis; sugars and red meats being restricted, high proteid cereals and vegetables being allowed freely. His medical treatment consists of sodium salicylate or aspirin alternately with sodium bicarbonate, this interrupted medication being continued for months.

It is well known that potassium iodide has pronounced value in rheumatic conditions, therefore, when we treat these cases of bronchial asthma with the iodides are we not in reality removing the underlying lithemic condition, the result being the same as when aspirin or soda are given?

REFERENCES.

I.   A. SACHS. Bronchial Asthma. Western Medical Review.

II. VON NOORDEN. Beitrage Zue Pathologie des asthma bronchiale. Ztschr. f. klin. Med., 1892.

III. BILLINGS. Marked Excess of Eosinophiles in the Blood. New York Medical Journal, May 22, 1897.

IV. HIRSCHFIELD, H. The White Blood Cells in Tuberculosis of Children. Monatschr, f. Kinderh, 1911, No. 10, p. 38.

V.   W. W. HERRICK. The Eosinophilia of Bronchial Asthma. Journal A. M. A., Dec. 2, 1911.

VI. HOLT. Diseases of Children.

VII. KERLEY. Treatment of Diseases of Children.

VIII. OSLER. Practice.

IX. HARE'S Therapeutics.

X.   TODD'S Clinical Diagnosis.

There is a stage in the development of every uterus when anteflexion is normal. If for any reason it is arrested or retarded at this stage, the anteflexion remains and becomes a pathological condition. Malnutrition, excessive mental activity or any infectious disease, shortly before or at puberty, frequently results in this arrested development.—*Int. Jour. of Surg.*

The very essence of a free government consists in considering offices as public trusts, bestowed for the good of the country, and not for the benefit of an individual or a party.—*John C. Calhoun.*

We are not skeptics, but know something. We are not on bypaths, but on the highway of humanity. We are in league with what will be holy and strong in the future.—*W. M. Salter.*

THE ANNOTATOR.

Preventive Medicine, Present Achievement and Future Field of Activity.[1]—

Bergey mentions some of the more important means employed in preventive medicine, isolation, disinfection, immunity, sera, vaccines, chemotherapeutic agents and the chemical, physical and biological agents used in the purification of water, sewage, and milk.

Isolation is often ineffectual owing to neglect or other fault on the part of doctor or nurse. Disinfection is often ineffectual because improper materials are used or efficient materials in too great dilution or for insufficient duration.

The prophylactic value of diphtheria and tetanus antitoxine is almost beyond question. The value of vaccine virus in preventing smallpox and the value of vaccine in controlling typhoid fever, cholera, plague and dysentery cannot be computed. The chemotherapeutic agents, quinine in malaria and salvarsan in syphilis, have proven inestimable in limiting disease and preventing death, and the laboratories teach us to hope that other great discoveries are imminent. The filtration of water and sewage and the pasteurization of milk have not only reduced the morbidity and mortality rates of the gastro-intestinal diseases but have also had an important influence in reducing the general mortality in many communities.

Diseases which are not yet under satisfactory control are scarlet fever, measles, pneumonia and tuberculosis but the proper application of preventive measures will sooner or later bring them under control.

Certainly no department of medicine has had a more brilliant record during the past few years than preventive medicine but we believe that record will pale into insignificance before that which will come during the next twenty five years, when the great workshops for the investigation of disease shall have perfected their methods of operation.

[1] D. N. Bergey, M. D., *New York Medical Journal*, April 13, 1912.

Infant Feeding With Undiluted Cow's Milk.[1]—

Handbridge tells us this subject has occupied his attention many years. He found that certain infants whom he had been called to see had been fed upon whole milk and had apparently thriven under it. By degrees he was led to investigate the matter practically and in his paper he reports thirty-five cases thus nourished with entirely good results.

He feels sure that the statements, oft repeated, that infants cannot digest unmodified milk is not true.

His observations convinced him that an average infant would be sufficiently nourished on one and three-quarters to two and a quarter ounces of undiluted cow's milk per pound weight in twenty-four hours.

The chief advantage in whole milk seemed to be that its abundant nitrogen must count for good development of the muscular system in infants thus nourished.

He concludes that if whole milk was good for the thirty-five sick babies thus nourished it must also be good for well babies with good digestive powers.

Feeding an infant only when hungry on this concentrated food seems to him a natural and rational procedure.

He begins with a small quantity, increases a little with each feeding, adding sugar, cream or lime water if circumstances demand it.

Many babies have survived and even thriven on a diet of whole milk, or even substances less well-adapted for an infant's stomach. Doubtless a great many more have succumbed under such nourishment, so the argument of the writer doesn't prove much except for the cases which came under his observation. He also fails to tell us whether he used the milk at body temperature or lower and whether the milk used was rich in fat or otherwise. To reduce the question of infant feeding to absolute simplicity has thus far been unattainable.

Milk, Typhoid Fever and Responsibility.[2]—

An editorial of exceptional

[1] W. B. Handbridge, M. D., *New York State Journal of Medicine*, April.

[2] *Medical Review of Reviews*, April, 1912.

force and logic notes that when municipalities receive milk that is forty to eighty hours old many difficulties are likely to arise which demand careful legislation in order to protect the public from infection or contagion from such a source.

Health departments now recognize their obligations to inspect carefully the farms from which milk is derived and to see that it is not contaminated from any source.

In 1909 an epidemic of typhoid fever in New York was traced to the milk supplied by one typhoid carrier and the Health Department was quite warranted in shutting off this particular supply from the city market.

If this had not been done, negligence could properly have been attributed to the Health Department and the heirs of those who had died from typhoid fever from this source would properly have held the city actionable in damages for criminal negligence.

Rochester has warned the people, on two occasions to boil the water supplied by the city in order to lessen the danger from infection, when the water supply was known to be contaminated.

Thus it becomes evident that people have the right to look to the municipal health authorities for information in regard to the healthfulness of these two most indispensable articles of daily consumption.

If a city is responsible for an unsafe sidewalk how much more should it be for the healthfulness of its food supply and a few suits for damages on account of neglect in this particular would soon show the importance of preventive health work in dollars and cents where now they fail to appreciate its importance in terms of human life.

These are facts which demand wide circulation, especially among physicians and the more alert they become to detect such sources of mischief in the community the more careful will boards of health become also, in safeguarding the public for which they are in large measure responsible.

Inoculation Against Plague at Nagpur.[1] —An editorial says the following conclusions were reached.

[1] *Therapeutic Gazette*, April 15, 1912.

1. Inoculation markedly reduces the occurrence of plague.

2. It also reduces the mortality.

3. It is quite harmless.

4. It is harmless even when the patient is in the incubation stage of the disease.

5. The temperature reaction is usually mild.

6. It has no bad after effects.

7. An attack of plague in an inoculated person is usually mild.

Inoculation is especially valuable for crowded towns and for those who live in dirty and crowded quarters. No preventive measure is so cheap and so effective.

The French Commission on Anti-Typhoid Vaccination.[1]— The report of this commission of the French Academy of Medicine is summarized as follows:

1. This method of procedure has been carried out on more than 100,000 soldiers in the English, German and American Armies.

2. The benefits of preventive inoculation are seen in the comparative statistics of typhoid mortality and morbidity. Only half as many of the vaccinated have had typhoid fever, as of the non-vaccinated.

3. Vaccination does not abolish typhoid fever, it diminishes its frequency, and the vaccinated who get the fever have it in a mild form.

4. Two or three inoculations with bacillary vaccine are better than one, and four will be necessary with antilysates of living bacteria.

5. Immunity lasts from one to four years, and hence revaccination is desirable.

6. Anti-typhoid vaccination is not dangerous. Dead bacilli when injected will cause fever and pain from twenty-four to forty-eight hours. An antigen of living bacilli will cause little or no pain.

7. Preventive vaccination should usually be performed before the appearance of the disease as an epidemic.

8. Vaccinated persons should not relax their precautions in the matter of food and drink for at least two or three weeks.

9. Soldiers and sailors may be vaccinated at their port of arrival if the dis-

[1] *Therapeutic Gazette.* April.

ease is not epidemic at that port at that time, otherwise the inoculation should be made about three weeks before leaving home.

10. Vaccination should be performed only on those who are free from all form of disease.

Those who are likely to be benefited by anti-typhoid vaccination are

a. Physicians, nurses and medical students.

b. Families in which there are bacillus carriers.

c. Those who have gone from salubrious localities to localities in which typhoid is endemic.

d. Dwellers in cities in which typhoid is prevalent.

e. Soldiers and sailors who are sent to colonies where typhoid is epidemic or endemic.

Surface Water Pollution.[1]— Wheaton thinks the chief causes of water pollution and winter epidemics are lost sight of by health boards and health experts. Streams from which the water supply of towns and villages are usually obtained are the natural drains of the tracts of land through which they flow, and constantly hold in suspension or in solution more or less solids and organic matter.

If the water flow is large the percentage of such pollution will not be dangerous to health and it becomes dangerous only when the water flow is lessened by excessive cold or prolonged drought.

In the latter case particularly the percentage of pollution often exceeds the power of the body to dispose of it or throw it off.

In very cold weather as crystallization and ice formation takes place at the surface the organic matter and other debris is crowded down, the condition becoming analogous to the mother liquor in a chemical solution. Such water taken into the pumping stations and then distributed is often unfit for household or drinking purposes.

If therefore during prolonged drought and during excessively cold weather as well the water supply is habitually boiled it will remove the danger of infectious disease from such a source.

The Cancer Problem Today.[1]— A. W. Blain quotes Crile as saying that there is no tie of sentiment between a man and his cancer. Enlightenment ought to be easy and effective. The medical profession and not the laity are responsible for the high primary and remote mortality of malignant disease and until the doctor, especially the general practitioner, assumes for cancer the same stand which he takes in strangulated hernia and appendicitis there will be little improvement in cancer statistics.

The points to be emphasized are:

1. Cancer has a pre-malignant state in which it is curable.

2. The time has passed for the profession to assume a passive attitude in suspicious malignant cases, since operative technic is so highly developed that there are practically no deaths from operations per se.

3. A large percentage of cancer cases are absolutely curable if the family physician is not the cause of fatal delay in his desire to obtain a positive diagnosis.

Instruction of College Students in Regard to Reproduction and Maternity.[2]— Elizabeth B. Thelberg thinks that the curriculum in colleges for women should contain instruction which shall fit them to be mothers and that without it they cannot be regarded as educated women. If not taught these matters right, adolescence will teach them wrong, and with a veil of sentimentality and false emotion which will hinder clearness of vision. They can best be taught by the physician who is in charge of the health of the college community. The writer in teaching physiology to the young ladies at Vassar College begins with the lowest forms of life and shows the progress of evolution in animal life. She shows the development of the reproductive organs in the female, and of the ovum by suitable models and by microscopic study. She also gives a course in public hygiene which embraces the communicable diseases

[1] T. C. Wheaton, M. D., *Medical Council*, April, 1912.

[1] *International Journal of Surgery*, June, 1912.
[2] *New York Medical Journal*, June 15.

including gonorrhea and syphilis and informs her students that a licentious man usually has an infected body and that the infection may be transmitted not only to an innocent wife but to children. She also lectures on constipation and menstruation.

At the close of the senior year she gives four lectures on reproduction, maternity and the care and feeding of children. They are also told about criminal abortion and abortion which is justifiable, also about heredity and eugenics.

Furthermore, models of the uterus and its appendages are shown, also the development of the uterus during pregnancy, and the various incidents connected with pregnancy and parturition are narrated. She admits that the subject is a difficult one to treat, but is impressed with its importance, and feels that an exact and wide knowledge of the subject is the first essential in teaching it. It is interesting to note the manner in which this important subject is treated in the pioneer American college for women. It is also interesting to note that Matthew Vassar, the founder of the college in arranging for the original appointments for the faculty stipulated that the resident physician should be a woman and that she should also be professor of physiology and hygiene.

The Regulation of Wet Nurses.[1]—An editorial observes that wet nursing has been constantly regarded as essential, in a measure for the preservation of human lives. But wet nursing has not only not decreased infant mortality, it has actually tended to increase it.

That is, while the children in private homes who obtain this nourishment are usually saved by it the children of the wet nurses usually succumb. In other words, the children to whom the milk belongs is robbed of their birthright. The children of wet nurses in general are those for whom breast feeding is most essential, while those for whom breast milk is stolen can, as a rule, afford all the requirements for preserving life without sacrificing the child of the wet nurse. Wet nursing thrives largely on immorality and a woman should

not be permitted to offer her breasts for money if her own child must be a sufferer thereby.

Of course it is proper if a woman's child have died, to sell her breast milk to the child of another. In some institutions in which babies are boarded wet nursing is permitted only if the wet nurse also nurses her own child. While wet nursing may not be suppressed regulative legislation should protect infancy and limit the employment of wet nurses. The high mortality rate of the children of wet nurses should be registered as due to the employment of the mother. The present form of wet nursing is a prostitution of motherhood and a sacrifice of infants.

Only when the maternal milk is superabundant should the mother be allowed to nurse an additional child in another home. This would seem like a very severe construction of a very important question. The sale of a woman's breast milk at the expense of the child to whom it belongs is undoubtedly wicked, but in how many cases the stimulus of an additional child at the breast means an additional supply for both which, as the records of maternity hospitals show, does not seem to work any appreciable harm to the nurse or to either of the children.

ETIOLOGY AND DIAGNOSIS.

The Diagnosis of Bowel Cancer.[1]—Paul, in the annual address on surgery before the 1912 meeting of the British Medical Association discussed intestinal surgery in general and drew attention to the fact that unfortunately we are still without means for recognizing cancer of the bowel in its really early stages. In fact, it sets up no symptoms at this period of its growth which would lead a patient to consult his doctor, except when low down in the rectum. Here it excites irritability, and attracts attention by the presence of blood and mucus, and so often allows an early diagnosis; but higher up we have almost invariably to wait until the growth has begun to impede the passage of feces before the patient is sufficiently alarmed to seek advice. Large ulcers without marked obstruction are chiefly characterised by intestinal toxemia, with elevation of the temperature, flatulent dyspepsia, loss of flesh, irregular colic with constipation or diarrhea and mucus

[1] *Medical Review of Reviews*, June, 1912.

[1] F. S. Paul, F. R. C. S. Eng., *Med. Press and Circular*, Aug. 7, 1912.

and blood in the motions—visible when the growth is low down, occult when higher up. A tumor may frequently be felt. The ring stricture usually causes less disturbance to the general health, but more colic and more obstruction. X-ray screen view of the behavior of a bismuth meal is useful if its limitations are recognised. It may inform us as to the site and the amount of constriction, though in regard to the latter atony or tonicity of the bowel must be taken into consideration. In no circumstances can it indicate either the extent or the malignancy of the growth, nor can the ready passage of a bismuth meal be regarded as a contra-indication to operation. If the disease is within the reach of the sigmoidoscope, this treatment may be of considerable assistance in the diagnosis of growths situated in the pelvic colon, where they frequently escape touch when examined either by the rectum or the abdomen.

———

Remarks on the Etiology of Enuresis.[1]—In considering his subject, Allan emphasizes the importance of studying the origin and causes of this condition. At the outset it should be remembered that enuresis is merely a symptom, and that every case should be thoroughly investigated for some underlying cause. It is generally customary to classify enuresis as one of the functional neuroses, but Miller has taken the bold step of including it under the diseases of the bladder in order to emphasize the fact that the condition is frequently due to local causes. With regard to causation the affection may be roughly divided into five groups: (1) genito-urinary; (2) nervous; (3) malformations; (4) general; (5) idiopathic. As regards the first the urine may be at fault: there may be hyperacidity or excessive alkalinity, or there may be bacteriuria. Inflammation of various parts of the genito-urinary tract, calculi, new growths, etc., may be responsible for the disorder. The nervous causes are very numerous and many are reflex in character, such as balanitis, vulvo-vaginitis, worms, etc. Malformations of the spinal cord or of the genito-urinary organs may be accompanied by urinary incontinence, and treatment in such cases is particularly hopeless. As general causes may be mentioned rheumatism, thyroid insufficiency, diabetes, etc. Still found enuresis associated with rheumatism in about 5 per cent. of his cases. Williams is the great apostle of the thyroid insufficiency theory. His contention is that in many cases there is deficiency of the thyroid gland secretion, and that if carefully looked for many of the stigmata of cretinoid degeneration will be found in these patients. Particular stress is laid on the following in this connection: (1) a persistently subnormal temperature; (2) a deficiency in height and weight; (3) abnormalities of the skin and its appendages, more especially the hair, not only of the head, but also and particularly of the superciliary region. The evidence submitted in his able and interesting brochure is certainly of a convincing character. It should be pointed out that he does not maintain that this theory holds good in every case, as some subsequent investigations would apparently have us infer. In this connection Williams also advances the theory of thyroid insufficiency as a probable cause of adenoids, and he believes that the association of adenoids and enuresis is not a mere coincidence. I think this statement requires to be considerably modified. In the first place adenoids may be present in children who do not suffer from enuresis: in 850 adenoid operation cases that have come under my notice during the past two years not one showed incontinence of urine. Some little time ago when I was connected with a large hospital for children, and had the opportunity of seeing many cases of enuresis, I found these two conditions associated in a small number of cases only, and the percentage of cures after removal of adenoids was infinitesimal. The last group of cases —the idiopathic—accounts for a large number of the cases of enuresis. There are two distinct classes in this group; (a) those in which there is lack of tone of the external sphincter; and (b) those in which there is hypersensitiveness of the bladder. The above is not to be taken as a full discussion of the etiology of enuresis, but it will serve to render more clear various points in treatment which will now be dealt with.

———

The Etiology of Renal Infection.[1]—In the course of a most interesting symposium on kidney diseases, Stokes contributes a valuable paper on surgical kidney and in referring to the etiology of kidney infection states that it has two main sources, either from the blood stream itself, and in the direction of the urinary secretion, or second, through the urinary tract against the stream of urinary secretion. Both conditions have been observed, perhaps, about equally. The origin of hemogenous infections has been observed from metastatic infection following pyemia, asepticemia, ulcerative endocarditis, less frequently following measles, scarlet fever, smallpox, dysentery, typhoid fever, through small wounds in the skin and mucous membrane of the respiratory, digestive, and genital tract. When the infection is of hematogenous origin it always begins as small multiple abscesses in the substance of the kidney.

The urogenital infections of the kidney of the male genital apparatus follows gonorrhea of the urethra and bladder, bladder infection following urethral stricture and prostatic hypertrophy. In the female genital organs following gonorrheal cystitis, bladder catarrh during pregnancy, and puerperium. Much experimental work has been done to determine the character of the infection and the direction of their incidence. Particularly favorable are the micro-organisms introduced into the urinary tract during a course of gonorrheal infection. Rarely, if ever, does the gonococcus itself travel

———

[1] J. Allan, M. D., *The Prescriber*, Aug., 1912.

[1] A C. Stokes, M. D., Omaha, Neb., *The Med. Herald*, Aug., 1912.

to the kidney. But the urogenital infections are secondary infections upon a mucous membrane changed by the action of the gonococcus. The most common bacteria affecting the kidney in the order of their frequency are as follows: The bacillus coli communis, staphyloccus, the streptococcus, and from that on a number of rare affections, such as proteus vulgaris, the pneumococcus, typhoid bacillus.

Infections may be either pure cultures or mixed infection. The bacillus coli communis occurs very frequently as pure culture. It does not precipitate the urinary salts and renders the urine acid. The presence of the urine does not seem to have untoward effect on the growth of the bacillus coli. Schmidt and Aschoff state the following: If there is no ammoniacal decomposition of the urine and still pus be found, the cause may be either tuberculosis or colon bacillus.

Most of the cocci produce a very rapid ammoniacal decomposition of the urine. The streptococcus practically never reaches the kidney by means of the urogenital tract, but always through the blood stream. The staphylococcus may enter by either route.

Whether the gonococcus can produce an infection of the kidney in pure cultures is very questionable. They probably present themselves very rarely in pure culture but frequently in mixed culture and it is probable that all cases of pure gonorrheal infection of the kidney are of hematogenous origin.

The Albumin Reaction of Sputum in Diagnosis of Pulmonary Tuberculosis.[1]—In a comprehensive article on the subject, Fishberg describes this test as follows: a three per cent. solution of acetic acid is added to the sputum, which is then thoroughly shaken. During ten or fifteen minutes the bottle is allowed to stand, and repeatedly shaken during this time. It will be observed that the mucus is coagulated by the acetic acid, and when it is then filtered through paper into a test tube, the filtrate appears as a clear fluid. Occasionally all the mucus is not coagulated with the first attempt, and this is easily ascertained by adding a drop of acetic acid to the filtrate, which in such cases again shows flocculi collecting as a precipitate. The process is then repeated, until a clear filtrate is obtained. The clear fluid is then boiled over a Bunsen burner, or an alcohol lamp, and while boiling, some crystals of common salt, or a concentrated solution of sodium chlorid is added. If albumin is present there results a cloudiness, or a curdy precipitate which, on standing, settles to the bottom of the tube. Roughly speaking, the amount of the precipitate gives us an idea of the amount of albumin present The most important precaution to be observed is that nothing but a curdy precipitate can be considered as positive, because

the presence of mucus, which the acetic acid does not always dissolve completely, may also give a cloudy precipitate on boiling. But this reaction is not curdy, nor does it settle on standing. Of course, any of the other tests for albumin may be used on the filtrate, but the above procedure has given me satisfactory results.

The author draws the following conclusions:

1. The albumin reaction of sputum is a useful test in cases suggestive of pulmonary tuberculosis and will often be of assistance when the microscope fails to reveal tubercle bacilli.

2. A positive albumin reaction is not always decisive, because many diseases, not at all tuberculous in character, may show albumin in the sputum.

3. A negative reaction, when repeatedly found during several examinations, from specimens of sputum carefully collected, excludes tuberculosis.

4. In cases of tuberculosis, in which the albumin reaction was positive but has become negative for some time, we may conclude that the process of cicatrization of the pulmonary lesion is progressing favorably, even when the physical signs are slow in disappearing.

5. The albumin reaction has a prognostic value. It gives us an opportunity to follow the progress of the tuberculous process. Whenever albumin makes its appearance in a case in which the reaction was negative for some time, there is surely to be found an acute exacerbation, or an extension of the lesion in the lung.

6. In pulmonary emphysema a positive albumin reaction appears to be an indication of cardiac dilatation, thus indicating the proper treatment to be pursued.

Grocco's Sign in the Diagnosis of Pleuritic Effusion.[1]—In a scholarly article Brown states that this sign is a triangular area of dulness, paravertebral in position, situated on the side of the chest opposite the effusion; he has found that in cases with free fluid in the pleural cavity, or in which an encapsulated effusion lies along the spine this sign is practically constant in its presence. When the patient lies upon the affected side, diminution or disappearance of the triangle is noticed (except when the pleural cavity is enormously distended), reappearing when the patient assumes the sitting or standing position, or reclines on the other side. A more pronounced triangle is present in right sided effusions. The hypothenuse of the triangle is usually a curved line, especially at the upper portion. The size of the triangle varies with the amount of pleural effusion, except that right sided effusions usually present a somewhat larger triangle. The presence of this triangle is not pathognomonic; it may exist in subphrenic conditions accompanied by a fluid accumulation.

[1] Maurice Fishberg, M. D., Archives of Diagnosis, July, 1912.

[1] M. A. Brown, M. D., Lancet-Clinic, June 15, 1912.

TREATMENT.

The Therapy of Cold.[1]—According to Blackader the effect of cold air on the body is twofold. First, there is an actual extraction of heat which is rarely desirable, and as far as possible should be prevented. The body loses the largest amount of heat through conduction and this should be prevented by proper clothing. Much more important than the abstraction of heat from the body is the stimulating action of the cold on the delicate sentient nerves of the periphery. Both respiration and circulation are strengthened, oxidation is increased, and nutrition becomes more active. There is also a powerful stimulation conveyed to the medullary centers by the effect of cold air on the nasal mucous membrane. Cold, provided it be not excessive, has a markedly stimulating action on the digestive system. Cold also seems to stimulate the blood-forming organs. As a result of these factors, the resisting powers of the body against toxins and its ability to respond protectively to the assault of infection is greatly increased. These benefits of cold depend, however, on the power of the individual to react and this varies greatly and seems to be dependent on the vasomotor tone. Those suffering from any interference with the free passage of air through the nostrils do not react well to cold air. Inflammatory conditions of the larynx and trachea may be subjected to additional irritation by cold air. To benefit from a winter in the north, the intestinal tract and the kidneys should be in good working order. Extreme cold is not desirable for those suffering from gout, arthritis or neuritis. For those suffering from advanced degeneration of any organ, for those advanced in years and for the very young extreme cold may be distinctly harmful. It cannot be too strongly emphasized that all the benefit to be derived from a residence in the north will depend on the completeness with which an outdoor life is lived.

The Treatment of Flat Foot.[2]—Judson, in a notably brief and comprehensive article, gives the following salient points in the treatment of a condition that is surprisingly common:

1. Advise the patient that, as a rule, the only use of the uppers in a shoe is to keep the leather sole under the foot, according to the old saying that to a man with shoes it is the same as if the world were covered with leather. Therefore prescribe a wide and flexible sole, with slight if any elevation under the heel, and let the uppers simply retain the foot without making much pressure along the sides or over the instep. Soles and uppers should be made comfortable and convenient with not too much regard for fashion or the exigencies of the trade.

2. Advise him that the arch of the foot is flexible and sustained by the dynamic action of the great muscles of the calf rather than by the static resistance of the ligaments of the foot, and that as the tendons have the difficult task of changing from the vertical to the horizontal direction on their way to the anterior part of the foot, they should never be hindered by artificial constriction above the ankle. Prescribe, therefore, either very loose lacets or low shoes, with the warning that walking will necessarily be painful for a time after the ankles and feet are released from compression, to be followed later by comfort and increased ability. Note: It is difficult to conceive of the weight of the body as sustained alone by the balance of forces in so small an arch composed of bone and ligament.

3. Advise him that, of all the parts of the body, the feet are the hardest worked, and the most sure to wear out. Therefore prescribe frequent rest for the feet.

The Treatment of Dogbites.[1]—Lesser considers the subject in detail and recommends the following course of procedure:

1. The wound should be allowed or encouraged to bleed as freely as possible for several minutes. If a large vessel be severed, it needs to be controlled earlier, of course, than if there were capillary bleeding.

2. After the wound has bled sufficiently, a wad of cotton saturated with a mild antiseptic solution, such as equal parts of alcohol and water with a small percentage of iodine, should be applied with as moderate pressure as may be required to control the bleeding and protect the wound from further infection. The wad should be kept moist (not too wet) with a similar application, but with as little interference with the wound as possible.

When the area is small after the bleeding has been controlled, an application of an antiseptic wool-fat ointment may be found of advantage. The selection of the application or ointment must be left to the physician, but it should consist of ingredients well calculated to soften the tissues, favor absorption of the active antiseptic, and at the same time stimulate the area to encourage different action of the tissue fluid. A properly prepared lanum, lanolin or kindred medium will be found to serve well.

3. If the wound does not bleed, a suction pump (similar to a cupping pump) should be applied, but where there is none at hand cautious suction with the lips could be made. This may be done by the patient if he can reach the part, or it may be done by an attending person without injury to himself or the patient, if proper precautions are followed. It has been demonstrated that a perfectly healthy person may swallow snake poison or septic material

[1] A. S. Blackader, Montreal, Can., reported in J. A. M. A. Society Proceedings. Aug. 10, 1912.
[2] A. B. Judson, M. D., Medical Council, Aug., 1912.
[1] A. M. Lesser, M. D., American Jour. of Surgery, August, 1912.

.without any harm whatsoever, their poisonous properties being made innocuous by the healthy digesting fluids, particularly fresh human saliva and gastric juice. Still, the uncertainty of health and a possible abrasion on the lips or in the mouth make precaution advisable. The suction should therefore be made by holding in the mouth an alcohol, water and iodine solution above mentioned, while the lips are held over the infected area, so that the solution may play around the wound and protect the mouth from infection. In experimental work a properly prepared acidulated pepsin solution has also been found very serviceable for this purpose, but the alcohol seems to stimulate free bleeding and, as said, also protects the wound from possible mouth infection.

4. When the suction does not produce bleeding it indicates that the blood capillaries were not injured and the poison is carried in the lymph channels. In these cases an application of the antiseptic wool-fat ointment should be made. While these antiseptic applications may exert no immediate special influence upon the internal portion of the wound, they keep the parts pliable and permit the exit of the virus, while by natural processes the tissues endeavor to eliminate, or they at least aid in limiting or localizing the septic process.

Indications for Operation in Chronic Disease of the Middle Ear.[1]—Leslie, in a very complete and valuable paper, gives the following ten indications for performing a mastoid operation in cases of chronic aural suppuration:

1. Continued pain in an ear which is discharging, or on that side of the head.

2. When the discharge has lasted three months in spite of attention to the ear, throat, and nose.

3. If there is bleeding, blood stained, or brown discharge coming from the ear.

4. If the perforation in the drum is enlarging. (This means that the membrane is being destroyed).

5. If there is polypus or a bulging membrane, with a perforation draining the cavity.

6. If there is increasing deafness, giddiness, or permanently blocked Eustachian drainage.

7. If the discharge is foul smelling or abundant in spite of the use of drops.

8. If there is facial paralysis on that side.

9. Optic neuritis, fits, mental derangement.

10. Evidences of tubercle or diphtheria in the discharge (miscroscope) may demand a radical operation.

GENERAL TOPICS.

American Association of Clinical Research.—The fourth annual meeting of this body will take place in New York, at the Academy of Medicine, on November 9, 1912. The sessions

will be held from 9 a. m. to 1 p. m., from 3 p. m. to 6 p. m., and from 8 p. m. to 10 p. m. The evening session will be open to the public. Notable contributions on the Negri bodies, on certain fluids for tubercle bacilli in the urine, on adjustment and function, on psychoanalysis and *traumbedeutung*, on a pandemic of malignant encapsulated throat coccus, on the single remedy, on indicanuria and glycosuria, on disease conditions expressive of correct diagnosis, on biochemical problems, on the two most far reaching discoveries in medicine, and others are to be given. Every member of the association is cordially invited to contribute a paper. The title should be sent at once to the permanent secretary, so that the programme may be completed. As soon as completed, the programme will be mailed. Members will please make an effort not only to contribute a paper, but to be present at the coming meeting, to bring friends, and to assist in the most important movement of medicine as represented in the aim of this association, the systematic, scientific investigation and advancement of medicine by conclusive clinical and clinically allied methods. Friends should be invited to become members, and their support will be cordially appreciated.

The Fallacies of Drug Nihilism.[1]—Meltzer, in a scholarly address, replete with statements concerning the underlying principles of medical practice that will appeal to cultured physicians calls attention to the fact that in medicine there is human life and happiness at stake, and one ought to recognize the undeniable fact that some claims may be true, even if our methods have not yet been able to prove them. The history of the use of iron in the treatment of chlorosis ought to be a lesson. While every physician could tell from his own knowledge that, say, Blaud's pills act in these cases like a charm, great laboratory men like Bunge and Schmiedeberg denied persistently that inorganic iron can be absorbed and thus capable of supplying the iron deficiency of the anemic patient. The struggle lasted nearly a quarter of a century. The trouble with the men, trained exclusively in laboratories, is twofold. First, they do not seem to see that a medical fact, observed critically by a capable physician, deserves as much credence and consideration as a fact developed by laboratory methods, and, second, that the laboratory man offers here positive opinions in a field in which he has had no experience.

Great physicians, like Traube and Kussmaul, who were busy general practitioners before they entered on their brilliant scientific clinical careers and whose training has been more in the experimental laboratory than in the deadhouse, were never infected with therapeutic nihilism, though they dwelt then in the midst of this mental epidemic.

---

[1] F. A. Leslie, Ph. B., M. D., Toledo, O., *New York Med. Jour.*, August 10, 1912.

[1] S. J. Meltzer, M. D., *Jour. A. M. A.*, Aug. 24, 1912.

American Medicine

H. EDWIN LEWIS, M. D., *Managing Editor.*

PUBLISHED MONTHLY BY THE AMERICAN-MEDICAL PUBLISHING COMPANY.

Copyrighted by the American Medical Publishing Co., 1912.

| New Series, Vol. VII., No. 9. Complete Series, Vol. XVIII., No. 9. | SEPTEMBER, 1912. | $1.00 YEARLY In advance. |

The increasing number of charity depots for certified milk and their increasing popularity among those too poor to buy in open market, are certainly very desirable conditions if our aim is to preserve by half-charity the types of people unable to preserve themselves. The amazing result of this movement is in fact the creation by these artificial means of a species of domesticated man who cannot exist without aid from society. We are all dependent upon society for existence, for we cannot live without that organized protection, but the ideal of the fittest for survival has been those who can earn enough to buy the necessities of existence, and this new type cannot. From time immemorial there have been men who couldn't do even that, but they perished sooner or later unless they parasitized on abler men. It is now a recognized policy that such people must not be allowed to die, but must be preserved by the voluntary labor of abler people in charity organizations. Milk of proper grade is out of the reach of these inefficients—so we spend money to get it to them.

The death rate of infants is being reduced as was never thought possible. There has been a spirit of exultation and self-congratulation among the workers; but what will the harvest be? Is the nation to consist of self-supporting country peasantry, and the cities to be crowded with people who cannot exist unless the rest are taxed to feed the babies? Taxes will be necessary in time, for these milk depots cannot exist on voluntary contributions forever—and taxes, no matter how we disguise them, can invariably be traced down and down until we see them coming from the whole people. We hope the milk movement will continue, for when the burden of raising the incompetents becomes insupportable, we will be forced into an eugenic law preventing any further reproduction of types unfit to support themselves. Infanticide was universal for these reasons in the past, but what is to replace it when the semi-paupers are too numerous to support? England by very vicious poor-laws formerly allowed paupers to breed in work houses, but stopped it when the appalling burdens of this sentimental charity were fully realized. We are allowing them to breed in slums and model tenements erected by sentimental rich people, and we too will stop their breeding when the numbers become too great for support. We are committing the same blunder as that of the poor-laws of England a century ago. But the modern problem is different.

What shall be done with pauper parents who deliberately bring into the world a lot of babies for the public to raise in whole or part? Shall we sterilize the whole lot to end the geometrically increasing burden? It certainly would check begging if every beggar, man or woman, were at once operated upon. England did not go that far, but now wishes she had. How much worse will be our condition, after our charity folks have raised another generation from the European failures who now patronize our milk depots to raise their babies for them. May the milk depots flourish and raise every worthless brat they can, for that is the only way we can possibly create a public opinion which will condemn the man who cannot feed his own babies. In other words, prevention nowadays replaces the infanticide of old, and we must mend our ways accordingly. What shall we do?

The physician's responsibility for the cocaine and morphine evils is charged in the report of the Chicago Vice Commission. The facts certainly warrant a house cleaning, and we had better clean our house voluntarily before we are compelled by neighbors. It is stated that most of the cocaine and morphine used by depraved people is obtained on physicians' prescriptions for which a good fee is paid. Much of the drugs used is obtained from druggists at a price for the mere asking. Drug clerks even send solicitors into the dens to get orders, but the larger bulk is issued on prescriptions of more or less respectable "doctors." Luckily, many of the prescriptions are known to be ill-written self-evident forgeries and though that clears our skirts a little, it makes matters worse for the druggists. Luckily too, there are only a very few physicians who stoop to such a degrading practice as furnishing what they know will kill the victims, and perhaps there will always be black sheep in every fold. But the point is, that this tiny percentage of the medical profession has created an impression that we are all bad. The commission itself has evidently been deceived, for it fails to emphasize the fact that the wrong doers are too few to stigmatize the whole class. They should know that as long as the law exempts prescriptions, there will always be a few men to abuse it, but these few do not warrant us in revoking a law which does deter the wrongful sale more or less.

The real causes of drug habits are not even mentioned in the commission's report. Indeed medical literature itself is strangely defective in that line, for it is assumed that anyone will be a victim if the materials are handy, and the only thing to do is to keep them out of reach. It is true, that physicians furnish a larger percentage of cases than any other calling, but the vast majority of doctors never have the slightest temptation to use them—and we may say the same of druggists and the manufacturers. The tendency to use such harmful drugs is almost invariably an indication of some profound constitutional weakness, and that is why the failures in civilization are so prone to use cocaine or morphine—the prostitutes and criminals. The laws making it difficult to obtain the drugs merely make the price higher, but have not necessarily reduced the number of victims or prevented new ones. We do not advise revoking the law, but we do advise an investigation as to why certain classes will get it in spite of all laws. The consumption of cocaine and morphine in America is something beyond belief and is constantly increasing. We will not check this awful plague until we remove its cause, and it is right there that we are hopelessly in the dark. We have much to learn, but no reason to be discouraged. Our fire department does grand work, but does not prevent conflagrations though it will reduce them to a negligible number in time. We are facing conflagrations of drug use, and we are not even reducing them, but we too will succeed. So let us get at it.

The proper disposal of sewage is such a vital matter, that it would be a good plan to have medical societies devote some of their meetings to it. All physicians are really specialists and can not be expected to devote study to matters out of their sphere, so that as a class they have been rather reluctant to enlist in the present crusade, especially since they are ignorant of its finer points. But there is no earthly reason why they should not be made aware of the general principles on which sanitarians are conducting the movement for clean municipal habits. Indeed, the profession are rather looked upon as the proper instructors of laymen in all questions of public health, though as a matter of fact, laymen are the leaders to a degree rather uncomfortable to our professional pride. Already a public opinion is forming to the effect that each community must dispose of its wastes in some other way than throwing them in the water of streams, lakes and harbors, to be thence carried to neighbors. In addition there is a growing demand that all waters be restored to the original clean condition in which they were when we obtained them from their former owners—the Indians. As this state of purity is a remote necessity and can be approximately obtained by means now known, the sooner we wake up the better.

The Bronx Valley Sewer Report of the Metropolitan Sewerage Commission of New York is of such vital interest that we wish we had space to print the essential parts. From these we may accept it as proved that New York harbor is in a dreadful state of pollution from the discharge into it of wastes in far greater amount than can be oxidized. A certain percentage merely sinks, largely near sewer outlets, though the floor of the whole upper harbor is now covered to considerable depths, except where the currents scour it out in spots or channels and deposit it elsewhere. None of it reaches the ocean, as it is deposited long before the current could carry it that far. The harbor is in fact a septic tank which works so inefficiently as to constitute a cesspool needing periodical excavation. Further increase of pollution is intolerable, and we must devise ways of preventing present discharges. The problem is simple in the Bronx project, for by well known methods the sewage can be purified and then emptied into its own valley at moderate cost.

New York City's sewage problem is extremely difficult, but it can be solved and must be. This report shows the utmost necessity for the experimental sewage stations we have previously urged. We have no precedents from abroad, for no city in the world has anything like our difficulties—with our millions of people piled almost ten deep on a little island with nowhere to pour their filth. We must learn how to separate the waste material from the water, and then destroy it or carry it away without offense. With a little money and time our engineers will solve the problem, for they have solved far more difficult ones. In the meantime, the community owes a debt of gratitude to the Sewage Commission for its outspoken words. We hope there will be a change in the law so that all such matters will be under sanitary control, as the present helplessness of the authorities is civic folly. More amazing still is our supineness as a city when neighbors proposed to defile our front yard. Bad as we are, we should have objected to further nuisance.

The septic tank seems to be losing favor with sanitary engineers, because they are finding that the substances thus formed are more difficult to oxidize later in the "contact" or filter beds. The "tank" is being replaced by mere "settling" reservoirs in which the grosser materials may be separated and removed, the raw sewage passing on to the filter for destruction of its suspended and dissolved impurities. There is a suspicion that these settling basins can be built on Manhattan and can be made so efficient in removing impurities that the harbor waters will be able to dispose of the balance. Of course the whole shore line will thus be a polluted sewage disposal plant, but it will be far better than the present cesspool condition. It seems that the system will be the first step towards the perfect method to be devised at sewage experiment stations. It is quite evident that we must cut down the amount of these waters as much as practicable at once—street dirt, for instance, must be swept up and not left for the rains to wash into the harbor. Nevertheless, at the rate at which population is piling up on the island, the time is surely coming when the harbor waters cannot dispose of this semi-purified sewage, even if they can do so now—a matter of much doubt. Then it

will be necessary to build tunnels under the harbor to conduct the sewage to distant filters. The cost will not be prohibitive, the unearned increment of real estate values will easily bear the tax. We might as well begin thinking in these huge terms instead of those of house drains, now that the water-engineers are solving far more colossal problems.

Our fresh water courses must also be purified, and here is where the up-state medical profession can do a world of good, for it seems their special sphere. Our silly cheap-John sewage habits have well nigh ruined water supplies worth untold millions, and even rendered it unsafe to live at places which should be paradises of health. The financial folly should appeal to everyone even if they ignore health and life. If it were safe to drink water from any fresh stream we would save enough in bottled waters to change all the sewage systems in the state. Then think of the lessened death rates and sick rates which always follow upon clean water. *Let every medical society take up the cry for clean water courses* and for each community to dispose of its own filth.

————

Eugenics must surely at last be coming into its own. By the time that any innovation gets real acceptance in England it must have amply justified its existence in other countries. And eugenics has been having great innings there lately. In the first place Sir James Barr devoted his presidential address before the British Medical Association to that subject, and while he said nothing that can be regarded as altogether new, neither did he say anything that was not more or less true. A more important matter was the meeting at the University of London, from July 24th-30th of the First International .Eugenics Congress under the presidency of Major Leonard Darwin, which was attended by over six hundred people. At the inaugural banquet the Right Honorable Arthur Balfour, M. P., reviewed the subject with that clarity of vision and expression which has made him a man of mark in both science and statesmanship. This is explained, perhaps, by his putting into practice the principle expressed by him on this occasion that the future progress of mankind in most departments must be based upon the application of scientific methods to practical life. He pointed out that most common of all logical fallacies, the use of words in two quite different senses. "We say that the fit survive. All that that means is that those who survive are fit—fit because they survive and survive because they are fit"—the naturalistic definition of the word fit, which, as Mr. Balfour rightly said "adds nothing to the facts." The Eugenist, however, he pointed out, does not admit that mere survival indicates fitness. When he speaks of fitness "he means he has ideals of what a man ought to be, of what a state ought to be, of what society ought to be; and these ideals are not being carried out because we have not yet grasped the true way to deal with the problems involved."

Professor Van Wagenen of the Eugenics section of the American Breeders' Association, threw out the very valuable suggestion that out of the Congress might grow a small permanent body, of international composition, to be the medium of communication between forces representative of the eugenic idea throughout the civilized world; while the President, Major Leonard Darwin, carefully cautioned that as conditions in different countries varied greatly, the laying down of extensive and very definite programmes of reform suitable for all could not be expected to form part of the proceedings. In his presidential address, also, on the following day Major Darwin gave expression to the salutary warning that the knowledge of the laws of heredity, however perfect it might become, would be of comparatively little use as a method of insuring the progress of mankind until it had become actually incorporated in the moral code of the people. The practical application of the work of the Congress would seem to be, then, in the direction of a general educative campaign looking towards an encouragement of the marriage of the fit, with careful legislative restriction of the marriage of the unfit; bearing always in mind, *first*, that to obtain a workable law, the facts of heredity must be first determined and their interpretation be generally agreed upon by scientists, and *second*, that no rash and ill considered heroic measures shall be hastily adopted when the required ends can be attained without revolting the moral sense of the people. Otherwise the refining work of civilization on centuries of primitive impulses may be undone.

A final proof of the permeation of eugenic principles, even in slow moving England, is to be found in the presidential address of the Archbishop of York at the Congress of the Royal Sanitary Institute, held at York the last week in July. Not only did the Archbishop approve the principles of the Government Mental Deficiency Bill which prohibits marriage to mental defectives and provides for the segregation in institutions of such as are not properly cared for at home; but he went to the extent of declaring himself in favor of an amendment to the marriage law, which should render null and void any marriage in regard to which it was shown within a certain time that facts disclosing insanity, epilepsy or venereal disease had been withheld when the marriage was contracted.

Antityphoid vaccinations are causing considerable discussion in France—in marked contrast to the apathy in America and England. It is difficult to understand the absence of opposition among the English speaking nations, and the bitterness of it in France. The process is now a routine in the American and English Armies, as though its safety and efficacy were proved so completely as to need no further comment. If there are any English military physicians opposed to it, they have carefully concealed the fact and the civilians do not seem interested at all. The opposition in France seems to center around Metchnikoff, and the reason may be the fact that he is at the head of the method of inducing immunity by injecting mild strains of *living* organisms. The essential of the typhoid prophylaxis is that the bacilli must surely be dead or they will multiply and, no matter how attenuated, will cause a disease and perhaps create a dangerous carrier. The human tissues do not seem to be able to manufacture antibodies to kill off these bacilli as promptly as in the case of the attenuated organisms derived from animals with rabies or variola. These unknown organisms are evidently in an entirely different class than bacilli and do not behave the same. Hence the French physicians are bitterly opposed to Metchnikoff's plan to immunize with living bacilli of typhoid.

Metchnikoff's reasons for opposing typhoid prophylaxis with dead bacilli have not been fully reported in English medical literature, so it is not possible to form any conclusion as to their value. As far as we can read between the lines, he seems to think that immunity can not be produced unless there are myriads of organisms to make the poisons the presence of which gives rise to the tissue reaction. These poisons must be manufactured very slowly at first, but by constantly increasing numbers of living organisms. We can not introduce at one time a sufficient number to do the work, or we would overwhelm the person. So we must inject a small number and let them increase—moreover they must not be virulent ones. To his mind therefore, immunity cannot possibly be created by the injection of three doses of the poison, as it is wholly insufficient and if the doses were large enough to be effective they would kill the patient. He seems to make some kind of an analogy to the way people immunize themselves to morphine and arsenic by beginning with minute doses and slowly increasing to huge amounts after a long time, and that this is really the way it is done by attenuated organisms of rabies and variola in a shorter time.

The need of more definite discussion is evident, for Metchnikoff is too big a man to dismiss by the simple statement, "he is too old a dog to learn new tricks." The method with dead bacilli cannot be accepted as standard until his objections are proved baseless and his own way shown to be useless. It should be settled soon too, because we may

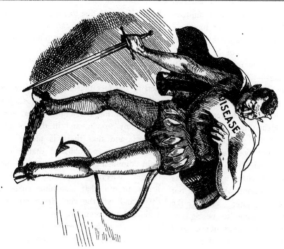

A New Patient

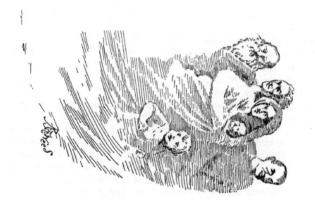

be postponing a great method of improving public health. On the other hand we must not allow its acceptance by default not only because it may not be very efficacious but it may increase susceptibility to other things—tuberculosis for instance, as in one report. We hope that this matter will receive more comment in the future—the hotter the better. There has not been sufficient time to find the real value of the statistics so far published and statisticians have not been convinced of the value of the methods. To be sure very few get typhoid within a few months but that is not significant, as it does not tell us what they get later. So far, the evidence of figures seems to be against Metchnikoff. His intolerance has created a bad impression even if he is later shown to be right. He has put the method under indictment, that is certain. The worst feature is the early fading of the protection and the necessity for a repetition every 2 or 3 years, and this will be intolerable if resistance to an incipient unrecognized but healing tuberculosis really is lessened by each inoculation. The profession is evidently very wary and does not care to repeat the sad history of tuberculin.

***

Outdoor treatment of puerperal infections lessens the mortality of severe cases by nearly twenty per cent. (Young and Williams, *Boston Med. and Surg. Jour.*, Mar. 14, 1912). Currettage increases mortality ten per cent—one intra-uterine douche of salt solution seems best; while serums and vaccines have no effect for good. Here we have another epoch in therapy, and another illustration of the incalculable value of cool air. Yet we are sorry to see the authors drag in the old dogma that the general benefit and the increase of

hemoglobin are due to sunshine as much as to fresh air. They can convince themselves of their error by putting the patients out in the sun some noon-day when the thermometer is about 100° F. in the shade. In the meantime let us call attention to the fact that Lawrason Brown has only recently shown (*J. A. M. A.*, June 1, 1912) that his consumptives do worst in the sunny season, and in the hottest and coldest, and that there is plenty of evidence elsewhere published that too much light diminishes the hemoglobin or its oxygen carrying capacity. Until they bring proofs that sunshine cures their cases and not the cool fresh air, as explained by Brown, we must deny the accuracy of their observation, and suggest that if on very sunny days the patients are shaded outdoors the improvement will be greater and that hot air will only do injury. In the literature of the last few years there has not been presented, as far as we know, one single bit of evidence that sunshine is beneficial to us except where it is used locally to irritate or destroy, as in lupus or open infected ulcers. Nevertheless, several articles have repeated parrot-like this old baseless unproved dogma of the need in all conditions of plenty of the sunshine which always irritates or destroys, and from which nature does her best to guard us by pigmentation.

***

"Home work" for school children has been condemned so thoroughly by both teachers and physicians that it is not a little surprising it should still be the routine practice in so many schools. The medical objection is based on the fact that the evening—the only time a child can do the work—is the period of greatest fatigue in the twenty-four hours. Results are obtained only at great expense of energy with the inevitable exhaustion. In addition, the fatigued brain does not retain impressions well if at all, but in the morning hours when the brain is fresh more can be accomplished and remembered in a mere fraction of the time spent when tired. Evening is "story-time" the world over, and to deprive the little hungering minds of this delight is nothing short of a crime and a cruel one at that. The enjoyment of stories or games is highly recuperative and if not carried to excess, it is the best possible preparation for a sound sleep all night,—nature's sweet restorer. Night work often irritates the brain so greatly that sleep is impossible and the child has to be taken from school for that reason alone.

Home work for high school students is a subject we have not cared to attack because of their greater age and the impression that a little home work was really necessary, though the same principles apply as with the younger children. We are now delighted to know that the Newark High School has tried the plan of having the "home-work" done in the school house with results so good as to be beyond the wildest dreams of the advocates of the new system. Not only have the students made better progress than ever before, but from reading between the lines of the reports it is safe to assume that they are in far better health both physically and mentally. The system seems destined to become universal, but why was it not tried out long ago? We have known for years that "half-timers" who had to work for their living half of every day, made more progress than the full timers who had not the recuperative benefit of a half-day's ex-

ercise. Schools seem too quick to take up fads but too slow to correct defects in the system. Now let us go a step further and try to induce college and university students to give up night work and go to bed so they can get up early to work in the mornings when they will be able to do more in half the time without any drain on the nervous system.

· **Criticisms of our hospitals** are far from uncommon, but it has remained for a recent medical visitor to our land to precipitate a discussion for and against our hospital system that has undoubtedly attracted more attention than any for many a day. Dr. Henri Neumann, the critic in question, is able to speak more authoritatively than most men, not alone because of his very considerable experience in hospital administration but also because of the careful study and investigation he has just made of our leading clinical institutions. In a way, the discussion—conducted in the main in the daily press—has been very amusing and our distinguished visitor in laying emphasis on the value of autopsies was quoted, for example, to the effect that patients who went into European hospitals thoroughly understood on entering that a post-mortem examination would be made; that it was a rule of every institution, a matter of routine and patients had grown to expect it! It is perhaps facetious on our part to point out that a post-mortem examination is the very last thing that patients expect in entering our American institutions. And if autopsies are few and far between in the routine of our leading hospitals, is not this fact a matter for congratulation? Does it not offer a very significant as well as gratifying comment on the efficiency of our methods? Finally in

472   AMERICAN MEDICINE
Complete Series, Vol. XVIII. }   EDITORIAL COMMENT   { SEPTEMBER, 1912.
New Series, Vol. VII., No. 9.

saving a patient from the autopsy table—snatching, as it were, "a brand from the burning"—are we not approaching closer to the ideals of hospital treatment? But enough of this. Dr. Neumann undoubtedly simply intended to convey the idea that European patients felt quite differently toward autopsies, and unlike our American patients have been taught the desirability of post-mortem examinations when unavoidable conditions make them possible. Therefore, in spite of the ambiguity of Dr. Neumann's remarks—for which his interviewer must be blamed—his real intent is plain. Post-mortem examinations most assuredly are not pursued as they should be in our charitable institutions. While this is largely attributable to the widespread sentiment in opposition to post-mortem mutilation, and the consequent difficulty of inducing relatives to allow autopsies, it must be admitted that few of our leading clinicians exert themselves very strenuously in this direction. That post-mortem study is of great value no one will deny. As far as the people are concerned, autopsies are largely a matter of education, and as the benefits to science are emphasized their acquiescence is much more easily obtained. But the profession itself is very lethargic in this direction and until more zeal and ambition develop for post-mortem study, this important and highly productive field of investigation is bound to be neglected. It may be true, as some point out, that surgical progress has brought the various internal organs under such frequent scrutiny that autopsies are becoming less and less necessary. But the careful painstaking study of a cadaver offers opportunities for acquiring information, leisurely and thoroughly, that surgery can never supply. Some one has said

that autopsies are disappointing, they so seldom corroborate our diagnoses! Could a more eloquent argument be made in behalf of post-mortem examinations? Dr. Neumann has done us a real favor in showing this particular lack of our hospitals, and pointing out that in neglecting to secure an autopsy whenever possible we are losing one of the principal advantages of our public medical institutions.

Hospital efficiency very naturally came in for its share of consideration in Dr. Neumann's discussion and our methods of administration, system of medical service and general management suffered severely in his comparison with the methods and systems in vogue in European institutions. While in these matters we are inclined to feel that our learned critic is perhaps somewhat prejudiced, and that the relative efficiency of American and European hospitals may very properly be looked upon as open to controversy, we are quite ready to admit that a great majority of our foremost American clinical institutions deserve criticism on more than one count. If our memory serves us right, moreover, the recollection of conditions noted only a few years ago in more than one prominent hospital in Europe leads us to believe that there may also be room for improvement in some of these institutions that Dr. Neumann considers so superior to our own. The fact is hospitals the world over are not measuring up to their highest efficiency, and while European institutions may be better conducted in some respects, and their administration generally be more satisfactory, in certain definite details they are no nearer perfection than those in this country.

One thing is certain, we are under no delusions as to the conditions that obtain in the administration of American hospitals. No smug complacency blinds us to urgent needs of improvement, and this recognition of the situation promises real substantial progress. The great drawback to greater efficiency, in this country at least, has been lack of public interest. In many communities the hospitals have been looked upon as institutions provided mainly for medical benefit and convenience. This has largely come from the fact that in small cities the hospitals have usually been organized by medical men and kept alive by professional interest. Of course there are many exceptions and most institutions have sooner or later attracted the attention and received the support of certain public spirited men and women of each community. But there is no denying the fact that the people at large have not taken the interest that they should in their local hospitals nor familiarized themselves with the ways and means of raising their efficiency to the highest. Until our hospitals become more public, in the sense that they must be better appreciated, their advantages more thoroughly recognized and more general and consistent support be given them, they are bound to fall short of accomplishing the good they can.

When we see how some of our hospitals have to struggle on with support so meagre that it is sometimes a marvel how they continue to exist, there can be little surprise that they have failed to measure up to every ideal. The real wonder is that they have done so much, have been conducted so well, and have been so free from gross abuse. It is a high testimonial to the medical profession of America that our hospitals have done what they have for the people in the face of opposition, prejudice, ignorance and indifference. The people are just waking up to what has been accomplished by earnest medical men, and while dissatisfaction with our hospitals is a good sign and augurs well for the interest and cooperation that is so essential to future progress, it should not be overlooked that most institutions have been seriously handicapped. Let us be tolerant therefore with the shortcomings of our American hospitals, and while welcoming the splendid prospects that promise such substantial improvements all along the line, never fail to realize the good honest work that has been done day in and day out for years—and this in spite of indifference, ignorance and deep rooted prejudice on the part of many who instead of upholding and aiding the hospitals of their communities have been most active in opposing them. Criticism is good if kindly and well intentioned. But in criticising the hospitals of America let us be fair enough to realize that the lack of efficiency we deplore has many times been due to conditions that have been unavoidable. As the people grow in intelligence and judgment many of these conditions are certain to disappear and on these grounds alone we have every reason to expect a gratifying increase in hospital efficiency—but it all rests on the people.

———

The short professional life of trained nurses has long been known, but it seems to be attracting more attention recently. The trend of the remarks partake of the nature of a charge that young women deliberately regard the calling as a stepping stone to matrimony. It is further stated that this attitude makes it impossible for them to take their work seriously or in that altruistic way necessary for success. Commercialism is said to be replacing humanity, and love of man destroying love of mankind. Well, perhaps this is largely true,—girls will be girls,—but is it so black as painted? Boys enter a calling as a life work, to be able to care for a wife and babies later. That's nature. The girl's nature is matrimony too; that is, the healthy girl's. Can she be expected to be so unnatural as to live an isolated life? Experience shows that the strain of self-support is too great for female nerves and physique and early breakdown results. In very few callings do we ever find women of middle age who show anything like the comparative vigor of men of the same decade of life. As far as we know, every class of female labor is considered a temporary employment and not a life calling. It is almost invariably exchanged for the more normal family life—if the right man comes along.

The advantages of a short professional nursing life are so great that we need not worry over the early desertions. In the first place it is a most unnatural life. Woman always is the nurse to be sure, but the patient is a relative for whom she is willing to make enormous sacrifices. It is asking rather too much of them to make similar sacrifices all the time for strangers, as our altruists imply they should. Though they are instinctively the best fitted for the duty it is one which in natural family conditions lasts but a few days or weeks at a time, and requires a long period of rest. If it is kept up, collapse is the invariable rule. The physique can not stand it. Many professional nurses do break down, and many more stop because they feel the break coming. For these reasons the work should be in the hands of the young and vigorous who can bend to the strains and not break. Then again, the elderly woman has not the necessary quickness of perceptions and the ability to act promptly in emergencies. She does not need them after the child bearing period and by ordinary biologic laws she loses them. The woman of 20 in spite of her ignorance, is far better able to raise her baby than the woman of 40—the end of the period of childbearing in primitive times when our physique took its present form and rates of decay. So we must have young hands, and nerves and bodies for the work, and it is not at all an unmixed evil that nurses leave us just when their experience and wisdom are at the maximum. We would like to have them stay with us awhile longer than they do, but an average of four or five years is as much as we can expect, and the schools must have under training at least one-fourth as many as are in professional work. So let them drift back to their true profession of being a woman and let us stop worrying over their womanliness. Of course the nursing profession is a temporary one and of course the nurses will marry; but it is good to have young aids even if one of them, now and then, is a wee bit flighty and inexperienced. As for pay, they must live; and the remunerations are so pitifully small for the intermittent work of self-supporting people that the charge of commercialism is ridiculous. If it were any less, the ranks would be restricted exclusively to those who live at home, supported by parents and who took up the life for charity or pin money—both types utterly beyond discipline or dependableness.

ORIGINAL ARTICLES.

CALVIN AND SERVETUS: AN EPISODE IN THE HISTORY OF RELIGIOUS PERSECUTION AND SCIENTIFIC SUPPRESSION.

BY

JOHN KNOTT, A. M., M. D.
Dublin, Ireland.

The quiet French town of Vienne has, I understand, utilized the opportunity afforded by the coming of the quarter centenary anniversary of the birth of its celebrated and illfated (naturalized) medical citizen Michael "Villanovanus" by erecting a dignified monument to the memory of the most *deservedly* famous of the past makers and masters of medicine. For some twelve years, or so, of the mesial segment of the restless sixteenth century, a singularly studious, and somewhat peculiarly secluded, Doctor of Physic exercised, within its precincts the functions of his profession —under the special patronage and protection of its genial Archbishop, Pierre Paumier. He was known to the general public as Dr. Michel Villeneuve. He had, very evidently—and very fruitfully, taken all knowledge for his province; and continuously cultivated every accessible portion of his chosen domain with the most devoted industry. He was an intensely earnest student of both science and literature, and made many original and important contributions to the common funds of each. Like other men of that unusual type, he was rather solitary in his habits. But he loved his profession, and his patients loved him; for nobody questioned the superiority of his skill and attainments, while his unvarying kindness and unfailing attention were the common property of both rich and poor, when visited by bodily affliction of any kind. Of his early history and antecedents nothing appeared to be known. He was not a native; he was not even a Frenchman. The Archbishop —as a junior ecclesiastic—had made his acquaintance in Paris, where the young physician, after an exceptionally brilliant curriculum, had made himself disconcertingly conspicuous in the eyes of the senior dons, of theology as well as of medicine, by a somewhat aggressive originality of thought. This liberal-minded dignitary of the then much-agitated church did not, however, hesitate to make the brilliant young foreigner his bosom friend and trusted medical adviser. Accordingly, when opportunity offered, he imported him to Vienne; and made him a partaker of his own palatial residence. And seldom, indeed, has a more curiously interesting, and strangely isolated individual trodden the thorny pathway of science, in the pilgrimage from this world to that which is to come!

It was only at the close of this series of years of apparent happiness and relative worldly prosperity that the repose of Dr. Villeneuve's existence was—very abruptly, and very alarmingly—interrupted; and, as subsequent events far too definitely demonstrated, brought to its final termination this world. On March 16, 1553, Dr. Villeneuve was sought by certain judicial functionaries of Vienne; and subjected to a searching "interview" and cross-examination, on the subject-matter of very important documentary evidence which had been placed in their hands by the officials of the Inquisition—who had themselves been placed in possession of the same by the automatic intervention of a Geneva correspondent. After a series of laborious preliminary inquiries, a solemn meeting of Council was convened within the Archiepiscopal Chateau of Roussillon, which included: Cardinal Tournon, the Archbishop of Vienne (Paumier, the old-standing friend and patron of Villeneuve), two Grand Vicars, Matthew Ovy (Cardinal Tournon's specially-trained Roman agent; *Pénitencier du Saint Siége Apostolique, et Inquisiteur général du Royaume de France et dans toutes les Gaules*); and a number of prominent ecclesiastical officials and doctors of divinity. At the close of a searching scrutiny and debate, with the unanimous concurrence of the members of this Assembly, orders were issued for the immediate arrest of Michel Villeneuve, physician, and Balthasar Arnoullet, bookseller; to answer for their faith regarding certain charges and informations to be placed in evidence against them.

And now for a digression—of which the preliminary move is in the direction of coincidence. Historians and biographers who have read themselves deeply into the depths of their special subjects of research have often been struck by strangely interesting coincidences of dates, in connection with the life-histories of individuals of communities, of nations, and of races. So have astronomers, and meteorologists, and general physicists. Even those who are least disposed to recognize the interference of the supernatural in matters physical or mundane must admit the temporal coincidence, in many striking instances, of events otherwise utterly unconnected, and their subsequent development of mutual influence to a degree which savours of the mysterious. And among the curious record of matters anthropological and ethnological must be reckoned some of those connected with birth and death. We are

told that Virgil was born on the day on which Lucretius died; Cervantes and Shakespeare died on the same day; Robert Boyle was born in the year which saw the death of Francis Bacon; Isaac Newton first saw the light in the course of the same annual cycle which produced the final extinction of the long-faded glimmer that dimly guided the closing years of the earthly pilgrimage of Galileo Galilei.

The trial of Dr. "Villeneuve" brought before the public eye some very unexpected revelations. It was ascertained that his original name was Miguel Serveto. He gave Tudela (of Navarre) as the place of his nativity, and his age as 42. This would make 1511 the date of the latter. But he subsequently (at Geneva) declared that he was born at Villanova (in Arragon); and having regard to the name which he had adopted, and the removal of inducements to prevarication, that statement seems far more likely to represent the biographical fact. The date given on this latter occasion was 1509; which may, I think, be also safely assumed to be the correct one. Now this same year of 1509 witnessed the birth, in the old French province of Picardy, of another individual who, like Miguel Serveto, was predestined to have much influence on the future progress of European thought and intellectual enlightenment. This contemporary (and future telepathic correspondent) of Miguel Serveto bore the name of Jean Chauvin— one which unquestionably secured the world-wide attention of contemporaries and of posterity in its Latinized version of Johannes Calvinus. John Calvin was the son of a cooper, resident in the French village of Noyon; Michael Servet appears to have been the son of a jurist—probably of the Spanish town of Villanova, although certainty in this matter does not appear to be attainable; and the subject of the inquiry gave, on other occasions, the respective names of Tudela and Saragossa as the seat of his nativity. Each was gifted by nature with the restless activity of genius, and each displayed throughout life the very characteristic feature of every—or almost every—bearer of that doubtful blessing: the native incapacity to limit his mental exertions to the locality and direction of a single groove; to expend the resources of his intellectual capacity while working in a rut, after the manner of most "practical" and "common-sense" members of the various sections of modern civilization. The educational adolescence of Jean Chauvin was devoted to the profession of law, the pursuit of which he elected to abandon for that of theology; Miguel Serveto appears to have been originally destined to the church, a choice which yielded pretty early to the attraction of law; the latter succumbing in its turn to that of the broader and more sympathetic inducements offered to the curious and philosophical student in the limitless mazes of the fascinating domain of medicine. Neither was blessed with robust health; great students seldom, if ever, are; Calvin's whole life was one long disease, and Servet, who appears to have been the subject of a congenital—or early developed —hernia, was naturally endowed with the energies of a student rather than those of the athlete. Let us not, however, regard them as unfortunate on such account: each had been liberally supplied with the gifts of the *mind*, not those of *matter*.

On two successive days, April 5 and 6 of that memorable year of 1553, Dr. Michel "Velleneuve" was arraigned before the representative officers of the Inquisition; and gravely questioned—upon "Gospel oath"—regarding his personal identity, his especial antecedents, and his gravely doubtful theological opinions. His neighbours and patients at Vienne then, for the first time, learned something of the early history of their highly-gifted physician. His father was a notary, of hereditary legal descent; his mother's family, Revés by name, was of French origin; his ancestors on both sides of the house were "d'ancienne race, vivants noblement." Having received the conventual education of early boyhood, he entered the University of Saragossa, which then occupied the zenith of contemporary classic and scientific fame; whence he emerged in time to enter the school of Toulouse as a law student. He there pursued his studies with characteristic industry and insatiable variety of mental appetite; and, among other new intellectual experiences, made his first acquaintanceship with the text of the Old and New Testament. The cross-fertilization of legal and theological germs which the productive mind of Servetus displayed under the influence of his varied reading is often displayed in his writings. A curious—and personally characteristic instance may be noted here: he points out that in the covenant between Jehovah and Abraham we have the earliest recorded case of one of the four forms of unindentured contract—then known to legists as the *Facio ut facias*. From Toulouse he entered—presumably as secretary—the service of the Franciscan friar, Juan Quintana, who was then confessor to the Emperor Charles V; whom he accompanied to the Imperial coronation ceremony at Bologna, and thence to the Diet of Augsburg. Both these uniquely interesting experiences must have greatly influenced the receptive mind of Servetus, and the skilled reader may easily recognize in many of his writings of after years vivid reflections of the impressions then received. That conveyed by the Papal section of the great historic proceedings at the crowning of Charles was decidedly unfavorable, and some of his comment thereon could be taken as representative of Martin Luther in his most emphatic paroxysms of vituperation. So we are not surprised to find him soon, after the great Ausburg meeting, emerging, in his hankering pursuit of evasive truth, as a free lance among the most noted of the Swiss reformers. His queries and expressed opinions had come to prove a source of spiritual trouble to 'Œcolampadius, who found them sufficiently important to bring under the notice of his confreres (Bucer, Bullinger, Zwingli, &c.) at a meeting in Baste in 1530—when Servetus had just reached his majority. And even the usually tolerant and fair-minded Zwingli emphatically expressed his horror at the dissemination of such views as those reported of the young Spanish enthusiast: "ein unleydlichen Sach in der Ryrchen Gottes." A more definitely tangible error was perpetrated by our restless enthusiast in the following year; for a printed volume appeared which bore on its title-page: *De Trinitatis Erroribus, Libri Septem. Per Michaelem Serveto, alias Revés, Ab Aragonia, Hispanum, 1531.* The printer and publisher, each respectively more wise in his generation than the single-minded knight-errant of imprisoned and tortured science, had judiciously avoided the production of their names. The impression made by the contents of the book may be fairly surmised when we learn that Bucer,

usually one of the most gentle and humane of the reformers, after denouncing it and its author from the pulpit, declared that the writer of such a volume deserved to be disembowelled and hewn into pieces. The appearance of the work hopelessly wrecked his chances of ever finding favour in the eyes of the Swiss Reformers; and, accordingly, after the issue of a small appendicular booklet, *Dialogi de Trinitate,* we find him shaking off the dust of the Alpine stronghold of religious and political freedom, and emerging directly in the midst of the university of the brilliant French metropolis with all the symptoms of his incurable intellectual *bulimia* as thick upon him as ever. The professions of law and of theology having been laboriously explored and conscientiously sounded, further voyaging on their troubled waters was—for the present, at least—definitely abandoned; in case of the former probably through loathing, in that of the latter probably in despair. Our adventurous student was duly registered in the Paris University as Michel Villeneuve (of Saragossa!)—which surname was retained down to the date of his examination before the authorities of church and state in Vienne. He entered as a student of mathematics; after a two-years residence (1532-4) he left for Lyons—probably influenced by needful finance—and worked there, with his usual untiring application, as "proof-reader" to the printing-house of the famous and scholarly Trechsels; as editor of some of their most celebrated new editions; and as original author. Another important event may have tended to determine a temporary retirement from Paris; he there for the first time cannoned against the evil genius of his career, the Reformer of future world-wide fame, his contemporary John Calvin.

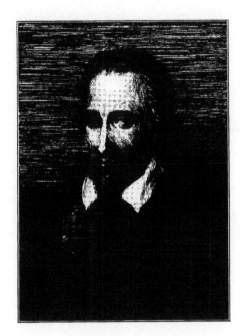

Michel servetus

It will easily be conceived by those who have studied the respective records of those two enthusiastic and self-willed seekers of truth that a collision was inevitable. After some preliminary private debates, a public discussion was agreed on, but Villeneuve failed to appear—so that Calvin scored a silent victory. His opponent pretty surely recognized that he could not defend his special opinions without exposing the au-. thorship of his notorious *De Trinitatis Erroribus,* which at that date would inevitably have doomed him to the fate of a heretic. So that he then, at least, proved that he possessed sufficient discretion to adopt the better part of valour.

One of the engagements of Servetus with the Trechsel firm was the preparation of a new edition of Ptolemy's *Geography* (1535). This famous work included, of course, a section descriptive of *Judaea.* The whole work was very carefully annotated by *Michael Villanovanus;* and one of the outlets of his indiscreet zeal for scientific truth is displayed in his comment on the physical characteristics of the "land flowing with milk and honey":—"Know, however, most worthy reader, that it is mere boasting and untruth when so much of excellence is ascribed to this land; the experience of merchants and others, travellers who have visited it, proving it to be inhospitable, barren, and altogether without amenity." (*Willis's version*). And this same note in the fateful future furnished effective material to the *fiery* zeal of John Calvin, by whom it was put forward in evidence at the trial of the writer for heresy in Geneva: as an incriminating document which not merely impeached the veracity of Moses but "grievously outraged the Holy Ghost!" The general comment at the time too, must have displayed an unusual degree of em-

phasis; for the portion of this note which might be regarded as dangerously unorthodox was cancelled by Servetus when preparing the next edition (1541).

No further event of the private or public life of the Viennese physician appears to have attracted special notice down to the date of the unexpected attention of the officials of the Inquisition; an attention which, as already mentioned, was elicited by special information forwarded from Geneva —the then city of refuge of the victims of religious persecution, from all the countries of Western Europe! And the thrillingly morbid interest associated with this probably unique event is based upon the how, as well as the why and wherefore, of the supply of this damning information: from a denizen of the favored fortress of religious and political freedom to the active agents of an institution which was unanimously denounced by the refugee dwellers in that Alpine stronghold as the most uncompromising and ruthless enemy of both. An examination of these questions necessarily involves the exposure of the principal details of what is regarded by the present writer as one of the foulest transactions which stains the dark pages of the criminal history of the human race.

We have seen that Servetus, as a junior enthusiast, had made himself personally known to (one at least of) the leaders of the Reformation in Switzerland; and utterly objectionable to all teachers of Western Christendom—both orthodox and heretical—by his printed opinions on the subject of the Trinity. Also that he had immediately afterwards, in Paris, come into personal (and controversial) contact with the future "Protestant Pope," John Calvin. There is no doubt that the heretical opinions of Michael Servetus ever after stuck deep in the soul of John Calvin; and the unnecessarily, and insolently, contradictory tone which was usually adopted by the former in his disputatious correspondence with the spoiled and morbidly sensitive Geneva leader, fanned the glowing temperature of the unsurpassable *odium theologicum* of the latter to a sizzling white-hot degree beyond which the readings of the ethical thermometer can furnish no record. Just a little over seven years before the arrest of Servetus, Calvin had forwarded to that detested rival and troublesome correspondent a copy of. his representative work, *Institutiones Religionis Christianae,* as the most comprehensive and satisfactory reply to the complex queries with which he was pestered. The volume was in due course of time returned, with copious—and evidently hypercritical—marginal annotations; in the language of Calvin to a confidential correspondent: "there is hardly a page that is not defiled by his vomit." And in strict accordance with this growing display of celestial charity, we have his letter of that period to his trusted coadjutor Farel (dated Ides of February, 1546), which includes the following sentences: "Servetus nuper ad me scripsit, ac literas adjunxit longum volumen suorum deliriorum, cum thrasonica jactantia, dicens me stupenda et hactenus inaudita visurum. Si mihi placeat, huc se venturum recipit. Sed nolo fidem meam interponere. Nam si venerit, modo valeat mea authoritas, vivum exire nunquam patiar." (As Englished by Willis: "Servetus wrote to me lately, and beside his letter sent me a great volume full of his ravings, telling me with audacious arrogance that I should there find things stupendous and unheard of until now. He offers to come hither if I approve; but I will not pledge my faith to him; for

did he come, if I have any authority here, I should never suffer him to go away alive"). Such was the unspeakable travesty of Christian charity and forbearance which was taught and practised by the "Pope of Geneva"—himself a fugitive heretic whose life had been long under the ban of the authorities of the Catholic Church.

The opportunity for which Calvin had so long yearned and prayed came to him at last—in the early months of 1553. His friendly bookseller, Arnoullet, had printed for Servetus, with all imaginable precautions of secrecy, a volume bearing the title:

"CHRISTIANISMI RESTITUTIO. Totius Ecclesiæ Apostolica est ad sua limina vocatio, in Integrum Restituta Cognitione Dei, Fidei Christi, Justificationis nostræ Regenerationis Baptismi, et Cœnæ Domini Manducationis Restitutio denique nobis Regno Cœlesti, Babylonis impia Captivitate soluta, et Antichristo cum suis penitus destructo."

And to give further dignified emphasis to the paramount theological importance which our Viennese physician evidently attached to his anonymous volume, there was subscribed a motto—beneath the above title—in Hebrew, and in Greek. Did the coming events cast their shadows before, when poor Servetus chose the quotation: Καὶ ἐγένετο πόλεμος ἐν τῷ οὐρλνῷ. The date, MDLIII, concluded the contents of the title page of one of the most interesting volumes known to the annals of (at least, uninspired) authorship and of typography; which thus presented neither the name of author, publisher, or printer; nor the address of any of the same. In mysterious secrecy and silence this book was ushered into existence; in flaming publicity and explosive execration it was soon whisked out of the world—with a completeness of (approximate) annihilation which has hardly ever been paralleled.

In order, as one might be easily led to think, that the theological sponge of Calvin's gall and vinegar might be soaked even to supersaturation, the volume contained thirty epistles to that uncompromising doctrinaire —representing, with approximate exactness, the documents which had been from time to time furnished, during their years of contradictory controversy. And in addition to the full elucidation of the author's up-to-date views and solutions of his special theological theorems, the text included many pregnant incidental allusions to illustrative (scientific as well as historic and logical) data. To one of these I will afterwards invite the special attention of all readers. The question which now requires elucidation is: How came the evidence against Dr. Michel Villeneuve into the hands of the officials of the Inquisition? There exists a *Vie du Calvin* by a surviving contemporary, Dr. Bolsec, who had had the temerity to enter the theological arena with the uncompromising Reformer of Geneva. Calvin did not fail to have his opponent indicted of heresy; and had so far succeeded as to have secured the conviction of Bolsec on the minor counts—which meant death by decapitation—when the "Libertine" section of the Genevese authorities suggested that before pressing controversy so far as to adopt the methods of martyrdom, the unanimous votes of the Swiss Reformed Churches should be obtained. Accordingly, Berne, Zurich and Neuchatel were respectively questioned, and they all voted against extreme measures. The prosecution accordingly collapsed; Dr. Bolsec *won by a neck!* In his Life of Calvin, this his surviving opponent states that the latter wrote with his own hand to Cardinal de Tournon, informing him of the damnable opinions fostered and privately propagated by his neighbour, Dr. "Villeneuve"; and that his Eminence laughed to scorn the idea of receiving from an arch-heretic information against a questionable culprit of minor magnitude. Bolsec would appear to be the only available authority for this statement. Accordingly, the friends and advocates of Calvin have repudiated his evidence, in this particular—as largely biassed, if not absolutely invented. They have surely some plausible grounds for the soft impeachment —when Bolsec's hair-breadth escape and the usual trend of human passions and feelings are simultaneously considered! But whatever the original fact may have been, the accusers of John Calvin may let this count of their indictment go; if he did not do what Bolsec says, he, most assuredly, did what, in the classic phraseology of a former Lord Mayor of Dublin, was "aiquilly worse"; for—being skilled in the controversial tactics of law, as well as in those of theology—he *forced* his evidence under the notice of the agents of the Inquisition in such a way that they were obliged—as representative agents of an official body—to give it their fullest consideration: and the way he did it was this. There was then resident at Geneva a refugee from Lyons, who, as a Calvinistic convert, had placed himself—for protection, both physical and spiritual—under the wing of his great leader. This individual, who rejoiced in the name of Guillaume Trie, maintained a correspondence with an orthodox cousin at Lyons; who continually reproached him with his lapse from the true faith, and as continuously urged on him the necessity of his return to the straight and narrow path from which he had so unwisely deviated. At the season which we have now reached, Trie wrote to this cousin (whose name was Arneys) a memorable letter, which includes a ponderous retort, and explicit information:

"As to what you say about there being so much more of freedom, or latitude of opinion, with us here than with you, still we should never suffer the name of God to be blasphemed, nor evil doctrines and opinions to be spread abroad among us, without let or hinderance. And I can give you an instance which, I must say, I think tends to your confusion. It is this: that a certain heretic is countenanced among you, who ought to be burned alive, wherever he might be found. And when I say a heretic, I refer to a man who deserves to be as summarily condemned by the Papists, as he is by us. . . . The man I refer to has been condemned in all the Churches you hold in such dislike, but is suffered to live unmolested among you, to the extent of even being permitted to print books full of such blasphemies as I must not speak of further. He is a Spanish-Portuguese, Michael Servetus by name, though he now calls himself Villeneuve, and practises as a physician. He lived for some time at Lyons, and now resides at Vienne, where the book I speak of was printed by one Balthasar Arnoullet. That you may not think I speak of mere hearsay I send you the first few leaves as a sample for your assurance. . . . ."

The leaves referred to in this precious document were the four printed ones which had been forwarded to Calvin by the too impetuous—and too confiding—author, Michael Servetus. It is quite needless to trace the intermediate steps of their transference. The good and orthodox Arneys immediately consulted his confessor; the letter and enclosed printed matter were communicated to Ory, the representative of the Inquisition, and to Bautier, the Canon of the Cathedral of Lyons. Hence the interview, the examination, and the consignment to durance vile, of the generally unobtrusive physician of Vienne! How closely the proceedings at this city were watched from the Geneva refuge is well shown in another letter written exactly a month later (February 26—March 26), which may safely be held to distance its forerunner in its unsurpassable combination of hypocrisy and malignity. After some introductory observations it proceeds:—"But as you have shown to others the letter I meant for yourself alone, God grant that it tend to purge Christianity of such filth, of pestilence so mortal to man! If your people are really so anxious to look into the matter as you say, there will be no difficulty in furnishing you, besides the printed book you ask for, with documents enough to carry conviction to their minds. For I shall put into your hands some two dozen pieces written by him who is in question, in which some of his heresies are set prominently forth. Did you rely on the printed book by itself, he might deny it as his; but this he could not do if his own handwriting were brought against him. In this way the parties you speak of, having the thing completely proven, will be without excuse if they hesitate further, or put off taking the steps required. All the pieces I send you now—the great volume as well as the letters in the handwriting of the author—were produced before the printed work; but I have to own to you that I had great difficulty in getting these documents from Mons. Calvin. Not that he would not have such execrable blasphemies put down; but that, as he does not wield the sword of justice himself, he thinks it his duty rather to repress heresy by sound teaching, than to pursue it by force. I importuned him, however, so much, showing him the reproaches I might incur did he not come to my aid, that he consented at length to entrust me with the contents of my parcel to you. . . At the moment, I fancy you are furnished with evidence enough, and that there need be no more beating about the bush, before seizing on his person and putting him on his trial."

Dr. Michel Villeneuve accordingly was, as we have already seen, "put on his trial": thanks to the single-minded charity and Gospel purity of John Calvin. But the proceedings, formidable looking enough during the first few days, soon showed a tendency to hang fire. And, accordingly, an opportunity will be afforded us, bye-and-bye, in this connection, of comparing and contrasting the ways and means of the "bloody" and "fiery" *Inquisition,* at this period of its (necessarily) greatest activity and incessant irritation, with those adopted in a season of favourable opportunity by the zealous Reformer of Geneva. It need hardly be said that the heretical inmate of the Dauphinal prison of Vienne was personally know to—and respected by—his gaoler, who freely allowed him to take exercise in the garden of its enclosure. And on the morning of April 7, he actually arose at 4 a. m., and asked for the key of the garden door—which he received as a mere matter of ordinary civility. A raised terrace and shed abutted on the inside of the garden wall; while a buttress supported its outer side, which there limited the court-yard of the Palais de Justice. The sloping architecture of each easily lent itself to the facilitation of ascent and descent, respectively. Michael Servetus availed himself thereof on that special occasion, and the interior of the prison of Vienne saw him no more! Curiously enough, he was first missed by the wife of the gaoler, who in her paroxysm of distraction clambered about the roofs in the emission of a jeremiad which bewailed the breaking of the previously unsullied record of that model establishment. Then the alarm was followed up by the action of the authorities; every nook and cranny of Vienne underwent scrutiny of the most critical kind on that April morning; but the person of Dr. Michel Villeneuve (*alias* Serveto, *alias* Reves) was nowhere to be found. And, as the Inquisitorial authorities of that date possessed the proverbial reputation of being able to discover a lost needle in a bundle of hay, it is surely unnecessary to ask the reason why.

As soon as the culprit had escaped, his trial began to proceed as rapidly and satisfactorily as such procedure can; the missing heretic was convicted, sentenced, and burned at the stake—in effigy; the condemned *Restitutio* enjoyed its share of the combustion—to a degree of plenitude which probably remains unequalled in the fate of any doomed volume known to bibliographical history; the demands of orthodox equity would appear to have rested satisfied; and—the fiendish malignity of the espionage of John Calvin seemed to have badly missed its mark. And yet that enthusiastic Reformer ever continued to hope and to pray!

Michael Servetus was now at large to tread the thorny pathways of a world all (nominally, at least) thoroughly hostile to his person and to his cherished opinions. He had, however, slipped from between the jaws and fangs of the deadly Inquisition. And be it remembered by all interested readers, too, as a chain of associated facts of great historical and critical importance in the estimation of the various agencies of religious terrorism and persecution in that restless and ruthless generation, that France was then governed by King Henry II; Henry II was governed by *Diana of Poictiers;* while the latter was, in turn, governed—economically, even more than religiously—by Cardinal de Tournon and the representative agents of the Inquisition; *the principal perquisite of her private exchequer being furnished by the proceeds of the disposal of the confiscated goods of (and fines levied on) convicted heretics*—which had been graciously made over to her by a special mandate of her royal and devoted lover. Accordingly, the advocates and defenders of the Reformation would seem to have some solid grounds for their representation of the orthodox mechanism of the Gallican Church Government of that period as approximating to the worst possible, and crying aloud to heaven for a cataclysmic process of purification. Yet our heretical Spanish-Portguese saved his person—very easily too—from its most active representatives, during his long sojourn, and final trial and imprisonment, at Vienne. We shall now have an opportunity of contrasting his experience of the latter locality with the subsequent developments at Geneva which were initiated and carried out to their completion in that city of general refuge by the refugee heretic, John Calvin.

Miguel Serveto had already explored the pathways of all the principal sciences, and had made his own distinctive mark on each of their most important domains— and this proved to be, in many cases, a highly noticeable and important one. He had mastered, and exploited the mysteries of mathematics and of astrology; had done record work in geography; had added to contemporary medical knowledge in his work on *syrups;* had displayed profound powers of discrimination in the departments of textual criticism and theological dogma in his edition of the Bible; and much—far too much—boldness of speculation and originality of thought and point of view in his theses on the subject of the *Trinity,* and (most recently, and most fatally) in the pages of his *Christianismi Restitutio.* He would seem, pretty evidently, to have felt that there remained but one champion of controversy still unconquered who was really worthy of his intellectual steel. Accordingly, with the characteristic instinct of the true (or fabulous)

knight-errant—or of the intellectual parody of the pugilistic prize fighter, he could not rest till he had definitely measured his weapons and his skill against those of the redoubtable heresiarch of Geneva. How little did his simply confiding, and most unprophetic, soul foresee or suspect the moral capabilities of the latter! So the escaped and exiled votary of science, divine and human, after some weeks of apparently irregular and fruitless wandering bent his steps to the great central European city of refuge, to which had already thronged in that very troubled generation so many thousands of the votaries of State-persecuted religious systems; and so many, too, of the most expert and depraved of criminal outcasts, and of the specialized experts in the most advanced types of luxurious vice and license who could not bear the restraints imposed by the respectability of home life, or that of any well-united and well-governed community. The "Protestant Pope" was then at the zenith of his theological fame and civic influence. The devoted practice and application of his inflexibly rigid system of faith and morals undoubtedly did a great deal to restrain the explosive movements of the chaotic nuclei of which Genevan life was then so largely composed. Many of the prominent native citizens who thoroughly detested the man, and never missed a discreet opportunity of deriding his sanctimonious pretensions and self-selected apostolate, were only too glad to encourage his presence among them as a restraint upon the boisterous movements of the refugee martyrs and criminals who formed so considerable—and so very active—a proportion of the population of Geneva at that date. Calvin's undoubted devotion to what he regarded as the call of duty could not fail to win confidence and respect in any community of men, and one of the special results was that the representatives of the municipal government of the city availed themselves of his advice and assistance in the preparation of a reformed legal code—even long before he had himself been formally admitted to the citizenship of Geneva. And a very significant—and all to highly prophetic—fact is presented by the record that, while he made many and mostly very judicious changes in the direction of encouragement of religious thought and freedom of (well-ordered) individual action, he secured a conspicuous exception by retaining the old standard of punishment for major heresy —that of burning alive at the stake. The future *Pope of Geneva* had been originally trained for the legal profession—which he abandoned when he found that he was called by the spirit to the exercise of a loftier mission. He began his new career, as reformers are always sure to do, by appealing to the latent sense of justice and mercy of collective humanity. And he must be credited with enthusiasm and ardent application to the pursuit of what he had succeeded in persuading himself was the object of duty's call. After the inevitable preliminaries of misery and persecution he succeeded in attaining a position which can be paralleled by very few of the records collected in the history of the progress of human thought and opinion. Then he assumed the reins of spiritual power and the whip of scorpions associated therewith, and unquestionably utilized the latter with a degree of unblinking attention and ruthless vigor which has probably never been surpassed. By the time of the visit of Servetus to Geneva, Calvin had established his power therein—and therefore

—on so firm and secure a foundation that its influence radiated from that centre with phenomenal effect to every point on the circumference of European Christendom. No contemporary European monarch exercised so great an influence on men's minds, whatever may have been the comparative effect on their bodies. His theological opinions have elicited the comment —*pro* and *con*—of every considerable thinker of his generation. And he had on more than one occasion broken (paper-and-ink) swords with Michael Servet, who continued to remain one of the very few—I incline to think, indeed, the *only* controversial contemporary from whose intellectual panoply his arguments and assertions ever and anon recoiled in quite ineffective—if interestingly boomerang-like —fashion. Forgiveness was—at least it had certainly come at that stage of his career to be—no part of the theological theory or practices of John Calvin. He was more a disciple of the Hebrew *Torah* than of the Greek *Testament,* as every prominent opponent was made to feel.

(*To be continued*).

THE THERAPEUTIC DOSAGE OF X-RAY AND APPLICATION.[1]

With Special Reference to Subcutaneous Dose Calculation.

BY

WM. H. MEYER, M. D.,
New York City.

Of the various periods through which the medical art has progressed, none have been more productive of real advancement and benefit to mankind than that of the present

[1] Read before the Medical Society of the Borough of the Bronx, June 12, 1912. Preceded by a presentation of cases in illustration of the article.

generation. Of all the discoveries, it must be admitted that few are of greater importance than that of Prof. Roentgen; few can show more rapid advancement.

Yet several years' experience in the field of X-ray and electrotherapy, have convinced me that the merest tolerance of the subject is often all that can be expected.

No doubt there are numerous reasons why this is so. At the very outset, the discovery of the Roentgen ray was met with doubt and scepticism, until by actual test each had satisfied himself that a valuable new discovery had been made. Our ideas of things opaque were completely upset, and it took no little strain to change these notions.

Following the period of doubt came one of wild conjecture and almost endless imaginings of the wonderful possibilities of this apparently law upsetting agent.

Extravagant claims of the overenthusiastics soon brought about a period similar to the first; only that to doubt and scepticism has been added an undeserved condemnation.

One phase has been no less extreme than the other and it is from the last of these periods that I believe we are now recovering.

There are as earnest workers in the field of X-ray as there are in any other branch of medicine—quiet, unassuming but steadily searching the truth. Thanks to these men the improvement and advancement in roentgenology has well kept pace with surgery, chemistry, and biology, as witness alone the recent rapid strides in intraabdominal diagnosis. On the other hand this paper has not to do with the diagnostic value of the X-rays, but with their therapeutic value. Before entering upon greater detail, however, I cannot suppress a few

words concerning the ill repute to which roentgeno-therapeutic procedure has, in some respects fallen.

What but evil results can be expected when the janitor, pharmacist or orderly becomes the X-ray operator? And what can be expected even under the guise of medical supervision, can be judged as this article continues.

Undoubtedly much harm has been done the cause of roentgenology by some physicians who do X-ray work simply as a side line. With insufficient data and faulty technique they fail to produce the desired effect and both the patient and his numerous acquaintances become ardent enemies of a therapeutic and diagnostic procedure which when properly handled, is capable of the greatest good.

In an article of this size it is not possible to go deeply into the scientific side of the question, so one must be content only with a general description of the why and wherefore of roentgeno-therapy.

The bitter experience of the early workers with the X-rays led to more guarded experimentation concerning the action of this agent; so that today we have a fair working knowledge of its use and limitation.

It has been found that exposure to the rays brings about certain changes in living tissue which vary, not alone, according to the time and strength of irradiation, but also according to the resistance of the cell structures exposed.

One of the earliest conditions noted, among those engaged in the manufacture and testing of X-ray tubes, was sterility. The more exposed portions of the body became reddened or tanned; the hair fell out; the skin became shriveled and atrophied; while the most intensely rayed areas became inflamed and underwent degeneration and destruction.

It has been noted that the more highly organized structures are the earliest to be affected; thus is it possible to cause epilation and check secretion without damage to the remaining epidermis; likewise to affect the lymphatic and other glands without injuring surrounding tissues.

Time and space forbid a lengthy description of the actual pathological changes but enough has been said to show that the X-rays seem to have a peculiar selective action; yet it is preferred not to credit the ray with a faculty of selection, but to state that certain cells show a greater resistance to the devitalizing and destructive action of the ray than others.

The action of the X-ray may be roughly summarized as primary *stimulating,* in larger dosage *inhibitive,* still larger dosage causing *devitalization* with final *cell death* and *tissue destruction.* This is considering the X-rays as a whole, including whatever effect may be credited to electrical discharge. On the other hand attempts have been made at ray isolation; and there are times, when limited superficial action is desired, that the interposition of screen or filter to absorb the rays of low penetration are successfully employed.

Recalling the variance of cell resistance it is but natural to suppose that *any cell foreign to its surroundings would have the less resistance*—thus, *if it is possible to give a sufficient dose of X-radiance to devitalize and destroy a foreign cell element, without injuring the surrounding normal tissues beyond repair,* then do we establish a cure in every sense of the word. Likewise, because *special cell structures have been found to exert reduced resistance,* it is possible to mitigate glandular overactivity and

check secretion—with or without actual destruction; according to dosage. This then is the fine line which the successful roentgeno-therapist must draw. It explains why the (side line) radiologist fails, why the (hurry up) routine system of hospital cases is unsatisfactory, and why the employing

FIG. I.—SCHEMATIC ILLUSTRATION OF RADIOMETER OF HOLZKNECHT.

Scale for Sabouraud.

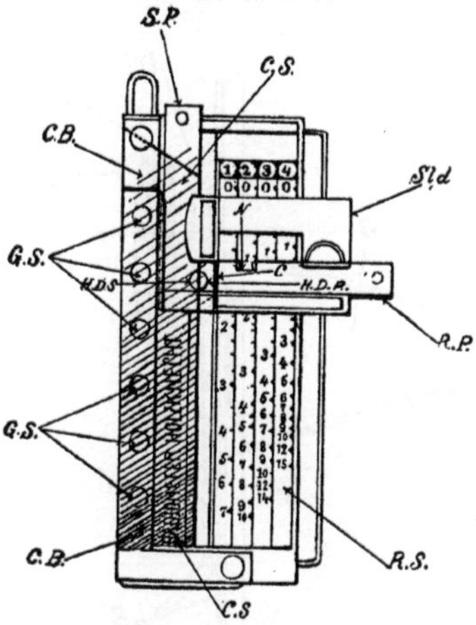

Fig. 1.—One-quarter Original Size. R. P., reaction or measuring piece. S. P., scale piece; both of these are seen inserted in the slider (Sld.) of the instrument. Sld., slider. C. B., color band or scale. C. S., continuous scale. G. S., graded scale. R. S., reading scale. H. D. R., half disk of platino-cyanide of barium at end of reaction piece. C., transparent piece of celluloid covering H. D. R. (2 and 7, Fig. 2). H. D. S., half disk of platino-cyanide of barium at end of scale piece. N, notch on reaction piece where reading is to be taken.

of untrained and nonprofessional radiologists is an insult to medical science.

Permit me to tax your patience with the more practical side of the qustion. We hear and read so much of what 10 minutes of X-rays, repeated so and so often, can do, that I cannot refrain from showing how little this means and that such statistics are worse than useless and should be banished from print.

Two systems of dosage are generally in vogue. In this country the ampere and milliamperemeter are apparently preferred; while in Europe the pastel systems of Holzknecht, Sabouraud, Kienböck, and others are the methods of choice. A word of ex-

pensive and have to be imported and further, they record only superficial dosage and give no clue whatever of the penetration of a given ray. In attempting the treatment of lesions beneath the surface, if it were true that greater intensity meant proportionate increased penetration then this system would be ideal, but this is not

Fig. II.—Schematic Illustration of Author's Gauge.

Side   Front

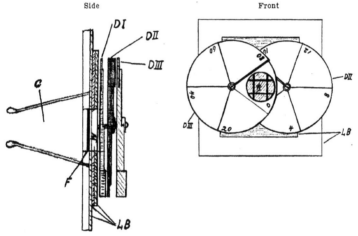

One-quarter Original Size.

(D 1) Disk 1; which is behind disk 3, has 4 consecutive thicknesses of metal ranging from ½x to 3x. Each 1x equalling the approximate thickness of 1 inch flesh. (D 2) Disk 2; ranges from 4x to 16x while (D 3) Disk 3, ranges from 20x to 80x.

These disks can be revolved so that any consecutive number of thicknesses can be brought before the window (W); this window being cut through a sufficient thickness of brass and lead (LB) to effectually obstruct the rays over the remaining area. The window itself is backed with a fluoroscope; (F) Fluorescent screen,—(C) Box.

The whole is mounted on an adjustable stand.

planation concerning the latter may be acceptable.

The pastels consist of sensitized films which react to the X-rays and are compared to a graded color standard—and at given distances are supposed to register the dosage. Among the difficulties encountered in this method are, that the films deteriorate rapidly and become inaccurate, they are ex-

the case. It has long been known that, under like excitation, a low vacuum tube would cause an X-ray dermatitis much quicker than a high tube; yet the latter has by far the greater penetration. Again a tube which through use, has become partly discolored, has had its bulb so altered that it emits a greater amount of soft rays than when new, irrespective of vacuum; thus a hard tube may be made to give soft ray effects; while still further discoloration again tends to reduce the intensity. From this it becomes apparent that the character and structure of the tube wall have a bearing on the kind of ray emitted. (In further substantiation of this it has been recently found that tubes blown of Strontium glass are very rich in soft rays).

There are other factors that have an influence on the quality and quantity of X-radiance and besides the *time* and *distance, current* and *frequency, tube vacuum* by estimating the degree of ray absorption, by various thicknesses of one metal, as compared to that of a fixed thickness of another. "In this latter instance it is necessary that the degree of ray absorption of the first metal vary proportionately with the number of thicknesses"—and that the second fixed standard offers a constant degree of opacity to rays of any quality. Such a meter is that of Benoist.

Yet with both pastels and penetrometers the dosage problem is not entirely solved. True the first gives us surface intensity and

Fig. III.—IMPROVED BENOIST PENETROMETER.

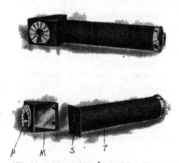

(P) Measuring piece backed by fluorescent screen; (M) Reflecting mirror; (T) Tube made to revolve so that examining slot (S) can be brought to expose different portions of the image of (P) on the mirror (M).

and *structure,* may be added the *size, shape* and *material of the target.*

Considering all this it becomes clear that any pastel system no matter how accurate of superficial dosage, gives no idea of penetration. For this purpose one must employ a penetrometer. The principle of all penetrometers is practically the same; namely the measuring of the penetration of a given ray by finding the number of thicknesses of a standard unit thickness of metal through which radioactivity is demonstrable or lost; (such is the author's gauge)—or the limitation of superficial dosage; but the latter gives only the penetration and not any idea of the intensity at various depths of tissue.

Experience with pastel dosimetry, or the knowledge of what constitutes the dermic limit of tolerance to X-radiance, is what is necessary for the satisfactory treatment of those superficial conditions, amenable to this mode of therapy.

In those cases where the maximum X-ray effect is desired just beneath the skin and where it is possible to ray only from one direction, then one must resort to filters to protect the epidermis from the effect of the soft rays and from the electrical discharge.

The filter I use in such cases consists of a thin sheet of aluminum backed by a sufficient thickness of leather to approximate the thickness of the overlaying flesh. The aluminum is used to form contact with the diaphragm and protective lead, the whole being insulated from the patient and grounded.

In this way though the skin receives the first impact of the filtered rays, yet greater dosage is possible and experience has shown that in this manner a sufficient degree of X-radiance, to be of value, can be brought to act upon subcutaneous lesions without seriously affecting the skin.

Thus, as far as superficial conditions are concerned the technique seems well enough but when considering deeper situated lesions then some other method becomes imperative for there is no doubt that failure in this line has been entirely due to the lack of internal dose estimation.

At this point it may be well to state the law to which the X-rays are reputed to conform, namely:

"The *intensity* of X-radiance varies *inversely* as the *square* of the distance from its source."

Quantitively speaking this is probably correct but only so far as surface intensity is concerned and providing the surface under bombardment does not itself become radioactive. But qualitively or when considering depth or penetration then this law does not hold.

A rule which seems to answer the purpose as far as the body is concerned and to which I have found that the X-rays seem to conform with but slight variance, is as follows:

"The penetration of X-rays vary *inversely* as the *square-root* of the distance from their source." As proof of this I offer the following chart and plate:

Experiment to verify the statement that (The Penetration of X-rays vary *inversely* as the *square-root* of the distance from their source).

N. B.—The set of 9 small plates were cut from one plate. The standard unit thickness of the 9 gauges are all the same with only a change in arrangement and size for convenience. The tube was a med. high taking 4 Mil-amp. with coil prim. at 16 Amp. Time ¼ minute. Development continued for 10 minutes. (All exposed at once).

DATA.

Exp. No.	1	2	3	4	5	6	7	8	9
Dist.	4"	7¼"	9"	12¼"	16"	20¼"	25"	36"	64"
Penet.	12*	9*	8*	–7*	6*	–5½*	–5*	4*	3*

N. B.   Dist. = Distance from target in inches.
Penet. = Number of thicknesses of penetration (last visible).

Example—A glance at the plates and chart data will show
that at 9 inches the penetration was 8*.
and at 36 inches the penetration was 4*.

Thus according to the above statement
Law 2 $\sqrt{9} = 3$ inverse $= \frac{1}{3}$.
and the $\sqrt{36} = 6$ inverse $= \frac{1}{6}$.

Therefore if $\frac{1}{3} = 8*$.
then $\frac{1}{6} = 4*$.
And since this example holds true with any of the above figures the law is verified.

Keeping both laws in mind; it will be noticed (according to my findings by the 2nd rule) that the increase of penetration, for instance, from 16 inches to 9 inches is but 2* yet the increase of intensity (according to the 1st law) is as $\frac{1}{256}$ is to $\frac{1}{81}$ respectively; thus if at 16 inches with this particular tube it would take ½ hour to produce an X-ray erythema, the same tube, with a gain of but ⅓ in penetration at 9 inches would produce a like dermatitis in less than 10 minutes—and at 4 inches but

2 minutes would elapse ere the danger point would be reached. (In this last instance it will be noted that the penetration is double what it was at 16 inches but the intensity is 15 times greater).

At first glance the value of a law of penetration may not be relevant; yet I have found the penetrometer backed by a law of penetration of considerable value; it has

the source as unity the following would be true:

Distance in inches	4″	9″	16″	25″ etc.
Intensity proportion	1/16	1/81	1/256	1/625

Second, according to the rule of penetration:

Distance in inches	4″	9″	16″	25″ etc.
Penetration proportion	½	⅓	¼	⅕

In order to better explain the interrelation of the two laws let us cite a specific in-

Fig. IV.—Schematic Illustration of Plate to Prove Penetration at Various Distances.

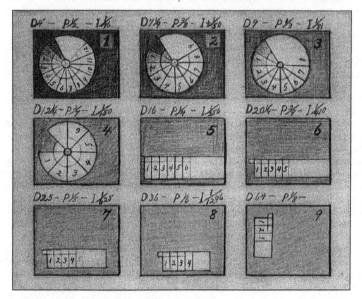

One-half Actual Size.

(D)=Distance from target in inches. (P)=Penetration proportion. (I)=Intensity proportion.

The small figures of the gauges indicate the number of thicknesses of penetration; each unit equalling 4x on author's gauge.

made it possible to predetermine results under any conditions and at any distance. Given a tube the ray intensity and penetration of which are known at a given distance it is possible to determine both the intensity and penetration at any other distance: First, according to the law of intensity, counting

stance; a case that recently came under my observation, one of inoperable cancer of the right side of the abdomen, involving the ascending colon.

The problem is as follows: How to calculate the dosage reaching a tumor approximately 3 inches beneath the surface, it being possible to ray the growth from different positions without the superficially rayed areas overlapping?

Supposing it is decided to keep the skin surface at a distance of 9 inches from the target with a diaphragm opening of 4 inches in diameter.

Supposing the tube selected, under known excitation, has a penetration of 36* on author's gauge at a distance of 9 inches from the target; also the erythema dose of the tube is known to be 30 minutes' exposure at the same distance.

Since the unit of measurement of the author's penetrometer (1*) offers practically the same resistance to X-radiance as 1 inch of flesh—then the penetrating power of the X-rays would be reduced 3* in passing through 3 inches of human flesh.

Since the penetration at the surface in this instance is 36* at +9 inches, it would be reduced to —31* at +12 inches without the added resistance of the body—and the interposition of the 3 inches of flesh reducing the penetration by 3*, leaves a penetrating power of 28* at the tumor site.

By referring to the (law proportions) it will be found that, without the interposition of flesh resistance, the penetration would not be reduced to 28* till —16 inches of space intervened.

At this distance (16 inches) the intensity has been reduced to $1/_{236}$ of its source and this is approximately ⅓ the intensity imparted over a like area at 9 inches, thus a 30 minute exposure under the above conditions would deliver ⅓ an erythema dose at 3 inches beneath the surface. Since in this case it is possible to ray the mass from 3 different positions a full erythema dose can be delivered at the tumor site, without serious injury to the overlaying structures. Numerous tests have convinced me that such calculations can be made at any distance or depth, under any conditions, with any tube, that can be held reasonably constant.

On the other hand I do not believe that the X-rays are justifiable in any case that will not permit of full dosage at the site of disease.

Without going any further into the detail of technique let me mention, not from hearsay nor from statistics, but from personal experience, of what I have found the X-rays capable, i. e.—that the rays can and do, check and cure epithelioma, superficially located cancer, lupus vulgaris, and other tubercular skin affections, sometimes with the surgeon's aid, but frequently much better without.

That in the so-called precancerous stage in breast adenoma, etc., the timely use of a few, properly graded X-ray applications, might well supplant the knife, or render its use much safer.

The logic of tying off arteries in exopthalmic goitre is lacking when the inhibitory action of the X-rays are considered and not alone have I seen the symptoms abate, but under persistent treatment the enlarged thyroids have been markedly reduced and remained so.

Again in cervical adenitis I have yet to fail in reducing the glands when adenoids or scalp inhabitants were not to be considered.

Chronic eczema and ringworm of the most stubborn character have yielded to the rays and if I would delve into literature this list might be still further continued; but the foregoing has been the extent of my experience, and though I have not the 10,000 cures to make a medical axiom, nor has it all been glory, yet it has been enough to convince both myself and those with whom I have had the pleasure of working that under proper manipulation we have in the X-rays an agent that ranks high in the armamentarium of human therapy.

In closing suffice it to say that I have attempted to verify my introductory remarks and permit me to repeat that such work belongs only to the *physician* who is willing to devote his time to the details of this interesting but trying and none too lucrative specialty.

391 East 149th St.

ON THE OCCURRENCE OF SYPHILIS AND GONORRHEA IN CHILDREN BY DIRECT INFECTION.[1]

BY

ABR. L. WOLBARST, M. D.,
New York.

Consulting Genito-Urinary Surgeon, Central Islip State Hospital; Genito-Urinary Surgeon, People's Hospital, West Side German Dispensary and Hospital, and Beth . Israel Hospital Dispensary, etc., etc.

The subject of this paper, though it applies directly to children, has a distinct and immediate bearing on the men and women of the future, for the diseases we are about to consider, do not leave their young victims without a lasting heritage.

Of the two diseases we are about to deal with, as affecting childhood, syphilis is the only one which may be transmitted to the child in utero, as a constitutional taint. The manifestations of hereditary syphilis are known to all, and do not concern us at the present moment. We shall devote ourselves exclusively to the study of these diseases, acquired by direct infection. By direct infection, I mean the infection of a child born healthy, with the active principle of the disease, either through negligence or with vicious intent.

Gonorrhea is the more common of the two diseases, both in the adult and in the child. This disease may attack an infant at birth or immediately thereafter, usually selecting the mucous membrane of the eye as its nidus. The infection is carried to the infant while it is passing through the vaginal canal of the mother, which has previously been the seat of the disease. As the infant passes through the parturient canal, pressing with its head against the walls and putting them on the stretch, the vaginal secretion containing the infectious gonococci, among its other bacterial flora, is squeezed into the infant's eyes and there sets up an acute inflammation. Any mucous surface may be attacked; and there are not a few cases on record in which the genitals of female children were involved, with the production of a typical vulvovaginitis.

During the past decade, much has been said concerning the occurrence of gonococcus opthalmia in the infant, with its attendant blindness. Let us give this subject a moment's consideration, in view of its well nigh unbelievable frequency and its terrible consequences. From the standpoint of child hygiene, ophthalmia neonatorum of gonorrheal origin, is perhaps the most important single factor we have to deal with. First, because of its great frequency: it is said to occur in about one in two hundred of all births, rich as well as poor; second, because it is the most common cause of blindness: fully 25% of all the cases of blindness in the world to-day, are said by responsible authorities to be due solely to gonococcus ophthalmia; thirdly, because it is largely preventable and usually curable, if proper measures are

[1]Read before the Third Section of the IV International Congress on Hygiene and Demography, held at Washington, September 23-28, 1912.

adopted in time to avoid permanent damage.

In his classic work on this subject (Ophthalmia Neonatorum, Its Etiology and Prevention, Trans. Obstet. Society, of London, 1905, xlv), Stevenson showed that about two-thirds of all cases of ophthalmia in the newly born are due to the gonococcus. In the United States alone, according to the last census, there are fully 7,000 men and women who owe their blindness entirely to this disease.

The exact time of inoculation of the infant's eyes with the infectious maternal secretion is not known, but it may occur at any moment after the rupture of the enveloping membranes. In few cases, the inflammation is well advanced at birth, but it usually does not make its presence known until 12 to 48 hours after birth. Cases are recorded in which the children were born with well advanced destruction of the cornea of both eyes, and Phillips mentions an extraordinary case in which the eyes were found infected and filled with pus when taking the child from the abdominal wound after Caesarean section (N. Y. Med. Jour., July 23, 1912). It is not stated whether or not gonococci were found in this pus.

Bathing the infant soon after birth has been the means of transferring the infection to the eyes. Unless extreme care is employed, the infectious vaginal secretion adhering to the skin of the infant's body may be washed into the eyes, thus producing the inflammation. Such a bath surely merits the term "Giftwasser," applied to it by Schirmer.

In all the mass of evidence as to the awful nature of this infection, the important thing for us to remember is that much, if not all of this blindness and con-sequent misery can be prevented. Prophylactic measures were first suggested by Créde, of Leipsic, in 1882. During the three decades that have passed, eyes innumerable have been saved from perpetual darkness, by this method of prophylaxis. Its value may be judged by the statistics offered by Kösling. In 17,000 cases of childbirth in which preventive measures were *not* used, 9.2% of cases of ophthalmia neonatorum developed; on the other hand, in 24,000 cases in which the Créde method *was* employed, the percentage of cases of ophthalmia was reduced to 0.65%. Surely, a convincing argument in favor of the method. Nevertheless, in spite of the teachings of bitter experience, there are still 25% of our blind, who have been permitted to become so through carelessness or negligence.

Here then, lies a great field of endeavor for the humanitarian—the abolition of blindness through the universal adoption, by law or by custom, of the Créde method of prophylaxis.

Next in importance, though greater in frequency, is the occurrence of gonococcus infection of the genitals in children. It is far more common in girls than in boys, and for obvious reasons. The anatomic arrangement of the female genitals especially in childhood, presents a soil that is highly favorable to infection from without, and this alone would appear to account for the greater frequency of the infection in girls than in boys. Another plausible reason is perhaps found in the fact that the tendency for adult males to tamper sexually with female children is greater than for women to have relations with male children; hence the greater risk of infection. In female children infection spreads rapidly from adult to child or child to child, by the mere handling of toys, wash-cloths, towels, urinals, etc. Anything, in fact, that comes in contact with the child's genitals may carry the infection.

It should be borne in mind, however, that every case of vaginitis or vulvovaginitis is not necessarily caused by the gonococcus, but it should be looked upon with suspicion and the diagnosis positively made; for even though the gonococcus may not be detected in the early stages of the infection, the purulent discharge increases and the specific bacteria appear, after several days.

This disease is not limited to the children of the poor, though filth and congestion are favorable factors in its causation; it may be found among the well to do, as well, in boarding schools and in private homes. In these instances, the infection may be brought into the home by maids and nurses or playmates. R. E. Kimball, speaking of this feature of the disease, states that one of the worst cases of gonorrhea he ever saw was in a child eight years of age, and was acquired in a fashionable school in New York.

Among the poor, where crowding and congestion and lack of privacy are synonymous terms, the disease is almost endemic. Stella refers to the occurrence of gonorrhea among the little children of the Italian population of New York (*Med. Rec.*, May 2, 1908) and laments "the hundreds of young girls of five and ten reeking with pollution accidentally communicated to them through bedding and towels and lack of sanitary conveniences in overcrowded tenements," and Charles H. May wonders that gonococcus infection of the eye is not more frequent, in view of the frequency and persistence of these genital affections in female children. It is quite likely that eye infection is rather unusual in these cases, owing to the fact that the virus reaches the eye in a somewhat attenuated form.

Children who sleep in the same bed with the mother are frequently the victims of infection. Here we have a link in a vicious chain, which deserves our most serious consideration. The immigrant reaches this country alone, as a rule, leaving his wife and children in Europe, until such a day as he shall have established himself firmly in his new home. In the meantime, likely as not, he is infected with gonorrhea, and when his family arrives to share his prosperity, his faithful wife is made to pay the penalty in the form of a gonococcus infection from which she rarely recovers entirely, and which she often transmits innocently to her children. In a study of this subject made in one of the largest hospitals in this city, I was enabled to show (*N. Y. Med. Jour.*, Oct. 16, 1909) that about one-third of one per cent of all the male immigrants who applied for treatment in its dispensary, were suffering from venereal disease, mostly gonorrhea, acquired during the absence of the wife. Ultimately, the wife and children are infected, and thus the endless chain progresses.

In institutions and asylums, the gonococcus infection has often run riot and assumed terrible proportions. Not alone the genitals, but other parts of the body are affected. Kaumheimer (*Munch. Med. Wochen.*, May 3, 1910) has dwelt on the occurrence of rectal gonorrhea in young girls, the result of contagion by direct infection from the vaginal discharge. The symptoms of this condition are often so slight that it passes unnoticed, but he expresses the opinion that this may be the means whereby the infection spreads so rapidly and insidiously in hospitals, institutions and asylums where many children are congregated. He also wisely suggests that on this account, the temperature of a child suffering from genital gonorrhea should never be taken per rectum. His data have received full corroboration through the earlier observations of Flügel, (*Berl. klin. Wochen.*, March 20, 1905), who found the rectum involved in 11 of 56 cases of vulvovaginitis, or 20%. In adults the proportion is greater—about 30%.

These children are also apt to be crippled for life, when arthritis supervenes as a complication of the vulvovaginitis. In 1905 Holt found 26 cases of gonorrheal arthritis, single and multiple, in the Babies' Hospital, New York, in a period of 11 years. He states, in this connection, that "a pyemic arthritis in a young infant, I believe, is much more frequently due to the gonococcus than to the streptococcus or any other pyogenic organism."

Nor is this the most serious complication to which these little victims are endangered. Inguinal adenitis and abscess formation are not unusual; less common, fortunately, is the occurrence of an infection of the peritoneum, local or general, with the grave possibility of a fatal termination. Sterility in after life, may also follow the infection, particularly if the uterus and the tubes have been involved.

Lastly, I wish to mention a source of infection in young girls, which is of considerable sociologic importance. I refer to that form which follows sexual contact with adult or youthful males. This phase of the subject has been carefully studied by Pollack, of Baltimore, with startling results. She reports 184 cases of gonorrhea in young girls, varying between one and fifteen years of age. She estimates that there must be from 800 to 1000 such cases each year in the city of Baltimore, these figures being considered a conservative estimate. She believes the cause of most of these outrages upon children to be due to the superstition among many peoples, that a person suffering with gonorrhea or syphilis may get rid of the disease by infecting another of the opposite sex, preferably "an untouched virgin." Thus a defenseless child is the most natural victim. She does not agree with the oft expressed view that these attacks are the result of sexual perversion. In her cases, nearly one-third of the victims were between three and six years of age. This superstition is quite prevalent in many European countries and among the southern negroes, and is alluded to in the works of Havelock Ellis and Kraft-Ebing, as a prolific cause of sexual attacks on young children.

The reported experience of W. T. Gibb, physician to the Children's Society of New York, is of interest in this connection. In 15 years he examined over 800 girls ranging from 8 months to 16 years of age, on whom rape and other crimes had been committed. Almost 13% of all the children examined suffered from venereal disease; 10% had gonorrhea, 2½% had chancroids and the remainder had syphilis. The rarity of syphilis was probably due to the examination having been made but a short time after the commission of the crime, when the time elapsed had been too short for the characteristic symptoms of the disease to have appeared. He believes that the number of cases seen by him is but a small proportion of the actual number of such crimes, as the great majority of children never tell what has happened to them.

In boys, gonorrheal infection is far less common than in girls. Infection spreads with less facility, owing to anatomic reasons above mentioned, but once the infection has been established, the victims are subject to all the dangers and complications that have been previously discussed. It has been my privilege to have studied 41 cases of gonococcus infection in boys ranging in age between 18 months and 14 years, as follows: 2 years or under, 5 cases; 4 to 7 years, 17 cases; 8 to 10 years, 4 cases; 11 to 14 years, 15 cases. The largest percentage is found among boys between 4 and 7 years, and those between 11 and 14. The former age is the most favorable for the practice of the superstition already mentioned, and the latter includes the boys who are old enough to have learned the possibilities of the sexual function and the means of its gratification. In one of my cases, the victim was a boy of four, who was "assaulted" by a precocious girl of twelve, who was found to have attacked and infected many young boys of the neighborhood; she had previously been infected by a youth of twenty. A somewhat similar case is mentioned by Wilson (*Buffalo Medical Journal*). A boy, aged nine, was infected with gonorrhea by a girl aged twelve. On examination, the girl was found to have gonorrhea. The infection seemed to be prevalent in the neighborhood among the younger children and further investigation revealed its source to be a women of public affection and of nymphomaniacal tendency.

Still more serious, in my opinion, because far less excusable, are the cases of young boys, infected with gonorrhea in public hospitals, through the use of unclean catheters. I have seen eleven such cases. These children were sent to the hospitals for various diseases of childhood and in the course of their illness it was necessary to empty the bladder with a catheter. In this manner gonococcus infection was carried to these innocent children, with dire results. This is nothing short of a criminal act, which ought to be unheard of in a civilized community. This form of infection can be done away with, by the simple expedient of using a new catheter for each new patient. The Supreme Court of Washington (Helland vs. Bridenstine) recently decided that damages may be recovered for alleged malpractice consisting of the use in and on the plaintiff of unclean and unsterilized instruments whereby the disease of gonorrhea was communicated to the plaintiff. This leads me to wonder whether these victims by catheter infection in hospitals could not also recover damages under this ruling of the court.

In boys, the disease is apt to run a more virulent course than in girls. Arthritis is more common, as is shown by the figures of Holt, above quoted. Of the 26 cases of gonorrheal arthritis, 19 were in boys and 7 in girls; most of the cases reported by Kimball were also found in boys.

Coming now to the subject of acquired syphilis in children, it is apparent that this form of the disease is quite unusual, though not rare. It is not so readily transmitted as gonorrhea and those who suffer from it are not always in the infectious stage. Pollack, in the paper referred to, saw 36 cases in girls with the double infection of gonorrhea and syphilis. Seven were in the primary stage and 29 in the secondary. Stella, also quoted above, tells of "the many mothers of the poor who take children from institutions to nurse them and who have been inoculated with the poison of syphilis"; and he further mentions a case in his own experience where the infection was not recognized on account of its extragenital origin, and was communicated by the mother to four of her children, her husband and a sister.

Some years ago, I saw a frail little Polish immigrant boy, not more than two years old, with a primary lesion on the lower abdominal wall; secondary symptoms which were present made the diagnosis unmistakable. It has also been my fortune to have seen recently a little boy of five, who had a typical genital chancre, with extensive secondary symptoms. How these children are thus infected, it is difficult to say, but surely there must be some way of saving them.

To recapitulate:—Children are frequently the victims of gonorrhea and (less often) syphilis; girls are more often infected than boys; the infection spreads with great rapidity and assumes a terrible virulence when introduced into hospitals, asylums and schools; girls are often the victims of perverts and superstitious immigrants trying to rid themselves of their own disease; complications sometimes follow, which are far more serious than the original disease, among these being blindness, arthritis, proctitis, adenitis, peritonitis, and sterility in later life; congestion, crowding and lack of privacy lead to precocious sexual knowledge and facilitate the spread of infection; the male immigrant is a frequent agent in carrying infection to his wife and children; male children are often infected in hospitals through unclean catheters; they are subject to all the dangers and complications of the adult; both sexes are equally liable to infection

with syphilis, but it seems to be more frequent in male children; lastly, the combined effort of intelligent men and women, having the welfare of childhood at heart, is needed to combat the unfortunate conditions that make these diseases possible; suitable prophylaxis and attention to hygienic principles can minimize to a marked degree, the disastrous effects of syphilis and gonorrhea in children.

113 East Nineteenth Street, New York.

CHRONIC CATARRHAL COLITIS IN CHILDREN.[1]

BY

LEGRAND KERR, M. D.
Brooklyn, N. Y.

Visiting Pediatrist to the Methodist Episcopal (Seney), The Williamsburg, The Bushwick and the Swedish Hospitals in Brooklyn, N. Y. Consulting Pediatrist to the Rockaway Beach Hospital, the Industrial Home for Children, etc.

Chronic catarrhal colitis in children is by no means a similar proposition to the disease as it occurs in adult life. Of course there are the marked differences which are dependent upon the dissimilar anatomy and physiology of the colon in childhood and adult life, but this very dissimilarity brings with it other factors which cannot be disregarded.

Thus we cannot expect the child to co-operate readily in any feature of the treatment and in many instances it is difficult even to get the parents to realize the necessity and importance of certain features.

The child's natural constitutional preference for the various infections adds another element of complication and the fact that

[1] Read before the Williamsburg Hospital Staff Association Jan. 4, 1912.

all children, irrespective of their disease, stand hunger, pain and depletion very poorly, adds other difficulties to the management of this disease.

Now, it is not the intent of the writer to discuss this matter fully or even orderly, for everyone is more or less familiar with most of the problems involved. However, there are several points upon which there is abundant room for discussion and it will be my aim to bring a consideration of some of these as they have appealed to me after a close observation and some experimentation; in other words, I offer my personal experience and personal experiences are always discussable. Chronic colitis is divisible into several other forms, but we are to deal with chronic catarrhal colitis which is sometimes called mucous, muco-membranous, psuedo-membranous, or more incorrectly, membranous. It is a simple catarrhal inflammation with the mucous membrane swollen, reddened and thickened. Naturally it is characterized by the appearance of mucus in the stools which is usually noticed on the surface of the fecal mass and not mixed with it. Atrophic colitis is not common in childhood, being usually reserved for adult life, and consequent upon neglected cases in youth. Syphilitic colitis is not within the realm of this paper.

Now such a condition is not infrequent in young children although it is commonly overlooked and thereby is laid the foundation for the continuance of the disease throughout adult life in a more or less aggravated form and with its unpleasant and painful sequelae. It is because the subjective symptoms are so slight or absent that the disease is overlooked and as the rebellion of the child is naturally against restraint, its continuance in its normal activities is commonly looked upon as an evidence that it cannot be ill. If the child be young enough, the old diagnostic soporific "teething" is used to lull to sleep the anxiety of the parents and to quiet the conscience of the physician, while the infant may go on to chronic invalidism. We find therefore that the recognition of the disease is simplified if the etiology is remembered and the onset of the chronic consequence suspected rather than if we wait for a definite symptomatology. After all acute affections of the large intestine and in every instance of prolonged fecal stasis, repeated examinations should be made to determine the presence or absence of this chronic consequence.

With subjective symptoms, trivial or absent, what must we look for? First, the examination of the stool is of great value and it need not of necessity be more than a gross examination at first because we only aim to determine the presence or absence of mucus which is sufficient in amount to appear grossly and which is coated over rather than mixed with feces. After this is determined, the examination of the abdomen is undertaken. In chronic catarrhal colitis, it is sunken and never becomes markedly distended with gases, except under the influence of some acute condition. Pressure reveals the fact that the large intestine is sensitive, although it may not be painful. If the disease has been long standing the thinned out abdominal walls, allow one to easily demonstrate on deep palpation, cord like masses which have a consistency of rubber and which correspond to the moderately thickened and contracted colon. Palpation over these masses may cause considerable pain. Practically all of the cases are recognized by such an examination, and the wonder is that so many cases are overlooked. It is only in rare instances that microscopical examination is necessary and the demonstration of cylindrical cells, leucocytes, red blood cells, crystals of cholesterin, oxalic acid, uric acid and increased bacteria an essential factor in the diagnosis. It is a clearly established fact that in the treatment of mucous inflammation, irrigation is probably the most important factor. But all mucous surfaces are not so easily accessible and the colon is one of these. It has been the custom to attempt to imitate direct irrigation in the cases of wholly or partly inaccessible mucous surfaces, by giving by the mouth substances which will partly cleanse the inflamed surface. In adults this may be practical but during childhood its application is often impossible or actually harmful.

But since mucous membranes contain such an abundance of secreting glands, they need when inflamed, more frequent cleansing than does the skin. This is the more essential because their moisture makes them more attractive to bacteria. Then again, their permeability permits the penetration of bacteria and their toxins to the blood stream and body fluids, thus making a constitutional out of what was originally a local disorder.

Now if we study the anatomy of the colon in the child, we will soon see how utterly hopeless it is to attempt to completely cleanse its mucous surfaces. Irrigations are certainly overdone and frequently are the cause of the persistence of the symptoms or the addition of complications. It is practically impossible to use a long tube without its doubling and yet it is easy to be deceived in this matter. Tubes which are thought to be well introduced into the bowel can almost always be shown to have doubled upon themselves and are ineffectual if not positively harmful. Several experiments with the X-ray have demonstrated the fact that the long tube is practically an impossible

proposition for bowel irrigation that is to be effective. With such uncertainty regarding the long tube or rather the almost inevitable failure of its efficacy, we should turn to the short tube which is certain because it is short and can be made of more inflexible material. The short tube placed well within the rectum will accomplish more than the long tube and accomplish it better. H. T. Machell in an experiment covering some 200 cases of irrigation, concluded that irrespective of age or weight, the short tube was capable of introducing a larger amount of fluid; that it was retained longer; that the amount permanently retained was larger and that the fluid found its way higher in the bowel than with the long tube. These experiments were substantiated in several instances by the X-ray (*Archives of Pediatrics*, October, 1911). Personally, I do not feel that merely as a cleanser in this disease, irrigation accomplishes anything more than the mechanical evacuation of the rectum with subsequent progress of the fecal mass from above into the emptied rectum. But if it is used as it always should be with the idea uppermost that absorption of the injected fluid is to be accomplished rather than mere cleansing of the bowel, its value in selected instances may be great indeed. Elimination is assisted by small enemata of saline, given slowly, given hot, and given without force and this is all that we may hope to accomplish by its use in chronic catarrhal colitis, for remember we are not dealing with conditions which are similar to acute processes in which the superficial layers of the membranes are alone affected but are combating a condition in which the deeper layers are most affected; a condition in which elimination is more effective than surface cleansing alone. I mention drug treatment at this point not because of its importance, but to avoid repeated references to some things that have been mentioned in regard to local irrigation.

For instance, the quality of permeability of the membrane makes bacterial invasion of deeper structures probable and this same quality influences to some extent the local actions of some drugs. The mucous membrane being more sensitive than the skin would seem to make sedatives more desirable and this is so, but it must be remembered that the permeability renders the stronger ones unnecessary. In the matter of drugs there are two types that may be indicated. Either there may be a need for the antifermentatives and antiseptics, or the intestinal ferments to carry the food beyond the reach of putrefactive organisms. No ferment is needed when inspection of the stool shows that digestion is complete. There is but little doubt in the writer's mind that peristalsis is the very best intestinal antiseptic and that drug action as such is of doubtful utility. Of all that we have used within the last few years, iodine has most uniformly given good results, although its prolonged use is impossible. By far the most important element in treatment is the diet and what diet is best suited for each individual case cannot be decided by any system or scheme or pet theory of which the writer knows. Diet lists are usually more attractive on paper than on the table and what will prove efficient in the management of one case will prove an absolute failure in the next one, unless the elimination of one or more articles of diet is based upon something more reliable than past experience in a few cases or a study of caloric or proteid needs. If these cases are to be dieted effectively, the stool must be frequently inspected. The appearance of undigested or only partly digested residues is an indication for elimination of the offending articles. I know of no more satisfactory method of diet control than frequent stool inspection by the physician. Time and time again, I see cases in which the child's diet has been restricted and restricted until there is very little left that it is allowed and yet conditions get worse and worse. Of course they do, it is only natural that they should. The child is being slowly starved and children bear hunger and starvation badly. The simplest diet made up from a text-book without regard for the individual factors in the case under observation may have in it some offending material that aggravates the chronic condition. To further cut the diet under such conditions is unnecessary. The child has a greater chance for health if the offending article is eliminated and other articles added. Generally speaking, I am convinced that more harm is done in these cases by unnecessary restriction of diet than by liberal feeding suited to the studied individual needs. Some of the failures in the early correction of this disease are undoubtedly due to the fact that these children do not appear ill and therefore go about unrestrained in their activities. Rest in bed for a week or ten days as an adjunct to the other methods of management will often produce the results which are unobtainable without it. Many cases of chronic catarrhal colitis are treated as instances of intestinal intoxication or the latter is considered as being the most important element of the disease. There are fashions in pathology as in manners and in dress and signs are not lacking that intestinal intoxication is given too much importance. Its progress is like any other uncontrolled movement; the outcome is uncertain and like the gossip of every-day life, one thinks

502   AMERICAN MEDICINE
Complete Series, Vol. XVIII.   ORIGINAL ARTICLES   SEPTEMBER, 1912.
New Series, Vol. VII., No. 9.

about it, another suggests it and another states that it is so. The almost continuously sunken abdomen of chronic catarrhal colitis shows that this factor is not a large one. Give these children proper hygienic surroundings; give them a diet selected after your personal inspection of several stools and not handed out from a text-book diet list, give them a few days' rest in bed in the earlier stages of the disease and you will begin to get results. But you must have patience, a tremendous amount of patience, for one of the difficult features may be the absence of prompt results. But prompt results are not necessarily good results and if after one year you have very materially improved a child with chronic catarrhal colitis, you are well on the way to reduce the army of adult chronic invalids by at least one.

THE PRESERVATION OF THE TEETH.

BY

NORMAN ROBERTS, A. B., M. D.,
Washington, D. C.

For several years past the dental profession and certain commercial interests have been waging an admirable publicity campaign on the desirability of constant cleanliness and systematic early repair of the teeth. (If the medical profession had done as well in proportion to its opportunities, we should today deservedly stand far higher than we do in the public estimation). This toothbrush crusade is indeed very opportune; but there is something far better along the same line, of which today we hear scarcely a whisper, least of all from the dentists, who of late years, by reason of intensive but narrow special training have been allowed to assume a position of authority in a field which still rightly comes under the more comprehensive domain of the physician.

Clean teeth are of course not so *apt* to decay as dirty ones; but *strong* teeth can hardly be *made* to decay—a strong statement, but amply justified. To prevent decay by cleanliness alone, the mouth would have to be kept constantly aseptic, a practical impossibility; but strength can be secured with certainty if systematically worked for from childhood up. The obvious way to secure strength is by physiologic use, i. e., by chewing something with adequate resistance and with sufficient taste to stimulate the impulse to chew. The enormous consumption of gum shows the instinctively-felt need of civilized humanity for *more chewing,* but gum lacks resistance; what is needed is something like a fibrous root containing, and when chewed slowly yielding, a nourishing and agreeably-tasting salivary extract, preferably containing much carbohydrate (for the reason that carbohydrate more effectively than anything else physiologically stimulates the flow of the saliva and the impulse to prolonged mastication). The structure of the human teeth, and the known manner of life of many primitive peoples shows that human teeth were evolved mainly for just such use; hence they are best to be kept in condition by such use, rather than (though not at all to the exclusion of) such artificial measures as oral asepsis. Moreover, such natural use of the mouth (with the resulting long-continued flow of alkaline saliva) is far more efficient in reducing the numbers and virulence of tooth-destroying bacteria than any *practical* system of artificial oral asepsis; and the slight but sufficient individual motion of the teeth during vigorous and prolonged mastication is in the long run far more effective and less damaging than silk or toothpick in dislodging fermenting material from between the teeth—although of course artificial aids are not to be despised when especially indicated.

A familiar substance that meets the requirements of proper consistency and normal physiological stimulation is *licorice root*. A set of fairly strong teeth can safely break off the sticks into the proper lengths (about an inch) and soon reduce them to a fibrous coherent pulp, which on continued chewing yields the carbohydrate *glycyrrhizin* and other agreeably-flavored extractives during ten or twenty minutes' moderate chewing. If the teeth are too weak to break up the stick, it may be taken in a safer "fine-cut" (*not ground*) condition, which may be chewed as vigorously or as gingerly as desired. Besides licorice, there are doubtless many other suitable substances already known; and if there were a demand, much better ones could be provided.

The best way to use licorice for this purpose seems to be to chew a comfortable mouthful (swallowing the saliva, of course) until the sweet taste is replaced by slight astringency and the pulp begins to disintegrate and irritate the pharynx. One or two helpings after each meal is sufficient; but no harm is known to result from keeping it up for several hours a day, although of course the salivary glands may be depleted more or less if there is no intermission before meals. The habit may with great advantage be substituted for the use of tobacco; it is beneficial instead of harmful; it gives one "something to do while doing nothing"; it does not interfere with most kinds of work; and it molests no one except a few selfish and supersensitive souls who are irritated at the sight of others quietly enjoying themselves. The main drawback to its extended use by large numbers of people seems to be that it is largely controlled by a soulless trust, who mix a little good root with a great deal of bad, and who would probably boost the price out of sight if the demand were much increased.

There are obvious "medical" as well as "dental" grounds for advocating such a partial return to primitive habits of eating. Modern soft, bland foods do not stimulate the act of mastication or the secretion of saliva enough to cause the carbohydrates to be adequately digested in the stomach during the half hour or so that elapses before the hydrochloric acid becomes so concentrated as to kill the ptyalin, and digestion of carbohydrate is hence delayed until the amylopsin of the pancreatic juice reaches it in the intestine. This delay often results in fermentation and heartburn, which (in at least my own case) is quickly relieved by chewing the licorice. The salivary glands, even in their present neglected condition, secrete much more of the starch-splitting ferment than does the pancreas, and should for every reason be given opportunity to contribute it at the proper time. Of course it would be better if the carbohydrate ration could all be taken in such form as to require prolonged chewing; and some day such will be the universal custom; but until then it will materially help to take even a small part of it in the manner described.

Certain Sunday-paper evolutionists are prone to amuse themselves and turn an honest penny by prophesying the future physical condition of the race when civilization and evolution shall have made us a finished product. We shall be hairless; our limbs will be delicate tentacles of use only to manipulate electric organ-keys controlling the machinery that is to obviate all need for gross physical exertion; our sense-organs will be superseded by infinitely more delicate electric receiving apparatus, and will atrophy for want of use; our women will simply ·ovulate as the frogs do, the product of conception being cared for in the womb of some lower animal (or in another of the omnipotent machines) until maturity; and we will live somewhat as the amoeba does, by absorption through our delicate skins of predigested nourishment from a bath, our digestive apparatus having faded entirely away, especially the teeth, against which these great scientists seem to be as violently prejudiced as they are against the hair. Now this tapeworm-like existence may seem highly to be desired by a few people with tapeworm-like minds, but it does *not* appeal to the undersigned or any other normal human being; and as Man will undoubtedly soon completely control evolution throughout the world, it is a foregone conclusion that he will take care of himself in a way to recover the organs and faculties that he has lost, rather than submit himself to further mutilation. Undoubtedly "superfluous" parts and powers make a human being a less tractable and less highly-specialized producer of wealth for his "betters" (hence please note the rising volume of protest from the *influential* against the higher education of the masses, and the substitution of vocational training in the schools); but producing wealth for one's betters is rapidly losing popularity. Soon ·the practical application of correct economic principles (now opposed by the shortsightedly selfish) will convert Machinery and System from cruel tyrants over the bulk of humanity to efficient servants of the whole race. Once before, in Ancient Greece, an entire people was free, though they lived on the labor of alien slaves; and all free citizens delighted to house their splendid minds in perfect bodies. Even more so in the golden future, when all living things shall be free and only machines shall slave, man's animal body will be as perfect as his godlike mind—not a flabby, helpless parasite, to be swept out of existence by the first accident to the sheltering machines, but a real king of the earth, the physical as well as the mental superior of any other live thing on it.

And so we shall keep all our parts and powers, including our teeth; and this rather by intelligent use of them than by coddling and tinkering, although for the next few years or maybe generations the coddling and tinkering may have to be kept up (decreasingly) to atone for the follies of the past. We shall recover all that we need of what we have lost; we shall not need teeth for weapons, nor even for tools, hence we shall be as far removed from projecting tushes and prognathous jaws as from chinlessness and the likeness of spoon-fed senility.

The right time to begin to recover the lost ground is at once. Five cents' worth of licorice root will start any one person (or two or three) on the right track, if he has any serviceable teeth left. Young children should especially be gotten into the practice, as it will not only conserve their already-erupted teeth, but will favor the proper eruption of the later ones, normally develop the whole lower part of the head (bony, muscular and glandular), and tend to break up thumbsucking and mouthbreathing and prevent the development of adenoids and enlarged tonsils.

Is it too much to hope that someone with time and influence now less profitably employed will take this matter up and give it the *initial impetus* that it deserves?

TRANSLATION.

A STUDY OF INFECTIOUS DISEASES OF THE LABYRINTH.[1]

BY

DOCENT HEINRICH NEUMANN
of Vienna.

Translated with Docent Neumann's permission

BY

IRVING WILSON VOORHEES, M. S., M. D.,
New York City.

The results which aural surgery has achieved in the last decade depend chiefly upon the growing knowledge of the pathogenesis and diagnosis of the endocranial complications of otitic processes. These advances maintain in the entire field of aural surgery, but chiefly that chapter of the same which has to do with suppurative diseases of the labyrinth. The lively interest which labyrinth suppuration has engendered has been brought about both through the physiologic importance of this organ and through its relation to other vital organs. Suppurative diseases of the labyrinth offer both from a pathologic-anatomic and from a clinical viewpoint a rich field for study which is governed by the kind of middle ear disease causing a given complication, by the path of infection which was followed, and by the spreading out of the suppuration into the labyrinthine spaces. The complicated structure of the labyrinth and the fine functional differentiation of its constituent parts can cause an almost inconceivable variety of clinical symptoms of labyrinthine suppuration. The diagnosis and therapy of labyrinthine suppuration have the fixed purpose of retaining labyrinthine function and protecting the suf-

[1] Translated from the Monatsschrift für Ohrenheilkunde und Laryngo-Rhinologie. XLV. Jahrgang, 5 Heft. Festschrift für Professor Victor Urbantschitsch.

ferer from the highly dangerous intracranial complications of labyrinthine origin. In spite of the current interest in this highly important chapter of ear disturbances, all questions are not sufficiently answered with respect to indications for treatment. The exceedingly variable clinical course of labyrinthine suppuration is doubtless in great part responsible for this condition. The nature of such suppuration is just as variable as the beginning and course of the same. Disregarding the kind of labyrinthine suppuration whether acute or chronic, circumscribed or diffuse, it may result in death in a few days, or may go on to complete healing after months have passed by with or without operation. The results of purulent invasion into the labyrinth may be set down as follows:

(1) Recession of all symptoms and *restitutio ad integrum*.

(2) Recession of all symptoms except the loss of labyrinth function, which may remain completely destroyed.

(3) Increase of symptoms and death from diffuse meningitis or brain abscess.

The anatomic changes on the inner wall of the tympanic cavity do not suffice to determine the extent and the course of labyrinthine suppuration. They simply help one to decide whether suppuration has attacked the entire labyrinth or only part of it. Even severe lesions of the labyrinth wall, such as caries and necrosis, do not guide us to the assumption of a complete destruction of the labyrinthine function (Ernst Urbantschitsch). Experience teaches that under certain conditions the endosteum of the labyrinth possesses sufficient resistance to prevent penetration of infectious material into the interior of the labyrinth. Experience also teaches us that suppuration may remain limited to only a part of the labyrinth. These observations suffice to establish the following generally recognized rule:

The clinical picture of labyrinthine suppuration can only be understood if a careful investigation of the changes found on the inner wall of the tympanic cavity are considered together with an exact functional test. This picture consists of symptoms which may be traced back either to irritation or to loss of function in the nerves of the mechanism. The symptoms elicited from the cochlear apparatus have little or no pathognomonic significance, since the cochlear apparatus may already have been injured in its function through the middle ear disease. Disease of the cochlea asserts itself in a more or less diminished hearing power, or what is more frequent, in complete deafness accompanied by subjective noises. These disturbances show the usual character of labyrinthine deafness. The tone of a tuning-fork placed upon the skull is conducted toward the better ear and the bone conduction is markedly shortened. For the determination of the shortening of bone conduction, the following method may be carried out:

The middle fork is placed upon the mastoid process of the investigated ear. If bone conduction is absent the tone of the tuning fork is not changed if the external canal of this ear is stopped with the tip of the finger; but if the good ear is closed, then the tone of the tuning-fork is heard in the sound ear. This method of investigation makes it possible for us to decide how much of the vibration is perceived through the resonance in the diseased ear and how much is perceived through resonance in the sound ear. The tuning-fork test by air conduction is only of value in the diagnosis of labyrinthine deafness when we find that the high tones show an apparent increase of the duration of hearing on the diseased side, for the higher the tuning-fork, the better is the tone heard on the sound side.

Deafness caused by labyrinthine suppuration may usually be recognized by the relatively short time of its development. In general, extreme rapidity of development may be expected in acute middle ear diseases or acute exacerbations of chronic middle ear diseases. As to latent chronic middle ear inflammations, the pathologic-anatomic substratum such as cholesteatoma, polyps, or tuberculosis may alter the cochlear function long before the suppurative process has attacked the labyrinthine spaces. If we further take into consideration that many pathologic changes in the cochlea are, under certain circumstances, capable of receding, then it is not sufficient to base our operative procedure upon alteration of the cochlea alone, but we must try to determine also the capability of return to normal. A functional test of the vestibular apparatus is unreliable in which we merely concern ourselves with the manifest vestibular symptoms such as dizziness, nystagmus, disturbances of equilibrium and vomiting, we must also examine the vestibule for excitability to caloric, mechanic and turning irritations. With respect to the peculiarity of the symptoms caused by a vestibular lesion, it must be remembered that the dizziness possesses a turning character. The patient believes either that he himself turns or that the objects about him turn, and in the direction of the quick component of the nystagmus. Disturbances of equilibrium are strongly pronounced only in the beginning of the disease. They assert themselves usually in a staggering toward one or the other side. In total destruction of the vestibular apparatus the swaying is usually toward the diseased side, in circumscribed lesions to the sound side. In the later stages the disturbances of equilibrium may only be determined by special investigations, such as the goniometer or walking backwards or jumping with the eyes closed. It must be remembered that the rotatory type is the most frequent form of nystagmus in labyrinthine suppurations in which the quick component is directed to the sound side at the height of the disease upon looking in any given direction. In the later stages of the disease this rotatory nystagmus is manifest, however, only upon looking in the direction of the quick component of the nystagmus. Since all these symptoms vanish after a shorter or longer time it is obvious that in the latent form of the disease, only an exact functional test of the vestibular apparatus can show the changes which have taken place in this organ. Here we must mention that the anamnesis is not of special importance since the vestibular apparatus can lose its function without causing dizziness, nystagmus or disturbances of equilibrium. The various methods of investigation for eliciting the function of the vestibular apparatus depend upon the fact that the apparatus can be excited not only through physiologic irritations but also through caloric and galvanic tests, as well as through compression and aspiration of air in the external ear. The vestibular apparatus does not react to such irritations if it has completely lost its function through disease of the end-organ. Reaction to such irritations through pronounced nystagmus, dizziness, and disturbances of equilibrium, and the manifestation of these symptoms during our manipulations makes it possible for us to determine the condition of the vestibular apparatus even in the absence of other symptoms. If we assume the fact, which although not yet experimentally proven,

seems to be established through clinical experience, that the nystagmus is always produced in the irritated ear, then it is not difficult to determine the nystagmus in a given labyrinth through thermic or galvanic irritations. Since the cathode increases the excitability and the anode diminishes the same, we may take for granted that in an excitable labyrinth the nystagmus must be directed toward the cathode if the vestibular apparatus which is under the influence of the cathode is still excitable. If, on the contrary, the anode is applied to the investigated ear, then the nystagmus must be directed, in a still excitable labyrinth, to the opposite side. Much more reliable are the thermic tests for the determination of the excitability of the vestibular apparatus. If an ear is irrigated with cold water the nystagmus is directed toward the opposite side; by using warm water, the nystagmus will be directed toward the irrigated ear, which means that the vestibular apparatus is still excitable. A labyrinth which is not excitable to caloric and turning irritations may under certain circumstances, still show a slow movement of the eyes (if any excitability at all is retained) upon compression and aspiration of air in the external canal. This method of examination, which is called "the fistula test," makes possible in many cases the determination of a circumscribed lesion on the labyrinthine wall. The differentiation between circumscribed and diffused labyrinthine suppuration is exceedingly difficult; for in those cases in which an invasion of pus into the labyrinth takes place in a relatively short time, not only that part of the labyrinth is diseased which is attacked by the suppurative process, but the other parts of the labyrinth may also be disturbed in their function. Upon this ground a diffuse labyrinthine suppuration may be diagnosed when in reality a circumscribed suppuration is present. On the contrary, in those cases of labyrinthine suppuration in which the disease of the labyrinth has progressed gradually, the suppuration may remain localized to one place while the remaining parts of the labyrinth are still intact. It is, however, a very important clinical fact that circumscribed labyrinthine suppurations which have remained localized for a long time to one part of the labyrinth may become generalized through an acute exacerbation. Such acute exacerbations may be brought about through a simple rhinitis, or what is more important, through intra-tympanic operations, such as the removal of polyps, extraction of the ossicles or upon operative exposure of the middle ear spaces. A fact which is not to be lost sight of in studying the indications for operation is that not every circumscribed labyrinthine suppuration must become diffuse; for the parts of the labyrinth which are still intact may remain protected by firm adhesions (Alexander) till the diseased part of the labyrinth is spontaneously and completely healed. In order to make this possible, it is necessary to bring the causative inflammation in the middle ear to a standstill.

The condition of the facial nerve is likewise to be considered in labyrinthine suppuration, for paralysis of the nerve may represent the advance of the suppuration from the middle ear to the labyrinth. With respect to the frequency of facial paralysis in labyrinth necrosis, Bezold gives a percentage of 8.3. While in uncomplicated middle ear suppurations this takes place in only about one per cent. of the cases, labyrinth necrosis may also run its course without facial paralysis if only a small part of the labyrinth is affected by the necrosis.

In this manner a complete exfoliation of the cochlea or of the semi-circular canals without facial paralysis may take place. If in such cases, however, a facial paralysis does take place, then this chiefly depends upon the pressure of a sequestrum or is produced through erosion of the demarkating granulation formation. While the facial nerve in a considerable number of cases, in spite of intensive inflammation in the region suffers no loss of function, the acoustic nerve shows on the contrary quite a different tendency. From these facts, one must conclude that facial paralysis is to be considered of labyrinthine origin when total deafness is present, and the vestibular apparatus is no longer excitable. The otoscopic findings very seldom give exact hints as to the presence of an existing labyrinthine suppuration. If such are present, then the diagnosis is probable, if, besides the fistula or granulations in a circumscribed spot on the promontory, a nerve deafness exists at the same time. If there are no carious or necrotic changes on the promontory wall, a diffuse granulation mass which fills in the oval and round windows and covers the entire tympanic labyrinthine wall may mean an existing or a beginning labyrinthine suppuration. The diagnosis is otoscopically certain if from the oval window or another opening pus wells up, or if the probe reveals the presence of sequestra.

Neither the clinical picture nor the otoscopic examination are important criteria of the labyrinthine suppuration, but the findings on the labyrinthine wall at the time of the radical operation are a great aid. In most cases a fistula is found on the horizontal canal, more seldom on the anterior vertical canal, which is discolored and covered with pus or granulations. Not seldom one finds on the posterior surface of the

·pyramid a deep extra-dural abscess, which may originate either from a carious invasion of the posterior vertical canal or from an empyema of the saccus endolymphaticus. If the tympanic labyrinthine wall is seen to be intact at operation, then the tedious course of healing and the slight epidermization of the operative cavity may give important diagnostic points. Many authors consider the formation of granulations during the process of healing in many places on the labyrinthine wall as a valuable symptom of labyrinthine suppuration, but if we remember that such granulation formations may also take place in simple carious erosions of the labyrinthine capsule, that they may develop as a result of many middle ear suppurations, then we must consider the same as having only a limited otoscopic value. The diagnosis of labyrinthine suppuration is assured, therefore, by means of the labyrinthine changes taken together with an exact functional test.

In considering the indications for operative opening of the labyrinth, the question is of special importance whether the labyrinth operation in a given case shall be carried out simultaneously with the middle ear operation, or whether the opening of the labyrinth shall be undertaken some time later, since at the time of the middle ear operation, no definite reason may seem to necessitate this. The labyrinthine operation is indicated in all those cases in which a diffuse suppurative disease of the labyrinth has already been determined. If, however, this question cannot be decided with certainty, then the presence of intracranial complications of labyrinthine origin are sufficient reason for an attack upon the labyrinth. In circumscribed disease of the labyrinth, the necessity of opening the labyrinth depends chiefly upon the question

whether the circumscribed lesion after carrying out the middle ear operation is capable of spontaneous healing or not. In order to determine the indications for labyrinthine operation in individual cases, I demonstrated a table in the year 1906 before the meeting of the German Otological Society in Vienna. Those factors were taken into consideration which are decisive for the operative attack upon the labyrinth.

' First, one must consider the cochlea; second, the vestibular apparatus, and third, the pathologic-anatomic changes on the inner wall of the tympanic cavity. If one varies these three elements: cochlea, vestibular apparatus and pathologic-anatomic changes, that is to say fistula, seven combinations are possible. Clinical experiences have taught us that the statements made by me at that time were not merely theoretical, but are of use in actual practice.

NEUMANN'S TABLE OF INDICATIONS FOR OPERATION
UPON THE LABYRINTH. SLIGHTLY MODIFIED.

	Cochlear Function	Vestibular Function	Fistula	Treatment
I	+	+	+	No operation or do a radical mastoid.
II	—	+	+	No operation or do a radical mastoid. Labyrinthine op. rarely.
III	+	—	+	ditto.
IV	+·	—	—	No operation or do a radical mastoid.
V	±	—	+	Radical and labyrinthine operation.
VI	—	—	—	ditto.
VII	—	+	—	Radical mastoid ± Labyrinthine operation.

The first possibility is as follows: the patient hears, the vestibular apparatus is excitable, and on the inner wall of the tympanic cavity a fistula is seen at operation. This is not rare. Very frequently, one can determine a defect in the labyrinthine wall, when the vestibular apparatus is still excitable, before operation by means of the so-called fistula test. The negative result of this test has no diagnostic significance. A positive result on the contrary is of diagnostic value in so far as we can assume with certainty that the defect on the inner labyrinthine wall is not merely an erosion but a complete fistula. Under no condition is a labyrinthine operation indicated in these cases of middle ear suppuration. It must be mentioned that in such cases, after exposure of the middle ear spaces, an acute exacerbation may set in which generalizes the previously localized lesion and makes necessary the opening of the labyrinth at a second sitting. This secondary labyrinthine operation is, however, only indicated if the generalization caused by the acute exacerbation has produced a suppurative inflammation of the labyrinth but not a serous condition of the same. In the latter case, serous labyrinthitis, we are opposed to opening the labyrinth. According to my experience, the differential diagnosis between serous and suppurative labyrinthine inflammation is very frequently almost impossible. We now possess points for the differentiation of these two forms of labyrinthine suppuration (Bondy), and recently exact functional tests and experience have shown us that suppurative inflammation of the labyrinth leads to complete destruction of labyrinthine function, while serous inflammation is not usually followed by this result. Remains of function may still be retained; for example, hearing for tuning-forks through air or bone conduction, presence of hearing for conversation voice, in-

excitability of the vestibular apparatus to thermic irritations in the presence of still retained excitability for compression, or even increased excitability for turning irritations. A moderate increase of temperature is of value for the diagnosis of suppurative diseases of the labyrinth if other causes can be excluded. In other words, our task is to determine in post-operative extension of a circumscribed labyrinth disease whether the labyrinth to be opened has still any function left or not.

The second possibility is cochlear apparatus destroyed, vestibular apparatus excitable and a defect on the inner labyrinthine wall. Here simultaneous operation on the labyrinth is not strictly indicated. For my part, I open the labyrinth as a result of my experience that the operative attack on the vestibular apparatus has no very disadvantageous results, but I do not deny that a contrary opinion is to be entertained. The complete labyrinthine operation is, in the first place, no indifferent matter; but in the second place, deafness may be the result of toxic degenerative disease of the same. In this case, if we can determine the cause of the deafness, the opening of the labyrinth is not indicated, since through the anamnesis the history of the development may also frequently help in its determination. But if the deafness has developed in a relatively short time, and if the possibility of an isolated suppuration in the cochlea exists in spite of the excitable vestibular apparatus, vestibular symptoms being present; then the labyrinth operation is absolutely indicated.

Those cases, on the contrary, in which the causes of deafness can not be determined with certainty are to be operated upon, because a circumscribed diseased vestibular apparatus not merely hinders post-operative epidermization but frequently makes it impossible. Not rarely the sufferer from circumscribed disease of the vestibular apparatus complains of attacks of dizziness until the circumscribed diseased spot heals or until the entire vestibular apparatus is consumed in the circumscribed disease. The third form of labyrinth disease is that in which the cochlear function is retained, the vestibular apparatus is not excitable and in which there is a defect on the inner wall of the tympanic cavity. Immediate opening of the labyrinth is not indicated in this case because, according to our experience, an endo-labyrinthine inflammation which leads to complete destruction of the vestibular function leaves the cochlea not uninfluenced. However, if in the course of the after treatment, deafness be added to the already present inexcitability, then the opening of the labyrinth is indicated. The same data obtain also for the combination of cochlear function retained, vestibular function gone, and no evidence of a defect on the labyrinthine wall. This fourth eventuality is to be distinguished from the last mentioned only through lack of a positive demonstration of a labyrinthine wall defect. This is, however, not reliable since as above mentioned, such a condition may be present. It is merely not demonstrable. The vestibular apparatus is inexcitable and the fistula not accessible to the eye, since it can have its site in the niche of the oval or round window. If, on the contrary, both the cochlear and vestibular apparatus are without function (fifth possibility) and there exists on the inner labyrinth wall a visible defect, then immediate labyrinthine operation is strictly indicated since we have to do with a so-called diffuse labyrinthine suppuration. Failure to operate may be accompanied by deleterious consequences,

while the post-operative acute exacerbation may lead to infection of the endocranium, and we must open the labyrinth secondarily when the cranial complication is manifest, which may be too late. We hold the same opinion for eventuality six where the cochlea and vestibular apparatus are without function but a labyrinthine defect is not demonstrable. The possibility must be taken account of that the labyrinthine function has become destroyed through a nonsuppurative disease of the labyrinth, or if a suppurative inflammation was the cause of the destruction then there is the possibility of a complete healing of this inflammation and the operation would be superfluous. Since we have no certain data to determine this in such a contingency, it is better, after my opinion, to carry out the exenteration of the labyrinth for the same reasons as are set forth in eventuality five.

Ruttin made the observation at the March sitting of the Austrian Otological Society in the year 1911 that "compensation" of the labyrinthine excitability is sufficient to answer this question. I myself, in the discussion at this meeting, made the remark that in such cases one must be guided by other circumstances, such as the presence of a deep extra-dural abscess, marked pneumatic structure of the pyramid, etc. Professor Alexander, on the contrary, believes that sleeplessness and headache are signs of beginning cranial complications.

Eventuality seven is to be recognized through deafness, excitability of the vestibular apparatus and absence of labyrinthine wall defect. If the deafness has gradually developed, the necessity of opening the labyrinth is not present. If, on the contrary, the cochlea has become functionless in a relatively short time and if symptoms are present in the vestibular apparatus, one must think of an isolated inflammation of the cochlea and carry out the labyrinthine operation. The reason for this attack is exactly the same as in eventuality two, since the two forms are only to be differentiated through the presence or absence of the labyrinthine wall defect.

Labyrinthine operations may be divided into tympanic and retrolabyrinthine. The tympanic method, as practiced by Hinsberg, Bourges and Botey consists in opening the middle ear as is done in the radical mastoid operation, and then with a chisel or curette taking away the prominence of the horizontal semi-circular canal which in most cases is already fistulous. After careful cleansing of the promontory region, by removing the anterior margin of the oval window with a chisel or with a curette, after previous extraction of the stapes if it is still present, a counter opening is made. In this manner we make an opening in the lateral pyramid wall.

The bony canal of the facial divides this into two unequal parts. The smaller part of the opening is found above the facial; the larger part, which corresponds to the vestibule, below the facial. This method of opening the labyrinth is easy and is usually not dangerous. In this operation it is very important to protect the facial which can be easily wounded, especially so since the bony canal which seals it may be fragile, as a result of chronic inflammation. This method opens only the labyrinthine spaces. It makes possible the emptying of the contents, but does not prevent the spreading out of the infection along the posterior pyramid wall into the interior of the skull. Still it discloses any pathologic process which may have developed in these spaces.

If we take into consideration that cerebellar abscess causes symptoms similar to labyrinthine suppuration, it is clear that we have to exclude labyrinthine suppuration first and then decide upon the presence or absence of cerebellar abscess. This operation, however, does not assure the exclusion of the labyrinth in the diagnosis of the labyrinthine cerebellar abscess. Much more reliable in this connection is the retrotympanic opening of the labyrinth. The operation begins by exposure of the dura of the posterior fossa in front of the lateral sinus. We then proceed to remove the posterior surface of the pyramid. Although the exposure of the dura of the posterior fossa makes easier the carrying out of the operation, it is not always necessary in every case.

In those cases in which the mastoid process lies quite deep and is filled with air cells, the labyrinthine spaces may, as I have done it in a great number of cases, be opened through removal of the posterior pyramid wall without exposure of the dura of the posterior fossa. By chiselling parallel to the posterior pyramid wall two openings are made. The upper one corresponds to the cross-section of the crus commune of the anterior and posterior vertical canals, and the lower opening to a cross-section of the posterior canal in the region of its ampulla. Both openings are circular, are situated near the middle of the labyrinth wall, and the probe shows that they are not the shortest ways into the vestibule. Further removal of the posterior pyramid wall by means of the chisel discloses a third cavity somewhat oval on cross-section about in the middle of the two previous openings but lying somewhat more externally. This latter is a cross-section of the horizontal semi-circular canal. By means of a hooked probe it may shown that this opening is the shortest route into the vestibule. By gradually increasing the size of it the vestibule is opened from behind. By taking away the bone on the posterior pyramid wall, the lateral boundary of the inner ear is removed little by little, and the inner ear itself is exposed. This is of especial importance since the histopathologic investigations of Politzer have shown that suppuration not seldom can be concealed in the depths of the internal ear without showing any symptoms whatever. In all these manipulations it is very necessary to keep parallel to the posterior pyramid wall. A deviation upward from this direction is very dangerous to the superior petrosal sinus. A deviation downwards threatens the juglear bulb. A removal of the posterior pyramid wall externally may endanger the facial nerve. The occasional unavoidable wounding of the dura of the posterior fossa in the retrotympanic opening of the labyrinth is only dangerous if it is too small. The operation is ended by opening the promontory in which care must be taken to avoid wounding the facial, the carotid and the juglear bulb. After the operation is finished one can introduce a curved sound from the posterior pyramid surface into the tympanic cavity, in order to show that the greatest part of the labyrinth has been removed.

Following the operation, it is important ɔ investigate whether the dura has been injured, for if so, then it is always best to widen the small opening. The retrolabyrinthine cavity is loosely tamponed with strips of iodoform gauze and left open. Healing requires usually only a short time, for the freely exposed dura shows great inclination to granulation formation. In a relatively short time, the granulations extending out from the dura fill up the cavity and the wound may now be closed by sutures, if there is no reason to prefer an open granulating wound.

CORRESPONDENCE.

VANISHING SECTARIANISM.

To the Editor
AMERICAN MEDICINE:—

For the reason that this letter pertains to "medical politics," it is without my usual signature.

One evening I was called to my telephone by a prominent merchant of my home town and asked whether I would meet with an osteopath at his residence in consultation. I replied that I would be most happy to do so at any time. The consultation was soon over. I made certain suggestions as to diet, and actually prescribed a simple medicinal preparation for the patient, all with the warm approval of my colleague. The osteopath evinced such decided symptoms of surprise at my treatment of him that, on leaving the house, I ventured to inquire,

"What made you hesitate to send for me to-night?"

"Because I had been turned down by several others, and we never dreamed that you would respond to the call!"

"Well," I replied, "here is a suffering man whose condition falls within the range of my specialty, and I have always supposed that one of my professional duties was to relieve suffering."

"Yes, but you know how much prejudice you regulars have against osteopaths and homeopaths!"

"As wearers of a sectarian designation, yes; as men of science, you are absolutely wrong. Everything to-day must go into the hopper of science and be run between the millstones of practical experience. The scientific test alone can stand the light of modern experience and every day practice. Sectarianism must of necessity warp and twist facts to conform to theory, whereas science treasures the facts and allows the theories to look after themselves. Come into the medical profession, throw your nuggets into the melting pot and trust the rest to the tests of the official assayer. Whether we like it or not, evolution is the supreme law of medicine. Ephraim McDowell did not perform a perfect ovariotomy, but he blazed the trail for all time.

514   AMERICAN MEDICINE
Complete Series, Vol. XVIII. }   CORRESPONDENCE   { SEPTEMBER, 1912.
New Series, Vol. VII., No. 9.

"You have mistaken the attitude of real men of science. Write up one of your fairly illustrative cases for AMERICAN MEDICINE and submit it to the editor for publication. I agree with you that the medical profession has a great deal to learn, but it is always more than willing to learn of useful things."

In this connection, I suggest for the serious consideration of the officers of our National and State Medical Societies the propriety of extending invitations to the officers and members of sectarian bodies to unite with us in the presentation and discussion of scientific problems, and to extend to those accepting the invitation a courteous welcome and a serious hearing.

It may be said without unkindness that the end of organized sectarianism is in sight. Apparently prosperous colleges in Chicago, St. Louis, Louisville, Cincinnati, Denver and other places have died, others are slowly dying, and it must be apparent that the end can not be long delayed. Some of the remaining schools are well equipped, have large endowments, and a respectable list of alumni who remain loyal to the old colors because they dread the supposed stigma of having been graduated from a "dead college."

I shall not be personal, recalling an old adage. That Samuel Hahnemann was a profound thinker and a true reformer we have the testimony of no less an authority than Sir John Forbes, as well as thousands of lesser fame. Why not the "Hahnemann College of the University of ————?" The idea is worth considering.

Just how much longer organized medical sectarianism shall exist, depends largely, I think, upon the attitude of the medical profession. Within recent years the prestige of the profession has grown enormously in popular esteem. It will continue to grow. Even persons of low intelligence understand the value of trained medical skill.

In short, I hope that the organized profession of medicine will maintain its honorable position of broad-minded hospitality to all sects and factions, inviting them to the first table, and accepting whatever they may have to reveal in the way of helpful suggestions for the benefit of our common humanity. Sectarianism can not thrive in such an atmosphere, and science will be the gainer.

            MEDICUS.

ANTI-TYPHOID VACCINATION.

To the Editor
   AMERICAN MEDICINE :—

About six years ago the writer began to use vaccines in the treatment of typhoid fever. Since that time he has thus treated more than one hundred cases and has obtained numerous articles upon the same subject written by physicians in various parts of the world. It seems possible, however, that some may have escaped notice. He also realizes that many of the profession may have treated some cases without reporting them. A paper upon the subject is now in the course of preparation. In this it is earnestly desired to incorporate reports from a large number of cases, good, bad, and otherwise. He accordingly makes the following request to the readers of this journal:

Will any one who has used vaccines in the treatment of typhoid fever, whether but one case or more, kindly communicate to him that fact accompanied by name and address of the reporter. If the results have already been reported, a note of the journal in which they appeared will be sufficient. If they have not been reported, a short blank form will be sent to the physician to be filled out. Due credit will be given in the article to each person making a report. If any physician happens to know of other confreres who have any such cases, it will be appreciated if he sends their names, as they may not happen to read this note. It is hoped that by this means a sufficient number of cases may be collected to somewhat definitely settle the now mooted question whether vaccines are or are not of benefit in typhoid therapy.

Reports of cases will be accepted at any time in the future but preferably by November or December of the present year.

Kindly communicate with Dr. W. H. Watters, Director of the Department of Pathology and Bacteriology, Evans Institute for Clinical Research, Boston, Mass.

     Respectfully yours,
           W. H. WATTERS.

THE ANNOTATOR.

Out-door Life for City Children.[1]—A. Friedländer in a review of the recent literature upon this subject first quotes Ayer who tells of the forest school at Charlottenburg near Berlin, which was started in 1904 as an adjunct to the treatment of tuberculosis. The first schools of that kind in England and America had a similar object in view. The open-air idea now applies to anemic and badly nourished school children, and indeed it is thought that all school children would have better health if part of the school hours were spent out of doors. In such schools for healthy children the school schedule must, of course, receive first attention.

Open air schools in cities may be located in parks, or city play grounds, or upon the roofs of school buildings.

Questions of especial importance in such annexes to schools are such as relate to suitable provisions for elevators and fire escapes, and to protection from storms, wind, dust, sun, heat, and cold.

Furthermore if the window sashes in school rooms were removed except in bad weather the scholars would practically be out of doors. Williams writes that in the open-air campaign for schools in Sheffield attention was also given to the cleansing of the children, their teeth were looked after, their meals were served out of doors, and physical exercise was enforced.

It was noted that the influence of such procedures upon the parents of the children was also beneficial and instructive. Wood reported that open air schools resulted in increase in weight and in hemoglobin and in the general physique of the children. Cope reports that Boston is endeavoring to cultivate the bodies as well as the minds of its school children, and with equal care. Thousands of deaths among children from preventable diseases would not occur if the physical development received the same care as the mental, and the ultimate result would be a higher type of citizenship. Hertz declares that problems of school hygiene should always be under the control of the boards of health. School sanatoria, open air schools and clinics for the care of school children are demanded everywhere.

Carr speaks of the disadvantages of city life to children both in their homes and in the schools and pleads for open air treatment. Opportunities for physical exercise for school children must be multiplied. Meylan endeavors to prove that abnormal city children when given the chance of the life out-of-doors improve greatly, both physically and mentally.

Symposia like the foregoing are of immense value in fixing upon the mind of the public the fact that the duty of government does not end with providing school accommodations and educational privileges for its children.

The best ultimate results cannot be expected from a child who gets no chance at the sports and games of childhood and youth any more than from a plant which is forced in a hot house. Man, as an animal, was designed to live out of doors.

Neosalvarsan.[1]—E. Schreiber tells us that neosalvarsan bears the laboratory number 914, and represents work additional to salvarsan or 606. It is derived from salvarsan by condensation of that substance with formaldehyde sulphoxylate of sodium. It is a neutral yellowish powder, and dissolves readily in water. It is much less toxic than salvarsan and 1.5 grams corresponds with 1 gram of salvarsan. When prepared for intravenous use it is poured from the containing ampoule into freshly distilled sterile water, is shaken gently and is then ready for use. The dosage is 1.5 grams for men and 1.2 grams for women, but one should begin with about half that quantity. Clinical results occur with great promptness and there is very little collateral disturbance. It will often be advisable to administer mercury or mercury and potassium iodide in conjunction with neosalvarsan. The contraindications are the same as for salvarsan.

The following may be considered a summary of its advantages.

1. It is more readily soluble than salvarsan and has an absolutely neutral reaction.

[1] *Interstate Medical Journal*, July, 1912.

[1] *Medical Times*, July, 1912.

2. It is better tolerated than salvarsan and can be given in larger doses.

3. Its therapeutic activity is at least as great as that of salvarsan.

4. It is better adapted for intra-muscular injection than salvarsan.

The Nervous Child.— Whether presented in the form of the typical, or in the guise of the child prodigy the cause of a child's differentiation from the normal is nearly always traceable to a nervous condition says Barbara Allen, in a recent issue of *American Motherhood.* Nervous children constitute the great mass of the earth's misunderstood, and they are doomed, through our ignorance of their needs, to a pitiful isolation in a dark and distasteful atmosphere. And in direct ratio with the child's losses does mankind lose. The musician in embryo is treated as a dunce in the school of mathematics to which he is assigned by his parents. The child who lacks poise and develops temper is submitted to a will breaking process by his family that results in his loss of all self control rather than the power to exercise the same. The child who is visionary, who has, like William Canton's "W. V.," an invisable child playmate that she sees, and can describe, and whose loss causes her exquisite pain, is not recognized as a genius, a child possessing vivid imagination of the construction type which may be turned into the channels of literature, of drama. She is, rather, looked upon as a changeling, a personality out of tune with her environment.

If the nervous child continues to be the misunderstood child, if he grows up in an unsuitable environment and is improperly educated, either of two results may take place; as in Birton's case his nerves snap and instead of a useful member of society he becomes a burden to himself, or his nervous system develops at variance with his surroundings. There is eventually forced to the surface an unreal, a weaker personality, a composite self, unstable, and having the elements of dementia. From this soil springs the criminal and the degenerate.

A child's nervous system, the network of telephone and long distance telegraph and wire cables with which he is equipped and by which he established connections and relations with life is a remarkably fine and sensitive system. The wires are unusually slender and keenly attuned to their business of transmitting sensations to the unwritten plates of the new brain. Through their means the little child slowly, wonderingly, feels his way from the border land of birth to the crowded, noisy machine world in which he must learn to co-ordinate and poise, and adjust himself to unknown conditions.

There is so much that we can do to help him in this process of place finding, of nerve stimulation. When a nerve system is wrecked, doctors are of little avail, but the child who shows signs at three or four years of differentiation from type must be studied and not misunderstood, that his greatest usefulness as a member of society may be brought about.

"Putting yourself in his place" is the primary line in the home nerve prescription. We have been adults so long that we forget how a child feels. We misconstrue his aims and intentions. We neglect the gentle art of growing down to his level. The child who is normally afraid of the dark is to be pitied, not urged to a heroism of which he is nervously incapable. Back of him are lined up centuries of ancestors who were continually surrounded by real fear, terror of the hunt, of persecution, of martydom. As he goes upstairs alone in the dark, his ghosts are the spirits of the Inquisition. The flaming eyes that he sees at every landing are the same fiery eyeballs that gleamed out of the gloom of jungle and fores as the cave dwellers laid down their heads for the night. The creatures beneath his crib are the mobs that stoned the prophets. A child's terrors are very real and may wreck him nervously. They are neither a matter of fancy nor a whim, but such a force for evil in themselves, they form a special phase of child study.

One wise mother took her children into the dusky outdoors every evening as an antidote for their night terrors. She taught them the bedtime habits of birds, insects, and stars. She showed them the marvellous expanse of night sky, and told them stories about the star world. Then each child provided with a candle and mother leading the procession, they trailed upstairs to bed and after they were tucked up, just before the candles were snuffed, mother opened the windows wide, and pulled back the curtains that the children might have the stars for company when she had gone downstairs. It is well worth while to help children to overcome fear. The task alone is too nerve racking for them.

The child who is shy needs help as well, over the difficult sea of self consciousness. The social training of the kindergarten will prove to be his best school, and all semblance of "showing off" should be avoided in his home life.

The apparently naughty child forms a nerve class by himself. Perhaps he belongs to the type of perverted will phychologists tell us really exists. Certain lines of conduct exacted of him suggest to his nerve cells exactly opposite reactions. The force with which we tell a child who sobs in an apparent agony of temper to stop crying really makes him continue. We tell him that there are matches in a certain forbidden spot and he will be burned if he lights them, but in so doing we start an inexpressible longing for experience on the part of the child, a tingling nerve system that demands, exacts this novel sensation of being burned, and he touches the forbidden fire sticks, and through wilfulness, but as a nerve reaction because of our suggestion.

Every kindergartner and many mothers know the agony of the nervous child's first school day. He throws himself upon the floor, has hysterics, perhaps, and is so exceedingly naughty in the eyes of the grown ups—but it really is not naughtiness at all. There is a mass of new sensations crowding along his nerve telephone system—the crowds, the new environment, the unknown adjustments which are expected of him. He suffers keener agony than we know, and we scold him for his apparent bad behavior.

Early years of childhood are not only the most impressionable, but because of their very plasticity the most dangerous ones, along the line of nerve strain. A little child is a wonderfully emotional animal. He is quick to smiles and quicker to tears. He needs a depth of sympathetic study, and a wealth of tenderness. Modern life is full of just the stimulants that a child's brain should not have—late hours, moving pic-

ture entertainments, comic supplements of Sunday papers that shock his eyes with their glaring colors, and overstimulate his imagination with their suggestions, the mechanical toy, and the indulgence and unmeant cruelty of misunderstanding parents.

There is no medicine to cure the soul ills of the nervous child. What he needed from babyhood was Rousseau, and rompers, and bare feet, and God's good outdoors. The nervous child, at large, unhampered by the conventions of society, and unfettered by the "don't," and "do" of worrying parents will outgrow his nerves. His toys should be garden tools, and balls, and bats, and a velocipede, and a gay express wagon. He should be in the open every day of the year, and sleep there too, if possible. Fresh air used to be looked upon only as the tuberculosis antidote. Now it is the elixir for diseased nerves. Life in the open, as far as possible from the haunts of the city dwellers, combined with wise and patient study of the individual emotional needs of the nervous child will accomplish the desired results, and put him back where he belongs with the sane, nerveless, healthy child.

Human Conservation.[1]— An editorial states that conservation of child life is one of the foundation stones of the republic of the future, and that the ravages of enteric diseases among our infants will be felt in the generation to come. Pure milk will lower the death rate immediately and permanently, and it can be obtained as easily as impure milk. Stricter legislative enactment and vigorous prosecutions of the men who control the milk supply will do much toward bringing pure milk into our cities.

Montclair, N. J., a city of twenty-two thousand inhabitants went at the milk question in a very positive and strenuous fashion and all of Montclair's milk is now pure. During the hot spell in July, 1911, only one baby under twenty-four months of age died in Montclair from gastro-intestinal disease. If this plan had been followed in other cities the mortality from summer diseases among the babies could have been similarly reduced.

[1] *Medical Times*, July, 1912.

What Montclair can do every city in the country can do. If infant life is worth preserving, physicians and boards of health should hear opportunity knocking and bid him enter.

This sounds nicely, but what about the crowded tenements imperfectly ventilated, and the wretched conditions of life generally in the larger portion of the poor and ignorant in our cities?

Pure milk will not relieve such conditions valuable and indispensable though it be. The axe must be laid at the root of the tree and social conditions be changed in order to produce such ideal results as were obtained in Montclair.

———

ETIOLOGY AND DIAGNOSIS.

Fractures, Dislocations and Sprains—Their Differential Diagnosis.[1]—In the course of a series of articles on fractures that for trite, practical information are the most notable that have appeared for many a day, Colcord gives the following terse points for differentiating certain conditions liable to confuse in diagnosticating fractures.

1. *Dislocations.*—This is especially true in fractures of the upper end of the humerus, either of the anatomical or surgical neck with marked displacement of the lower fragment. Here the sharp edge of the lower fragment may be felt under the skin and the upper one in the axilla.

Dislocation of the elbow in adults is often accompanied by a fracture. Here the X-ray is usually necessary to clear up the diagnosis.

Dislocation of the wrist may simulate Colles' fracture. Feel for the styloid processes of both radius and ulna and compare with those of the sound side. Feel for the point of sharp tenderness on the outside of the radius just above the lower end.

Dislocation of the hip should not be difficult to differentiate from fracture.

2. *Sprains.*—The most difficult sprain in my own experience to differentiate from fracture has been that of the ankle. In this sprain, if severe, something gives way and it is always the weakest thing. The ligaments only may be torn, constituting a simple sprain, or a ligament may come away at its insertion, carrying with it portions of its bony attachment. Often there is fracture of one or both malleoli. Look for points of tenderness over the malleoli, keeping away from the margin, and follow well up to the fibula. Many fractures of the malleoli give no crepitus.

Sprains of the elbow may simulate fracture even to joint crepitus, which is frequent in babies. When you find crepitus in a baby's elbow, see if it is not also in the other one.

Sprained wrist with much swelling along the tendon sheaths may simulate Colles' fracture, but the classical points in the diagnosis of the latter should clear up most cases.

3. *Contusions.*—A contusion severe enough to injure the periosteum may closely resemble subperiosteal fracture. Absence of a point of tenderness on the opposite side of the bone will usually exclude fracture, as where a heavy body has fallen on the dorsum of the foot, we may try pressure on the sole of the foot over the point of a suspected metatarsal fracture.

In contusions of chest where fractured rib is suspected, apply pressure with each hand over the ends of ribs, keeping well away from the contused area. If there is fracture we get sharp pain at the point of the break. Or we may use a stethoscope over the rib and often elicit crepitus with movements of breathing.

A contusion of the scalp may feel to the touch like a depressed fracture from the hard rim of swollen tissues around it.

A contusion of a joint of the finger or thumb, transmitted from a blow on the end of the finger, is often difficult to tell from a fracture of the joint surfaces. From the frequency of this injury to those playing the "national game" the writer has called it "baseball" fracture. X-ray examinations will show quite a large proportion of these cases to be real fractures, as the annexed skiagram will illustrate. In my opinion, all that present large joints afterward have been real fractures.

When in doubt in regard to the diagnosis of any fracture, give the patient the benefit of the doubt and take an X-ray picture, treating the case as a fracture until the diagnosis has been made.

———

The Clinical Diagnosis of Renal Insufficiency.[1]—Fulton, in a paper of extraordinary interest and merit makes the following statements:—

The physician should, in bedside work, consider the subject from the functional standpoint rather than as a pathologist.

It does not matter how badly damaged a kidney is so long as it performs its functions: nephritis may exist without renal insufficiency.

Renal insufficiency may be marked even when albumin is absent from the urine.

The use of the sphygmomanometer, ophthalmoscope, stethoscope, and physical examinations, give more reliable data than do the urinary findings.

Physiological tests of the kidney functions are unfortunately of dependable value only in surgical nephritis: in other forms of nephritis they show too great variations.

The measurement of the urea output is of undoubted value, *if the intake of food substances is known.*

[1] A. W. Colcord, M. D., *International Jour. of Surgery*, June, 1912.

[1] J. S. Fulton, M. D., Los Angeles, Cal., *Interstate Med. Jour.*, July, 1912.

TREATMENT.

Asthma in Children.[1]—True asthma is a paroxysmal respiratory neurosis, characterized by attacks of intense dyspnea with bronchial catarrh, returning at intervals, more or less prolonged. It is very common in children of all ages. In 75 cases collected by Comby the first attack showed itself in 9 under 6 months old, in 15 between 6 and 12 months old, in 36 between 1 and 3 years, in 9 between 3 and 6 years, and in 10 over 6 years old. Children predisposed to the attacks often suffer from eczema, which comes on in the early months of life, persists for months and years, to end in asthmatic attacks. In these cases the eczema takes the place of the asthma. Comby does not believe that true asthma can be looked upon as caused by the presence of adenoids, nor can it in any way be deemed a symptom of tubercle. The etiology of the attacks is the same as in adults; they are more frequent in winter than in summer, and are influenced by the wind, dampness, etc. Certain diseases provoke a return of the attacks. Influenza is often followed by them in asthmatics and the same is the case with indigestion. Usually the attack is quite sudden. The child, which went off to sleep well, is seized in the middle of the night with a dry cough. Breathing is hurried, and the child sits up in bed. Respiration is very noisy and auscultation easily reveals sonorous râles, musical and sibilant, and a *bruit de tempête.* The special character of the bronchitis is very musical. The face shows great distress, and the lips are cyanosed. The pulse is at the rate of 120 to 140. There is a slight rise of temperature to about 100.4° F., but never so high as in the case of pneumonia and broncho-pneumonia. During the attack there is complete anorexia, distress, and insomnia. The condition lasts for some hours up to a day, but after this it all disappears. The asthmatic attack is done, but in some cases some bronchial catarrh remains for some days. Asthma is more catarrhal in the child than in the adult. As a rule the interval between two attacks increases the farther the first attack is left behind. Frequent and violent attacks give rise to fears of pulmonary emphysema appearing. Comby insists upon the special syndrome of nasal asthma. The children have spasmodic sneezing and nasal catarrh is very marked. With asthma may be associated laryngismus stridulus, spasm of the glottis or general convulsions. The diagnosis of a first attack is often difficult. The sudden onset and the fierce intensity of the dyspnea are as a rule enough to prevent confusion with broncho-pneumonia, which may end in this way, but never begins so. The musical character of the breath sounds are also quite distinctive enough. Spasm of the glottis is a short and apneic attack. The stridor and stertor have not the same character. The only diagnosis which may be difficult to set up is that between infantile and glandular asthma,

but the latter has not the abrupt onset and the sudden ending of an asthmatic attack, it has no definite fit with musical bronchitis.

The treatment consists in giving plenty of air, putting a mustard plaster on the back and front of the chest, or applying dry cupping. No nitre fumes, or anti-asthmatic cigarettes, or inhalations of ether or chloroform should be given. Comby gives every two hours in a teaspoonful of water a powder composed of 1 gr. of Dover's powder and 8 gr. of sugar of milk, 1 gr. of Dover's powder should be given per diem, and for each year of age. Instead may be given in a teaspoonful of sweetened water, five to ten drops, three or four times a day, of the following:—

. ℞ Tincturæ Aconiti,
    Tincturæ Belladonnæ,
    Tincturæ Droseræ,
    Tinturæ Grindeliæ,
    Tincturæ Lobeliæ..............aa Mxv.
    Extracti Opii....................gr. viij.
    Misce.

If necessary, an hypodermic injection of morphia (gr. $\frac{1}{32}$ to $\frac{1}{12}$ according to age) may be given.

In the interval between the attacks the child must live in the open air, have cold douches, and be well rubbed. The food must be eaten slowly; it must consist very sparingly of meat (which must never be given in the evening), but must be largely vegetable. For drink, water only is allowed. According to the case, a stay by the sea or in the mountains is recommended. Internal treatment is thus to be carried out. For 10 days, before the two chief meals, a teaspoonful of a solution of potassium iodide in water (4½ grains to ℨj.) is to be taken. For the next 10 days this is replaced by a teaspoonful of a solution of arsenate of soda, gr. ⅛ in ℨj. The iodide is begun again after a further period of ten days. In the case of bronchial catarrh a claret-glass full of sulphur water from Labassére is to be taken at early breakfast.

Bites of Insects.[1]—Neal states that he has found the following procedure very useful:

Take one ounce of Epsom salt and dissolve it in one pint of water, wet a bath cloth so that it will not drip and rub the body well all over, and not wipe afterward but dress, and flies, gnats, fleas, bedbugs, mosquitoes, etc., will never touch you. If one is exposed more than usual, being near water, or in a forest, then make a somewhat stronger solution, wet a cloth and rub the face, neck, ears and hands well—do not wipe, but allow it to dry; it will leave a fine powder over the surface that the most bloodthirsty insect will not attack. Besides, the solution is healing and cleansing; it will heal the bites, subdue the consequent inflammation, and cure many diseases of the skin.

[1] *Jour. des Practiciens.* April, 1912.

[1] H. D. Neal, M. D., *China Med. Jour..* March, 1912.

GENERAL TOPICS.

Frazier says that ipecac will abort typhoid fever. It is given in six successive single daily doses, the first day 30 grains, and each day 5 grains less. It is administered in salol coated capsules, so that it will not act in the stomach and cause vomiting.

Dirt and Disease.—Dr. Charles Wardell Stiles makes the statement (*Lancet-Clinic*) that the United States is seven times dirtier than Germany and ten times more unclean than Switzerland, and that the lack of interest in preventive measures against disease is slaughtering the human race. Not race suicide but race slaughter is Dr. Stiles' diagnosis of our national census report. Too many children are allowed to die. Tuberculosis still claims an annual death toll of 5,000,000, and typhoid fever probably costs the nation an annual loss of $300,000,000. With the new powers granted to the public health service at Washington will undoubtedly come an awakening of the cities and States to their responsibility in these matters. The Federal Government can investigate and recommend measures to bring about better conditions—in the case of epidemics it may even put certain regulations into effect, but the regular routine arrangements to care for health must be made by the local community.

OBITUARY.

DR. MAURICE H. RICHARDSON—A FAMOUS NEW ENGLAND SURGEON.

It was a shock to the profession of America when the news was flashed the country over that Maurice Richardson was dead. In the whole galaxy of new world surgeons who have made American surgery something other than a by-word in the great medical centers of Europe, Richardson deserves a place second to none. Fortunate in his associations and his connection with a famous institution, Dr. Richardson had the ability to measure up to his opportunities. Thus he became early in his career one of the foremost surgeons in one of the country's recognized medical centers, and for years has enjoyed this distinction.

An article in the *Journal of the American Med. Assn.* (Aug. 10, 1912), states that Dr. Richardson was found dead in his bed in Boston, July 31, aged 60. He was born in Athol, Mass., Dec. 31, 1851, the son of Nathan Henry and Martha Ann (Barber) Richardson. He attended the public school of Athol and Fitchburg High School, and entered Harvard University in 1869 from which he graduated with the degree of A. B. in 1873. After a four-years course in Harvard Medical School he

was graduated in 1877. During his last year in medical college, Dr. Richardson was assistant in anatomy under Dr. Oliver Wendell Holmes, occupying this position for two years. He was then made demonstrator of anatomy and served until 1887, and thereafter was assistant professor of anatomy until 1892. From 1883 to 1887 he was assistant in surgery; in 1895 he was made assistant professor of clinical surgery; in 1902 associate professor of clinical surgery and from 1903 until his death was Mosely professor of clinical surgery.

He had been a member of the staff of the Massachusetts General Hospital since 1881, and was made surgeon-in-chief in 1910. Among his other hospital appointments were those of district physician and physician to the Boston Dispensary; surgeon to the out-patient department of the Boston City Hospital and Carney

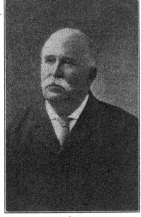

DR. MAURICE H. RICHARDSON.

Hospital, and physician to the House of the Good Samaritan.

His society membership included the American Medical Association; American Surgical Association, of which he was president in 1902; American Academy of Medicine; Southern Surgical and Gynecological Association and Boylston Medical Society, of which he was once president.

Dr. Richardson was a prolific contributor to the literature of surgery and contributed sections to Park's "Surgery by American Authors" and Dennis' "System of Surgery."

Everyone who knew Dr. Richardson loved him, for he had a kind and lovable disposition. Although his clientele was known to include the wealthiest residents of his community and people from all over the country sought his advice and skill, he did an enormous amount of charitable work. Indeed, it is doubtful if another man of Richardson's calibre and standing was doing more work for which he received no remuneration. A remarkably dexterous operator, and consequently often able to achieve results that a less skillful surgeon would find impossible, Dr. Richardson was nevertheless exceedingly conservative. Never would he undertake an operation for the sake of doing a brilliant piece of work. The first, last and constant consideration with him was the best interests of the patient. He held very positive views along these lines and never neglected an opportunity of condemning surgery that had any other incentive than a patient's needs.

The world misses such men and American surgery has lost one of its noblest and most capable practitioners. For many years Dr. Richardson gave the best that was in him to the service of humanity. He was successful from every standpoint, but in the gratitude of the thousands of patients he has been able to restore to useful lives, he doubtless found his most satisfactory reward.

Now that he has journeyed on to that "bourne from which no traveller returns," genuine as will be the personal sorrow felt at his demise, there will come a real feeling of appreciation that it was given to Dr. Richardson to carry his work to fruition for so many years. It is good that such a man has been permitted to devote his talents to surgical science.

We can hardly grasp the influence he has had on surgical progress. It will take the perspective of another decade to realize the magnitude of his work. But when the history of American surgery is written the full stature of Maurice Richardson as a great surgeon will be very evident.

DR. JOHN J. TAYLOR—PHYSICIAN, EDITOR, CITIZEN.

Every now and then the ruthless hand of Death plucks from our circle some one who in his life and work has become so integral a part of the world as we know it—such an essential fixture in the social mechanism—that adjustment is never possible, a new order must be evolved. This is exactly the situation created by the death of Dr. J. J. Taylor, editor of the *Medical Council* of Philadelphia. Quiet, gentle and unassuming he had nevertheless fitted himself into his field of activity and become so useful in his own particular way to every one fortunate enough to come in contact with him, that his passing has meant a loss that can never be replaced. As Time, the Great Comforter, reconciles us to the void forced upon us, others may take up the essential or fundamental portion of Dr. Taylor's work and carry it forward efficiently and successfully, but it is no reflection on them when we say that henceforth it will be their work—not his. It is out of the question to expect that anyone could fill Dr. Taylor's place, or fight life's

battles in the exact way that his distinctive personality made possible. Perhaps it is better to have it this way, but this constitutes the real loss after all, when men like Dr. Taylor lay down their labors. Their work, constructively and substantially, goes on. It is a testimonial to their craftsmanship that it is always too valuable and important to allow it to lapse, even temporarily. But something that gave it charm and made it attractive along special lines, is gone, and no matter what progress it makes or what success it achieves there is a lack, a genuine loss that can never again be restored. New interests and new personalities will undoubtedly safely preserve the substance of Dr. Taylor's work and impart new features that will strengthen it and increase its usefulness as the years go on. But with Dr. Taylor there has vanished an intangible something that went hand in hand with our association with him, and though memory is rich with choice recollections of his fine character, his noble deeds and his thousand and one acts of loyal friendship, it is the sense of losing forever those indefinable qualities that were so woven into the fabric of Dr. Taylor's personality that brings home this bereavement that time may rob it of its present poignancy, but can never efface.

Dr. Taylor was born in Indiana, November 24, 1853.

He came East early in his career to study medicine. While a very successful practitioner, still, having the literary bent that is the mark of an Indianan, he found his natural sphere in medical journalism.

Nothing need be said of his twenty-five years of work for the medical profession in this field. It is known to all.

A member of the Medical Club of Philadelphia, the Philadelphia County Medical Society, the Medical Society of the State of Pennsylvania, the American Medical Association, the American Medical Editors' Association, the American Academy of Political and Social Science, the American Society for Advancement of Science, many social clubs, including the Masonic Order, as well as other organizations, Dr. Taylor had a host of friends and an extended sphere of influence and usefulness.

A man of even and judicial temperament, tolerant, of irreproachable integrity, fine feeling, sympathetic manner and high ideals, Dr. Taylor was one who devoted much time and heart-interest to many lines of human uplift and the cultivation of an ideal professional and home life. He was one who realized in his own life, and made others to realize, that "All the way to Heaven is Heaven."

He died of exhaustion, at his summer home in Ocean City, N. J., on August first.

In closing these few words of tribute to a friend, we cannot refrain from saying that Dr. Taylor exemplified in every act or deed the best and truest principles of modern medicine. With his ear tuned to every note of genuine progress, he was yet conservative enough to appreciate the methods and measures that have stood the test of time. Never would he forsake or discard the old until he was thoroughly convinced that he had something better. Like all good men, loyalty was one of the foundations of his character. No one ever suffered injury at the hands of John J. Taylor. It was a well known fact that his kind and trustful disposition often led the unscrupulous and tricky to take advantage of him. But even when confronted by some act of deceit, dishonesty or meanness, he was ever ready to condone the offence and try to find some excuse for the culprit. Indeed, he was always ready to place the burden of blame on himself for not recognizing the situation, or being astute enough to avoid the circumstances that made him a victim! Few men ever had a larger supply of the milk of human kindness.

Kind and gentle as a woman but with all the virile force of a man who knew the strength of his own intellect and will, it seems too bad that he should be taken away from us while in his very prime. But deeply as every one must regret the withdrawal of this fine and noble man from the human stage, there yet must remain a wealth of gratitude that it was given to us to know and be with him as much as we have. He was a force, an inspiration, and no man who ever knew John J. Taylor can have failed to receive some measure of benefit from the acquaintance. Fortunate, indeed, were those who were thrown into intimate relations with him, for there were no weak or uncertain spots in his character. He was white clear through, and there was never a time when he failed to ring true to every clean sentiment or proper demand. As physician, editor, citizen, man of affairs and true gentleman Dr. Taylor never shirked a duty or dodged an issue. Men knew where to find him, and while never dogmatic, he could always be relied upon to hold sound and stable views on every important question.

It is platitudinous to say that the world is better because such a man has lived. There is hardly any good and honest man who does not leave the world better than he found it. The strength of Dr. Taylor's life is the help and inspiration he has been to other men. The desire that he has planted in the breasts of countless of his colleagues to do more and better work, to discount difficulties and obstacles, and to cultivate poise and self-mastery, has borne abundant fruit, and though Dr. Taylor in the last few months of his life showed men how to die nobly and with courage sublime, it is the aid he has been to his fellowmen in helping them to live useful, well balanced lives that makes his own life stand out as such a conspicuous success.

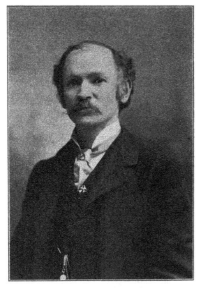

DR. JOHN J. TAYLOR.

American Medicine

H. EDWIN LEWIS, M. D., *Managing Editor.*

PUBLISHED MONTHLY BY THE AMERICAN-MEDICAL PUBLISHING COMPANY.

Copyrighted by the American Medical Publishing Co., 1912.

| Complete Series, Vol. XVIII., No. 10. New Series, Vol. VII., No. 10. | OCTOBER, 1912. | $1.00 YEARLY in advance. |

The Congress on Hygiene and Demography recently convened in Washington was one of the most important conventions ever held in this or any other country. The daily newspapers and the various weekly publications have given unusually complete reports of the principal addresses and their discussions. Probably no meeting of scientists ever excited greater interest or received more earnest attention generally than this Congress on Hygiene. So much has been written and published that we feel it unnecessary to give more than the brief but comprehensive report that will be found on another page (575). At the same time so great was the success of the meeting and so far reaching have been its lessons and results that we cannot refrain from expressing a few words of commendation, not only for the splendid work of the Congress itself, but also for the high order of executive and organizing ability that played such a conspicuous part in the direction and management of its affairs. The opinion was freely voiced that this large convention of scientists from all over the civilized world was organized, directed and carried through to adjournment with better system, less confusion and closer adherence to modern business-like methods than had ever before been witnessed. More than this, it was the universal sentiment that this great Congress on Hygiene was certain to exert more profound influences on the welfare of the people than had any of its predecessors, owing to the remarkable publicity that had been systematically obtained, not only for many days previous to the convention but throughout its sessions. A good many individuals contributed to the success of the Congress, many whose only reward will be their own knowledge of the aid they gave. But there is one man who deserves more than passing mention, for it is a pretty well established fact that to him more than to any other one person, the extraordinary success of the Fifteenth International Congress of Hygiene was due. It is hardly necessary to say that we refer to Dr. John S. Fulton of Baltimore, the Secretary of the Congress. Dr. Fulton has long been known as an organizer and executive of exceptional ability. Many large affairs have been placed in his hands from time to time during the past ten or fifteen years, and always their direction and outcome have added to his reputation. But in all his career, Dr. Fulton never won laurels more fully deserved than those that have come to him for his splendid services in organizing and directing the Congress on Hygiene. It is not our purpose to be fulsome in our praise or to embarrass a modest gentleman by excessive adulation. But there is an unfortunate tendency in connection with enterprises like this International Congress on Hygiene to exalt those who present important contributions in the shape of addresses, reports of discoveries, new theories, important conclusions, etc., and overlook those who have done the routine, and often arduous work of organizing and preparing the meeting itself. This is hardly fair, and ample recognition should always be given to those whose efforts make possible every successful or eventful convention. Referring to the Congress on Hygiene, too great credit cannot be given to Dr. Fulton. Realizing that the strength of the meeting would be the educational influences it would exert on the whole American people, this keen, strong man instituted a campaign that was thoroughly modern and progressive, in that it included the latest and most approved publicity methods. Systematically the interest of the intelligent classes was stimulated and the objects and purposes of the Congress spread broadcast. Without the slightest exaggeration it can be truthfully said that never was a scientific convention exploited so widely and aggressively. With all the aggression and activity of his campaign, however, it never lost its dignity and earnestness. As a consequence, Dr. Fulton had the satisfaction of directing a Congress that was not only extraordinarily successful from every standpoint, but one that probably impressed the American people more and left a deeper imprint on their daily lives than any other that has ever been held in this country. Those who followed the work of the Congress and noted the really wonderful interest that was taken in its deliberations from day to day will readily agree with the foregoing. As a matter of simple justice, therefore, in recognizing the great and lasting good that has been done by the Fifteenth International Congress on Hygiene and Demography for humanity at large, let no one forget the unostentatious and unassuming labors of the man who more than any one else laid the foundation for its success and permanent benefits.

The segregation of defectives is not so far off, now that we are able to detect arrested mental development so accurately. Ever since we found out that Lombroso was not correct in his estimate of the large number of criminals who were physical degenerates, we have been inclined to view the majority of offenders as mere weaklings lacking inhibition, but now that the recent pyschological tests have shown such a high percentage of them to be cases of arrested mental development, mere grown-up boys and girls all their lives, we must shift our viewpoint quite markedly. We have been deceived by the very excellence of the results of the training in juvenile penal institutions which report that about three-fourths more or less can be made into fairly good, though childish, citizens if they are taken soon enough. Many, of course, are merely cases of slow development, requiring many years to mature, whereas the average normal person stops his mental development sometime before eighteen and a few much earlier who are really normal. Only the exceptional persons keep up mental growth longer, a few even until 35 or 40. Some of these later developers are as well or farther advanced at 16 to 20 as those who stop at those ages. The juvenile criminals are almost invariably subnormal, so we are told, and range all the way down to the border line of imbecility in which mental growth is checked in early childhood. The idiot, whose development stops in infancy and most imbeciles, have not enough sense to devise crimes except of the purely animal type and are early segregated. The later cases must now be put under restraint, as they are the ones who are constantly recruiting the underworld, utterly unable either physically or mentally, to endure the strains of making an honest living. The Rosenthal murder has shown what the type can do if at large.

The effects of the environment loom up larger than ever by these new psychologic revelations. Gutter-life of the slums has hitherto been considered more in the light of bad training of otherwise fair material. Nevertheless we have frequently called attention to the fact that though the parents of our unfit are able to make a respectable living and raise a family, it is generally a poor living and an indifferent raising. Something has happened to them to push them to the poverty line or over. This something has continued to act in the next generation, and it is our task to discover this something or these somethings. The prospects of prevention are very bright. If we are not greatly in error, every one of these decayed lines springs from perfectly good ones, and every perfect branch is occasionally sending off a defective twig. Every man has some remote relations he regrets to own, and no line is wholly bad. The few very bad lines which have been worked up, have given a very false idea as to the inevitable heredity of badness, for those families have many living excellent citizens, who dare not declare their relationship. For their sake the family is hidden under such an assumed title as "Jukes." The eugenists are showing that feeble-mindedness and epilepsy do stick in families many generations, but that both tend to disappear by proper marriages of the best of them. Yet even these must have a start-

ing point somewhere in normal families. Adam and Eve weren't such, even if one boy became a murderer,—a typical story, by-the-way, of what we see now.

The first step in preventing crime is to test all convicted offenders and detain each one until he does develop and if he does not improve, confine him for life in appropriate colonies as unable to make a living—the same rule we propose in the case of tramps and drunkards. This will surely reduce our dreadful record. Then we will be able to look into the causes of such failures of normal heredity and apply preventive measures. Mere punishment for crime is barbarous and behind the times. Conviction should merely be an order to experts to cure the offender or care for him the rest of his days,—deliberate unprovoked murder alone excepted.

Experience shows that nothing but death acts as a deterrent for this crime and that it does deter even if all these men are subnormal, though not sufficiently so to warrant confinement beforehand. So let us hurry up colonies for all who are unable to make their living. Epileptics, insane and the senile are cared for, but we must turn our prisons into hospitals, as we did our bedlams, and treat our tramps and drunkards like the invalids they are. They are only three per cent. of the population, so we are informed, but these three million are costing the other 97 million too much to be allowed liberty any longer. Besides we may soon reduce the unfit to one per cent., and less than that in time, if we get at the causes of their unfitness.

The use of hair seems a very academic matter, but it begins to appear to be a very practical hygienic one, and not beneath the dignity of a physician's notice. We all once thought it trivial, though we should have known that nature is never a trifler. There is no doubt now that in our primitive hatless stage head hair developed over the cerebral cells to shade them from the disinfecting powers of sunlight, by which the nerve cells would be killed as surely as bacterial cells. If the hair is removed or so arranged as to lose its shading effect, all people instinctively restore the shade by opaque head dresses. Visitors from India have been shocked at our carelessness in this respect in our short summers, which are just as hot and light as their longer ones. It is said that because of this carelessness we suffer more from the effects of light and heat than tropical residents. If all this is true—and we see no reason to doubt it—would it not be well to warn against the fad of going hatless in the sun? In addition, the head-gear the world over, for man or animal, is opaque, and yet some of us have been wearing summer hats so gauzy as to give no protection whatever. Those ladies, who wear huge mounds of other folks hair, of course, are properly protected outdoors, and can remove the wads at home when not needed, or too warm—another instance of the universal rule that good can be found in every evil, if we search for it.

The disappearance of body hair seems on the road to explanation. Prehistoric engravings recently found show that primitive man was well covered with short hair, and its subsequent disappearance was quite puzzling until it was found that naked-skinned types were the fittest to survive rapid changes of temperature.

They could be cooler in very hot surroundings and clothe themselves in cold. By ordinary selection they replaced the hairy specimens. Attention has recently been called to the fact that the least hairy race—Mongols—exist where there are the greatest and most rapid changes in temperature, and that our Indians seem to be descended from such Asiatics. All this confirms theory, and has the practical corollary that to be healthy we must vary our clothing to suit conditions and do it far more frequently than has been our custom. Some people seem to think they should wear the same kind of clothes the year round. Perhaps we may find in that habit, the reason for much illness, for, as we have frequently mentioned, we are clothed too much in winter, too heavily for hot houses and too scantily for cold streets. In summer our garb is idiotic whereas if we could hang our fashion makers we might be clothed so as to approach—if not actually reach—comfort every day and every hour, and be healthier for it.

The use of the beard has also been explained at last. Many a soldier has let his beard grow in forest or brush campaigning because he found it a great protection from injury. This one fact shows why it developed in man during the hunting stage of culture, but not in women, and why it disappeared by reversed selection when no longer of use to Mongols and others who wandered to the steppes and plains. There are some apparent exceptions to this generalization, but they may be migrants in whom the process has not had time to occur, as it evidently requires thousands of years. The forest living Ainus had big beards, but their Mongol conquerers (the present Japanese) had none, and still have little, except where Ainus mixture is suspected. The beard, like every other character, may persist long after its use is gone, providing it is not harmful. It now seems a mere ornament which may be useful in very exceptional cases. It is entirely outside the realm of sanitation, if it is kept clean and not a garbage receptacle. A dirty beard is another matter,—a germ carrier. A clean beard cannot be a vital protection to the larynx as once thought, because men in the coldest countries do not have beards, as a rule. To shave or not to shave is then a matter for individual esthetic taste. Men are healthy with it in cold places and hot, light and dark, indoor or out, and at sea level or on mountain tops. It is an enormous relief to find some toilet fad of clean people, which hygienists may conscientiously ignore as none of their business.

The finding of an alleged white race among the Esquimaux proves to have been greatly exaggerated. Mr. V. Steffensson, who made the discovery, now reports that he saw no blue eyed specimens, though he heard of some. The men whom he did examine, resembled the Esquimaux very much, so closely indeed, that they would have been taken for Esquimaux were it not for a reddish color of hair and beard. Steffensson thinks that they are remnants of Norwegian blood introduced centuries ago. His opinion was based on the discovery of certain words which were apparently of Norwegian origin. If all this is true it confirms the old theory that the whole Esquimaux race is, in fact, a mixture between European intruders and North American Indians. They have the long head of the European stock and the broad face of the American, a disharmony never found in pure races. Nevertheless, there are spots in Northern Asia where the natives have reddish hair and beard and the phenomenon has never been explained. There certainly is no evidence that it is due to an admixture with blonder types, but seems to be on the same order as the reddening of the hair of black horses exposed to intense sunlight, such as exists in the Arctic summers. If it is really due to Norwegian blood the climate very quickly eliminated those of fair skin, blue eyes and yellow hair. In time they will undoubtedly be as dark as any other Esquimaux. This is the way blondness has been eliminated from the Aryans, who invaded India, and the French who invaded Louisiana. The facts of the story, as far as known, merely confirm what has already been established as to the effects of climate in modifying an intruded type to perfect adjustment.

The excess of births over deaths is a universal phenomenon the world over, and is generally considered a good sign, but it may be the forerunner of disaster. Unless the surplus can find food, they must move out or die. Scandinavia, for instance, has witnessed such an emigration for thousands of years. Sometimes the surplus piles up for famines to wipe out as in India and China. Only in the last century have factories absorbed many who there earn the wherewithal to buy the foods imported from places where a man can raise more than he needs. Formerly many of the babies were deliberately slaughtered and are yet for that matter here and there. Even where not deliberately killed they are allowed to perish from avoidable infections and malnutrition. Consequently we can not determine the sanitary value of a large birth rate, unless we know what becomes of the babies. What complicates the matter in regard to the city, is the rapidity of the changes of its population, from a constant moving in and out.

It may well happen then that a large birth rate is a bad sign, for it is highest in New York City and progressively lessens with population in smaller cities and is the least in the country. The result in a large city may be a mere increase of deaths from children's diseases, and of no permanent social benefit.

The comparative wholesomeness of city and country life can not be determined, therefore, by birth rates and death rates, but it can to a certain extent by finding out what becomes of the babies born in each. As far as known, the country baby still has by far the best chances of surviving vigorously to old age, though as before mentioned we are on the way of evolving types better off in the city. Recent statistics show that the country has more deaths from accident, suicide, influenza and typhoid and almost as many murders, all of which kill people a little later in life, while the city kills them earlier by infantile diseases and reduces the average length of life. The death rate gives us no information as to what we want to know,—how long and how vigorously people live.

The normal death rate is exceedingly variable, and if people could die only of old age it would be only slightly less than the birth rate, for the world's population increases very slowly. Some localities have waxed and waned, but have not appreciably altered the course of human events. The enormous increases in Europe and America in the last century are merely temporary phenomena due to finding new food supplies, and cannot continue forever—or very much longer—counting in centuries or even decades perhaps. What the birth rate will be reduced to, no one can guess except in a very general way. When North America is so crowded that it uses up its own food and all it can import from South America or Asia, each of which too might have use for all of its own, and when there is no place to which to move as the Scandinavians have been doing, we can rest assured that women will refuse to bring forth babies to die early. In primitive times when the average life was only ten or less and no one lived more than 40 years or even 35, all women were productive, and the birth rate was probably 200 per 1,000, but now with an average life of 50 and with many too old to have babies, the normal birth rate even with many to each family can not be over 40, and it is lowest in the country partly because there are more old people there. It is destined to go down far below 20, probably to 10, without the least danger of race suicide. When that happens the death rate will be low and most of the deaths will be of adults or even the aged. We cannot reduce the death rate much below 16 now unless we reduce the birth rate, and even if we could, the surplus would have to move somewhere also, for they cannot pile up indefinitely without food.

———

The study of brains of eminent men will soon be an accomplished fact, if we may judge from the trend of opinion as to the disposition of the dead. Our text books of anatomy have often been illustrated by pictures of our lowest types, criminals, paupers, etc., as they were the only ones obtainable for the dissecting room. The more eminent a man, the more impossible it was to obtain his brain for study. Thus it happens as we have previously remarked, that the organ which enabled man to obtain supremacy over every other species of living thing, has received the least study of all. We are completely in the dark as to why the low races cannot raise themselves in culture, nor why they cannot sustain a culture thrust upon them. The matter seems destined to be cleared up in the near future. Many anatomists are taking up the study, and several associations are carrying on a propaganda to induce all men of exceptional intelligence to will their brains for postmortem study. The latest man to comply was Dr. W. J. McGee, the eminent Washingtonian anthropologist, lately deceased. We hope it will become the vogue for everyone who has accomplished anything at all, to permit the world to know why he was able to do it. Perhaps the most valuable of all brains for such study are those of men who have never been noted for originality, but who have succeeded in life in any calling, and have raised a fair number of children in health, and started them as good citizens. The study is not purely academic, for it will result in advancing practical psychiatry.

The American Anthropometric Association of Philadelphia has devoted itself largely to this end. Its collection of brains is now in the care of Dr. E. A. Spitzka, Prof. of Anatomy, Jefferson Med. College, from whom we expect important discoveries, as he has made many in the past. We certainly urge all to do as did Dr. McGee, and make it certain that their brains will be preserved for future study.

––––––––––

The home of plague has been definitely determined to be in Thibet. According to Dr. Paul Preble of the Public Health Service, the permanent host of the *bacillus pestis* is the tarbagan (arctomys bobac) an hibernating rodent or marmot related to our woodchuck and ground squirrel but larger than the rabbit. It is used both for food and its fur, like the marten and sable. This is good news and bad, for though it shows the possibility of exterminating the disease by killing off its host, it also shows that until we do this, there will be a succession of epidemics through the migration of the few bacilli which occasionally escape in fleas to the bodies of rats and travel around the world. The more we develop means of transportation, the more frequent these escapes. The bacillus seems to be as harmless to the tarbagan as the colon bacillus is to us. The animal is of value to the natives and they will surely object to its extermination. Nevertheless there is a hope that we can convince the Chinese that they owe this duty to the world, and will permit Europeans to go in to do the work, if Thibetans refuse. A small fraction of the money spent in a decade fighting our epidemics, if spent exterminating the rodent, would lessen the epidemics if not prevent them forever. Of course if we had no rats we would have no plagues, but the extermination of rats depends solely on a condition of cleanliness which starves them to death and we will not be that clean for a long while yet. The crusade against the rat must be continued—it would be folly to stop—but the only really effective prevention is a crusade against the tarbagan.

The menace of Thibet is one more instance of the way nations are not only dependent upon each other, but influence each other. For thousands of years Thibet has been periodically sending out death to humanity—in all, a matter not of millions of deaths but billions. Have we not a right to tell her to, stop it? If she refuse, what man will say that a war to compel decency will be unjustifiable? Sanitation is no longer a household matter or a city or state or national, but is international and world wide. It looks as though nothing but force will prevent this disease—and yet some short sighted men are trying to cripple our navy which must take part in this distantly future sanitary crusade. Force itself may not be needed, its mere existence is what the oriental heeds, but if we have no force to back up our demands for cleanliness, they will be laughed at. The world is also serving notice on the nations which keep yellow fever in existence, and if they themselves wish to survive they had better heed the notice. This is one of the reasons why Cuba can never be considered independent—she would not be sanitary and we reserve the right to intervene when necessary. If she becomes a hot-bed for cultivating yellow fever and plague to kill us, she may die as a nation. Indeed no nation can expect to live if it harms all the rest. Our central American hot-beds of yellow fever had better sit up and take more notice. We cannot be guarding against their diseases forever. The ideal quarantine is at the ports of exit and not at those of entrance, and the ideal is not at all unattainable. It should be possible quite soon.

This year's Nobel Prize has just been awarded to Dr. Alexis Carrel of the Rockefeller Institute for Medical Research. While this award comes as more or less of a surprise, it will evoke no adverse criticism. On the contrary it will meet with genuine approval, for among those who know something of Dr. Carrel's work, his studies and researches are recognized as epochal. But brilliant as Dr. Carrel's achievements have been and far-reaching in effect as they surely will be, so quietly and modestly has he pursued his work that only a vague indefinite conception is had generally of the things he has actually accomplished. It is characteristic of the man that his discoveries no matter how astounding and almost miraculous they have been, have never been spread broadcast for the delectation of the public. It is very evident that the splendid researches and investigations of this remarkable man have been presented to his colleagues with no other thought than to give a true and faithful report devoid of all sensationalism or exaggeration. No one, consequently, can read Dr. Carrel's statements outlining his results without being impressed with the modesty and humility of the man. In this day of extravagant claims and hasty conclusions it is refreshing to find such a spirit as Dr. Carrel has shown in all his undertakings. It is this modesty that has kept so many, even of his colleagues, ignorant of the really marvelous work he was engaged in. Among those who know, however, it is felt that few discoveries since Harvey's concerning the circulation have exerted more far reaching influences on medicine and surgery than Dr. Carrel's investigations in connection with blood vessel surgery, the transplantation of limbs and organs, and the preservation and growth of tissues outside of and away from the body. As more becomes known of his wonderful skill and daring in experimental

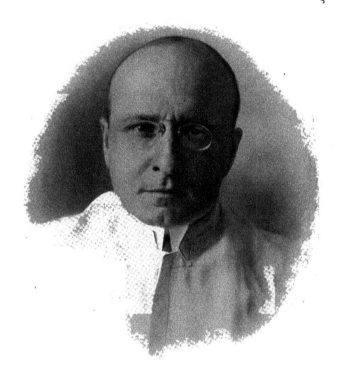

530

ALEXIS CARREL, M. D.
Rockefeller Institute of Medical Research

Recipient of Nobel Prize, 1912

Supplement American Medicine

surgery and the manipulation of living tissues, the infinite possibilities he has opened up for the future will be readily seen. At the present time Dr. Carrel's results are so startling, and so far removed from the accepted order of things that it is hard to view them in proper perspective. Indeed, it is not uncommon to hear the opinion expressed that while the things he has done, and is doing, are undeniably wizard-like, they are highly impractical! One surgeon has gone so far as to term such experimental work "acrobatic surgery." Such criticisms and remarks are most unfair, however, and born of a lack of imagination. Many of Dr. Carrel's scientific researches, to be sure, are so unique, so original and so at variance with established teaching that it is hard to grasp their significance and estimate their true worth. As one studies his humble and modest reports, however, the brilliant character of his attainments begins to appear and soon it is easy to understand the greatness of his work. No wonder, indeed, that Dr. Carrel's associates are such enthusiastic admirers, for they have had a chance to observe his genius. No one can come in contact with this master workman and note, not only the earnest, whole-souled purpose that dominates the man, but the wonderful technical skill that he is able to command, without acquiring a respect for his character that is only equalled by the admiration his dexterity inspires.

It is altogether fitting, therefore, that this earnest, capable physician should have been made the recipient of this year's Nobel prize. That he is not a native American makes no difference. The bulk of his work has been done in this country, and the opportunities and resources of an American institution have made his studies and investigations possible. Science knows no country or nationality. When humanity's interests are at stake, there is no thought of country, race or nativity. At the same time, there is great satisfaction felt throughout the United States that the Nobel prize comes this year to a man who has been singled out for this great honor because of scientific achievements brought to fruition under the auspices of an American research institution that every citizen can well feel proud of—the Rockefeller Institute for Medical Research.

To be fair and honest in everything we say, is our earnest purpose. If we fail, it is due to mistaken views or misunderstanding, never to intent. Above all do we aim to be fair to every one. To no one will we do an injustice, if we know it. And if we should, through ignorance or error, misjudge or misquote any one, we will invariably try to be first in making correction. To this end we wish to make a statement supplementary to the remarks that appeared in our August issue relative to the political situation and the attitude of the different presidential candidates to the Pure Food and Drug Law. We stated that owing to Colonel Roosevelt's frank support of the movement for organization of all public health agencies under one head and his advocacy of stringent pure food laws we believed him to be the candidate the medical profession could best support. We further based our opinion on the fact that Governor Wilson was non-committal on these subjects so highly important to medical men. At the time this was true to the best of our knowledge and belief. But since then we have learned that Governor Wilson has come out very strongly for effective health laws and in every way takes as high stand concerning pure food and drug legislation as Colonel Roosevelt. In all fairness, therefore, there is no reason to fear that these questions that mean so much to medical men will suffer in any way should Governor Wilson be elected. We say this because we have too great respect and admiration for Governor Wilson to wish to do him the slightest harm or injustice. That our personal regard and affection lead us to hope for Colonel Roosevelt's election does not blind us to the ability and manly strength of the Democratic nominee. Governor Wilson has shown himself to be a fine American gentleman and if the votes of the American people place him in the presidential chair on election day there will be no rancor or ill feeling in our breast. We can only say that the country is fortunate that the candidate of each party is a man that we can all point to with pride as a fine type of American citizen.

The attempted assassination of Colonel Roosevelt is reported as we go to press. Happily the mysterious hand of Fate again manifested itself and this strong man is saved to the country that needs him. In all history there have been few more striking examples of how Destiny marks a man, carries him through war and danger, protects him against foe and assassin, moulds him, develops him, showers honors upon him, and makes him the pivot of many striking events. Never was a man closer to instant death—only a spectacle case and a number of sheets of manuscript saved him! An inch to one side and the bullet would have passed obliquely up through the auricles of the heart and the aorta. In less than a minute Colonel Roosevelt would have been dead!

Can any one consider every phase of the affair and not be impressed with the fateful character of Colonel Roosevelt's deliverance from instant death? With all the reverence that comes from our sense of a Higher Power's intervention, we say —thank God, for sparing this great American!

There's a lesson— yes, many of them in this awful deed and the events immediately connected with it. There can be no question at all that the vicious vituperation and frightful attacks that have been hurled at Colonel Roosevelt in the daily press have created an enmity and hatred against him that is little short of terrible. Intelligent people can discount these slanders and calumnies, and realize their exaggeration, but among the illiterate and weak minded they work incalculable harm, for they engender a sense of wrong and injustice that is all too apt to lead to violence and crime.

It is really inconceivable that people can become so bitter against those who do not agree with them politically. In the old days, religious controversies led men to hate each other with the most fearful animosity. But as mankind has grown mentally, morally and spiritually, one would suppose that men had become more tolerant of each others views, and no longer allowed differences of opinion to arouse hatred and bitter feeling. Apparently we have not grown as much as we had hoped, for strange as it may seem, the few words we had the temerity to express in response to requests for our political views, brought down on our innocent heads some of the foulest, most vulgar and most indecent execrations it has ever been our misfortune to read—and these, too, from American doctors, supposedly cultured gentlemen! Happily these vicious epistles were very few compared to the many courteous letters that reached us. We are glad and proud to say that less than a dozen out of several hundred communications were vile and discourteous. The great majority were letters from real gentlemen, and even those differing from us—with the exceptions mentioned—were kindly and courteously expressed.

This is as it should be. We lay no claim to infallibility of judgment, nor have we any extraordinary wisdom or powers of deduction. We are just plain American citizens, proud of our splendid country, and deeply appreciative of the right to think for ourselves. We aim to be right just as much as we possibly can. But if we are wrong—according to *your* views— we are not necessarily vicious or dishonest. Just think that we may be mistaken.

The world is growing better, after all. When Colonel Roosevelt was shot, it was gratifying to see the wave of sincere regret and sympathy that swept over the country. President Taft and Governor Wilson were among the first to express their sorrow and hearty good wishes for his speedy recovery. Both immediately held up their engagements and refused to continue on the stump since Colonel Roosevelt was obliged to withdraw. Such conduct is splendid. It plainly shows that there is something actuating our leaders other than mere desire to win. The best feature of the whole situation, moreover, was the tacit approval which the people as a whole gave to the courteous, manly and Christian-like acts of President

Taft and Governor Wilson. There are some probably who will attribute their course to political expediency and shrewd tactics. But to the great majority it was simply followed because it was right, and it was right because it was playing the game fair and square without the slightest effort to take unfair advantage of someone's misfortune. Every one of the candidates of the three leading parties proved his manhood when the test came. And no matter which one of the three is elected our next president, we know that he will be a man to trust, honor and respect.

In previous issues we have expressed our preference for Colonel Roosevelt. We still feel that the great questions that confront us call for his personality, aggressive, fearless and strong. The country needs him at the helm. His great grasp of the people's needs, his courage, and in spite of what his enemies say, his forgetfulness of self will enable him to solve the great social and national problems of the United States as we hope to see them solved. The following from *Collier's Weekly*, a publication that has fought fearlessly for pure food and drugs expresses our ideas splendidly: .

A MAN.

Theodore Roosevelt is a fairly close presentment of what this nation likes to call *a man*. Such faults as fault-finders like ourselves have been able to descry in him are faults of the highly tempered, hasty, and not always reasonable nation which selected him to govern it. No man probably could have risen so high in American politics and emerged as stainless from his early struggles. No man could have used his power with a larger moral usefulness to his whole people. And we doubt whether any man in history has undertaken late in life as high an unselfish venture in the field of politics as the Bull Moose. It is fortunate that those who value lightly the important things of life—courage, personal honor, and the well-being of those about them, and who guard closely safety, comfort, and their pocket-books—are almost the only Americans cynical enough to disbelieve in the honesty of Theodore Roosevelt's words within five minutes of an attempt upon his life:

Friends, I want to say this about myself: I have too many important things to think about to pay heed or to feel any concern over my own death.

Just one word in closing, however. Nothing we have said is intended to swerve any of our readers from their honest convictions. We have expressed ours honestly, and we have no quarrel with anyone who thinks differently. Our only admonition is to let no hatred or unwarranted dislike create unjust prejudices against any man. Let every man study things carefully, look at the various questions from every standpoint, form his own conclusions and true to himself, act on them. And finally, no matter who gets his vote, let him not fail to vote for someone.

Whoever wins we may rest assured that the country will have a president that every man may trust and respect.

The terrestrial origin of life is being asserted with more and more confidence. The latest is the Presidential Address of Prof. E. A. Schaefer to the British Association for the Advancement of Science. He shows how impossible it is for life to come from other planets or stars and he asserts that such substances must have been evolved on earth from simpler and simpler forms. There could not have been a jump from inorganic compounds to the modern complex molecule of protoplasm. It was a very long process by very small steps. These ideas were put forward in these columns several years ago and have been appearing frequently in other journals also, but they have been considered too speculative to come within the sphere of science. Now that the sober minded scientific bodies are discussing the matter seriously the subject is definitely taken from the domain of pure speculation. All this does not mean that we are to create an actual living molecule soon, if ever, but it does mean that it will not be long before we find out the actual steps by which nitrogen gas entered into those unstable but complex groupings, whose functions we call vital, merely because they are so vastly different from the functions of stable compounds.

The scientific use of the word soul is the startling innovation of Schaefer's address. He rightly calls theologians to task for confusing the words soul and life. He shows that the vast majority of living things do not even possess intelligence. On the other hand what is known as mind, exists in bodies which are not supposed to possess a soul. The human mind is only a highly developed form of that of lower animals. By making these clear cut distinctions Schaefer is removing all discussions of vitality from the domain of theology. As a result the clergy have received his article with wonderful equanimity, in marked contrast to the denunciations of a half century ago. Evidently they have made up their minds that it makes no difference to theology how living substances were created. It deals with the soul which enters into the most intelligent form yet evolved. It begins to look as though the old warfare between science and religion is coming to an end, through the realization of both, that they have nothing in common. One is based on facts and the other on faith. It does seem that each is the stronger for tolerating the other.

ORIGINAL ARTICLES.

LIGATION OF THE INTERNAL ILIAC ARTERIES[1]

for

1.—Hemostasis in extensive extirpation of pelvic viscera for cancer.

2.—To prevent recurrence of apparently completely extirpated cancers of the pelvic viscera.

3.—To retard the growth of inoperable cancers of the same viscera.

4.—To arrest hemorrhage in inoperable cancers, chiefly of the uterus. With Report of Six Cases.

BY

IRVING S. HAYNES, Ph. B., M. D.,
New York City.

Uterine cancer is the most insidious and fatal disease by which women are attacked.

Three out of every four cases coming under observation, in Germany, are absolutely inoperable and beyond all hope of cure; the percentage is much higher in this country.[2]

Combining the statistics of Wertheim, Hannes, and Schindler we find that their average mortality was 22.92% and their absolute cures according to the formula of Werner is 14.06%. In a similar manner considering the statistics of the simpler vaginal operation as carried out by Schuchard, Schauta, Standa, Hannes, Doederlein, Glockner, Zurhelle and Olhausen we find that the average mortality is 10.64% and the absolute cures after five years after Werner's formula is 16.75%.[1]

The radical operation formerly performed by Wertheim is not necessary. The reason is that recurrence was thought to be in the pelvic lymph nodes, hence their removal was obligatory. Further experience shows this is not true, much to our surprise. In four out of five cases of recurrence the growth returns in the vaginal scar. In one case out of 104 did a recurrence take place in an *iliac* lymph node and in only two cases in the *inguinal* glands.

It is absolutely impossible for anyone to determine during the operation whether the lymph nodes are involved or not. If not involved their removal is not necessary, if

---

[1] Presented at a meeting of the Eastern Medical Society, May 10, 1912.

[2] Of the cases subjected to operation by various surgeons of international reputation we find the following figures hold. Regarding operation by the abdomen according to the so-called Wertheim method (although this was practiced and described by Werder, and was modified from the older methods of Ried, Strumpf and Clark).

Operability of Cases of Uterine Cancer.

Operator.	Cases.	Inoperable.	Operated.
Hocheisen	1,706	1,538	168
Schindler	588	471	117
Zurhelle	253	168	85
Stauda	156	52	104
Hannes	361	216	145
Doederlein	151	78	73
Wertheim	400	232	168
Totals....	3,615	2,755	860

Percentage of operable cases, 23.8.

[1] Operations, Cures According to Weiner's Formula.

Abdominal route.	Primary mortality.	Cures.
Wertheim	22.50%	24.7 %
Hannes	32.6 %	14.3 %
Schindler	13.67%	3.18%
Average.......	22.92%	14.06%
Vaginal operations.		
Schuchard	9.6 %	20. %
Schauta	10.8 %	12.6 %
Hannes	8. %	28.8 %
Standa	20. %	23. %
Doederlein	16.4 %	15.8 %
Glockner	8.46%	9.72%
Zurhelle	4. %	14. %
Oldhausen	7.7 %	10. %
Average, vaginal..	10.64%	16.75%
Average, abdominal	22.92%	14.06%

Difference in favor of the vaginal route, 12.28% less mortality, primary.
Greater percentage of cures, 2.69%.

they are involved their removal is useless for there has been involvement beyond the field of possible removal.

Schauta, who made most extensive investigations along this line concluded that in 43.3% there was no lymphatic involvement, hence the operation (the extreme radical) was unnecessary; in 43.3% the glands were so extensively involved beyond the field of possible removal that the operation was useless; and in only 13.3% were the accessible nodes involved. But the attempt to extirpate these few possibly involved nodes is not justifiable when there is an immediate mortality of the extremely radical operation of 66 to 72%. For these reasons Wertheim and other leading surgeons have abandoned this extreme operation.

Indeed the reaction has been so marked that some of the former radical advocates have concluded that as good permanent results can be obtained by the so-called palliative measures, as a thorough curettement followed by local applications of the actual cautery, zinc-chloride, fuming nitric acid, formalin and probably best of all the acetone treatment advocated by Gellhorn.

Close analysis of these palliative measures gives one a real surprise. We are so accustomed to think that nothing but wide excision in cancer alone gives any hope that the figures offered by these various operators cause us to sit up and take notice. Chrobak treated 408 cases with fuming nitric acid. His patients lived from 3 to 5 years, one even for 22 years and one for 20. The primary mortality is probably not more than that due to the anesthetic plus 1 or 2% from peritonitis following perforation of the uterus by the curette. These palliative measures are used by Lomer, Mond, Roessling, Fleischmann, Zacharias,

A Reeves Jackson, Chrobak, Webster, Gellhorn and others. Czerney has recently revived this treatment and it has received the favorable commendation of Murphy.

The preceding statements are based upon a comprehensive article by Dr. John B. Murphy and Dr. Frank W. Lynch in the VIII volume of the American Practice of Surgery by Bryant and Buck.

Inasmuch as hemorrhage is one of the frequent accompaniments of the actual cautery method, and as we know that starvation of the cancerous bearing tissues is a potent factor in not only aiding a cure but also in preventing a return of the growth I am led to advocate the ligation of both internal iliac arteries as a preliminary step in the treatment of these cases with completion of the operation by a thorough curettage and the use of the acetone treatment after the method of Gellhorn. Ligation of the internal iliac produces definite anemia of three distinct pelvic systems. (Byron Robinson, *Annals of Surgery*, Vol. 35, p. 189). 1. The lower part of the ureters, the bladder (and in the male the prostate), and the urethra. 2. The uterus and its adnexa, the vagina and the vulva. 3. The lower portion of the rectum and anus. I would therefore advocate the use of this ligation in the following conditions:

1. All inoperable pelvic cancers attended with hemorrhage, profuse and recurring, more especially from the uterus.

2. As a preliminary procedure to prevent hemorrhage and recurrence in all such operations as extirpation of the bladder, prostate and urethra; hysterectomy with or without removal of the upper portion of the vagina; excision of the rectum and anus, or vulva.

3. As a preliminary step in the so-called palliative operations upon the uterus and

vagina, in connection with the later technic of Gellhorn.

I should claim that it was a wise procedure in all cases of suspected or actual malignant pelvic growths.

If the suspected case ultimately proves to be positive it will tend to delay if not actually prevent a return. In the actual case it serves to arrest hemorrhage and delay growth.

The comfort, rapidity and ease with which extensive pelvic operations can be performed would in itself justify the performance of this operation as a preliminary step in many instances. This contention has been fully demonstrated in my own cases and especially by one very recently, April 27, in the practice of Dr. Furniss at the Red Cross Hospital. At the doctor's request I assisted him in the operation of ligation of both internal iliacs preliminary to total extirpation of the bladder in a woman. There was none of the very active bleeding and troublesome oozing. We would have had a practically bloodless field had we ligated both ovarian arteries. Their free anastomosis with the uterine vessels furnished the only vessels we had to ligate. A running catgut suture in the other tissues effectually controlled all the others.

The effect of the ligation upon uterine hemorrhages in the otherwise inoperable cases is positive and immediate. How long such arrest is maintained I am unable to state.

The ligation of the arteries, so far as my experience goes, is attended with no bad effects, immediate or remote. The only complaint has been of a heavy tired feeling, which was present before the operation, in one case that lasted for about two weeks.

Ligation of the internal iliacs was first performed by Dr. W. Stevens of Santa Cruz, in 1812. (Keyes, Bryant and Buck, Vol. IV, p. 508).

Pryor (*Am. Jour. of Obs.*, June, 1896) records 34 cases of malignant disease of the uterus treated by ligation of the internal iliac arteries, with one death.

Bainbridge (*Woman's Med. Jour.*, April, 1911) reviews the subject of arterial ligation for various conditions and especially for irremovable cancer of the pelvic organs.

Ligation of the internal iliacs by the transperitoneal route is usually an easy operation. Difficulties may arise from the filling up of the pelvis by the growth or from its extension to the pelvic tissues covering the arteries, or from a low course of a very tortuous external iliac artery. The internal iliac is found by incising the peritoneum in line with the course of the artery, and below the level of the pelvic brim at a distance of an inch and a half from the mid-line. The ureter will be seen attached to the under surface of the outer flap of the peritoneum; it must not be disturbed. The artery is covered by the pelvic fascia which needs to be divided in the line of the peritoneal incision. Blunt dissection exposes the artery and a double ligature of No. 3 plain gut is passed by the carrier from within out, being careful to lift the artery away from the vein while insinuating the ligature carrier beneath the artery. Before tying the ligature, have some one get the femoral pulse, if it is not arrested by traction on the ligature, tie the latter and close up the peritoneal incision by a running catgut suture. On the left side the mesentery of the sigmoid may add a little to the operative work. I have found it best to firmly draw the sigmoid to the left and proceed as above. Keyes (ibid) mentions gangrene of the limb, peritonitis and secondary hemorrhage, as the chief dangers. If sepsis is present or follows, such possibilities might occur. But one would not perform the operation in septic pelvic conditions and sepsis is such a remote contingency in previously clean cases that I consider such dangers too remote to be seriously considered. So far as my experience goes the operation has been followed by no bad effects, immediate or remote. Pryor in 34 cases of malignant disease of the uterus, had one death.

Kelley (*Operative Gynecology*, Vol. II, p. 331) testifies to the value of this procedure in such conditions as the following:

·"When there is much lateral infiltration the embarrassment from the hemorrhage in cutting through the infiltrated tissues is sometimes so great that the operator has to abandon all ideas of operative relief, and finish the operation the best way he can. I operated upon a case of this kind. As the operation proceeded, it was found impossible to extirpate the disease in the broad ligaments and to check the free oozing from the diseased tissue which was cut; in order, therefore, to control the entire blood supply of the part, I ligated both internal iliac arteries. After the ligation all pulsation in the pelvis on both sides ceased. The patient made a good recovery and suffered in no way from the artificial pelvic anemia, and the disease returned so slowly that she lived over two years after the operation."

I have operated in the following six cases without operative mortality, with such freedom from hemorrhage as to be of the greatest value to the patient and assistance to the operator in rapidity and ease of the work.

From my experience, I would further advise that in all cases where the genital or urinary tracts are involved and after ligation of the internal iliacs that both ovarian arteries should likewise be tied whether extirpation of the organs is contemplated or not. The free anastomosis of the ovarian with the uterine furnishes too much blood to the latter and unless ligated before division would interfere with the operation.

CASE I.—A. G., German, aged 38. Admitted to Harlem Hospital, Feb. 24, 1908. Discharged, March 24, 1908.

Family history.—Negative.

Past history.—Has had 3 children. For the past 5 weeks has lost weight rapidly. Feels she is growing weaker. Has pain over the lower part of the abdomen.

Physical examination.—Is a medium sized woman, thin, anemic and cachectic.

Abdomen is retracted, scaphoid, tense but not rigid. No masses can be felt.

Vaginal. Perineum is relaxed, cervix hard and the seat of a large ulcerating cauliflower growth. The uterus is enlarged and fixed in position. No masses can be felt in the fornices. T. 98. P. 92. R. 18.

Urine, Feb. 28, showed trace of albumin, otherwise negative. Feb. 29, operation.

The upper third of the vagina was dissected free of the bladder and the rectum. In performing this separation the base of the bladder was opened into. This was sutured and healed promptly, causing no subsequent trouble.

The abdomen was then opened, both internal iliacs ligated with No. 3 plain gut at a point about an inch below the bifurcation of the common arteries. The uterus with the appendages and broad ligaments was removed. The peritoneum was closed transversely in the pelvis. The ventral wound closed in layers. Iodoform gauze strips were placed into the vagina.

By March 4 the gauze packing was all out. Primary union took place in the abdominal wound. The patient was out of bed on March 18.

The highest T. P. R. occurred on the day following the operation and were 101. 120. 26.

March 24, discharged. T. 99½, P. 78. Apparently perfectly healed. This extensive extirpation was rapidly carried out as I did not have to stop for troublesome hemorrhage and all oozing was easily controlled at last by continuous gut sutures.

Final result.—Patient died about six months later from local return of growth.

CASE II.—Mrs. L. W. Private patient referred to me by Dr. Neff. Stout woman of 60. Married. Admitted to the Red

Cross Hospital, June 1. Discharged, June 20, 1910.

Complains of very severe pain in the back over the sacrum.

Married 22 years, never been pregnant.

Three weeks ago began to have sharp pain in the left hip. Hemorrhage from the vagina for the past 24 days.

Physical examination negative except for the pelvic region. The uterus is generally enlarged, more especially on the right side. It is quite firmly fixed by an induration extending more especially into the right broad ligament but some into the left side. The cervix is not enlarged, and there seems to be no vaginal or rectal involvement.

Positive diagnosis not ventured.

Operation.—June 2. Curette removed masses of tissue unmistakably cancerous.

Abdomen opened. Uterus so far involved that the cancerous tissue showed through the peritoneum. Both broad ligaments extensively infiltrated. Radical operation impossible, therefore the internal iliacs were ligated with No. 3 plain gut and the wound closed in layer sutures.

Highest T. P. R. on the day following the operation, 101, 100 and 28. Wound healed by primary union. Sat up in bed on the 10th day and was out of bed on the 11th day. She went home on the 18th day. In spite of this extensive carcinoma this patient recovered, the growth was held in check and she did her own housework for over a year after the operation and only died March 4, last, 1912.

CASE III.—Mrs. I. C., private patient, 45 years of age, married, has one child 17 years old. In the summer of 1910 she flowed freely for 5 weeks. She was curetted and the uterine scrapings submitted to one of the best laboratories in the city. The diagnosis then was adenocarcinoma. She was so discouraged and disheartened that she did nothing for herself, expecting to die very soon. However as a year passed without death having come, and as she was in constant pain she determined to seek relief, one way or the other. She consulted me April 4, 1911. Thorax and abdomen were negative. No glands palpable. The uterus was slightly enlarged, very tender, freely movable. The cervix was red but not eroded. There was a thin watery non-irritating vaginal discharge.

I operated at the Red Cross Hospital, April 7, accepting the laboratory diagnosis, and believing I had a very slow growing cancer to deal with.

Both internal iliacs were easily ligated and a total removal of the uterus, upper part of the vagina, tubes and ovaries carried out. The appendix was also taken out.

The pelvic condition was extremely interesting. Especially in view of the laboratory diagnosis under which I was working. There was a small amount of pale straw fluid in the pelvic cavity. All the blood vessels leading into and from the pelvic viscera were deeply injected. A more "angry" looking condition I have never seen. This appearance confirmed, in my mind the correctness of the previous diagnosis. However an examination of the specimen removed showed that the uterus was the seat of a general fibroid change, without any evidence of cancer.

The patient was out of bed on the 10th day and left the hospital at the end of three weeks. Of course she has remained cured until the present time.

CASE IV.—G. B. Admitted to Harlem Hospital, Nov. 17, 1911. Discharged, Feb. 7, 1912. Widow aged 48.

Last August, after sexual intercourse, first noticed a burning and frequent urination. Slight discharge. In October noticed that the vaginal orifice was hard, contracted and tender, especially on the left side. She enters complaining of pain in the back and frequent and painful micturition.

Physical—Thin anemic nervous woman. Inguinal glands are palpable and very hard. Nothing found in the abdomen or chest. There is a hard indurated mass involving the anterior part of the vaginal orifice, urethra and clitoris, larger on the left than right, but on both sides firmly attached to the ischio-pubic rami. Gonococci found in the vaginal discharge.

W. B. C. 17000, Polys, 70%.

T. P. R. normal.

Nov. 25. Both internal iliacs were ligated with No. 3 plain gut in continuity. There seemed to be no pelvic growth apparent. The abdominal wound was closed and the entire vulva with the clitoris, the urethra up to the vesical sphincter and the lower half of the anterior wall of the vagina was excised.

Patholgical examination showed that the growth was an adenocarcinoma originating from the glands of Bartholin on both sides. The T. P. R. the day after the operation were 101, 102 and 24. There was primary union in the abdominal wound and quick healing in the perineal gap. Patient was out of bed on Dec. 16.

There was a return of the growth in the shape of a small nodule at the left of the vesical sphincter. This was enucleated and thoroughly cauterized on Jan. 4 by electric cautery.

At the time of her discharge, Feb. 7, 1912, there was no recurrent growth apparent.

She was placed in a home for incurables. At the present, April 20, I am informed by her sister that there is a nodular recurrence at the site of the original operation which has begun to ulcerate. She is in a very debilitated condition.

CASE V.—M. G., Bohemian, 53 years old, married, entered Harlem Hospital, Jan. 22, discharged, Feb. 6, 1912.

Patient had good health up to 6 months ago when she was taken with a profuse leucorrhea, occasionally blood stained. Her menstrual history began at 14, was always irregular and painful. Has had two children, the last 22 years ago.

Sept. 8 she was admitted to one of the large city hospitals and some vaginal operation performed, its nature was not explained to her. She was in the hospital 13 days. Three weeks ago she again went to the same hospital, was there for a week and discharged with nothing operative having been done.

Her present complaint is excessive bleeding with constant pain.

Examination shows a large uterus and cervix, deeply indurated; the vaginal walls, bladder and rectum all being involved. There are irregular hard nodules in and about the cervix. Diagnosis made of inoperable uterine cancer.

January 23. Both internal iliacs were tied with No. 3 plain gut in continuity. There was some difficulty experienced in finding the left artery as the uterus was much enlarged and had become firmly attached to the sigmoid and the mesentery of the gut was greatly thickened and shortened.

In order to make sure of the artery about which the ligature was passed it was necessary to have an assistant feel for the femoral pulse. Twice was the ligature placed about the external iliac, which from a low bifurcation of the common iliac and a low course of the external iliac simulated the position of the internal. This precaution, however, served to finally secure the right artery.

The wound healed by primary union.

The highest T. P. R. on the day following the operation, were 101⅘, 124, 28.

No reaction whatever. Patient out of bed on Feb. 2, eleven days after the operation. She left the hospital on the 6th of Feb. There were no more hemorrhages from the uterus and the patient said she felt greatly relieved.

CASE VI.—Mrs. G. K. Private patient. Referred by Dr. Upton. Large stout German woman of 46.

Menstruation regular and painless. Has had 2 children and 6 misses. Last pregnancy 10 years ago.

For the past month has had a vaginal discharge of blood, coming in a regular gush and lasting for an hour or two, every day. Last menstruation was 4 or 5 months ago and was normal. No trouble with bowels or urine. Examination is negative except for pelvis. There is an excavating ulceration in the cervix which has disappeared. There is apparently no infiltration present. The uterus is generally enlarged and freely movable without pain. No glands enlarged.

Diagnosis of cervical carcinoma in an early stage made. A total hysterectomy after ligation of both internal iliacs with removal of tubes, ovaries and upper part of the vagina made. The appendix was also removed. April 19 at the Red Cross Hospital, examination of the specimen shows that the cervical growth was benign papilloma.

The patient is making a satisfactory recovery. The condition not being proved malignant really does not interest us, except to demonstrate that the operation of ligating the internal iliac arteries was easily performed and has been attended with no unfavorable result.

The subsequent history showed that the clinical diagnosis was correct. Recurrence of the cancer took place in the vaginal scar and progressed very rapidly, terminating in the death of the patient during the past summer.

SPLANCHNOPTOSIS.

BY

HAROLD BARCLAY, M. D.,
New York City.

Consultant in Gastro-Intestinal Diseases at the General Memorial Hosp. Asst. Attending Phys. J. Hood Wright Hosp.

By splanchnoptosis literally is meant a descent of the entire abdominal viscera. I have used the term to designate a class of cases where ptosis of the abdominal organs exists in varying degrees rather than to describe accurately the anatomical condition.

Splanchnoptosis, as we see it in the adult, presents two forms; the first acquired, the second congenital.

The first, or acquired, is the type most frequently met with. It may be the result of pregnancy, of wasting disease, or of prolonged mental or physical strain. In fact, any condition which results in a rapid loss of weight.

The degree of ptosis is seldom excessive and yet may be productive of profound mental and physical disturbance.

The commonest form of ptosis is the prolapsed stomach. This is generally associated with varying degrees of the kidneys, especially the right, and in consequence of the weakening of the muscular support there is a tendency of the lower half of the abdomen to bulge forward. The true essential type is characterized by certain underlying constitutional defects. The patients give a general impression of frailness, expressed in the contour of the form and often in the features. It is characterized by the stooping shoulders, scant adipose tissue, flabby musculature, and barrel-shaped chest, somewhat flattened anteroposteriorly, with the upper ribs widely separated, the lower ones slanting downward, and being close together, form a costal angle which varies from sixty to eighty degrees in the well developed type.

The abdominal walls lack resistance and again there is the same tendency for the lower half of the abdomen to bulge forward. Stiller called attention to the barrel-shaped chest and unattached tenth rib to which he gave the term habitus enteropticus. In other words, there is a distinct picture of a defective development.

Recently W. J. Butler and Richard Smith, in an examination of some two hundred children, noted that the characteristic conformation of the enteroptotic habit began to make itself apparent about the twelfth year.

In this congenital class we have many predisposing factors, conducive under slight provocation, to a descent of the abdominal organs, such as the diminished thoracic abdomen, loose ligamentous attachments and a general muscular insufficiency, so that it requires but a slight exciting cause to bring about the change of position in the viscera.

Lane, of London, has demonstrated and explained the mechanism of the changes brought about as a result of the various ptoses. When the viscera begin to drop they exert a drag upon the mesentery. This results in the formation of bands so thick and strong in some cases as to form supplementary mesenteries which support the bowel and tend to prevent dropping. These "adhesions" are entirely non-inflammatory in origin, they are brought into being as the result of preternatural strain. If these adhesions were uniformly strong in all parts the viscera would be held up uniformly and all would be well, but unfortunately, they are often strong in some places, weak or absent in others, and consequently the bowel is held up in some places and allowed to sag in others, thus producing kinks which often lead to some degree of obstruction. The points where these kinks are most often encountered are at the ileo-cecal junction hepatic splenic flexures and at the sigmoid flexure and the rectum.

I have personally studied splanchnoptosis in 410 cases. Of these 273 were of the acquired type, 137 of the congenital. The difference in the general appearance of these two classes is a very striking one. In the first class they present a broad costal angle, and generally are well developed physically. There is generally some diastasis of the recti especially where the abdominal wall has been distended as in pregnancy.

Apparently the chief etiological factor in the vast majority of cases was the result of the parturient state. The costal angle was measured in all cases with a calipers and the degree of its angle noted.

In the first, or acquired, class it varied from 90 to 120 degrees. In the second class, from 60 to 90 degrees. Cases between 85 to 90 degrees I have regarded as being on the border line.

The position of the stomach was in all instances ascertained by inflation with sodium bicarbonate and tartaric acid. The position of the kidney was noted and the degree of their excursions on deep inspiration. The colon was inflated to determine its position, and where possible an X-ray

was made. In the lesser degrees of ptosis of the small intestine it is practically impossible to make any diagnosis without an X-ray.

To be brief, it may be said that in the first type the most characteristic feature was gastroptosis, associated with increased movability of the right kidney, so that on deep inspiration the kidney could be palpated over two-thirds of its entire length. The left kidney was only palpable in a small percentage of cases. The colon, as a rule, was held fairly well in position.

In the second or congenital class, in which there were 137 cases (126 female and 11 male), the costal angle varied from 60 to 85 degs. Stiller's detached rib was present in about one-third of the cases.

An X-ray examination of the colon in twelve of these cases showed a decided coloptosis, in addition to the gastro and nephroptosis; hepatic flexure sagged from two to three inches with the consequent descent of the transverse colon. Whether this condition is more characteristic of this class of cases I cannot say. In about one-fourth the left kidney could be palpated from one-third to one-half of its distance.

In none of my patients have I seen a case of ptosis of the spleen or liver, or at least I could never satisfy myself of their presence.

A whole volume could be written on the symptomatology of splanchnoptosis. I shall consider it solely from the standpoint of gastroptosis.

The gastro-intestinal symptoms are largely due to the degree of atony. For example, in making a routine examination of the abdomen, it is frequently surprising to note the extreme degree of gastroptosis that can exist without producing symptoms. It is after the onset of motor insufficiency that these patients complain of digestive symptoms. These symptoms are especially characterized by epigastric distress, or a bloating sensation immediately after eating often with a marked excess of gas both raised and passed. Its immediate onset after food seems to me to be especially characteristic of this class of cases, in contradistinction to the discomfort and distress that occur one or two hours after eating due to hyperacidity, as in the chronic ulcer or the chronic appendicitis.

The patients attribute this to some dietetic indiscretion and gradually eliminate one article of food after the other until in extreme cases they are practically limited to tea and toast. With the reduction of the diet and consequent loss of weight and nutrition the degree of gastrointestinal motility is further lowered, and the nervous element more pronounced. Nausea is occasionally present, vomiting seldom unless it is induced to obtain relief. Constipation is the rule. These, I believe, are the cardinal symptoms which are directly referable to the gastro-intestinal tract.

J. J. Nutt in a yet unpublished monograph calls attention to many cases of chronic backache due to weakness of the abdominal muscles. He shows that when the abdominal muscles are weak, support is maintained by keeping the gravity-plane back of its normal position, by increasing the normal anterior curve of the spine and tilting the pelvis downward. In consequence of which there is constant action and strain felt by the anterior common ligaments of the vertebrae and the sacro-iliac ligaments of the sacro-iliac joints.

The retroflexion of the uterus so frequently met with in these cases may be accounted for by the pressure of the pro-lapsed intestines in the utero-vesical pouch.

In the physical examination in addition to the above findings, the cecum is frequently found enlarged and can be distinctly palpated. In rubbing it under the fingers a scrunching sound can be elicited denoting a condition of atony, and at times considerable tenderness was present. The atonic and dilated cecum results in more or less intestinal stagnation. This stagnation is, I believe, in some instances responsible for an appendicular involvement. In five of my cases it seemed advisable to remove the appendix, and although that organ in every instance showed a distinct lesion, I must confess the patients were not benefited by the operation to any appreciable degree, the general condition remaining unchanged. The examination of the stomach contents, other than the estimation of the degree of gastric motility, does not yield great practical results, as far as prognosis or treatment are concerned. Allowing five and a half to six hours as the average time in which a normal stomach empies itself after an ordinary meal; in the atonic stomach this time will be retarded to seven, eight, nine, and in two instances, to twelve hours, although subsequent observation showed there was no pyloric obstruction. One hour after an Ewald test breakfast, viz., an ordinary baker's roll and a glass of water in the nonatonic stomach 30 cc.-40 cc. will be extracted of a homogeneous, well chymified material. Where a motor insufficiency exists the quantity will be increased to amounts varying from 60 to 180 cc. depending on the degree of atony.

In 377 examinations of the stomach after a test breakfast in the above series of cases, I have tabulated my results as follows:

In 313 the acid was practically within normal limits.

Fifty-three showed hyperacidity; in 11 it was diminished. The quantity extracted varied from 60 to 180 cc. There was complicating gastritis in three cases.

Examination of the stools frequently showed the presence of mucus generally in small amounts.

Treatment:—Treatment divides itself into mechanical, hygienic, dietetic and medical.

The mechanical treatment consists in the correction of postural errors and in so far as possible the support of the prolapsed viscera by a belt or corset.

The corset on the whole has given me far more satisfaction that the belt. In addition to the support these people require careful training which should be carried out by an experienced teacher under the supervision of a doctor. They should be taught the proper position in standing, and have such exercises as will develop the muscles of the abdomen, not only of the abdomen but of the entire body. An excellent guide to such exercise has recently been published by J. C. Miller, entitled "My System."

Dietetic:—The improvement of the general nutrition by means of a good full nutritious diet. The feedings should be small in amount and repeated at frequent intervals, so that the patient receives six meals a day instead of three. The meals should be dry—that is, solid food, and liquids such as water being allowed only between times. Fats in the form of cream and butter are especially desirable. The diet, when constipation exists, should be as laxative as possible. Milk should be used infrequently as it invariably increases the general discomfort.

Some simple hydrotherapeutic measures are often of great benefit, as a warm bath with the addition of sea salt, followed by a cold spinal douche, and a brisk rub. Recently I have been giving my patients what I term a salt glow, viz., the patient is allowed to stand in the bath tub filled with warm water; two or three handfuls of salt are put in a bowl of warm water and the nurse beginning at the head gives the entire body a vigorous rubbing. The patient is then allowed to immerse herself in the bath and wash off the salt. This is followed by a spinal douche with a spraying nozzle or by pouring a pitcher of water varying in temperature from 80 to 65 degrees down the spine and over the chest. By these means I have been able to obtain excellent results, and the patients invariably feel invigorated after such treatment. The daily activity, as far as practicable, should be curtailed, so as to avoid any undue fatigue, and when possible a rest in bed in the afternoon should be insisted on.

Medicinal Measures:—The medicinal measures which have given me the best results have been strontium bromides given three or four times a day, in amounts varying from five to fifteen grs. This relaxes the nervous tension, which is almost invariably present, and in consequence the appetite improves and the amount of discomfort following food is lessened. A mild degree of chlorosis is a frequent accompaniment of these cases, and as almost any form of iron seems to increase their constipation and abdominal distress, I have latterly tried sodium cacodylate by hypodermic injection with apparently good results.

The question of constipation is often very troubling. I have gotten my best results from the use of cotton-seed oil given in the knee chest position at bed time. I have used from four to eight ounces having the patient retain it if possible over night. This if necessary can be followed by a soapsuds enema in the morning. General massage over the abdomen is often a very valuable adjunct.

In the extreme cases of splanchnoptosis where marked prostration and subnutrition exist, a well conducted rest cure is of the greatest benefit, often being productive of results where other measures have failed.

68 E. 56th St., N. Y.

THE TREATMENT OF CLEFT PALATE.

BY

WILLIAM FRANCIS CAMPBELL, M. D.,
Brooklyn, N. Y.

From the varying age at which this defect is sent to the surgeon for repair it is obvious that there is as yet no definite standard of treatment upon which the profession is agreed. This is to be regretted since the old traditional dictum of operating on hare-lip at the third month and cleft palate at the third year is physiologically irrational and surgically unnecessary.

As Lane observes, "the treatment of cleft palate has been a matter of creed and tradition and has not been arrived at in any reasonable manner." Fortunately surgeons are beginning to appreciate that the old dictum of delay has nothing to commend it. It is fallacious in premise and conclusion. It is obvious that cleft palate is a serious menace to the nutrition of the infant since it is impossible for the child to suckle or satisfactorily swallow the food introduced into the mouth. The food often regurgitates through the nose and endangers respiration. *Children with cleft palate should be fed in the upright position so that fluid will gravitate directly into the pharynx.* Later, articulation and phonation are seriously compromised—the defective nasopharyngeal wall permits the air current to escape through the nose and makes the distinct articulation of consonants impossible. *The tools of speech must be normal in order to have correct speech.* Not only this, but unless the mouth and nasal cavities are separated early in life normal physiological function is impossible; hence, normal development is seriously compromised, vital capacity is impaired, the physiognomy is altered, and the individual is physically and intellectually a defective.

If the normal development of the nasopharynx and the surrounding structures depends upon its normal physiology it is obvious that the nose and mouth cavities should be separated as early as possible. The child cannot develop so long as its supply of air and food is deficient.

The proper time to operate for cleft palate is as soon after birth as possible. Nothing is gained by delay except the consequences of faulty nutrition.

The plasticity of the new-born tissues, their capacity for repair, the trifling hemorrhage, the slight risk to life, the possibility of obtaining a broad, well-vascularized flap before the teeth have begun to encroach upon the mucous membrane combine to make early infancy an opportune time for repairing this defect (Fig. 1).

The author has no hesitation in commending the "Lane operation" as the most satisfactory for all varieties of cleft, providing the operation is done early. It is ingenious, rational and satisfactory, and far superior to the older plastic methods or the complicated method of Brophy, who approximates the two superior maxillary bones by means of silver wire and adjusts the vivified edges of the cleft with sutures.

The principle of this operation is "to close in the interval between the edges of the cleft by muco-periosteum in the case of the hard palate, and by mucous membrane and submucous tissue in case of the soft palate." The features of the operation are the breadth of the flaps and the ingenious method of overlapping them so that the fissure is closed in by a curtain of tissue on which there is no tension and in which the play of the muscles is unimpaired. If hare-

methods can be given, which must be modified to suit the individual needs.

One of the greatest difficulties we have found is to get the child in a stable position for operating. This has been solved by Miss Dorothea Göthsen, Superintendent of Trinity Hospital, who has devised a satisfactory sling, by means of which the patient is held in a position, which while adjustable, does not shift (Fig. 2). It consists of a sheet pinned about the child's body from the neck and extending beyond the feet so that the weight is borne at the shoulders and the lower part of the sheet fastened to

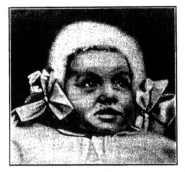

Fig. 1. Case of hare-lip and cleft palate, operated at third week—result at end of nine months.

lip exists the defect is repaired at the same time as the cleft in the palate.

Lane under no circumstances ever removes the intermaxillary bone or performs any operation upon it with a view of displacing it backward. "The pressure which is exerted upon it by the lip after its continuity has been effected is quite sufficient to bring about its backward replacement."

It is obvious that in the closure of any particular cleft the surgeon must be largely guided by his experience, and that only the principles and a general description of

the operating table. Thus the child becomes a part of the adjustable portion of the table, and gives the operator a steady field on which to work.

The operation as described by Lane is as follows: "The mouth gags are placed in position and the tongue drawn forward by a ligature so as to give free access to the cleft in its entire length. If the soft parts underlying the edges of the cleft are thick and vascular a flap is cut from the mucous membrane, submucous tissue, and periosteum of one side, having its attachment or base along the free margin of the cleft. The palatine vascular supply is divided while the flap is being reflected inward, and it depends for its blood supply on vessels entering its attached margin.

"The mucous membrane, submucous tissue, and periosteum are raised from the opposing margin of the cleft by an elevator, an incision being made along the length of the edge of the cleft.

"The reflected flap with its scanty supply of blood derived from small vessels in its attached margin is then placed beneath the the posterior palatine has been excluded, and which pivots on a base formed by the margin of the cleft. Here we have a mobile, well-vascularized flap, which can be thrown as a bridge in any direction and can be superimposed on the flap of the opposite side, the closure being necessarily rendered complete by flaps from the edges of a harelip."

The method may be best illustrated diagrammatically as indicated in Fig. 3, which represents the roof of the mouth with a cleft extending through the hard

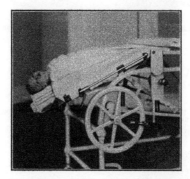

Fig. 2. The "Göthsen Sling" used in cleft palate operations.

elevated flap, whose blood supply is ample, and it is fixed in position by a double row of sutures. In this manner two extensive raw surfaces well supplied with blood and uninfluenced by any tension whatever are retained in accurate opposition.

"If, on the other hand, the cleft is too broad to admit of its safe and perfect closure in this manner, one flap, comprising all the mucous membrane, submucous tissue, and periosteum on one side, is raised except at the point of entry of the posterior palatine vessels, while the soft parts on the opposite side are raised in a flap from which and soft palates. The alveolus is indicated by AAA.

The operation consists in introducing a reflected flap on one side beneath a raised flap of the opposite side as follows:

The *reflected flap* is made by the incision *ab*, which extends from the anterior limit of the cleft forward and outward through the mucoperiosteum to beyond the outer surface of the alveolus; *bc* runs along the outer surface of the gums at the junction of the cheek and alveolus; *cd* extends along the free posterior margin of the palate to the uvula. This flap is carefully raised

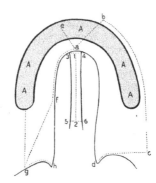

Fig. 3. Lines of incision for repair of a median cleft in infancy. (Lane).

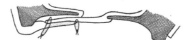

Fig. 4. Showing the method of fixation of the reflected flap beneath the elevated flap by a double row of sutures. (Lane).

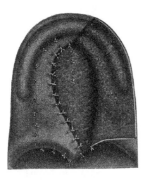
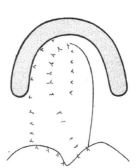

Fig. 5. Flap sutured in position for repair of median cleft.

from the underlying structures, the posterior palatine vessels and nerves being clamped and divided. Its attached border is the edge of the cleft on one side, and as it is reflected over the cleft its mucous surface looks upward.

The *raised flap* is made by an incision *af* extending on to the alveolus; the incision *af* courses along the free margin of the cleft and is continued as *fg*, obliquely outward and backward along the upper surface of the soft palate. The incision *gh* extends along the posterior free margin of the palate to the top of the uvula. The mucoperiosteal flap *afg* is now raised from the bone, the soft palate freed from the posterior margin of the hard palate, and the mucous membrane on its upper surface turned outward.

The completion of the operation consists in introducing the reflected flap of one side beneath the raised flap of the opposite side and the two fixed in position by a double line of sutures as shown in Fig. 4. The completed operation with dotted suture lines is shown in Fig. 5.

If the septum presents a free margin which extends to the level of the cleft (Fig. 3), an additional incision (1-2) is made along the middle line of the septum through the mucous membrane and periosteum with two transverse incisions (3-4 and 5-6).

These two narrow flaps are turned down laterally and the reflected flap denuded of its mucous membrane along the area of contact is sutured to the superimposed flaps and the margin of the septum (Fig. 5) (Lane).

A natural objection to this operation is the large area of raw surface which is left. It is surprising how rapidly this surface is covered over by new tissue and the normal appearance of the mucosa restored.

This general principle of superimposed flaps is applicable to every variety of cleft palate, it is modified as the individual needs and ingenuity of the surgeon suggests.

After-treatment—For the first twenty-four hours give only sterile water. Do not give milk until the injured mucosa is sealed up by the products of repair, since milk is a good medium for bacteria, and the mouth is difficult to cleanse.

Keep the child quiet and try to prevent crying.

Milk diet may be given on the second day. Always follow the feeding with sterile water to wash away the milk remnants.

No mechanical cleansing of the mouth is practical in small children.

On the seventh day the sutures should be removed.

THE NEWER TREATMENT OF GOUT.

BY

GEORGE MEYERS, M. D.,
New York City.

Some years ago one of the British journals, *The Practitioner*, devoted an entire issue to the subject of gout. At the close of the series of articles the final editorial comment was: Gout is a disease which we do not understand.

About two years ago the same journal devoted another issue to the same subject, and at the close of that series the editor again commented as follows: In our last special number we concluded with the words: Gout is a disease which we do not understand and even now (July, 1909) it is impossible to avoid admitting that concerning the real nature of gout our knowledge lacks completeness and is still wanting in regard to accuracy.

In the few minutes allotted to me this evening, I desire to bring out for discussion some of the newer forms of treatment of gout which rest on the scientific bases established by the more recent experimental and laboratory endeavors.

In order to comprehend the rational treatment of this disease it is necessary to understand what are the disturbances in the physiology and pathology of the metabolism of the new nucleoproteins which characterize this clinical picture. The nucleoproteins form a distinct food class, distinguished from other proteins, and having their own special processes of disintegration and elimination. They are the mother substances of the well-known uric acid. They enter the body as one of the large components of certain foods. Those foods richest in these substances are the glandular organs (liver, pancreas, thymus) numerous varieties of fish and their roes, and some classes of vegetables.

This compound proteid is split up in the digestive tract into an easily assimilable proteid portion, and into the nucleic acid radicle. This latter by oxydation processes, taking place throughout the body, is transformed into purin bases, and then by further oxydation into the end product, uric acid. In this process special ferments called oxydazes or uricolytic ferments, are for the most part employed. The oxydazes exist in the liver, muscles, and in various parts of the body, having been actually demonstrated there in perfusion experiments on the lower animals.

Physiologically a normal man ingesting a large amount of nucleoproteids will have no difficulty in excreting the end products of their metabolism within 24 or 48 hours. The urine is found rapidly to contain the excess in the form of uric acid. The blood rapidly frees itself from the superabundance retaining only its normal traces. On the other hand, the picture is entirely altered in a gouty person. There the urine, which continually shows a lessened amount to be present shows after the ingestion of a large amount of nucleoprotein only a slow and prolonged excretion of the excess. The blood and tissues are surcharged with the effete products, a uricemia results. This uricemia seems to be caused by:

(1) A disturbance in the oxydizing enzymes.

(2) By the formation of a uric acid salt, which is excreted through the kidney with great difficulty.

(3) Some change in the kidney itself; which seems to be affected by the disease, and scarcely able to excrete the salt, the result being a retention.

The gouty person cannot even care for the nucleoproteins of an ordinary mixed diet. On such a diet his urine always shows less excreted uric acid than that of a control person. He eliminates his uric acid with difficulty. His blood frequently shows more of this substance than it should. His tissues are surcharged with an overabundance of the purin bodies and of uric acid. The acute paroxysm or gouty attack consists of the precipitation of much of this excess uric acid in the smaller joints of the body in the form of insoluble urate salts.

Now in the light here shown the difficulty of the gouty person to use up and excrete the end products of this particular protein, the therapeutic indication is clear. He must avoid in his diet not so much all protein food but this particular class of protein, the nucleoproteins. He must for long periods be directed to eliminate from his intake the sources of this food, the so-called exogenous source of purin substances, thus reducing him to the necessity of metabolizing the normally present nucleoprotein of his body (the so-called endogenous source).

These, of course, will always appear in the urine, as the result of the normal wear and tear of his own tissues. He must not eat foods rich in nuclear contents. Glandular meats are forbidden; pancreas, liver, thymus, anchovies, sardines, herring, pork, beef, lamb, squabs, deer; among the vegetables, beans, peas, barley, cauliflower, and turnips. The diet should consist of the most part of fruit, eggs, milk, cereals, bread, onions, white cabbage, cucumbers and salads.

Having maintained the patient upon such a purin free diet, and established a tolerance we may then begin with small amounts of food containing purins. We have thus rested his ferments, protected his kidneys, and eliminated his retained and excessive, stored-up uric acid. This method of treatment follows closely the lines laid down in the modern treatment of diabetes.

The presence of a sodium salt is the greatest factor in precipitating out soluble quadriurates, converting them into the insoluble crystalline biurate. This takes place where the sodium content of the fluid is the highest, namely, in the synovial fluid and in the cartilages nearest the joints, these containing .5 to .8% of sodium, while liver and other internal organs contain .1 to .2%.

The therapeutic indication to be taken from this is toward an achloride or salt free diet, but not as against any other salt than sodium. Any medicament containing sodium is forbidden, and potassium is substituted. Common salt is inhibited in the diet to the greatest degree. So too, concerning the mineral waters, and watering places. While the waters may be useful, especially those containing radium, as we may later demonstrate, it is absolutely necessary that waters with high sodium content be prohibited.

From what has previously been said we have noted that one of the factors in the faulty metabolism of purins is connected with the ferments. For the most part they are oxydizing ferments, breaking down the purins to uric acid. It is evident that in giving a purin free diet we are resting these enzymes, and allowing them to reaccumulate their strength and vigor.

Just a word about radium: It seems that radium has some effect upon these conditions. The nature of its effect is not known—but I myself have seen a case in which so-called radium water was administered to a gouty patient with very good result. What the future may bring forth in this direction it is impossible to predict, but it is well to remember that radium is one of the things which alters those formations in the body which are connected with the metabolism of the purins.

After all, the newer treatment of gout, based as it is on scientific and accurate laboratory research, merely bears out and corroborates the empirical treatment of the older school of clinical physicians.

MEDICAL HINTS.

A warm vaginal douche should be at least four quarts in amount and of a temperature of from 110 to 120 degrees F., usually 115 degrees F. It is well to add a heaping tablespoonful of common salt to each two quarts of a simple douche. This should always be given at a time when the patient can remain in the recumbent position for at least an hour.

CALVIN AND SERVETUS: AN EPISODE IN THE HISTORY OF RELIGIOUS PERSECUTION AND SCIENTIFIC SUPPRESSION.

BY

JOHN KNOTT, A. M., M. D.
Dublin, Ireland.

(*Concluded*)

When Servetus arrived at Geneva he lay in quiet retirement within his lodging for three whole weeks. He would seem to have been looking forward to an earnest, but quietly convincing, *tête-a-tête* theological tournament with the most notable and unflinching of living controversialists. Then came another Sunday, and as the religious element was strongly developed— and always assiduously cultivated in the nature of the refugee physician (and amateur theologian) he determined to absent himself from public worship no longer; and accordingly, attended Divine Service in the evening. The Argus eyes of Calvin and his agents (informers and spies) saw, criticized, and identified every new immigrant, as well as settled resident, of his stronghold city of refuge. The presence of Michael Servetus—and his assured identity were notified to the Reformer immediately after the conclusion of the period of worship, and the possessor of the patience which had for so many years lain in wait for an enemy of divergent Christian opinions saw that the opportunity for which he had so long wished and prayed had at last flown into his arms. Without loss of a moment the presence of a malignant (and convicted) heretic was notified to the responsible public official, the necessary warrant was issued, and Michael Servetus was arrested on the *Sunday* night of his first walk

abroad in the republican stronghold of civil and religious liberty!!! John Calvin appeared in court on Monday morning to conduct the prosecution, armed with a series of thirty-eight articles of indictment —the number and complexity of the subjects therewith associated being so great as to lead critical observers to express the opinion that he must have sat up all night in preparing them. The details of the prolonged trial cannot, of course, be even glanced at; I will just indicate that the principal items of evidence were those furnished by the private letter which had been written by Michael Servetus to John Calvin, and the few printed (specimen) leaves of his recent book. (One of the articles of indictment—to which I have already referred—was specially interesting, too, from the point of view of the modern natural historian: in his edition of Ptolemy's famous geography, which had been published eighteen years before, Servetus had drawn an unfavorable picture of the physical aspects of Palestine. Such an exercise of the liberty of speech was denounced with fiery energy by Calvin—as not merely an impeachment of the veracity of the divinely inspired Moses, but an act of foul blasphemy against the Holy Ghost, at whose dictation the "land of milk and honey" had been originally so described). The "Libertine" party in Geneva were (naturally) strongly opposed to Calvin's vigorous discipline and gradually progressive assumption of dictatorial power, so that they threw every obstacle in the way of his conduct of the trial of Servetus for major heresy—with prospective sentence of the stake—in a city which harbored the refugees from similar proceedings from all the countries of Western Europe. But they had no *personal* interest in poor Servetus, and the *burning* zeal of his prosecutor never flagged for an instant. The opponents of Calvin in the ranks of the governing municipal body grew apathetic and careless in attendance—with the result that his perseverance was rewarded in October by the attainment of the requisite majority of two-thirds, and Michael Servetus was burned at the stake by a *slow* fire on the day after the passing of the sentence. Owing to *hepatic indisposition* John Calvin was unable to treat himself to the luxury of attendance at the execution, but he and his friends took care that the arrangements were so carried out that he was able to gratify himself by inspection of the final scene from his bedroom window. Such are the manifestations of the *charity* which has been so frequently displayed by the self-elected apostles of various improved versions of the teaching of Christ. The most accomplished physician, the most original scientist, and the most earnestly devoted explorer of Nature's mysteries in that restless sixteenth century, thus ended a truly benevolent and inoffensive career as the victim of the religious—Christian (!!!)—zeal of the most ardent "Reformer" of his generation. In this quarter centenary anniversary of the birth of Calvin and (probably of) Servetus, the memory of this remarkable pair of men may well be made the vehicle of a profitable, as well as humiliating, lesson—to the philosopher and the philanthropist, as well as to the zealously expert physician, and the zealously enthusiastic amateur theologian. What makes the horrible sacrifice of the life of poor Servetus of so enthralling interest to every devoted member of the one profession which was practised and blessed by Christ himself during the whole period of his Divine mission to

mankind lies in the fact that a copy of his last book—of which the contents so largely contributed to the sealing of his earthly doom—was tied to his thigh and burned with him at the stake, and that volume contains a description of the circulation of the blood, printed exactly seventy-five years before the publication of William Harvey's celebrated "discovery!"

This little-known fact is one of the most interestingly important, as well as melancholy, in the whole history of the healing art—indeed it may be said, with a reasonable claim to truth—of the history of the advancement of man's physical comfort. For it must be universally admitted that modern scientific medicine—in the departments of both diagnosis and therapeusis—dates its birth from the promulgation of the doctrine of the circulation of the blood. Servetus introduced the subject merely in way of illustration—incidentally—but his *extremely brief* description of the *pulmonary* circulation is quite complete, and far more lucid—with all reverence be it written—than the somewhat muddle-headed one placed before the reader, in copious verbiage, by the famous physician whose more fortunate privilege it was to make the mystery of the circulation known to the world at large. He doesn't push the *systemic* circulation to its conclusion—physical or logical—he follows the blood to the extremities, and leaves the return to its own care, or that of the guiding Providence with which he was immediately concerned in his great theological disquisition. It would take us too far and too long to discuss the date of the recognition of the systemic circulation, but I will take the opportunity of pointing out that the etymological suggestion so usually made that the (unwise) predecessors of Harvey believed that the *arteries* carried *air*—*only* displays a sad deficiency of reading and reflection. They *did* not recognize and teach that those vessels contained a *spirit:* so do the moderns, and call it *oxygen!* That the leaders of ancient Greek thought, medical and philosophic (Hippocrates, Plato, and Aristotle) knew that was a *systemic* circulation is perfectly proven to every discriminating reader of their works; and to deny that Galen knew that arteries conveyed blood—and *from* the heart—is too preposterous for serious contradiction in presence of the fact that he describes the operation of deligation of those vessels in cases of hemorrhage. The *one link* in the systemic circulation of which the ancients do not seem to have formed a clear conception is the maintenance of a *continuous* current in the *veins*—*towards* the heart. They do not seem to have ever estimated at its true value the significance of the presence of the *valves;* and, accordingly, allowed the blood to wobble therein upon occasion—backwards and forwards, as well as collaterally by divergent branches and anastomotic channels. The valves are beautifully figured in the magnificent folio of Fabricius ab Aquapendente, who was professor of anatomy at Padua, "nursery of arts."

It is difficult to realize how and why their function could have escaped him, having regard to the mechanical and artistic attainments of Italy in his generation. Still his text seems to indicate that it did. Nevertheless, historic evidence goes to show that the secret had been revealed. We have the testimony of Johannes Leonicenus to the fact that it was fully known to the restless genius, Fra Paolo Sarpi, the famous historian of the Council of Trent. That he would have kept this knowledge from "the general" is by no means unlikely; the authorities of the Church had never displayed a proneness to cast scientific pearls before swine, and the learned Servite had suffered but far too much from the consequences of his natural leaning towards public discussion. Anyway, Padua was then universally recognized as the anatomical focus of Christendom; its University was the one institution in existence in which a mastery of the mysteries of human anatomy could be attained. Thither, accordingly, William Harvey directed his steps for the purpose of completing his medical education—as did the more ambitious candidates for the medical profession from every other centre in Europe. He saw the *valves* demonstrated by the foremost of living anatomists. But he was not taught their function, and could not guess it; so he returned to England without the attainment of this most important item of information. Soon after his return, and with the subject still fresh in his mind, he discussed the curious intra-vascular items with an *engineering* friend, who at once suggested the inevitable use to which they must have been assigned by the formative hand of Nature. So the missing link was at last supplied! And William Harvey had *discovered* simply—*nothing* at all!!! Such is reputation. Well may the Iagos cynicize! And a supplemental illustration of the crucifixion treatment which has evermore been meted out to important discoverers and innovators was in time supplied by the ruinous effect which Harvey's publication of his so-called *"discovery"* had on his private practice—and public peace of mind. His professional brethren behaved, in the mass, as the proverbial mob has always done, whether learned or unlearned. The professional popularity of the discoverer sank below the horizon, from beneath which it never again emerged. For the remainder of his life he lived "a man forbid." Such is a typical specimen of the origin and mode of procedure in cases of scientific martyrdom! The scientists have always done as the theologians did—so far as their power extended, or could be made to stretch.

Thus came the "discovery" of William Harvey to arrive at its place in the public eye, exactly three-quarters of a century after the *original* one of Servetus had been extinguished, with the life of its author, by the procedure which had been inspired and maintained by the religious zeal of John Calvin—in the promotion of his own special edition of Christian doctrine, and the maintenance of his own authority, as one and indivisible, in the promulgation of the same. The newly printed edition of Servetus's *De Christianisme Restitutiono* was seized and committed to the flames on the arrest of its author, in accordance with the inquisitorial procedure which had been made necessary by the elaborate—and legally-skilled—conveyance of incriminative evidence by the enthusiastic Reformer. Only a few copies were retained (by Calvin's instructions) for the special purpose of supplying the necessary evidence of major heresy. But two are definitely known to have survived. One of these which bears demonstrative evidence of having been that used by Calvin himself in the preparation of the articles of indictment, and the conduct of the prolonged prosecution, is now preserved in the *Bibliotheque Nationale* in Paris. The other is in the Imperial Library at Vienna. The extinction of the book (and its lonely author) was so complete, and the special physiological group of sentences was so obscurely imbedded therein that there is some reason for surprise that the latter was ever disinterred. Thus John Calvin in his

zeal for the salvation of his fellowman, and for the security of his own position as the theological dictator of the radiating movements of the Reformation and its apostles, successfully arrested the hand of the dial of physiological science for three-quarters of a century! I venture to assert that no case of persecution can be disinterred from the annals of the much-reviled Inquisition which displayed so malignant a spirit of personal vindictiveness and malignant treachery!

I trust that the curiosity of every reader who is a devoted disciple of his (truly "divine") profession has been sufficiently awakened to call forth a desire to see the *verba scripta* of the physiological (illustrative) digression which contains the original description of the circulation, and has formed the inspiring "text" of the present communication. They are these:

"Ut vero totam animæ et spiritus rationem habeas, lector, divinam hic philosophiam adjungam, quam facilè intelligas, si in anatome fueris exercitatus. Dicitur in nobis extrium superiorum elementorum substantia esse spiritus triplex, naturalis, vitalis, et animalis. Tres spiritus vocat Aphrodisæus; veré non sunt tres, sed duo spiritus distincti. Vitalis est spiritus, qui per anastomoses ab arteriis communicatur venis, in quibus dicitur naturalis. Primus ergaest sanguis, cujus sedes est in hepato, et corporis venis. Secundus est spiritus vitalis, cujus sedes est in corde, et corporis arteriis. Tertius est spiritus animalis, quasi lucis radius, cujus sedes est in cerebro, et corporis nervis, in his omnibus est unius spiritus et lucis Dei energia. Quòd a corde communicatur hepati spiritus ille naturalis, docet hominis formatio ab utero. Nam arteria mittitur juncta venæ per ipsius fœtus umbilicum: itidemque in nobis postea semper junguntur arteria et vena. In cor est prius, quàm in hepar, a Deo inspirata Adæ anima, et ab eo hepati communicata. Per inspirationem in eos et nares, est veré inducta anima: inspiratio autem ad cor tendit. Cor est primum vivens, fons caloris, in medio corpore. Ab

556   AMERICAN MEDICINE }
Complete Series, Vol. XVIII.   ORIGINAL ARTICLES   { OCTOBER, 1912.
New Series, Vol. VII., No. 10.

hepate sumit liquorem vitæ, quasi materiam, et eum vice versa vivificat: sicut aquæ liquor superioribus elementis materiam suppeditat, et ab eis, juncta luce ad vegetandum vivificatur. Ex hepatis sanguine est animæ materia, per elaborationem mirabilem, quam nunc audies. Hinc dicitur anima esse in sanguine, et anima ipsa esse sanguis, sive sanguineus spiritus. Non dicitur anima principaliter esse in parietitus cordis, aut in corpore ipso cerebri, aut hepatis, sed in sanguine, ut docet ipse Deus. Genes. 9. Levit. 17, et Deut. 12.

"Ad quam rem est prius intelligenda substantialis generatio ipsius vitalis spiritus, qui ex aëre inspirato et sublilissimo sanguine componitur, et nutritur, vitalis spiritus in sinistro cordis ventriculo suam originem habet, juvantibus maxime pulmonibus ad ipsius generationem. Est spiritus tenuis, ut sit quasi ex puriori sanguine lucidus vapor, substantiam in se continensa quæ, aëris et ignis. Generatur exfacta in pulmonibus mixtione inspirati aëris cum elaborato sublili sanguine, quem dexter ventriculus· cordis sinistro communicat. Fit autem communicatio hæc, non per parietem cordis medium, ut vulgo creditur; sed magno artificio a dextro cordis ventriculo, longo per pulmones ductu, agitatur sanguis subtilis: a pulmonibus preparatur, flavus efficitur, et a vena arteriosa in arteriam venosam transfunditur. Deinde in ipsa arteria venosa inspirato aëre miscetur, et expiratione a fuligine repurgatur. Atque ita tandem a sinistro cordis ventriculo tolum mixtum per diastolem attrahitur, apta suppellex, ut fiat spiritus vitalis.

Quòd ita per pulmonis fiat communicatio, et præparatio, docet conjunctio varia, et communicatio, venæ arteriosæ cum arteria venosa in pulmonibus. Confirmat hoc magnitudo insignis venæ arteriosæ, quæ nec talis, nec tanta facta esset, nec tantam a corde ipso vim purissimi sanguinis in pulmones emitteret, ob solum eorum nutrimentum, nec cor pulmonibus hec ratione servinet: cum præsertim antea in embryone solerent pulmones ipsi aliunde nutriri, ob membranulas illas, seu valvulas cordis, usque ad horum nativitatis nondum apertas, ut docet Galenus. Ergo ad alium usum effunditur sanguis a corde in pulmones hora ipsa nativitatis, et tam copiosus. Item, a pulmonibus ad cor non simplex aër, sed mixtus sanguine mittitur, per arteriam venosam ergo in pulmonibus fit mixtio Flavus ille color a pulmonibus datur sanguini spiritusco, non a corde, in sinistro cordis ventriculo non est locus capaæ tantæ et tam copiosæ mixtionis, nec ad flavum elaboratio illa sufficiens. Demum, paries ille medius, cum sit vasorum et facultatum expers, non est aptus ad communicationem et elaborationem illam, licet aliquid resudare possit. Eodem artificio, quo in hepato fit transfusio a vena porta ad venam cavam propter sanguinem, fit etiam in pulmone transfusio a vena arteriosa ad arteriam venosam propter spiritum. Si quis hæc conferat cum üs quæ scribit Galenus, lib. 6 et 7, de usu artium, veritatem ponitus intelliget, ab ipso Galeno non animadversam.

"Ille itaque spiritus vitalis a sinistro cordis ventriculo in arterias totius corporis deinde transfunditur, ita ut qui tenuior est, superiora petat, ubi magis adhuc elaboratur, præcipue in plexu retiforme, subbasi cerebri sito, in quo ex vitali fieri incipit animalis, ad propriam rationalis animæ accedens;....
. . . ."

The above scintillation of the vital spark of heavenly flame, which was destined to be so soon extinguished by the theological authority provided by the Protestant Pope of Geneva, is surely one which should be permanently photographed on the mental retina of every physician who is devoted to his profession, as every medical man worthy of his sacred calling must always be. Michael Servetus died the death of a martyr to science—to the ideal *philosophy* of the ancient Greeks, who carried the term which in itself presents so convincing an item of testimony to the unparalleled brilliancy of the Hellenic genius in the brightest ages of its luminosity. His life had been devoted, perhaps more completely than that of any other student known to the annals of science, to the pursuit of knowledge for its own sake. He rather coveted seclusion, as public display would necessarily prove a heavy tax on the time which was his great asset, and the occupation of any public position would mean not only a curtailment of invaluable—and irreplaceable—time, but would also mean the imposition of a serious drag on his liberty of thought and on his consuming desire to convey to his contemporaries and to posterity every item of the message which he believed that he had been divinely commissioned to deliver. I have already emphasized some most important facts in the history of the slow evolution of the discovery of the circulation of the blood—the great central fact in human physiology, and that on which all scientific medical practice is necessarily based. I have affirmed the ancient Greek familiarity—to an approximate degree of accuracy—with the systemic circulation. And Greek science remained unexpanded till the advent of the Renaissance—the dawn of all "modern" science and literature, with all their splendid qualities and (without offence be it added) their irritating defects. Most readers have sometimes revelled in the pages of the roystering Rabelais, perhaps few have taken mental note of his physiology:

"The Intention of the Founder of this Microcosm is to have a Soul therein to be entertained, which is lodged there as a Guest, with its Host, it may live there for a while. Life consisteth in Blood, Blood is the Seat of the Soul; therefore the chiefest work of the Microcosm is to be making Blood continually. At this Forge are exercised all the Members of the Body; none is exempted from Labour, each operates a part, and both its proper Office. And such is their Hierarchy, that perpetually the one *borrows* from the other, the one *lends* the other, and the one is the other's *Debtor*. The Stuff and Matter convenient which Nature giveth to be turned into Blood is *Bread* and *Wine*. All kinds of nourishing victuals is to be comprehended in these two, and from hence in the *Langue Goth* is called *Campanage*. To find out this Meat and Drink, to prepare and boil it, the Hands are put to work, the Feet do walk and heat up the whole Bulk of the Corporal Mass; the Eyes guide and conduct all; the Appetite in the Orifice of the Stomach, by means of the little sourish black Humour (called Melancholy) which is transmitted thereto from the Milt, giveth warning to shut in the Food. The Tongue doth make the first essay and tastes it; the Teeth do chaw it, and the Stomach doth receive, digest and chilify it; the Mesaraick Venis suck out what is good and fit, leaving behind the Excrements, which are, through special conduits for that purpose, voided by an expulsive Faculty; thereafter it is carried to the Liver, where it being changed again, it, by the Virtue of that new transmutation becomes Blood. What joy, conjecture you, will then be founded amongst those officers, when they see this *Rivulet of Gold*, which is their sole Restorative? No greater is the Joy of Alchemists, when after long Travel, Toil and Expense, they see in their Furnaces the Transmutation: then it is that every Member doth prepare itself, and strive anew to purify and to refine this Treasure: The Kidneys through the emulgent Veins draw that Aquosity from thence which you call Urine; and there send it away through the Ureter to be slipped downward; where in a lower Receptacle, and proper for it (to wit the Bladder), it is kept, and stayeth there until an Opportunity to void it out in his due time. The Spleen draweth from the *Blood* its terrestrial Part. viz., the Grounds, Lees, a thick Substance settled in the bottom thereof, which you term *Melancholy:* The Bottle of the Gall subtracts from thence all the superfluous *Choler:* whence it is brought to another Shop or Workhouse to be yet better purified and refined, that is the Heart, which by its Agitation of *Diastlolick* and Systolick Motions so neatly subtiliseth and inflames it, that in the *right side* Ventriclet is brought to Perfection and through the Veins is sent to all the Members; each Parcel of the Body draws it then into it's self, and after it's own Fashion is cherished and alimented by it: Feet, Hands, Thighs, Arms, Eyes, Ears, Back, Breast, yea, all; and then it is that who before were *Lenders*, now become *Debtors*. The Heart doth in it's *Left-side* Ventricle so thinnify the Blood that it thereby obtains the name of Spiritual; which being sent through the Arteries to all the

Members of the Body, serveth to warm and winnow or fan the other Blood which runneth through the Veins: the Light's never cease with its Lappets and Bellows to cool and refresh it; in Acknowledgment of which good the Heart through the Arterial Vein imparts into it the choicest of it's Blood: At last it is made so fine and subtle within the *Rete Mirabile* that thereafter those *Animal Spirits* are framed and composed of it; by means whereof the Imagination, Discourse, Judgment, Resolution, Deliberation, Ratiocination, and Memory, have their Rise, Actings, and Operations."

The occasion of an allusion to Rabelais in his rarely recognized capacity as a medical writer of the foremost rank in his own generation may well be utilized for the purpose of calling the attention of the reader to the restlessly inquiring spirit of the newly-awakened age of that very remarkable man, when the recent introduction of printing and the exodus of Greek scholars and Greek manuscripts from Constantinople, which was the direct result of the capture of the capital of the Eastern Empire by the Turks, had sown all Western Europe with dragon's teeth. Indeed, it may be pointed out parenthetically that the impetus supplied by the penetration of Europe by the adjacent portion of Asia would seem to have been transmitted across the southern margin of the former continent, and during a temporary arrest on arriving at the Atlantic border to have generated the momentum which transmitted the Spanish expedition to the shores of the Western World. The group of co-incidents which were focussed by the mysterious guidance of Providence in that epoch is surely the most remarkable—and has proved the most fertile of any known to the history of human civilization and human opinion. The series of seismic waves of thought—political, social, philosophical and theological (moral and im-

moral)—which rapidly followed could not fail to produce so great a degree of mental friction in all directions as to raise the temperature of the intellectual (and political) atmosphere of Western Europe far above the boiling point. And, as necessarily occurs during every process of violent ebullition, a large proportion of the veriest intellectual dregs was brought to the surface, and for a considerable period constituted the principal portion of the topmost layer of floating scum; many wondrously and fearfully inspired bubbles were ejected therefrom to a great height, and were seen to flash forth richly artistic and iridescent hues before they burst or disappeared; while the really nutritious and valuable portion of the liquid medium was that which remained excluded from the general gaze. Francois Rabelais was born in the year 1483, the same year in which Martin Luther first saw the light; and he died in 1553, the year in which Michael Servetus was burned alive at the stake for heresy at the prosecution of John Calvin—another curious brace of items in the history of rare coincidences! The average reader, who goes to the works of Rabelais for the enjoyment afforded by a perusal of the buffoonery and obscenity in which, unhappily, they far too largely abound is rarely cognizant of the fact that the author was one of the most learned medical men of his generation; that, like the great philosophic reformer, Lord Chancellor Bacon, he had "taken all knowledge for his province"; that he had turned from the theology and law which he had earnestly tried (and found wanting) to the study of medicine, as offering the widest field of general knowledge obtainable for cultivation in this world; and that his coarse buffoonery and gross indelicacy are, probably, in every instance but the reflex of the contempt and scorn for the cant and corruption which he saw everywhere around him. The inspiration of his indescribable work was assuredly quite similar to that displayed on a parallel occasion by the "English Rabelais," Jonathan Swift. The heroic deeds of Gorgantua and Pantagruel grew from the same intellectual germs as did the veracious travels of Lemuel Gulliver. . But even medical men who while away an occasional evening hour over the fantastic pages of Rabelais seldom notice, or rarely think the fact worth the trouble of remembering, that the quotation which I have above given contains the best compendium of the general—up-to-date—philosophical knowledge of that time which has descended to us. A comparison of the contained sentences (which I have copied from a Dublin reprint of Ozett's celebrated version—published in 1738 by Philip Crampton, one of the historic booksellers and publishers of the Irish metropolis) with those of the quotation from the last work of poor Servetus will prove to every discerning reader what seven-league strides the victim of Calvin has passed beyond the attainments of the best informed of contemporary physiologists and what a loss the world suffered by the sacrifice of his book and its author. The quotation from Rabelais shows that the author had very definite ideas of the continuous processes of waste and repair, of absorption, assimilation, and elimination, as they go on in the human body. Also that he had a perfectly clear notion of the *continuous* movement of the blood within the vessels, which formed the sole vehicle of the requisite pabulum for the tissues—and also of the transudation which gave each of these structures the opportunity of

making its own selection of appropriate nutriment and material for repair. So that, although he cannot be said to have made the current of the blood precisely "circular," he has unquestionably placed on record sufficient testimony to show that his physiological ideas were not so much behind those of William Harvey as most medical men of the present generation have been taught to think. It is interesting to notice how the scientific enthusiasm of both Servetus and Rabelais induced each to place in the context of a literary masterpiece devoted to a subject and domain of thought wholly unconnected with either medicine or any of its ancillary or germanic sciences a perfectly polished gem of medical science and medical history—each of which specimens seems to look out with Argus eyes on every illuminating area of contemporary knowledge, and to reflect from a superfocus of myriad facts rays which individually convey to the mental retina of the skilled reader in every instance a flood of light on the various aspects of the progress of human scientific research, and opinion, and attainment. And a comparison of the two summaries of the physiology of the vital fluid as presented to the minds of the two most brilliant medical geniuses of the sixteenth century shows precisely how far Servetus had outrun all his contemporaries and what an unspeakable loss the world suffered by the most malignant murder known to authentic history—successfully carried out, under the auspices of religion and the aegis of law, by the "saintly" John Calvin. The circumstances of the closing scenes of the tragedy of the life of one who was naturally disposed, and scientifically qualified to prove the greatest (physical) benefactor of the human race always recall to the mind of the present writer a brilliant parallel of character which appeared in print a couple of decades ago from the pen of that switching stylist, Mr. Belfast Bax.

"William Morris once said to me that he looked upon John Calvin as quite the worst man that ever lived. I would pair with the name of John Calvin in this distinction that of Maximilien Robespierre. The old French province of Picardy assuredly deserves the merit of having produced at an interval of two hundred years, two of the most exquisitely developed scoundrels the world has ever seen—Calvin in the sixteenth, Robespierre in the eighteenth century. Both alike were redolent of cant; Calvin sniffed the theological cant of the sixteenth century, with its Christian bigotry and asceticism; Robespierre the political cant of the eighteenth century with its Rousseauite intolerance and affection of Roman austerity. Both alike were bloodless, villous, blear-eyed abortions—crosses between the fish and the human—who owed the reputation they obtained with simpletons for clean living, purity, and incorruptibility to this very fact. Shakespere must surely have had those two precious Picards in view of his prophetic soul when he spoke of the 'treacherous, kindless villain.' Poor Anacharsis Clootz had the misfortune to fall into the jaws of the second of these monsters, as did poor Michael Servet into those of the first."

Another item of duplex interest in its special associations with both medicine and literature may here be submitted to the attention of the reader. As already indicated, the physiological position which had been attained by the giant strides of the combined enthusiasm and genius of Servetus was absolutely unique; while that of Rabelais represents the thoroughly up-to-date attainments of the first class theorist and scientific practitioner of the same generation. The fact of this common proprietorship is emphatically demonstrated by a hasty summary of the cir-

culation and nutritive functions of the blood which has been placed on record by England's "immortal dramatist".—which represents, to a startling degree of resemblance, the concentrated essence (a convex-mirror reflection it might be very appropriately styled, I think) of Rabelais; more expanded word-painting. I refer to the following:

"True is it, my incorporate friends," quoth he,
"That I receive the general food at first,
Which you do live upon; and yet it is
Because I am the store-house and the shop
of the whole body; but, if you do remember,
I send it through the rivers of your blood,
And through the cranks and offices of man,
The strongest nerves and small inferior veins
From me receive that natural competency
Whereby they lived."

The two great critical and exegetical parties of Shakespearians and Baconians have, I believe, not yet quite agreed as to the extent of the acquaintance of the author of *Coriolanus* (from the text of which the above quotation has been made) with the quaint contents of the fantastic work of Rabelais. But they must admit (at least all of them, as I think the reader will agree, who are capable of forming a sane opinion on any textual question) that the ideas of those inspired authors on the subjects of digestion, nutrition, and the (? circulatory) movements of the blood in the human body display a degree of convergence which closely approximates complete parallelism, and even simulates absolute coincidence. Thus the lay text of the "inspired" dramatist represents the attainment of a plane of physiological equipment and culture which, most assuredly, was *not* the common platform of the medical faculty of Great Britain at that date—when Padua was the cosmic centre of medical light and treating. The only objections to the identification of the source of Shakespere's most remarkable up-to-date-ness in this interesting particular are, I think, that: there may have been access to a common source; or, the old and oft-repeated story that the tracings of the pencil of genius have often been observed to display closely similar—and even precisely coincident—curves, even when the guiding hands had been separated by an entire quadrant of the earth's circumference, and their inspired respective owners were utterly unconscious of one another's existence.

Thus, above the sixteenth century highwater mark indicated by the lines of the dramatist above quoted the tide of English scientific knowledge of the facts and conditions of the circulation of the blood failed to rise by even the fraction of a degree, till William Harvey imported his inspiration from the "nursery of arts." The discovery of poor Michael *"Villanovanus"* —if ever revealed by him to anybody—lay forgotten during a period of three-quarters of a century. Indeed the wonder is, considering the lonely position of the author during life, and the almost complete extinction of his book, that the passage was ever discovered—or, having been discovered, came to be publicly discussed. And, having regard to the fact that all scientific medicine is necessarily founded on the bed-rock of a knowledge of the movement and nutritional function of the blood, and bearing in mind the almost electric velocity of the progress of hygiene and preventive medicine during the past half century, it can hardly be said to be too confident an expression of opinion to state that were it not for the effects of the fiery zeal of John Calvin, the epidemic diseases would now be known to the citizens of civilized communities only by historic record and by the reported experience of travellers. Surely

then, the name of the cruelly martyred Miguel Serveto should be engraved on the most sacred tablet of the memory of every true physician, and held up to the devoted respect and admiration of every professed follower of Christ the healer of the sick, and of Luke the physician; and as an inspiring example to every devoted philanthropist and every true *philosopher*— who devotes his life and talents to the *pursuit of knowledge, for its own sake, alone!*

TYPHOID AND TYPHOID-LIKE INFECTIONS, TOGETHER WITH A METHOD FOR THE ISOLATION OF THE RESPECTIVE BACILLI.

BY

T. A. STARKEY, M. D. D. P. H. (London)
Montreal, P. Q.

Although using the customary term "Typhoid" in the above title, simply for the sake of preventing misunderstanding, it would be as well at the very outset to enter a plea for the substitution of the term "Enteric" as being more correct scientifically. "Enteric" is strictly applicable to those diseases caused by the *B. Entericus* and "Enteric-like" to those caused by the other members of the "colon-typhoid" group, variously named *paracolon, paratyphoid A*, and *paratyphoid* B, and the "Gartner Group."

To obviate confusion, I advocate the use of the following scheme, which not only does away with the groups arbitrarily named, but gives an approximately correct position in the scheme, by means of a number, to any organism of the well-known "colon-typhoid" group, at the same time furnishing most valuable information as to the probable clinical picture caused by such an organism. The scheme as first set forth in the *Journal of the Royal Sanitary Institute,* 1911, may be shown graphically (Fig. 1): The terms paracolon, Gartner, etc., are put in to show where these groups would fall into the above plan.

The bacteriological characteristics of the bacilli, their virulence, and the clinical picture caused by them, together with the duration of the disease, all gradually advance upon an ascending scale beginning almost at zero, at the colon end and reaching the maximum at the typhoid end.

I maintain that endless varieties exist between the two extremes of the scale from 0-10, but for practical purposes it is quite sufficient to give to an organism its ap-

nently necessary. It is at this juncture however, that a tremendous difficulty crops up under the old terminology. Any disease not closely simulating true enteric fever could hardly be notified as such, and as we know that the bacilli about the middle of this big "colon-typhoid" group cause a disease only slightly resembling true enteric, such cases are rarely if ever reported to the authorities, and no steps are taken to safeguard the public.

During the last few years I have met with quite a number of the milder infections, and the fact that various terms have been used by practitioners to designate them, e. g., intestinal grippe, dysentery, gastro-enteritis, etc., has been most interesting.

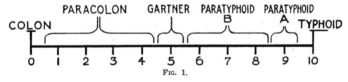

FIG. 1.

proximate position; for instance, it would not matter seriously if an organism whose true position lay between 6 and 7 were designated by either number; an approximation is all that is really requisite.

Again, as all these enteric-like diseases are just as infectious as true enteric fever, although less fatal it is true, still notification of their occurrence is equally important from the public health aspect, if we ever hope to combat their spread and so stamp them out.

I have within recent years repeatedly called attention to these diseases which generally occur on this continent in conjunction with true enteric fever. But occasionally any of them may have an epidemic "all to themselves" so to speak, and as the collected evidence goes to show that they are nearly always waterborne, their notification to the health authorities is therefore emi-

I recall one very remarkable instance of an outbreak in a fairly large town, which gave rise to about 200 cases, all mild in character. Some diarrhea and fever were noted at the commencement; but there were no spots, and recovery about the 10th or 12th day was the usual history of each case.

The authorities, much puzzled as to the actual nature of the outbreak, nevertheless suspected the water supply; and I was able to isolate an organism which would come in our scale somewhere about No. 7.

Further investigation showed that the drinking water reservoir was being slightly contaminated by seepage from a farm privy close by.

Under the new scheme of classification suggested such a situation would be handled vigorously, and in reporting such a case of enteric-like infection, the medical practitioner would simply enter up on the requisite notification form:

Enteric or enteric-like disease, Nos. 10 or 7, as the case might be. No. 10 would indicate a case of well marked enteric fever of the usual 21 days' duration, whereas No. 7 would signify a disease of about 10 or 12 days' duration. It is only right to point out at this stage that the isolation of these organisms of the colon-typhoid group can be easily accomplished by the method described in the *American Journal of Medical Sciences,* July, 1906.

Not only are the organisms easily isolated, but the method has the additional recommendation that the organisms can be graded from the colon end right along to the typhoid end of the scale.

Such results are not easily obtained by the ordinary enrichment methods wherein the search for the *colon bacillus* is the predominating feature. Surely we are in a stronger position, particularly with reference to the examination of water supplies, if we can ascertain the presence—or absence—of members of the colon-typhoid group of organisms, especially those towards the typhoid end, which undoubtedly are capable of causing disease of more virulent character in man. At the same time the method is equally useful to those workers who pin their faith upon the presence and numerical strength of our old friend, the colon bacillus.

After several years working with this method, I have personally found it sound practice to condemn a drinking water sample if I find any members of this colon-typhoid group from the middle to the typhoid end, quite regardless of the numerical strength of the colon bacillus.

The cultural characteristics and morphology of this colon-typhoid group are so well known that no difficulty ought to be experienced in definitely deciding whether or not a bacillus belongs to this group; this being so, the placing in the scheme is then quite a simple matter.

Several bacteriologists have suggested to me that other bacteria causing particular diseases are intimately associated with this group, e. g., bacteria causing some forms of food poisoning, etc. I quite fail to understand the difficulty; it is only befogging the issue unnecessarily; as I have said before, most workers can agree as to whether or not a particular bacillus is fairly comprised within the colon-typhoid group. If it is, allotment in the scale is easy; if it is not, keep it apart even though some of the clinical features of the disease produced may simulate in some respects those caused by the bacilli of the colon-typhoid group.

TRANSLATION.

LUMBAR PUNCTURE.
(Rachicentesis).

BY

P. RAVAUT, M. D.,

Translated from the French; with Notes and Additions

BY

O. L. MULOT, M. D.,
Brooklyn, N. Y.

When in 1890, Quincke proved that the subarachnoid space could easily be reached in the lumbar region, and with a simple needle some of the fluid withdrawn, practically without danger, no one, not even Quincke himself realized the vast extent to which medicine, diagnostically and therapeutically, had been enriched by this very simple operation. Every physician, be he surgeon, specialist or general practitioner should be ready at any moment to perform it.

Immediately after its announcement, this procedure was applied in the treatment and diagnosis of affections in the course of which, high tension of the spinal fluid seemed to play a part and in the various affections of the meninges, especially the tubercular form. Unfortunately, the results did not come up to expectations, and it came to be looked upon simply as a palliative measure for emergency use. Undoubtedly it would soon have sunken into oblivion, had not some few, working along different lines, proven its great value to the clinician. In 1900 as a result of the work of such men as Widal, Sicard and Ravaut, reports on the diagnostic value of examinations of the spinal fluid began to multiply and the various methods used in these examinations were made known. It was Sicard who first showed that this procedure could be utilized for the introduction into the subarachnoid space, of substances to produce, either anesthesia, or to act directly upon the nerve centres or the coverings, in disease. From the many reports of the revival of this operation, we learned many interesting phenomena important for us to know. Many of these facts, at first considered simply as curious, became the subject of further study and as a result of all this the indications for lumbar puncture gradually became clearly defined.

The withdrawal of several cc. of spinal fluid, may be followed by a variety of results; it may modify symptoms of cerebral or meningeal origin; it may act upon organs that are directly in communication with the spinal fluid, as the eye or the ear, or its action may be observed at some distance, probably through the action of the vasomotor system. Of this nature are the results from lumbar puncture observed upon the skin and upon blood pressure. The very complex therapeutic mechanism of lumbar puncture can often only be explained by the relation between arterial pressure and the pressure of the spinal fluid. Richet,[1] Franck,[2] and Cushing[3] have experimentally proven the relation between these two systems. In a very recent study, Parisot[4] has shown the parallelism between the two systems and insists upon the lowering of the arterial tension in certain cases as a result of the abstraction of cerebrospinal fluid by lumbar puncture.

These facts incited experimenters to study the question of tensive relations between the two systems with the hope of accurately determining a number of points; it is important to know how the one tension is effected, when the other is experimentally lowered or raised and the lapse of time necessary for the reestablishment of the equilibrium; to determine the role of the vasomotor system in transmitting to the arterial system, the variations in pressure in the cerebrospinal fluid.

Pagniez in a course of experiments which one of the authors outlined for him, failed to get precise and constant results, but just as in other questions where unstable results were obtained in experimentation, recourse must be had to the results of the clinic, and the sudden modifications observed in animals are entirely different, to the slow and progressive effects of disease in man. The only group of effects which can be of value are derived from certain conditions in the human clinic; these alone can be guiding. We cannot accept as valid for all clinical purposes, the observations recorded in cases of injuries to the skull, for here the symptoms of hypertension of the cerebrospinal fluid very promptly appear and are justly comparable to the conditions that can be produced in the animals in the laboratory. In such cases it is very easy to understand how the abstraction of a sufficient quantity of liquid will relieve the brain and spinal centres compressed by the excess of fluid and the operation bring about a rapid lessening of the phenomena of hyper-

Technic.

Instruments.— A trocar needle from 8-10 cm. (4½ to 5 inches) in length, but not over one millimeter in diameter, made of steel or iridio-platinum. In excitable, nervous and restless subjects, the platinum needle is to be preferred for while it will

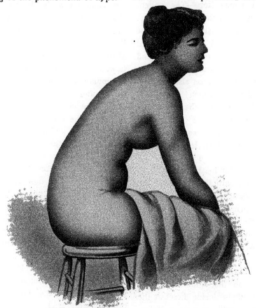

Fig. 1. Showing posture best adapted for lumbar puncture in adults. Curving the spinal column as indicated insures maximum spread of the lumbar interspaces.

tension. Still more typical is the behavior of the pia-mater to certain injections.

It would be interesting to group the results which are about to be described according to their pathogenic interpretations, but all cannot be so grouped and it therefore seems preferable to adopt a purely clinical classification.

bend and become useless, there is no danger of breaking and a broken fragment being left behind. The steel needle pierces better and can be replaced at a small cost; the platinum needle soon loses its edge and therefore an entrance may not be so easily effected with them, and in use these become bent and twisted. Whatever be the metal, the needle should have a stiletto; both ground to a bevel and provided with a pin and slot to maintain the bevels of the stiletto and the needle exactly alike.

It is well to collect the liquid in a gauged receptacle in order that the quantity withdrawn may be exactly known.

Technic of the operation.—The patient may either be lying on the side or sitting; but whatever be the position chosen, the spine must be well curved, for in the curved condition the muscles are on the stretch and anatomical landmarks stand out more prominently, and this position also enlarges the openings through which our needle must pass. We may enter the 3rd or 4th intervertebral space of the lumbar region or by the lumbo-sacral space which is just a little below a line, level with the crests of the ilii. With the fingers of the left hand, the operator locates the crest of the left ilium and with the thumb of the same hand he locates the spinous process directly at or just below this level and punctures a little below the middle of the space between this spinous process and the one next below. It goes without saying that the very strictest asepsis is to be observed. The operation may also be performed laterally to the landmarks given above. A jet of ethyl-chloride direct at the point of puncture will produce sufficient anesthesia. If the lateral entrance is chosen, we plunge our needle slightly upward and inward about a half an inch to the side of the median line and a little above the spinous process below that of our landmark. At a little more than two inches the needle will be felt to come upon the resistance of the laminary ligament, pushing through this the needle will be in desired cul-de-sac; by giving the stiletto a motion like the piston of a syringe we assist the flow of the liquid and it should now flow when the obdurator is entirely withdrawn. If the puncture is made in the median space the needle should be directed slightly upward but without any lateral deviation; the same resistance of the ligaments is felt but not as deeply as in the lateral operation. The lateral operation is most commonly practised because it gives a little more liberty. If on withdrawing the obdurator, blood, instead of cerebrospinal fluid should flow, this can often be overcome by slight manipulation; either withdrawing the needle a little and then forcing it a little deeper; but if then blood still flows, it is better to withdraw the needle entirely and make a new puncture. If the liquid does not flow, replace the stiletto to clear the tube of any material that may obstruct its lumen and rotate the needle on its axis, if then the fluid still does not flow, it is very evident that the needle is not in the cul-de-sac; *aspiration is entirely unnecessary and is dangerous,* for if the needle is properly within the cul-de-sac the fluid will flow of itself. The puncture completed and the fluid gathered in a graduated vessel, the needle should be withdrawn and with a quick motion and the skin at the sight of the puncture should be touched with tinct. of iodine. To avoid any possible bad after-effects, the patient should be kept in bed for 24 hours after the operation, and if there be any malaise, he should not be allowed to resume his usual mode of life until this has entirely disappeared; a small dose of opium may advantageously be administered after the operation.

(The bibliographic references, from 5 to 14 inclusive, are the principal works upon the general therapeutic value of lumbar puncture).

Traumatism of the Skull and Spine. Meningeal and Cerebral Hemorrhages. Meningeal Reactions After Injections. Aseptic Meningitis.

(A) Traumatisms of the skull and spine.— In the course of the various

fices to explain many of the symptoms. Further, the resorption of the extravasated blood can be the cause of certain other morbid phenomena, such as coma and delirium, for according to Tuffier, the blood is toxic to the bulb and gives rise to changes in pulse and temperature. It is this fact

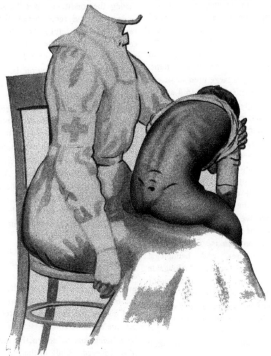

Fig. 2. Proper posture for lumbar puncture in children.

traumatisms to the skull and spine and particularly in fractures, the effusion of blood into the meningeal sac, is one of the chief determining causes of the clinical picture. The presence of blood and the various meningeal reactions which this incites, suf-

that enables us to interpret the good results of lumbar puncture reported by so many good observers who have recorded the notable amelioration of the clinical signs. Therefore in considering fractures of the skull, it is evident that puncture acts upon two different groups of symptoms; but is in the main upon the first group, those general signs of meningeal reactions that are benefitted by the abstraction of cerebrospinal fluid.

In most cranial traumatisms, headache, vomiting and frequently coma, are observed; these symptoms may vary in degree, from simple drowsiness to prolonged and absolute loss of consciousness; the vomiting may be very rebellious and difficult to control and the headache severe and tenacious. Upon all of these symptoms, puncture, verified by a large number of observations has a manifest and rapid action. Sometimes a single puncture suffices to greatly relieve, and even cause them entirely to disappear, but generally several abstractions are necessary, but progressive diminution of the evidences of hypertension accompanies each puncture.

The second group of clinical signs in traumatisms of the skull are nervous and are referable to the compression of the centres; thus we see developed the convulsive phenomena of Jacksonian epilepsy or the generalized convulsions; more or less extensive contractures, and hemiplegic paralyses are very frequent. Alongside with these we must range oculo-motor troubles, whether these involve only the external muscles of the eye, producing strabismus, or also involving the internal musculature structure and giving rise to mydriasis so commonly observed in skull injuries.

In the psychic troubles, as delirium and disturbances of the intellect and those other troubles the pathogenesis of which seems complex, as dyspnea, slowing of the pulse, be they attributed simply to compression or to bulbar intoxication, upon all of these accidents which are directly or indirectly due to the effusion, puncture has a happy influence. Therefore when in a case of fracture of the skull, evidences of hypertension occur, lumbar puncture should without hesitation be performed and it may replace the necessity of trephining which formerly was the only means at our command of relieving the condition. But it must be well understood and remembered, that if as a result of the fracture there be a flow of cerebrospinal fluid from the ears or the nose, puncture is not useful.

Another contraindication is, when as a result of the fracture, the sinuses at the base have been injured; for here the abstraction of fluid would have as an immediate result an outpouring of more blood into the subarachnoid space. It is difficult to fix the quantity of fluid to be evacuated, for this varies with the degree of hypertension and the quantity of effused blood. What is important though, is to repeat the evacuation frequently and in amounts of medium abundance, particularly if there be any reason to suspect that the hemorrhage has not completely ceased.

Fractures of the skull do not get well without leaving some sequellae. Poirier,[15] and then Rochard[16] insist upon the frequency of rebellious headache, persisting for months; these they have often relieved and cured by repeated punctures. Paralyses due either to compression of the centres by a hematoma or destructive changes, are also observed. Only in the former can any hope be entertained that puncture may have a good effect and then only when the hematoma is of recent formation. The importance of lumbar puncture in the treatment of fractures of the skull has been shown by the reports of Poirier, Rochard, Chevrier,[17] Quenu,[18] Potherat,[19] etc.

L. Tixier[20] who has especially studied the symptomatology resulting from long standing traumatisms of the skull, insists upon the role of the hypertension of the cerebrospinal fluid in the pathogenesis of the various sequellae and claims that repeated puncture is often very efficacious in their treatment. He reports Abadie's case, in which 7 years after the injury there appeared a very severe headache and attacks of Jacksonian epilepsy and there was a beginning papillary edema; a single puncture rapidly relieved the compressed centres and brought about a cure.

sion and irritation of the medulla. Paraplegias, troubles of sensibility and disturbances of the sphincters are seen in the course of these injuries and these symptoms reveal the presence of an intervertebral hematoma. To evacuate this, puncture should be systematically practised. Generally the results are as good as in fractures of the skull and a series of punctures usually brings about a cure. The first improvement is seen in the sensibility and the motor functions then undergo a change for the better. The medullary lesions that may be present are not influenced by punc-

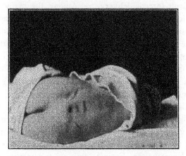

Fig. 3. Posture for lumbar puncture in children unable to sit upright.

He cites another personal observation, of a case where 5 years after the injury, the patient presented headaches and an amblyopia due to papillary stasis, in which a series of punctures resulted in a definite cure. But these are fortunate cases and from them Tixier does not conclude that puncture is always of absolute curative value, for he argues that it can only be of temporary avail against irritative lesions of the meninges.

In traumatisms of the spine, phenomena of a meningeal order are less generally evident; on the contrary the symptomatology is more that of signs of local compres-

ture. Kiliani,[21] Albertin[22/23] and Mauclaire[24] have reported cases that clearly demonstrate the advantages of puncture in these traumatisms.

(B) Meningeal and cerebral hemorrhages.— Side by side with fractures of the skull and spine can be placed certain meningeal hemorrhages, in which lumbar puncture acts in the same manner. A clear distinction must be made between the meningeal hemorrhages of the new born, and those occurring in the adult.

The former result from an external mechanical cause, a traumatism, and most frequently due to the application of the obstetric forceps. There is then an effusion; the abstraction of fluid relieves the compression of the centres and is followed by an abatement of the symptoms. These facts have been clearly established by the work of Dutreix [25] and Devraigne.[26/27] The latter reports a case in which the withdrawal of 5 cc. of blood from the spinal canal yielded a prompt relief of the symptoms with an immediate fall of temperature from 104 to normal. In other cases, the same author recommends that the operation be repeated from 2 to 4 times and he further advised that in cases after apparent death after difficult forceps delivery, the operation be performed to determine the presence or absence of meningeal hemorrhage as a cause of death.

In the adult on the other hand, meningeal hemorrhages indicate a diseased condition of the arterial system or an inflammatory process of the meninges. In these cases it is not simply a question of hypertension but of a complex lesion; puncture from a therapeutic point, not only gives but a transitory result, and sometimes not even this, but it may be dangerous. Nevertheless, Froin[28] recommends it on the ground, that besides its decompressing action upon the centres, it will drain from the high and dangerous zone of the brain the fluid loaded with dead blood cells, drawing this into the lower and more spacious region of the spine, where the irritating and toxic effects of this fluid are much less dangerous. We must not however, forget that in the adult we also encounter traumatic meningeal hemorrhages and in these puncture may be of as great utility as in the cases reported of the new born.

In the course of cerebral hemorrhages, particularly those in which there occurs a flooding of the ventricles, the results of puncture are ephemeral and give only a transitory diminution of the contractures. In summing up, we may say that in the adult, outside of traumatic meningeal hemorrhages for which the indications for this operation are very precise, lumbar puncture in hemorrhages of the cerebro-spinal system should be undertaken with extreme caution. We believe that in the early stages its use should be confined to the relief of deep coma and violent contractures and convulsive phenomena.

(C) Meningeal reactions to substances aseptically injected.— *Aseptic meningitis.*—Among the many things which throw a light upon the therapeutic value of lumbar puncture, those resulting from spinal anesthesia, are by no means the least interesting. In the first efforts in this direction, a 1% muriate of cocaine solution was used and these first attempts were regularly followed by severe headache, vomiting, elevation of temperature to 102 and even 104 and in some instances Kernig's sign was present; these symptoms usually persisted for several days and then subsided without leaving any traces. Ravout and Auberg[29] have shown that these symptoms were due to a violent irritation of the meninges and were accompanied by a leucocytosis sufficient to cause turbidity of the liquid with the presence of fibrin and sometimes blood. In collaboration with Giunard,[30] these authors proved that these results were due to the lack of isotonic harmony between the injected solutions and the cephalo-spinal fluid and that by modifying their technique and using solutions rendered isotonic by the addition of sodium chloride these symptoms were avoidable and this has become the general practise in spinal anesthesia.

But what is still more interesting is that in these aseptic meningitis resulting from the injection of cocaine in hypotonic solutions puncture and the evacuation of some of the fluid caused a rapid disappearance of the symptoms. The fluid spurted from the needle and the evacuation of 20 to 30 cc. (½ to 1 ounce) of fluid was necessary to reestablish the normal pressure. After

The importance of these facts cannot be overstated. They show the remarkable and rapid influence of lumbar puncture upon the headache, vomiting, pyrexia, and even Kernig's sign by which irritation of the pia-mater betrays itself. The results can favorably compare with those obtained by punc-

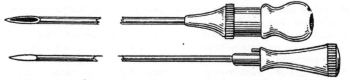

Fig. 4. Trocar for lumbar puncture, natural size, length approximately 5 inches.

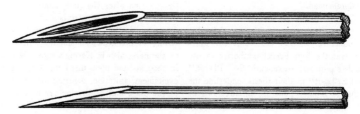

Fig. 5. Enlargement of needle and obturator points to show necessity of fitting accurately.

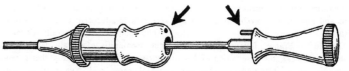

Fig. 6. Trocar enlarged showing device for insuring parallel bevels of obturator and needle.

such an evacuation the headache disappeared almost instantaneously, often diminishing during the outflow of the liquid, the temperature became normal within a few hours, the vomiting ceased and the marked agitation that was present gave way to calm.

ture in meningeal hemorrhages due to traumatism.

Widal[31'32] has isolated a group of cases of acute meningitis in which while the liquid has a purulent aspect, the cellular elements are intact, but there are no microorganisms present; in other words aseptic.

In these, without any specific treatment, other than repeated lumbar puncture, a cure always was obtained and all the symptoms disappeared when the fluid returned to its normal state.

Meningitis and Reactions of the Meninges.

In the preceding we have studied the facts revealing an irritation of the meninges and those of hypertension, two conditions commonly occurring together. In those conditions the therapeutic mechanism of lumbar puncture was easy to understand. Now we proceed to a series of affections, revealed by signs of a much more complex pathogenesis and in which the mode of action of this operation is not nearly so easily comprehended.

(A) Acute meningitis.—It is especially in cases of acute meningitis that the value of puncture has been best observed. Marfan was the first French authority to use lumbar puncture therapeutically. Blavot,[33] and Pellagot[34] in their thesis, underline the value to lumbar puncture in affections of the meninges. Numerous other authors have published observations of the same nature and Netter[35] in a series of communications strongly insists upon the efficacy of puncture in the treatment of acute meningitis and especially in cerebrospinal meningitis.

Outside of France, following the first works of Quincke, the observation of Lenhartz, Neurath, Tobler and several others, all speak favorably of its action in meningeal conditions. In all the literature cited, emphasis is laid upon the indications for puncture in cerebrospinal meningitis and the same is true in all the acute forms.

There should be no need to insist upon the absolute necessity of lumbar puncture in every case in which there is even only a slight reason to suspect a meningitis, not only for diagnostic but for therapeutic purposes as well. All the authors who have published their experiences with this operation in acute meningeal conditions, are agreed that these results are due to two things: 1st, the relief of compression of the centres; and 2nd, the drainage of the toxic and infectious elements in the cerebrospinal fluid. The first puncture therefore should be as abundant an evacuation as possible and the more purulent the fluid more abundant should be the amount withdrawn. The German authors report cases from which they evacuated 60 and 80 cc. at a single operation. It would seem more prudent to be content with smaller quantities. Often after the first diagnostic and therapeutic puncture there is a decided improvement in the clinical signs; such as lessening of the headache and the stiffening of the neck, also in Kernig's sign. Netter in 1899 insisted upon this latter fact. The excitement, agitation, delirium, irregularity of the pulse and respiration are influenced for the better; sometimes even the stupidity and the coma may be lessened but the effect upon these is less marked than upon the other signs. The symptom of inhibition is probably of a toxic order and is usually seen only in advanced stages of the disease.

The temperature, generally elevated in acute meningitis, often falls decidedly after puncture. Canuet[36] in his thesis reports several cases and lays particular stress upon one case in which the fall of temperature was not followed by any subsequent rise. Tarrade cites an analogous case but he believes that this is not the rule and that the lowering of the temperature is temporary and necessitates the repetition of the operation. We observed the same thing in a patient suffering from cerebrospinal meningitis; the temperature fell 2 or 3 degrees centigrade after each puncture. In certain cases the puncture has a marked influence upon the backache and the articular pains. In very young children, meningitis is often attended by convulsions and distension of the fontanelles and Netter and Debre[38] have lately shown that puncture very favorably influences these symptoms. Enough has been shown of the advantages which may accrue from this operation in meningitis, but the good results are rarely derived from one single puncture. Upon this fact, Mackenzie, Bokay,[39] Biltay, Rayboud. Blavot, Pellagot, Babinski[40] and more recently still Netter, Hudelo, Merle and Comby[41] insist and all conclude that the operation should be repeated whenever the agitation or the headache reappear or the respiratory troubles and the temperature increase.

These authors recommend that it be repeated every three or four days and until the fluid becomes absolutely limpid. Armand Delille reports the case of a child cured of cerebrospinal meningitis in which 400 cc. were withdrawn in a series of daily punctures. In the present state of our science the treatment of cerebrospinal meningitis does no longer consist in hot baths and lumbar punctures, but to these has been associated the injection of antimeningococcic serum. Each injection should as far as possible be preceded by an evacuation of the purulent fluid and as a rule the amount withdrawn should exceed by several cc. quantity of serum to be injected. During the first three or four days of the disease each puncture should be followed by a serum injection; after that the puncture should be repeated when the symptoms demand it and for the purpose of ascertaining the condition of the fluid which should be examined

as to its cytological and bacteriological contents. If purulence persists, an evacuation followed by a serum injection is to be practised. Sometimes the extreme purulency of the liquid makes it difficult to withdraw enough of the fluid to make room for the injection of serum, but the latter should nevertheless then be injected without hesitation, a fact upon which Comby strongly insists.

Lumbar puncture should be performed only during the active and acute stages of meningitis, that is to say while the symptoms are at their height, but also during the period of decline for these cases often present for a long period, sometimes for months, a series of minor symptoms such as inequality of the pupils, Argyll-Robertson pupil, headache, amblyopia, exaggeration of the reflexes, apathy and pulse disturbances and upon all of these symptoms puncture acts efficiently and in these cases it will be found that the cerebrospinal fluid still presents a lymphocytosis. Widal and Philibert[42] report such cases and in them they practised puncture over a period of several months before these clinical signs entirely disappeared and a cure does not occur until the fluid has become normal.

The effect of puncture upon the complications and sequellae of meningitis are dependent upon the nature of these; only those which are directly or indirectly due to intercranial hypertension are affected. This is the case in hydrocephalus following acute infections of the meninges but this will be discussed further on: When papillary stasis and labyrinthic troubles are due to hypertension and pressure, benefits from puncture may be expected, but nothing should be expected from it except the paralyses. The good effects which we have shown to follow puncture in acute meningitis may also be expected in other varieties, but we wish to insist upon the value of this operation in the acute meningitis which sometimes occurs in the second stage of syphilis and the meningeal reactions which may occur in hereditary syphilis; of these we will speak in detail under their own heading.

(B) Tuberculous meningitis.— Despite the gravity of their aspect, the acute meningites have not the grave prognosis of the tubercular variety, for here we have no therapeutic procedure to check the cause and all are agreed upon the inefficacy of puncture except as a palliative means. For the time being it will give some relief from the headache, delirium, somnolence, convulsions and contractures, in children, and the fontanelles are relieved from their distension, the pulse takes a more normal character, but all the symptoms very soon return for the relief is only transitory. Marfan[46] who was the first to systematically try puncture in this form of meningitis, credits it with only very small therapeutic value and his opinion is shared by many others. Nevertheless, Schlesinger[47] advises its use even if only to lessen the distressing picture.[1]

(C) Serous meningitis and pyrexial meningeal reactions.—This is not the place to discuss the nature of that clinical entity to which Dupre has given the name of meningism and which Hutinel calls serous meningitis; these are undoubtedly always infectious, but often of a mild clin-

ical aspect. While the fluid rarely contains definite cytological elements, it is often albuminous and excessive in amount, thus producing hypertension, nevertheless pathological elements have been found. These meningeal reactions are frequent complications in the course of pyrexial diseases, but in no other disease are they so common or pronounced as in the pneumonias, especially broncho-pneumonia in children or alcoholics. In these it may give rise to a very definite meningitic syndrome, with Kernig's sign, convulsions, delirium and headache. Under such conditions puncture becomes imperative, not alone therapeutically, but a knowledge of the state of the cerebrospinal fluid is indispensable, for there may be an invasion of the meninges by the pneumococcus. The therapeutic results generally are good; it may be a case of infection of the meninges, but if the liquid is limpid and devoid of cellular elements, just albuminous and in excess we are able to diagnosticate a serous meningitis and puncture calms the symptoms to which this state has given rise. The same train of symptoms may be observed in certain cases of whooping cough and Dopter[45] in an article with a wealth of references describes the condition as occurring in mumps and fully describes the microscopical and bacteriological picture of the cerebrospinal fluid. In many instances it is relieved by a single puncture.

In the course of gastrointestinal disturbance in children, a train of meningeal symptoms is often observed and sometimes true meningitis is present as a complication and the clinical indications are for puncture. Quincke and Carl Beck have described cases in which these serous meningitis have merged into acute hydrocephalus, with distended fontanelles and later there occurred enlargement of the head; against this punc-

---

[1] In the light of the progress that has been made in the preparation of tuberculous sera, there is some reason to hope that the withdrawal of fluid, followed by a spinal or intra-ventricular injection of a serum, may give this operation more therapeutic value in the future in the treatment of tuberculous meningitis. The technique of intra-ventricular puncture will be discussed further on. (Note of American Editor).

ture should prove an effective procedure of prevention.

In all pyrexial diseases regardless of their etiology, meningeal and nervous symptoms may appear and Rocaz and Firmin Carlos[48] record their disappearance after puncture. These symptoms have been especially noticed in typhoid fever in children and in the adult the same symptoms may render a puncture advisable to positively eliminate meningitis or to reveal its presence as a complication; in all events puncture has a beneficent influence on the symptoms. Neurath has observed the benefits of puncture upon the meningeal conditions accompanying grave scarlatina. Tarrade reports a number of cases of acute rheumatism with cerebral symptoms which were relieved by repeated punctures and L. Tixier has treated the same cerebral symptomatology, with good results in the same manner. More recently Comby[49] has attributed the nervous phenomena observed in the course of many pyrexial conditions, as seen in pneumonia and in whooping cough, not to meningeal reactions but to irritation of the brain proper and bases his opinion upon normal condition often found in the fluid withdrawn in these cases and the sequellae of cerebral sclerosis, idiocy, epilepsy and spasmodic hemiplegia. But these are the cases in which puncture is not followed by a relief of the symptoms and there is no hypertension of the fluid. Whenever the latter is present, puncture is of avail. This is a wide field and most clearly shows how important it is that every physician should be prepared at any moment to perform this simple operation.

(D) Insolation.—The nervous symptoms of sunstroke must be considered to be of meningeal origin. Dopter[50] who has studied the cytology of the spinal fluid came to the conclusion that in the mild cases there is simply a hypertension, but in grave cases there is blood, albumen with, at first, a polynuclear leucocytosis which later on changes into lymphocytosis, which persists. The headache and somnolence which sometimes amounts to coma, and the convulsions which are at times observed in cases of sunstroke are indications for puncture and upon which it frequently has a favorable action; De Massary and Liau.[51] Good results have been reported by many observers; the condition is probably very much of the nature of an aseptic meningitis, of which we have previously spoken; Dufour.[52]

In summing up our study of lumbar puncture in the course of meningeal conditions in the widest and broadest sense, it shows this procedure to be of the utmost importance to the diagnosis and it is to be a therapeutic measure which in certain forms suffices in itself to bring about a cure and in other forms an adjuvant of the very highest kind, while even in the incurable tubercular form it is a means of alleviating the sufferings of the patient.

(To be continued).

CORRESPONDENCE.

THE FIFTEENTH INTERNATIONAL CONGRESS ON HYGIENE AND DEMOGRAPHY.

BY

OUR SPECIAL CORRESPONDENT.

The Fifteenth International Congress on Hygiene and Demography, held at Washington, D. C., from September 23d to 28th, while emphatically a success, was perhaps chiefly remarkable for the extraordinary interest it aroused in the lay press throughout this country. Besides the medical publications represented at the daily sessions of the Congress, all the greater newspapers of our larger cities also despatched their representatives to get at first hand the pith of the papers read by the most famous scientists ever assembled from thirty-two foreign countries and from each of the forty-eight States of the Union.

As such it was fairly a Representative World's Congress. Some idea of the magnitude of the ground covered will be had when we state that upwards of 240 papers exhaustively showing the startling progress made by modern hygienic research, were read at this mammoth conference.

The subjects treated were divided into nine sections, as follows:

Section I.—Hygienic Microbiology and Parasitology.

Section II.—Dietetic Hygiene; Hygiene Physiology.

Section III.—Hygiene of Infancy and Childhood. School Hygiene.

Section IV.—Hygiene of Occupations.

Section V.—Control of Infectious Diseases.

Section VI.—State and Municipal Hygiene.

Section VII—Hygiene of Traffic and Transportation.

Section VIII.—Military, Naval and Tropical (Colonial) Hygiene.

Section IX.—Demography.

Under Section I, six papers were read by men long pre-eminent in bacteriology, and two by Dr. Anna W. Williams, of the Research Laboratory, Department of Health, New York City. The one on Salmonellosis (Paratyphic Bacillus B, Bacillus of Food Poisoning, etc.), by E. Sacquépée, was of especial interest to the profession generally.

Under Section II, the harmfulness of some, and the harmlessness of various substances used in the preservation of foods; the influence of the ingestion of food upon metabolism; nutrition and bone growth; the role of proteins in growth; the roles which common salt and water assume in nutrition; the choice of foods in disease; diet and metabolism in fever, etc., were all brilliantly discussed.

Section III brought out thirty-four separate papers, comprising briefly: Hygiene of the teacher, of the pupils, and of the school-room; breathing exercises and open-air instructions in schools and colleges; transmission of disease by books; syphilis and gonorrhea in children from direct infection; disinfection of schools; the relation of physical inability and mental deficiency to the body social; protection of children against tuberculosis; the relation of the employment of mothers to infant mortality; prevention of mental disease; and dental hygiene, and the necessity of care of the teeth.

Under Section IV, the fatigue effects of temperature and humidity, the fatigue factors in certain occupations, the deleterious effects of unnecessary noise, and the various occupation neuroses, were all thoroughly gone into. Also, under this head were discussed: Caisson disease, prophylaxis of labor in compressed air; the effects of exposure to intense heat on the working organism, and accidents and diseases of miners, and of tunnel and iron workers. Next, the injuries caused by electricity were enumerated, and ways to avoid them indicated.

The Effects of Industrial Strain upon the Health of Working Women, and Infant Mortality in Relation to Factory Labor, were titles of two extremely interesting papers. In the latter paper the startling conclusion was reached, through actual statistics, that "the infantile mortality among the class of working mothers exceeded that of the domestic class by 43 per cent."

Finally, means to prevent many of the occupational diseases, including mercurial, lead and other poisonings peculiar to special occupations, were pointed out.

The Attitude Sanitary Authorities Should Adopt toward Bacillus Carriers, and The Relative Importance of Aerial and Contact Infection, were the first two papers read under Section V. Antityphoid vaccination, community immunization against typhoid, small-pox vaccination, and the dangers from flies, mosquitoes, fleas, vermin and domestic animals as germ carriers, were discussed also under this head.

Under Section VI, papers were read on: The purification of water, the best disposal of city refuse, rural hygiene, the prevention of inebriety, ventilation, proper handling of perishable food in transportation, sanitary control of local milk supplies, and practical eugenics.

Sanitation of Street Cars, by Mr. J. C. Halleck, was the first paper under Section VII; and this was followed by remarks on the ventilation of sleeping cars; food, water and ice supplies in railway stations and on railway trains; the disposal of sewage into tidal waters; and problems of immigration from a hygienic standpoint.

A large part of Section VIII was devoted to the prophylaxis of venereal diseases in the army and navy. Other subjects treated under this head were: First, treatment of wounded in sea battles; some sanitary problems on hospital ships; influence of high temperature in the stokeholds of ships in the tropics; restriction of malaria; dissemination and prevention of yellow fever; prophylaxis of sleeping sickness; hygiene in the field and methods of disinfection; and vitiation of air in submarines.

Under Section IX were comprised: The present status of infant mortality, and possibilities of the world-wide effort to diminish it; statistical comparison of the mortality of breast-fed and of bottle-fed infants; infant mortality in the City of New York; statistics of divorces and marriages; criminal statistics; eugenics and demography; workingmen's insurance; and the role of women in industrial life.

Afterward, under joint session of Sections I and V, a paper was read by Dr. Netter, a French physician, on the Etiology of Poliomyelitis, and Prophylactic Remedies. Then, under joint session of Sections I and VIII, hookworm disease was viewed from all angles in several papers.

The Demography of Industries and Professions, by M. Lucien March, was read under joint session of Sections IV and IX; and under the same session, Dr. Jacques Bertillon discussed the relation existing between phthisis and alcoholism.

The Municipal Control of Plague, by Surgeon-General Rupert Blue, was a timely and interesting paper, under joint session of Sections V and VII. Other topics under this joint session were: The Relation between Traffic and the Spread of Bubonic Plague; the Prevention of the Spread of Cholera over Maritime Transportation Routes; the Supervision of the

Migration of Tuberculous Patients; and the Intercarriage of Typhoid Infection between Urban and Rural Communities.

Throughout the Congress, the prevention of disease, as was to have been expected, was the key note. Physicians have long realized that few organic diseases can be cured absolutely; weaknesses often remain, complications ensue, and usually some permanent disability follows. Therefore, to prevent disease, and reduce as far as possible all contributing or predisposing factors very properly constitute to-day a large part of the modern physician's duties.

The large audience of eminent men and women at the Congress evinced great interest in all papers pertaining to the problem of the child, such as the education of physically and mentally deficient children, the hygiene of infancy and childhood, and the prevention of infant mortality. Again, papers were closely followed which discussed the bearing of the employment of mothers on the infant death rate.

Relegated to a dark past is the theory that children are born "cussed." We believe now that their upbringing and the influences of their environment generally make them bad, (when they are so) rather than that their ancestors are solely responsible. Nearly all children are naturally good, and they remain good until evil influences corrupt them. Hence, when we solve the problem (if, indeed, we ever do) of preventing these evil impressions, then, and not till then, will the child develop into the good citizen which we all wish him to be.

But, to return to our subject, Dr. Henry P. Walcott, of Massachusetts, President of the Congress, opened the meeting by presenting William Howard Taft, President of our United States, who made an eloquent and forceful address, in which he suggested, to the delight of the American delegates, that the splendid Public Health Service be taken as a nucleus for a New National Health Department.

On the whole, we feel justified in saying that America can well feel proud of the showing she made at this Fifteenth—but, in this country, First—International Congress of Hygienists; for, although more than two hundred of the most eminent scientists of Germany alone were present at this meeting, American physicians proved themselves to be well in the van of the triumphant march of progressive medicine, at least in so far as hygiene and preventive measures against disease are concerned.

THE ANNOTATOR.

A Common Abuse in the Practice of Gynecology.[1]— W. A. Wade considers that curettage is performed with unnecessary frequency. He believes it has been amply demonstrated that the uterus cannot be curetted thoroughly, and that a pathologist can only rarely find in the scrapings a difference between normal and inflamed endometrium. In view of the changes which take place in the endometrium in connection with the menstrual cycle it is easy to understand that normal changes in the mucosa have frequently been mistaken for hypertrophic and interstitial endometritis.

Curettage when the uterus is actually inflamed is dangerous to life.

In chronic endometritis hysterotomy, followed by excision of the diseased glands with a small sharp curette, is proper practice. Erosions of the cervix are best treated by the actual cautery or by amputation of the cervix.

Curettage prior to plastic operations on the cervix and perineum is wrong, both in theory and practice.

The curette should not be used for the delivery of portions of placenta or fetus in post partum and post abortum cases, rather should one use the gloved finger, a sponge holder, or placental forceps, and this should be followed by the light packing of the uterine cavity with gauze moistened with tincture of iodine diluted one-half. Curettage is not indicated for such conditions as congestion of the endometrium resulting from ovarian activity.

The curette is of assistance in making a diagnosis as to malignant disease of the uterus, but as a therapeutic agent it has little value.

Probably few gynecologists of experience will agree with the opinion which has been thus expressed.

Undoubtedly the curette has been shamefully abused and many crimes have been committed with it, but in the hands of one who is skillful and experienced there is no instrument in the gynecologist's armamentarium which could be less readily dispensed with. It is well to sound a note of warning, certainly, to the unskillful and the injudicious who have done much damage by their rashness. The unfortunate teaching that curettage is a simple operation which anybody can do, has led many ignorant and unskillful physicians to attempt it, often to the undoing of their patients.

The Bacteria of Digestion and Intestinal Antiseptics.[1]— An editorial states that changes produced by environment have much to do with the bacterial factor in normal and abnormal digestive processes.

Bacteria abound in the soil and greatly influence its fertility, and they are fed to domestic animals.

On the other hand, Arctic animals digest their food without their presence.

Certain bacteria are advantageous to man under proper conditions.

The upper portion of the digestive tract does not depend upon bacterial action in the digestive processes, but rather upon chemical and ferment action.

In the lower intestinal tract bacteria assist digestion. Colon bacilli may prevent undue development of more harmful bacteria. This goes to show that we should not strive to make the bowel sterile but rather to modify bacterial action.

Cellulose can be split up by certain bacteria, but cannot be acted upon by sterile digestive juices. We should therefore conserve the processes of nature before we depend upon drugs to limit the number of bacteria in the gastro-intestinal tract.

We should maintain peristalsis with as little use of irritating antiseptics as possible. We should limit the prolification of bacteria in the mouth and nasal passages and prevent the use of food which is bacterially contaminated.

Dietetic care will do more than drugs, and antiseptics seldom accomplish much when the trouble is primarily with the

---

[1] *International Journal of Surgery*, May, 1912.

[1] *The Medical Council*, June, 1912.

stomach. In the intestines antiseptics may be useful the same as is true of cholagogues. Bismuth, salol, calomel and betanaphthol are regarded as the best intestinal antiseptics, but they must not be used to the point of producing intestinal irritation.

It is desirable to have a few drugs to call upon for antiseptic treatment of the intestines, and if we remember these four and forget all the others we will be equipped for most requirements.

The Vaccine Treatment of Typhoid.[1]—

W. Engelbach gives an analysis of sixty different scientific papers representing the entire recent literature of this subject. He speaks of the rapid advances which have been made during the past two years in immunization which teaches unerringly that it will be only a short time before this treatment will be accepted for active typhoid.

Prophylactic treatment of typhoid by vaccination and the treatment of chronic local lesions in typhoid carriers and contact-carriers by vaccines is now well established.

Investigations as to the conditions in the last mentioned individuals prove that specific immune bodies can be created by vaccine treatment, hence the only requirement for the treatment of active typhoid is an abundant production of antibodies early in the history of the disease.

This necessitates improvement in the preparation, dosage and administration of vaccine. The methods of treatment in the United States army are given in some detail and the conclusion is advanced by the surgeon-general that the protection against typhoid will compare favorably with that against small-pox.

Home Hospitals for the Tuberculous.[1]—

An editorial questions the optimism which looks for the wiping out of tuberculosis. It is plain that only the upheaval of our present social system will eliminate the economic and social causes which are as efficient factors in the development of the disease as is the bacillus.

As long as the tuberculous roam about freely, distributing the bacilli, there will be tuberculosis. As long as invalids with the disease are without proper care and nursing, infections within the family will continue.

Hospital facilities for all grades of the disease are still inadequate.

The New York Association for the Improvement of the Condition of the Poor is attempting to improve matters by transporting entire families to tenement houses which may be regarded as home hospitals. There they will receive medical care, nursing, proper food, fresh air and sunshine and other necessities.

This is certainly fine if it can be carried out. Patients will not be allowed to work except by permission of their physician and the family will be under supervision until the wage-earner is restored to health and the family is made self-supporting again. The children will be educated in open-air schools.

This is all in accord with modern sanitation and hygiene.

An attack is thus made not only upon the diseased individuals, but upon the conditions which brought about the disease.

Teaching Hygiene for a Better Parenthood.[1]—

T. D. Wood thinks that the teaching of hygiene is of supreme importance with reference to parenthood.

The affectional basis of marriage should be preserved, but the sentimental and emotional elements should be supported and guided by appreciation of all the factors necessary for parenthood. If human beings subordinated their interests to the welfare of future generations as perfectly as do the animals which are controlled only by instinct there would be a more enduring type of family life and a more perfect type of parent-craft.

This can be accomplished by the development of controlling ideals, supported by reason and intelligence, and also by ethical impulse and religious motive.

Teaching hygiene will contribute to better parenthood when broad and comprehensive, taking into consideration the

[1] The Inter-State Medical Journal, June, 1912.
[2] Medical Review of Reviews, June, 1912.

[1] New York Medical Journal, June 29.

psychic social and moral, as well as the physical nature of the young.

Appropriate education relating to reproduction and parenthood is necessary in the development of every young person.

The parent is the child's logical teacher of sex and parenthood.

Class-room instruction in sexual matters is not yet feasible in the public schools, the public not being educated up to it, and the teachers lacking the intelligence, wisdom and tact to teach it successfully.

Such instruction should be given in universities, colleges, normal and private schools. The basis of successful teaching of sexual matters is companionship and confidence between parent and child. .

More important than the knowledge of sex hygiene are the motives which should control thought and action.

Important, indeed, is it that the parent should communicate knowledge of sex matters to the child, but if the parent is ignorant or lacking in tact how is it possible for him to do so?

It should be a part of the education to have the imparting of such information in view.

Typhoid Vaccination and the Widal Reaction.[1]—A. Maverick remarks that it is important for a physician to know whether his patients who have been vaccinated for typhoid have been rendered immune or not, inasmuch as vaccine which has been kept too long, or a faulty thermostat in the manufacturer's laboratory may render the vaccine valueless. The results of vaccination being found in the blood no opinion can be formed from the local and general symptoms of the patient after inoculation.

There is usually no general reaction, but the skin in the area of vaccination may appear normal, but the bactericidal elements of the serum are increased.

The Widal reaction is the blood test used, the agglutinins being equally abundant whether the vaccine has been given subcutaneously, within the muscles, or by high intestinal injection.

It is noticeable in five to ten days after the first dose, grows stronger with the

[1] *New York Medical Journal*, June 15, 1912.

second and third, and is strongest in ten to thirty days after the last inoculation. The reaction may persist one or two years; if it is persistently absent or weak it signifies a bad prognosis.

An absent or weak Widal reaction after typhoid vaccination suggests slight resistance to typhoid infection, and a very severe attack should infection occur. Those who have had typhoid fever usually show pronounced symptoms after vaccination. This seems paradoxical as an attack of typhoid usually confers life immunity against re-infection.

The Importance of Physical Health in Childhood.—Physical efficiency, says A. E. Schelin, in a recent issue of *Life and Health,* is the foundation of all efficiency. In order to be a strong race, we must give more attention to physical development. A man's physical health is like the foundation of a house. The better the foundation, the more can be built upon it. If it is weak, its burden will crush it, and all will go down together. .

If children were thoroughly taught the value of physical development, their capacity for intellectual development would be far greater. Many children grow up with the impression that they can endure almost anything, and as a consequence they tax their physical organs in many foolish ways. When a wagon is new, it will stand much rough usage without breaking down; but the effects of this rough usage will show as it gets older. If children could comprehend this; if they could be made to know that every wrong use of the body, every careless indulgence, every excess, is that much in preparation for an early breakdown; if they could understand that later efficiency depends on the economy of their powers in youth, they would be more careful not to misuse them.

The child should be made to realize that without good health one can not make the best use of an education. In fact, no one can consider himself truly educated who does not understand what is necessary for the proper care of his body and the development of all his powers.

If at school and at home our children were taught the value of hygiene; if, in addition to these theoretical lessons, cleanliness and personal hygiene, mastication, deep breathing, and physical exercise were encouraged, rewarded, and if necessary enforced, we should soon have a nation of healthy—and therefore happy and efficient —people.

Advocates of moral reforms will make the greatest advancement when they begin by teaching the importance of physical reform. When we have more walking and less car-riding, more careful mastication and less gluttony, more natural living and less following of fads and fashions, we shall have an excellent foundation on which to build up great moral reforms.

And the place to begin such reforms is with the children. Those who have fixed habits of life do not often change, much as they may appreciate the desirability of change. The time to work a reformation in habits is in the plastic period of childhood, when the mind and the habits, like the bones, may be molded into almost any shape.

There is much agitation for a national department of health. Such a department will be of great value in many ways; but meantime every family should establish its family department of health. So far as the home and the well-being of its inmates are concerned, such a department will be of far greater value than a national department.

In establishing such a department it will be necessary to make use of reliable health books and health magazines. Also the services of the family physician, as personal adviser and counsellor in health, will be invaluable. Remember that the early health habits formed by the children, and the lessons learned by them regarding the care of the body, will be of incalculable value throughout life.

The Training of the Nervous Child.— In his admirable address on the Care of the Nervous Child, Dr. Barker, according to *Life and Health,* states that, above all, it is important to overcome the tendency to give way to emotions. Children should early be given to understand that they must control themselves before they can get what they want. The child must learn that it is more apt to get what it seeks if it controls itself than if it gives way to an emotional outbreak. Beginning later in life, it will be found almost impossible to control this emotional instability.

Vacillation is another characteristic which must receive especial attention in childhood. Parents should see that the child finds in them no example of this failing. While a few children of the "hair-trigger" type need to be taught deliberation in making decisions, most children should be encouraged to make a decision and stick to it.

Another matter parents must guard is the criticism of neighbors. Such criticism favors a malevolent spirit, which has a most pernicious effect on the nervous system.

But the child should not be protected from everything which might stir his emotions. He needs such experiences in order to learn self-control. While a hot temper is bad for the child, it is less damaging than a habit of holding a grudge, which grows by degrees into the persecutory ideas of the paranoid state.

But at best sudden outbursts of emotion or passion, if frequently repeated, are very deleterious to the nervous system. The attempt to avoid or overcome these attacks either by petting or by punishing is not apt to end well. As a rule, it is best to ignore the attacks, and, as far as possible, forestall them. To older children one can explain the lack of dignity and senselessness of giving way to anger. Such lessons given during the seasons of calm will often have the desired effect.

A mistake often made by parents, and oftener by nurses, that of frightening children with stories of the bogy man, the policeman, etc., is apt to set up nervous disturbances which last through life. One must learn how to deal with the fear of being alone, the fear of the dark, and the fear of thunder and lightning. Certain of these fears are easily overcome, especially by an example of courage on the part of older persons.

Sometimes fear is a symptom of disease, and the child should be examined by a physician. Night terrors, for instance, may indicate the presence of adenoids.

But we must not think that a lack of feeling is desirable, or that it protects against disease. We should not forget that the emotions have very much to do with the child's future nervous make-up. The elevating emotions are constructive, helping to build up a strong nervous system; the depressing emotions, if long continued are damaging, and have the opposite effect.

The child should be given the highest development possible, but always at a suitable age. It is a mistake to give children experiences at an age when they can not be appreciated. "The child's childishness is its greatest asset."

One of the greatest pleasures and the best protection is the joy of work, but avoid overwork. The best tonic is enjoyable work. The country is a more favorable place in which to rear nervous children than is the city.

Nervous children should not be sent to school too early, and should not be pushed ahead too fast. Competition is dangerous to the nervous child. Sleeplessness is a danger-signal. In children it is often due to indigestion, mental overstrain, or premature sexual excitation. If it persists a physician should be consulted.

Outdoor Life for City Children.[1]—
For the first five or ten years of a child's life he should do little else but play, says Dr. Walter Lester Carr in the *Archives of Pediatrics*, if we are to insure for him the best physical and mental development. Some of this play may be directed by competent nurses and teachers, but the best of all play is spontaneous in character, with constant change of action. Barrie, the novelist, recognizes this desire for change that is part of the physical and mental development of child life.

A walk on Fifth Avenue or in Central Park with the restrictions of police regulations cannot make up, in any way, except for an opportunity to be in the open air, for the free use of the muscles such as is enjoyed by children who can play out-of-doors regardless of police, nurses and clothes.

[1] *Archives of Pediatrics*, June, 1912.

One of the greatest difficulties with which a teacher has to deal in the management of young pupils is the desire for change and the natural predisposition to physical activity which always accompanies childhood and youth. Lane emphasizes this succinctly as follows:

"For the so-called normal condition of the skeleton it is necessary that during growing life the individual shall combine attitudes of activity with attitudes of rest, and that the attitudes of activity as well as those of rest shall be varied in character."

The school hours of children in kindergarten and primary classes should not exceed two hours for the former and three for the latter. Such classes can be held in open air schoolrooms and on roofs with beneficial results to the children, both from the standpoint of increased vitality as well as from a lessened danger from contagion. The stimulating influence of open air classes for children who are below the average but who are not tuberculous is shown in "Reports of Defective Children." These children gained in weight during the school year, although they showed an almost entire absence of gain during the summer months, probably due to home conditions. Their appetites improved during the school session, the hemoglobin was increased and there was also an improved mental condition as well as a gain in bodily tone and vigor.

ETIOLOGY AND DIAGNOSIS.

A New Method of Kidney Palpation.[1]—
Zerlaut says that the method taught him by Dr. Gaubeau and to which he attaches Gaubeau's name as the originator gives far better results than the method of Guyon, or that of Glenard both of which are practised in the dorsal decubitus. He further claims for it better results than can be obtained in the lateral or in the sitting positions. He describes it as follows:—For the examination of the right kidney, the physician stands on the left of the patient, passes his left hand under the patient and beyond the patient's spinal column; the right hand is placed on the anterior surface of the abdomen. With the left hand in this position the left kidney can be much better pushed up and its surface brought to the

[1] Dr. A. Zerlaut, *Journal des Practiciens*, May 21st, 1912.

touch of the right hand. For the exploration of the right kidney the position is reversed. The doctor stands on the left side and the right hand is placed beneath the back, while the left hand goes to the surface of the abdomen. Of course the knees are raised as they are in all examinations of the abdomen when the patient is in the dorsal position.

Diagnosis of Duodenal Ulcer.[1]—Folsom gives a clear description of the symptoms which may lead one to suspect the presence of this condition. There is usually a definite history of a very uniform array of symptoms about as follows: These patients will tell you of their trouble having extended over a various number of months or years, consisting of pain or some kind of discomfort in their stomachs, coming on from one and a half to three hours after eating. This pain or discomfort usually getting worse and at times accompanied by a gaseous distention of the stomach. Almost without any exception they will explain that the pain appearing thus can be almost instantly relieved by taking some kind of food into the stomach. These patients usually go to bed with a cracker or something to eat near the bed, and usually about 1 or 2 a. m. they are awakened by the appearance of this pain or discomfort and after eating the cracker or drinking a glass of milk or even of water, they are relieved entirely and go back to sleep, not to be disturbed until the usual time following the morning meal. In addition to the hunger-pain and the relief afforded by eating they tell of persistent and recurring sour stomach, and have usually been given a diagnosis of hyperacidity, acid gastritis, etc. Moynihan goes so far as to say that "Repeated and persistent hyperchlorhydria is duodenal ulcer." To Folsom this seems extreme, and yet to disprove it would be difficult. By hyperacidity Moynihan means a subjective and not an objective hyperchlorhydria, for when those patients complain of sour, acid stomach an analysis of the gastric contents shows a hyperacidity or even an anacidity. The condition with which duodenal ulcer is most likely to be confused is gastric ulcer, though gallstones or appendicitis may cause confusion. In gastric ulcer there is the same pain or discomfort coming on after meals, but the time of the appearance of this pain is not the same. It comes on immediately or very soon after the meal and is never relieved by taking more food into the stomach, but rather made worse. Vomiting occurs early rather than late, and is a more constant factor, usually relieving the pain or discomfort, and more frequently containing blood. There is, however, the same history of definite attacks, lasting from a few weeks to months, separated by interims of comparative comfort.

[1] A. B. Folsom, M. D., *Texas State Jour. of Med.*, July, 1912.

TREATMENT.

Treatment of Catarrhal Jaundice.[1]—Lereboullet places hygiene and diet first in his recommendations as to treatment, ordering the patient to bed and putting him on milk diet. Intestinal poisoning is thus combated. About three quarts of skim milk daily are prescribed, but kefir or yaourt may be substituted. Full diet is resumed very gradually, eggs being cautiously added and only the white meats used at first. Grapes are thought to be a powerful hepatic stimulant, and lemon juice has its partisans. Plenty of water is given to help diuresis; this is important, and mild mineral waters may be used. Cold enemata, twice a day, are advised. Benzonaphthol and salacetol are given to combat the intestinal sepsis; a calomel purge follows at the end of the first week, then opotherapy by means of half a dozen daily capsules of bile. Pills of extract of liver are sometimes substituted. At the end of the third or fourth week, urotropin and sodium salicylate are indicated. If the liver remains enlarged the patient is ordered to one of the mineral spring resorts, or a powder may be given of sodium bicarbonate, eight grammes, sodium phosphate, four grammes, dry sodium sulphate, two grammes, dissolved in a quart of hot water and taken three times daily one hour before meals. Remember that jaundice is often a sign of infection. If it persists, repeated calomel purges are given, the bile opotherapy is continued, also the cold enemata. As to secondary symptoms, itchiness of the skin is best combated by very hot lotions containing alcohol or vinegar or dilute carbolic acid, or by zinc oxide ointment containing a small proportion of menthol. Hemorrhage is met with calcium chloride and the opotherapy already mentioned. Prognosis should always be guarded, although the majority of cases terminate favorably.

Methods of Facilitating Labor.[2]—The question of what in the way of remedies and general measures may be safely and conservatively employed with a view to stimulating a tardy or non-progressive labor is a rock on which many opinions divide. As a rule, physicians attempt to maintain a "masterly inactivity" and let the labor proceed in its own good time and way. The man who is engaged in this work year after year learns in time that certain agencies and certain conditions in which the woman is placed favor and facilitate the progress of labor, while conversely other things retard it. If the first stage of labor has set in, then it is that the accoucheur must map out his line of procedure. Much may be learned from the history of the case, provided she has previously borne children. It is not a sure criterion, of course, but a woman who

[1] Pierre Lereboullet, M. D., *Paris Medicale*, Sept. 14, 1912.

[2] Editorial *Charlotte Med. Journal*, Oct., 1912.

has a tough labor once or twice is probably not going to get through in a jiffy at the next confinement. Certain families are also conspicuous for tardy labors. The woman's pelvis, her muscular development, her general health and many other things must be weighed and considered for what they are worth in estimating the probable character and duration of the labor.

After being many years at the game I am fully convinced that ordinarily it is best to keep the woman on her feet or knees a goodly portion of the time until the labor is well advanced. In this position—the pelvis upright—we get increased pressure and wedge-like action on account of increased cephalic and hypostatic congestion. There is seldom a contraindication for the woman stirring about.

Labor is often retarded by a weakness of the general or peripheral circulation. Every woman seems instinctively to know that the pains are in a measure futile if the feet are cold. A pediluvia in mustard water and a drink of hot tea often turns the course of a stubborn labor into one that is gratifying to all parties concerned. Sitting over steaming water is a remedy of our grandmothers and one not to be despised. It aids in relaxing the soft parts and in some manner seems to add strength to the pains. The sitz bath is highly useful in stubborn labors but it must be used thoroughly—an hour or more—to get certain results from it.

If the dynamics of the uterus are not all that may be desired a few full doses of quinine may set things right. Strychnine hypodermically is occasionally of value. If the pains seem to be held back on account of gas on the stomach a hypo of apomorphine may clear matters up. I have often terminated labor by a capsule of ipecac. The woman will attribute her sick stomach to the natural course of events.

Nearly everything is "good for" rigid os. After all I doubt whether much of anything can supersede morphine and chloroform and perhaps occasionally apomorphine. Very often a tardy condition attributed to rigid os may be due to a full rectum and an enema may in such work wonders. Chloroform has given me good results in nine out of ten cases when used to blunt the woman's suffering and encourage normal labor. It should not, as a rule, be employed until the uterus is well along in the act of dilating or it may possibly bring on a state of passivity in that organ. On the other hand I have found a slight dilatation which persisted for hours to be at once improved by a little inhalation of chloroform. The woman who has been given the beneficent effects of a certain measure of anesthesia in one labor will call for it in subsequent labors.

Rupture of the membranes is a procedure that is usually unnecessary, as the "bag of waters" ordinarily serves a useful purpose. Often, however, it is necessary to rupture the membranes in order to allow the head to engage and the uterine expulsive forces to exert themselves to any advantage. A large quantity of amniotic fluid precludes the descent of the presenting part and if neglected or left to nature to rectify may allow the labor to go on without results for hours.

The physician should see that his obstetrical armamentarium is full and complete before attending a case of labor. Take along the whole thing except the murderous craniotomy forceps. You will have time to send for such instruments while you are getting other doctors on the ground. Besides you will probably never be compelled to engage in a procedure so hideous.

———

Veratrum Viride.[1]—This is an important agent in medical practice says A. J. Crance, and has always held a conspicuous place in my medicine case. I have invariably found it to be one of positiveness in action, always doing good when properly indicated. It is preeminently a drug for sthenic conditions; the more pronounced this picture the more actively it may be pushed to effect; when this has been accomplished, it should be discontinued, or the dosage very materially reduced. It is usually called for during the onset or early periods of acute febrile movements, when the circulation is active and the vessels overcharged with blood, as evidenced by the full-bounding pulse, obstructed capillaries and congested facial expression.

Whilst veratrum is classed as a poisonous agent, its toxic features are but rarely manifested, owing to its property of exciting the vomiting centers and otherwise in non-toxic doses opening the avenues of elimination for its removal, therefore is non-cumulative. Medically, veratrum viride is primarily a radio-vascular depressant and sedative, with antispasmodic properties as a secondary result. On the heart, it reduces its pulsations and lowers the tension; on the arterial circuit it causes a relaxation with softening of the pulse. The combined influence serves to lessen the temperature of the body in febrile states. In exalted action of the circulatory system its power over the momentum of the heart is readily demonstrated by the exhibition of the agent in five to ten-drop doses of the specific tincture given hourly or halfhourly for a few repetitions. It is unwise to employ the drug in this manner, except we have a definite object of accomplishment in view, as occurs particularly in convulsive diseases and especially of a puerperal nature. Ordinarily the fraction of a drop or two-drop doses, repeated once hourly or even two hours, will best serve the purposes for which veratrum is usually employed. Thus given, its action over the circulatory apparatus is regular and steady, gradually overcoming the rapidity of the heart's impulse, reducing the tension of the arterial vessels, relieving the engorgement of the capillaries and inducing transpiration from the skin; which in the aggregate brings about a physiological state of nature approximately that of health, or places the systemic

[1] A. J. Crance, M. D., *Eclectic Med. Journal*, Aug., 1912.

forces in a receptive mood for auxiliary treatment.

It is understood when speaking of veratrum in controlling the rapidity of the heart's action that it applies in direct opposition to the use of digitalis for the same purpose. The digitalis heart is rapid and feeble, whilst the veratrum heart is rapid and hard or bounding. The inconsistency of a combination of these remedies, which I have now and then seen, is clear, and the practice is extremely illogical. The symptomatic condition calling for veratrum is in some respects the same as that for gelsemium, which is frequently indicated in combination, and thus united are workers in harmony, owing to a synergistic influence contributed by gelsemium.

The Management of Sciatica.[1]—Watson divides the affection in the following manner:

A. Primary group: (1) Sciatic neuralgia. (2) Sciatic perineuritis. (3) Sciatic neuritis.

B. Secondary group.

The primary group includes sciatic neuralgia. This is supposed to be a functional trouble not associated with definite inflammatory change in the nerve trunk, the condition being purely functional. It occurs most frequently in flabby, anemic, debilitated women, being apparently an expression of nervous exhaustion. Occasionally it is associated with dysmenorrhea, or irregular menstruation. He has seen it alternate with facial neuralgia. The pain is intermittent and the patient may be quite comfortable between the attacks.

Sciatic perineuritis or neuritis is a disease of adult life, and in the writer's experience four times as common among men as women. There is almost invariably a gouty or a rheumatic history. In fully developed cases there is muscular atrophy, paresent, with diminution of tactile sensibility, areas of anesthesia and hyperesthesia, tinglings, pins and needles, formication, etc.

The exciting cause of the hyperacute attacks is usually exposure of a limb to cold and wet.

The secondary group of cases includes all those in which the condition is due to involvement of the sciatic nerve, by pressure or the spread of inflammatory processes. Hence the importance of making a complete and systematic examination before diagnosing primary sciatica. It is stated that a rectum overdistended with scybalous masses sometimes exerts sufficient pressure to give rise to sciatica, but whether this be so or not, it is at any rate quite sufficient to aggravate the condition if already present. It includes those cases of sciatica due to tuberculous or osteoarthritic disease of the spine, bones of the pelvis or hip-joint.

As to treatment, rest in bed is essential and a water-bed is advisable, the sheets being either of wool or cotton and not of linen. Woolen socks and pajamas should be worn. He fixes the limb with a long Liston splint,

which adds greatly to the comfort of the patient when he has become accustomed to it, and does away with the startings, which are such a painful feature of the disease. Should this prove unsatisfactory, it should be slung in a fracture cradle. The limb should be kept very warm, preferably swathed in cottonwool. A dose of calomel should be given, followed by a saline in the morning. Salicylates in combination with the bromides and tincture of gelsemium answer well. Aspirin appears to have a specific effect in relieving the pain of fibrositis; and pyramidon, exalgin, acetanilide, and phenalgin are worthy of mention. Potassium iodide is a most valuable remedy, more particularly in chronic cases, especially when combined with glycerophosphates. Tonics are very necessary when the acute symptoms have subsided.

Regarding local treatment, many pin their faith to fly-blisters; the disadvantage of these is that if not effective they interfere in a measure with the adoption of other methods of treatment. Hot linseed poultices, antiphlogistine, a canvas bag containing mustard bran, electra cloth applied along the course of the nerve, are all good methods of counterirritation.

Anodyne colloid is excellent for relieving local pain, and morphine is given when required. Cocaine is extremely valuable administered hypodermically in doses of 1-10 to 1-2 grain. It should be injected at the seat of pain, but not into the nerve. The balneological and electrical treatment receive detailed attention. High frequency and sinusoidal current are indicated without very clear indications as to the selection of each, as are massage and douching and passive movement. Stretching is advocated as a last resort. As to further treatment, the patient is especially cautioned against sitting on a cold seat of a draughty water-closet, he is advised to use a felt cover.

———

Treatment of Fever.[1]—The treatment of fever due to infection or microbian intoxication, the only one referred to here, should be essentially pathogenic and symptomatic when it is not specific.

The treatment of infectious disease, says Dr. Luc Vital, rests on four fundamental principles:—

(a) Annul the action of the pathogenic microbes.

(b) Annul the action of their toxins.

(c) Lower the high temperature.

(d) Enable the organisms to resist the infection.

To act directly on the microbes, internal antisepsy was tried, but beyond quinine in paludism, mercury in syphilis, salicylic acid in rheumatism, that method gave little results.

To annul the action of the toxins, the only aid to their elimination may be found in purgatives, diaphoretics, diuretics, hence, exception being made of the above specific injections,

———

[1] A. Watson, *British Medical Journal.*

[1] *Med. Press and Circular,* Oct. 9, 1912.

the therapeutics of fever are purely pathogenic and symptomatic.

The principal symptoms of fever are: Thirst, oliguria, hyperthermia, acceleration of the pulse, adynamia.

For the thirst the patient should be given abundant drinks, not only to relieve the inordinate thirst, but as the best means to provoke diuresis and diaphoresis, necessary to the elimination of the toxins.

A patient suffering from infectious disease should consequently drink largely. Lemon water (two lemons cut up for a quart of boiling water), apple tea, etc., are agreeable drinks. Citric lemonade is particularly indicated in acute rheumatism:—

Citric acid syrup, 3 oz.
Water, 1 quart.

In affections of the intestine lactic acid might be prescribed:—

Lactic acid, 2 dr.
Syrup, 3 oz.
Water, 1 quart.

For oliguria lactose might be given to increase the diuresis; two ources in a bottle of Evian water.

To aid in the elimination of the toxins, purgatives should be given, castor oil, or sulphate of soda:—

Sulphate of soda, 1 oz.
Lemon syrup, 1 oz.
Water, 9 oz.

Calomel is useful both as a purgative and a diuretic, two grains every hour for four hours.

Enemas of cold water also favor diuresis (8 oz.).

Hyperthermia.—There is no special treatment for hyperthermia as long as the temperature does not exceed 102° F.

One of the most active means of acting against it is cold water; cold baths (77 deg., ten to fifteen minutes), lower the temperature by one degree. Their further effects are: increase of the diuresis, elimination of the toxins, and stimulation of the organism. Cold compresses on the abdomen should be prescribed in the interval of the baths, while a stimulating mixture should be given before and after the bath:—

Tincture of cinnamon, 1 dr.
Syrup, 1 oz.
Brandy, 1 oz.
Water, 3 oz.

Where cold bathing is refused or not possible, cold effusions may be practised every two hours; spirit of lavender may be added to the water.

Antithermic drugs are of little use; however, phenacetine might be given:—

Phenacetine, 6 gr.
Citrate of caffeine, 2 gr.

for one wafer; one to two a day.

Tachycardia.—The pulse should always be the object of careful attention as it furnishes important indications on the state of the heart and the degree of resistance of the patient. Where the pulse is small, depressible, and exceeds 120, a cardiac tonic is required: small and repeated doses of sulphate of sparteine (½ gr. three times a day) fulfil the indications.

Adynamia.—The strength of the patient should be kept up as much as possible, but only by liquid food: milk, vegetable soups, decoction of cereals, lemonade mixed with a little wine, weak coffee. Hypodermic injections of camphorated oil repeated frequently or injections of strychnine form the medical treatment.

————

Treatment of Tonsillitis.[1]—Medical treatment is commenced by Griffith by giving calomel grain ⅛ or grain ¼ (grams 0.008 or 0.016) tablets, one every thirty minutes until 2 grains (gram 0.130) are taken, or until the patient's bowels are well moved; so keep regulated thereafter. When first seen a hot mustard foot bath is given (heaping tablespoonful of powdered mustard stirred up in a pail of hot water), having the patient wrapped in a blanket in which he is afterward put to bed The diet should be light and meat is better wholly refrained from. In cases accompanied by prostration, home-made meat juice may be employed. The course of treatment is planned to extend over a period of one, two or three days to suit requirements of acute attacks of tonsillitis. The specific treatment consists of quinin bisulphate (used because most soluble) grains 2 (gram 0.130) with Dover powder grains 5 to 10 (gram 0.333 to 0.666) when the patient is first seen, then administered night and morning thereafter during the course. Separate and distinct is the following treatment, which is directed to be regulated according to the amount of purulent exudate dripping from the infected tonsils, for it is these throat droppings, absorbed down in the stomach and intestines, which cause the exacerbations of systemic reaction in tonsillitis. To combat this Griffith gives drops 1 or 2 (c.c. 0.05 or 0.1) of pure phenol, stirred into a quarter of a glassful of cold water, to be administered from two to eight times a day of twenty-four hours as required.

Local cleansing of the throat may be employed by the patient with a mild gargle and oily spray, which latter does good by aiding suspension of the falling exudate. Hydrogen peroxid Griffith finds too harsh for use. The throat and tonsils may be gently wiped over once every one to three days by a solution of tannic acid, one part, in glycerin, four parts, or one of tincture of chlorid of iron, one part, in glycerin, five parts. Throat lozenges containing guaiacum grain 1 or 2 (gram 0.066 to 0.130), or made up with camphor, grain 1/10 (gram 0.006), menthol grain 1/10, and cocain hydrochlorid, grain 1/32 (gram 0.002), may be administered at the rate of six or eight a day. Lumps of cracked ice may be sucked to relieve thirst and lessen local inflammation. An ointment or hot poultice application to the neck under the angles of the jaw when lymphatic glandular involvement is manifested by swelling and pain, may be used. Marked mechanical obstruction to breathing is to be met by a

---

[1] F. Griffith, M. D., *N. Y. Med. Journal.* Sept. 7, 1912.

linear slash with a guarded bistoury through the bulging tonsil; one organ offending more than the other by its prominence is the rule. One or more cuts are to be made as necessary, reliance in this method depending on shrinkage obtained by blood depletion and sacrifice of the least amount of tonsillar tissue. Griffith does not object to a proper shortening of an elongated uvula, provided it is causing a symptomatic cough.

Tonic treatment, as of the hypophosphites, is employed subsequently if necessary. Excessive diarrhea, or the pressure of smoky urine, calls for reduction or cessation of the phenol medication.

Diagnosis and Treatment of Pruritus.[1]— There are no specifics for itching, says Dyer, but there are medications in particular diseases which may apply for general use, of course individualizing the case in hand. Arsenic is the prime treatment for the nervous basis of the disease, and its administration is largely corrective of the itching. The derivatives of wheat and oats may aid in these types and the tincture of avena sativa (wild oats) is of special usefulness, given in conjunction with the arsenic. Where there is no neuropathic cause or association, the arsenic not only does no good, but it may actually do harm by local over-stimulation. Strychnin serves excellently in the vasomotor disturbances with itching. Zinc phosphid acts similarly, and is of special service in chronic itching diseases. Cannabis indica, in the fluid extract, may be used every hour in five-drop doses; as soon as the acute itching is controlled, the dose may be reduced and the period of administration lengthened to every three or four hours. Chlorid of calcium is of service in senile pruritus and in all itching where there is any suggestion or evidence of lowered coagulability. Freshly prepared chlorid of calcium may be administered in 5 to 15 grain doses, well diluted and repeated every three or four hours. Antipyrin and salicylate of soda, used in combination, serve best in gouty subjects or in uric acid cases. The use of the sodium and potassium citrates, at the same time, materially aids in the treatment. Gelsemium, odein, veratrum viride, bromids, choral hydrate and chloroform are among the antispasmodics which have good effect in stopping the paroxysms of itching, but any and all of these may be relegated until the above named drugs have been first essayed. The too free use of morphin for itching should be condemned. With all cases of pruritus, mild laxatives, diuretics, mineral waters of alkaline sorts, diet restrictions and limitations by injunction, habits, etc., should be carefully weighed and considered where indicated.

The local treatment of pruritus is of considerable importance and needs to be suited to the particular case. General baths are of supreme service in the treatment of itching,

and these should be taken as hot as can be comfortably borne. Such baths may be employed in all diseases or conditions in which itching is general. The baths may be plain or may carry such emollients as starch, marshmallow or bran (in bags), or alkalies may be added, such as carbonate of soda ($\bar{3}$ss to $\bar{3}$i to 30 gallons of water), household ammonia ($\bar{3}$i, $\bar{3}$ii to the 30 gallons), or suphuret of potassium ($\bar{3}$ii, $\bar{3}$i to the bath), the last named being especially indicated in all parasitic diseases, vegetable or animal. Wet dressings may be substituted for the general bath, when the itching is so localized as to permit of such. The dressings should be kept wet with saturated boracic acid solution, 1-5,000 to 1-10,000 mercuric chlorid solution, 1 per cent. phenol solution, 1-5,000 potassium permanganate solution, or 1 or 2 per cent. solutions of resorcin, in water always. Fixed dressings of coal tar made into a felt with superimposed cotton may be applied and left in place for days at a time. Even dry cotton may be firmly bound in place, when such a dressing can be so fixed that the patient cannot remove it easily.

Oily substances may be employed and the old-fashioned carron oil may be used, or camphor and chloral hydrate. Cocoa butter and cocoanut oil are excellent protective applications when the skin is dry. An oily substance of excellent antipruritic value in small areas may be derived by combining phenol, menthol, camphor and chloral hydrate, and this may be diluted with any of the simple oils. Itching of the anal area is frequently relieved by ergot, used either in ointment made with the fluid extract or in suppository with the solid extract. Intestinal parasites should be excluded or removed. Genital pruritus is often helped with weak resorcin solutions. The use of the high frequency spark over the sacral plexus is an excellent adjuvant for genital pruritus and a systematic general effleuve will often aid when other remedial agents fail. All cases of pruritus should be studied as individual types, and the etiology should be determined when possible; then the way to cure will be easier.

Fracture of the Patella.[1]—The method that the author outlines is as follows: First, a mold is made of the sound knee by taking poroplastic material, 1½ feet long by 6 inches broad, which is softened in boiling water, and then firmly placed on the sound knee. In this way a perfect mold of the knee-cap is taken; this is used as a splint for the fractured patella, the fragments being viced in the cap of the splint. A little cotton-wool is placed in the cap and sufficient to pad the rest of the splint, which extends above and below the knee-joint. Prior to fixing the splint the fragments are strapped into position by adhesive plaster and longer strips are placed immediately above and below the patella and drawn in contrary directions to pull the upper and lower fragments together.

---

[1] L. Dyer, M. D., *Jour. of Arkansas Med. Soc.*, Aug., 1912.

[1] J. F. Maclachlan, F. R. C. S., *British Med. Jour.*, July 29, 1912.

Lastly a plaster-of-Paris bandage is put over all. In three weeks the plaster-of-Paris bandage is taken off. The splint is kept on for two weeks, passive exercises begun, and a knee-cap worn for two months, when it is discarded.

A Simple Method of Appendicectomy.[1]—Van Hook states most sententiously that every surgeon of some experience, and even those who are comparatively new in the work, can carry out the following suggestions for removing the appendix, at first in uncomplicated cases, and later in complicated ones:

1. Make an oblique incision ¾ of an inch long over the appendix; carry the incision through the aponeurosis of the external oblique muscle, which is recognized by the fact that it can be felt with the left forefinger as well as by the knife point with which it is scratched.

2. Separate with the left forefinger and an artery forceps, held in the right hand, the fibers of the external oblique, internal oblique and transversalis muscles, keeping in mind the direction in which their fibers run. Do not cut these fine fibers, but merely separate them.

3. Push a hole through the peritoneum with the left forefinger or, if the connective tissue and peritoneum are too tough, lift them with an artery forceps and cut a hole in the peritoneum with scissors.

4. Find the appendix with the finger-tip by touch. It feels somewhat like a fishing worm. Lift it with an artery forceps passed down by the side of the finger. If you do not close the artery forceps too tightly you will not crush the organ.

5. Having drawn out the appendix, crush and ligate the mesenteriolum.

6. Cut off the appendix between two pairs of artery forceps, and whip over the cut stump of the appendix with a silk or catgut suture.

7. Having removed the forceps from the stump, turn in, with intestinal sutures, the peritoneum about the wound in the cecum.

8. With the left forefinger in the wound, feel for the slippery peritoneum, draw up its edge by friction with the finger, grasp it with an artery forceps, and lift it up into the wound far enough to stitch together with a catgut suture.

9. Lift the muscles of the abdominal wall in the same way, and insert catgut stitches in two layers.

10. Close the outer wound with two silkworm stitches.

11. Patient to sit up next day after operation, if there is no wound complication, and leave hospital in six to ten days.

Treatment, the Paramount of Practice.[2]—In an address of extraordinary value and interest

---

[1] Wesley Van Hook, M. D., *Med. Council*, July, 1912.

[2] S. J. Meltzer, M. D., *Jour. A. M. A.*, Aug. 24, 1912.

for the young practitioner, Meltzer very properly states that those who are in the practice of medicine, and those whose task and duty it is to make the practice efficient, ought to become imbued with the idea that the treatment of the patient is the paramount object of the practitioner. The very fact that great stress is to be laid on treatment will assist greatly in the development of its efficiency. The enlistment of men of genius in behalf of therapeutics brought us in recent years the marvelous new facts and principles of the serum treatment and chemotherapy. The actual curative remedies are still small in number, but on the basis of these principles more may be expected. But the prevention of the fatal outcome of a grave disease is not the only aim of therapeutics. Treatment covers a variety of objects, to be attained in various ways. The patient must be made comfortable even in hopeless diseases. Self-limiting diseases must be attended in order to obviate errors of nature or of attendants, and an attempt must be made, where possible, to accelerate the recovery. All sufferings, even of only temporary nature, must be alleviated. Our old clinicians had and have too much contempt for the treatment of symptoms. Salicylates which surely relieve rheumatic pains should be given even if they do not accomplish a cure, or even if the rheumatic fever would have gotten better without salicylates—if the sufferer could have waited long enough. Of course, no treatment should be given which could diminish the patient's chances of recovery, and no such treatment should be given which increases the patient's suffering and discomfort without having reliable evidence that it increases his chance for life. It is an interesting psychologic phenomenon that some medical men who are drug nihilists would insist on giving cold baths to typhoid patients who beg to be left alone, with flimsy statistics as the only proof for the usefulness of the method. I hear that some of our confrères became milder in their requirements after they had to take a dose of their own medicine. The story repeats itself in the cold-air treatment; an ardent advocate of the method recovered from his pneumonia without its aid.

Picric Acid as a Skin Disinfectant.[1]—In the *Annals of Surgery*, August, 1911, a report was made from this laboratory upon the germicidal and osmotic properties of picric acid. At that time, picric acid solutions had been used in 19 cases in the service of Dr. F. G. Nifong at the Parker Memorial Hospital. The laboratory tests were so pleasing that the action of picric acid as a disinfectant for the skin seemed promising.

Up to the present time the picric acid solutions, in the main 1 per cent. alcoholic solutions, have been used in 78 cases. Commenting upon its use, Dr. Nifong writes me as follows: "During the last year I have used it in

---

[1] By O. W. H. Mitchell, M. D., *Annals of Surgery*, April, 1912.

practically all of my cases. When a patient can be prepared over night he has the usual shaving and soap and water scrub, with a saturated watery solution of picric acid applied over the field. Before operation he is washed again with soap and water and the alcoholic solution is applied. In cleansing a scalp or sterilizing an infected wound I have found it most efficient and reliable, which is no doubt due to its high germicidal action and its great power of penetrability, as you have shown by your experiments. I have had no case of wound infection since I have used the method. The only objection I have to it is the intense and tenacious staining, and on two occasions when I did not have my wound edges perfectly coapted there were one or two small points of delayed union due to small coagula of serum between the edges of the wound. These coagula were cultured and found to be absolutely sterile. This high power of coagulating serum makes it necessary to make close and perfect approximation of wounds and leave no pocket of serum which will be coagulated with a very small quantity of the picric acid and hinder union mechanically."

Shortly after the publication of the uses that have been made of the picric acid solutions here, Fontana published his results. The review appearing in the *Journal of the American Medical Association* is as follows: Fontana uses a 1 per cent. alcoholic solution of picric acid for sterilization of the field of operation, and extols its advantages over other methods. It is as effectual, his tests seem to show, as the tincture of iodine method, while it is much more convenient for sterilization of the hands. Both of these do away with the long scrubbing indispensable with other technics, and which is so liable to chill the patient.

The solutions of picric acid can be depended upon as germicidal and are to be recommended for skin disinfection because of this property and the one of penetrability. Picric acid is cheap and efficient, and deserves a prominent place among the substances used for disinfecting the skin before surgical intervention.

HYGIENE AND DIETETICS.

The Hygiene of Pregnancy.[1]—Cragin in his admirable paper outlines his plan of treatment as follows: First, as to the care of the kidneys. There are two certain indications in the care of the kidneys during pregnancy which may well be impressed upon the laity. In the first place the kidneys during pregnancy have more to do than in the non-pregnant state, as they are called upon to excrete waste products both of the mother and child. This excretion is favored by keeping the urinary tract well flushed out with large draughts of water, and it is hindered by anything irritating the urinary tract, such as alcohol.

[1] E. B. Cragin, M. D., *N. Y. Med. Jour.*, June 8, 1912.

It is Cragin's custom to advise his patients to drink if possible six glasses of water each day between meals: one before breakfast, two in the middle of the forenoon, two in the middle of the afternoon, and one at bedtime. At the same time he forbids the use of all alcoholic drinks.

Of all the criteria of the condition of a woman during pregnancy, none is so available or so trustworthy as the frequent examination of the urine. It is not enough to have the urine examined once, and if it is found normal to rest assured that it will remain so. Within a week conditions may change entirely, and examination of the urine may show that the woman is in grave danger. The urine should be examined as often as every two weeks, even if the woman is feeling perfectly well, and the woman who does not send regularly to her physician a specimen of her urine is running a risk which, in the present days of enlightenment, is unjustifiable.

The elimination through the skin of the woman during pregnancy is a process which certainly should not be neglected. For this reason frequent bathing is not only a comfort, but a safety. The temperature of the bath may be determined largely by one's habits, and where a woman has always been accustomed to a cold bath in the morning, Cragin asserts he has not found that its continuance during pregnancy does harm. One or two warm baths each week just before retiring, in addition to the regular morning cool baths, will prove of value in increasing perspiration and thus favoring elimination. An extremely cold bath for one not accustomed to it should be avoided. On the other hand, a very hot bath should not be taken.

In the care of the breasts during pregnancy, cleanliness is to be maintained by frequent general bathing. The cleanliness and toughening of the nipples obtained by bathing them daily with a saturated solution of boric acid in 50 per cent. alcohol has seemed in his experience to add greatly to the comfort of the woman during the nursing period which follows.

The elimination of both maternal and fetal waste products, through respiration, and the need of fresh air are often overlooked by the pregnant patient until she finds herself in a crowded room where the air is bad. She then realizes that she needs fresh air and plenty of it, and that she soon feels faint if she does not seek it. Sleeping with open windows and spending a part of each day in the open air are almost essential to a high standard of health during pregnancy.

During pregnancy the mental condition of the woman is usually that of high tension and unstable equilibrium. There are numerous causes for this. She may have found herself pregnant unexpectedly, perhaps unwillingly. Her plans for the year or two to come may have to be entirely rearranged. She may feel like secluding herself from her friends and abstaining from occupations she enjoys. She may feel wretchedly from the nausea which, although made light of by her friends, is disagreeable enough for her. She may dread the ordeal of her labor; and last, but by no means least, she may be suffering from a form of poisoning resulting from the lack of elimination of waste products from the body, the results of this poisoning showing themselves chiefly in the nervous system.

Adenoid Growths in Children.[1]—These growths are responsible for more of the complaints of childhood than many people are aware of. If the child suffers from an obstinate catarrh, in nine cases out of ten on examination the cause will be found to be adenoid growths of the vault of the pharnyx, and, in fact, the majority of throat, nose and ear diseases have a like origin. This has been well exemplified in the report of Dr. F. Willcocks, who was sent down recently by the City of London to inquire into the health of the children at the Hanwell Schools. He found that no less than thirty out of the eighty-two examined were suffering from adenoids. A prominent pediatrist, writing on this subject makes the following interesting remarks: "Every observer must have been struck by the curious fact that the actual amount of obstruction to nasal breathing in a child produces very varying amount of symptoms in different cases. It is not by any means rare to find a boy, and a boy oftener than a girl, I think, the picture of robust health, with perfect hearing, a fully developed thorax, no excessive tendency to cold-taking, even a good runner and foot-ball player, and yet with his mouth habitually open, and his sleep broken only by his school fellows' shoes and other missiles, gentle hints that he should modify his furious snoring. Such a boy is, I confess, more liable to ordinary cold-taking than he should be, and may at such times suffer from more or less deafness. Still I maintain that even these are not infrequently absent even with a remarkable quantity of adenoids. On the other hand, we know the other picture: the stooping, thin, and anemic child, undersized with contracted thorax, and deaf, always in the state of general catarrh, whether of nose, ears, or stomach, taking cold with every change of atmosphere, peevish and capricious in temper, tossing about in sleep, with voracious appetite, but easily fatigued. Such a patient may have either a large or a small amount of adenoids; the amount of buccal respiration may be conspicuous or insignificant; the snoring may be habitual or only noticed when fresh cold is contracted. And yet in the latter case, irrespective of the actual quantity of growth, operation is absolutely imperative, while in the former case the only good reason for interference would be for the sake of improving the articulation; indeed, if this is not very faulty, we should not be erring, if we advise the postponing of an operation until symptoms should arise, or if the boy is sixteen or seventeen years of age, waiting to see if nature would not

take the case out of our hands by inducing spontaneous atrophy of the growths in the course of the next two or three years." We agree with the author that in the first case operation is not absolutely imperative, but at the same time it appears that he has overlooked a rather important point: that even though a person be robust and healthy and has adenoids, that in the event of his contracting certain diseases, his chances of recovery are considerably prejudiced by the presence of these growths.

SOCIETY PROCEEDINGS.

THE EASTERN MEDICAL SOCIETY OF THE CITY OF NEW YORK.

Regular Meeting, October 11th, 1912.

EXECUTIVE SESSION.

The preliminary report of the Committee on Annual Dinner was received and it was decided to hold the Annual Dinner and Dance at the Hotel Astor, on December 3rd, 1912. The Chairman of the Dinner Committee announced that a most imposing array of dinner speakers would address the society.

SCIENTIFIC SESSION.

A. Report of Cases.

Report of a Case of Caesarean Section. By Dr. E. K. Browd.

Report of a Stomach Case. By Dr. Harris Weinstein.

B. Papers.

1. Use of the Secondary Blood Clot in Mastoid Surgery. By Dr. R. Johnson Held.

2. Symposium on the Practical Application of Bone Transplantation.
   (a) In General Surgery. By Dr. A. A. Berg.
   (b) In Mastoid Surgery. By Dr. Milton J. Ballin.
   (c) In the Special Surgery of the Nose. By. Dr. William W. Carter.

3. The Surgical Treatment of Meningitis. By Dr. Irving S. Haynes.

4. The Sluder Operation for the Removal of Tonsils. By Dr. Charles J. Imperatori.

The discussion was participated in by Drs. Robert T. Morris, Wendell C. Phillips, Duncan Macpherson, Seymour Oppenheimer, Otto Glogau and others. The Scientific session then adjourned.

The members and guests of the society partook of the usual collation.

The papers which were presented at this meeting will appear in the next issue of AMERICAN MEDICINE with the exception of the paper of Dr. Irving S. Haynes which has been already published.

---

[1] Editorial *Pediatrics*, March, 1912.

5^{q}

American Medicine

H. EDWIN LEWIS, M. D., *Managing Editor*.

PUBLISHED MONTHLY BY THE AMERICAN-MEDICAL PUBLISHING COMPANY.

Copyrighted by the American Medical Publishing Co., 1912.

Complete Series, Vol. XVIII., No. 11.
New Series, Vol. VII., No. 11.
NOVEMBER, 1912. $1.00 YEARLY in advance.

The recent convention in New York City of the Clinical Congress of Surgeons was one of the most notable gatherings ever held in this or any other city. Too great commendation cannot be extended to the men who made this great meeting not only a brilliant success, but what is more important, so productive of substantial, far-reaching results. We are reliably informed that at least three thousand surgeons came to New York and attended the various clinics.

That great benefit resulted from this Congress has been evident and it can be truthfully said that the whole affair went far and away beyond the expectations of those originally responsible for the organization of the movement. This year's meeting was the third annual gathering and much satisfaction has been felt that New York was chosen this time. New York is so large and people get so in the habit of conceding big things to the metropolis, that there is constant danger that the real excellence of its institutions will be overlooked in viewing them too exclusively from the standpoint of size. It was extremely gratifying that so large a feast of surgical material could be placed before visitors so capable of appreciating its diverse as well as interesting character. Without the slightest desire to be egotistical, we believe that no city in the world today enjoys more or better surgical facilities than New York. It is only when attention is focussed on the opportunities afforded, as during the Congress of Surgeons, that realization is had of the splendid work New York surgeons are doing. Day in and day out, as matters of daily routine, surgical operations of the most advanced and modern character are being performed, without hue or cry, or the slightest attempt to win the plaudits of the multitude. There is something fine and noble about this kind of work, and the people of New York should take genuine pride in the high grade character of the surgery that is working so modestly yet earnestly for the welfare and efficiency of the community. This recent Congress served to pull aside the veil of professional reticence and gave even the local medical profession a surprise. Hundreds of New York physicians were unaware of the enormous amount of surgical work that was being done in the city. It was a revelation to many and gave new cause for appreciating this great American community.

The executive details of the Congress were admirable. Under the skillful direction of Mr. A. D. Ballou the problems of registration and the thousand and one other matters pertaining to the organization of the Congress were carried out with precision and a uniform courtesy that gave the utmost satisfaction. It was pleasant to hear the frequent words of praise extended to those charged with the general management, as the usual drawback to these great meetings is the inability to find any one who knows anything or can give any information. This Congress was a new experience to those who frequently attend large conventions, and the efficiency shown in meeting the members' and visitors' wants will not soon be forgotten.

The clinical conferences held each night were splendidly attended and the interest shown was most stimulating. Important problems were discussed by men of prominence who could speak with knowledge and authority.

Two great questions were given especial attention and the results bid fair to be very far-reaching. It is safe to say that no scientific convention has ever accomplished more practical results than this Congress, and a high mark has been set for other gatherings.

The first great problem attacked was the early necessity of establishing a surgical degree. It was recognized that too many operations are performed by the illy prepared or inefficient, with the result that surgery suffers immeasurably. If special courses were established leading to a degree indicating special efficiency in surgery it was the opinion that surgical science would receive a wonderful impetus. A committee of the country's leading surgeons were entrusted with the proposition.

The other great problem was the evolution of ways of educating the women of the country to the significance of early symptoms of cancer of the uterus. The following resolutions tell the story:

Be it Resolved, That the time has arrived when, if the surgeons of America are to do their duty to the citizens of this country, a campaign of publicity should be at once undertaken to bring to the attention of every woman in this country the early symptoms of cancer of the womb and to point out that if the cancer be detected in its early stages it can often be cured.

Be it further Resolved, That this society at once appoint a committee of five, to be named by the President, to disseminate this information.

And, further, That this committee be instructed to write or have written articles to be published in the daily press, the weekly or monthly magazines, as may prove most expedient.

And, further, That they report their progress for the year to the next annual meeting.

Dr. Edward Martin, President of the Congress, appointed this committee to act in accordance with the resolutions:

Dr. Thomas S. Cullen, Baltimore, Md., Chairman; Dr. Howard C. Taylor, New York City; Dr. C. Jeff Miller, New Orleans,; Dr. F. F. Simpson, Pittsburgh, and E. C. Dudley, Chicago.

Every one reading these resolutions cannot fail to grasp their humanitarian importance.

It cannot help but be a source of pride, not alone to those who managed and took part in this Congress, but also to the people of the whole country, that such a convention could be held in this day of hustle and hurry. While it is true every one in attendance derived great and lasting benefit, the results that are bound to accrue to the people at large emphasize again the unselfish, earnest and conscientious work that is being done by the physicians of our country. May the Congress of Surgeons go forward as surely as its good works promise.

The arrogance of expert witnesses—of the medical variety particularly—was never better exemplified than during the past few days at the trial of a New York lawyer for murder. Evidence was given that the deceased had remained in the water two days; eight hours after recovery of the body it was embalmed; burial followed; and fifty-three days thereafter the body was exhumed and an autopsy performed. From the conditions and anatomical relations which the physicians performing the autopsy claimed to have found, the opinion was advanced unequivocally that death had resulted from strangulation produced by external pressure on the throat at the time the deceased fell or was thrown into the water! It hardly seems conceivable that medical men of the unquestioned experience and ability of those who performed this post mortem examination would be willing to go into court and swear that death was thus caused. One might advance such an opinion as his belief, according to his best knowledge and observation. But to offer such an opinion as an absolute fact, with the life of a human being at stake, is incomprehensible. Such cock-sureness always runs the danger of being made ridiculous. To have men of recognized intelligence and skill swear to pathologic deductions and deny the possibility of error does not tend to create confidence, either in the opinions expressed or in the persons making them. Ordinary intelligence teaches the fallibility of human judgment, and human events are constantly presenting instances of faulty or mistaken observations and deductions, even on the part of the most trained and careful investigators. All this makes the medical expert who claims that his deductions and conclusions are absolutely correct and essentially infallible, little less than ridiculous. The very arrogance of his statements robs them of strength and too often destroys their credibility. Every one knows how frequently the most conclusive opinions in regard to the cause of death have been shown to be erroneous. History is full of mistaken verdicts of coroners' juries based

on misinterpreted autopsy findings. This is not to be wondered at, for our knowledge concerning pathologic conditions and post mortem changes is far from absolute, despite the great progress that has been made in recent years. But the myriad variations that may occur in appearance as well as anatomic location and relation, the result of the infinite variety of modifying factors that may exert their influence post mortem, make it impossible in any obscure case, for any medical man however experienced or capable he may be to tell from the autopsy findings alone, the sole, exclusive and incontrovertible cause of death. Note that we state "from the autopsy findings alone." Obviously, information gleaned from a post mortem examination united with facts from other sources may supply a chain of evidence that will be practically absolute. But, for example, finding cyanide of potassium in the body of a supposed suicide would not necessarily indicate that this was the cause of death. It is possible that a person murderously killed by some other poison might have potassium cyanide placed in the mouth shortly after death, and the bottle from which it was taken arranged to give the appearance of self administration. This may be a highly improbable situation, but it is presented for illustration only, to emphasize that conclusive as the presence of cyanide might be, its simple determination in a dead body would prove nothing. Without corroborative evidence it would not be more than a presumptive cause of death. The average expert would be satisfied, however, and nothing could swerve him from the opinion that death had been caused by poisoning with potassium cyanide. That another observer had gone further and found, for instance, unmistakable evidence of progressive arsenical poisoning, extending over a considerable period, and the purchase and administration of arsenic by the suspected murderer was definitely proven, would not alter his belief that cyanide was the causative factor. The determination of its presence in the body, and the fact that the individual was dead, would be enough. So it has been with many expert witnesses. The facts as they have observed them have been all sufficient, and once having formed a conclusion everything opposed to it has been denied or ignored.

What has been the result?—Just this, that lawyers, judges and intelligent people in general have discounted medical expert testimony and to a large extent lost confidence in medical witnesses. Among the legal fraternity it is a common expression, "you can get some doctor to swear to anything." Referring to the case that suggested these remarks we have a very pretty illustration of the evils of medical expert testimony. Hardly any physician who has had any experience in autopsies, especially on bodies of persons drowned, or in connection with exhumed bodies will deny the great variations that may exist in the changes and relations of the soft parts. To be able to state from an autopsy fifty-three days after interment of a body that had remained in the water two days and then been embalmed with formalin, that death was due to strangulation produced by external pressure, is not possible. A physician might state this as his opinion, that conditions as he found them led him to believe that death had been so caused. But in the interests of justice and fairness he ought to be as willing to admit that post mortem changes, the effects of two days' immersion, the manipulations of the undertaker and finally the contractions occasioned by formalin might produce

alterations in the appearance and mechanical relations of the muscles and tissues of the throat that would be similar to those found. At any rate, however conclusive the conditions determined from the autopsy, the physician performing same should be careful to point out that his deductions, while certain to him, were founded on personal opinion and belief, and that the conditions described might exist, however improbably to him, as the result of other causes than strangulation or external pressure on the throat. This attitude would have been the scientific one, the attitude of the earnest, God fearing physician anxious to do his duty to the state and at the same time to do no injustice to a fellow being. Let the prosecuting attorney fasten the crime if he can, and make as damning deductions as he deems necessary. Let him take possibilities and weave a chain of evidence as convincing as lies within his power. It is his duty to interpret the facts and draw the most positive deductions possible in order to link the accused as closely as he can to the assumed crime. The very nature of his work makes the prosecuting attorney a violent partisan. But the medical expert should not be a partisan. His duty is to supply facts and point out the truth. When he becomes a partisan his usefulness is lowered and his testimony weakened. There are three reasons for partisanship on the part of a medical expert, price, pride or personal animosity. Little need be said of these for few will deny their evil tendencies. That a medical man will go into court and prostitute his calling by testifying along a certain line solely because of what he is to receive is detestable. That a physician would take a certain position and hold to it because he disliked to admit a limitation of knowledge or inability to answer positively is more comprehensible, but none the less to be deprecated. Finally, that a medical man would allow personal likes or dislikes to determine the character of his testimony is a sad reflection on human as well as professional decency.

It is difficult in connection with the trial we have made reference to, to understand the apparent partisanship of the experts for the prosecution. We are not denying the possible accuracy of their conclusions. The ultimate cause of events may show that their contentions as to the cause of death are right, but in the presence of any possibility of their deductions being wrong— we have not questioned their .findings for at least two are remarkably expert pathologists—it is a matter for regret that so positive a position—partaking so much of partisanship, and therefore the manifest evils of medical expert testimony—has been taken.

Certain it is that such instances add still more to the disrepute into which medical witnesses have ·fallen. The only bright side is that they hasten the day of reform, the day when medical men of established ability and probity will be appointed by the State to give medical expert testimony. Then may it be expected that the truth will be advanced and determined by the medical witness, and not obscured and befogged as is so often the case under our present system.

The transmission of disease by telephone has been a subject of much discussion, and many alarmist statements have been uttered in regard to its possible frequency. Tuberculosis especially has been mentioned, but according to some experiments recently undertaken in London at the instance of the Postmaster General, there appears to be little likelihood of its trans-

mission in that manner. Dr. Harold Spitta, bacteriologist to the Royal Household, conducted the experiments. Mouthpieces were taken not only from public 'phones, but also from 'phones exclusively reserved for the use of consumptives in a sanatorium. After washing the mouthpieces and the discs in a very little sterile water, this water was injected into a number of healthy guinea pigs. Notwithstanding the fact that these investigations were repeated very many times during several months, in not a single instance was tuberculosis developed in the guinea pigs. Dr. Spitta thereupon concluded that "the transmission of tuberculosis through the medium of the telephone mouthpiece is practically impossible." Assuming adequate care and accuracy in the experiments, it must at least be conceded that such transmission is so very unlikely as to fail to justify any widespread alarm. We should be disposed rather to regard the possibility of syphilitic infection from mucous patches as more likely in the case of those careless people one occasionally sees, who bring their mouths into actual contact with the mouthpiece. There is no necessity whatever for the mouth of the speaker to be brought into contact with the mouthpiece, for those who have tried it find that when one speaks across the mouthpiece at the distance of a few inches, provided the enunciation is clear, every word is distinctly audible.

All possible vigilance, however, should be exercised in regard to possible methods of conveyance of disease. The subject of carriers of disease is a most important one, and certain diseases, such as typhoid and diphtheria, are now recognized as being spread to a very appreciable extent by persons who, while themselves not presenting any of the signs of the disease, harbor in their bodies the germs which, however, innocuous to themselves, are potent for evil when disseminated by them to be taken up by others. To the diseases thus occasionally propagated it would appear likely that plague must now be added. On July 25th a boy, aged 7 years, was admitted for operation into the Royal Infirmary, in Liverpool, with a diagnosis of appendicitis. But an enlarged gland which was removed was found to contain plague bacilli, and this is said to have been confirmed by the Laboratory of the Local Government Board. One would hardly expect a disease of such usually fulminating severity as plague to be found among those that could be harbored in this way; but now that attention has been drawn to the matter all cases of enlarged glands should be regarded as suspicious, and be carefully observed in localities affected by plague. After all, if due recollection be had of the fact that the resultant disease is a product of two factors, the seed and the soil, there is no reason why the most active of seed should not lie dormant on a really sterile soil, as seeds of less vigorous character do.

The dietetic theories of the doctrinaires were vigorously combated at a conference on School Diet recently held in London at the Guildhall, under the patronage of the Lord Mayor, himself a highly respected octogenarian physician. While the maxim, that one should leave the table feeling always that one could eat a little more, may be true as regards adults, it was emphatically contravened in the case of children, both by Dr. Clement Dubes, the medical officer to Rugby School, and by Dr. Robert Hutchison. Dr. Dubes said

that "while adults should rise from the table hungry, children should reach a sense of repletion before rising"; and Dr. Hutchison said, "I do not believe that you can habitually overfeed a healthy, growing child. Provide a sufficiency of good food and you may safely trust the child's appetite if it has not been debauched by tuck shops." Another important point insisted on by Dr. Dubes was that no child, boy or girl, should ever be called on to do work on an empty stomach.

The relation between morals and food, came in for its share of the discussion, and Dr. Hutchison vigorously opposed the idea prevalent with some vegetarians and other food doctrinaires, that the eating of meat has a demoralizing effect upon the spiritual and moral faculties, while *per contra* the exclusive use of a vegetarian diet has a humanizing and refining influence. In refutation of this theory Dr. Hutchison pointed out that some of the most bloodthirsty nations had been vegetarians. "It is not safe," he said, "to try to influence morals by playing about with food." As a matter of fact almost anyone can satisfy himself by contemplating his acquaintances, that oftentimes gross feeders are gentle of spirit, while many delicate feeders are of cruel nature.

The order in which food is taken is also another point of importance. Many people seem to think it a matter of indifference, but it is quite true, as Dr. Sim Wallace pointed out, that we often begin our meals at the wrong end. The importance of arranging the meals so that the mouth shall be left at the close in as hygienic a state as possible was insisted on. Foods he classed as "cleansing" or "non-cleansing" to the teeth and mouth. To the former belong fish, meat, lettuce, celery, bread crust, toast, fruit, tea and coffee. These, therefore, should be used at the end of a meal; while the non-cleansing foods, i. e., sweet biscuits, cake, bread and jam, milk puddings, porridge, preserved fruits, chocolate and cocoa, should never be taken last, according to Dr. Wallace. Looked at singly from Dr. Wallace's point of view, perhaps, this may be correct; but unfortunately feeding is far too complex a process to be regulated in detail from one point of view only, and many other factors have to be taken into consideration.

Small-pox in an insane hospital seems inexcusable and yet we are informed that fifty cases developed a few months ago in the State Hospital at Marion, Virginia. There was a wholesale vaccination inaugurated at once, and the health authorities, instead of finding out why this was not done before, are reported to have been wondering how the disease could have been introduced. If the patients and employees had been properly protected it would be immaterial whether small-pox was introduced or not. If physicians neglect vaccination of their helpless charges, can we wonder why laymen are so negligent? It is certainly a revelation that in any part of the country there are so many non-immunes. In Porto Rico some years ago, the whole population was vaccinated and small-pox temporarily eradicated—temporarily because a new unprotected generation would soon grow up to contract the disease if it were imported and we did not continue compulsory vaccination. At home, we allow anyone to do as he pleases because the voter is the ruler, but it is time to inquire whether heads of institutions are not legally bound to protect their charges.

Congratulations to our Department of Health! When this important bureau was established the yearly death rate was 36.31 per thousand. A reduction started which has steadily continued until it reached 15.13 per 1000 in 1911, and it is still going down. This life saving has been accomplished at a per capita cost so small as to be negligible in comparison to what every tax-payer spends on those few pleasures which are really harmful. The very men whose lives are thus saved have often obstructed the workings of the health bureau by unwise criticism, and opposition to the necessary appropriations. We hope now there will be an end of opposition and that everyone will do something to encourage the department and hold up the hands of Commissioner Lederle. Infectious diseases are well nigh conquered now, and children are being saved who were formerly slaughtered by bad feeding. Milk is practically safe, but to keep it so requires a small army of inspectors whose activities spread over several states. There is much more to be done yet, for perfection is never reached though we approach it all the time. How much further the death rate can be reduced depends largely on the birth rate and whether the population itself varies. Now let us get to work to see how long we can keep the babies alive. Let us continually strive to increase the average age at death—the real test of sanitation after all.

General hygiene as a required college course was discussed by Prof. Alan W. C. Menzies of the University of Chicago, in an address at Oberlin College (*Science*, Apr. 19, 1912). The purpose of the address was to show that many graduates are so ignorant of sanitation that they have no idea of the importance of a health department. We are much surprised at all this, as some of our high schools years ago gave excellent courses. The point is a good one, and must be taken up by our educators. The great campaign of publicity and education which sanitarians find they must constantly wage is too great a drain on their time and energies. It seems that they must give reasons for existence, whereas that should be taken for granted, and would be so taken if the colleges properly prepared students for citizenship. The excuse of lack of time from the already overcrowded curriculum is not only nonsense, but a confession of a badly arranged course of instruction. Omit a little Greek, and turn out fewer men who can quote ancient classics but do not know what killed off the classic writers. We then would not have to convince citizens of the vital necessity of destroying mosquito breeding places. Prof. Menzies is right—let Chicago University set us an example of common sense. Incidentally let us remark that more than one educator has protested against the extremes to which the elective courses have been carried in a few colleges—abusing a most excellent and necessary system. The average college boy does not know what he wants nor even at what he can make his living. He must be compelled to take more than he likes of some things—sanitation for instance—and confine his electives to the last year or two in preparation for his technical studies in the University.

One hundred thousand parents in New York City are unable to raise their babies! The Board of Health is reported as estimating that of the 250,000 children less than two years of age, 50,000 are in need of society's care, and we see no reason to doubt the accuracy of the estimate—indeed 43,000 are already reported as receiving assistance. What is to be the outcome of this wholesale preservation of incompetency? We may safely assume that the children when grown will be as incompetent to raise off-spring as their parents have been. Is society to be largely composed of people kept in existence by taxing the competent? It certainly looks so, as we cannot possibly permit the slaughter of the innocents by cold blooded refusal to help the health authorities. Nevertheless, we would like to ask the helping hands what they propose to do to the parents who are thus increasing public burdens through sheer lust? It is an evil, and every evil has a prevention. What is it to be in this case? Give it a thought please. It takes six hundred dollars a year to raise three babies, according to our social workers, so how would it do as a starter, to disfranchise the man with six children but unable to earn more than four hundred dollars a year? Is it not time to punish the men who let their babies go to school hungry? We do not refer to the children who are able to work for part of their living, for no common laborer can support them in any part of the world. If we force them to school, it is our duty to feed them. New conditions face us and new policies are demanded.

Abolition of small-pox quarantine seems to be getting popular. Boards of Health are apparently taking the view that the sick have some rights the healthy must respect. A small-pox patient is considered harmless to those who have been successfully vaccinated, and society has no concern as to those who foolishly decline to be protected. So it is decided here and there to allow the patient to stay at home under his own physician and nurse, and close up the pest house as a needless expense. The patient's house is, of course, to be placarded or flagged plainly to warn the public, but the inmates are to go out freely if they wish even if they do carry the infection. Society is tired of protecting those who will not protect themselves. It is another matter whether we shall carry this reasoning to its legitimate conclusion and permit unvaccinated children to come to school. They do not carry small-pox around with them, and if the disease appears in their homes, they are promptly down with it and will be kept from school until they are no longer dangerous. The kink in the reasoning is the fact that they might come to school with a mild case, and jeopardize the children whom we think have been protected but who in reality are not—a danger we all run as no human thing is perfect and we can not be sure that our operation has perfectly succeeded. This is a very nice question to decide and will undoubtedly be fought out in the courts. Already the anti-vaccinationists are taunting the health authorities with inconsistency—an amazing taunt from such illogical folks. Nevertheless courts are listening to their question, "If vaccination does protect your children, why are you so afraid of mine?" Unless we answer, the whole system of compulsion collapses as far as the school is concerned. Why would it not be a good plan to ignore the antis, and then if the unvaccinated children get small-pox, put the parents in jail for criminal neglect? These abnormal people have "fixed ideas," which cannot be eradicated. They resent force and

will ignore compulsory laws as they always have done. They have enough influence to defeat such bills in legislatures and the only thing to do is to insist on punishment when the neglect causes disease. Prevention has proved impossible.

————

The superior physical development of pupils of private schools is a fact, according to Dr. Sargent of Harvard, and perhaps it is due to inheritance from parents whose superior physique was a large factor in their success as money getters. In England the upper classes are notoriously better developed than the lower, and many are in families which established their fortunes by brawn as well as brain. In addition, the well-to-do are able to feed their children better than those nearer the poverty line, and this one factor of better nutrition is enough of itself to account for the differences Sargent finds. He is inclined to believe that public school boys do not work enough, but one would presume that they exercise more—particularly those who have real work in place of play.

The alleged superior mentality of public school boys is a difficult matter to explain and one is inclined to deny it as contrary to heredity. Perhaps Sargent is confusing mentality with scholarly acquirements, as it is notoriously true that the more pampered do not acquire "book-learning" as early or as well as the poor. Yet the delay of the former does not seem to do any particular harm and there is plenty of evidence that it does plenty of good. Besides all this, one of the best established facts of anthropology is the necessity for early mental maturity in lower species and races and the consequent rapid mental development of the young. A puppy six months old is the mental superior of a baby that old. Higher evolution has not only created a bigger and more highly organized brain, but one which necessarily is of slower development. Negro and Indian children always surpass whites, who seem positively stupid in comparison. This same law has been found among classes in any one race, and fully accounts for the poor scholarship of boys who subsequently do great things. Our universities could easily settle the matter by comparing the careers of students who, early brilliant in acquisition, with the achievements of those who were poor in scholarship at first but who found themselves later. We cannot believe that the most successful classes have the least intelligent children. Doing things for one's self and learning what others have done, are two entirely different matters, and divide the world into two classes—the history makers and history recorders.

Calcium starvation is the last of the systemic conditions under investigation by modern scientific dietetics. Excess or deficiency of lime salts has been blamed for all kinds of diseases—indeed there was once quite a fad in that direction, so the literature is voluminous. Yet every time we have apparently found a true indictment, some one has rushed to the defense with evidence establishing an alibi. There is so much lime in the ordinary foods, it is difficult to believe the small amounts in the drinking water have any effect one way or the other. Yet it seems to be proved by a German dentist that dental caries is less frequent in places where there is plenty of lime in the water. Perhaps other coincident factors have been overlooked. Caries was once quite defi-

nitely correlated with diseases which afflicted the child at the time those teeth were developing in the gums—long before eruption. We cannot settle such problems off hand, as there are too many factors in nutrition and development. To work on only one at a time warps us, so that we may ignore more important ones. Rickets, for instance, has many remote causes—even heredity has been blamed— and yet many believe lime deficiency in the food to be the sole cause. As for blaming such deficiency for tuberculosis, we had better go slow. We need have no fear of boiled water when typhoid is threatened. The few grains of lime deposited by the heat are made up in a glass of sterile milk —and besides boiling does not throw down all the lime.

The myth of Japanese medical excellence has at last been destroyed. Lieutenant-Colonel J. E. Kuhn, Corps of Engineers of the U. S. Army, who was with the Japanese during their late war, has recently said in a lecture at Fort Leavenworth: "In the matter of disease the Japanese were, after all, not so remarkably fortunate as popularly supposed." Cols. Hoff and Harvard, who were with the Russians, mentioned, in their reports, some excellent results on that side. Now come the official figures from both sides and published from time to time in the *Journal of Royal Army Medical Corps* of Great Britain. A comparison shows that the Russian deaths and sickness were about half those of the Japanese, and evidently the Russians performed some excellent surgery besides. In spite of all this, *The Military Surgeon* of July, 1912, says: "Any discussion of advances in military sanitation would be incomplete if no reference were made to the splendid work of the Japanese in the Russo-Japanese War." Some kind friend should whisper to the writer of the above, that it is time to wake up.

The arteriosclerosis controversy seems to be getting more complicated instead of clearing up the etiology. The latest word is a protest against misinterpretation of experiments. In *Science* not long ago, Klotz of the University of Pittsburgh takes vigorous exception to the conclusions of Levin and Larkin (*Jour. Exper. Med.*, 1911, xiii, p. 24) who state that "arteriosclerosis cannot be artificially induced in a previously healthy blood-vessel by a change in the blood pressure alone." He reminds them that the results in veins can not be compared to the arterial changes, and that compensation by new anastomoses quickly reduces high blood pressure resulting from joining an artery to a vein. Besides all this, it is suggested that intermittent high pressure as in man and horses is more effective than continuous high pressure. There is a general impression that increased pressure alone is fully competent to account for the condition, but it is now evident that we need considerable more evidence to settle the matter to everyone's satisfaction.

The toxic origin of arteriosclerosis has many adherents, but there is now a differentiation of views and only those poisons which increase blood pressure are generally considered as harmful. Indeed it is thought that fatigue poisons may be the cause in those who undergo undue exertion, and not the arterial tension during the exercise. It certainly is remarkable that the carnivorous cats and dogs rarely develop arteriosclerosis though pre-eminently subjected to intense activity, but that herbivora like horses and rabbits oc-

casionally have the condition "spontaneously." The facts suggest that a too great dependence on a vegetable diet may be a factor in men who have not led strenuous lives—though as a fact it is rare to find a case without a history of overexertion in early life, athletics to excess, or laborious employments, or the right radial thickening of blacksmiths, and the femoral of policemen. Old animals like old men, get thickened arteries far more often than the young, and we do not know whether this is the result of long continued strains or poisonings or merely due to the fact that the material is not designed for so long a use. That is, we may all live too long for our tissues.

The quality of our tubing is least often mentioned but it may turn out to be most important. There is a lot of evidence that the disease attacks the degenerate by preference. It is often accompanied by other congenital abnormalities showing that these persons are damaged by causes that are harmless to the average or normal. The matter deserves more consideration than it has received. Jacobi (*Arch. of Diag.* Ap. 1911) states that pulmonary hyperplasia with secondary cirrhosis is a frequent and frequently independent disease, and there are many who have similar views as to cirrhosis in other organs where high pressure is the usual explanation. There is such a universal belief that a diet of meats rich in purin bodies is the pre-eminent cause of high pressure and arteriosclerosis in man, that it is quite a shock to find that cats and dogs are free of it. But then, so many old hypotheses have been shocked to death in the last two decades, that we ought now to be accustomed to seeing these healthy brain-children join their fathers.

The fate of the dolicho-cephalic blond race is unnecessarily worrying our good friends of Europe. Prof. Retzins of Stockholm made the matter the subject of the Huxley lecture he recently delivered to the British Royal Anthropological Institute. It has long been known that this special type of man was evolved in a dark cloudy cold climate to which he is now so perfectly adjusted that he cannot migrate too far away from it with impunity. All this has been known for nearly a half century though our backward life insurance statisticians are just beginning to hear of it. When they found an inordinately high death rate in any place, they were inclined to stop doing business there or charge such high premiums as to be prohibitive. Now they are realizing that not all types are equally affected, and that the premature death of such men as the late Governor Johnson of Minnesota means something of business importance. Retzins is now alarmed over another fact known for a half century;—that these modern vikings cannot stand confinement of any sort, and that to flourish they must live in the open. Not only do such types disappear from cities which are always more brunet than the surrounding population even as far north as Glasgow, but also modern factory life is specially fatal to them. He finds that the brunet types are swarming in modern industrial conditions and is afraid that the poor blond is to be elbowed out of existence. He needn't worry, the blond type has enough brains to make a living in other and better ways than in such a confining specialty as standing before a machine, pegging shoes. They are instinctively clinging to the old normal village life by moving to the suburbs of every city and also taking up outdoor employments. As a remote consequence we find ships swarming with them, and recent observations show that northern armies are largely composed of them—even our own army

is essentially a blue-eyed one. In all parts of the world they are becoming more and more numerous as foremen, bosses and managers.

The management of blond patients is the practical point, particularly for physicians in the larger cities. A permanent cure of a case may be impossible if he is occupied in some confining city occupation. Change of employment or even removal to a village or country environment may be essential. The dreadful ultimate results in tuberculosis, for instance, might be prevented if we would not allow a "cured" or "arrested" case to return to the environment which broke down his resistance; while a case which ordinarily thrives in modern industrial conditions might be injured by sending him away. Why do not our specialists inform us what kind of cases are so easily cured at home as so frequently reported? Similarly in every other disease let us know the facts so that we can stop the blond mortality which Retzins and others have so persistently reported from adverse environments. Nevertheless, even if we do not succeed in checking the process no one need worry about the disappearance of these true Aryans as long as their birth rate at "home" is so enormous. They will find ways of surviving and there is no cause for worry. Moreover there will be an ample surplus to stream into America to replace the dead. All the blonds have died out from the original French population of New Orleans, but that city is full of blonds who have wandered in, later to disappear like the lamented late health officer of that city. The point of the matter to the blue eyed folks already here, is that they want to know what are the dangers which have done up their predecessors. The medical profession and particularly life insurance examiners can tell—if they only would.

November, 1912.
New Series, Vol. VII., No. 11. } ORIGINAL ARTICLES { AMERICAN MEDICINE
Complete Series, Vol. XVIII. 603

ORIGINAL ARTICLES.

THE TREATMENT OF PULMONARY TUBERCULOSIS BY MEANS OF GRADUATED REST AND EXERCISE.

BY

OLIVER BRUCE, M. R. C. S., L. R. C. P.

London, Eng.

The subject I have chosen, the treatment of tuberculosis by means of graduated rest and exercise, is one with which few are familiar, and since anything which adds to our knowledge of how to combat pulmonary tuberculosis to the best advantage must be welcome to all, I need offer no excuse for going into the subject in its minutiae.

Probably the bare outlines and general principles of the graduated labor system of treatment are known to most physicians, but an intimate knowledge of the means by which it acts is only arrived at after some experience and is absolutely essential before one can hope to apply it practically with any success. For though not, perhaps, an exact science, yet it has an entirely scientific basis and not merely an empirical one.

Before one can obtain this knowledge, however, it is necessary to study to some extent the subject of immunity and the action of bacteria on the blood. In diphtheria we do not make a prognosis of any case on the local condition alone but far more on the extent to which the diphtherial poison is invading the blood stream. Or again in a pus infection or abscess, although we attend with scrupulous care to the locality of the infection, yet it is only with a view to preventing if possible the invasion of the blood stream by the pus organisms, in other words

blood poisoning, and it is on this we base our prognosis, our expectations of the course the disease will pursue. And yet in pulmonary tuberculosis, likewise a bacterial infection, how many physicians rely solely on the local condition and on what they hear through the stethoscope!

You are all doubtless aware that the blood consists of a fluid substance, the plasma, which holds in suspension millions of little cells, which give the fluid its characteristic color, and white cells or leucocytes. It is with the action and properties of these latter cells that we need now concern ourselves. These cells are, so to speak, the scavengers of the body, for the part they play in the metabolism of the tissues is the removal of all noxious substances which may happen to gain access to the body and amongst these are bacteria of all kinds.

Inflammation of any part is due to a flushing of that part with blood which contains a large number of these white cells and the pus which forms consists simply of millions of these little cells for which the poison has been too strong and has destroyed them. They are ameboid in movement, surround the offending object, ingest and destroy it. On account of this action they have been given the name phagocytes and the phenomenon of the destruction of offending substances has been termed phagocytosis.

It was at once evident that an immensely important part was played in disease by these minute cells, especially in bacterial disease. In fact, it was at first thought by Metchnikoff and his school at the Pasteur Institute that these cells were the only factor in the destruction of germs; that it was merely necessary for the cells to be brought into contact with the germs to take them up and destroy them. But that this idea was an entirely erroneous one was proved beyond question by Sir A. E. Wright in his researches at St. Mary's Hospital, London. There he showed, and his results have been since confirmed by other observers, that a third substance was necessary for the phenomenon of phagocytosis. White cells and bacteria mixed together *in vitro* and incubated give rise to no phagocytosis, but add to them some blood serum and we get the desired effect. If we examine a film of this latter mixture under a microscope we shall find numbers of the bacteria lying within the bodies of the cells whereas in the first instance they all lay outside the cell walls. Now the germs and white cells were common to both experiments, therefore, there is some substance present in blood serum which acts on the white cells in such a way as to enable them to take up and destroy the germs, an action they do not possess of themselves. This chemical substance Wright after many experiments discovered and named opsonin. Carrying his researches still further he was able to demonstrate that the amount of opsonin present in the blood serum of healthy individuals was always the same. For on mixing a definite number of white cells and germs together with one healthy person's serum the number of germs eaten up by the cells would be approximately the same as on mixing the same number of cells and germs with the serum taken from another person in good health. Not so, however, if we substitute the serum of a person suffering from a bacterial infection, such for instance as tuberculosis. We shall then find that the 100 cells have eaten up either a greater or lesser number of the germs than in the case of the healthy serum, and the ratio of one to the other may be called the opsonic index, an indication as to the amount of this substance opsonin present

in a person's blood. Thus if 100 cells under the influence of the healthy serum phagocyte 310 bacteria and under the influence of the infected serum 425 bacteria the opsonic index will be $425/310 = 1.37$ compared with a normal index of 1.00. Obviously then this opsonin is a protective substance which helps the body to eliminate invading germs by means of its action on the white cells. The experiment of the estimation of the opsonic index opens up a very valuable aid to diagnosis, for anyone having an index outside the normal limits should be strongly suspected, at least, of infection. Now, though theoretically speaking, a normal index should always be at 1.00, yet in practice it is found owing to the delicacy of the technique, to vary within certain limits. These have been set at 1.20 and 0.80 and any index outside these figures is considered an abnormal one. At the same time it must be pointed out that in itself one negative result is of little value for at some time or other even infected people's serum will contain a normal quantity of protective substance. Two or more observations should be taken. The first sample of blood should be drawn while the patient is at rest; then some form of exertion should be taken, such as a walk, and another one or two samples of blood drawn some time after the exertion. Then if all three or four samples be within normal limits the assumption is that no disease is present.

Wright discovered during the course of his researches that it was possible to remove all the opsonin for a certain organism from a sample of serum by saturating it with that organism for a considerable time; at the end of that time he found that if he mixed that sample of serum with some white cells and an emulsion of that organism, no phagocytosis took place. If, however, he substituted some other germ he found that phagocytosis did occur, showing that such microorganism has its own specific opsonin. The property of this substance, however, which concerns us most in the study of pulmonary tuberculosis and its treatment by means of graduated labor is that the amount present in the blood serum of an infected person can be made to vary at will by certain means. It is as has been shown a protective substance and makes for health and so it is obviously desirable to raise the quantity present in the serum of all infected people. Wright found that certain things affected the opsonic index and in a specific way. For instance in the case of a gonococcal joint, massage and movement will bring about a strong local reaction accompanied by pain and fever. This reaction moreover is attended by a drop in the opsonic content of the blood to below normal. All bacterial diseases are due, not so much to the actual presence of the germs in the tissues but to the fact that the germs throw a poison into the blood stream. But this is not the only action they perform, for this throwing out of toxin, if the dose be not too great, stimulates the tissues to manufacture this antitoxin or opsonin. Thus massage in the case of joint disease, and exertion in the case of a lung lesion cause the germs to throw out a dose of poison, this tends to excite the tissues to manufacture more opsonin and so we get the variations in the index. It is exactly analogous to what happens in vaccination for smallpox or inoculations with tuberculin. As Wright pointed out a certain train of events follows whether it be an artificial inoculation by means of a syringe or an artificial autoinoculation by means of massage or exercise. Immediately follow-

ing the administration of the dose he observed a drop in the opsonic content of the blood and this he termed the negative phase. At a greater or lesser interval according to the size of the dose, a positive phase followed during which the opsonic index was above the normal. This in time gave place to what he termed a phase of maintained high level during which the index returned nearly to the point whence it started.

Graduated labor is a service of artificial autoinoculations. Now a patient with advanced disease, showing a high temperature every evening in spite of being at rest in bed is undergoing a series of excessive autoinoculations accompanied by a fluctuating opsonic index. This means that the dose of poison thrown out by his germs into the blood stream is so great that an insufficient amount of protective substance is formed. If the opsonic index of such a patient be examined at certain intervals over a period of 24 hours it will be found that when his temperature is high his opsonic index is low and vice versa. The opsonic index in other words varies inversely with the temperature. This is a most important point which was brought to light in the course of over 300 blood examinations performed by Dr. A. C. Inman and myself at the Brompton Hospital. For in regulating the amount of exercise to be prescribed in graduated labor, some guide is necessary, some indication as to the amount of protective substances which are being elaborated as the result of the exercise. It would be found far too laborious a task to have to take the opsonic index as a guide and this knowledge enables us to substitute for it the temperature chart. The clinical symptoms and feelings of the patient, however, must be very carefully studied at the same time.

There has been much controversy as to the reliability of the opsonic index, but in a paper such as this I cannot, of course, go into so vexed a question. I should like, however, to describe a certain experiment which more than anything else impressed me with its value. When Dr. Inman and I started our work at the Brompton Hospital the physicians were very sceptical about it and tried in every way they could to trap us. They sent us for examination amongst other samples of blood those of three cases of bronchiectasis in which no tubercle bacilli had been found by the house physicians. We estimated their opsonic indices and made two of them abnormal to tubercle and one normal. We then proceeded to examine the sputa in each case by carbolizing and centrifugalizing it and by these means were able to demonstrate the undoubted presence of the tubercle bacilli in the two abnormal cases, finding none, however, in the normal case.

We have then two main facts to work on, that the amount of opsonin or antibody in the blood can be raised by exercise and that the temperature chart and feelings of the patient are a sufficient guide to an experienced observer as to whether the amount of exercise prescribed is too great or too little.

Paterson has fixed the danger mark, the point signifying excessive autoinoculation, at 99° F. in the case of men and 99.6° F. in the case of women. Our first object therefore in every case is to reduce the temperature to below these points and this, of course, we do by rest in bed. Ordinary rest in bed will usually attain this object, but it is an interesting fact discovered by Paterson and Inman, that if what is known as "absolute rest" is prescribed the temperature will return to normal more quickly still. By absolute rest is meant the treatment prescribed in typhoid fever where the patient is not allowed to move for any purpose whatever. Now when this point has been reached and the patient's temperature has been continuously below the normal for ten days we know that excessive autoinoculation has been checked and that his output of antibodies is sufficient to cope with his poisons. It is at this point that other methods of treatment stop short. For if nothing more than rest and forced feeding be prescribed there will be no stimulation of the tissues to form antibodies in excess of poisons. This point too was clearly shown during the course of our investigations. We examined the blood of many patients while at rest or on unchecked walking exercise at the Brompton Hospital and again the same patients while on strict graduated labor at the sanatorium. In every case on the former treatment the opsonic indices were low, and in every case the latter treatment raised them high above normal. This is why graduated labor is so far superior to other methods. Our object then is to raise the patient's opsonic index above the normal line and it has been shown that this can be done by means of exertion. The exertion, however, must not be too great or the output of toxins will swamp the tissues and an exactly opposite result to that which we desire will occur.

It is my practice to prescribe as the first step, an hour a day out of bed, sitting in a chair. If no rise of temperature occurs, on the third day I allow the patient to dress himself for the hour he is up, as the act of dressing after a long period in bed is a trying one. Still keeping a careful watch on the temperature chart and feelings of the patient I gradually increase the number of hours spent out of bed to two, four, six, eight and ten hours with an interval of two days between each increase, until finally the patient is getting up for the whole day, though doing no more than rest in a chair. If from time to time we examine such a patient's opsonic index, we will find it is tending to rise, but not to any very great extent. We are gradually immunizing him to larger doses of poison but we want to carry it further still and raise his opsonic content as high as we possibly can. This we can only do by giving him bigger doses of poison and so the next step is to order him walking exercise which must be very carefully graduated or the dose will be too great. I start my patient at half a mile a day, walking quite slowly and preferably over gently undulating ground. The distance is gradually increased until finally he is walking six miles a day.

The patient should lie down for an hour after each period of exercise and this "rest hour" should be as vigorously enforced as is the exercise, for it is then that the positive phase should take place and the protective substances be elaborated. Any rise of temperature to the "danger mark" or over indicates excessive exertion and should be dealt with accordingly. The point has now been reached when the patient is walking six miles a day without any rise of temperature. During all this time, however, he has only been using the muscles of his lower limbs and as the muscles of his arms and trunk have more effect on the expansion of his lungs some form of exercise which will bring these into play should be the next step. It is from this point that the real "labor" part of the system begins and I think I cannot do better than tabulate shortly the various grades as performed at the Brompton Hospital Sanatorium. In all the grades the work is carried on for four hours a day.

Grade I.—Small baskets. A weight of about 10 pounds of mould or other material is collected into baskets and carried a distance of about fifty yards, total weight carried about 8½ cwt.; distance traveled about 7 miles. For this may be substituted such tasks as light weeding, potting, picking out seedlings, picking off dead flowers, watering plants and painting. Time spent on this grade one week.

Grade II.—Larger baskets. A weight of about 18 pounds is carried a distance of about 50 yards; total weight carried about 15 cwt.; distance traveled about 7 miles. For this may be substituted weeding with hand fork, planting out in open ground, cutting vegetables and watering plants. Time spent on this grade one week.

Grade III.—Sweeping paths and grass, cutting grass edges, chopping firewood, hoeing, painting with large brush and cleaning windows. Time spent on this grade one week.

Grade IV.—Using a small shovel or digging with a small fork. Five men can pull a hand cart containing soil or stones, mowing grass or rolling. Time spent on this grade two weeks.

Grade V.—Using large shovel or pick axe or digging with large fork. Pulling down trees and trenching ground 3 feet deep, hauling stones, etc., in cart, using wheelbarrow and doing general heavy navvy work. Sawing and planing. Time spent on this grade three weeks.

Grade VI.—Similar to Grade V, patients working for six hours a day instead of four.

The work for the women should be slightly modified. Small baskets should carry a weight of 8 pounds and large baskets 15 pounds. Besides this they can sweep paths, do light gardening, clean out small chicken houses and prepare food for the chickens. Their final grade should consist in scrubbing floors and such heavy work as they may have to perform at home.

Naturally such a routine as I have sketched here will be found too ambitious for a small sanatorium containing but 30 or 40 patients. Moreover the different conditions which prevail in Canada, especially in the winter months, will necessitate a modification of this routine and some difficulty will be experienced owing to the land being snowbound. Much of this difficulty will disappear, however, if one considers that any work will serve the same purpose provided the amount of energy expended be proportionate.

At the Byron Sanatorium during the winter months I instituted the following forms of work: Collecting small wood into heaps for kindling purposes, sawing trees into lengths with a cross-cut saw for burning in the various furnaces, and shovelling snow. Now more outdoor work is possible and the men are employed in various forms of gardening such as cutting out and digging up new flower beds and manuring them, hoeing, weeding and raking, also painting gates, fly screens, etc. The women in removing stones from ploughed land, weeding and hoeing. Dumbbell exercises and skipping too have proved a very useful form of exercise for both sexes as an adjunct to outdoor work.

The patient should be gradually immunized to harder forms of labor until finally he is able to work for 6 hours a day at the most strenuous exercise that can be found for him without any rise of temperature. At the same time the work, if possible, should always have some aim and object apart from its curative function or it will become uninteresting and tedious.

When Paterson originated the graduated labor system of treatment he had no knowledge of the scientific basis which was the real cause of its success. Wright's epoch-making work had not then been given to the world and the action of bacteria on the blood was but very imperfectly understood. Paterson instituted it from merely common

sense motives for he said clearly that previous methods did not go far enough towards raising the resistance of patients and making them fit for work. It would be necessary for all his patients to return to work at the conclusion of their treatment and he knew that after a regime of rest and milk they would very soon break down again. His idea, therefore, was to raise their muscles to such a high state of resistance that they would be able to perform the hardest work without detriment. He had noticed that many of his cases had been working hard right up to the day of admission to the sanatorium without harm. "If consumptive persons under adverse circumstances and without any medical guidance could act in such a way, ought they not to be able, under ideal conditions and with the work carefully graduated to suit their physical condition, to perform useful labor?" In these words he sums up his reasons for the great change he intended to make in the treatment of the consumptive. A few years later Wright published his work and Inman's investigations put the whole system on a thoroughly scientific footing.

Our examinations of the bloods of the Frimley patients went to prove that all Dr. Paterson's conclusions and theories were correct. Were we to ask him for the blood of a patient with a high opsonic index he was able to pick one out, or if that of a man with a low index, again such a patient was found and invariably he was right. From this it can be seen that though the opsonic index is the best guide to the amount of protective substances each patient is elaborating in response to the exercise, yet with experience the temperature chart and clinical symptoms of the individual can be made to take its place. This scientific knowledge however has been of inestimable value in another direction as well. Up to this time Dr. Paterson had been obliged to work very carefully in increasing each patient's exercise for fear of an overdose. These fears were then proved groundless and as a result the same number of beds can now accommodate 40% more patients in the year than when graduated labor had to stand on its own merits with no scientific proof at its back.

The blood examinations afforded convincing proof that the work actually did result in autoinoculations with the patient's own antibacterial products.

It was a striking feature of these investigations the very high indices the majority of the patients showed as the result of the labor and moreover it was noticed that the harder the work performed the higher rose the index.

There were, however, some patients who were apparently marking time. Although in good condition they did not appear to be deriving the full amount of benefit from the particular grade of work they were on and in some cases even they had occasional rises of temperature. Dr. Paterson thought that perhaps what this type of patient needed was still harder work. Accordingly they were promoted to a yet higher grade with a successful result and when we investigated the bloods of these patients the reason for this was made manifest. The first grade of work had not been sufficient to excite a satisfactory stimulus on the part of the tissues to manufacture antibodies and their indices were low. On putting them onto the higher grade, however, the resulting stimulus was sufficient. There was a corresponding increase in the amount of opsonin formed and a rise in the index. This

rule has in consequence been followed ever since with success.

The effect of over-exertion was well shown in the case of several patients who on account of feeling so much benefit from the work become over-zealous and did too much against orders. These patients all had rises of temperature accompanied by a drop in the opsonic index as revealed by blood examinations. The same thing was recorded in the case of a musical patient who played the piano before he was in a fit state to do so. His temperature chart showed a rise to 101° and his index a drop to much below normal. This latter case emphasized the fact that rest is just as important as the work and should be rigorously enforced.

The next fact that was revealed by these investigations, perhaps the most interesting of any, was that whereas patients on the higher grades of work showed very high indices, the same patients when on the final grade and ready to be discharged had indices which never varied from the normal, however hard the work. The reason for this is that when the final grade is reached their lesion is so shut off from the blood stream by fibrous tissue that no toxins can be poured into the circulation and consequently there is no need for the formation of antibodies above the normal amount. Such patients are in the true sense of the word cured and may be discharged with confidence. It would be an ideal state of affairs if at the conclusion of the treatment of every consumptive person a series of indices could be taken to determine if the hardest work was having any effect at all on his antibacterial output or not. If any of the indices proved to be abnormal, then further treatment would be indicated, but if not, then the patient might return to his occupation without fear.

After the Brompton Hospital Sanatorium had been opened some 18 months and further experience gained, it was seen that many patients who had a rise of temperature to 99° F. as the result of over-exertion, were not only none the worse for it, but in most cases actually better. This is explained by the fact that though the over-exertion had produced such a dose of toxin as to cause a marked negative phase, yet the response on the part of the tissues had been correspondingly great in the formation of opsonin and so good had resulted instead of harm. Such cases, however, cannot be too carefully watched and if headache or malaise accompany the rise of temperature, stringent measures must be taken. If on the other hand the rise of temperature is the only indication of over-exertion, after a few days walking exercise, the patient may be allowed to resume work in the grade in which he suffered from the temporary setback. Some patients even go so far as to say that they date their real improvement from one of these slightly excessive auto-inoculations.

There is, however, another side to the graduated labor system, and that is the mental and moral effect produced by the work. Patients are apt at first to be sullen and discontented when made to work, but as soon as they feel the great benefit which accrues their demeanor completely changes and they take to it with great zeal. For this reason it is often advisable to give them some occupation while they are confined to bed unless they are on "absolute" rest, for it prevents them from continually brooding over their ailment. As a certain eminent physician once put it, "no *fool* was ever cured of consumption," and it is a fact that the more determined a patient is in his own mind to get well the better will his progress be.

The conditions prevailing at the Brompton Hospital Sanatorium are obviously very different to those in any similar institution in Canada. To begin with it has its own hospital containing some 300 patients at its back, and therefore only the very best cases are picked out for treatment at the sanatorium. More important still is the fact that all patients, early and advanced cases alike, can be watched at the hospital, and any that improve can be selected for graduated labor treatment.

A sanatorium not having a hospital at its back must refuse all advanced cases, and yet we know that many of them could be cured if given the chance. In these days the extent of the disease is not so important a factor as it was considered to be in times past, for it is recognized that a man may have an advanced lesion extending over some years and at the same time may have a good resistance. Such a man will do better than one with a small and early lesion, but a poor resistance. There is, we know, a percentage of early cases, though happily a small one, on which no treatment will have any effect, however early it be instituted. There are probably two factors bringing about this state of affairs, a lowered resistance and a virulent type of organism. A hospital acts as a sifting ground for all these different types of cases, whereas a sanatorium acting by itself has to do its own sifting and it is impossible for the medical officers' prognosis to be always correct.

The patients at the Brompton Hospital Sanatorium number some 125 and this, added to the fact that there are very few patients confined to bed, enables them to undertake more ambitious work than can be done in most sanatoria in Canada. For example the patients have completed, entirely by their own labor, a reservoir capable of holding 500,000 gallons of water. For this purpose they cleared the land of trees, excavated it, mixed all the concrete and laid all the blocks of granite. A skilled engineer is kept on the staff for the special purpose of instructing them in the work and under his guidance they are now engaged in building an open air chapel and a Dutch garden.

It is found then that rules and regulations have to be most vigorously enforced. The patients are not allowed to abstain from work on account of inclement weather or indeed on any pretext whatever, save that of illness, for Dr. Paterson very rightly thinks that to work one day and not the next is harmful and opposed to the success of the system. Certainly it is a striking fact that despite periodical soakings the patients at Frimley are remarkably immune to colds and pneumonia and yet they may be seen working in all weathers.

A system of punishment for infringement of orders has been instituted. Passes are issued to patients on certain of the higher grades which permit them to take walks in the country instead of doing their ordinary work on one or two afternoons a week. If, however, any trouble is experienced in making them perform their allotted tasks, their next pass is suspended and as the privilege of these outings is very much appreciated it is seldom that the punishment has to be repeated. In order that the system may be successful it is absolutely necessary to have in force very stringent rules and regulations though they need not be quite so rigorous in this country as in England where the class of patient is somewhat different.

It should be explained to every patient on admission in what the system consists and that he will be ordered a certain amount of rest and a certain amount of work, and that this is now more important than any medicine, and is in itself a form of treatment and nothing else. Further, it should be pointed out that as he himself will not know how much exercise should be taken at any time, he must be guided absolutely by the medical officers' orders, for while too much exercise will result in harm, too little will not secure the amount of benefit required.

At the Byron Sanatorium I also give the patients short lectures at intervals, explaining how the system works, and I find that it gives them a greater interest in their cure, besides making them see it is for their own benefit and not for the benefit of the institution.

To sum up, the graduated labor system of treatment is an effort at the scientific cure of the consumptive. It aims at raising the amount of antibacterial substance in his blood to as high a degree as possible and keeping it there by gradually increasing doses of his own tuberculin.

BINET'S TESTS FOR BACKWARD CHILDREN; CRITICISM AND IMPROVEMENTS.[1]

BY

SIEGFRIED BLOCK, A. M., M. D.,

Brooklyn, N. Y.

As far back as 1877, H. C. Wilbur read a paper before the Association of Medical Officers of American Institutions. In part he said: "Do we not need some effective form of description of our cases,

[1] Read before a stated meeting of the Brooklyn Neurological Society, Feb. 7, 1912.

some generally recognized tests of physical and mental conditions that will show the starting point in the pupil's career, to which reference can be made from time to time to test their absolute or relative progress? Do we not need some mile posts along in the educational path to the same end?" (Barr).

Until recently there has been no way of speaking and writing of a case of mental deficiency in exact terms, without giving a full description or going into minute details. Even then, one observer would call a case very defective, another would say mildly so, a third might simply say backward or retarded; thus it remained for the late Professors Binet and Simon to invent a scheme of classification and gradation. They used the various ages as mile posts of the degrees of intelligence. Now when one speaks of the "intelligence of a six year old child" in a general way we know what is meant, no matter if physiologically the child is twelve.

For this purpose they have devised eleven groups of tests, each group applicable respectively to one year of the ages ranging from three to thirteen. If the child succeeds in correctly answering the questions in the test for his age, the child is normal. If he can answer only those intended for an individual a year younger he is a year behind for his age, likewise for two, three or more years. If more than three years behind he is called defective.

Binet has adopted a few rules, as: "A subject has the mentality for the highest age, for which he has been able to answer all the tests in a group but one. For example, if a boy answers all the tests in the eight-year group save one, and all the nine-year group except one he may still be

credited with nine-year mentality. There is another arbitrary rule Binet used, let a child's mentality be properly fixed, he is to be advanced a year for each five higher tests in which he succeeds, two years for each ten, etc. For instance, if John is nine years old, and he fails in two of the nine-year tests he would be mentally only eight. But if he succeeds in three in the nine-year test, and three of the ten-year making six in all, he is advanced a grade and called nine, or normal.

This seems most artificial, but Binet claims to have "tried it out." I will read you briefly the original tests without comment (Goddard's Translation) except to emphasize the fact that these are only tests not material for teaching purposes. They have and still are continuing to take like wild-fire. If wanted for scientific purposes however, they should not be undertaken by anyone except an experienced psychologist. They may aid in giving the general man some sort of an idea of a child's mentality, but for anything like exactitude only such persons as I mentioned should be entrusted for a result.

CHILDREN OF THREE YEARS.

1. Where is your nose? Your eyes? Your mouth?
One of the best signs of awakening intelligence in young children is the comprehension of spoken words. We test this by asking these questions which can be answered by a gesture.
2. Repetition of sentences of six syllables.
It rains. I am hungry (6 syl.).
Experiment proves that it is easier for a child to repeat words than to speak a word of his own.
If a child does not respond one may try him with two syllables (mamma), then four, etc.
A child of three repeats six syllables but not ten. There must not be a single error.

3. Repetition of figures. "6-4" figures. Figures require closer attention than words because they mean nothing to him. Pronounce the figures distinctly, one-half second apart and without emphasis on any one figure.

4. Describing pictures.

A picture is shown to the child with the question, "What do you see?" The pictures must be chosen with some care. Each one must represent some people and a situation. Binet used three pictures. The first is a man and a boy drawing a cart loaded with furniture. The second a woman and an old man sitting on a bench in a park in winter. The third a man in prison looking out of a window; a couch, chair and tables. A child of three names the things— enumerates. He does not describe any actions in the pictures.

5. Name of the family.

All children of three know their first name. They sometimes know the family name but not always.

CHILDREN OF FOUR YEARS.

1. Sex of child. Are you a little boy or a girl? (of a boy—reverse for girls). Children of three do not know. Children of four always do.

2. Naming familiar objects.

One takes from his pocket a key, a knife, and a penny. The answer should indicate that a child knows what each is. This is more difficult use of language than naming objects in the pictures; there the child chose his own object to name; here we say, "What is that thing?"

3. Repetition of three figures. "7-2-9."

4. Comparison of two lines. "Which is the longer line?"

Draw two parallel lines three centimetres apart, the one five centimeters and the other six. Hesitation is failure.

CHILDREN OF FIVE YEARS.

1. Comparison of two weights. "Which is the heavier?"

Use weighted blocks of wood of equal size and appearance. Compare three grammes with 12 grammes and 6 grammes with 15 grammes. Note the curious and interesting errors that are made.

2. Copying a square.

Draw a square of three or four centimeters. Have child copy it with ink—

not pencil. Pen makes it harder. It is satisfactory if one can recognize the square.

3. Game of patience with two pieces. Cut a visiting card diagonally. Place a whole card on the table. Nearer the child place the two pieces with the two hypothenuses away from each other. Ask the child to make a figure like the uncut card. One child in twelve fails.

Be careful (1) that child does not fail because he is too indolent to reach out and try; (2) that one of the pieces does not get turned over—because then it is impossible; (3) that you do not show by a look whether the child is right or wrong.

4. Counting four pennies.

Place four pennies in a row. Insist that the child count them with his finger.

At three years a child does not know how to count four; at four, half succeed; at five all succeed.

CHILDREN OF SIX YEARS.

1. Right hand. Left ear.

One says to child "Show me your right hand" and when that is done "show me your left ear." There are, in the main, three kinds of response. (1) Does not know right and left. Shows right hand because of natural tendency. Shows right ear also. (2) Knows but is not sure. Shows right hand, then right ear but corrects himself at once. (3) Knows and without hesitation touches right hand and left ear. (2) and (3) are considered satisfactory. If child touches one hand with the other in such a way that one cannot tell which hand he means, ask him to hold his right hand up high. Be very careful in this test to give no hint by look or word. At four years no child points to left ear: at five half of the children make a mistake; at six all succeed.

2. Repetition of a sentence or group of sentences of 16 words.

Prepare sentences of familiar words, e. g., "Boys work on the farm: Girls work in the house; boys and girls go to school." Half of the children of five years do this: all do it at six.

3. Aesthetic comparison.

"Which is the prettier?"

Binet uses six heads of women in three pairs. the one pretty and the other ugly or even deformed. Fig. 1.

Care is taken that the pretty one is now at the left and now at the right. At six all choose correctly; at five, about half.

4. Definition of known objects. "What is a fork? A table? A chair? A horse? A mamma?"

There are three kinds of response. (1) Silence, simple repetition or gesture, e. g., "A fork is a fork," or pointing says "That is a chair." (2) Definition in terms of use, "A fork is to eat with." (3) Definitions better than by use. This includes all answers that describe the thing or even begin with "It is a thing," "It is an animal," etc., all of which expressions are not so childlike as the simple "use" definitions. In deciding which type of answer we shall credit to the child, we accept three out of five. At four years half the children define by "use"; it increases a little at five and at six practically all define this way. Not before nine do the majority give the definitions that are "better than by use."

5. Execution of three simultaneous commissions. "Do you see this key? Put it on that chair. Then shut the door. After that bring me the box that is on the table. Remember, first the key on the chair, then close the door, then bring in the box. Do you understand? Well, then, go ahead." Such are the directions. They must all be done without further help, hint or suggestion. At four years almost none can do this; at five, about half; at six, all, or nearly all succeed.

6. Age. "How old are you?"

Not until six do the great majority of children know their age.

7. Distinction between morning and afternoon. "Is this morning or is it afternoon?" It should be remembered that a certain type or child will always answer the last of two alternatives. Therefore, if the time is afternoon, it is well to put the question, "Is this afternoon or morning?" Not before six do children know this.

CHILDREN OF SEVEN YEARS.

1. Unfinished pictures. One shows four sketches of such as Fig. 2. Ask the child "What is lacking in that picture?" Child must answer three out of four correctly. At five years none are correct; at six errors number two-thirds, at seven the great majority are accurate.

2. Number of fingers. "*How* many fingers on your right hand? How many on your left hand? How many on both hands?"

Answers to all three questions must be given without hesitation and exactly right without counting. At six years only half the children know the number of their fingers.

3. Writing from copy. "The little Paul" or some sentence having two capital letters. The child is to use pen and ink. This is a test in which training enters, but the deviations from copy show much about the intelligence of the child. The test is "Passed" if the sentence can be read by one who is ignorant of the copy.

4. Copying a diamond.

Draw a rhombus about the size of the square used for age five. Have child copy this with pen. The result is satisfactory if it would be recognized as intended for a diamond shaped figure.

5. Repetition of five figures. "4-7-3-9-5." Same method of procedure as given above, age 3. Only three-fourths of the children succeed.

6. Description of a picture. Same picture as used in age three. Child now describes things instead of simply enumerating.

7. Counting thirteen pennies.

Pennies must be placed in a row and counted with the finger. Finger must touch the piece at the same time that the child names the number. No piece must be counted twice and none omitted. The number thirteen must be given exact. At six years two-thirds fail; at seven they make no errors.

8. Naming four common pieces of money—penny, nickel, dime, quarter.

This is the hardest of the seven year tests, but a great majority know the four pieces. At six hardly any know them.

CHILDREN OF EIGHT YEARS.

1. Reading for two "memories."

This test marks the limit between imbecility and feeble-mindedness. It is by a test of reading that we find out if a child is imbecile or feeble-minded. (Provided the effort has been made to teach him to read).

"Three Houses on Fire."

"New York, September 5th."

"A big fire in Hastings, last night, destroyed three large houses in the center of the village. Seventeen families are without shelter. The loss exceeds thirty thousand dollars, while rescuing a child in his cradle, a barber's boy has had his hands very seriously burned."

This test has a triple purpose. It assures us that the child knows how to read; measures the rapidity of reading and makes sure that he understands and retains a little of what he reads. The average time of reading these 53 words is as follows: Child of eight years, 45 seconds; nine years, 40 seconds; ten years, 30 seconds; eleven years, 25 seconds.

2. Count nine cents or stamps.

3. Compare two things from memory. "What is the difference between a butterfly and a fly?" "Wood and glass?" "Paper and pasteboard?" "Or cloth?"

The question may be differently put so as to make it intelligible as possible, e. g., two at least out of three pairs should be answered correctly. If it takes more than two minutes it is a failure.

At six a third of the children do this test; at seven, nearly all; at eight, all.

CHILDREN OF NINE YEARS.

1. Name the day of the week, the month, the day of the month, and the year.

The test is passed even if the day of the month is as much as three days wrong. Children least often know the year.

2. The days of the week.

These must be given in order without omission within ten seconds. Most persons would expect that this could be done before age nine, but it cannot.

3. Make change. Nine cents out of twenty-five.

Play store, using real money. If child's cash consists of twenty-five pennies, 5 nickels, and two dimes, interesting degrees of intelligence will be discovered by noticing the coins he uses in making change. Child is store keeper. One buys something that costs nine cents. Child must actually give sixteen cents as well as say it.

At seven no one can do this test; at eight a good third succeed; at nine all do it.

4. Definition better than by "use."

This was explained under age six. At ages 7 and 8, half the children give definitions of this kind. At nine they all do.

5. The six "memories" from reading.

See under eight years. At eight hardly anyone has six "memories."

6. Arrangement of weights.

Use five wooden cubes of same size and appearance but loaded so as to weigh 6, 9, 12, 15, 18 grammes. "Metal pill boxes may be used. Place the five boxes on table in front of child and explain that they do not all weigh alike and he is to lift them one at a time and put them in order from the lightest to the heaviest. (The initial of each weight written on the bottom of each box makes it easy to see if they are right). Record the exact order in which the child has placed them. Three trials are made. Two must be absolutely correct. The whole operation must not take over three minutes.

CHILDREN OF TEN YEARS.

1. The months of the year. Recited in order within fifteen seconds. Allow one omission or transposition.

2. Naming nine pieces of money.

3. Using three words in a sentence.

4. Questions of comprehension. First series. *What ought one to do:*

(a) When one has missed the train?

(b) When one has been struck by a playmate who did not do it purposely?

(c) When one has broken something that does not belong to one?

At seven and eight half respond correctly; at nine three-fourths; at ten all. If two questions out of three are answered correctly the test is passed.

SECOND SERIES.

a. When he is detained so that he will be late for school?

b. What ought one to do before taking part in an important affair?

c. Why does one excuse a wrong act committed in anger more easily than a wrong act committed without anger?

d. What should one do when asked his opinion of some one whom he knows only a little?

e. Why ought one to judge a person more by his acts than by his words? Allow at least twenty seconds to each question.

Three of the five must be answered correctly. At seven and eight no one responds to a majority of this second series; at ten half are successful; it is therefore a transition between ten and eleven years.

CHILDREN OF ELEVEN YEARS.

1. Criticism of sentences.

These are sentences that contain some absurdity or ridiculous expression. Binet explains that formerly he used sentences like "is snow red or black?" but he found that many bright children fell into the trap, and others through confidence in the questioner failed to look for an absurdity. Therefore, he has changed the plan and now says to the child: "I am going to give you some sentences in which there is nonsense; you listen carefully and see if you can tell me where the nonsense is?" Then he reads the sentence very slowly.

These are the sentences:

a. An unfortunate cyclist has had his head broken and is dead from the fall; they have taken him to the hospital and they do not think that he will recover.

b. I have three brothers, Paul, Ernest and myself.

c. The police found yesterday a body of a young girl cut into eighteen pieces; they believe that she killed herself.

d. Yesterday there was an accident on the railroad, but it was not serious; the number of dead is only forty-eight.

e. Some one said: "If in a moment of despair I should commit suicide, I should not choose Friday, because Friday is an unlucky day and it would bring me ill luck"

The test should last about ten minutes; three at least of the questions should receive good answers. At nine years hardly any child gets them; at ten, scarcely a fourth; at eleven, a half.

2. Three words in a sentence (given under age ten).

At eleven all succeed.

3. Sixty words in three minutes.

"Say as many words as you can in three minutes; as table, board, beard, shirt, carriage," we tell him that children have named two hundred words.

This test gives a splendid opportunity to appreciate the intelligence of a child. At least sixty words must be given.

A. Abstract definitions.

"What is chastity, justice, goodness?"

Two good definitions must be given. It is often somewhat difficult to decide if the definition is passable. If it contains the essential idea it must be accepted however badly it is expressed. At ten years a third succeed; at eleven they are generally successful.

5. Words to put in order.

"Make a sentence out of these words. Hour, for, we, good, at, park, a, started, the.

To, asked, exercise, my, have, teacher, correct, my, I.

A, defends, dog, good, his, courageously, master."

Place the printed words before the child. He gives the sentence orally. Time limit is one minute for each sentence. At least two must be given correctly.

CHILDREN OF TWELVE YEARS.

1. Repetition of seven figures. 2, 9, 4, 6, 3, 7, 5, 1, 6, 9, 5, 8, 4, 7, 9, 2, 8, 5, 1, 6, 4.

Tell the child there will be seven figures. Give three trials. One success is sufficient.

2. Rhymes.

Explain what is meant by one word rhyming with another. Illustrate. Then ask for as many words as the child can think of, that rhyme with a given word, e. g., day or spring or mill.

One minute is allowed. Three rhymes with one word should be found in the given time.

3. Repetition of a sentence of 26 syllables.

This should be done without error.

4. Problem of various facts.

(What is it?)

1. "A person who was walking in the forest at Fountainebleu suddenly stopped much frightened and hastened to the nearest police and reported that he had seen hanging from a limb of a tree a ——— (after a pause) what?"

2. "My neighbor has been having strange visitors. He has received one after the other a physician, a lawyer and

a clergyman. What has happened at the house of my neighbor?"

Both questions should be answered correctly.

The answer to the first is "a dead man." Some object to this story as too gruesome. Others say that children are not so sensitive to such things as we think. Aside from that question it would seem that the picture is hardly familiar enough in America to make the answer certain. A substitute better be found.

CHILDREN OF THIRTEEN YEARS.

1. Cutting out.

Get the child's attention and let him see you fold a sheet of paper in four. Then with the scissors cut a small triangle from one edge—the edge which does not open. Ask him to draw a picture of the paper as it will look when unfolded. Do not unfold or allow another sheet to be folded. It is a difficult test. If a child does it the first time always ask him if he has seen it before.

2. The reversed triangle.

Cut a visiting card along the diagonal. Ask child to describe the resulting shape if one of the triangles was turned about and placed so that its short leg was on the other hypothenuse and its right angle at the smaller of the two acute angles.

3. Differences:

Ask the difference between:

Pleasure and honor.
Evolution and revolution.
Event and advent.
Poverty and misery.
Pride and pretension.

Such are the tests. In practice the examination should be conducted in a quiet place, the child being taken alone and as free from distraction as possible. The examination should not and need not last long enough to fatigue the child.

Begin with the tests corresponding to the age of the child or below according as the child seems average or dull.

It is very desirable when feasible, to have an assistant who records "verbatim" everything that the child says, as well as makes notes on what he does during the examination. When this is impossible the examiner must keep his own notes but care should be had that they be made as rapidly as possible, consistent with accuracy, so as not to keep the child waiting. This spoils the game. As said above, constantly encourage the child; continually tell him he is doing splendidly.

While examining the child forget all your preconceived ideas. Regard him as an unknown quantity, an x which is to be determined.

Finally, while tests of Binet and Simon seem to have been worked out with great care and are the result of large clinical experience so that they seem to be almost mathematically exact, yet they must be used with judgment and intelligence.

I believe they are the most valuable contributions yet made and in the hands of the reasonably intelligent teacher or parent will be found of great help in "measuring" the intelligence of the child and determining whether he is in need of special treatment. When such need is indicated even to a possibility he should be taken to an expert whose large experience with such children enables him to confirm the suspicion or to show why it was founded.

The reader who is at home with French should read the original articles of Binet and Simon, L'Anne, the article containing discussions in psychologique, 1908, part of which we have here condensed. The rest of suggestions we hope to resume at another time. (Some of the translations are not exact).

Almost everyone who has worked with the tests for a length of time finds fault with them. The greatest fault perhaps is that a knowledge or training are neces-

618   AMERICAN MEDICINE
Complete Series, Vol. XVIII. }   ORIGINAL ARTICLES   { NOVEMBER, 1912.
New Series, Vol. VII., No. 11.

sary, some schooling as reading, is essential for the older tests. The tests are useless for the blind, deaf or dumb, and it is reasonable to suppose that they cannot be carried out well in persons with partial defects as stutterers, cross-eyed, poor hearing, choreics, etc.

Another serious error on which almost all observers agree is that the tests for the lower ages are too easy while those for the later ages are by far too difficult. Prof. Lewis M. Terman, of Stanford University, much too severely sums up his results on four hundred trials of the tests. He says Binet's data were of very limited extent and rather carelessly elaborated, the scale is far too limited in extent, it is very far from accurate at least for the average American children. He condensed the tests in "nine age groups."

To the writer's mind this same critic repeats the errors. He adds such things as the interpretation of fables, vocabulary tests of 100 words, a test of judgment as finding a lost ball in a circular field. These very additions require training in language, good eyesight and other things, special criticism, I feel, falls on the vocabulary tests, two of the greatest errors of the original Binet scale.

A series of tests were tried at all the elementary schools of St. Cloud, Minn., 784 pupils were tested. A series of definitions of graded words were used as at 6. What is a fork, table, chair, etc., at 8 difference between paper and cloth, a butterfly and a fly, glass and wood; at 11, what do you mean by charity and justice, goodness; at 13, the difference between welfare and pleasure, event and prevent, pride and pretension, evolution and revolution, poverty and misery.

These tests you can readily appreciate are valueless for age classification. If I were to try them on the members of this society, some might regard them as difficult for adults. My main objection to words—is children of foreigners do not hear a large vocabulary at home and in many cases on the street. How often do they talk in the foreign language, or even when talking English a foreign word is substituted for want of the English—we are all familiar with the German child's "gies-can" for watering can, or the Hebrew word "psores" for worry—or of "gini" or "dago" or "wop" for an Italian, or "Mick" for an Irishman. It is surprising how many children know these words and hundreds of others without knowing the true English expression. The same may be said of baby talk which even in some of the best qualities exists until the children have reached a mature age.

A third observer, Dr. J. E. Wallace Wallin, of Stanton, Iowa, gives some modifications and variations to the tests which has its faults, as follows:

TESTS FOR IDIOCY—MENTAL AGE ONE TO TWO YEARS.

1. Move lighted match slowly before S's eyes (or ring bell from behind S.) Mark + if eyes follow or S. listens. Watch for incoordinated eye movements. Light is necessary—muscular paralysis must not be present.

This seems to me a good test for six months, not one year.

2. Place small block (cube) in palm of S's hand with statement, "Here is something for you," and + if S. grasps and handles. Prehension from tactual stimulation. I tried this nine times on what I thought normal children, four did not grasp the cube and two actually drew their hands away as if frightened—only one-third had it correct.

3. Move colored ball or cylinder, suspended by string, slowly before S.'s face (eyes) or hands without touching; + if S. grasps and handles. This may or may not be of value, I do not know. The writer is inclined to favor it but thinks it is a test for six months not one year.

AGE 2.

Hold before S. or place within S's reach a piece each of candy (or cookie) and wood of equal size. Avoid favored positions for either. At two years child is likely to place either in his mouth, at 3 to 4, only cookie.

Wrap paper about candy in S's sight, and hand packet to S. + if S. removes paper before eating. That is good if child has sight, but many children will not remove paper at three years without retardation.

Imitations.

E. extends hand for greeting as S. enters room. "Do as I do;" or "do this way." E. clasps hands, hands in front, on head, or shoulders; rises on toes, etc.

Commands:—(by gestures or words); "Sit down," "Stand up," "Shake hands," "Pick up" (object purposely dropped by E.). "Give me that book." + if S. imitates simply movements or executes simple commands. Watch out for failure through negativism or stubborness. Again sight and hearing are necessary and the test is of importance only when the parents or brothers or sisters do it. Too young for co-operation with a stranger. The rest of the tests are substantially the regular Binet's tests.

Thus we may continue the more persons who have worked with these tests, the more variations and differences of opinion we find. In many persons when the question comes up, the blind, deaf, dumb, etc., they must give results which are useless. Many of these children are bright and it is not fair to class them with the mentally deficient.

Binet, himself, expected criticism on this point and wanted information to overcome it. Some are crippled in speech, sight or hearing from physical defects, accidents, perforated drums, trachoma, gonorrheal ophthalmia, and from a thousand and one other causes. Is it fair to class all these with a crowd of feeble-minded because they cannot make good in Binet tests?

Many teachers of these children have asked to have a new set of tests. Miss Farrel, who is in charge of all these classes in Greater New York, and Miss Hamilton, who does the same work in Jersey City, have asked the writer to make tests with more motions, actions, deeds. Tests that show what the child can *do, comprehend,* or imagine, *without* training, especially if one or more of the special senses are absent.

Hence the attempt to improve the original scheme. The writer has more tests than are given here, but many were subject to the same criticism as the original ones. A few are left. So far no adverse criticism has appeared against these. Language, sight, training, speech or audition are not entirely but practically unnecessary, while correlation of judgment, memory, response to external stimuli and working with a purpose toward a definite result are tested.

The children who attend public school are automatically tested. It is those in private, parochial schools, etc., and ¼ to 10 who do not attend school at all, for whom these tests are especially designed.

You will note that one of the main departures is the use of solids. These are the things we encounter in daily life. Nowhere in literature could I find any case where the form sense was absent, and the individual variations are such as we would find in personal variations of most faculties. Persons differ in everything but the individual differences always come with a certain maximum and minimum to be classed normal variations.

I have paid special attention to get tests of two kinds, one such as every child might strike in daily life, the second the kind no child is likely to encounter daily. Most of my questions have come from the mothers of normal children, getting the averages of what they could do at certain ages and not a year earlier.

In general my tests are:

EIGHTEEN MONTHS.

1. In eight minutes can be taught to place a small handkerchief into a large pocket of its clothes.

2. Ring a small bright colored bell and move before child's face, see if he turns toward it, or if child tries to grasp it.

TWO YEARS.

1. In five minutes a child of two can be taught to place a small handkerchief into a large pocket of its clothes.

2. Where are your eyes, open your mouth, put your finger on your nose.

3. Does not soil clothing (barring disease).

4. Can remember one thing for an errand for 15-20 minutes as a pound of sugar, etc.

5. Place sphere and cube on table—say, give me the ball or touch the ball, or pick up the ball—must be perfect.

THREE YEARS.

1. Can use handkerchief properly.

2. Can partly dress self.

3. Can differentiate straight sided figure from ellipse.

4. Can remember two things on an errand as one pound of butter, and one dozen eggs—or a broom and one pound of sugar. (Somewhat associated).

5. Can differentiate pear and apple in board forms.

FOUR YEARS.

1. Can dress himself completely, if all the clothes button in front or on the side.

2. Are you a little boy or girl (of boys) reverse for girls.

3. Length of two sticks—give me the longer stick 3½"x4", one inch apart.

4. Can remember two things to purchase on an errand, as one pound of sugar and a quart of potatoes (very different kind).

5. Differentiate triangle, square, circle, ellipse and rectangle—must be perfect. Also can replace circle and ellipse correctly—a wrong attempt is an error.

6. Animal heads—must be perfect.

FIVE YEARS.

1. Tell some difference between summer and winter.

2. Can differentiate two weights of similar shape and size (pill boxes).

3. Can remember three things on an errand as one pound of sugar, one pound of rice, and a broom.

4. Make triangle with three sticks of wood, the sticks must almost touch at the angles.

5. Can replace square and rhombus; a wrong trial is an error.

6. Put articles in bed room (from board) or landscape (trees and house).

SIX YEARS.

1. Is this morning or afternoon? Reverse terms in the afternoon.

2. Place two triangles so as to make figure (square). If wrong replace piece in triangle.

3. Can tell circle is more like a sphere than a square is like a sphere.

4. Show on your fingers or by these pieces of wood how old you are, or tell the age, or when is your birthday? (Any one correct).

5. Repeat four actions or movements of the body (three considered correct).

6. Replace two triangles with different bases.

7. Can remember four things on an errand at store, somewhat related, as butter, eggs, salt and pepper.

SEVEN YEARS.

1. Make square with four pieces of wood (sticks).

2. Replace two ellipses different. (A wrong attempt is an error).

3. Make rhombus out of four sticks of wood, must differ from one.

4. Replace funnels properly (or hang clothes on line). Two minutes allowed.

5. How many brothers and sisters have you? Show on fingers if you do not know number. (One error allowed if over four).

6. Should be able to replace fowls in boards.

EIGHT YEARS.

1. Place of birth or ages of brothers and sisters (at least know their order of birth and one of the ages about, guess if you were not told).

2. Can remember five things somewhat related on an errand—as, "Go to the corner grocery and buy three eggs—one pound of butter—100 clothes pins, and one quart of apples and five cents' worth of pepper (same store). (Repeat order if necessary).

3. Should be able to arrange in order sand paper of three different grades and a piece of satin (no error allowed).

4. Should differentiate pentagon and hexagon in board (a wrong attempt is an error).

5. Make five actions of body (or motions). Should be perfect although order may be changed.

6. Replace star and envelope in squares for them in the wood.

NINE YEARS.

1. Can differentiate a series of five weights of the same appearance but different weight.

2. Can name the days of the week (if deaf, write the question; if dumb, child should in some way indicate). (Answer must be perfect).

3. For what is a doctor, a teacher, a police-man, a lawyer, a king or a president? (Must be perfect). "Judge may be used if lawyer is incorrect."

4. Can replace sectors in circles—I do not think that this can be done before nine with one attempt.

5. Can replace figures of persons in form board.

6. Two eight pointed stars in ¼ minute (at once) a wrong attempt an error.

TEN YEARS.

1. Can differentiate *something* about the four seasons.

2. Can name months of the year perfectly.

3. Tell 1c, 5c, 10c, 25c, 50c pieces (must be perfect).

4. Age or place of birth of at least one parent *about* (country for place of birth sufficient). Guess at the age if you do not know. (Approximately is good enough).

5. Can make square out of three pieces of wood, right triangular divisions of square (in two minutes) at eleven years at once.

6. What is a cousin, an aunt, a nephew, a niece, an uncle, a brother-in-law, a sister-in-law? (Five out of seven enough for a correct answer).

7. Replace three triangles, acute, obtuse, and right angle of same base and altitudes at once, no error permitted.

ELEVEN YEARS.

1. Can remember and concentrate four separately ordered actions—as sit down on this chair. (1) Carry that book on the table over to the floor near the door. (2) Sit down again, pull up the shade. (3) Sit down again. Go over to the far corner of the room and touch the wall with one finger. (4) Sit down again, take this ruler and place it on the window sill. (Three enough if done exactly as directed).

2. What is the latest possible hour on a clock at night before it is morning. (Half past twelve or a quarter to one is called correct).

3. What is electricity? (Something that makes a car go or gives a shock, etc., O. K.). If such an answer, How does it differ from steam? (Don't accept I don't know any difference. O. K.).

4. Replace sails in ships (one error allowed) two minutes.

5. Replace trapezoid and two right triangles without error at once.

6. How much do you love your mother —or father—or guardian? "A whole lot, or very much" should be followed by the question, "How much is that?"—the answers show very much.

TWELVE YEARS.

1. Here is a triangle with a piece out. Now what would the square look like if

622   AMERICAN MEDICINE }   ORIGINAL ARTICLES   { NOVEMBER, 1912.

Complete Series, Vol. XVIII. }   { New Series, Vol. VII., No. 11.

the same triangle were cut out of it? Draw the figure or make it with the sticks.

2. What is some difference between a liquid and a solid? (make a guess).

3. Here is a square piece of paper, fold it as nearly as possible to the same shape and size as this triangle (piece of wood 8"x 8") (two minutes allowed).

4. Make star of pieces of wood (not in its form board—this should really be at thirteen years).

THIRTEEN YEARS.

1. Concentration and memory for five different acts or positions of body—(one alteration in order allowed).

2. Here is a triangle with a piece out now; if I took the same piece out of both of the other sides what would be left? Draw it or make it out of sticks (approximately is perfect) really too difficult.

3. If there are twenty-four hours from nine o'clock in the morning until nine o'clock the next morning, how many hours are there till nine o'clock that same night? (Very few have this correct).

4. What is a dream? If unknown, what is meant by escape, or if unknown tell me first a "truth" then an "untruth"? The choice is so great that "vocabulary objections" can be omitted.

In summing up we must acknowledge the real contribution Binet and Simon gave to science. It was Binet's plan that made a clear, simple, and practical classification possible. As to my own modifications as aforesaid, nowhere in literature have I been able to find a positive statement regarding the "form sense."

People differ in this sense about as much as they do in others, but marked deviation from normal inappreciation by sight, touch, and muscle sense and form sense naturally means poor comprehension and weak judgment, hence, deficiency of a general mentality can be presumed with tests especially designed to be the counterpart of facts one is liable to meet in daily life. Solids mean much more than figures of one or two dimensions. As to the answers of state-

ments of accidents, fire, ludicrousness, etc., these tax the adult's judgment so much that I cannot conceive of a natural reply from a child showing anything in intelligence that disproves feeble-mindedness.

For instance:—In institutions where fire had taken place one of two things has occurred. Either all acted like mad men, howled hideously and ran as fast as they could from the scene, or automaticaly not using their own judgment, but following rules they have been taught, formed fire brigades and assisted in putting out the fire. Any of these children I have here tonight might have answered the questions in some way and I defy anyone to tell me which answer makes one proof of feeble-mindedness or even defect. As I have before mentioned definitions require training. Instead of number memories I use memories of *actions* or deeds. To one unacquainted they mean more and there is no chance of practice effect.

I have kept some of the original test questions because I so far had no better. My method of marking is a slight modification of Binet's. I count 100% if all questions for a given age have been answered perfectly. 80% passes the age in question. If only 60% are answered correctly and 50% of the age above it still leaves the age in question. It is about the same as Binet's, only I believe more exact mathematically. There should at least be from 10 to 20 questions for each age.

In conclusion the writer will be very grateful to anyone suggesting more tests that require only the form sense, muscular sense, memory and comprehension of things, child's judgment, not adult's, (as rhombus, feel or see it, and make it out of sticks). Things that a normal child should be able to do and know, whether it ever went to school or not, omitting as much as possible reading, writing, etc. Before closing I desire to impress upon you that in a child's imagination those forms mean much more than to an adult—hence, I feel this point so prominently brought out and emphasized is not *unnecessarily exaggerated.*

C. Stanley Hall has well said "We prehend everything in about the same manner, but we certainly handle everything in a special manner; a glass, an axe, a pen, a spade, etc.

Prehending has only one object, obedience or it is for the direct use of the child; but handling is, we may say, always a willed action having reference to things, to persons, to feelings, and to combinations of these innumerables. The hand is the best servant of man, the best instrument of work, *the best translator of thoughts.*

The mutual assistance of the eye, to the hand, and the hand compelling the attention of the eye, results in a mental development logically the sequence of physiological training.

Oppenheim states in the "Development of the Child," "the clear appreciation of numbers and the use of mathematics, are unquestionably as abstract as plainly to be outside the scope of the elementary school child. Young children learn numbers by rote, just as they can learn any other arrangements of sounds."

Sequin states, in another place: "Our main object is the intellectualization of the muscles."

Finally: There is no well conducted educational institution where Sloyd, manual training, physical exercise, and the associated studies are omitted, their purpose being to complete or round out and make real the more theoretical work of a school

room. Hence, we must all recognize the importance of these practical tests.

848 Greene Ave.

THE TRANSPLANTATION OF BONE FOR THE CORRECTION OF NASAL DEFORMITIES.[1]

BY

WILLIAM WESLEY CARTER, A. M., M. D.,
Assistant Surgeon Manhattan Eye, Ear
and Throat Hospital.
New York City.

The scope of this paper based entirely on my own clinical experiences, will not permit me to enter into a scientific discussion of bone transplantation, nor will the time allotted me permit me to review the work of others who have labored in this field of surgery.

I have adopted the autoplastic operation, i. e. the transference of bone from one part of the body to another, for the reason that it gives the quickest and best results. It has been shown by numerous experimenters in general surgery that the homoplastic operation, i. e. the use of bone from another animal of the same species, and the heteroplastic operation, i. e. the use of bone from an animal of a different species, are difficult, and that even when the primary operation is successful, the bone is soon absorbed.

The use of bone for the correction of nasal deformity is a different proposition from that of transposing it for the purpose of filling in defects in the long bones or in the bones of the skull. In the former instance the bone is introduced into the soft tissues, where its surroundings are foreign to its natural environment, and where it is dependent for its nutrition, at

[1] Read at a meeting of the Eastern Medical Society, Oct. 11th, 1912.

least at first, upon the fluids that surround it.

Personally I feel that I cannot accept without reserve the views of McEwen, who regards the periosteum merely as an envelope, the chief function of which is to limit the growth of bone. I am quite certain that in the young the periosteum has much to do with the growth of bone, while in the adult this function is limited or lost, and no doubt at this period of life this firm, inelastic sheath under certain

tic conditions from one part of the body to another. I feel that in my work I have demonstrated the correctness of this view. The transplanted bone will die and be absorbed if the technique is imperfect, it will suffer a similar fate if it is transferred from another person, for in this instance there is a difference in the molecular constitution of the two bodies, and this chemical incompatibility, so to speak, causes the death of the bone and its subsequent absorption.

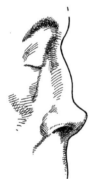 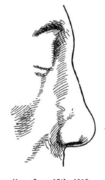

Fig. 1. Traumatic Deformity. Operation June 15th, 1912.

circumstances limits the growth of bone as suggested by McEwen. In my own work, I have used bone both with and without periosteum, and as far as I can observe there is no difference in the results obtained, so that at present I no longer preserve this covering except in the very young.

It is my firm belief that cells and groups of cells possess an inherent, independent vitality of their own, and that this vitality is not destroyed by the immediate transference of tissue under proper asep-

The use of bone for the correction of nasal deformity was suggested to me by the limitations of the bridge-splint operation for restoring a depressed nasal bridge. This latter procedure, with which I presume many of you are familiar, was devised by me several years ago. Briefly, it consists of a combined bridge and intranasal splint which is applied to a recent fracture or to an old deformity after the bony framework of the nose has been thoroughly mobilized by suitable means. This method presupposes that there is enough bone left in the nose to hold it in proper position after the support of the bridge has been removed. The cases which are not amenable to this method are those of depressed deformity in which, owing to disease or injury, there is left little or no bone to support the nose. Here the use of bone grafts is indicated.

Cases suitable for this operation may be divided into:

(1) Traumatic. (2) Congenital. (3) Those due to destructive diseases, such as syphilis, atrophic rhinitis, etc.

addition to all this I have on two ocasions applied the "bridge-splint" in order to give needed support. In all cases a Wassermann test should be made, and under no circumstances should the operation be done when this is positive, or when there are any signs of active syphilis, until after a thorough and effective course of treatment. Most of those who need this operation are poorly nourished and should be given suitable tonics until we are reasonably certain that the general condition of the patient will favor the reception of the bone graft.

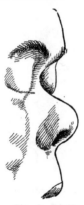
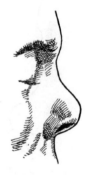
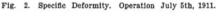

Fig. 2. Specific Deformity. Operation July 5th, 1911.

In traumatic cases, as a rule, the nasofrontal process, the nasal spine, and a portion at least of the nasal bones and the nasal processes of the superior maxillæ remain and can be utilized as a support for the bone graft. In these cases a single strip of bone is all that is necessary. In congenital cases and those due to disease, there may be entire absence of bony framework; in some of these it may be necessary to construct a V-shaped pier for the support of the dorsal strip, by introducing two additional pieces of bone. In

My reasons for using the rib are: (1) It is easily removed. (2) The patient suffers little or no inconvenience and the rib is quickly regenerated. (3) Its shape is convenient, and it is thickly studded with minute nutrient foramina, which favors its nutrition after transplantation.

Preparation of the patient.—In this operation the strictest antiseptic and aseptic precautions must be observed. Primary union is the sine qua non. Even if an accidental infection is subsequently controlled without expulsion of the bone graft, the latter is dead and will either slough out or be absorbed. It must be remembered that the staphylococcus pyogenes albus has been frquently found in the deepest layers of the skin, and while its own virulence may be slight, its tendency to invite a mixed infection is great; therefore every effort should be made to effect a complete, penetrating sterilization of the entire operative field. The nasal cavities too should be thoroughly cleansed and kept clean after the operation. Most of these patients have ethmoiditis and

collodion and the nasal chambers are irrigated with Dobell's solution.

Operation.—A curvilinear incision, convexity downward, is made from the inner extremity of one eye-brow to that of the other. This cut extends to the periosteum but not through it. A special sharp elevator is introduced through this incision and the skin and subcutaneous tissue elevated over the dorsum and sides of the nose, and in some instances for a considerable distance beyond the nose under the cheeks. The semi-

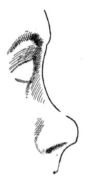 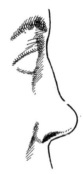

Fig. 3. Congenital Deformity. Operation June 21st, 1910.

atrophic rhinitis with foul, purulent discharge. The bone graft is placed in close contact with the nasal chambers, and it is possible that infection may reach the operative field by penetration from this quarter. This I believe has occurred in my experience.

Several hours before the operation the skin over the nose and over the ninth rib, (preferably the right side) · should be scrubbed with green soap and water, followed by alcohol and bichloride 1-5000. This area is then painted with tincture of iodine. The eye-brows are covered with

lunar flap made by the first incision is then lifted up, and a short transverse cut made through the periosteum over the naso-frontal process. The periosteum above this incision is elevated for about ¼ of an inch. This wound is covered with sterile gauze, and we proceed to the second step in the operation, the resection of the rib. A straight incision four inches long including the periosteum, is made directly over the ninth rib. The rib is then shelled from its periosteum by means of a curved elevator and two inches of the bone removed with the costotome. This section of the rib is then split in its transverse diameter, and from one of the halves (usually the outer), all of the medullary tissue is scraped with a sharp curette. This piece is shaped to suit the deformity, and in the following manner is slipped into the place previously prepared for it in the nose. The semilunar skin flap is held upward out of the way with

The wound is closed with horse hair sutures and a sterile dressing applied. If all is well this dressing is not disturbed until the seventh day when the sutures are removed.

The action of the bone strip in reducing the deformity is that of a lever, the short arm of which is anchored under the periosteum. The naso-frontal process or

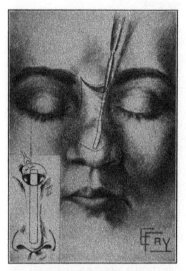

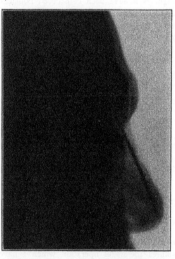

Fig. 4. Bone transplantation for nasal deformity. The central figure shows method of elevating skin and subcutaneous tissues; the insert figure shows the bone in place.

Fig. 5. X-ray plate showing transplanted bone in position.

a tenaculum, the strip of bone is introduced and the end pushed nearly to the tip of the nose. The upper end is passed through the slit in the periosteum and anchored in contact with the frontal bone. We now observe whether or not the deformity has been corrected; if it has not, one or two strips of bone are superimposed on the first.

nasal bones act as the fulcrum and the long arm of the lever which reaches nearly to the tip of the nose does the work of lifting up the depressed bridge. In doing this a wedge-shaped cavity is created beneath the bone-graft which immediately becomes filled with a blood clot. Upon the sterility of this clot and its subsequently becoming organized depends to a large extent the success of the operation.

Results.—A detailed account of the cases operated upon would prove tedious and would serve no useful purpose. Therefore I will consider them collectively.

I have transplanted bone for nasal deformity fifteen times. Two of the cases were congenital, five traumatic, and eight syphilitic, one of the latter having no nose. All were cases of extreme deformity. Some might well have been considered hopeless by any method of treatment. The ages of the patients ranged from six to forty-seven years. My first operative case is of two

remained for two weeks. A flap including the bone was then made, the arm was bound to the head and held in position by means of a plaster bandage, after the flap had been sutured into a proper position on the face. After circulation was established (which took about two weeks), the flap was severed from the arm and shaped into a nose. The result in this case is very good.

The results in these fifteen cases may be briefly summarized and classed under three heads:

(1) Failures.

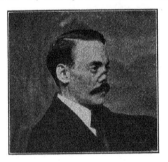

Fig. 6. Specific deformity before operation.

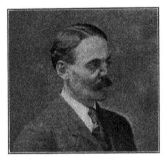

Fig. 7. Specific deformity after bone transplantation. Operation July 31st, 1911.

and a half years standing. In two instances the usual operation which I have previously described, was elaborated by the introduction of two additional pieces of bone, which were placed in the form of an inverted V-shaped pier to support the dorsal strip. In two instances the bridge-splint was applied to lend additional support to the reconstructed nose, one of these cases having had the pier modification of the operation.

In the case of the woman who had no nose, the bone graft was first placed in the subcutaneous tissue of the arm, where it

(2) Successful correction of deformity with probable absorption of original bone graft.

(3) Successful correction of deformity with retention of bone, the vitality of same having been preserved.

There were two failures: In one the bone from another patient was used. In the other unsuspected syphilis was the cause of the deformity and had not been eradicated at the time of the operation. In both of these cases the bone grafts had to be removed. The condition of these patients was not made worse by the attempted correction of the deformity.

Under the second heading, successful correction of deformity with probable absorption of the graft, two cases may be classed. In both of these cases after primary union and a seemingly perfect result had been obtained, on the tenth day there was a bulging at the point where the bone was introduced. The wound was opened and there was an escape of dark blood, showing that the clot which filled the wedge-shaped cavity beneath the bone had broken down. The bone graft was free and no doubt it was dead. After several irrigations, the wound closed without the loss of the bone. A recent examination of these cases shows that the deformity remains corrected, but that the bone has been almost completely absorbed, and in its place is tissue that feels very much like cartilage. It is possible that new bone is being formed in place of the original transplanted bone. There were two other cases in which there was a similar breaking down of the clot. I have been unable to examine these recently, so cannot say whether or not the bone has been absorbed.

In the remaining nine cases, some of which I still have an opportunity to observe, and one of which I show you tonight, the condition seems to have remained the same as at the time of the operation, and I feel reasonably certain that the bone remains alive and that it has taken part in the local process of repair.

My experience in this work leads me to the following conclusions in regard to the fate of the bone: (1) The bone may die in the process of transposition. (2) The tissues of the patient may not have sufficient vitality and reparative energy to receive the bone, nourish it and incorporate it. (3) Infection will invariably cause death of the bone. (4) If for any cause the bone dies even if it is not expelled it will be absorbed.

On the other hand, it is my belief that if the technic is perfect, and the clot which immediately surrounds the bone becomes organized, that a covering of connective tissue will form about the transplanted bone which will nourish it and cause its retention as a part of the living tissues of the nose.

I may add that I have not hesitated to attempt the most difficult cases, many of which would seem impossible of correction by any means. I therefore feel that this method has been subjected to a fair test and that the results obtained, while not always perfect, should warrant its adoption for the treatment of a class of patients for whom little or nothing has hitherto been done.

69 West 50th Street.

REMARKS ON THE USE OF BONE TRANSPLANTATION IN GENERAL SURGERY.[1]

BY

A. A. BERG, M. D.,
New York City.

At the outset I wish to call attention to the microscopical section of a fetal bone in order to recall the processes of bone growth and development. You probably all remember this early picture in your histological studies in which the first evidences of bone formation consist of a re-arrangment of the cartilage cells. In the primal state the cellular structure of the cartilage

[1] Read at a meeting of the Eastern Medical Society, Oct., 1912.

lies irregularly distributed. The first evidences of ossification in the cartilage consist of a re-arrangement of the cells into longitudinal columns around a so-called center of ossification. It has been believed that it is around this center that bone commences to form, and on this, McEwen has based his hypothesis of bone growth. But bone does *not* commence to form around these cartilage cells. On the contrary, if we take a picture of the perichondrial covering of the bone, we will find that a sprout of periosteal cells occurs at this point of ossification. Inside of this sprout, there is a little blood vessel. This sprout-like process carrying on the inside a small blood-vessel, is covered on the outside by osteoblasts. These sprouts penetrate inwardly and the osteoblastic cells begin to form new bone. The longitudinal arrangment of the cartilage cells has nothing to do with the formation of bone. The bone comes from the osteogenetic or osteoblastic layer of the periosteum which projects inwardly from the periosteum. The little cavities within the sprouts form the future Haversian canals. The cartilage cells become marrow cells or are lost in the circulation.

We will find in adult life that, as the structure has developed in the fetus, it will develop in the adult. When we have removed part of an organ, it will always reform as in the fetal organism. The bone will reform from the outside inwardly as in the fetus and we will find that is actually the case in studying sections of transplanted bone.

There are three layers, the periosteal layer, the solid, compact or spongy layer, and the inner or marrow canal layer. The periosteal layer carries on its inner side osteogenetic cells which will form new bone only. The marrow consists of cells which may have been originally cartilage cells and also cells which may have been carried into the bone by the finger-like sprouts from the periosteum.

History of bone transplantation in the human being.— Away back in 1859, Ollier, a great French investigator, experimented on bone transplantation. After very careful experiments, made without the microscope, he concluded there is a fundamental difference in the results from bone transplantation depending on whether the transplant is taken from the same individual—autogenous—or another individual and whether it has a periosteal covering or not. When he transplanted the bone from another individual it died; but if he transplanted a bone into the same individual, that transplant lived; he thought both the transplanted compact bone and the periosteum lived. He concluded it was best to use bone from the same individual and to have it covered with periosteum. This view was accepted until the Radzimowsky and Bonome found that living periosteum when transplanted remained viable, but that the compact bone always died, their proof of this being that the bone cells in the compact bone lost both their staining property, and their cell configuration. They concluded that the bone must be taken from the same individual in order to live; that, however, of the transplanted bone the periosteum lived but the bone itself died. This conclusion held up to the time of Barth in 1893.

Barth came to the conclusion that all the parts of the transplanted bone, whether taken from the same individual or not, whether covered with periosteum or not, died, the transplant becoming a foreign body and encysted. The transplanted bone acted only as a splint. He maintained that as all parts of the transplant died, it was immaterial whether we use living bone or dead bone, bone from the same individual or another, whether the bone is decalcified or not; as long as we use something which will act as a splint, we will be able to hold the parts in position until new bone will hold the neighboring and surrounding structures. These conclusions were accepted by the entire fraternity and resulted in the use of various kinds of amalgam, iodoform paste, chicken bones, etc., with very unsuccessful results. In Germany at the Surgical Convention on Bone Transplantation, the surgeons decided that the use of the decalcified bone cells for filling up cavities was unsuccessful. On his return home, Pick in Germany, put Axhausen to work on the subject. He came to the conclusion that the fundamental law of Ollier was right, that in the healthy living bone covered with periosteum, the periosteum remains viable but the bone died; that it made a great deal of difference whether the bone was transplanted into the same individual or a foreign bone was used; that for successful transplantation, we must use healthy living periosteum covered bone. All this was proven by the most accurate and careful microscopical and histological studies and the surgical world has accepted it.

Following this teaching of Axhausen, the most successful transplantation of bone has been achieved.

We have, however, a year ago, been met by the position of McEwen who comes back to the principles of Barth. McEwen's work was all judged by macroscopical appearances. His work is experimentally insufficient. It has attracted considerable attention, however, from the surgeons in New York City. McEwen does not bother himself with the viability of bone or whether it is taken from the same or another individual. He says it is not periosteum which produces bone, but bone cell reproduces bone cell; that the periosteum has nothing to do with the formation of new bone cells. Now it has been proved that bone cells die when transplanted. Secondly, McEwen must settle with the fact that bone in the fetus does not produce bone, but that bone comes from the finger-like processes carrying with them bone as they enter into the cartilage. McEwen has proven none of his facts microscopically or histologically.

I now exhibit twenty-three X-ray plates showing results obtained in bone transplantation operations. The cases demonstrated comprise tuberculosis of the metacarpo-phalangeal joint, osteosarcoma of the end of the clavicle, osteosarcoma of the lower end of the jaw, an ununited fracture of the two bones of the forearm which had failed under all other previous methods of treatment, osteosarcoma of the lower end of the humerus and an osteosarcoma of the upper end of the shaft of the humerus. These plates showed the formation of bone and the transplanted portion becoming gradually absorbed, and the periosteum spreading underneath the transplant. All the transplants that were used were taken from the same individual (autogenous), and the bones used for filling the defect were the rib (three), the tibial crest (twice), the fibula (twice).

REMARKS ON BONE TRANSPLANTA-
TION IN THE POST OPERATIVE
MASTOID WOUND.[1]

BY

MILTON J. BALLIN, M. D.,
New York City.

Encouraged by the excellent results of
bone transplantation of the general surgeon and especially of Dr. A. A. Berg,
who read a paper on this subject at the
Academy of Medicine last winter, the idea
occurred to me of filling the post operative
mastoid wound with a bone transplant. I
did not know at that time whether this
was feasible, but I thought I would give
this method a trial, and was gratified to
see this belief substantiated by the excellent result which I am presenting here this
evening.

This patient entered the hospital on a
Thursday. Two days later I did the ordinary Stacke operation. Five days later
I took out the packing and found the
wound filled with healthy granulations.
Two days later I repacked the wound. A
few days after this I did a bone transplantation, taking a piece of bone with the
living periosteum from the crest of the
patient's tibia. This I transplanted into the
patient's mastoid wound. I did not touch
the bone, did no scraping but simply closed
up the mastoid region with the exception
of a small opening at the inferior angle of
the wound in which I left a small gutta
percha drain. At the end of the second
day I removed this and allowed the small
opening to close. Five days after the
bone transplantation the wound had closed
and the entire time consumed was twelve
days.

[1] Read at a meeting of the Eastern Medical
Society, Oct., 1912.

I performed the operation as above described on July 6th, and the wound has remained perfectly closed since, this being
Oct. 11th, a period of three months. In
other words, this is a case of bone transplantation of the mastoid wound with an
absolutely perfect result. The closure
shows merely a post-auricular curved
linear scar with no cosmetic deformity.
This I believe is the first case in which
bone transplantation has been performed
in the mastoid wound.

The experiments of Ollier, Axhausen and
others carried on as early as 1858, proved
that to make a bone transplantation successfully we must take the living periosteum along with the bone. I have tried
this method in several other cases with
fairly good results, but I am not prepared
as yet to express a decided opinion on this
subject. I expect in the course of the
next few months to publish a paper in
which I will describe the technic in detail
and report the results in other cases.

I do not advocate this procedure as a
routine, but think it advisable to adapt it
in cases in which we have a clean granulating wound, for, if we succeed, we not
only obtain a very good cosmetic result and
hasten the time of healing, but relieve the
patient of the necessity of packing and re-
packing the wound, which is usually tedious and generally associated with more or
less pain.

SURGICAL HINTS.

A small erosion of the trachea may give
rise to a distressing hemoptysis which differs from a hemorrhage from the lungs in
that there are no lung symptoms, no loss of
weight or constitutional symptoms and in
that the bleeding occurs in small lumps of
clotted blood.—*Amer. Jour. of Surg.*

"TWO TALES OF A CITY—TETANUS HEMORRHAGE."[1]

BY

H. SEYMOUR HOUGHTON, M. D.,
New York City.

About the middle of May, 1906, one of those innocent sounding summons to "stop in during your rounds this morning," which one jots down in his notebook, without the least realization of the tragedy which may be impending, took me to see a Mrs. H., a young married woman in her early thirties, a patient who had originally been referred to me by Dr. McGinnis. She was a woman of excellent health, had borne three children; was of slight but wiry build, and intellectually rather above the average. Her home environment was congenial and happy, the only disturbing element, and one which might have been a factor in lowering her resistance, was the distress which came a short time previously in the failure of her husband who was caught in the steel slump which occurred that year. Her reason for asking me to come in was due to the fact that while dressing that morning she had felt, and subsequently in the mirror had seen, a peculiar lump, which would every few minutes thrust itself up from somewhere behind and below the tongue.

Careful inspection of the fauces, using a spoon as a tongue depressor, failed to show any sign of any lump or other abnormality, and after repeated examinations, I was beginning to wonder in what diplomatic language I could convey this, my view of the situation to her, when she remarked that she felt the lump coming up. Quickly looking into her throat, there was, sure enough, a small round nodule, about

the size of a small marble, resting on the base of the tongue, and from it extended downward toward the larynx, a fine thread-like pedicle. In a moment it quickly slipped back. It so happened that while we were discussing the subject, she took occasion to speak of something else which bothered her, and showed about the middle of the left forearm in its dorsal surface a small pigmented flat mole. Partly from habit, partly because of its tendency to itch a little, she had for some time been scratching and picking at it, so that it had become somewhat irritated. Advising her to leave it alone and apply some slight protective dressing, I suggested that we go down to Dr. Coakley's office and see about that growth in the throat. If my memory serves me right, I recall that Dr. Coakley also failed in his first inspection to see anything and manifested symptoms of poking fun at me, but very shortly the irruption took place, and the growth again came into view. It was then a small matter to grasp it with forceps and cut the pedicle. Slight as the operation was it seemed to leave an extraordinary amount of pain, and the patient felt faint. Taking her home she was advised to remain quiet and spray the throat frequently. That evening I saw her again, and was astonished at the amount of pain she declared was still present. On the following morning she was unable to get up on account of the pain, and in addition the whole lower jaw felt stiffened. I am ashamed to admit that being so obsessed with the operation of the previous day as being the cause of these symptoms, it never occurred to me to think of the real cause, and it was only in speaking of it to Dr. Dowd at a meeting that evening, and his suggestion that I was dealing with a case of tetanus that the

[1] Read before the Hospital Graduates' Club, April 25, 1912.

situation dawned upon me. Dr. Dowd was immediately invited to see the case, and on the day following, the condition was plain enough; the pain still present, the rigidity of the lower jaw, and beginning but marked stiffness of the neck muscles. On the 25th of May the record of the nurses begins, and notes a temperature of 98.4, pulse 84 and respiration 20 with pain in the neck, back and chest, very restless, nauseated and with frequently recurring paroxysms, and of giving two hypodermatic injections of morphia, a quarter grain each. On the 26th the temperature began to rise, maximum 100.6, pulse 108, and respiration 26, with restlessness and irregular sleep; frequently recurring paroxysms, pain and numbness in the right leg, a disposition to expel the good steamship Enema, and such difficulty in swallowing that she was fed by rectum, and ice bags were applied to the spine with chloral by rectum.

On the following day after consultation with Dr. Park, the first injection of antitoxin was administered by Dr. Dowd and repeated by me twelve times between this date and the second of June. I do not recall the amount in cubic centimetres given each time, but it was the regulation dose as given by Dr. Park. During this period the temperature remained at about 100, pulse 92, respirations 22, the nourishment which could be swallowed, fluids, and the medicine, codein, chloral and bromide. The patient was very nervous and restless, expelled much flatus and by this time had developed the full picture of tetanic paroxysms including opisthotonos, and thus far no apparent beneficial effects of the serum were apparent, except that she could sleep more quietly and at longer intervals and had less pain.

It was at this time that she began to secrete a thick tenacious mucus, having the greatest difficulty on account of the condition of the throat, in expelling it, and giving her no end of trouble for many days thereafter. And also at this date, June 1st, the temperature began to rise, reaching 104 and pulse 150, respirations 32, with great exhaustion and beginning delirium. At the suggestion of Dr. Le Fevre, who saw her at this time, she was given hypodermatically 1/100 gr. each of eserine salicylate and atropine. The temperature then gradually lowered ranging between 100 and 101, with pulse 96 to 112, until the 10th when it again rose to 102 and 103 and 104 with pulse at 132 and respirations 40, until the 15th when it went down to 101, the patient during this time being restless and very irritable with periods of delirium, but with a very marked diminution of the paroxysms. She was being given five minims of strophanthus. The general condition was rather serious, the pulse weak and irregular, the delirium marked, sleeping fitfully and incessantly talking when awake, a persistent cough with inability to expel the mucus, and frequent cyanosis, with involuntary passing of urine. This condition of restless talkative delirium, red dry tongue, tight sticky cough, inability to properly swallow food, and the temperature ranging between 101 and 102, continued for two days when it was noted that she seemed somewhat more rational, slept better with the spasmodic state diminished, the tongue very dry, but a tendency to perspire profusely set in. The strophanthus had been increased to ten minims. She slept better and the bromide was discontinued. By the 19th the temperature had come down to 99, pulse 90, respirations 22; her mind was clear at intervals, but would later wander with a desire to get out of bed, the perspiration and coughing still continuing until the twentieth when the temperature became normal. For the next few days with temperature normal, she was very delirious, irritable and talkative, sleeping poorly, veronal seeming to have an exciting rather than a somnolent effect. Digitalis ten minims was added to the strophanthus. The delirium and excitability continued with lucid intervals until the 29th when she was able to sit up for a short time, so that by the fourth of July she had practically recovered, making about seven weeks of a most stormy and threatening siege, the latter four weeks of which had been under the entire charge of Dr. Le Fevre on account of the necessity of my being out of town.

The noteworthy features of the case were the development of the disease without any definitely known cause, its initial symptoms bringing to light this small pedunculated growth in the larynx, the existence of which had never been previously suspected, the evident efficient effect of the serum from the laboratory of Dr. Park, given as it was when the disease was in full bloom and not at a period prior to its development. The high temperature with evidence of lung congestion and finally the wild delirium, so that after the acute manifestations had subsided, she was absolutely insane. It was my own opinion, one I think shared in by the others, that the infection took place in the black mole on the forearm, following her nervous habit of scratching at it, and made possible, as Dr. Le Fevre thinks, by previously handling vegetables and other market produce. That would seem the only natural explanation in the complete absence of any his-tory of traumatism. Of course, it might be possible that the laryngeal growth was in some way connected with it, but at the time of its excision in Dr. Coakley's office, there was nothing about its appearance in the way of erosions or ulceration to suggest this as a means of entry.

In one previous case of tetanus which occurred in the Third Surgical Division at Bellevue during my service as interne, there had been the classic symptoms following the usual course in a boy of fifteen, a lacerated wound of the palm from the blank cartridge of a toy pistol. Here there were no mental symptoms, the mind remaining clear up to his death, and preceded only a short time beforehand by a marked rise in temperature.

The second story I have to tell, bears on the case, the specimen from which I presented before this Club in January last, it being a fibrinous cast, so-called "bronchial tree" which came from a case of profuse bronchial hemorrhage. The patient, J. D. R., kindly referred to me by Dr. Kerley, is a woman in affluent circumstances, about 43 years of age, with two children, no miscarriages and a normal family history, particularly as regards both syphilis or tuberculosis. She had had one similar attack in the early summer of last year while abroad on the shore of the Mediterranean. She had supposed the previous attack, as in fact she thought this one, to be one of hemorrhage of the stomach, and upon my hasty arrival, on seeing some ten to fourteen ounces of blood in the basin, I took the same view of the matter. I assumed, on general principles that I had a gastric ulcer, possibly a varicose ulcer of the stomach, to deal with. While she had herself no history or evidence of tuberculosis whatever, it is a remarkable fact in this connection, that her husband, while an active and apparently healthy man, is now suffering, and has been for the past three years, from a cough, and considerable expectoration containing— from the report of Dr. Sondern—tubercle bacilli, and with an area of infiltration over the right upper lobe. There is nothing about his appearance to suggest a sick man, and his excellent general health has unfortunately created in him a disposition to treat the matter lightly. He feels that his open camp life in the Adirondacks in the summer, during which time he gains weight, is amply sufficient to meet the situation. The only condition in his wife which led up to this hemorrhage on the night of January 18th, was a slight influenzal cold to which she paid no attention, and the fact that she had just finished her menstrual period. Although the amount of blood in the basin was considerable, she failed to show much pallor, her pulse was normal and her temperature 98.4. A careful palpation over the stomach failed to reveal any tenderness or flatulence, and it was thought that a little bismuth and codein with absolute quiet would help matters. The patient however, was much alarmed for fear it would happen again, and for this reason I remained during the night. In the course of a couple of hours her maid said she was having another hemorrhage from the stomach. I watched this performance with considerable interest, and at once was struck with the fact that there was no nausea or actual vomiting, on the contrary the blood came slowly and as the result of a slight hacking cough, also coming in foamy masses and with some effort to expel from the mouth. After a time it subsided and all was quiet again until in the early hours of the morn-

ing when the blood started again in the same way. This time I determined to test matters and had her drink two glasses of hot water. There was no return of the water and no nausea or vomiting, but the blood continued in the same way. Listening over the lungs, some diminished breathing and many medium coarse rales could be made out on the right posterior aspect.

The next day she was quiet but with a slight rise in temperature and a nurse was sent for, a recurrence being feared. The recurrence took place promptly in the evening, and after three hemorrhages of ten, thirteen, and ten ounces respectively, Dr. Le Fevre was asked to see her; he arrived right in the middle of one of them, and it was on this occasion that he picked out the bronchial tree which was shown at this meeting.

Diffuse coarse rales could be made out pretty generally distributed throughout the chest. During that day and the next the temperature ranged 102.5 and 103, with pulse 116 and respirations 22 to 25, subsiding to normal on the fifth day.

The treatment consisted of morphia hypodermatically one-half grain every four hours with gelatine in which was placed powdered suprarenal extract. Lactate of calcium was also given regularly. The solution of adrenalin, either hypodermatically or by mouth seemed to have absolutely no beneficial effect, and was discontinued. Her fluid nourishment was retained as there was at no time any nausea. The record of the amount of blood exclusive of the first night which must have been nearly a pint, was on Thursday 23 ounces, on Friday 17 ounces, on Saturday 16 ounces and Sunday six ounces, in spite of which there was only comparatively slight pallor, some weakening of the pulse and only a moderate drawn look to the face. The hemorrhages ceased entirely after Sunday morning, and her recovery was prompt and uninterrupted.

Now what lay back of this condition of affairs it is difficult for me to say. I have unfortunately mislaid an article which bears on these hemorrhages, spontaneous in their character, taking place not only from the bronchii but from the nose, mouth and uterus. In that article the view was advanced that the hemorrhage results from the toxic effect of the influenza bacillus in the capillary vessels of the mucous membrane. As a matter of fact the only evidence of an exciting cause in this troublesome case, was the history of previous cold, possibly an influenza, and the fact that her menstruation had ceased only a day or two before. There was nothing then or since to give ground for the belief that she is infected with tuberculosis, although her husband's condition would suggest an easy explanation of possible contamination.

301 W. 88th St.

TRANSLATION.

LUMBAR PUNCTURE.

(Rachicentesis).

BY

P. RAVAUT, M. D.,
Translated from the French; with Notes and Additions
BY
O. L. MULOT, M. D.,
Brooklyn, N. Y.

(*Continued from October issue.*)

Intoxications.

From the results obtained by lumbar puncture in meningeal conditions it was quite natural to seek the same good results in the nervous manifestations occurring in certain intoxications; in uremia and eclampsia good results have been obtained.

(A) Uremia.— Puncture has not been restricted entirely to the type with the severe cerebral manifestations but also has been used in the milder cases, in which the headache, ringing of the ears, and vertigo reveals the high tension. Uremia presents a series of symptoms of two types: those attributable to high tension and those attributable to the intoxication. While in practise it is not always possible to separate these, both seem to be influenced by puncture. The symptoms which may make one think of performing a puncture are very variable, from rebellious headache, with dizziness, ringing of the ears, cloudiness of vision and intellect, to convulsions with coma and Cheyne-Stokes respiration.

The liquid obtained under such conditions is very variable; it is generally under high tension but it is difficult to establish a relation between this and the severity of the clinical symptoms. Widal[53], Froin and Carriere[54] have studied this fluid chemically and insist upon the gravity of the prognosis when it contains in the neighborhood of two grammes (30 grains) of urea to the liter. It is difficult to say just exactly how much liquid should be withdrawn; in some cases 6 to 10 cc. have sufficed to produce a decided and permanent amelioration of the symptoms, while in other cases it was found necessary to withdraw 30 cc. and more. There seems to be no definite relation between the amount withdrawn and the results. The results are not constant and it has its advocates and its opponents; but this is a serious condition and if, by its employ we can save a case from going to

convulsion and coma, it certainly merits
a place in the treatment of uremic cases,
particularly since the *pro* and *con* camps
are about evenly divided.   Marie and
Guillain[55], Legendre[56], Vigouroux[57], Carriere[58].

(B) Eclampsia.—The results obtained
by puncture in certain uremic cases led
to its trial in eclampsia. Kronig's[59] results
were indifferent; as were also those of
Henkel[60]. It is during the convulsions
when there is a high tension that it will
do good by rapidly lowering this; and
Audelbert and Furnier[61] have used it with
success under such conditions.   Villard
and Tixier[62] used it to advantage but as
there was considerable cloudiness of the
fluid in their case they argue that there
may have been autoinfection.   The
number of cases reported *pro* and *con* are
still too few to permit of a definite conclusion as to the value of this operation in
this condition; but there is sufficient evidence to warrant its use. It may here be
mentioned that in infantile convulsions,
which, like the eclampsia of the adult are
of a toxic nature and clinically much resemble each other, it sometimes gives good
results, but the operation must usually be
repeated in a few days.

**(C) Diabetes; Lead Poisoning; Alco-
holism.**— In all of these cases there are at
times marked signs of nervous reactions;
such as convulsions and coma, it is therefore natural to try to affect these by lumbar puncture but so far there is not a single
case reported that permits us placing this
procedure among the valuable means of
meeting these conditions. In delirium tremens the results have been most ephemeral
and inconstant and while Tixier reports
good results for it in this condition it cannot be considered as a means of treatment
of this condition.

Seegelken reports the cure of a case
saturnine encephalopathy by this means;
Mosny denies ever having observed the
least benefit from it; nor is this surprising
in view of the fact that the cerebral symptoms in this condition are due to deep
seated lesions in the brain substance itself, and of which the nervous phenomena
are only the expression.

ABSCESS AND TUMORS OF THE BRAIN.

The value of puncture in these conditions is still under discussion; some favor,
some condemn, and this is due to the accidents which have been observed following its employment in such cases, making
it a delicate and sometimes dangerous operation, the results of which are but passing
and only palliative. For this reason it is condemned by many who in these conditions
prefer craniectomy.   We will be content
simply to show on what symptoms it may
have some influence, to report the results
obtained by its partisans and give the
arguments which they who prefer trephining, advance.

(A) Cerebral Tumors.—We will not
here trace the clinical picture of cerebral
tumors, but it is useful to recall that the
symptoms which characterize them are of
different kinds, some revealing their location in the brain; these are the least constant. Other symptoms depend upon the
compression within the skull while the
third group refer to the cortical irritation.
In certain tumors of a syphilitic, tuberculous, or sarcomatous origin involving, the
cortex and the meninges, there is hypertension.   The symptomatology of brain
tumors is very complex; but whether the
diagnosis is established upon symptoms
that localize it or upon the others above
mentioned, the question of the nature of

the intervention becomes most important. In the solution of this problem one symptom is of the highest value; that is the papillary stasis. The presence of this justifies the suspicion of tumor and at the same time serves as an indication for the therapeutic course to be followed. All the punctures that have been practised in cases of cerebral tumors have been undertaken with the object of relieving the hypertension, whether that hypertension was itself well. marked or simply revealed by other symptoms such as papillary stasis and violent headaches. All authors are agreed in its efficacy in relieving hypertension irrespective of its cause.

Widal[63] reports a case of cerebellar tumor, with pains, vertigo, vomiting, tinnitus aurium, and ocular troubles, in which in the course of several months, 17 punctures were performed, each time withdrawing from 10 to 30 cc. of fluid and each operation was followed by a decided and prolonged amelioration of all the symptoms. DeLapersonne[64] reports another case, in which the abstraction of a small amount of fluid brought relief from a severe headache that had resisted all previous treatment, and this is confirmed by the observations of Babinski[65]. Roux[66] reports a case of epilepsy supposed to be due to a tubercle, in which each puncture brought so much relief that the patient himself asked for the operation whenever the symptoms grew in severity. There are many cases reported in which good results have been obtained, but all the authors—Moindrot[67] —Schereyder[68]—are agreed that the good effects are transitory and for that reason it must be frequently performed in these cases. While these results warrant us in employing this operation and give it a recognized place in the treatment of brain tumors, still we must not be hasty in accepting it. It has given valuable results but there are many who prefer craniectomy, especially in cases where the symptoms are intense; for in brain tumor cases puncture is to be practised with prudence. In these cases we must never withdraw more than 5 or 10 cc. of fluid at a time; the patient should always be in the lateral decubitus and with the head lower than the rest of the body. If the liquid does not flow, *never aspirate;* the patient should keep to the bed the day before the operation and remain there at least two days after it, with such precautions it is fairly safe in these cases, but even under such excessive caution sudden death has occurred—Sicard. Of course such accidents are often due to defective technic, such as a too abundant withdrawal of fluid; sitting posture during operation or a cerebellar location of the tumor, which latter seems particularly prone to give such disastrous results. The ever present possibility of such deplorable accidents and the ephemeral character of the relief causes this operation to be rejected by many neurologists—Chipault[70], and surgeons Dubarry and Guillot[71]—and in justification of their attitude they advance the argument that much valuable time may be lost during which damage is done, against which later on the more radical measures fail to give a cure. Whenever the location of a brain tumor is possible, craniectomy is the operation of choice,—Babinski[69/72]—but until this is possible or while the diagnosis is still uncertain, we may give some relief by this operation, but otherwise it is strongly to be condemned.

(B) Abscess of the Brain.—What has been said about lumbar puncture in brain tumors, also applies here with all its force;

the drainage to be obtained is entirely inadequate to stay the ravages; and trephining alone can accomplish this. If the meninges also are involved then it may act favorably and the question of its use in mentation of the cerebro-spinal fluid, its very nature argues that lumbar puncture, should prove of benefit. It has been practised in the various types of this disease, but with varying results; in some the

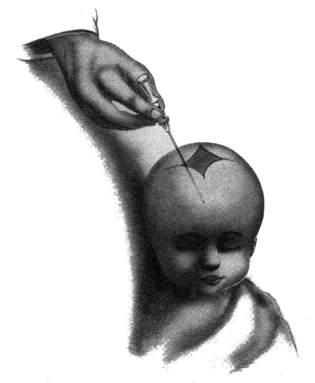

Fig. 7. Showing insertion of trocar through anterior fontanelle to reach the ventricles. Note introduction at angle of fontanelle.

connection with the other might be considered.

Hydrocephalus.

If we recall the nature of this disease, of which the primordial symptom is an augmentation of the cerebro-spinal fluid, its results were very encouraging while in the others disappointing, so that we believe a detailed study to be warranted. The conditions for its use cannot be deduced from the classical characteristics distinguishing the various clinical types. A case of hydrocephalus may run an acute course, during the whole of which time, meningeal symptoms dominate the picture. In another case the hydrocephalus is as it were post-meningitic and is a sequellæ of that disease. In these forms the disease develops under ·the eye of the physician. The pathology is not always identical, especially in the congenital forms; these latter may be due to an anomaly of development but more commonly are due to some meningeal lesion occurring during fetal life and when such a lesion is of an exudative nature, it may obliterate the communicating openings between ventricles and the arachnoid space. All fetal infections may determine a meningitis and in this particular, syphilis seems to be the most potent. The congenital form may be accompanied by malformations and lesions and is simply mentioned here as an explanation, why in the congenital form of the disease we may not get uniformly good results from this operation. Therefore for purposes of study we must divide hydrocephalus into two groups: 1st, established hydrocephalus; 2nd, hydrocephalus in evolution.

(A) Established Hydrocephalus.—Quincke[73] was the first to use this operation in the relief of this condition, but without success. Neurath and Gebhardt[74] also failed but Grober[75] reports two successful cases. One of his cases he punctured 25 times and the other 12 times, and in both obtained a notable diminution of the skull and a persistent re-establishment of cerebral functions. Other successes and failures have been reported but in some of the cases reported as successful, it is a question whether the good effects claimed, were not more upon the secondary symptoms, rather than upon the hydrocephalus

itself. Tobler in a critical review of this procedure says that he has not been able to observe any decided and durable improvement and refuses to attach to it any value in the treatment of hydrocephalus, when this disease is once established. His opinion is shared by many good observers and its employ in this condition has been very generally renounced. [The increasing number of favorable reports of the auto-curative power of ascetic and hydrocele fluid, suggests the trial of this procedure in hydrocephalus. There is certainly nothing contra-indicative to the re-injection under the skin of the hydrocephalic, of 10 or 15 cc. of the fluid obtained by lumbar puncture. This is a simple procedure and properly done under aseptic precautions, is free from danger, and certainly seems worthy of a fair trial.] (Suggestion of the translator.)

(B) Hydrocephalus in Evolution.—In this condition on the contrary, every indication is in favor of its use. When hydrocephalus occurs in the course of any acute meningitis, it must be regarded as due to the hypertension usual to meningitis and this does .not occur with nearly the same intensity in the ventricles, as the enlargement of the cranium and the distension of the fontanelles proves this. But acute hydrocephalus may have other causes than acute meningitis; hereditary syphilis is not to be forgotten, nor infectious phlebitis, obliteration of the 4th ventricle, serous meningitis and digestive auto-intoxications. In all such cases there is some ventricular distension; it is now generally admitted that an inflammatory process may start in and be almost exclusively confined to the ventricle—Merle and Weissenbach[76]. Against these conditions except the last mentioned cause, occlusion of the communicating openings, puncture affords a therapeutic means, for we have very nearly the identical indications as those we studied under the head of meningitis and therefore need not repeat them here. The results are usually favorable, but there are cases where these fail to be realized, which can be explained by obliteration of the communicating orifices between the ventricles and the arachnoid space.

The purely post-meningitic hydrocephalus are only seen in children in which the sutures have not yet knit and give rise to that peculiar head deformity of the exaggerated cranium, with the small face. In these latter cases it has not been systematically practised except in a small number of cases and in these it has been attended by good results. Rocynski reports 5 cases with decided amelioration in two; and Bokay reports even more encouraging results. Shilling insists upon its value and in one of his cases he obtained a good result by puncturing the ventricle. [It may be proper here to give some of the details of ventricular puncture and injection for the injection into the ventricles has been practised in some cases; in children before the fontanelles are closed this is quite easily reached by inserting the needle at the outer corner of the fontanelle, about an inch from the median line; the direction of the needle being from without toward the center and it must enter a depth of from ¾ to 1½ inches, see figs. In performing this operation preparatory to making an injection, it is best to withdraw a quantity greater than that to be injected. In the adult a trephining at about the same place, known as Kocher's point must precede the entrance of the ventricles. In connection with this question it is interesting to review

Barr's experiments. He was able, in a case, dead of cerebro-spinal meningitis, practically to wash through the ventricle into the cerebro-spinal canal; he connected the needle in the ventricle, with a tube through which ran a carbolized fuchsine solution and one minute later this trickled from a needle which he had previously inserted in the lumbar region. He afterwards applied this method in a case of streptococcic meningitis, using a streptococcic serum as the washing fluid; the case at the time of operating was in coma and died. This is therefore not a fair case to warrant any conclusions. Barr claims that this operation was well borne and insists upon its practicability.—Barr[44] Fischer[43], Dopter[45].] (AMERICAN EDITOR.)

Tobler reports good results in similar cases, and among others, in a case of post-meningitic idiocy with slight hydrocephalus. Hydrocephalus may also be a manifestation of a chronic meningitis, which in the adult is betrayed by headaches, due to hypertension of fluid in the cranium and some stiffness of the neck; in this form, puncture has been attended by good results. Brusch[77] reports that in some forms, the quantity withdrawn has been as high as 50 and even 100 cc. at a time:—Freud[78] —it has also been practised in the meningitis following gastro-intestinal troubles and brought a prompt end to the convulsive seizures—Merklen and Devaux[79].

Among the most interesting forms of the disease is that occurring in the course of syphilis and this is favorably influenced by lumbar puncture. Ravout[80] studying the spinal fluid in cases of hereditary syphilis, found that in hydrocephalus of this type there was always a lymphocytosis. These children presented convulsions, distension of the superficial veins

November, 1912.
New Series, Vol. VII., No. 11. }   ORIGINAL ARTICLES   { AMERICAN MEDICINE
Complete Series, Vol. XVIII.   643

of the skull, enlargement and distension of the fontanelles.—Ravout and Darre[81],—sometimes attended with stiffness of the neck and Kernig's sign. In 28 cases of this nature, puncture proved a valuable adjunct to the regular mercurial treatment and was accompanied by a steady recession of the lymphocytosis; the systematic measurement of the skull also proved conclusively, the abortive and retrogressive action of this plan of treatment. Even in cases where the head did not actually diminish in size as it frequently does not, it remained stationary, indicating a stay or arrest of the process. What has been said in these paragraphs applies to children in which the sutures are not knit. In the adult the increase in cerebro-spinal fluid cannot manifest itself by an increase in the circumference of the skull, but the same pathological process occurs, causing headaches, torpor, papillary stasis, etc., and the puncture is as effective in the adult as it is in children, of course, in conjunction with the specific treatment, to which it must always be but an adjunct in syphilis.

Syphilis.

Of all of the symptoms of this disease, it is the headache, against which puncture has the most manifest action. Headache is one of the numerous symptoms that indicate that the disease has reached the nervous system and it may occur during any period of the disease. The syphilitic origin of a headache, often cannot be definitely asserted, except after a lymphocytosis of the cerebro-spinal fluid has been revealed by a microscopic examination. The studies of Ravout[82], Widal and Sicard have shown the necessity of this. But it is from a therapeutic point, against the nocturnal headaches of the secondary stage,

Marie and Guillian[84], that puncture is most valuable and all who have practised this operation therapeutically for these headaches, are in accord in the favorable results obtained. Milian, Crouzon and Paris[83].

During the tertiary period, the headache may be due to quite different causes; it may be due to an irritation of the meninges by a gummatous or sclerous process, and under such circumstances, puncture may still do some good—Oettinger and Hamel[85]—but in a much less degree than in the secondary stage. If the headache be due to an osseous or periosteal lesion, puncture will be absolutely without effect. In the acute meningitis, which often occurs in syphilis and makes its appearance anywhere from the third to the tenth month, puncture is of high value and each operation has been followed by a notable amelioration of the symptoms. Babinski[86] reports a case of paraplegia of the lower extremities, with disturbances of the sphincters, in which the spinal fluid was blood stained and fibrinous; this case was favorably influenced by repeated lumbar puncture in connection with the classical mercurial treatment.

Syphilis may attack the cranial nerves, especially the optic and so cause a neuritis, most frequently of meningitic origin; but this will be more fully discussed under the head of ocular troubles.

The importance of meningeal lesion in determining parasyphilitic accidents—Gilbert Ballet[87]—and complications, such as general paralysis—Clergier[88]—and tabes, warrants the hope that in these, puncture may prove of some value, if there is hypertension,—Debore[89]—but good results are only to be hoped for in the very early stages. Milan[90] reports 25 cases in which he used this means for the relief of the pruritis of tabes and in a certain number obtained some permanent good.

Psychoses. Idiocy. Epilepsy. Incontinence of Urine. Neuralgias. Tetany. Chorea.

As a therapeutic measure lumbar puncture has been tried in this very diverse series of affections and it has been practised many times in different types of psychoses. The results have been inconstant, sometimes ephemeral and always difficult to judge. However, Moty cites a case of long standing lypemaniac stupor, cured by twice lumbar puncturing; Obregia and Antonin obtained a cure in a case of melancholia and in two cases of dementia precox.

Merklen and Devaux report their observations on a case of a child suffering from idiocy with convulsions but not hydrocephalic; after the second puncture the convulsive crises were less frequent, milder and of shorter duration and the child began to walk. Beyond these cases the action of lumbar puncture is useful only in those cases of idiocy which are due to encephalo-meningitic process and even in these it is not always palliative.

In the essential type of epilepsy puncture has been tried but with uncertain results. Still Pichenot and Castin think it may be useful to lessen the intensity and frequency of the crises. Donath has recorded similar observations and has priority in this belief over the before mentioned authors.

Some cases of incontinence of urine have been markedly benefitted and Babinski and Boisseau report cases in children who were cured by two punctures. In three cases of organic incontinence (2 spasmodic syphilitic paraplegias and 1 of tabes) prolonged amelioration was obtained; the above named authors are unable to explain clearly the mechanism. Sicard records similar facts.

The neuralgias following herpes zoster zonalis, have sometimes been treated with signal success by puncture. Abadie obtained a cure in a case of post zonal neuralgia which had lasted several months. Sicard insists upon the therapeutic effect of the abstraction of cerebro-spinal fluid in certain cases of trigeminal neuralgia.

Gilbert and Villaret report the cure of a case by puncture, of symmetrical gangrene of the lower extremities, with sciatica and tactile disturbances.

In tetany puncture has not given manifest results; still some authors counsel its use and Hutinel thinks that it may be usefully associated with other methods of treatment. He recommends the abstraction of a few cubic cc. of fluid every three or four days.

The results of puncture in chorea have been much discussed; but to its value, the different forms of chorea in which it has been practised would have to be clearly defined. Bacciali and Bozzolo derived benefits from puncture. Donath obtained a good result from it in a case of Huntington chorea. Allaria in 6 out of 10 cases obtained encouraging results. Hutinel on the other hand never saw any benefits from it in the many cases in which he tried it and Lesue agrees with Hutinel in this after having given the operation a very systematic trial in a series of cases of chorea.

(To be continued.)

THE ANNOTATOR.

Scientific Medical Inspection at Ellis Island.[1]—A. C. Reed says that physicians must not only diagnose and cure physical ailments, but they must apply their intellects to the diseases of society, of politics, and of industrial life.

There are few questions which so concern the future of this country, from social and economic points of view as the influence of immigration.

Physicians know what immigrants are desirable and they must inspect them.

During the fiscal year 1911 there were 1,052,649 immigrants to this country, and 749,642 landed at Ellis Island.

Of the 33,000 inmates of the state insane hospitals 8,000 are aliens.

It is not easy to recognize the feebleminded infants and young children.

The work which is done on Ellis Island is far better than might be expected in view of the existing facilities.

The tests for intelligence are the so-called Binet-Simon tests which compare the mental age with the physical; those who are below this standard are classed as feeble-minded, imbecile, or idiotic.

Each group of tests forms an index of the mental status of a normal child for the corresponding age. This system is not applicable to immigrants on account of the varying conditions in different nations, hence a standard of normal intelligence for each race or nation is requisite.

The investigation which is made on normal illiterates is only to establish the minimum standard for each race or nation, all who are below this standard being defective.

A large percentage of insane immigrants were stopped at Ellis Island during 1911, but such people are often adroit in concealing their mental disease.

Those who have become insane within three years from the time of landing, from pre-existing causes, are often difficult to discover, and legal reasoning may nullify a case entirely, a layman's reasoning being superior to a physician's even in the face of the mandate of the law.

[1]*Medical Review of Reviews*, August.

Anthropological investigations of value are being made at Ellis Island, many cases showing defective physical and sexual development as to age, especially among immigrants from southern and south-eastern Europe.

The hookworm disease now excludes four per cent. of the immigrants at Ellis Island, while in 1911 six thousand trachoma patients were examined. All of this special work is performed by the Marine Hospital and Public Health Service.

The Binet-Simon tests for standardizing intelligence consists in a series of three to eight questions which were asked of two hundred normal French school children between the ages of 3 and 13.

Different degrees of intelligence were shown in the different social classes.

The results of investigations with these tests in England, France, and America have been quite uniform and permit reliable determination with regard to the intelligence of the person examined. The questions are very simple and plain. All of which shows the importance of combining the physician, as psychologist, with the teacher.

Immunity.[1]—J. C. Shaw states that every physician is asked why he so seldom acquires the infectious and contagious diseases to which he is exposed.

An answer is not always easy to give. In general he is obliged to say that he is not very susceptible to them or that he has greater or less immunity which enables him to resist them. Natural immunity to bacterial infection is often a natural quality of a race or individual, its opposite being natural susceptibility.

Natural susceptibility may be transformed into acquired immunity by an attack of disease or by inoculation with vaccines or sera. We can account for these facts by heredity and a gradually acquired immunity through long continued ancestral exposure to infections. The blood serum is the great factor in the human organism which enables it to resist infection so successfully.

[1]*International Journal of Surgery*, August.

The antitoxic substances in the healthy body are identical with those which are found in actively immunized animals.

Our protective immunity comes from the bactericidal substances in the blood which are called alexins by Buchner and defensive proteids by Hawkins. Metchnikoff claims that immunity comes from phagocytosis, that is the leucocytes have the power of taking up, rendering inert and digesting micro-organisms encountered in the tissues. In other words, susceptibility or immunity is the struggle between invading bacteria and resisting leucocytes. Immunization increases the opsonins or the substances which act upon bacteria preparing them for the phagocytes or leucocytes.

From this arises the theory of the opsonic index. The ductless glands exert controlling influence over many of the metabolic activities of the tissues which is shown by the results following their removal or pathological involvement.

Such glands have an internal secretion which is essential to growth and function.

Furthermore, glands which have ducts also secrete substances which are taken up by the blood or tissues for the benefit of the entire organism.

It is thought that the important discoveries along these lines should be received with an open and impartial mind in the hope that they may soon be arranged in their proper order and proportion. At the present moment there is no little bewilderment at the obscure and sometimes conflicting statements which are made from time to time by investigators in this most important field.

Bewilderment indeed! and many of us, the majority of us are compelled from the pressure of that which occupies our daily lives to confess ourselves agnostics who are waiting until the waters have settled and crystallization has taken place.

Excluding the Mentally Unfit.[1]—An editorial remarks that control of mental defectives and prevention of their increase is one of the most vexatious sanitary and

[1]*New York Medical Journal*, August 17, 1912.

medical problems which confronts New York.

More than 80 per cent. of the insane or mentally defective immigrants are bound for New York, and more than 25 per cent. of the inmates of the state hospitals for the insane are aliens.

In the New York schools there are 7000 feebleminded children and an equal number of imbeciles and idiots who are not in school, there are also many more who are morally defective. Thirty per cent. of this number are the offspring of aliens or naturalized citizens who were admitted because Congress has failed to provide facilities for mental examination at Ellis Island.

The state board of alienists makes the following recommendations to the state commissioner in lunacy:

1. That the transportation companies should be fined $100 for each insane person brought over.

2. That alienists from the Marine Hospital be detailed at all ports of entry to make mental examinations of immigrants.

3. That aliens who have been improperly admitted or who have become public charges from causes which existed prior to their landing may be deported within five, instead of three years as at present.

4. That deported patients requiring personal attention shall be provided with it at government expense.

5. That it shall be a misdemeanor for a steamship company to refuse passage to any alien in a public institution who was brought here by that company if he can travel unattended, and if he is attended the government shall pay for such attendance.

The Causes of Pain in the Upper Right Quadrant of the Abdomen as Determined by Miana of the Roentgen Rays.[1]—G. E. Pfahler draws the following conclusions upon this subject:

1. Practically all pathological conditions in the chest which may cause pain in the right upper quadrant of the abdomen can be demonstrated by the Roentgen rays.

[1]*New York Medical Journal*, May 18, 1912.

2. Subdiaphragmatic abscess can usually be demonstrated.

3. Biliary calculi can be shown in some cases.

4. Duodenal, gastric and colonic adhesions can practically always be demonstrated by their effects on the position and movements of these organs.

5. Gastric ulcer can be shown only when it has perforated, and can be suspected by spasmodic contractions which may be present in the stomach.

6. Duodenal ulcer may be suspected if spasmodic constrictions are present in the duodenum.

7. Gastric carcinoma can almost always be demonstrated.

8. Renal calculus can be demonstrated in about ninety-eight per cent. of the cases.

9. Renal abscess can often be demonstrated by combined cystoscopic and roentgenoscopic examinations.

10. Perinephric abscess can be demonstrated when it is large enough to produce a palpable tumor, or when it displaces neighboring organs.

11. Colonic kinks and constrictions can be demonstrated.

12. Each of these conditions requires careful technic and study in the sequence of the various steps during the examination and usually requires not only a fluoroscopic examination but a number of plates.

The Prenatal Care of the Infant.[1]—E. P. Davis thinks the time will come when we will be aroused to the necessity of safeguarding the natural increase in population, beginning our task with childhood.

Factors which will help in this direction are the giving of a living wage in order to permit early marriage, the abolition of tenements and the substitution of model houses.

Only recently have the nations begun to appreciate the necessity of lessening infant mortality, this fact appearing in the study of eugenics and in care over prenatal influences. More attention than ever is also being given to the care of the pregnant mother, and to the elimination of the violence culminating in miscarriage

which often follows the physical strain of domestic and industrial work. The dangers of modern locomotion and travel are found responsible for many of the abortions and premature births.

Efforts to prevent alcoholism and syphilis are becoming more and more significant and will have their influence upon the pregnant women of the near future.

The nutrition of the pregnant woman, especially with the view of avoiding the toxemia of pregnancy is another problem which is being assiduously studied and this means that subjects relating to hygiene must be carefully considered; it means frequent examinations of the urine during pregnancy, pure milk at a low price, instruction in cooking and the establishment of markets where fresh fruits and vegetables can be obtained direct from the farmer.

A prematernity ward in the hospital will furnish opportunity for considering the anemia of pregnancy with the various lesions of the heart and bloodvessels which accompany it, and will thus save many lives both of mothers and their offspring.

Obstetric surgery is gradually becoming available in treating the surgical lesions of pregnancy, including those of the kidney, the appendix, the liver, and the gallbladder, not to speak of the lesions of the genital passages, and timely attention to such matters will mean the safe delivery of many children.

Hand in hand with the physician is coming the helpful assistance of the visiting obstetric nurse and the sociological worker.

All these factors promise much for the democracy of the future, and nobody will play a more important part in the coming reforms than the doctor.

A Review of the Dangerously Poisonous Snakes of the United States.[1]—H. Tucker in a beautifully illustrated article gives the following suggestions in regard to treatment, the article being written for the assistance of the physician.

1. Don't lose your head, death from snake bite rarely occurs in this country. Most of the so-called poisonous snakes

---

[1]*Therapeutic Gazette*, September 15.

[1]*Therapeutic Gazette*, May 15, 1912.

are harmless, while the poisonous varieties are usually found in places remote from civilization. More than two punctures at the seat of injury would be a strong indication that the wound was innocent. The head of the snake should be kept for identification if possible.

2. If the bite is upon an extremity, tie one or more ligatures, preferably a rubber band above the injury, to prevent the poison from entering the general circulation.

3. Incise the wound deeply, cutting across the puncture for at least an inch and beyond the depth made by the fang. Then wash in running water and encourage free bleeding. Or suck the wound as there is no danger in taking the poison into the mouth unless there is a break in the mucous membrane. Then rinse the mouth thoroughly with potassium permanganate solution.

4. Wash the wound thoroughly with the potassium permanganate, or inject a 1 to 100 chromic acid solution. Be sure and infiltrate not only the wound but the surrounding tissues.

5. Don't administer ammonia but stimulate with small doses of whiskey, remembering that more people have been killed by large quantities of whiskey than by snake bite.

6. Take the patient to a good surgeon as quickly as possible.

7. If you are sure that the poison has been removed from the wound loosen the ligatures cautiously, the one nearest the heart first, but do not remove them as it may be necessary to tighten them again. The patient must have the best surgical care, and the wound must be kept open by packing with wet antiseptic gauze, as sepsis and local gangrene often follow the injury.

———

Intravenous Injections to be Used With Care.[1]—An editorial remarks that the importance of this subject is not fully recognized. The saline solution is often prepared by an incompetent nurse and the working formula which is given her is not accurate. She is usually directed to add a teaspoonful of salt to a pint of water, the teaspoonful being an uncertain quantity and the salt being seldom sterilized. In Locke's modification of Ringer's fluid we have a solution in which the normal saline ingredients of the blood are present in the proper proportions. If a saline solution of less than 0.9 per cent. is injected into the body of a human being osmosis of the salts of the body will result until the injected fluid is isotonic with the tissues, while if a solution stronger than 0.9 per cent. is injected it will abstract fluids from the tissues until the two liquids are isotonic. Any considerable variation in the tonicity of the fluid may produce serious functional and organic changes in different organs of the body.

Hart and Penfold have observed that fever, rigors, sub-normal temperature, intestinal hemorrhage, Cheyne-Stokes breathing, convulsions, and death have followed intravenous injections, and these symptoms can readily be produced in animals. Various observers have noted in animals, after intravenous injections glycosuria, vacuolation of liver cells, injury of red cells, and degenerative changes in the heart muscles, the kidneys, and the walls of the capillaries.

It has also been observed clinically that large quantities of fluid cannot be injected into the circulation without throwing a heavy burden upon the kidneys and perhaps upon the heart. Death has resulted even when saline solutions have been injudiciously used by the rectum or subcutaneously. But it is not denied that when saline solutions are properly prepared, are of proper strength, and sterile they may be used within certain limits with great advantage.

In cholera hypertonic saline solutions are advantageous because in that disease anything which diminishes the amount of fluid which is poured from the body will be advantageous.

———

Practical Eugenics.[1]—An editorial quotes an opinion that every person before marrying should be compelled by law to undergo a private and confidential medical examination, just as one must pass an examination before obtaining a policy for life insurance.

———

[1]*Therapeutic Gazette*, May 15, 1912.   [1]*The Medical Times*, June, 1912.

While such an examination might cause more serious thought upon the subject of physical fitness at the time of marriage, it is recognized that when two people are determined to marry, the doctor's views as to their physical condition will not have much weight with them.

The department of vital statistics would be benefited by such a plan and the classification of married people from the physical standpoint would be a matter of important record.

In the course of years this would result in the accumulation of valuable data affecting many obscure problems of heredity.

It is admitted that no one is competent at present to say who is fit to marry and who is not; it would be an extremely difficult matter to draw the line beyond which marriage should not receive public sanction.

A public requirement of this character is worth striving for as it would be an incentive to acquire good health especially if the certificate of the highest grade were refused to those who were not physically well developed. It would enable the state medical service to watch over the children of degenerate parents and give them the best possible chance. A symposium on this subject is also reported in this number of the *Medical Times*, a series of very interesting and valuable contributions being made by clergymen and doctors. The opinions expressed were all but unanimous that a law requiring a certificate of health prior to marriage would be a valuable law, but that it might not be easy to enforce it, at least not until public sentiment caught up with it.

The Doctor and Public Health Education.[1]—G. T. Palmer writes that there can be no doubt that popular medical education should come, in part at least, from medical men.

Of course, this cannot be brought about unless some doctors get their names in the newspapers. We must not forget that popular medical education now thrives under the guidance of fakes and humbugs and quacks and this will continue until they are displaced by those who are properly qualified to teach the public.

[1] *The Medical Times*, June, 1912.

People are as much interested in their livers and kidneys as they are in their hearts and souls and will satisfy that interest with misinformation unless there is a readily available supply of truth. It is recognized that peculiar literary talent is required, in addition to a knowledge of preventive medicine to dress the solid and unromantic facts of health conservation in a form to compete with fiction. It would therefore seem to be entirely fitting that those who have this talent should use it for the public welfare.

No Marriage License Without a Physician's Certificate of Freedom from Venereal and Mental Disease.[1]—W. J. Robinson thinks that woman is now awake to the fact of her independence and that she demands the right to dispose of her body as her own, and not her husband's property.

She desires to know what is to become of her body when she becomes married.

She is becoming foolish enough to refuse to be a victim to man's ignorance and brutality, and to ask for a guarantee that the marriage bed will not soon be converted into an invalid's bed, and that the wedding march may not be a prelude to an early funeral march.

The miseries which come to women soon after marriage with infected husbands could be eliminated if each male applicant for a marriage license were compelled to furnish a physician's certificate of freedom from venereal or mental disease.

A law which required this could be passed if public sentiment demanded it.

Of course, the law must apply to all the states and must be uniform.

Such a law would make young men very careful in their sexual relations, or would impel them, if infected, to use all proper means to get cured.

A requirement of this kind would be in line with that which is made by many parents that a man proposing matrimony to their daughter should take out a policy of life insurance in the daughter's favor. The requirement of a similar certificate from a woman need not be insisted upon since the chances of venereal disease in

[1] *American Journal of Clinical Medicine,* June, 1912.

the woman are far more remote than in the man.

This is in the line of the advanced thought of the times and means that important social changes are imminent, in fact that some of them have already taken their place on the statute book in Indiana and elsewhere. Logically, if a certificate of physical well being is required of a man it should be required of a woman also, and probably very few women who were proper subjects for matrimony would refuse it if it were exacted from both sexes alike.

ETIOLOGY AND DIAGNOSIS.

Diagnosis of Surgical Diseases of the Stomach.—Vomiting in any of the above lesions is extremely variable, and apart from the presence of blood is of no aid in arriving at a differential diagnosis. In many cases it depends not so much upon the actual disease as upon the consequent mechanical change. Thus, in a large number of cases of chronic gastric ulcer there may be no actual vomiting, although eructation and regurgitation of acid material may be present. In other cases vomiting occurs at the height of pain, which is immediately relieved. If there is any constriction of the stomach, either in the body (hour-glass) or at the pylorus, large quantities of decomposing and fermenting material may be vomited.

In carcinoma, again, the character of the vomiting depends upon the presence or absence of obstruction of the gastric outlet. If there be no obstruction there is early flatulence and regurgitation of bitter and foul material, while later actual vomiting occurs. In either case it may be associated with slight hematemesis. The amount of vomited material is generally small and, as a rule, it does not give relief, as in chronic gastric ulcer. If there is pyloric obstruction the characteristic type of vomiting found with a dilated stomach occurs early and does not differ from that of obstruction due to gastric ulcer.

In duodenal ulcer vomiting is rare. Moynihan has shown that it is a constant symptom only if stenosis of the duodenum had supervened from constriction of the ulcer. In an otherwise typical case of a duodenal ulcer vomiting points to the coexistence of a gastric ulcer, gall stones, or chronic appendicitis.

When gall-stones are producing severe pain, vomiting is common. It is followed by relief, which, although definite, is not generally so marked as in the case of chronic ulcer.

In chronic appendix gastralgia vomiting is frequent, and often is the most marked symptom. It is most evident during the exacerba-

---

[1] A. J. Walton, M. S., F. R. C. S., *Brit. Med. Jour.*, Oct. 5, 1912.

---

tions of the symptoms, but may even be present between the attacks.

It will be seen that in many cases it is possible to arrive at a diagnosis from a careful consideration of the history, but there are so many exceptions to the common types that it is impossible to diagnose with certainty from this aspect alone. Further evidence can be gained from a careful examination.

In most cases anemia is present. In chronic ulcer this may be due to the loss of blood or to the underlying toxemia, for this is often marked when there has never been any visible loss of blood. Anemia may also be present in chronic duodenal ulcer, gall-stones, appendicitis, or carcinoma of the stomach.

Emaciation and cachexia are likewise useless as a means of diagnosis. In carcinoma they appear late, and they may be present in chronic gastric ulcer.

The ordinary methods of palpation, percussion, and auscultation are of limited value. In gastric and duodenal ulcer there may be an area of deep tenderness of limited extent, and its position may aid in the differential diagnosis between them. Again, in chronic cholecystitis there is generally deep tenderness over the gall bladder, which may be best shown by Murphy's sign. The enlarged gall-bladder, or a tumor of the stomach, may be easily palpable. These last two symptoms are, however, often absent, and a palpable tumor in the stomach points to the disease being far advanced although not necessarily inoperable.

Hertz has shown that percussion and auscultatory percussion are useless to determine either the size or position of the stomach. (*Review*, 1911, p. 295). This is, indeed, what one would expect, for even if distended the stomach may contain solids and no gas. Radiography of the stomach and duodenum after administration of a bismuth meal, may be of considerable value, but there is difficulty in interpreting the results. It has been shown that the stomach is not a simple sac, as was believed, but is divided into a cardiac part, which is more or less saccular, and a tubular pyloric portion separated by the incisura angularis. In an atonic and distended stomach the division may be lost. Care, therefore, must be taken not to mistake a normal stomach for one with an hour-glass deformity.

In every case of doubt a test meal should be given. Active HCl is nearly always increased in gastric and duodenal ulcer, whilst it is markedly diminished in gastric carcinoma. There are, however, many exceptions, and, as Sherren has shown, too much stress must not be attached to the test meal. He found that, "in those cases in which most help is needed, namely, those with many years' history, which may be chronic ulcer or may have overstepped the line and become malignant, no information is given of any value."

With the gastroscope an admirable view of the gastric mucosa can be obtained, but the two stomach lesions which are most difficult to distinguish are chronic ulcer and gastric carcinoma, and not uncommonly it is impossible to recognize them. Moreover, in most cases the passage of the instrument necessitates general anesthesia and since, in careful hands, the sole danger of an exploratory operation is the small one of the anesthetic, the patient will thereby be exposed to the same risk in return for much less information.

The final and most certain method of diagnosis is exploratory laparotomy. But as in all the above lesions the only satisfactory treatment is an operation, the laparotomy is not performed for the purpose of diagnosis alone. It is the first step in the operative treatment. In the majority of cases a careful investigation will lead to the diagnosis of one of the above lesions. There are a few cases in which one can say with certainty that one of the lesions is present, but it is impossible to say which. Exploratory operation is then desirable, or rather operative treatment is demanded, but the exact nature of the operation can be determined only after the abdomen is opened.

The most important reason for operation is the possibility, even if remote, of carcinoma. This in the early stage is curable, but then the diagnosis is difficult. W. J. Mayo states that "gastric cancer itself does not give rise to diagnostic symptoms during the curable stage." The other lesions are, however, not only so intractable to any other form of treatment and are so readily relieved by surgical measures, but if left are so likely to be associated later with severe or fatal complications that valuable time should not be lost. The indications for operative treatment are as follows:

1. Any case where the symptoms are such that one of the above lesions can be diagnosed with tolerable certainty.

2. Any case commencing after the age of 35, which is not markedly relieved by a few weeks' adequate medical treatment.

3. When symptoms have recurred after previous attacks relieved by medical treatment, especially if the symptoms have changed from those typical of a chronic gastric ulcer.

4. Any case in which the stomach shows definite evidence of distension, whether the symptoms are those of ulcer or carcinoma.

5. Any case in which a tumor is present suggesting any of the above conditions.

6. Any case with repeated hemorrhage.

The writer lays special stress upon the fact that if rapid progress is not made under adequate medical treatment operation should early be resorted to. It affords the only certain method of diagnosis and cure, and if undertaken early many of the more hopeless complications can be prevented. Also in these cases no operation must be considered complete unless the stomach, duodenum, gall-bladder, and appendix have all been examined.

The Significance of Acute Abdominal Pain.[1]
—The following practical points are taken from the teaching of Mr. Sampson Handley at Middlesex Hospital and deal in a helpful manner with the difficulties and doubts arising in the case of a patient who, suddenly seized with acute abdominal pain, sends for his doctor. One of the main points upon which stress is laid is that tne pulse and temperature may be found normal in the presence of an abdominal disaster. A palpable appendical abscess may be present without pyrexia. An appendicitis of the most deadly character may commence merely with acute general abdominal pain, no other symptoms appearing for six or eight hours, during which the pulse and temperature remain normal. Complete intestinal obstruction, if not accompanied by strangulation, and especially if there has been previous incomplete obstruction, may persist for several days without producing any marked quickening of the pulse. In perforated gastric ulcer, after the first shock has passed off, and before the fever of peritonitis supervenes, there may be a deceptive lull, in which the depressed temperature returns to normal and the feeble pulse resumes its steady beat. If the pulse and temperature, especially the latter, fail as criteria of the seriousness of the case, a most important point to remember is that in perforation, during the stage of reaction, when other signs are sometimes absent, muscular rigidity of the abdomen can nearly always be detected. If, however, morphia has been given all the symptoms are masked; and, therefore, in abdominal crises morphia must be withheld until some diagnosis is made, no matter what the distress of the patient. Small doses of belladonna are, perhaps, allowable during the period of doubt. If a case of acute intestinal obstruction be allowed to reach the stage of fecal vomiting, operative treatment has hardly any chance of success. Fecal vomiting is not to be regarded as a symptom of intestinal obstruction, but as a herald of approaching death. If flatus and feces both fail to pass during a period of twenty-four hours, in spite of repeated enemas, the diagnosis of intestinal obstruction is established, and should be acted upon immediately. Another reason for prompt action is that patients who would bear moving in the the earliest stages of acute abdominal disease may at a later stage be killed by the process of transport. This applies especially to appendicitis, and even in the earliest stage no case of appendicitis should be moved except upon an ambulance. If a diagnosis is impossible, the best line of treatment is to place a nurse in charge, with instructions to take the pulse and temperature hourly, and the case should be seen frequently. The administration of an enema repeated if necessary, should be a routine measure. Within from eight to twenty-four hours it will usually be possible to arrive at a working diagnosis, and, failing this, if the patient's condition is not improving, an exploratory operation will probably be advisable.

The Action of Salvarsan and Neosalvarsan on the Wassermann Reaction.[1]—McDonagh

[1] The Practitioner, London, July, 1912.

[1] A. McDonagh, M. B., L. R. C. P., Brit. Med. Jour., June 8, 1912.

gives his observations on the value of the Wassermann reaction as a guide to the treatment of syphilis. In the primary stage, when the reaction is negative before treatment is commenced, most cases give a positive reaction afterwards. This reaction is most marked about the forty-eighth hour. In some cases on the other hand, the reaction does not become positive until the fifth day. Although it may remain· positive for several days, the degree diminishes generally about the third week, until · it becomes negative before the eighth week. If the reaction is only slightly positive after the injection, it becomes negative much earlier. If the first injection gives rise to only a weak reaction then three or four more will undoubtedly suffice to make the reaction permanently negative; if, however, the reaction is strong, then the patient is in the secondary stage, and will require at least 3 grams of salvarsan or neosalvarsan before the desired effect is obtained. In the secondary stage when the reaction becomes strongly positive after an injection, and in cases in which it is markedly positive before treatment is commenced, no blood tests need be made until before and after the fourth injection, as in McDonagh's experience the four injections are the minimum likely to be required to produce a permanent negative result. In the tertiary stage the Wassermann reaction behaves much in the same way as it does in the primary and secondary, except for one peculiar phenomenon, which is occasionally to be noted—that is, a case with a strong positive reaction before treatment may become negative immediately after an injection and remain so from twenty-four to seventy-two hours, and then becomes quite positive again. Patients who have had syphilis and give a negative Wassermann reaction are either cured or in the latent stage which of the two can only be ascertained by giving a provocative injection of salvarsan and then testing the blood. As an injection of salvarsan will not give rise to a positive reaction in a non-syphilitic, one must regard the occurrence of such as indicative of the presence of disease, and efforts should be made to bring about a cure. Taking all stages of syphilis, McDonagh has found that three to seven injections are necessary to cure most cases of syphilis. There is no doubt that many cases in the tertiary stage can be cured with neosalvarsan which failed to be cured with salvarsan. Liable to change as these conclusions may be, he cannot but admit that the alterations in the Wassermann reaction as the result of treatment are most constant, and when tested at short intervals, give a much safer guide to regulate treatment than by saying that just so many injections will be required, or, as the old syphilologists used to teach, that a three years' pill treatment was sufficient for all cases alike. As there is a possibility of fallacy, he advises his patients to have a provocative injection of neosalvarsan six months or a year after they have been discharged, and the blood tested forty-eight

hours, the seventh, fourteenth, twenty-first, and twenty-eighth day after that injection. ·

TREATMENT.

The Inunction Treatment of Measles.[1]—According to Connolly the method of treatment employed by Dr. Milne is given, as follows, in his book: "For the first four days in a scarlet fever case—and presumably also in a measles case—commencing at the earliest possible moment, I have pure eucalyptus oil gently rubbed in all over the body, morning and evening, from the crown of the head to the soles of the feet. Afterwards this is repeated once a day until the tenth day of the disease * * * *." "The tonsils, however, I always swab with 1-10 carbolic oil every two hours for the first 24 hours. Only on rare occasions have I found it · necessary to swab the tonsils for a longer period than 24 hours, and never when commenced early. My method is to make a firm mop of cotton-wool on the end of a pair of forceps, thoroughly soak the wool in the carbolic oil, and then swab the tonsils and the pharynx as far up and down as possible. It is advisable, however, to use a tongue depressor and depress the tongue as far as possible * * * The mop used should be rather larger than the last joint of the patient's thumb. The wool should thoroughly cover the end of the forceps (or lead pencil), while a fresh swab is used on every application."

In Connolly's cases, the Milne method, just described, is followed in the main, with, however, some modifications. As soon as the child is received into the special ward assigned to measles, a hot bath is given. Then follows a thorough application of the eucalyptus oil to the whole of the body, with the exception of the hands and the part of the face round about the nose, mouth, and eyes. The mouth is irrigated twice daily with weak alum lotion, and glycerine and borax if applied to the interior of the mouth and to the gums. The throat (tonsils and fauces) is treated with carbolic oil (1-10) morning and evening, in a similar manner to that described by Dr. Milne. Every day for the following four days the child is blanket-bathed morning and evening, and again rubbed all over with eucalyptus oil, the throat and mouth having the same treatment as on admission.

It will thus be seen that a more determined attack is made upon the mouth and throat. In most of the cases, it was found that the gums were very red and more or less swollen, and often quite definite ulceration was present on the inner side of the cheeks and lips, much larger and whiter than Koplik's spots. Further, it was believed that by attacking the mouth and throat one was striking at one of the chief strongholds of the virus. Connolly is of the opinion that the moist spray and particles,

[1] D. I. Connolly, M. B., Ch. B., Manchester Eng., *London Practitioner*, Nov., 1912.

coughed out by the patient, are highly infectious to a susceptible person. In those cases in which broncho-pneumonia is already established, the statement holds true to a greater degree.

As regards the thorough rubbing in of the eucalyptus oil, some local effect would, doubtless, be produced, but the main idea was to get the vapor inhaled into the air passages. If the virus were dwelling in the skin or the subcutaneous tissues, it seems reasonable to suppose, too, that direct conflict would take place between the eucalyptus absorbed and such virus as might be present. The face area was omitted, because of the irritation caused to the eyes by the vapor, and it was not thought necessary to apply the oil to the hands.

***

Treatment of Asthma in Children.[1]—McClanahan states that in the treatment of the asthmatic paroxysm care should be taken to have the room warm and to exclude draughts. If the child's bowels are distended with gas, a warm enema should be given. If the paroxysm comes on soon after a hearty meal, an emetic will give relief. Epinephrine solution (one to 1,000) hypodermically in doses of three to five minims proved quickly beneficial in two of the author's little patients, but in others was without effect. Other cases were relieved, respectively, by 1/30 grain of morphine sulphate, three grain doses of chloral hydrate, and inhalations of nascent oxygen. Where cough, wheezing, and dyspnea on exertion persist after the paroxysm proper has been subdued, the use of heroin in a syrup of hypophosphites will often benefit. Antipyrine given at bedtime will sometimes allay cough that tends to disturb the child's sleep. For dry, teasing cough, one teaspoonful each of creosote and oil of eucalyptus may be added to a pint of water and the mixture inhaled, with the use of an improvised croup tent, for one half hour at a time two or three times daily.

As for the treatment of asthma during the intervals, McClanahan points out the necessity for proper protection of the child's chest, neck and lower extremities against cold, and advises that a diet poor in meats, but rich in vegetable proteids be generally ordered. In asthmas induced by bowel trouble, green vegetables and fruit juices should be included in the dietary. Since acute bronchitis frequently precedes an asthmatic paroxysm, appearance of the former should be the signal for prompt confinement to bed, restriction to liquid foods, and administration of an active cathartic and hot drinks.

In cases which fail to respond, a change of climate, or sometimes merely a change in location of a few miles, is necessary. Anemia or a history of rheumatism should suggest appropriate treatment. Pulmonary gymnastics in the form of daily exercises in deep breathing, with emphasis upon complete expiration, or the wearing of an elastic binder around the chest,

light enough to exert constant light pressure, are strongly recommended by the author in asthma of children.

Where catarrhal bronchitis persists after the paroxysms have been subdued, sodium iodide, in doses of two to four grains, three times daily, after meals, is of decided benefit. It should be given for several weeks.

***

The Treatment of Diabetes Mellitus.[1]—The carbuncle of diabetes mellitus, of all carbuncles, says Kolipinski, should never be operated upon by excision. Diabetic coma is always imminent. Far better is it to cure this infection of the skin by means of precipitated sulphur, applied as a powder into the points of suppuration, or ulceration, or used as an ointment with a cacao-butter base (1 to 8). Equally efficacious to render a carbuncle innocuous is the constant application of a compress wet with a solution of calcium creosote.

Extensive gangrenous phlegmons must be incised and then thoroughly dressed with the same applications.

Diabetic cataract, when in its incipiency may clear up under the antidiabetic diet.

Albuminuria, where faint and incipient, may likewise entirely disappear. Where it is an essential part of subacute or chronic nephritis, an attempt to cure these may be made with a diet consisting of curds or schmierkase. When the albuminuria has practically disappeared, the artificial milk is added to these two foods. The artificial milk consists of a modified formula of a series of liquid foods imitating milk chemically, devised by the writer and described in the *Medical News*, New York, December 21, 1901. It is prepared as follows:

1 broken raw egg.
2 teaspoonfuls of malt extract.
4 teaspoonfuls of olive oil.

Beat up in a bowl with a spoon or egg-beater for five minutes. Add gradually while stirring 1 pint of drinking-water. Season to the patient's taste with table salt. In hot weather add crushed ice.

Cows' milk cannot be used in treating diabetes or the succeeding nephritis. With a milk diet it is possible in the nephritis of diabetes to remove the urinary albumin entirely, as well as the dyspnea and anasarca, and very rapidly to increase the strength and weight of the patient; but soon after the glycosuria, previously very much reduced or for a time even absent, will reappear. With this the diabetic dyscrasia returns in its full intensity. A meat diet now produces a fresh albuminuria, the sugar again receding, and death finally results. It may occur as a result of both diseases—gangrene of a lower limb and uremia.

Milk has been allowed as a food in diabetes by many practitioners, and has been approved as proper in the diabetic form of nephritis, but not wisely, as it is agreed that the ingestion of lactose in diabetes increases

***

[1] H. M. McClanahan, M. D., *Amer. Jour of the Med. Sciences*, June, 1912.

[1] A. Kolipinski, M. D., *Monthly Cyclopedia*, Aug., 1912.

the glucose in the blood. In the abandoned skimmed-milk treatment of Donkin, the singular error was committed of taking away useful food substances and allowing sugar of milk, a harmful one, to remain.

Gangrene, when superficial, heals spontaneously or with boric acid compresses or baths.

Deep or complete gangrene of a limb gives a heavy mortality after operation. In such cases the prognosis is always unfavorable unless the patient reacts to the proper diet, which alone can save the life that is in jeopardy. Gangrene, like albuminuria and all other complications, never appears where dieting has permanently rendered the urine normal.

The pulmonary tuberculosis of diabetes is insidious, never chronic, rapidly fatal, with deep sepsis and enormous wasting of the body. Hemoptysis may be the first evidence of a disease already established. Equally as fatal as tuberculosis, and sometimes a part of it—at other times after a croupous pneumonia—is pulmonary gangrene. The antidiabetic diet always eliminates the grape sugar in the urine, but never retards the rapid progress of either of these diseases.

True glocosuria occurring in the course of typhoid fever requires no treatment until the temperature is normal and convalescence begins. The sugar, as is known, disappears in four or five days from the onset of the fever, reappearing when the disease has run its course.

Syphilis, secondary and tertiary, should be treated as in the non-diabetic. Antisyphilitics, like all other well-known remedies, have no power to alter the state of glycemia, and lues, present or past, or its treatment, neither aggravates nor mitigates the associated disease.

Beginning acidosis may vanish, and the acids and fat derivatives found in the urine in cases near to a fatal ending will likewise be removed together with the sugar under the influence of diet; but where great weakness, drowsiness, labored breathing, and beginning stupor herald the oncoming of diabetic coma, the case is a lost one. Perhaps the discovery of a suitable antidote for acetone and diacetic and oxybutyric acids in the blood, or of an eliminant, will eventually lead to success, or else, by transfusion or the introduction of enough water into the stomach to dilute sufficiently the poisoned blood, better results may be obtained than those now achieved; but as yet the coma of diabetes is still the most rapidly fatal of all the dangerous complications to which its victims are exposed.

HYGIENE AND DIETETICS.

The Fallacy of Fumigation.[1]—The recent International Congress on Hygiene and Demography at Washington arrived at the conclusion that disease is almost invariable conveyed by contagion and not by infection, that is to say, by contact, either direct or indirect, with

[1] Editorial New York Med. Journal, Oct. 19, 1912.

a patient suffering from the disease in question. The method of direct infection is obvious; indirect infection is caused mainly by the inhalation of dust acting as a vehicle for the pathogenic organisms diffused by an infected person.

This conclusion, in conjunction with the appointment of a joint committee of this congress and of the International Congress of Applied Chemistry with the object of defining a simple method of testing disinfectants, may have a far reaching effect upon the health of the nation. At first sight the appointment of this joint committee may appear to be of little more than academic interest. Such, however, is not the case. At the present time, in this country, there is no accepted method of controlling the sale and manufacture of disinfectants, and the result is the use of many preparations which are disinfectants in name only. When once a workable test has been decided upon, this abuse will come to a speedy end, and users of disinfectants will be able to assure themselves in advance that the preparations which they employ are capable of performing the work required of them.

An illustration of the unsatisfactory condition of disinfection in this country may be found in the practice of fumigation by means of formaldehyde. Contrary to the generally accepted notion as to the use of formaldehyde for fumigating rooms, this disinfectant does not act in the form of a vapor or gas; In practice, it is dissolved in the minute droplets which result from the condensation of steam, in the absence of which formaldehyde has no bactericidal action whatever. Water will take up in solution forty per cent. of formaldehyde gas, in which form it is known officially in the United States Pharmacopia as "formaldehyde solution," the Rideal-Walker coefficient of which is 0.3, i. e., it has about one-third the efficiency of pure carbolic acid. If we take one part of carbolic acid in twenty parts of water as our standard of efficiency, to prepare a solution of formaldehyde capable of doing the same work, one part must be mixed with six parts of water.

We now see the difficulty of obtaining uniformly trustworthy results when working with formaldehyde. If too much steam is admitted into the chamber the ultimate dilution produced may be too weak, and if too little steam is admitted, part of the formaldehyde will be unavailable, i. e., it will remain in the gaseous form, which, as already explained, has no bactericidal action. Compare with this the ease and accuracy with which a standardized disinfectant can be prepared and applied in the form of a fine spray.

The British Medical Journal for November 3, 1894, referring to the disinfection of rooms by fumigation, stated: "On the ground even of economy there is no comparison between this obsolete process and a disinfectant spray; and while cases of renewed house infection are familiar to almost every medical officer in this country, we have Dr. Dujardin-Beaumetz's authority for saying that where the disinfectant spray has been introduced they are practically unknown in France."

Japanese Rules of Hygiene.[1]—The Japanese Government has recently issued for free distribution to the people a code of rules for hygienic living. These rules are of particular interest for their peculiar amalgamation of persistent Oriental with Occidental ideas. Most of them are essentially the same as those of all civilized people; some are even in advance of Western practice; others could hardly be recommended for general guidance. The first eleven of these rules are as. follows:

"First: Spend as much time out-of-doors as possible. Bask much in the sun and take plenty of exercise. Take care that your respiration is always deep and regular.

"Second: As regards meals, eat meat only once a day, and let the diet be eggs, cereals, vegetables, fruits and fresh cow's milk. Take the last named as much as possible. Masticate your food carefully.

"Third: Take a hot bath every day and a steam bath once or twice a week if the heart is strong enough to bear it.

"Fourth: Put on roughly-woven underwear (cotton fabrics are preferable) and clothes; a comfortable collar, light hat of any material and well fitting boots.

"Fifth: Early to bed and early to rise.

"Sixth: Sleep in a very dark and very quiet room, with windows open. Let the minimum of sleeping hours be six or six and one-half hours, and the maximum seven and one-half hours. In case of women a rest of eight and one-half hours is advisable.

"Seventh: Take one day of absolute rest per week, on which you must refrain from even reading and writing.

"Eighth: Try to avoid any outburst of passions and strong mental stimulations. Do not overtax your brain at the occurrence of inevitable incidents or of coming events. Do not say unpleasant things, nor listen, if possible, to disagreeable things.

"Ninth: Be married! Widows and widowers should be married with the least possible delay.

"Tenth: Be moderate in the consumption of even tea and coffee, not to say tobacco and alcoholic beverages.

"Eleventh: Avoid places that are too warm, especially steam-heated and badly ventilated rooms."

The injunctions about food and sleep are especially to be noted, particularly that not to take too much of the latter. With regard to matrimony, however, and the use of tobacco, the rules are not so cordially to be commended. It is significant that the Japanese appreciate so well the hygienic effect of conduct and temperament.

THE DOCTOR'S AUTOMOBILE.

When It Cries for Oil.—When a cylinder is becoming overheated, either from a stoppage of the oil supply or any other cause, it in-

[1] *Boston Med. and Surg. Journal.*

variably makes the fact known by a scraping, grating noise at each stroke of the piston caused by the dry metals rubbing against each other. A loss of power can also be noted whereupon the driver should get down at once and ascertain what the trouble is. To keep on forcing the engine to run after these warnings may result in giving it a badly scored cylinder as well as a seized piston along with the many difficulties resulting therefrom.— *Am. Med. Compend.*

To Prevent Skidding.—There is little doubt but what the relative position the body of a motor car bears to the road wheels has a considerable influence upon the tendency or otherwise to skid. When the early motor 'buses were designed little attention was paid to the length beyond the hind axle, and to this doubtless may be attributed the erratic action of many of those old vehicles. The same argument holds good with the pleasure car, I was forcibly reminded of this recently, when following an overhanging car. Of course the driving cannot be ignored, and all have learned to recognize the fact that the sudden application of the brakes accentuates side movement; but another often forgotten factor is that when descending a hill the car should not be allowed to run free, but instead the engine should be used as a brake, by closing the gas inlet valve to the cylinders and drawing air through the exhaust-pipe. Although purely mechanical in action it is certain in practice; the only objection that can be raised to using the engine in such a way is the danger of drawing in any foreign matter with the air into the cylinders and choking the valves. On the other hand, although the air is super-heated by passing through a warm exhaust-pipe it is colder than exploding gas, and so has a cooling effect. With engines which, owing to their construction, are not suitable for such a procedure, the throttle can be closed, and one of the low gears engaged; almost any gradient can thus be descended in safety without using the brakes, if action is taken in time. Again, extra care is necessary when the tires have begun to show signs of wear, for the older they are the less is the adhesion to the road surface they afford. The luggage grid behind a pronounced over-hanging car is bad policy. With the horse the rule has always been to keep the load as near the active agency as possible, and for even and economical running and a straight course there is nothing to beat the same principle with the self-moving vehicle.—*Am. Med. Compend.*

In the Tool-Box of the Automobile.—Besides the special tools given with each make of car, and usually adapted especially to its particular parts, there are always a few handy things of general usefulness which the motorist can with profit carry. A small pocket electric torch is extremely convenient, for examining the amount of "gas" in the tank at night, for instance, and can be bought for a dollar or less. A small monkey wrench, such as is made for use on bicycles, is often convenient, as it is but half as thick in the jaws as the regular style, and will fit some places which would otherwise take only a thin "spanner." A small funnel, probably of copper, tinned inside, is useful for filling the oil tank. With the equipment of the car comes usually an oil can which is often too large for ordinary use. For "touching up" such places as the spark and throttle levers and oil holes in various places a small oiler such as is used for sewing machines and other light machinery will be found of considerable value. Special benzine cans, approved by the boards of fire underwriters, are sold for the use of tailors, printers, etc. The one-pint size to carry gasoline for cleaning hands, spark-plugs, and anything else will be found of the greatest convenience. It is safe as regards the risks usually incident to gasoline and is most readily accessible. No one who has once carried this accessory will ever dispense with it.— *Medical Record.*

Going Like a Crab.—While driving a car backward is not recommended as particularly fascinating form of amusement, nevertheless, it is a very valuable accomplishment and should be practiced by every man who takes control of a motor car. In many cases speedy and skillful manipulation of the reverse gear is the means of preventing a serious accident. The ability to steer backward becomes of great value if through the fault of the operator the motor should stall while ascending a steep hill or when loose brakes refuse to hold the car on the incline. In this connection it might be stated that sometimes you can manage to climb hills that are otherwise too steep even for the low gear, by running the car backward, for the gear ratio of the reverse is even lower than that of the first forward speed. —*Motor Print.*

SOCIETY PROCEEDINGS.

THE EASTERN MEDICAL SOCIETY OF THE CITY OF NEW YORK.

Regular Meeting, November 8th, 1912.

EXECUTIVE SESSION.

Nominations for officers for the ensuing year were made as follows:

For President,
Dr. Joseph Barsky,
Dr. Joseph Bieber.
For First Vice-President,
Dr. Nathan O. Ratnoff.
For Second Vice-President,
Dr. Gustav G. Fischlowitz.

For Recording Secretary,
Dr. Samuel J. Scadron.
For Corresponding Secretary,
Dr. Harry E. Isaacs.
For Treasurer,
Dr. Herman Lorber,
Dr. Joseph F. Saphir.
For Chairman of Committee on Ethics,
Dr. Samuel W. Bendler,
Dr. Joseph Bieber.
For Chairman Committee on Legislation and Public Health,
Dr. Moses Keschner.
For Chairman Committee on Physicians Aid,
Dr. Abraham Rongy.
For Chairman Committee on Admissions,
Dr. Meyer Rabinovitz,
Dr. Isaac S. Hirsch,
Dr. Samuel Spiegel.
For Trustee,
Dr. Emil Altman.

Ninety-eight members of the society were expelled for non-payment of dues.

The President announced that the Annual Oration would be delivered by Dr. Joseph C. Beck of Chicago, Ill.

SCIENTIFIC SESSION.

A. *Report of Cases.*

    1. Cases Showing Operations Upon the Rectum, Under Local Anesthesia, Dr. J. F. Saphir.

    2. Report of a Case of Sinus Thrombosis—Operation—Recovery,
Dr. I. Grushlaw.

    3. (a) Case of Intestinal Intussusception.

        (b) Persistent Hiccough following Appendicitis.

        (c) Femoral Hernia Simulating Strangulated Hernia.

        (d) Saphenous Varix Simulating Strangulated Hernia.
Dr. L. B. Meyer.

    5. Case of Tumor of the Brain, Simulating Paresis.
Dr. I. Strauss.

    6. Case of Retro-Peritoneal Cyst with Probable Diagnosis of Cyst of the Right Suprarenal Gland.
Dr. G. A. Friedman.

B. *Papers.*

    1. Remarks on Intrathoracic Resection of the Esophagus, with a plea for early diagnosis.
Dr. Willy Meyer.

    2. What Shall the General Practitioner Know of Orthopedic Surgery?
Dr. P. William Nathan.
Discussion by Dr. Virgil P. Gibney.

The general discussion of the program of the evening was shorter than usual but interesting.

After adjournment, the usual collation was served to the members and guests.

American Medicine

H. EDWIN LEWIS, M. D., *Managing Editor.*

PUBLISHED MONTHLY BY THE AMERICAN-MEDICAL PUBLISHING COMPANY.

Copyrighted by the American Medical Publishing Co., 1912.

Complete Series, Vol. XVIII., No. 12.
New Series, Vol. VII., No. 12.

DECEMBER, 1912.

$1.00 YEARLY in advance.

Salaries for medical practitioners have been discussed quite often in these columns, but always as a possibility in some distantly future socialism when men will be different. We have frequently mentioned the constantly increasing percentage of us who are under salary, but always with the idea that the increase was so slow that we of to-day need not bother about it, but could go on making huge fortunes in private practice—if we could. We are therefore justified in saying that we were greatly startled by the news from Great Britain, that the medical profession there was discussing ways and means of putting everyone on salary right now—immediately. Is the socialistic millennium right here in time—there in space—and no one at the gate to give it welcome? We have always held that the captain who salves a million dollar ship is entitled to a bigger fee than he who salves a ten dollar row-boat. But now our British brethren are taking the stand that if a doctor saves the life of a Pasteur, his labor is worth just as much to society as if he saved the life of a drunken worthless tramp, and will receive the same pay. No, no! The levelling of democracy can't go that far. We've still the right to struggle for life and buy the best help we can afford, and the best of us can rest assured that no law can yet compel a millionaire to accept the advice of the worst of us. The law of supply and demand is natural and no human law has yet upset nature. The man with exceptional medical ability can no more be deprived of the right to sell it to the highest bidder than can the man who has exceptional ability to manage a bank. We will all be put on equal salaries when a bank president gets the same salary as the night watchman. Private practice will last a long time yet.

The advantage of public salaries is solely for those who answer public calls from those who cannot afford to hire anyone. Lawyers have long ceased to give advise to those who cannot pay for it, and if a pauper is in urgent need of advise the court assigns counsel and sees that he is given a living wage for the work done for criminals. Yet when it comes to the doctors, the lawyer says that public welfare demands that we give our labor freely to the pauper without fee, and let our own children go barefoot. So we tax our rich patients more than we otherwise would, or we couldn't live. Well, an end will be put to that system. Services to the poor are public duties to save society the expense of caring for men who would otherwise cease to be self-supporting, and society must pay the bills, not the sick rich. It is nonsense to say we are remunerated by the increased experience for that rule does not apply to counsel assigned to crim-

658   AMERICAN MEDICINE
Complete Series, Vol. XVIII.   EDITORIAL COMMENT   DECEMBER, 1912.
New Series, Vol. VII., No. 12.

inals. Time spent in public hospitals and dispensaries must be paid for, and will be. Already our larger hospitals and colleges are discussing the advisability of placing all the staff on salary to save them the necessity of spending so much time making a living, and to secure their whole time and best thought. And of course the salaries must range in accordance with the value of the services, as in banks and railroads, or the best men will not serve but remain in private practice. A good man leaves public service every time when he is assured more outside.

The proposed English system of fees seems therefore to be in line with the progress of events on this side of the ocean. They have been giving old age pensions to everyone, but we confine them to old soldiers. So we will delay both pensions for civilians and fees for public medical service to them, but not for very long. Lodge practice will disappear because the lodges will be able to hire only the worst of us —the best will be public servants or in more remunerative private practice. The dreadful evils of the insurance system will have to be eliminated for want of funds, and the pay for doctors will lessen the tax on the rich but increase that on the poor —just as the lawyers' fees do now. It seems inevitable. Nevertheless there is one thing which shows that the whole business is premature and will act as a check upon its too rapid adoption. Reports from Germany show that by reason of state insurance, workmen are giving up to ills and injuries they formerly ignored, and by sheer idleness are sinking into a disabling introspective neurasthenia, whereas work formerly cured them of "nerves." Actual sickness has increased, and minor ailments which formerly cured themselves are now the subject of paid attention of public servants. Unless penalties are devised, the nation will make malingering a fine art— and a well paid one too. It's just as well we are going slow.

———

Underfeeding at boarding schools seems inconceivable and yet we are informed it is a fact in England because the "master" is better paid if he is economical. It is said that the boys are abnormally hungry, that is, chronically. A boy who is not ravenously hungry at proper intervals is sick or starving. The craving for sugar —an easily oxidized fuel—is normal, and a mere continuation of the infantile appetite for the only carbohydrate it can digest—milk sugar. When this craving becomes insatiable and leads to habitual over indulgence it is an invariable sign of pathological exhaustion. For this reason there is a movement to investigate the question and find out exactly what kinds of foods should be supplied and how much. Nor is the question of serving to be neglected, for it is an exploded idea that food can be dumped down before a child like swill to a pig. Such coarseness actually repels the delicately nurtured. Perhaps we had better look into the question in America, and see if the child has an abundance of properly cooked and served nitrogenous foods. The baby is carnivorous in a sense, for milk is an animal product, and the child is essentially carnivorous for years after. The avidity with which a toothless tot will gum a bone is almost puppy-like, and shows the craving for building materials. There is a suspicion that we supply too much starch to the neglect of meat and fat. A famous writer has well said that they do not need bread and butter—we must give them butter and bread. Perhaps they really suffer from starch indigestion. We must also recognize the fact that the child is guided by appetite much more powerfully than adults. Over feeding with normal food is rarely if ever seen in health, as the healthy child stops eating almost automatically the moment hunger is satisfied. We love to call them "little gluttons," but they are not. Only those who are underfed the year round are apt to gluttonize at Thanksgiving and Christmas and then it is generally of foods they should not have. So let us be more generous. The Hospital of London is taking the matter up seriously and our dietitians might do so here.

The etiology of nephritis should certainly be cleared up, but as there are many kinds of nephritis there are many kinds of causes, and we regret the tendency of certain investigators to group all cases together under a common cause. A large white kidney and a small contracted one, are so different that they apparently have nothing in common. The work "Nephritis" (1911 Cartwright Prize Essay) by Dr. Martin H. Fischer of Columbia University is an epoch making investigation, but it is to be regretted that he has made such a sweeping generalization—"all the changes that characterize nephritis are due to a common cause—the abnormal production or accumulation of acid in the cells of the kidney." If true, it confirms the opinion of many of our best pathologists that an interstitial nephritis is merely a later stage of parenchymatous, the connective tissue taking the place of degenerated cells. There must be an added cause which makes some kidneys harden, and that cause

is bound up with the coincident sclerosis of the arteries and other organs.

The use of neutral salts in nephritis is advocated by Fischer on the strength of experiments showing that they do prevent the cloudy swelling cause by acids. He also shows that nephritics in coma with anuria have recovered after rectal injections of solutions of sodium carbonate and sodium chloride. Here is opened a great big field whose existence was not known except in a very general way. An excess or deficiency of certain unknown salts has been proved or suspected to be the cause of so many diseases, that we must now get back to first principles. Here is where our specialists in protozoology and protobotany can make themselves famous by discoveries leading to prolongation of human life and efficiency. We must consider the body cells as marine animals bathed in a very salt ocean or floating in it. We already know that very minor changes in the dissolved salts make profound changes in some unicellular marine organisms but the facts have not yet been sufficiently classified for some genius to make the necessary generalizations. Surely we are on the verge of great things for the good of mankind, and our chemists must work hand in hand with physiologists. The curse of nephritis must be eliminated.

Another cancer microbe has been announced, and though we have been much inclined to believe that the evidence once pointed to a living cause of this cell-anarchy, we are now much more afraid that the extremists are creating an Ananias club of germs. The present evidence inclined towards a non-vital cause, which starts certain cells with a mania for reproduction and weakens the resistance of the others. Nevertheless the known facts are so contradictory that no one is justified in forming an opinion one way or the other. All investigators seem to be at sea and though most of them are apparently turning their backs to vital causes, none of them would be surprised if a parasite were found. If the internal secretions are wrong they accomplish even more wonderful results than cancer, consequently many a physiologist is fixed in that direction while the chemists are just as busy in their field to discover the cause in some chemical or the lack of it. Nor are the relations to senility being neglected. So while we must not reject the alleged discovery of Dr. Gaston Odin of Paris that he has found a living cause, we must not accept it until we have proved him right. Let us repeat that the chances are, that when recognized, the cause will prove to be so simple and evident that we will all be ashamed we were not able to see it. The man who makes the discovery may be, like Pasteur, totally outside the domain of medicine, and therefore able to size up the evidence without bias. Suggestions from extra academic sources must therefore, not be sneered at.

The carnival of murder in America seems to be growing worse every year. It has received the attention of sociologists and jurists with a view of applying remedies, but no one seems to know the cause. The dreadful pre-eminence of our southern cities has been shown to be due to the negroes who resort to violence and murder upon provocations which are ignored by higher races. Nevertheless the whites in the south do commit crimes more often than people of northern Europe. The Mediterranean races also are great offenders here as well as in their native lands. Southern Italy is a notorious hot bed of murder, in marked contrast to the north. All this does not explain why Americans of British descent resort to murder so much more frequently than Britishers at home. Even the Jews who have perhaps the cleanest record of all human beings, are now becoming as bad as the rest.

The cause of American murders seems to be something inherent in our institutions. We cannot blame the newness of the country for we have been settled long enough and have ample machinery for protection and for redress of wrongs. The machinery is not used for we are informed that only one-fourth of the murderers are detected and only one per cent are executed. In the early days before courts existed every man guarded his own life as in primitive times and had absolute liberty to kill those who threatened him. Indeed he had to resort to force to live. We cannot shake off this feeling that we are free to do as we please and the great chances of escaping punishment, remove all checks from those who would otherwise restrain themselves and depend upon the law. There is a still deeper cause which may take a long while to remove. The purpose of a trial in the mother country is the protection of the state, but in America the safeguards are thrown around the accused, and these safeguards have now become so numerous as to prevent conviction. Nothing short of a complete revolution of our legal procedure will end our dreadful habit of murder. Our jurists already know this and are at work discussing ways and means. The situation is not nearly so hopeless as many of our writers imply.

Public opinion instead of glorifying the murderer is demanding that he be executed or placed where he cannot repeat the offense. There is no justification for murder except self-defense from an actual attack, and as we have repeatedly stated, the man who deliberately murders must be executed, while he who commits a crime under provocations which the normal resist, must be deprived of his liberty until we are sure his inhibitions are strengthened.

The human physique, that of the female particularly, has ever been a controversial subject. Ever since mankind recognized the more or less intimate relation between physical development and personal efficiency certain ideals have existed concerning the physique and its proportions. Varying conceptions of efficiency at different periods of history have greatly modified these ideals. Thus during the days of hand to hand conflict when brute strength and bulk were all important, a massive chest and enormous muscles were necessary to excite admiration. As conditions changed the methods of warfare, and physical skill and agility were called for rather than great strength and size, a slender body with supple joints and lithe muscles became the ideal. So it has been. The social conditions of each epoch have defined the standard physiques, and natural laws of selection and heredity, substantially aided by environal forces, have all helped to produce the needed type. As civilization has extended and the evolution of machinery has greatly changed or decreased physical labor, one of the most potent factors in the development of physiques—routine muscular effort—has been eliminated. With an increase of mental effort and a decrease of systematic physical

exertion in the daily occupations of the masses, it has taken only a few generations to lower muscular development and reduce the male physique to a very commonplace level. There never was a time when physical development was on a lower plane or falling off more rapidly than it is today. Regretful as this may be from sentimental and esthetic standpoints, it must be accepted as one of the inevitable penalties of civilized progress. Happily, however, lack of muscular development does not mean loss of vitality, or ill health. But the enormous rush to urban living and a great increase of indoor or exertion-free occupations are having their inevitable effect, and there is little prospect of change. To be sure, there is a widespread interest in athletics, but a little investigation will show how very few actively take part in them after the school boy or student period.

Unpleasant as it is to admit, it must be conceded, therefore, that the male form has deteriorated and will continue to do so until more intelligent and systematic effort is directed toward correcting existing tendencies. The possibilities in this direction from systematic exercise are not half realized, but when they are, a new era of physical development will be at hand.

The female form has not been subjected to such diverse or potent influences, and as a consequence has maintained its primary characteristics more uniformly. Even when subjected to the modifying effects of prolonged or excessive muscular effort, the female physique has never developed as has the male. On the contrary, the natural lines and characteristics instead of being accentuated and strengthened as in the male, have been obliterated and destroyed. That this is largely due to anatomical relations and conditions can hardly be questioned. The female physique was designed for the one great purpose of child bearing. The contour of her osseous system, the arrangement of her muscles and her physiologic phenomena point unerringly to her fundamental place in the scheme of life. She was never intended for the arduous muscular pursuits that the male is fitted for. This does not mean that the female cannot engage in severe muscular effort, or that she cannot perform the hardest physical labor as satisfactorily as many men. But when she does she has to overcome special anatomical and physiological handicaps, and expend greater effort. Performing tasks for which neither the shape of her bones, nor the attachments and relations of her muscles are adapted, places an excessive burden on parts unable to meet the situation satisfactorily. The result is only what might be expected. Muscular development is irregular, compensatory growth and enlargement of muscles rarely or seldom used under ordinary conditions produce distortion or what may lead to marked deformity, and while it is true the female organs are admirably arranged to withstand physical injury, who can say how much their physiological efficiency is impaired by the unnatural abdominal tension and strain incidental to extreme muscular development and excessive or prolonged physical effort? The whole female body, for instance, is equipped for child bearing. The ready adaptability of the female heart and circulatory system supplies specific evidence of this, for under normal conditions these organs are quick to respond to the special demands of the pregnant state. If, however, through extreme or excessive physical exertion a woman has developed her muscles to a very marked degree, there is a corresponding development of the heart muscle. Now, if pregnancy takes place what follows? Hypertrophied as they are through excessive physical exertion the heart and blood vessels will obviously be unable to respond as they otherwise would to the immediate situation. The condition of the heart muscle may make it less susceptible to stimuli, or the condition of the nervous mechanism may be such that it is over sensitive to irritating impulses. Each case is a law unto itself, but it is a fact well known to obstetricians that cardiac and circulatory disturbances are more common during pregnancy in very large, robust and hard working women than in those who are distinctly feminine and more or less frail in comparison.

Failure of the heart to respond to the specific demands of pregnancy, may cause the mother little annoyance, for the condition may manifest itself in no other way than by palpitation on exertion and some shortness of breath. But all the time this failure to become exactly adjusted to the more indefinite or remote demands of the growing fetus, or to the circulatory needs incidental to metabolic changes in the liver, or the eliminative functions of the kidneys may be storing up trouble for the future. Not infrequently the health of the child is sadly influenced. Probably, therefore, the anomalous fact that the sturdiest and strongest mothers, those who boast of working up to "the last minute" in the most arduous occupations, often bear the puniest, most poorly developed children could many times be traced to a heart that had reached its maximum capacity before conception took place. On the other hand, it might be found that small, very feminine, and comparatively inactive women not infrequently give birth to large, beautifully developed babies because their hearts and circulatory systems are not abnormally enlarged and can respond to the requirements of pregnancy.

The foregoing have been brought forward to emphasize these truths: *First,* that the male was created to do physical work, that his physique requires a certain amount of physical labor or exercise to develop properly and approach physical perfection, and finally that his body will deteriorate if he does not get it; and *second,* that the female was not created to do the same work or to follow the same physical pursuits as the male, that her anatomy and physiology indicate that she should not undertake them, and finally, if she does, she not only impairs her physique, but develops conditions which may be fraught with the gravest harm, not alone to herself but to her unborn child.

The woman who must support herself presents a serious problem, therefore, though less from economic standpoints than from the physiologic and hygienic. Woman has shown herself equal to every task that man can perform. Her will, ingenuity and courage enable her to overcome her anatomic and physiologic handicaps, though the cost to herself and her own comfort is often very great. From the beginning women have borne their share of the struggle for comfortable existence. Enforced by the duties of maternity to remain at home while the husband and father fared forth for food, what more natural thing after her children were cared for that she should devote her time to making the home place clean and attractive against the return of the absent one? It is easy to see how the preparation of food, the repair of the clothing and many other duties early fell to her lot; and so she became the home keeper. That her efficiency in this direction has been one of the most potent influences in the evolution of society must be apparent. The home being the foundation of everything social, the more its benefits were appreciated and the more its value was understood, the more indispensable it became. Her maternal instincts and housewifely qualities created a sphere of activity, therefore in which she will ever be supreme. Civilization has had no factor of more far reaching influence on men's lives than the home-maker—the woman who without the stimulus or excitement of outside occupations, has gone about her work day in and day out cheerful and willing, always hopeful, never quitting no matter what her fears—a faithful worker, a true wife and a loving mother—proud of the home which her labors and her presence have made at once a haven of rest and comfort—a place to shut in love and repose and keep out strife and care. Such homes have provided satisfactory occupations for countless women and they always will. But as the social organism has grown in size and complexity many women from choice or necessity have sought other fields of activity than the home. Liberally endowed with mental qualifications women have fitted into every occupation—and made good. The problem of the working woman does not include the woman in occupations calling for brain work. She is abundantly able to solve any problems that concern her and her sisters —and solve them she will in her own good time.

But the problem we refer to concerns the working woman in factories, mills and shops, the woman who has to depend on her physical strength and skill to live and keep body and soul together. Poorly— often inadequately—paid, the conditions under which this class works call for careful thought and attention. Most of them young and inexperienced, working long hours in cramped positions, in poorly lighted and illy-ventilated rooms, it is little wonder they fall such easy prey to disease—and worse. Sad indeed is the fact that so many good, kind people are indifferent to the needs of the unskilled working woman. She needs help as do those of few other classes, help from the legislature, help from the local government, the social workers, the philanthropists—every agency that is trying in any way to better human conditions. Medical men in particular realize the menace that certain classes of working women too often offer to themselves and to society. Details are unnecessary but every community in striving to insure the prevention of disease, the protection of its youth, the elevation of its morals and the betterment of its social conditions must see to it that its working women labor under healthful conditions, no more than nine hours a day, for a living wage, and are provided with decent sanitary living places and opportunities for harmless wholesome amusement. Under such conditions, the unskilled working woman will become what she ought to be to her community, an asset—not a drag and menace.

What constitutes the perfect female physique is a question that is naturally suggested by the foregoing discussion of the effects of excessive physical labor on the male and female forms. The fact that the female body is more specialized than that of the male, i. e., adapted to a specific purpose, insures that certain characteristics will be maintained—as they have—and that it will hold closer under natural conditions to a uniform type. An examination of prehistoric skeletons of both

sexes shows that the female form has remained truer to type and been subject to much less variation as to size, weight, etc., than the male. In other words, the feminine physique has been more distinctive and therefore more easily identified. Environal influences have produced various changes but these have been individual and so much less persistent than the forces which give the female form its fundamental characteristics that the dominating tendency has ever been to revert to type. The male form, having no such constant and powerful stabilizer, has been infinitely more susceptible to passing influences and as a consequence shows much greater variation in size, weight and every other physical detail.

It would seem, therefore, much easier to establish a standard of perfection for the female body than for the male. Judging from the artistic ideals handed down from early times there has been a fair unanimity of opinion which the vagaries of feminine dress have not been able to change. The full chest, the curving waist, the broad hips and a general roundness without too much flesh have typified the ideal female form; the form that has been accepted as nearest to perfection because so manifestly natural and anatomically correct. Size has never been a quality. The real test of a perfect female form has ever been its symmetry and the relative balance of its anatomic features; that is, no matter what the size, a form approaches perfection to the extent that the chest, the waist, the hips and other parts bear a correct and symmetrical relation to each other.

The fallacy, therefore, of taking any one individual's physique as the perfect form can easily be seen. The latest mistake of this kind comes from a Cornell examiner who waxes enthusiastic over a maiden who weighs 171 pounds, is 5 feet 7 inches tall and who has a chest of 34.6 inches, a waist of 30.3 and hips of 40.4 inches! These dimensions may constitute perfection in the eyes of the examiner in question, but he will find many who will differ with him. In fact, the more one studies the question the more evident it becomes that all measurements of the female form are relative in their esthetic significance. With this so obvious to every one who considers the question other than superficially, it is apparent that the perfect female physique can never be described in the terms of the scales or tape measure.

———

Medical history teems with Romance and Tragedy. Indeed it is doubtful if the lives of any class of men contain more of that which brings us face to face with the real Drama of Life than the lives of the men who have contributed substantially to the history of medicine. Unfortunately, the nature of the physician's calling and the privacy that surrounds a large part of his work too often invest simple things with undue importance and keep the intei·· esting events, those that give real insight into character, hidden and obscure. It can readily be seen, therefore, how difficult is the task of any one who essays to write of the lives of medical men. Unless they are very, very fortunate they will have at their command nothing but a mass of trivial detail which will be sadly barren of the salient facts from which a comprehensive and authentic statement can be prepared. Those who have had any experience in this direction can doubly appreciate therefore, Robinson's *Pathfinders in Medicine*, one of the most thoroughly delightful books it has been our good fortune to read for many a day.

In going through this charming work one is impressed by many things. First of all, what a wealth of data the author must have had at his command and what an exceptional experience it must have been to delve so deeply into the intimate lives of these fine characters! Rarely, indeed, do such opportunities come to men nowadays, and if they do, seldom have we the good sense and judgment to seize and make the most of them.

Nothing of this kind, however, can be said of Robinson, and if he was lucky in having so much valuable and interesting material at his disposal, thrice lucky are those to whom he now presents it with the added charm of his own diction and inimitable powers of description.

In describing a work like *Pathfinders in Medicine* it is easy to become fulsome, for the literary talents and ability shown so unmistakably in its production are bound to command the liveliest admiration. In fact, one can hardly refrain from praising such a book in extravagant terms, for it is remarkable from many standpoints. For instance, the interest of the reader begins in the very first page—the first paragraph almost—an interest that never flags and is sustained to the last word. Only a true artist could take the lives of these medical men, great and famous though they were, and paint such intensely interesting word pictures of events that would be essentially commonplace in the hands of a less virile writer. Without being conscious of it the reader, however, quickly falls under the magic spell of the author and soon forgets everything but the scenes and tales his art conjures.

The story of each life with its intimate note is like a sojourn with some old and beloved friend. The details and events that are unfolded seem strangely familiar, and though actually it may be one's first introduction to them, there is a reality to each that makes the reader feel as though he was simply talking over old times and visiting old half forgotten places.

Pathfinders in Medicine is a book that will win a place for its author in the world of letters that will be secure if he never writes another line. No finer contribution to the history of medicine has ever been made and when countless other books on similar or kindred subjects have been read and forgotten, *Pathfinders in Medicine* will still remain a classic. Books of its quality are bound to endure, for aside from the pleasure they give they have a well defined mission which they never fail to perform.

Foreign born gunmen have again directed attention to the amount of crime committed by foreigners, and a great many unkind things are being said about this class of Americans which would not have been said had the writers fully realized that much more than half the population is foreign born or have foreign born parents. It would not be alarming if 65 or 70 per cent of crime were due to these people, for such a large percentage of them come from countries where crimes of violence, due to uncontrollable passions of emotional people, closely approximate normal acts. They have not been in America long enough to show the effect of the sobering influence of contact with the more quiet northern types, but the indications seem to prove that the second and third generations do not resort to violence to anywhere near the extent of the immigrant ancestor. A few, like the gunmen, seem to be made worse, but this is largely due to that transition period during which the old restraints have been weakened before new have been acquired.

What should worry us is the percentage of crime committed by the degenerate members of old familes, for here we are face to face with the evidence of serious decay of the stock as a whole, except where it is rejuvenated by new blood from Europe. In spite of our dreadful murder record, and in spite of the doleful remarks of pessimists, there is evidence that crime is lessening both here and in Europe, and has been decreasing ever since highway robbery was a gentleman's occupation, and drunkenness universal. Men are driven from public life and socially ostracized for acts which were scarcely considered wrong a century ago. Moral standards are higher and their violations less numerous even if we are very far from angelic. There is an awakened public conscience reflected by our juries which are now reluctant to release murderers on silly technicalities. The only ones who rejoice over failures of justice and make heroes of acquitted or executed murderers are newly arrived immigrants from places where oligarchic governments are oppressive and innocent men not infrequently accused. They are against all government acts. The older Americans are more on the side of law and order. It would be a cause for rejoicing if all our crime were due to the foreign element, for the amount committed by the old stock is really an evidence of degeneration which should be carefully studied by the medical profession. We do not here refer to the crimes of violence, but to the grafting, swindling, bribing of respectable people of good ancestry and often of rich families. These are the ones who have made our city governments so rotten, and we ought to find the causes. It is a medical matter not a purely ethical one. We as a profession ought to take more interest in such academic studies of social affairs and drop the habit of giving all our time to individuals.

The problem of poverty is one that is becoming more and more acute in all countries, owing to the fact that the development of material wealth is always accompanied by very unequal distribution thereof; consequently the more prosperous a country is as a whole the greater are the depths of poverty to be found within its borders. For some socialism seems to be the only promising corrective; to others this seems to sound the death knell of initiative and progress. Various are the plans that have been put forward to mitigate the disease of poverty with the result that all find earnest supporters and equally earnest opponents. In a little pamphlet by an English medical man* an attempt is made to give an explanation of the poverty and riches problem and to suggest a plan for dealing with it effectively, on individualistic rather than on socialist lines. Dr. Binnie Dunlop, starting from the postulate that the material basis of natural happiness is that a country should not have too many inhabitants for comfort or too few to provide for its safety against aggression, holds that the fundamental cause of unhappiness among fellow countrymen is unhappy competition for the means of healthy subsistence, which results in poverty and is due to dangerous overpopulation. A successful system of government must therefore check this tendency to overpopulation, by enforcing "the individualist law of parent responsibility," viz., that those who cannot afford to maintain children (in which maintenance is included elementary and occupational education, insurance against reduction or stoppage of wages by underemployment, unemployment, sickness, accident, or death) should not be allowed to beget them. The particular problem of the British empire, in his opinion, is too many Britishers at home, too few in the colonies. But as Britain's excess population is located principally in the cities they are for the most part useless as immigrants in the colonies. Dr. Dunlop, therefore, would propose the compulsory state emigration of all necessitous children—those, that is, who are persistently sent to school or work insufficiently fed, clothed, and cared for— the poor law authorities taking charge of them and the parents being made as a deterrent to contribute to the cost in proportion to their means. Experience has shown that even the slum-reared child may make an excellent colonist. Enforced state emigration of necessitous children, he thinks, would result in a rapid but humane elimination of necessitous stocks and would directly inculcate the lesson of parental responsibility. The application of such a principle in this country, would not, of course necessarily imply emigration over seas. We have uncolonized land enough at home.

Dr. Dunlop considers a country dangerously underpopulated, on the other hand, when it produces fewer inhabitants than it can support healthily and safely, and this condition must inevitably arise when an excessive portion of its resources are spent in the production of luxuries. The expenditure on luxuries would, if devoted to the production of necessities, increase and cheapen them so as to reduce the cost of living for all. If the use of luxuries could

*National Happiness Under Individualism, by Binnie Dunlop, M. B., Brasted, Kent, 1912. Price 3d.

be controlled, many persons of moderate means could afford to have families; many wage •earners could bring up properly the children they now have, and many bachelors could assume the responsibilities of married life, and parentage. Such a control of luxuries could be secured in Dr. Dunlop's opinion, by taxing them on their capital value. The taxes thus raised would suffice, he thinks, to support whatevery army and navy might be required for maintaining peace against aggression from without, so that a universal and uniform income tax would suffice· to pay all other costs of administration. As to what should be considered luxuries, he suggests undeveloped or underdeveloped land, taxation of which at its capital value would compel its being put to productive use in building or cultivation, numerous servants, two or more residences, yachts, pleasure horses and motor cars, many entertainments, all betting transactions, private collections of pictures, *objets d'art*, and jewelry, as well as numerous articles among drugs, drink, food, dress, and so forth. He protests, however, and as it seems to us with justice, against the taxation of wealth *per se* for the support of the poor, pointing out that it is not the possession of wealth, but the way it is used, that affects the well being of the community at large. One man may spend more injuriously to the nation his earned $5,000 than another does his unearned $5,000 or even much more. Luxury users are not solely the rich. Many by no means wealthy folk live more or less luxuriously, while, on the other hand, many very wealthy folk live comparatively frugally. Taxation of luxuries, therefore, on their capital value for the national defenses, would help to remove any economic injustice done to the really poor, and would benefit all by the removal of unnecessary taxation on living.

Many obvious difficulties present themselves against the accomplishment of this end, even if all· were agreed upon the principles enunciated by Dr. Dunlop. For instance, who is to define luxuries? What number of servants would constitute "numerous" servants? What kind of "entertainments" should be taxed? Recreation of some sort is a necessity for all, yet what would be recreation to one would be an intolerable bore to another. Again, how would it be possible to render effective a law that those who cannot afford to maintain children shall not be allowed to beget them? And what becomes of the natural affections under Dr. Dunlop's regime? It must be admitted that however undesired some children may be before birth, they are usually none the less dear after birth; and parental affection often, if not usually, becomes highly developed among those who find great difficulty in maintaining their offspring. Indeed it is often among that very class that it attains the highest degree of devotion. But however utopian Dr. Dunlop's ideas may be, it is highly desirable that medical men should realize that the problem of poverty is one to the solution of which the medical profession must contribute a considerable share, and the greater the evidence that medical men in their professional capacity are realizing the fact and seriously studying the subject, the more hopeful will the outlook become.

The decrease of insanity is the last bit of consolation extracted from a careful analysis of statistics. We have many times referred to the fact that the steadily increasing percentage of the general population in asylums, merely means that modern medical methods keep the cases alive longer. Certain alienists have shown that the admissions have also increased faster than the population, but now we have the statement of Macdonald of Concord, N. H., (*N. Y. Med. Jour.,* July 27, 1912) that 23.3 per cent of admissions in his state are readmissions of cases which had relapsed under the strains of liberty after an apparent cure in hospital. He also states it as his opinion that if we could deduct from the admissions, the descendants of these apparently cured cases which propagate their kind and then relapse, it would be found that really new cases are diminishing, "commensurate with our better habits of living and improved environment." All this is most comforting and in accordance with common sense. Modern stresses cannot be compared with ancient or medieval or even those of a century ago, and we must be the better for it. The rush and roar of modern life may be doing a lot of harm, but they are not driving us crazy.

The evil of liberating the cured insane is the new thought given to us by Macdonald and it certainly makes us take notice. That is, insanity is not cured nearly as often as the statistics of discharges from asylums would lead us to believe. They are too often cases in which relief from strains has quieted down the symptoms but not affected the disease. Some writers are becoming quite pessimistic over the large number of relapses and are unwisely jumping to the opposite conclusion that none are really ever completely cured. In the meantime the married ones reproduce their kind far more

than in former years, and are supplying cases for a few years hence. Any attempt to retain an apparently cured case is so bitterly resented by friends and relatives, that it seems hopeless to expect it. So what is to be done? Macdonald is quite sure that by keeping patients alive so long, we are unduly increasing the neurotic families which formerly perished. This is nothing new. Vaccination promptly stopped the slaughter of those most susceptible to smallpox, and the evolution of an immune race. Quinine is doing the same as to malaria. Surgery is ending the involution of the appendix, and instead of a race without this organ we are in time to be a race in which it must be removed. So with neurotics. And, by-the-way, he who lives 70 years, half of them in asylum, and leaves offspring able to survive by hook or crook, proves by that very token to be fitter for survival than the young giant who breaks his neck in foot-ball. The sole question with nature is who can survive, not who ought to. Eugenists say that we must extend this natural law and preserve what we want but who would otherwise die, and we must prevent the propagation of neurotics who will have families if we release them from asylums. It may not be practicable now, but they hope it will be in time. Man seems bound to become a domesticated animal—unable to survive by his own efforts and created in the form most useful to society and least burdensome.

———

The dangers of sunshine for babies have frequently been mentioned in these columns and several years ago, Grawitz of Berlin called attention to the neurasthenic conditions following light baths— particularly in children who had been unduly exposed at the seashore. An English physician is now reported as going a step further. He protests against the excessive use of white for the nursery, and the baby's clothes. He states that it is sheer cruelty to envelop the child in such a constant glare, which he compared to that of dazzling fields of snow, damaging the delicate retina, making the babies peevish, irritable and furious. He advocates subdued colors for walls, furniture, toys and outer garments—and he is right. If he has noticed such damage in London with its fogs and smoke, what must it be in sun cursed America? And how cruel to take the little sufferers out into our sunshine, or "protect" them with white sunshades, the glare of which is so painful. And what are we to think of those physicians who advise such cruelty? And of the architects and teachers who cannot see the irritation of over-lighted school rooms? What will be the ultimate results of the radiations from high frequency currents of a huge solenoid now proposed for the stimulation of school children?

——

The anti-noise crusade shows signs of renewed activity. This time the crusaders are not female "busy-bodies," but practicing physicians who have found that there is appreciable harm from noise and serious harm too. It is no doubt true that a normal nervous system can apparently adjust itself to all sorts of adverse circumstances, —we couldn't exist otherwise. Nevertheless the inimical agents make an impress, and, like water dropping on a stone, can overcome resistance in time. So we are finding many abnormal nervous conditions in those who have long been immersed in loud noises utterly unaware that any harm was being done. Heretofore we have strongly supported the crusade in the interests of the sick and nervous, and it is now a custom to surround hospitals with a zone in which noises are prohibited under deterrent penalties for the brutes who will not be quiet there from humanity.

Noise is harmful to the healthy so we now advocate a still further extension of the movement in the interests of the strong and healthy. Man's nerves and hearing apparatus were evolved in a comparatively quiet environment, to detect faint sounds warning him of danger or of the presence of game. Sudden loud sounds shock the system greatly—in childhood they may cause convulsions. In time we might evolve a race immune to noise, but it can only be done by killing off those who are most injured by it and these nervous people are often the very ones who are doing the most to advance civilization. So the only thing to do is to make the environment fit for them, and not kill them as unfit for the environment. The first step is to abolish unnecessary bells, whistles and street-cries, construct less noisy pavements, and give children play grounds where they can blow off steam to their dear hearts' content and not annoy anyone, not even long-suffering head-achy mamma. No wonder she is "cross" so often. Bless her, how she suffers because unable to turn the kiddies out into the back yard or cornfield. Then pray Heaven to send a genius who can still the noise of our dreadful subway and elevated cars. The world will call him "Blessed."

——

"Peribronchial Phthisis" is a term applied by Dr. Alfred C. Jordan, medical radiographer to Guy's Hospital and to the Royal Hospital for Diseases of the Chest, to cases of pulmonary tuberculosis in which the disease begins at the roots of the lungs and extends along the branches of the large bronchial tubes. He asserts that, so far from this mode of origin being a rarity, it is a more common form of the disease than that which, according to general belief, sustained by Allbutt and Rolleston's *System of Medicine,* has its initial lesion in "a small nodule or group of nodules situated somewhat below the extreme apex of the lung." Out of 150 consecutive x-ray examinations in cases— in which the diagnosis of pulmonary tuberculosis was clinically certain, including the finding of tubercle bacilli in the sputum, while there was no complication, purely apical disease was found in only 32 cases; the disease was confined to the region of the pulmonary roots in 59 cases (purely "peribronchial phthisis"); and in another 59 cases both the apices and the roots on one or both sides were affected.

Its importance is further greatly accentuated by the proposition that, according to Dr. Jordan, peribronchial phthisis may attain an advanced stage before any signs of its presence can be evoked by the usual methods of physical examination of the chest; for the lesion in the apical form lies near the surface of the body, while that in the peribronchial form is so deeply situated that it gives rise to no percussion dullness and to no alteration in the breath or voice sounds. The only available method of diagnosis in these cases, Dr. Jordan asserts to be the use of the Röntgen ray. His article, which is published in the *Practitioner* for February, is illustrated with radiographs that show very clearly the typical patches and nodules of tuberculous bronchopneumonia, with calcareous nodules in the bronchial glands, upon which he relies to prove his thesis. He further contends that the linear shadows seen in the lungs of healthy persons, and well known to all radiographers, which radiate downwards from the root of the lung and are usually described as "normal hilum shadows," are in point of fact pathological, being due to the previous entry of tubercle bacilli with the consequent fibrosis which is due to the reaction of the organism to render them inert.

The chief difficulties in radiography lie in accurate interpretation of the findings, and such accuracy can be attained for the new diagnostic aid of the x-ray, only in the same way in which it was laboriously attained for percussion and auscultation, viz., by the correlating of physical signs discovered *intra vitam* with the subsequent findings of the post-mortem room, a due appreciation of what is to be looked for being presupposed. This limitation is really essential, for, as Dr. Jordan points out, he has found by x-ray examination in a number of apparently healthy lungs obtained from the post-mortem room, calcareous deposits in the lymphatic glands, either at the roots of the lungs or along the course of the larger air tubes; and in no case had these calcareous deposits been noted at the post-mortem.

The serious import of Dr. Jordan's findings, if they are substantiated by other observers, lies in the fact that peribronchial phthisis, giving no abnormal signs in response to the ordinary clinical methods of investigation, may reach an advanced stage before the presence of tuberculosis is discovered. Even then, the flattening of the upper part of the chest below the clavicle, which is the result of the peribronchial activity, may be attributed merely to a slight apical involvement, and thus may be overlooked a massive fibroid disease at the root unless the x-ray is employed.

Dr. Jordan's statements add new force to the plea for an increased study of the chest by means of radiography. The encouraging features of peribronchial phthisis lie in its slower rate of progress and in the better fight made against it by the organism, which has a greater opportunity for surrounding the tuberculous nodules with leucocytes and overcoming their activity by fibrosis. If Dr. Jordan is right in his assertion, that the peribronchial form is nearly twice as frequent as the apical form, the routine use of the x-ray in all clinically suspicious cases should materially increase the proportion of cases of pulmonary tuberculosis detected in a curable stage.

———

The **"new phrenology"** seems destined to become really scientific. The brain has defied research long enough, for our ignorance is a blot on science. Man's wonderful works and supremacy over all other creatures are due solely to the size and organization of this organ, and yet it is so well protected and hidden away that we have little more than a hint as to what that organization is or how it works. The old absurd phrenology that assumed a surface localization for many or all mental qualities and further assumed these areas bulged out the bone, is of course outside the domain of science, but it was based on a few empirical observations and has kept alive the great idea that the brain may be a group of organs, connected for team work in an inconceivably intricate manner. This idea of localization has proved of practical

value in surgery of a few small areas, and our physiologists with some exceptions seem inclined to give it wide application to the parts of whose function we are ignorant. A few are bewildered by the fact that the enormous number and intricacy of the connecting fibers, permits the brain to act as one organ, though composed of specialized groups like an Army. It may be true that certain faculties are not localized at all, but the localizationists need not worry over that. Every baseball fan knows that the game is a function of the team, not of the players. The research work should be pushed, for there are innumerable problems of insanity waiting for solution. It is a work whose practical value to humanity is evident to every layman or could be made evident by a word or two. The harvest of neo-phrenology awaits the laborers, and we are glad to see them entering the field.

———

Facts Required by the New Postal Law.—
In accordance with the provisions of the law we have placed our sworn statement on file with the Postmaster General and with the postmaster at Burlington, and reprint it herewith:

STATEMENT OF THE OWNERSHIP, MANAGEMENT, ETC.

of American Medicine, published monthly at Burlington, Vt., as required by the Act of August 24, 1912.

Managing Editor—H. Edwin Lewis, M. D., 57 West 58th St., New York.
Business Manager—Wm. T. Hanson, 1576 Bergen St., Brooklyn, N. Y.
Publishers—American Medical Publishing Co., 84 William St., New York.
Owners—H. Edwin Lewis, M. D., 57 West 58th St., New York City.
     W. B. Howe, Free Press Ass'n., Burlington, Vt.

Known bondholders, mortgagees, and other security holders, holding 1 percent or more of total amount of bonds, mortgages, or other securities: None.

           H. EDWIN LEWIS,
               Managing Editor.
Sworn to and subscribed before me this 28th day of Sept., 1912.
         ROY F. STAHLBERG,
             Commissioner of Deeds of
               City of New York.

DECEMBER, 1912.
New Series, Vol. VII., No. 12. }   ORIGINAL ARTICLES   { AMERICAN MEDICINE
Complete Series, Vol. XVIII.   673

ORIGINAL ARTICLES.

DISEASE AS A FACTOR IN THE EVOLUTION OF THE HUMAN FAMILY.

BY

LAWRENCE IRWELL, M. A., B. C. L.,
Buffalo, N. Y.

Diseases may be divided into two classes: those which medical science is able to deal with successfully, and those which, in spite of medical skill, prove fatal. Unpleasant as the assertion unquestionably is, it is true that the latter class maintains the strength of the nation. When any disease of this class must be added to the former class, then there is danger of degeneration. This will be obvious to any observer who realizes that national efficiency depends upon the survival of those who are best adapted to the environment. The cause, however, of the danger referred to is not so much the disease as the advance of scientific knowledge which frees the individual from the necessity of combating the ills of life for himself. As an example of this we may take the adenoid growths which are often found in the throat during childhood, hindering breathing and preventing normal oxidation of the blood. If left to develop these growths would frequently be the indirect cause of death because they would reduce the power of the individual to fight any other disease that might attack him. It is now, of course, the custom to remove adenoids, and the operation in skilled hands is attended with very little danger. The result is often a great increase of vigor. But if we consider the interest of the race, and ignore that of the individual, the result is far from satisfactory. There is a milder environment than formerly; the physician with his new discoveries is part of it. In the milder environment, children need not be able to breathe freely and well without assistance. So long as they can carry on respiration in a suitable manner by the help of the surgeon's operation, all is well so far as they are concerned. They, however, have ceased to be self-dependent, have ceased to fight their own battle against disease, but are dependent upon aid from others.

To elimination of the weak by disease much of the physical strength of the English-speaking world is due. The circumstances of civilized life, it must be admitted, tend to foster a particular kind of stamina. The growing tendency under civilization is to live herded together, and there is consequently far greater risk of infection than in former times when the population was sparse, and the country was dotted with small villages or isolated habitations; when, in addition, the difficulty of traveling checked the spread of infection. The race has adapted itself to circumstances. Notwithstanding the large number of victims that are sacrificed to the various diseases of civilization, there is a rapid increase of population. When, on the other hand, uncivilized peoples are suddenly brought into contact with some disease which we have come to look upon without much alarm, the consequences are often astonishing. The fact, however, is easily explicable on the theory that it is only by constant elimination of the unfit that a race adapts itself to its environment. The weeding out through a long series of generations of those who are unable to fight a disease at length produces a race which, while not immune to that disorder, is able successfully to withstand its attacks so far as the majority of its members are concerned. A good example of this condition is the comparative immunity of Jews, not to tuberculosis, for many foreign Hebrews living in unhygienic surroundings in our great cities suffer from it, but to death as the result of it. It is correct to say that tubercular Jews usually continue to live, and death is, as a rule, due to some other cause.

Tuberculosis has long been at work in the civilized world, yet at all times it has been gradually but very slowly reducing its own power to destroy human life, for the microbe which causes it spares those who have no susceptibility toward this disease. As is well known, tuberculosis is responsible for from one-seventh to one-fourth of all deaths in the civilized part of our planet. As it is still so deadly, it might be argued that, after all, the white race is not becoming even partially immune to death from it through the working of *natural selection*. To this the answer is that the crowded life in the large cities of today makes the conditions very favorable to the germ. It is almost unnecessary to remind the reader that although the disease is spread by infection, heredity is responsible for some form of weakness which predisposes certain persons to the successful attack of tubercle bacilli. The prevalence of tuberculosis pulmonalis is undoubtedly accounted for by the circumstances of modern life, but if we wish to realize the progress made by our race in power of resistance to tubercle bacilli, we have only to contrast its limited activity in cities where the colored population is small with cities in which it is large. The white man having been an urban dweller for many years has, in some degree, undergone selection by tuberculosis; the negro having been an urban dweller for comparatively speaking, only a short period,

is still undergoing selection by the microbe of tuberculosis in a very decided manner, and the least resistant colored people continue to succumb in great numbers.

Consumption, smallpox and alcohol are three of the dangers which civilization usually brings with it. (It also brings the plague and venereal disorders). Against consumption, we white men have been fortified by a sweeping process of elimination in past generations; against smallpox and alcoholism we have been fortified by other means in addition to *natural selection*. But the unfortunate savage stands defenceless.

The microbic diseases, taken as a whole, are markedly decreasing, some in prevalence, others in virulence. To some extent science is warding them off, and to some extent the race is slowly rising superior to them. Such plagues as the "black death" are things of the past. Smallpox kills few people in our country; cholera and typhus are almost unknown in the United States. Speaking generally, diseases caused by microbes have become less terrible than they formerly were, and in the future they are likely to cause fewer deaths than they cause today. The question, therefore, arises: what diseases, if any, are taking their place? Deaths due to old age are not appreciably increasing, but chronic nephritis ("Bright's disease"), and disorders of the circulatory system are unquestionably on the increase. It may be, however, that the tendency shown by the non-microbic maladies to raise the toll which they demand is a result of the greater average length of life—it may be that longevity gives congenital defects time to tell. But this cannot be accepted as more than a very partial explanation of the facts, because our inordinate consumption of flesh foods (practically all over the United States) must necessarily produce diseases of the arteries and of the kidneys. With the possible exception of the Australians, we are, as a nation, the largest meat consumers in the world, and our death-rate after forty years of age is increasing more rapidly than is the mortality in England after that period of life.

It must be apparent to every investigator that science is causing a great change. It is relieving men of the necessity of fighting against death-dealing microbes allied with any constitutional defects which those microbes may discover. Microbes are being rendered innocuous; therefore, whatever a man may have of inherited tendencies toward certain diseases is likely to play its part in course of time unassisted by microbes. It is assumed that disease germs are most fatal in the case of those who have constitutional weakness. Indeed, if a broad view is taken this is beyond dispute. Even in these days, when the contagion theory of the cause of tuberculosis has been allowed to "run riot," it is admitted that defective chest development and other malformations predispose toward phthisis, and that perfectly healthy men and women never become tuberculous.

What effect, then, will the tendencies described above have upon the community? In other words, what part are diseases now performing in the evolution of the race? At least one fact is plain. Some congenital defects that formerly aided in the elimination of the unfit are rapidly losing their power, because they are compelled to work without the assistance of disease-producing microbes. Greater defect, wider deviation from the normal, will be possible without the fatal limit being reached. Persons,

therefore, having a lower standard of health and especially of physique will survive, and will leave offspring inheriting their abnormalities. It follows that there will necessarily be some lowering of the physical strength of our people generally. It is, no doubt, possible that this condition may be "screened" by the easing of the environment, so that relatively to that environment men may be stronger. But barbarous, or half-barbarous races sometimes become part of an environment, and then strength of the kind just mentioned is of little value. Our final decision as to the extent of the danger to the race (not to individuals, of course) in the present tendency to abolish microbic diseases—a tendency, which is beyond doubt permanent—must depend upon our belief or absence of belief in the cessation of *natural selection*, called by Weismann panmixia. If, by merely allowing disintegration, panmixia can bring about loss of whole structures, the masterpieces of organic architecture, imitating in the work of undoing the cumulative action of *natural selection* in building, then the loss to the race by the failure of microbes to eliminate the congenitally unfit is very great. That panmixia has worked among civilized nations with what appears to have been cumulative power, is shown by the great development of non-microbic diseases. Take, for example, all forms of what is commonly called rheumatism, which term, of course, includes several distinct diseases. It is hardly possible that when first the non-microbic forms of rheumatism, such as the lithemic form, appeared they could have had anything like their present malignity, for a very slight attack would have left a primitive savage at the mercy of his environment—

especially his enemies. Its power, therefore, has increased as generations have come and gone. And yet men have been selected, so far as selection has continued, not for rheumatic tendencies, but rather for their freedom from them. If, however, we deny that the cessation of selection possesses what is equivalent to cumulative power and only admit that it can produce instability of important race-characters no longer protected by *natural selection* in their full development, even then the danger of racial degeneration is not trivial.

In conclusion, we must never lose sight of a fact which the evidence brings out most strongly; there are certain organs which in civilized man must be sound, although not necessarily so efficient as in his barbarian ancestors. Among these we may count the heart, liver, muscles, nerves, intestines. On the soundness of these the general vigor of the individual depends. No artificial peptonising of food is ever likely to relieve the digestive system of the task of assimilating that food, so that certain diseases of digestion will continue to eliminate those who suffer from them. On the other hand, a man who is bald at thirty years of age, whose teeth are artificial, and who is markedly myopic may be vigorous and efficient under modern conditions. But we may feel sure that those qualities which are essential to general efficiency will die harder than those which, in their perfection at least, have become mere luxuries, if we may so describe soundness of teeth and keenness of sight. The former can at the fastest degenerate only at a rate proportionate to the general easing of the environment; the latter may have a velocity of their own, since they have ceased to rank among things of first-class importance.

THE SLUDER OPERATION FOR THE REMOVAL OF TONSILS.

BY

CHARLES J. IMPERATORI, M. D.,
New York City.

In the removal of the faucial tonsil, whether for hypertrophy of the gland or for a diseased condition—it is essential that the tonsil be removed completely—that is enucleated.

·The majority of enlarged tonsils are diseased. To leave a portion of a diseased tonsil, shows a lapse in technic.

The piece left behind may have few or many crypts, that are filled with bacteria and these under sufficient irritation can do much harm.

The mechanical obstruction produced by enlarged tonsils is of least danger to the patient.

The tonsil is the portal of infection in acute articular rheumatism, acute septic endocarditis and other diseases.

Poynton and Paine in their articles in the *London Lancet,* (pgs. 861 and 1524,) have demonstrated the same organism from the inflamed joints, pleura and endocardium, that was found in the initial sore throat.

Every operation or manipulation is decidedly a matter of personal equation of the operator, and what one man can do with a few instruments another under the same conditions would need a dozen.

The consensus of opinion is that there is no one operation for the removal of tonsils.

Every method used in the enucleation of tonsils has its advocate. Every method has its advantages and some disadvantages.

The Sluder method, devised by Dr. Greenfield Sluder of St. Louis seems to be one by which the tonsil can be removed completely in the majority of instances, with the least trauma to the soft parts and lessened shock to the patient.

As it is necessary to describe the manipulation in detail, reference and extracts have been made from Sluder's article that appeared in the *Journal of the American Medical Association,* March 25, 1911.

By this method the tonsil is moved "completely out of its normal bed—in the forward and upward direction and then utilizes one of the anatomic markings of the lower jaw as a vantage point in putting it through the aperture of the guillotine. This anatomic marking is the well defined eminence just above the mylohyoid line, produced by the last formed molar tooth, in its socket, which is rendered even more prominent in the mouth by the tissues of the gum. In childhood the posterior, unformed molar as it lies embedded in the alveolus helps to make the eminence."

This is called by Sluder the "alveolar eminence of the mandible."

The tonsil lies posterior and for the most part below the eminence; in children appearing much further back and much lower than in maturity. The instrument used is a modification of the Mackenzie, this in turn having been modified from one described by Physick of Philadelphia.

The instrument is described in detail in Sluder's article.

However, the latest instrument devised by Sluder has two fenestrae on either side situated 1½ cm. behind the aperture of the guillotine.

These holes have been placed there in order that more power might be applied to the cutting edge by forcing home the knife by means of a hooked bar, that has a right angle member. The hook being inserted in one of the holes and the right angled part

guided into the groove on the thumb piece; sufficient force can be applied to make the dull blade cut through the toughest fibrous tonsil.

Operation.— The patient should be in a recumbent position. Before commencing the anesthesia place mouth gag closed in patient's mouth. Anesthesia, ether or nitrous oxide. In selecting, which guillotine to use, choose the one that will fit the tonsil snugly. Usually the smaller of the two instruments will be used. When the patient is sufficiently under the anesthetic open the mouth gag; Sluder inserts a flexible wire between the jaws and stimulates the pharyngeal reflex, thus inducing gagging and the mouth gag can be readily adjusted. This is especially useful when nitrous oxide is used.

Examine the inner surface of the mandible posteriorly. Ascertain the buccinator ridge, then the alveolar eminence (Sluder) then the mylohyoid line.

The reason for doing this is to ascertain the "angle of slant" of the internal surface of the mandible below and behind the alveolar eminence and also its breadth.

In the young the angle is greater—"60° outward and backward from the antero-posterior axis and even more than 60° downward and outward from the transverse; while in maturity these angles may be less than 45° in one or both directions."

In order to properly apply the guillotine in this operation it is necessary to ascertain this "angle of slant."

This area is bounded by the sulcus mylohyoideus, posteriorly-inferiorly and by the linea mylohyoideus, antero-superiorly. It is triangular shaped, with the apex pointing toward the foramen mandibulae.

Having ascertained the anatomical conditions present and decided on the size of the instrument,"the operator approaches the tonsil at an angle approximately 45°, which requires the shaft of the instrument to cross the mouth from the opposite side. This necessitates the distal side of the shaft being applied to the tonsil. At the same time it has the advantage of leaving the lateral portion of the field of operation wide open for view and the use of the other hand. Assuming that the surgeon uses his right hand for both tonsils and stands at the patient's right: for the right, he faces the patient's head; but for the left, he must turn around so that he faces the patient's feet and stands somewhat beyond (above) his head."

"The guillotine, with the transverse axis of the aperture vertical, is introduced into the mouth at an angle of 45° outward and backward, passing back until the distal arc of the aperture is completely behind the tonsil."

The direction of the shaft is then changed to point downward in order to get the ring of the aperture under the lowermost part of the tonsil. The instrument at this moment may sometimes to advantage be rotated slightly by turning the handle downward (toward the feet). This tends to enlarge the field of vision. It is then pressed outward until the distal arc of the aperture has been pressed against the ramus of the jaw or in case the patient is not anesthetized, against the firmly contracted internal petrygoid muscle which is inserted here. It is now brought slightly forward and upward, but held firmly against the bone and muscle, when it will be seen that the lower distal arc of the aperture has acted very much like a scoop, having secured the lower part of the tonsil and brought it forward and upward into the neighborhood of the alveolar eminence. In case the shaft has been rotated to secure its lower part, it is now put back into its original position by turning the handle upward.

The upper portion of the tonsil is usually put into the grasp of the distal arc of the aperture by this rotation.

If the tonsil is not too large and flat (thin) it is usually secured, both lower and upper portions, in the first setting of the guillotine and no rotation is needed. The distal arc is now firmly held behind the posterior border of the tonsil and the instrument drawn forward and upward at an angle approximately 45°, which will be found to have pulled it upward and forward onto the eminence of the alveolus. The blade is now pushed down with the gentlest possible pressure, until the surgeon sees that it is in contact with the tissues.

It should not be pressed forcibly until the parts are engaged satisfactorily in the aperture.

The blade, being in contact with the tissue, prevents the portion of the tonsil which has gone through from slipping out again. At this moment the surgeon may perceive, that, although the distal arc of the aperture is entirely behind and external to the tonsil, a part of its anterior portion has still not gone through.

This is usually readily seen, but may be more definitely determined by feeling with the tip of the index finger of the other hand; and, at the same time it may be pushed through.

This is done by the gentlest massage—simply stroking it in the direction of the aperture with the ball of the index finger, and, at the same time pushing the blade very gently across the remaining portion of the aperture. "If all of the tonsil has gone through, the distal arc will be felt smooth and firm and to be covered by what seems to be a thick mucous membrane.

If a part of the tonsil has not gone through, it can easily be felt and recognized as a mass of tissue harder than membrane and usually irregular. All of the tonsil having gone through, the blade is now pushed across with all the power of the surgeon's hands. Great pressure is usually required because the blade has been made dull. If it is too dull or if it does not fit perfectly into the soft metal lining of the distal arc of the aperture, it will not cut altogether through.

The instrument must then be pulled forward a little and its ends stripped off with the finger of the other hand."

With these manipulations the tonsil, including its capsule will be found on the proximal side of the guillotine—the gland having the appearance of being turned inside out.

Advantages.— Useful in all classes of cases, but used to best advantage in large hypertrophied glands, that are either fibrous or soft.

No assistance excepting the anesthetist, who steadies the head. Time element must appeal to all. Anesthesia time is shortened, which necessarily lessens shock.

Trauma to the adjacent tissues is less, provided the gland has been removed with one stroke.

Resulting wound. The next day and following, the wound appears usually broader and flatter, possibly because of the snipping of the anterior pillar.

After effects—those of a properly performed tonsillectomy.

Hemorrhage is in most cases markedly lessened.

Instrumentation confined to mouth gag, tongue depressor and guillotine. No injury to posterior pillar, which is of most importance and also no injury to uvula.

Disadvantages.— The following are disadvantages encountered by the writer and it is possible that when a greater number of cases have been operated he will be able to overcome these difficulties as Sluder has himself.

Type of Tonsil.—The flat, that is the thin submerged type of tonsil or one bound down by many fibrous adhesions—successful results are not so apt to be arrived at, as by other methods.

Trauma.—Should it be necessary to make several attempts to remove portions of the tonsil—usually trauma of the parts is considerable, and hemorrhage is about the same as with other methods.

Snipping of the anterior pillar.—It is possible that sufficient can be removed to be followed by replacement with scar tissue and contractions.

The method is one that requires considerable practice before the enucleation of every case can be carried out successfully. The difficulty usually being with the right tonsil, assuming the operator is right handed.

However, when mastered the operation is a brilliant one and considering that the gland is enucleated, the short time of operation and lessened number of instruments plus lessened trauma, it should be the operation of choice in the majority of cases and particularly in children.

245 West 102nd St.

———

Lavage of the stomach preparatory to an operation for intestinal obstruction had best be done before anesthetizing. Performed during narcosis the procedure *may* cause alarming embarrassment of respiration and, if the throat *should* become flooded with mucus or stomach content, as occasionally happens, an aspiration pneumonia is very apt to follow.—*Amer. Jour. of Surgery.*

INTUSSUSCEPTION IN INFANTS.[1]

A PLEA FOR EARLY DIAGNOSIS AND OPERATION.

BY

L. MILLER KAHN, M. D.,

Assistant Surgeon, Lebanon Hospital,

New York City.

Intussusception in infants is a common affection which has in the past been attended by a very high mortality. It is confidently hoped that with a better appreciation of its early manifestations and a prompt resort to the certain relief of the invagination the malady will lose its terrors.

If unrecognized and untreated, intussusception in infants is a fatal disease and the very few cases in which recovery has taken place spontaneously through sloughing or otherwise, are of such great rarity, that it has been fitly said that recovery in this manner qualifies the patient to win the highest prize in the lottery of life. At the present time the treatment of invagination of the bowel has reached a high degree of efficiency and the results of the operative treatment are all that its most ardent advocates had hoped for.

In 1888 A. E. Barker (1) gathered together all the reported cases that had been operated upon for intussusception and the total number was 73. Of these 73 cases in patients of all ages only 12 recovered. There were 23 of the whole number in children and of these only 5 recovered. Even so late as 1895 Roughton (2) could only find 16 successful operations in infants. This is a little over 17 years ago but it seems a far cry from the discouraging facts of that time to the present when Clubbe (3) is able to report his latest series of 25 opera-

[1] Read before the Medical Society of the Borough of the Bronx, N. Y. City, Dec. 11, 1912.

tions in infants suffering with intussusception, with only one death and Roughton can show 14 consecutive operations without a death.

It will more than repay us to examine the methods by which such excellent results can now be achieved in a field of surgery of which as late as 1898 a writer in the American Text-Book of Diseases of Children said, "I am well aware that a few brilliant results have been recorded—but these cases should be regarded as surgical curiosities, showing what infants may sometimes safely endure rather than furnishing precedents for future guidance."

The chief factors in the reduction of the infant mortality in intussusception are the early diagnosis and immediate operation. Here rests the burden, and the record of present achievement is based on the accomplishment of these two absolute necessities in the treatment of this disorder. In Roughton's 14 consecutive successful cases all were operated upon within 36 hours of the onset and the greater proportion within 24 hours. Even more enlightening statistics are those of Harold Stiles (4) in which one may count exactly the cost in lives of each 24 hours delay. Of 33 children operated upon within 24 hours of the onset of the invagination 28 (85%) recovered; of the 7 operated upon during the second 24 hours five (71.4%) recovered; while of the 12 operated upon after 48 hours only 3 (25%) recovered. All the irreducible cases died. This experience of Stiles is typical and is to be duplicated in any hospital where these cases come for treatment.

Dr. Richard M. Pierce has recently said, "In the fields of observation chance favors the mind which is prepared." Indeed half the battle is won if the mind of the physician who first sees a case of intussusception is prepared to recognize it.

The diagnosis of acute invagination of the bowel is relatively easy for there is present in nearly all cases a definite group of symptoms which are, in a sense pathognomonic. The history given by the mother should be carefully listened to as it may be of the utmost importance. The child may have been in excellent health previous to the attack or it may have had slight diarrhea for a few days preceding the onset of the more serious symptoms. The disease is ushered in with screaming either intermittent or continuous, and other evidence of great pain, such as drawing the legs up over the abdomen as in cramps, and there is usually, even in very young children sudden blanching and depression. There is a history of having had one or more stools after the sudden onset, followed by passage of blood and mucus.

The constipation is then well marked and nothing is passed but blood and some mucus. There is almost always vomiting.

Here we have a typical history in the average case which if given indicates the probable diagnosis. Particular weight should be given the presence of blood and mucus which occurs in 85% of all cases [Adams (5)] and when these are passed without fecal material the probability of intussusception is strongly increased.

On examining the little patient we find usually a well nourished infant in a state of depression but I have seen several cases in which there was no evident shock or discomfort.

The abdomen may be soft or slightly distended and rigidity occurs late if at all. A well defined mass, rounded at either end and soft in its most prominent portion is to be felt through the abdominal wall

in nearly all cases. But its presence is not absolutely necessary to a diagnosis as may be seen in case 2. In most instances the mass described as sausage-shaped may be found at any point along the course of the large intestine but may be found in some instances in the middle of the abdomen. It is more commonly to be felt in the umbilical, right or left hypochondriac regions. If the invagination has progressed to great length the mass may be felt in the rectum.

Much harm has been done in the past by depending on feeling the mass per anum, for if one waits for this to occur the condition is already far advanced. Where the history is not straightforward and a mass is not to be felt in the abdomen the child should be given an anesthetic—preferably ether—and examined bi-manually, that is with a finger in the rectum and the other hand on the abdomen after full relaxation. This must, of course, not be done unless one is ready to operate immediately as the patient should not be given a second anesthesia where the first would have served. If after anesthesia no mass is to be felt but the history is clearly that of intussusception the operation must be undertaken as in case 2. Roughton had a similar case in his series. It may be stated here that each hour following the onset of the disease makes the work of the surgeon more difficult by increasing the edema of the invaginated section and thereby hindering the reduction.

In the differential diagnosis it may be necessary to exclude enterocolitis in which the blood and mucous are mixed with the fecal material and in which there is a history of diarrhea and an absence of the sudden onset and tumor. Here too, there is a great preponderance of mucus and the ileus is absent. Henoch's purpura with bloody stools has been confused with intussusception and in fact, these two conditions have been found in the same child simultaneously. If there are no other symptoms of the purpura present than the intestinal bleeding, it would seem impossible to distinguish them, but there are usually other evidences than the bloody stools to aid in making the diagnosis of an intussusception. This difficulty has seldom arisen. Enlarged mesenteric glands have been diagnosticated and operated upon as suspected cases of intussusception. In differentiating these conditions it is to be remembered that intussusception in infants usually has an acute history and that the mass is but rarely felt in the right iliac fossa or along the vertebral column as is the case in enlarged mesenteric glands.

The treatment of intussusception in infants has gone through various stages of development from studious neglect to active and really conservative surgical measures. The treatment of this condition by filling the large bowel with air, water, or oil under pressure has been extensively tried and while an occasional reduction has been accomplished the method has proven uncertain and unreliable.

The chief disadvantage of this method is its uncertainty for it is not possible to be sure that reduction has been effected and the loss of time, as has been shown, is a determining cause is increasing the mortality. Precious hours are lost and shock added to an already serious state of affairs. Ladd (6) concludes that the mortality of irrigation and palliation is high (70%) and that the mortality of surgical treatment is about 50% better than that of irrigation. Clubbe after an enormous experience has finally abandoned all methods of irrigation and says positively that the treatment of intussusception is laparotomy. Zahorsky. (7) has recently published a method of "Succussion and Taxis," in which he combines gentle pressure on the mass through the abdominal wall with inversion of and shaking the little patient. While an occasional reduction may be effected in this way the objections are the same as those to irrigations. Dr. John B. Murphy (8) reviewing this method says, "The open operation is much to be preferred. It should be performed early, and with the everyday surgeon has no dangers."

After observing the effect of palliation and delay in a considerable number of cases I agree with Ladd in the statement that, "Resection, especially in infants with intussusception is an exceedingly fatal procedure and should not and would not have to be resorted to nearly so frequently if the treatment recommended in various medical text-books was not so carefully followed."

It is not intended here to enter into a technical discussion as to the causative factors of intussusception nor the varieties of invagination, but merely to enumerate the simpler kinds. There are in the main four varieties: The ileo-cecal in which the ileo-cecal valve precedes the small intestine and heads the intussusceptum; the ileo-colic, in which the small intestine is invaginated into the colon and the cecum remains in place; the colic, and the ileal which require no explanation.

The operation in the early cases is simple in the extreme. The abdomen is opened in the median line with the umbilicus as the middle point of the incision. The mass is delivered, and beginning at the end nearest the rectum (aboral) is gently squeezed and "milked" towards the cecum and as the last portion is delivered it is permissible to make gentle traction on the intussusceptum. This last is to be done with great care. If reduction of the invagination is impossible after all possible coaxing, one of the several operations for establishing an artificial anus or resection will have to be done. Sometimes in delivering the incarcerated gut the peritoneum may be torn and patients have recovered with severe lacerations of the visceral peritoneum. Hot towels are applied to the exposed gut and all intestines brought out of the abdomen are to be protected in this way. If the appendix is highly inflamed or seems to have been the source of the trouble it should be removed if the condition of the patient warrants. The abdomen should be closed in layers with two or three additional through and through silk-worm gut sutures for additional strength.

Fairbanks and Vicker (9) using spinal anesthesia resected a piece of gangrenous gut in an infant 7 months of age and the child recovered. Spinal anesthesia has been used successfully in a number of cases and seems to greatly lessen the shock of operation.

The after-care really begins in the operating room, where before the operation the chest, limbs and back are wrapped in cotton batting. The operating room should be, if possible, overheated and every effort made to protect the patient from exposure. The bed is to be made warm to receive the patient and to be kept warm with hot-water bottles or as has been suggested with a lighted electric light bulb, covered so as to protect the patient against burning. The administration of hypodermoclysis is, I think, very valuable and in severe cases may be given almost continuously. The infant should be given food soon after recovering consciousness.

The two following cases will serve to bring out clearly the points made in this paper. They are taken from a number which have been admitted and operated upon at Lebanon Hospital in the service of Dr. Henry Roth, to whom I extend my thanks for permission to operate upon and report them.

W. C. Hospital Number 34896. Age 5 months. Admitted to hospital July 23, 1911. Discharged cured, August 6, 1911. History. Breast fed child. Had been in perfect health up to the day before admission on which day at 1 P. M. child vomited 8 or 9 times, dark brown fluid with no odor. After vomiting the child had one stool and succeeding stools contained blood. A physician was called and he advised sending the child to hospital.

Physical examination. Well nourished child, seemingly comfortable, not crying or giving other evidence of pain. A large mass is to be felt in the left hypochondrium—nothing abnormal felt on rectal examination.

Operation. Abdomen opened in the median line and the transverse colon delivered and found to contain intussuscepted gut. This was gently pushed towards the cecum and finally completely released. The appendix was found congested and was quickly removed. The ileo-cecal valve was in this case thrust into the ascending colon and the ileum then followed for a length of about 10 inches—ileo-cecal intussusception. The invaginated gut was of good color but slightly congested, otherwise normal.

Wound closed with layer sutures.

Child made a prompt recovery from the operation and two hours later was given the breast. No further complications ensued.

H. M. Hospital Number 38377. Aged 5½ months. Admitted to hospital Sept. 6, 1912. History. Breast fed child. Has never been well since birth. Has had "bowel trouble." Two days prior to admission patient began to vomit, had bloody and mucous stools, cried and "doubled up with cramps." For the last 24 hours has voided no urine. Temp. 102⅖F. Resp. 18. Pulse 92.

Physical Examination. A rather poorly nourished child with dark rings under the eyes. Very pale. Abdomen distended. Child does not cry when abdomen is palpated. No mass is to be made out and nothing abnormal felt in rectum. Child sent to operating room and ether anesthesia given. No mass was to be felt even on deep palpation but on acount of the typical history it was decided to open the abdomen.

Operation. Incision made in median line with the umbilicus at the middle of the incision. On opening the peritoneum straw-colored serum flowed out. Immediately on opening the peritoneum a loop of ileum was exposed with the peritoneal coat torn transversely around its circumference. There was no bleeding from the torn surface and the intestinal wall was very thin and distended. This was covered with a hot towel and I brought up the ascending colon containing a mass at the cecum. This mass was rapidly reduced by gentle pressure from above downward towards the cecum. The invaginated gut was squeezed out of the colon and found to have been about 4 inches in length with the meniscus shaped depression at its apex. The ileo-cecal valve had not been invaginated and we were therefore dealing with an ileo-cecal intussusception. The reduced gut was dark purple in color and edematous, although the peritoneal covering of this part of the ileum was still shiny. The appendix was congested, but had not been invaginated. Owing to the poor condition of the patient it was not removed. The tear in the peritoneum covering the loop of ileum was then sutured with Pagenstecher linen. The abdomen was closed by layers. The child left the operating room in fair condition and when seen an hour later the little patient was crying and seemingly in good shape. Four hours later the little patient became cyanotic and in spite of stimulation died a few minutes later.

The tear in the visceral peritoneum is interesting as it is, of course, difficult to say whether it resulted from too energetic palpation of the distended gut or whether it resulted from the violent peristaltic wave brought on by the obstruction. The edges of the torn peritoneum and the surface of the exposed area of gut were covered with a thin deposit of fibrin, showing that the damage was several hours old.

I have not seen in the literature a report of a similar tear in the peritoneum covering a loop of gut not involved in the intussusception and many inches distant from the cecum. That it might readily result from too sturdy palpation, one may readily believe and is to be remembered in palpating the distended abdomen of an infant. The repair of the damage took several minutes which could ill be spared. This child was operated upon more than 48 hours after the onset of the invagination. The temperature of 102⅖ F. is unusual as there is ordinarily no rise of temperature in these cases.

CONCLUSIONS.

(1) The treatment for intussusception in infants is laparotomy.

(2) Delay in the treatment of intussusception is fatal in direct ratio to the delay.

(3) Pallative measures have no place in the correct management of intussusception in infants.

(4) With an early diagnosis and prompt resort to operation a good prognosis can be given.

REFERENCES.

1. Barker, *Lancet*, London, 1888.
2. Roughton, *Lancet*, London, Vol. 1, 1895, and *Clinical Journal*, London, July 19, 1911.
3. Clubbe, *British Journal of Diseases of Children*, 1909, Vol. VI, page 311.
4. Harold J. Stiles, Article in A System of Treatment, London, 1912.
5. Adams, *Practitioner*, London, 1910, Vol. LXXXV, page 679.
6. Ladd, *Boston Med. and Surg. Jour.*, 1911, Vol. CLXIV, page 712.
7. Zahorsky, *Archives Pediatrics*, N. Y., 1911, Vol. XXVIII, page 380.
8. Murphy, Editorial Note, Surgery Vol., Practical Medicine Series, 1912.
9. Fairbanks and Vicker, *Lancet*, London, 1910, Feb. 3.

223 West 113th Street.

THE USE OF THE SECONDARY BLOOD CLOT IN MASTOID SURGERY.[1]

BY

R. JOHNSON HELD, M. D.,

New York City.

Visiting Otologist to N. Y. Red Cross Hospital;
Surgeon to Throat, Nose and Lung Hospital; Assistant Surgeon Manhattan
Eye, Ear and Throat Hospital.

In the various text-books and medical journals we read of the modern operation of mastoidectomy; how it has been developed by slow progression to the almost perfect operation as it is performed today by our well-known otologists.

While it must be admitted that the technique of the operation is such that complete eradication of the infection is invariably obtained, yet included in an ideal or perfect operation should be considered the healing of the operation wound in the shortest possible time, with as little possible pain and discomfort to the patient and with the least resulting deformity.

For some years efforts have been put forth with the view of improving the after treatment of the simple mastoid operation, and while many have been suggested not even a few have been chosen.

A long and tedious convalescence of from six weeks to four months is at its best exceedingly disagreeable, and so frequently means hardship to the individual or his family. Wearing the unsightly bandage, the pain and discomfort of the frequent dressings, and the loss of time to the patient during this long drawn out after treatment must be taken seriously into consideration. That form of after treatment which will result in rapidity of healing without additional risk to the welfare of the patient,

[1] Read at a meeting of the Eastern Medical Society, Oct. 11, 1912.

and will obviate the necessity of frequent and painful dressings and will produce an excellent cosmetic effect will surely be considered an advance in surgery and a joy to otologists.

Probably the most widely attempted operative procedure intended to overcome the objections enumerated, has been the primary blood clot dressing.

What are the objections to the primary blood clot dressing?

Fear of consequences of closing an abscess cavity filled with blood clot when it is practically impossible to render aseptic a wound so thoroughly septic, and especially so when the use of antiseptics to cleanse the wound has a deleterious effect upon the bactericidal properties of the blood serum.

That we have in the closed cavity ideal conditions for the growth of bacteria and spread of infection: heat, moisture, a good culture medium, and the bacteria present.

That there might be enclosed in the cavity microscopic particles of infected material.

That with the virulent infection and suppuration of the middle ear and mastoid cavity, more drainage for a reasonable time should be had than from the incision in the middle ear alone, and that the open posterior wound creates a counter opening; excellent surgical technique.

That during the virulency of acute mastoiditis and middle ear suppuration when the communication between the middle ear and the mastoid cavity is wide open, that the blood clot would immediately become infected via that channel.

In the method I am advocating tonight these objections are met.

Recognizing the advantages that would be gained by any form of after treatment in acute mastoid surgery which would shorten the long period of convalescence,

I conceived the idea of using the late blood clot treatment, or secondary closure of the original wound by allowing it to fill with blood clot.

Independently of me, this method has been advocated by others.

During the past 6 or 7 years it has been my custom when performing the radical mastoid operation to suture tightly the posterior wound and cut a flap which I turned upward so as to shut off the mastoid cavity from the exenerated middle ear. The middle ear was lightly packed and the mastoid cavity allowed to fill with blood clot. The results in these cases were uniformly excellent and applied in all cases with or without exposure of dura or sinus, excepting those with intra-cranial complications.

It occurred to me, with such results in the radical operation, that a secondary operation might be performed in the simple mastoid operation to suture the posterior wound and fill with blood clot at the time when suppuration in the middle ear had practically ceased and when the antral opening was closed, would probably result in a diminution in the time ordinarily required for healing. In September, 1910, I tried my first case in a person to whom time was of great importance. Eighteen days after the original operation the patient was anaesthetized, the old wound curetted lightly, the edges of the wound lifted from the bone and cartilage, the edges of the wound freshened and the wound sutured without a drain. Four days after, alternating sutures were removed, and two days later the others were removed. The result was excellent; a linear scar, no depression and the posterior wound healed and all bandages off in 24 days. Since that time I have performed this operation on all cases where the individual would allow a second operation,

and with especially good results, shortening the after treatment from three weeks to two months, and always without posterior depression. In several cases the secondary operation was performed under cocaine anaesthesia, with the same results. The cosmetic effect being so good, I began to use this method on all cases of permanent posterior opening and where there was any unsightly posterior depression. The results again were excellent.

I have used this method of closure twenty-seven times with uniformly excellent results, and believe it a mode of procedure which will lend itself toward shortening the time of after treatment in a large percentage of the average cases.

Regarding the manner of healing, experimental and clinical studies have shown that if any clean wound be filled with the patient's own blood, and safe-guarded from later infection, the blood clot tends to organize and new tissue, similar to that inclosing the clot, soon forms to replace the latter. The blood flowing into the wound cavity rapidly clots and the fibrinous framework of this clot constitutes a scaffolding on which the new tissue is built. Fresh granulations spring from the walls of the cavity and grow out into the clot, forming a new fibrous connective tissue, the nature of which is further altered to accord with the character of the surrounding cavity walls; that is, if the wound be made in bone, osteoblasts are sent out from the bony walls, or from the periosteum, to convert the fibrous substance into osseous tissue. The migratory power of these osteoblasts is limited, and they travel only a short way from their starting point, so that, in the case of a large cavity in bone, the newly formed bone does not extend far from the cavity wall, and the center of the new-formed tissue remains fibrous in character. It seems quite probable, however, that in a small cavity, such as we ordinarily make in the mastoid process, the osteoblasts, reaching out from all directions, may extend a sufficient distance to meet in the center and thus to complete the construction of a new bony process. Just how early this osteoblastic activity commences is not known, but such cells have been observed to form within forty-eight hours after the operation, and it is certain that granulation tissue grows more rapidly into a healthy blood clot than into space. It is plain, then, that Nature may be greatly aided in the reconstruction of destroyed tissue by providing an excellent framework on which to build and leaving her only the task of furnishing vascularity and new tissue cells (Reik).[1]

The Technique.—The technique of this procedure for the acute mastoid cases is as follows: Having decided that there is practically no further suppuration in the tympanic cavity and that the antral opening is about to close, the patient is anesthetized, the usual operative care as to asepsis and antisepsis being observed. The free edges of the wound have grown inward and are adherent. They are freed and together with the periosteum are lifted from the bone and auricle for from ½ inch in front to 1 inch above and behind. This is done so that when the edges of the wound are pared and freshened there will be no tension when they are sutured. In paring the edges of the wound sufficient tissues should be removed to assure proper coaptation. In some instances ⅛ or ¼ inch may have to be removed. With gauze covered finger the wound cavity is lightly rubbed to cause bleeding and stimulation of granulation.

Interrupted sutures are then used at very slight intervals. The more sutures the less tension on each individual one, so they are applied about ⅛ of an inch apart. The wound is then covered with plain gauze and bandage applied. At the end of 3 or 4 days alternate sutures are removed, and 2 or 3 days later the balance are removed.

In cases of posterior depressions the technique is slightly different. An incision is made well above the upper extremity of the depression and carried down through the center of the depression to terminate well below the lower margin. The skin and underlying tissue is now elevated all over the depression and for about ½ an inch around it. The wound edges are then brought together and sufficient tissue pared off so that when the opposing edges are sutured they will not dip into the cavity. The wound cavity in these cases is rubbed as in the former description. The remainder of the technique is identical with that described.

In cases of permanent posterior openings, plastic arrangement of tissue is done according to the character of the permanent opening, but after the tissues have been brought together and sutured, the cavity, like in the previous conditions, fills with blood clot and the suturing and after treatment is the same.

616 Madison Ave.

———

When resecting the cecum be careful not to tie the mesentery of the ascending colon too close to the bowel—the anastomosing loop of the ileo-colic and colica media lies very near the gut.

———

When dealing with a chronic bone abscess (and often, too, in acuter cases) it saves weeks of after-treatment to work with an osteo-periosteal ("coffin lid") flap, and close the wound completely.—*Amer. Jour. of Surgery.*

[1] Reik, H. O. The Johns Hopkins Hospital Bulletin, Vol. XXI, No. 225, April, 1910.

OPERATIVE HERNIA FOLLOWING SUPRA-PUBIC CYSTOTOMY.

BY

HOWARD CRUTCHER, M. D.,
Roswell, New Mexico.

In April, 1911, a farmhand, aged 54 (in appearance fifteen years older), was referred to me by Dr. D. H. Galloway. The patient complained of great distress in the hypogastrium and made frequent attempts to urinate, generally passing but a few drops at a time. Examination disclosed a series of strictures in the anterior urethra and an impassable obstruction in the membranous portion of the canal. I explained to the patient that his condition was mechanical in character and that only proper surgical measures would relieve him. He was "not much for surgical operations," in fact believed that a "good many people had been killed by them," which is doubtless true; he had also taken gallons of some notorious nostrum, "guaranteed to cure all kidney troubles," and really preferred to continue foundering in the bogs of quackery rather than accept the relief offered by modern scientific teaching.

I assured him that millions of well-meaning people had survived war, pestilence, famine and quackery, and that he was the judge of his own course of action. He purchased another supply of his precious nostrum and returned to his home.

Forty-eight hours later I received an anxious message from one of the patient's friends, saying that "something has got to be done; he's in awful bad shape, and can't make no water at all, except a drop at a time; no sleep last night; terrible pain." I directed that the patient be brought to Roswell at once and made preparations for an immediate operation.

On opening the perineum the urethra was found to be a mass of dense cicatricial tissue, tortuous and impossible to follow. The bladder was then opened through a high incision, the staff passed and the offending tissues divided freely as far as the prostate. The anterior obstructions were next dealt with, a congenital phimosis relieved, and the bladder wound closed with two layers of fine chromic catgut. The prevesical space was packed snugly with gauze, a drainage tube inserted through the perineal wound and the usual dressings applied. The drainage tube was removed the third day and sound passing instituted at once and continued for several weeks. The patient was up and about town within a week and I regarded the result as highly satisfactory. The suprapubic wound healed rapidly, the urinary stream was copious, and I was unprepared for any unusual after results.

In July, 1912, the patient returned to me, complaining of a swelling above his pubic bones. Examination revealed an operative hernia, the first I ever saw following such an operation. My impression is that the complication must be of extreme rarity, since I do not find it mentioned after an extensive search in many standard works on modern surgery. My patient doubtless returned to rough farm labor too soon after leaving his bed, and having never met with such a complication I took no means to prevent it. He now wears a comfortable pad, which affords perfect relief, in view of which I have not advised further operative measures.

It is pitiable if not shameful that infectious diseases of the male urinary organs should have been so grievously neglected by the general medical profession. Many men of sound training and ripe experience used to regard it as somewhat beneath their dignity to "dirty their hands with a case of gonorrhea." The pity of it. The result was a swarm of conscienceless, illiterate quacks not one in a hundred of whom could pass an examination on the crude anatomy of the parts involved. Years ago my old friend, G. Frank Lydston said to me, "Yes, quackery naturally takes to cover, and unfortunately the urethra shelters the largest crowd."

THE SIGNIFICANCE OF ABDOMINAL PAIN IN INFANTS AND CHILDREN.

BY

THERON WENDELL KILMER, M. D.,
Lecturer, Diseases of Children, New York Polyclinic; Asst. Attending Physician, New York Polyclinic Hospital,
New York City.

There is one fact to which more importance should be given by the physician and also by the laity, and that is, that when a child has persistent abdominal pain, there is something of sufficient seriousness brewing to either make a very careful examination of the abdomen, or as in the case of the laity, to at once call a physician.

Unrecognized abdominal trouble has been the death certificate of many an infant and child. It is to the various factors which may cause a persistent or even a temporary abdominal pain which I ask your attention for a few minutes this evening.

The laity interpret the abdomen of a child to be the volcano in which an eruption of any kind whatsoever may take place and still not injure the child in any way; the cause of a belly-ache in an infant is in ninety-nine out of one hundred cases put down as colic; a belly-ache in a child is believed by the laity to be due always to green apples or unripe fruit. Only a few years ago a popular air with fitting words was wrtitten and sung by all stagedom relating to a certain boy and his sister Sue who ate the peach of emerald hue and soon away to the angels flew, etc. In my own opinion this same boy and his sister Sue died of unrecognized appendicitis.

We as physicians should know a little bit more than many of us know at present, about the examination of a baby; it is the seemingly little things that count in this world, and the proper method of abdominal examination is one of them.

In the physical examination of any child, that child will fall under one of the three following classes:

1. The good child.
2. The nervous child.
3. The vicious (or spoiled) child.

The first class, the good child, will let you do about as you please. The nervous child will have to be approached tactfully and not with too great haste. The vicious child, well—waste no time on him but do your work at once and let him know from the start that you will in no way harm him and that you and you only are the boss of the entire situation.

In the examination of an abdomen the hands should be warmed as there is nothing that will tighten up the abdominal muscles like a cold hand placed on the abdomen; it is also liable to start the child to crying. While I am on the subject of the laying on of hands, let me dwell to a considerable degree upon gentleness; even my short experience in teaching has taught me that rather to submit a baby's abdomen to the examining hand of some, I would a great deal rather procure a blunt garden-rake and a paving-stone and allow their combined efforts to do their worst; some charming characters I have met with low, soft, well modulated voices and dispositions like a turtle-dove, yet when it came to palpating the abdomen of an infant, I surely expected to see at any moment, the index finger protrude through the spinal column.

A child's abdomen is best examined when he is in the dorsal position with his thighs slightly flexed on his abdomen. His absolute confidence is to be gained if possible and not abused after he has once given it to you. The distraction of his attention should also be sought; ask him questions about his play, his school, her doll, and in no way let it be known that the examination of the abdomen is your sole object.

While the hand is palpating the abdomen watch the face constantly for it is by its aid that many a momentary twinge of pain is indicated.

The various points of interest which I usually look for when I place my hand on an infant's or child's abdomen are as follows:

Fever: This is invariably detected by anyone who is constantly in the habit of feeling the skin of a sick child; long years ago at the Babies' Hospital we all used to make guesses at the degree of temperature of the various sick babies by placing the palms of our hands on their skin and one would be surprised at the accuracy of calculations as confirmed later by the clinical thermometer.

Rigidity: This is easier to detect in a child than in an adult except should the child be continuously crying, when rigidity can be determined by awaiting a deep inspiration during which the abdominal mus-

cles somewhat relax. Examine for a general abdominal rigidity or a local rigidity.

Breathing: While the hand is on the abdomen the character of the respirations should be noticed. Is the breathing abdominal or is it thoracic? The breathing normally is abdominal. Children whose abdomens are involved with inflammation generally show thoracic breathing.

Intestinal Tract: Notice whether the intestines are empty, full of feces, full of gas, is there abdominal distension? It is well to get accustomed to the feel of a normal abdomen for it is by the knowledge of the normal that enables us to distinguish the abnormal.

Liver: Always feel for the liver and notice whether it is palpable at or below the margin of the ribs.

Spleen: Feel if the spleen is palpable, which normally it should not be.

Tumor: Can any abdominal tumor be felt? Palpate for any small nodules such as are felt in cases of tubercular peritonitis.

Fluid: This should be very carefully examined for by placing one hand on one side of the abdomen and then gently tapping the opposite side with the finger; if fluid is present a wave will be felt as it strikes against the other hand.

Bladder: Is the bladder empty or distended?. This may be ascertained by both palpation and percussion of the bladder area.

Rectal Examination: This is of great value in abdominal palpation and I never venture a diagnosis of an abdominal condition unless I have supplemented the ordinary external abdominal palpation by a thorough digital rectal examination; and here let the word "gentleness" come forth once more.

Having gone over the examination of the abdomen, let us turn to the consideration of the causes of abdominal pain. There are some thirty-four various diseases or pathological conditions which will cause abdominal pain and in some of these, abdominal pain is the sole symptom.

Peritonitis: Here we either have a general abdominal pain or a local one, depending upon the situation of the inflammation. The pain of peritonitis usually is continuous and is accompanied by tenderness and rigidity.

Appendicitis: In disease of the appendix we also have pain either continuous or intermittent and colicky in character. It is too bad that so many physicians associate appendicular pain as occurring only at McBurney's point, for, in many cases it occurs on the left side of the abdomen and again high up under the liver. Pressure usually aggravates appendicular pain.

Intussusception: There may or may not be pain. In young infants with this condition pain was entirely absent in the cases which I have seen. On the other hand, in cases of intestinal obstruction in older children, pain may be quite a factor.

Gastric Ulcer: Although rare, is seen at times in older children; in these cases pain is usually referred to the epigastrium.

New Growths: Occurring in the abdomen, such as sarcoma of the liver or of the kidney, may or may not cause abdominal pain depending upon their situation. Pain is usually a very rare symptom.

Intestinal Colic: In infants is seen very often. The word "colic" should be used here as denoting a symptom only, as this condition is generally caused by some dietetic error such as too high proteid in the food. It is in just such cases as these that the careful examination of the ab-domen counts for a great deal, for in infantile colic we usually find a baby who cries intermittently, draws up his legs, and has a distended abdomen, all of which symptoms immediately stop when a dose of castor oil and an enema are given, relieving him not only of the colic, but also of a large, undigested and sometimes constipated stool.

Indigestion: Children both big and little have what is termed "indigestion"; here again is a word which covers a multitude of ills; it may be indigestion of fat or proteid or sugar in an infant, or of any sort of food whatsoever in an older child. I have seen youngsters of the runabout age whose stomach contents upon the nursery floor showed that their "indigestion" was due to an ingested chunk of meat which without chewing, no child could digest and at which any young stomach would rebel; so that when we use the word "indigestion" we must at least have some idea as to whether a proper or an improper food has been given the child. There is more or less pain accompanying all forms of indigestion and this pain may be referred to the stomach (immediately after a meal), or to further down the gastro-intestinal tract in the small or large intestine, from two to four hours after a meal. These obscure aches and pains are usually termed "gastro-intestinal," and clear up after a proper diet has been given.

Ileo-Colitis and *Summer Diarrhea:* The abdominal pain occurring during an attack of ileo-colitis or summer diarrhea may be severe, especially when there is tenesmus and passage of small, foul and bloody stools; this pain is general, intermittent and colicky in character, usually preceding a stool. The same applies to the pains accompanying colitis.

Constipation: May have associated with it abdominal pain not especially severe but rather of a dull nature and often accompanied by lame or sore back; this is seen in older children.

Impacted Feces: May give rise to abdominal pain which is immediately relieved by enemata or the removal of the rectal concretions with a suitable instrument or in an emergency, the handle of a teaspoon.

Pneumonia: Many have been the cases of pneumonia which at their onset were prepared for laparotomy; the abdominal pain occurring with pneumonia is severe and simulates appendicitis or a localized peritonitis closer than any other condition of which I know.

Hyperchlorhydria: In this condition we usually have some abdominal pain present, referred to the upper abdomen and occurring before meals; this pain is relieved by the administration of soda, calcium and magnesium.

Intestinal Parasites: Such as the tapeworm, the round-worm and the pin-worm often cause abdominal pain usually referable to the centre and upper abdomen. The only positive diagnosis is when you find the worm.

Malaria: Many children with malaria complain of left-sided abdominal pain, and upon examination, a large spleen can easily be made out.

Hysteria: The referred abdominal pain in hysteria, may be anywhere; just lately I saw a case in a boy of nine years who complained of an abdominal pain just as soon as he went to bed; this pain was never in the same spot but was always abdominal and cleared up immediately upon telling this boy that he would be severely punished if he had it again. He did not

have it again and seems to be very happy about it.

Tubercular Hip: Cases of tubercular hip in their incipiency often call attention to pain occurring at times in the iliac fossae.

Pott's Disease: Is also frequently associated with abdominal pain.

Abdominal Rheumatism: There have been several cases which have lately come under my care which I have termed abdominal rheumatism. These children were all of rheumatic history, had had attacks of undoubted rheumatism and presented nothing definite other than intermittent abdominal pain. Some days they were entirely free from pain, which was never severe while at other times they complained bitterly of deep abdominal pain unaccompanied by rigidity or rise of temperature. They cleared up nicely upon the administration of aspirin.

Cyclic Vomiting: May be accompanied or followed by seemingly intense abdominal pain; I remember one case in particular in a little girl where abdominal pain was a very pronounced feature of the attacks.

Epilepsy: Many child epileptics complain of abdominal pain as the first symptom of the aura preceding the convulsions.

Whooping Cough: During the spasmodic stage of pertusis, children will frequently complain of abdominal pain due to the excessive work of the abdominal muscles and diaphragm. They will often tell you that their stomach hurts so that they are afraid to cough. The abdominal pain and tension accompanying whooping-cough is entirely relieved when an elastic abdominal belt is worn during the course of the paroxysmal stage.

Menstruation: It should not be forgotten that girls between the ages of twelve and fourteen years begin to menstruate and some days before the first blood is seen they may complain of general abdominal pain usually intermittent and sometimes colicky in character.

"Growing Pains": I will speak for but an instant of abdominal so-called "growing" pains, only to say that I do not believe that they exist except in the minds of certain of the laity.

Herniae: Of either inguinal or femoral type, may be accompanied by slight pain in either groin.

Typhoid Fever: In this disease we have sometimes seen abdominal pain as a very prominent symptom; this is probably due to the distention of the bowel with gas or to intestinal ulceration. Abdominal pain, however, in typhoid fever is rather of rare occurrence.

Poisons: Irritant poisons of all sorts will have abdominal pain as a very prominent symptom.

Anal Fissure and *Rectal Prolapse:* Will both give at times, abdominal pain. I remember one recent case of anal fissure which gave abdominal pain on defecation as a sole symptom.

Poliomyelitis: During the past five years I have seen several cases of anterior poliomyelitis which were ushered in by vomiting, fever and a great amount of abdominal pain with no other abdominal symptoms.

Pathological conditions along the genitourinary tract frequently give rise to abdominal pain. Thus we have *renal calculi* (rare in children), *vesical calculi,* just common enough to keep one on their guard for this condition; *vulvo-vaginitis, phimosis, adherent clitorus* and *excessive acidity* of the *urine,* all causes of many of the obscure abdominal pains in children.

These then are the various diseases and conditions which will cause abdominal pain in infants and children and there is no symptom of more importance to the surgeon, the specialist, the internist or the pediatrist than the close and careful following up of *every pain* no matter of what kind or character when the seat of this pain is referred to the abdomen.

165 West 85th Street.

THE EXANTHEMATA.

BY

WALLACE C. ABBOTT, M. D.,
Chicago, Ill.

From all parts of the country come evidence that there prevails an extended epidemic of the exanthematous fevers, of considerable virulence. I propose here to discuss the question of the treatment of these maladies and submit to you if there is anything newer and better here than the so-called standard text-books may offer.

To a certain degree the indications and the dangers are similar, and the principles of treatment apply equally to all three. In the most malignant forms we may have with either a doudroyant ("lightning-like") outbreak, so intense that the little patient sinks under it and dies in a few hours, the vital forces being entirely unable to react against the shock of the invasion and display the necessary resistance. We have the initial chill or convulsion; the patient is cold, depressed, stupid, asphyxiated; and dies before the physician has time to get his remedies to work. Such cases are sometimes met during the height of an epidemic, in the debilitated denizens of the city slums, in weakly, depraved constitutions; with the influence of bad sanitation, personal, domestic and municipal.

694   AMERICAN MEDICINE
Complete Series, Vol. XVIII. }   ORIGINAL ARTICLES   { DECEMBER, 1912.
New Series, Vol. VII., No. 12.

The indication is to induce reaction, and stimulants are required, such as hot mustard baths, fiery draught of ginger, pepper, ether, alcohol, camphor, and other volatile oils being often employed. Far more effective weapons are to be found in the arsenal of modern science. The first need is to supply the brain centers with enough blood to enable them to perform their functions, and the quickest and strongest remedy is glonoin. Its effects being evanescent should be strengthened and prolonged by the addition of atropine; and the initial "shove," the electric spark that arouses the dormant powers into activity, is afforded by strychnine. The prescription is $\frac{1}{4}$ milligram, or gr. 1/250, of glonoin and atropine, and $\frac{1}{2}$ milligram, or gr. 1/134, of strychnine arsenate, preferably in hot solution, and this dosage should be repeated every five to fifteen minutes until reaction is evident.

Why not give a full dose at once, hypodermatically, since the need is so urgent? Those who have studied most closely the action of such remedies are aware that, when in times of great vital depression strychnine is administered in full doses, there may be an additional depression manifested. This corresponds with Crile's observations on shock, and with Mays' researches on the stimulant powers of minute doses and the sedation manifested by very large ones of the same remedies. *Primo non nocere.* Don't neglect the provision of pure air in unlimited quantities, and the benefits of direct sunlight. Don't add the paralysis of alcohol to the perils of the disease.

As reaction becomes established we have fever—lots of it. In scarlatina it may go to 112, in measles to 110. While this reaction is salutary and an evidence of the arousing of the bodily forces to resist the assault of the disease, it is nevertheless a peril if not restrained within safe limits. Rain is nature's means of refreshing the soil, but a cloudburst may not be especially desirable.

Claude Bernard first showed that vasomotor spasm was a constant feature of inflammation and febrile maladies, but not until late years has the profoundly significant nature of this discovery been recognized and utilized in practice. Burggraeve first put it to practical use by employing aconitine to relax this spasm and open the general circulation, to take away the surplus blood from the congested areas.

The existence of such surplus being granted in the conception of congestion or hyperemia, it followed that there must be relative vasomotor paresis in the engorged area, as the content of blood was greater than the normal, and that the balance between blood and vessels was lost, the latter being distended. Hence he united digitalin with the aconitine, and found that each affected that part where its action tended to restore vasomotor equilibrium. With the addition of veratrine when the case is sthenic or strychnine arsenate when asthenic, we have here the scientific treatment of fever, when analyzed into its pathologic elements.

The doses—aconitine, veratrine and strychnine, half a milligram, or gr. 1/134, each; digitalin a milligram, or gr. 1/67, each—should be administered every ten to sixty minutes as the case requires; and continued until the temperature falls and the pulse approximates the normal. There is little if aught to be feared from these remedies, for the maximum daily dose of either is about 100 times greater than that here recommended as a single dose. By their use the fever may be controlled with ease, and held within the useful and desirable limits.

Our next task is to eliminate from the case the element due to fecal toxemia. Those who have studied this factor most carefully attribute to it about 30% of the total symptom-complex in any fever. Subtracting this leaves the case in the category of mild or benign forms, easily managed and tending to speedy recovery without complications or sequels. We accomplish this by giving a centigram each of calomel and podophyllin, every half hour for six doses, followed by a laxative saline to sweep out the alimentary canal. Sometimes we find the symptoms of toxemia persisting, and have to repeat this medication and supplement it with repeated enemas. We keep on until the bowel is clear, and then disinfect it by a sufficiency of pure sulphocarbolates of zinc, soda or lime, to remove all abnormal odor from the stools. If the usual doses fail to render these quite odorless it is because there are still retained and decomposing fecal masses lodged somewhere in the bowel. Go after it.

During the epidemic of smallpox some years ago many reports were made indicating the power of calcium sulphide to check the progress of the disease, aborting its development and drying up the pocks in the vesicular stage instead of going on to suppuration. These reports were by many dismissed with the flimsy explanation that the advocacy of the drug was "commercial"; and it was forgotten until quite recently, when a notable paper by an American missionary in Syria, Dr. Ussher, in the *Medical Record*, directed attention anew to this matter. Dr. Ussher reported that by its use he was able to prevent or promptly cure typhus, smallpox and scarlatina; the immunity conferred by sulphide saturation in

smallpox infections being for the time quite equal to that of vaccination. Typhus patients treated with this salt recovered, those not so treated died. Scarlatina either failed to appear in those saturated, or appeared as an inconsiderable attack.

. Dr. Ussher wrote from a full heart. Alone in that far-away land, 1,000 miles by horseback from a supply of vaccine and similar stores, surrounded by that population of commingled races, the flotsam and jetsam of ten thousand years, with a large clientele, 600 children in the schools and a hospital with 50 beds and 70 patients, with no human aid near, he turned to that Being from whom all Christians draw their aid, and asked help in prayer. No man, however skeptic or even irreligious he may be, but will look with appreciation and respect on the simple belief and the courage of the man who in this age acknowledges such faith before the world. Some of us may believe with Dr. Ussher that the suggestion to use calcium sulphide was a direct answer to that prayer—and the rest of us wish we could believe it. At any rate he did use it, and with results that almost pass belief.

Saturation with sulphide is obtained by administering a small dose quite frequently, a centigram, or gr. ⅙, every half hour, until the perspiration exhales the odor of the drug. The period of acid digestion should be avoided as the hydrochloric acid decomposes the salt and annoying eructations of sulphydric acid follow. Saturation may be maintained indefinitely without harm. I have kept it up for weeks in some cases without the slightest unpleasant symptom, immediate or remote. The sulphide must be of good quality, fully up to the U. S. P. standard. Otherwise no such benefits are to be expected from it. And, unfortunately, most on the market is poor.

In measles at least, the leucocytosis usually manifested in fevers does not occur. In all these maladies it is worth while to reinforce these gallant little defenders by administering nuclein solution, in full doses of a dram each 24 hours; hypodermatically, or on the tongue to be absorbed from the mucous membrane of the mouth directly into the general circulation, without running the gauntlet of the portal system and the liver; or even the rectal route may be used. Nuclein can do no harm; it may and probably does do great good.

Heretofore we have considered these three diseases together, but we now reach the point where their history and the indications for treatment separate. Smallpox is apt to develop a tendency to scrofula, and elimination and restoration of the blood must go hand in hand. The vegetable alteratives are useful here, such as stillingin and xanthoxylin, and rumicin contains a form of iron that may be assimilated when none of the ordinary mineral salts will be taken up.

In scarlatina we have to watch the throat, and prevent diphtheritic complications that may show about the eighth day. These may extend to the nose, ears, malar bones, or any of the cavities communicating with the nasopharynx. Or chorea or rheumatism may develop. I have succeeded well by treating the mouth and throat with a saturated solution of salicylic acid, very frequently applied, as a preventive, whenever the mild angina begins. The urine should be tested often and a case never allowed to go out of our control as long as albuminuria persists. I still apply suet to the skin, not so much because I believe it prevents "catching cold," but because the children like it and say it relieves the itching and burning.

In measles we have to dread the occurrence of pulmonary complications. For these the old specific was ipecacuanha, but it too often induced nausea or even vomiting. Nowadays I employ pure emetine and get the benefits without the difficulty. Give a milligram every one to four hours, and tell me if any other remedy so completely controls the respiratory symptoms of measles.

The use of arsenic during the acute fevers we are treating deserves explanation. This remedy tends to induce fatty degeneration. Such an action is exerted upon the newly formed and as yet imperfectly organized products of morbid processes more effectively than upon the more resistant normal cells. Hence the use of moderate doses of arsenic favors the speedy disintegration and absorption of the debris of disease, and at the same time it affords a protective influence to the red blood cells that enables them to better resist the attacks of invading microorganisms.

If the stomach is weak we may give soda arsenate before meals; if there is fermentation or gastrointestinal mycosis we employ copper arsenite; during the fever stage quinine arsenate answers well; caffeine arsenate, is a useful diuretic and cardiac tonic, and in convalescence iron arsenate fills a useful place. Strychnine arsenate is the standard vital incitant.

———

After resection of the small bowel lateral anastomosis possesses several advantages, as to safety, simplicity and patency, over end-to-end union. The gut ultimately becomes a straight tube if the stoma is made near the closed ends.— *Amer. Jour. of Surgery.*

TRANSLATION.

LUMBAR PUNCTURE.

(Rachicentesis).

BY

P. RAVAUT, M. D.,
Translated from the French; with Notes and
Additions
BY
O. L. MULOT, M. D.,
Brooklyn, N. Y.

(*Concluded in this issue.*)

OCULAR AFFECTIONS.

At first, its use in this class of affections was restricted to cases of papillary stasis; but it has been extended to the ocular troubles which occur in the course of certain nervous and meningeal diseases and we will take them up in their order. (Frankel[102], DeRidder[103]).

It will be well, briefly to recall the connection and relations of the optic nerve. The nerve is enveloped throughout its entire course, from the brain to the Lamina cribrosa of the sclerotic coat of the eye, by the meninges, which form a veritable sheath; the nerve thus appearing as a root or spur of the brain. There is therefore around the nerve an arachnoid space. This continuity of membranes may be patent throughout its course and in places the membrane may be found to be adherent, but these adhesions are not complete and do not interfere with the circulation of the cerebro-spinal fluid which filters freely in either direction. Further, it has been proven that these coats of the nerve are entirely independent of the lymphatic circulation of the nerve; therefore this is a true meningeal sheath.

Now this little anatomical detail shows that the optic nerve is bathed in cerebro-spinal liquid and that here puncture may have a double action: 1st, by general drainage of the cerebro-spinal canal draw the fluid from the sheath of the nerve into the larger space and so directly or indirectly relieve the pressure on the venous and lymphatic circulation and this is the explanation of its effect in certain cases of papillary stasis; and 2nd, it may act by the withdrawal from the sheath of the nerve, the infectious and toxic products contained, and this in turn explains its good results in papillitis due to edema of the optic nerve. Besides this, puncture seems to give very good results in the amblyopias not accompanied by ophthalmoscopic lesion, but these we will discuss further on.

(a) Optic Neuritis.—This clinical term is applied to conditions, which by the ophthalmoscopic examination and etiological study can schematically be arranged into two groups. In the first, the examination of the fundus of the eye reveals hyperemia of the papilli, sometimes peripapillary hemorrhages and it is not rare to see the retina participate in the inflammatory process; these are caused by local inflammation and are mostly unilateral. In the second group, the ophthalmoscope shows the same lesions but besides this there is a prominence of the papilli characteristics of edema or stasis due to intracranial causes of a mechanical order; this group is bilateral. These two groups of optic neuritis still further differentiate themselves when we observe the effects of lumbar puncture; the papillitis of the neuritis of the first group are not at all or only slightly benefitted but it is of high value in the forms of stasis resulting from inter-cranial causes.

In the neuritis due to infections or other causes, the results of puncture are variable. This neuritis may occur as a complication in a number of infectious diseases, the eruptive fevers and certain intoxications such as lead and carbon dioxide, etc., and may be a simple optic neuritis or neuro-retinitis. In these, puncture can have only diagnostic interest and exert no therapeutic influence whatever on the local process. In the optic neuritis of syphilis, a most frequent variety, puncture gives no results, except there exists at the same time a meningeal reaction with a lymphocytosis and excess of the cerebro-spinal fluid. Moissonier[104], reports a case of post scarlatinous optic neuritis, cured by puncture and Morax[105], advises puncture in cases of bilateral infectious forms, for in these there is frequently a concommitant meningeal process.

On the other hand, in the optic neuritis of intracranial origin, puncture is often of great value; multiple causes produce this variety and according to the particular etiology, puncture has different therapeutic value. We cannot here go into full details of the entire etiology and discuss the pathogenesis and must be content to recall that papillary stasis is most frequently observed in tumor cases and sometimes in abscess. It may complicate fractures and grave cranial traumatisms, and if there be intracranial hemorrhage, papillary stasis may be present. We do not mean by this the unilateral stasis which occurs in severe, penetrating injuries of the orbit, such as in gun shot wounds. It may also occur in any of the meningites, acute, syphilitic or tubercular; or the serous form or in hydrocephalus. In all such cases, puncture is valuable and acts in two ways, first by relieving the pressure and secondly by the drainage of the infectious or toxic fluid. (Abadie[106], Dainoux[107]).

This operation has long been practised by many, against the edema of the papilli due to cerebral tumor, but the results are variable and only palliative. If the symptoms are mild, an improvement in the acuteness and an enlargement of the vision may occur; sometimes this is noticed even while the operation is in progress or it may not be observed until the next day or the day after, but the amblyopia after a time returns and the operation must be repeated. In cases of long standing and with marked symptoms, and more or less blindness, the efficacy of evacuating some of the cerebro-spinal fluid is still more uncertain, (Cabannes[108]), and if any amelioration at all occurs, it is very transitory and all the symptoms of compression soon return, with all, if not greater severity.

In the treatment of papillitis due to tumor, puncture has therefore only relative value; it may even be dangerous, as has before been mentioned; it is only a palliative measure and should not be used too long and trephining, which alone has a chance as a curative measure, should not be too long delayed. (von Hippel[109]).

The value of puncture is much greater in the papillitis of intracranial origin, not due to tumor and gives its best results in the stasis which follows grave traumatisms of the skull, particularly in fractures at the base. In these it constitutes an efficient mode of treatment, unless the symptomatology and localization imperatively dictate trephining. It may be followed by rapid and durable amelioration but may require to be repeated several times; the functional symptoms are the first to improve, then little by little the papilli become less engorged, the veins less dilated and exudates and hemorrhages become absorbed. Chaillous[110] reports a case of intense papillary stasis of long standing, in which a cure was effected by puncture; but such results must not be expected if atrophy of the papilli has already begun.

Optic neuritis, while comparatively rare in cerebro-spinal meningitis, is quite frequent in the tubercular form. The results of evacuation of spinal fluid have been generally good and Galezowski[111] reports a cure in a case of edema of the papilli, with marked visual disturbances, occurring in the course of a cerebro-spinal meningitis, but the prognosis in these cases must always be guarded, for as Terrien[112] has pointed out that the post-meningitic optic neuritis are exceptionally grave and very rebellious to treatment. In the tubercular type, the immediate results are prompt, but from the etiology we must realize that they are but transitory and the operation may have to be oft repeated. In the double papillary edema which occurs in the chronic syphilitic meningitis and in basilar meningitis, puncture gives excellent results. The edema, the cystological reaction of the fluid and its increase in albumen are often the very first signs of a meningitis; here puncture brings relief to the meningeal symptoms and those of high tension, while the amblyopia rapidly mends after one or two punctures and the lesions of the fundus of the eye recede; of course only in conjunction with the specific treatment.

The serous meningitis, irrespective of its pathogenesis, can by hypertension, which is their chief characteristic, cause edema of the papilli and in such cases the effects of puncture are remarkable; but the repetition of the evacuation until all signs of the disease process has disappeared, is imperative. Under this head must be considered the case reported by Widal[113]; that of sudden bilateral amaurosis with papillary stasis during typhoid fever; the edema was typical, with dilatation of the veins, but no hemorrhage; the liquid was under pressure, clear and without cytological elements; two punctures sufficed to bring about a cure.

In the optic neuritis of hydrocephalus, puncture is justified; in cases where the edema is of long standing, it will have no effect; but if the edema occurs while the hydrocephalus is in evolution, we may hope, in a large measure to diminish it. Babinski and Chaillous report a case of hydrocephalus with a bilateral neuritis of 8 months' standing in which, by puncture a cure was obtained and caused the disappearance of functional and ophthalmological signs.

Finally in sunstroke, edema of the papilli, which, with the headache may continue for a very long period, puncture brings rapid relief and is in fact the only treatment that so far has availed for this condition.

We will say only one word about atrophy of the nerve; here all hope in puncture is illusory.

The therapeutic value of puncture in edema of the papilli may be summed up as being depending upon the exact nature of the cause of the edema and as these are very variable, so naturally must be the results of this operation.

(b) Affections of the globe of the eye.— In the different affections of the membranes of the globe of the eye (choroiditis, retinitis, etc.) puncture has a diagnostic value only, but it is indicated if there is any suspicion of syphilis, for we must always bear in mind the possibility of a participation of the meninges in this disease and then puncture may bring relief to the headache.

(c) Motor disturbances of the eye.— Among the troubles of motility of the eye, we must distinguish between those due to nystagmus and those due to paralysis properly so-called. In congenital nystagmus, which is most frequently of ocular origin, puncture is of no value. In the acquired nystagmus due to cerebellar or cerebro-spinal lesion, the results are nil; but on the other hand, puncture may yield valuable results in nystagmus due to labyrinthian disease, for these belong to the reflex group. In these the essential element of the syndrome is hypertension and irritation of the labyrinth and this makes the mechanism of this therapeutics easily comprehensible. In oculo-motor paralysis dependent upon a concomitant meningeal process and this is by far most frequently the case; from what has been said before, we can understand that this operation may prove of real value. There can be no doubt or discussion about the value of this procedure in any condition referable to pressure due to an increase of the cerebro-spinal fluid; but we must place no hope in it, in conditions that are due to changes in the nerve proper, no matter what be their etiology.

(d) Glaucoma.—At the present time there is no record of a systematic application of puncture in primitive glaucoma, but it seems logical to expect some benefits from it in this condition. If we accept the conclusions of Vacquez[114] that the hypertension of the cerebro-spinal fluid is intermediary between the generally high blood pressure and the intraocular pressure, in this light then puncture becomes a logical procedure. Furthermore we

must remember that glaucoma usually occurs in those of advanced age and in arterio-sclerotics, and that high pressure is very common in both of these conditions. Besides these patients often present cutaneous troubles, Terson[115], such as urticaria, acute erythemas and other dermatosis; the effect of puncture on cutaneous conditions will be discussed under their proper heading. It is very possible that by acting upon the pressure of the cerebro-spinal fluid, we may influence certain forms of glaucoma.

(e) Amblyopias without lesion of the fundus of the eye.—It is particularly interesting to study the effects of puncture in these conditions. There exists a variety of amblyopias without apparent material lesions, in which the ophthalmoscope does not even reveal any edema of the papilli and which seem to be due solely to hypertension of the cerebro-spinal fluid. These appear in patients having high arterial pressure and also present a further complex clinical picture. Often these patients are arterio-sclerotics, with headache, vertigo, pruritus, and complain of loss of memory, cloudiness of intellect and a slow, progressive failure of vision, (Ravaut[116]). They sometimes present veritable crisis of hypertension, with violent headaches, attacks of pulmonary edema and troubles of vision; still the ophthalmoscope reveals nothing and there is no change in the tension of the eye balls. In such cases, puncture will do much good. The fluid is found to be under high tension, but clear, without cytological elements and containing no albumen. A puncture, with the withdrawal of from 10 to 25 cc. varying according to the case, brings marked improvement of all the symptoms, especially of the vision. An examination of the acuity of vision by test types shows the improvement; if this improvement takes place but slowly, two or three punctures may be required. The improvement will continue for a time and last from three to six months, after which time another puncture or series of punctures may be necessary.

The arterial tension, if high, as we have said, is promptly lowered; if it rises again, which it sometimes does, it is accompanied by the reappearance of the clinical symptoms.

AURICULAR DISEASES.

(a) Complication of Otitis.—There exists a certain number of clinical manifestations in diseases of the ear, which, while their primitive causes are lesions of the ear proper, they really are only complications. Of this nature are the infections resulting from otitis media, extending to the meninges and the brain and so causing acute purulent meningitis, cerebellar abscesses, or phlebitis of the sinus. Puncture has been practised in a large number of such cases. What was said under the head of meningitis and brain abscess applies here. Whatever good may be accomplished, is only by its effect upon the concomitant meningitis; (Chevasse and Mahn[117]), the sinus phlebitis is in no way affected, but there may be an aseptic or serous meningitis, (Rist[118]), in middle ear disease, and upon this, puncture will have a favorable influence. (Legue et Lapointe [119]).

(b) Auricular affections proper.— Babinski[120] was the first to draw attention to the therapeutic value of puncture in these. The symptoms against which it may be employed are the functional ones, and these are encountered in very diverse cases. They may depend upon chronic middle ear lesions, such as catarrh, sclerosis of the drum, ankylosis of the small bones, causing profound disturbances of auditive transmission and impression; again, there may be labyrinthian changes, which, whatever be their cause, their determination properly belongs in the sphere of the specialist. Clinically these patients present a more or less rich symptomatology; noises and ringing in the ears, loss of hearing, vertigo, typical of the condition, either labyrinthian or of Meniere type. The determination of the type of vertigo is of the first importance. Babinski[121], Meniere[123], Lumineau[122], all agree upon the relief obtained by lumbar puncture. In some cases they have obtained results that approach a cure. Weil's[124] case shows its value in the auricular vertigo accompanying chronic pharangitis and tubotympanic catarrh. Weil and Barre[125] report a case of ringing and whistling in the ears, sensation of falling, vertigo and amblyopia, which was perfectly cured by rachicentesis. Lermoyes[126] denies that puncture has any value whatever in cases of vertigo. Mollard[127] in a rather exhaustive study concludes as follows: "that it has an elective action on the ampullar system and that it represents the only therapeutics applicable to labyrinthian manifestations. The first results are upon the vertigo, and this is the only effect observable in advanced chronic labyrinthitis; but when the lesions are less complete and not of too long duration, a general improvement may occur. Several punctures of from 10 to 15cc., at intervals from 15 to 20 days, may be necessary to obtain lasting results and while the cure is not definite, still may last from 3 to 6 months, even a year and more."

Puncture may also be utilized in ear conditions dependent upon intra-labyrinthian hypertension, without lesions of the ear proper. The various methods of examination fail to reveal any lesions; still the patient complains of ringing of the ears, loss of hearing and nystagmus. Compression is the only explanation for such a symptomatology; the nystagmus is of the reflex mechanical order. Lemathee and Halpher[128]. Here the evacuation of cerebro-spinal fluid, by relieving the pressure, brings relief. Gastinel reports a case of this type; there existed the complete syndrome of hypertension, auricular and ocular. Two punctures brought about prompt relief for six months when all the symptoms returned and necessitated two further punctures. It may be well to note that there existed an accompanying high arterial tension which was decidedly lowered by each intervention. This is not a surprising fact, since there exists a close relation between the labyrinthian, cerebrospinal and arterial tensions. Laffite, Dupont and Maupetit[129] have studied this question and come to the conclusion that an augmentation of the labyrinthian and cerebro-spinal tension causes an increase of the general arterial tension and that a relief of the cerebro-spinal tension brings about a lesser arterial and labyrinthian tension.

CUTANEOUS CONDITIONS. ARTERIAL HYPERTENSION.

The peripheral nervous system and the vaso-motor apparatus may be influenced by puncture in certain cases. Here the action is not directly due to the withdrawal of toxi-infectious products or the relief of tension, but through a series of intermediaries is realized at a distance. This is the only explanation possible for the results obtained by lumbar puncture in certain cutaneous affections.

(a) Cutaneous affections.— Ravout with Thibierge[130/131] studied the curious and unexpected effect of this operation in the lichen of Wilson, lichen planus, in which the incessant pruritus disappeared completely. This discovery led to its employ in other prurigenous affections. This symptom is frequently benefitted by puncture but it is in the lichen planus that it is most manifest. After an evacuation of 6 or 8 cc. there is an amelioration, frequently even entire disappearance. Since then Ravout[132] has punctured many such cases and always with the same results. With the relief of the pruritus there is also an improvement of the local condition for this is no longer aggravated and infected by the scratching of the sufferer. In circumscribed lichen it also acts well but less so than in the planus variety. In other pruriginous dermatosis, according to Thieberge[133] its action is uncertain. The pruritus in a case of psoriasis was much relieved and the local lesions improved. The pruritus of diathesic origin in one case of six months' standing and in another case of one year's standing were completely relieved by one puncture in the first case and two punctures in the second case. In several cases of pruritus of eczema, improvements were noticed. One was a case of ano-vulvar pruritus with slight eczema. While the effects of puncture have been studied in a variety of other cutaneous conditions, the results in none have been as constantly good as in lichen planus and in this affection the best results are obtained when it is used early. The longer the existence of the trouble, the less definite and permanent are the results.

December, 1912.
New Series, Vol. VII., No. 12. }   THE ANNOTATOR   { American Medicine
Complete Series, Vol. XVIII.   703

While it is hard to determine exactly, all the cutaneous affections in which puncture will prove of use, it may legitimately be tried in any case of rebellious pruritus which resists all other therapesis. It may be well here to report the case of a woman, suffering from a moist eczema, which was very pruritic; she had marked amblyopia which prevented her from going about by herself; by one puncture her pruritus was completely calmed, her arterial tension lowered and her vision much improved as well as her dermatosis. After a time the symptoms returned and were again relieved by puncture.

These facts are of real interest since they seem to prove that this operation may have a very decided influence on the vaso-motor apparatus. It seems that the vascular system is influenced by the tension of the cerebro-spinal fluid. Attention has already been drawn to the effect upon the local lesions, but these are entirely transitory.

(b) Arterial hypertension.— The intimate relation between the tension of the cerebro-spinal fluid and the arterial tension has been mentioned; but all the facts concerning this are not known, Maupetit [134], and more work is still to be done along this line. That lumbar puncture does more than simply affect the vaso-motors of the custaneous system is certain. The proof of this lies in the fall of the arterial tension seen after it. This is most manifest in cases that at the time of the operation presented a high arterial tension and much less noticeable in cases where this is normal.

Parisot [135] has studied this question in diseases of the nervous system and found that the flow of spinal fluid when prolonged until its tension became normal or even subnormal, caused a lowering of the arterial pressure to the normal and this was sometimes attended or followed an acceleration of the pulse. These findings of Parisot have been confirmed by others; Babinovitsch and Prillard [136]. The effect is transitory and further study along this line is necessary before definite conclusions are permissible.

(Note.—This article is to be reprinted in book form, as it is the latest and most authentic consideration of lumbar puncture in any language. Lack of space makes it impossible to give the voluminous bibliography in our journal pages, but it will appear in the bound book).

THE ANNOTATOR.

Pedagogy and Medicine.[1]— An editorial remarks the increasing frankness with which the medical profession deals with the public in matters of sanitation, hygiene and prophylaxis, and it appeals, often convincingly, to the adult who has predilections and prejudices to be overcome, and vicious habits to be eradicated. Its task is difficult compared with that of public school teachers whose pupils are in the plastic stage, are subject to discipline, are seeking instruction and are good material for the propagation of sound sanitary and hygienic ideas.

But in order to inculcate such ideas the teacher must have adequate knowledge of sanitary laws and their consequences and hence there must come closer cooperation between such teachers and medical school inspectors.

It has recently been discovered that in only a few of our higher institutions is there any co-ordination between the schools of pedagogy and those of medicine, and inasmuch as many children who are deficient mentally owe their deficiency to their imperfect physical condition the importance of the training of teachers along physiological lines becomes only too obvious.

It has also been pointed out that many medical inspectors of schools are deficient

[1] New York Medical Journal, November 30, 1912.

in their knowledge of the pedagogic problems by means of which their medical ideas are to be enforced.

These facts emphasize the necessity of the correlation of the functions of the teacher and the medical school inspector, and the great improvement which has resulted both physically and mentally to multitudes of school children since medical inspection became a part of the school curriculum only inspire faith and confidence that still greater benefits are about to come in the near future.

Life Insurance of the Future.[1]—
G. W. Hopkins thinks that corruption, fraud, injustice and instability will be impossible in the life insurance of the future, but that it will not be government insurance.

The majority of men buy protection of this kind for their families only after being urgently solicited and this is not usually characteristic of government officials. The companies will be mutual, mutualized by legislation. They will maintain the full legal reserve on all policies, invested in solid, non-fluctuating securities.

Cash surrender values will be forbidden on new business, there will be no necessity to invest in fluctuating stocks and bonds, and policyholders' money will not be used to make or break prosperity, to influence legislation, or to injure policyholders and the country.

The surplus will be governed by law and the method of acquiring it will be equitable. Investment insurance will be abolished, the policyholder will know how much he is contributing for expenses each year, and the state will see that none of the money is squandered.

Expense charges will be uniform, not twice as much to a man of 50 as to one of 30.

Commissions paid will be as large for young men as for old men, for young men must contribute as much for expenses as the older ones since the management expense is the same in each case.

The policy of the future will pledge to return to the policyholder a definite percentage of the previous year's overcharge,

the balance to go to the surplus until the latter equals ten per cent of the reserve.

If a policyholder is defrauded he will be in a position to demand a receiver for the company.

The mutual companies of the future will be financed by small loans from many policyholders who will always conserve the policyholders' interests. The policyholders will have the privilege annually of electing disinterested actuaries to audit the companies' accounts and report directly to the policyholders in plain language. When these reforms have been obtained life insurance will be reduced to the lowest cost and the highest stability.

The Sanitary Control of Local Milk Supplies through Local Official Agencies.[1]—E. J. Lederle refers to the great importance to cities in general of the entire control of their milk supply.

New York is a conspicuous example of a city which exercises such control, from the cow to the consumer.

This includes the inspection of 45,000 farms of which 6,000 are outside of the state. Its control is based upon the sanitary code with supplemental rules and regulations, and with which no other department of the municipal government may interfere.

With regard to milk for infants the code requires that it must have proper nutritive value, and that it must be clean. The code recognizes infection of milk from tuberculosis, typhoid and scarlet fevers, diphtheria and tonsilitis.

Bovine tuberculosis may be transmitted by milk to children, while milk which contains the germs of the other diseases above mentioned is dangerous to persons of all ages. The importance of "carriers" of these diseases has been fully demonstrated. The problem of safe milk requires the following conditions:

(1) The prevention of adulteration by water or by the removal of fats, and the exclusion of all foreign substances.

(2) The production of milk, low in bacteria, involving the greatest cleanliness of everything which has any relation to it, from the time of its drawing to its con-

---

[1] *Medical Review of Reviews*, November, 1912.　　　[1] *American Practitioner*, October.

sumption. It also concerns the proper reduction of its temperature after it has been drawn.

(3) Freedom from pathogenic organisms, which means healthy animals and careful handling of the milk to prevent the entrance of infectious germs, flies and dust.

Inspections of dairies and creameries are elements of public control and should provide for the detection of contagious disease among those who handle the milk as well as the improvement of sanitary conditions. It should provide further for the inspection of stores and wagons for frequent chemical and bacteriological tests, and for resort to the courts when necessary. The magnitude of this task for New York city may be realized when it is stated that the daily milk supply is 2,500,000 quarts which comes from seven different states and from Canada, the longest haul being 425 miles.

It is dispensed at 14,000 stores while 127,000 persons are daily engaged in handling it. The method of dairy inspection was commenced in 1904 and there are now 56 milk inspectors, half of whom are engaged in the country, while the others inspect stores, wagons, etc., in the city. The code requires that no milk shall be sold in the city without a permit from the board of health. This necessitates the tracing of the milk to its source at the dairy or creamery. If permission to inspect these is refused the permit to sell the milk from such sources is revoked.

The question of authority over the production of milk from other states was settled by the supreme court of the United States which decided that such control was reasonable, valid, and not unconstitutional. The great need in a general milk supply suitable for people of all ages is a safe milk which can be furnished at a price within the means of the masses. No matter how complete or well-organized the system of dairy inspection it will not be possible to make ordinary commercial milk entirely safe when it is produced and shipped to a city from so large a territory as is comprised in the New York milk field. The only way in which sanitary authorities can meet these conditions is by requiring the pasteurization of all milk which is not of special exempted grades.

In New York the following plan of grading and labeling all milk was officially adopted in January, 1912:

Grade A for infants and children consists of (1) certified milk, (2) guaranteed milk, (3) raw inspected milk, (4) selected pasteurized milk.

Grade B for adults consists of (1) raw selected milk, (2) pasteurized milk.

Grade C includes that which is used only for manufacturing and cooking purposes. By this plan a farmer will know what grade he is producing and how he can improve the situation. Thus he will have an incentive to produce milk of the best quality.

Grading and labeling regulations will also furnish encouragement to honest dealers who are thus aided by official control. It is believed that no permanent reform in the sale of store milk can take place until there are milk stores in which no other commodities are sold. Under the administration of the board of health there are now 55 municipal stations for dispensing milk for babies, and there are also many similar private milk stations. The author believes that the ultimate solution of the infants' milk problem will consist in the production of special grades of milk suitable for infant feeding, and the placing of it in milk stores or with dealers where it may be obtained by mothers at reasonable prices. The municipal and other milk stations may then serve as centers for the education of mothers in the care and feeding of babies and in the care of milk in the home.

Senility and Its Management.[1]—McCorkle reminds us that many old people sleep more than they think they do while others sleep less than we think they do. The want of sleep in the decadent is a menace to comfort, well-being, and life. Pure air is a tonic to the aged but the bed should be warm.

A little alcohol in the form of hot toddy is a fine hypnotic for the aged and it is sometimes well to add to it a small quantity of chloral amide.

The senile heart calls for the most watchful care. It is usually accompanied with

[1] *Therapeutic Gazette*, October 15, 1912.

sclerosed arteries but not always with high tension. Digitalis is the drug par excellence, in the form of a tincture free from fat for such cases, but in small doses once a day, combined with potassium iodide or crythrol ternitrate. Opium in small doses is also a solace and comfort for the aged and infirm.

When given in such doses it is both a heart tonic and a gentle cerebral stimulant. The best results are obtained when it is given in the form of the gum. More and more the aged are receiving attention which will promote their comfort and their hopefulness. It is high time that this should be so.

The Health of School Children.[1]— An editorial writer thinks it is well to appreciate the fact that school children are not necessarily well children.

T. D. Wood gives the following statistics for the 20 million pupils in the schools of the united States.

a. Four hundred thousand have organic heart disease.

b. One million have or have had tuberculous disease of the lungs.

c. One million have spinal curvature, flat foot or some other deformity which interferes with health.

d. One million have defective hearing.

e. Five million have defective vision.

f. Five million suffer from malnutrition, which is due, in part at least, to one or more of the defects above enumerated.

g. Six million have enlarged tonsils, adenoids, or enlarged cervical glands which require surgical attention.

h. Ten million (and in some schools as many as 98 per cent) have defective teeth, which interfere with health.

Several millions of the before-mentioned have, each, two or more of these defects.

i. Fifteen million need attention for physical defects which are injuring their health and which are partly or completely remediable.

These figures mean that there should be more definite standards of school hygiene as to school construction, school furniture and the medical inspection of school children. Physical education should receive much more attention than it has. There should be adequate play grounds, special classes for defectives and cripples, open air schools, dental and medical clinics wherever there are children who require them.

Medical inspectors and school nurses should be selected with an eye only to their fitness for the task and the children and their parents should be educated in the matter of preventing and overcoming harmful physical conditions. Home and school should cooperate to obtain healthful physical conditions. These figures are startling in their significance. They demonstrate as nothing else can the possibilities of the next generation of American citizens unless this morbidity in the children can be overcome.

They also prove incidentally the great importance which attaches to the right kind of medical school inspection and the need for the right kind of inspectors.

A Practical Method of Prophylactic Immunization against Tuberculosis.[1]—H. J. Achard recounts the experience of Dr. Karl Von Ruck who has been studying the problem of prophylactic immunization against tuberculosis for more than eight years and who has never lost sight of this idea in his experiences with the employment of curative products of the tubercle bacillus.

His experience long ago convinced him that a sufficient degree of specific immunity could be conferred upon the non-tuberculous but predisposed subject to prevent possible harm from prolonged exposure to infection even amid favorable conditions of living which would diminish the power of resistance to the infection.

He succeeded in preparing a mixture of different proteid extractives, to which a minute quantity of fatty acid was added, with which he prevented the development of tuberculosis in guinea pigs, after having inoculated them with virulent tubercle bacilli which produced fatal general tuberculosis in control animals.

Dr. Von Ruck immunized 339 children, most of whom were inmates of an orphan asylum in Thomasville, N. C.

[1] *Medical Review of Reviews*, November, 1912.

[1] *American Journal of Clinical Medicine*, June.

Of this number 94 were suspected of being tuberculous, 85 were normal, 160 had signs of early tuberculosis in the lungs. The immunity of these children to tuberculosis infection was estimated by their blood alkalinity, by the serum agglutination of tubercle bacilli in a test tube, and by the complement fixation.

General improvement was noted in the immunized tuberculous children in from three to eight months.

There was very marked increase in weight, and in many cases enlarged lymph glands diminished in size.

The physical signs of tuberculosis in the lungs disappeared or nearly so.

An important observation was that the blood serum of immunized children would dissolve tubercle bacilli mixed with serum in a test tube and kept at blood temperature. The results which have been obtained are believed to be very significant and far reaching.

BOOKS OF THE YEAR.
1912.

Following our usual custom, we present herewith our annual list of books published during the current year. While this list does not include every book issued during 1912, it will be found fairly complete and comprehensive. Lack of space has prevented any discussion or statement relative to the merits of any book listed, but sufficient information has been given in every instance to enable the reader to learn the scope and source of each work. We trust that this list will prove as valuable for all reference purposes as those that have preceded it each year.

ANATOMY AND PHYSIOLOGY.
(Including Embryology, Etc.)

Practical Anatomy.—An exposition of the facts of Gross Anatomy from the topographical standpoint and a guide to the Direction of the Human Body.—By John C. Heisler, M. D., Professor of Anatomy in the Medico-Chirurgical College of Philadelphia. J. B. Lippincott Co., Philadelphia. Octavo 750 pages. 383 illustrations. Cloth, $5.00.

Manual of Practical Anatomy.—By D. J. Cunningham, M. D., D. S. C., LL. D., F. R. S., late Professor of Anatomy in the University of Edinburgh. *Fifth Edition.* Edited by Arthur Robinson, Professor of Anatomy in the University of Edinburgh, two volumes. 12mo, containing 1,321 pages, with 510 illustrations in black and colors. Flexible muslin binding, complete, $5.00. Wm. Wood & Co., New York.

Post-Mortems and Morbid Anatomy.—By Theodore Shennan, M. D., F. R. C. P., Edin.; Pathologist to the Royal Infirmary, Edinburgh; Lecturer on Pathology and Bacteriology in the College of Medicine of the Royal College Surgeons' Hall, Edinburgh, &c., &c. Large octavo, profusely illustrated by over 200 half-tones from original photographs. Muslin, $5.50 net. Wm. Wood & Co., New York.

The Comparative Anatomy of Vertebrates.—By J. S. Kingsley, Professor of Biology in Tufts College, Massachusetts. With 346 illustrations. Octavo. 410 pages. Cloth, $2.25 postpaid. P. Blakiston's Son & Co., 1012 Walnut St., Philadelphia, Publishers.

The Growth of Bone, Observations on Osteogenesis, An Experimental Inquiry into the Development and Reproduction of Diaphyseal Bone.—By William MacEwen, F. R. S., Regius Professor of Surgery in the University of Glasgow. Cloth, illustrated with 61 full-page halftones. Price, $3.75 net. (The Macmillan Company).

Human Embryology.—Written by Charles R. Bardeen, Madison, Wis.; Herbert M. Evans, Baltimore, Md.; Walter Felix, Zurich; Otto Grosser, Prague; Franz Keibel, Frieburg i. Br.; Frederic T. Lewis, Boston, Mass.; Warren H. Lewis, Baltimore, Md.; J. Playfair McMurrich, Toronto; Franklin P. Mall, Baltimore, Md.; Charles S. Minot, Boston, Mass.; Felix Pinkus, Berlin; Florence R. Sabin, Baltimore, Md.; George L. Streeter, Ann Arbor, Mich.; Julius Tandler, Vienna; Emil Zuckerkandl, Vienna. Edited by Franz Keibel, Professor in the University, Freiburg i. Br., and Franklin P. Mall, Professor of Anatomy in the Johns Hopkins University, Baltimore, U. S. A. J. B. Lippincott Company, Philadelphia. Imperial Octavo. Two volumes—$20.00 per set. Volume I, 548 pages, 423 illustrations. Volume II, 1,040 pages, 658 illustrations.

Aids to Histology (Students Aids Series).—By Alexander Goodall, M. D., F. R. C. P., Edin. 16mo, 135 pages, illustrated. Flexible muslin, $1.00 net. Wm. Wood & Co., New York.

Histology.—By George A. Piersol, M. D., Professor of Anatomy, University of Pennsylvania. *Ninth Edition.* J. B. Lippincott Co., Philadelphia. Octavo, 418 pages, 438 illustrations, many in colors. Cloth, $3.50. This edition entirely rewritten, reset, and reillustrated.

Manual of Human Osteology.—By A. Francis Dixon, M. B., Sc. D., Professor of Anatomy and Surgery, Trinity College, Dublin. 12 mo, 328 pages. Illustrated by 178 cuts, many in colors. Flexible waterproof muslin, $3.00 net. Wm. Wood & Co., New York.

Landmarks and Surface Markings of the Human Body.—By L. Bathe Rawling. Cloth. *Fifth Edition.* 96 pages, 31 illustrations. 1912. Paul B. Hoeber, New York. $2.00 net.

Malformations. A Clinical Manual of the Malformations and Congenital Diseases of the

Fetus.—By Professor R. Birnbaum, Physician-in-Chief to the Clinic for Women in the Royal University of Gottingen. Translated and Annotated by George Blacker, M. D., B. S., F. R. C. P., F. R. C. S., Obstetric Physician to the University College Hospital, London. With 8 plates and 58 other illustrations. Octavo. Cloth, $5.00 postpaid. P. Blakiston's Son & Co., 1012 Walnut Street, Philadelphia, Publishers.

Nutritional Physiology.—By Percy G. Stiles, Assistant Professor of Physiology in Simmons College; Instructor in Physiology and Personal Hygiene in the Massachusetts Institute of Technology, Boston. 12 mo of 271 pages, illustrated. Philadelphia and London: W. B. Saunders Company, 1912. Cloth, $1.25 net.

Outlines of Physiology.—By Edward Groves Jones, A. B., M. D., Professor of Surgery, Atlanta School of Medicine, and Allen H. Bunce, A. B., M. D., Associate Professor of Physiology, Atlanta School of Medicine. *Third Edition.* Thoroughly revised. 12mo, 111 illustrations, 372 pages. Cloth, $1.50 postpaid. P. Blakiston's Son & Co., 1012 Walnut St., Philadelphia, Publishers.

The Principles of Human Physiology.—By Ernest Henry Starling, M. D. (Lond.), F. R. C. P., F. R. S., Jodrell Professor of Physiology in University College, London. Octavo, 1,423 pages, with 564 illustrations, some in colors. Cloth, $5.00 net. Lea & Febiger, Philadelphia and New York.

A Text-Book of Human Physiology, Including a Section on Physiological Apparatus.—By Albert P. Brubaker, A. M., M. D., Professor of Medical Jurisprudence and Physiology in the Jefferson Medical College, Philadelphia. *Fourth Edition.* Revised and enlarged. With 1 colored plate and 377 other illustrations. Cloth, $3.00 postpaid. P. Blakiston's Son & Co., 1012 Walnut Street, Philadelphia, Publishers.

A Compend of Human Physiology.—By Albert P. Brubaker, A. M., M. D., Professor of Physiology and Medical Jurisprudence, Jefferson Medical College, Philadelphia, etc. *Thirteenth Edition.* Revised. 12mo, 256 pages, illustrated. Cloth, $1.00 postpaid. P. Blakiston's Son & Co., 1012 Walnut St., Philadelphia, Publishers.

Manual of Practical Physiology.—By John C. Hemmeter, M. D., Ph. D., Professor of Physiology, University of Maryland, Baltimore. With 55 illustrations. Octavo. Cloth, $2.50 postpaid. P. Blakiston's Son & Co., 1012 Walnut St., Philadelphia, Publishers.

CHEMISTRY (Analysis, Etc.)

Commercial Organic Analysis.—Volume 6, *Fourth Edition.* Organic Bases, Vegetable Alkaloids, Tobacco, Cocaine, Opium, Tea and Coffee, Cocoa and Chocolate, etc. Octavo, 735 pages. Cloth, $5.00 postpaid. P. Blakiston's Son & Co., 1012 Walnut St., Philadelphia, Publishers.

The Analyst's Laboratory Companion. A Collection of Tables and Data for the use of Analysts, Agricultural, Brewers, and Industrial Chemists. Including a number of Examples of Chemical Calculations and Descriptions of Analytical Processes. *Fourth Edition.*—By Alfred E. Johnson, B. Sc. (Lond.), F. I. C., A. R. C., Sc. I. 12mo. Cloth, $2.00 postpaid. P. Blakiston's Son & Co., 1012 Walnut St., Philadelphia, Publishers.

Methods for Sugar Analysis and Allied Determinations. A Concise and Valuable Book of Laboratory Methods.—By A. Given, formerly Chemist in the Sugar Laboratory, U. S. Dept. of Agriculture, etc. Illustrations. Octavo. Cloth, $2.00 postpaid. P. Blakiston's Son & Co., 1012 Walnut St., Philadelphia, Publishers.

Volumetric Analysis for Students of Pharmaceutical and General Chemistry. — By Charles H. Hampshire, B. Sc. (Lond.), A. I. C., Demonstrator in Chemistry at the School of the London Pharmaceutical Society. 12mo. Cloth, $1.25 postpaid. P. Blakiston's Son & Co., 1012 Walnut St., Philadelphia, Publishers.

A Manual of Chemistry. A Guide to Lecturers and Laboratory Work for Beginners in Chemistry. A Text-Book Specially Adapted for Students of Medicine and Pharmacy.—By W. Simon, Ph. D., M. D., Professor of Chemistry, College of Physicians and Surgeons, Baltimore, and Daniel Base, Ph. D., Professor of Chemistry in the Maryland College of Pharmacy and in the Medical Department of the University of Maryland. *New (Tenth) Edition,* thoroughly revised. Octavo, 774 pages, with 82 engravings and 9 colored plates of spectra and chemical reactions. Cloth, $3.00 net. Lea & Febiger, Philadelphia and New York.

A Manual of Clinical Chemistry, Microscopy and Bacteriology.—By Dr. M. Klopstock and Dr. A. Kowarsky, Berlin. This is a new edition brought up to date. The chapter relating to Typhoid Fever and to the Meningococci have been rewritten, and those dealing with the Spirocheta pallida and with the Wassermann Reaction are entirely new. $3.00. Rebman Co., New York.

General and Industrial Inorganic Chemistry. —By Ettore Molinari, Professor of Industrial Chemistry to the Society for the Encouragement of Arts and Manufactures and of Merceology at the Luigi Bocconi Commercial University, Milan. Translated by E. Feilmann, B. Sc., Ph. D. (Lond.) With 3 plates and 280 text illustrations. From the *Third Italian Edition,* carefully revised and brought up to date. Octavo, 720 pages. Cloth, $6.00 postpaid. P. Blakiston's Son & Co., 1012 Walnut St., Philadelphia, Publishers.

Public Health Chemistry and Bacteriology. A Handbook for D. P. H. Students.—By David McKail, M. D., D. P. H., &c., Lecturer of Public Health and Forensic Medicine, St. Mongo's College, Glasgow; Lecturer on Hygiene to Nurses, Glasgow Royal Infirmary, etc. Small octavo, 416 pages. Muslin, $2.50 net. Wm. Wood & Co., New York.

Practical Physiological Chemistry.—By Phillip B. Hawk, M. S., Ph. D., Professor of Physiological Chemistry and Toxicology in the Jefferson Medical College, Philadelphia. *Fourth Edition.* Revised and enlarged. With 6 colored plates and 137 other illustrations (12 in colors). Octavo, 495 pages. Cloth, $2.50 postpaid. P. Blakiston's Son & Co., 1012 Walnut St., Philadelphia, Publishers.

Digestion and Metabolism. The Physiological and Pathological Chemistry of Nutrition. For Students and Physicians.—By Alonzo Englebert Taylor, M. D., Rush Professor of Physiological Chemistry, University of Pennsylvania, Philadelphia. Octavo, 560 pages. Cloth, $3.75 net. Lea & Febiger, Philadelphia and New York.

The Preparation of Organic Compounds.—By E. De Barry Barnett, B. Sc. (Lond.), A. I. C. With 50 illustrations. Small octavo. Cloth, $2.75 postpaid. P. Blakiston's Son & Co., 1012 Walnut St., Philadelphia, Publishers.

DIAGNOSIS (Methods, Symptomatology.)

A Manual of Auscultation and Percussion.—By Austin Flint, M. D., LL. D., Late Professor of Medicine and of Clinical Medicine in the Bellevue Hospital Medical College, etc., New York. Revised by Haven Emerson, A. M., M. D., of the College of Physicians and Surgeons, Columbia University, New York. 12mo, 361 pages, illustrated. Cloth, $2.00 net. Lea & Febiger, Philadelphia and New York.

The Blood. A Guide to its Examination, and to the Diagnosis and Treatment of its Diseases. —By G. Lovell Gulland, M. D., F. R. C. P. E., Physician to the Royal Infirmary and to the Royal Victoria Hospital for Consumption, and Alexander Goodall, M. D., F. R. C. P. E., Lecturer on Physiology and on Diseases of the Blood in the Edinburgh Post-Graduate Courses in Medicine. New York: E. B. Treat & Co., 251-3 West 23rd Street. Large 8vo, 360 pages, many illustrations and sixteen colored plates. Cloth, $5.00 net.

Bronchoscopy. (Direct Laryngoscopy, Bronchoscopy and Oesaphagoscopy).—By Dr. Brunings. Translated by W. G. Howarth, M. A., M. B., etc. Octavo, profusely illustrated by numerous cuts in the text and by 26 full-page plates. Muslin, $5.00 net. Wm. Wood & Co., New York.

Clinical Diagnosis. A Manual of Laboratory Methods.—By James Campbell Todd, M. D., Professor of Pathology, University of Colorado. *Second Edition.* Revised and enlarged. 12mo of 469 pages with 164 text illustrations and 13 colored plates. Philadelphia and London: W. B. Saunders Company, 1912. Cloth, $2.25 net.

Diagnostic Methods. Chemical, Microscopical, and Bacteriological.—By Ralph W. Webster, M. D., Ph. G., Asst. Professor of Pharmacologic Therapeutics, and Instructor in Medicine, Rush Medical College, Chicago. *Second Edition.* Revised and enlarged. With 37 colored plates and 164 other illustrations. Octavo, 717 pages. Cloth, $6.00 postpaid. P. Blakiston's Son & Co., 1012 Walnut St., Philadelphia, Publishers.

A Dictionary of Medical Diagnosis. A Treatise on the Signs and Symptoms Observed in Diseased Conditions. For the use of medical practitioners and students.—By Henry Lawrence McKisack, M. D., M. R. C. P., Physician to the Royal Victoria Hospital, Belfast. Octavo, 601 pages, illustrated by 76 engravings in black and color. Muslin, $4.25 net. *Second Revised Edition.* Wm. Wood & Co., New York.

Differential Diagnosis. Presented through an Analysis of 385 cases.—By Richard C. Cabot, M. D., Assistant Professor of Clinical Medicine, Harvard Medical School. *Second Edition.* Octavo of 764 pages, illustrated. Philadelphia and London: W. B. Saunders Company, 1912. Cloth, $5.50 net.

On Gastroscopy. With a Description of New, Easy and Efficient Method of Oesophago-Gastroscopy, Combining Direct and Indirect Vision, and a Plea for Its Employment by Gastric Experts.—By William Hill, B. Sc., M. D. Small octavo, illustrated by numerous cuts and plates. Muslin, $1.25 net. Wm. Wood & Co., New York.

An Index of Differential Diagnosis of Main Symptoms.—By various writers. Edited by Herbert French, M. A., M. D., F. R. C. P., Assistant Physician Guy's Hospital. Octavo, 1,029 pages. Beautifully illustrated by over 200 engravings in the text and by 16 full-page colored plates. Muslin, $8.00 net; half morocco, $9.00 net. Wm. Wood & Co., New York.

Physical Diagnosis.—By Richard C. Cabot, M. D., Assistant Professor of Medicine in Harvard University. *Fifth Edition.* Octavo, 529 pages, illustrated by five full-page plates, one in color, and by 268 engravings in the text. Muslin, $3.00 net. Wm. Wood & Co., New York.

Physical Diagnosis.—By John C. DaCosta, Jr., M. D., Assistant Professor of Clinical Medicine, Jefferson Medical College, Philadelphia. *Second Edition,* revised. Octavo of 557 pages, with 225 original illustrations. Philadelphia and London: W. B. Saunders Company, 1911. Cloth, $3.50 net.

Atlas of Kilian's Tracheo-Bronchoscopy.—By Sanitätsrat Dr. Mann. Colored Plates Representing Pathological Preparations from Cases Examined During Life by Means of Tracheo-Bronchoscopy. Extra Buckram, large folio, $7.50 net. Wm. Wood & Co., New York.

Serum Diagnosis of Syphilis and Luetin Reaction, Together with the Butyric Acid Test for Syphilis.—By Hideyo Noguchi, M. D., M. Sc., Associate Member of the Rockefeller Institute for Medical Research, New York. J. B. Lippincott Co., Philadelphia. Crown octavo, 304 pages, 23 illustrations, 17 in colors. Cloth, $3.00. *Third Edition.*

Symptoms and Their Interpretation.—By James Mackenzie. Cloth. *Second Edition.* 304 pages, 18 illustrations. 1912, Paul B. Hoeber, New York. $3.00 net.

EYE, EAR, NOSE AND THROAT.

Outlines of Applied Optics.—By P. G. Nutting, Bureau of Standards, Washington, D. C.

73 illustrations. Octavo. Cloth, $2.00 postpaid. P. Blakiston's Son & Co., 1012 Walnut St., Philadelphia, Publishers.

The Hunterian Lectures on Colour-Vision and Colour-Blindness.—By Professor F. W. Edridge-Green. Delivered before the Royal College of Surgeons of England on February 1st and 3rd, 1911. Cloth. 76 pages, illustrated. 1912, Paul B. Hoeber, New York. $1.50 net.

Diseases of the Eye.—By J. H. Parsons, M. D., Ophthalmic Surgeon, University College Hospital, London, etc. *Second Edition.* Revised and enlarged, with 18 colored plates and 309 other illustrations. Octavo, 691 pages. Cloth, $4.00 postpaid. P. Blakiston's Son & Co., 1012 Walnut St., Philadelphia, Publishers.

A Handbook of the Diseases of the Eye and Their Treatment.—By Sir Henry R. Swanzy, A. M., M. D., Sc. D., Surgeon to the Royal Victoria Eye and Ear Hospital, Dublin, etc., and Louis Werner, M. B., F. R. C. S. I., Professor of Ophthalmology, University College, Dublin. 9 colored plates and 230 text illustrations. Small octavo, 652 pages. Cloth, $4.00 postpaid. P. Blakiston's Son & Co., 1012 Walnut St., Philadelphia, Publishers.

A Practical Handbook of the Diseases of the Ear for Senior Students and Practitioners.— By William Milligan, M. D., Aurist and Laryngologist to the Royal Infirmary, Manchester Surgeon to the Manchester Ear Hospital, etc., and Wyatt Wingrave, M. D., Pathologist to the Central Throat and Ear Hospital, London, and to the Polyclinic, London. Octavo, 596 pages, with 293 illustrations and 6 colored plates, gilt tops, $5.00 net. (The Macmillan Company).

A Manual of Diseases of the Naso-Pharynx. With Especial Reference to the Part Played by them in Diseases of the Ear, and the Treatment of These Conditions.—By Charles Adair Dighton, M. B., F. R. C. S., Hon. Assistant Surgeon Eye and Ear Infirmary, Liverpool; Hon. Ophthalmological and Aural Surgeon, Toxteth Infirmary, Liverpool; Hon. Ophthalmic and Aural Surgeon, Birkenhead and Wirral Children's Infirmary. Octavo, 181 pages, beautifully illustrated by 68 engravings and 5 plates in color. Muslin, $3.50 net. Wm. Wood & Co., New York.

The Ocular Muscles.—By Howard F. Hansell, A. M., M. D., Professor of Ophthalmology, Jefferson Medical College, etc., and Wendell Reber, M. D., Professor of Diseases of the Eye, Philadelphia Polyclinic, etc. *Second Edition.* 3 plates and 82 other illustrations. Octavo. Cloth, $2.00 postpaid. P. Blakiston's Son & Co., 1012 Walnut St., Philadelphia, Publishers.

Aids to Ophthalmology. (Student's Aids Series).—By N. Bishop Harmon, M. A., M. B., F. R. C. S. *Fifth Edition.* 16mo, 216 pages, 100 illustrations. Flexible muslin, $1.00 net. Wm. Wood & Co., New York.

Ophthalmic Therapeutics. According to the most recent discoveries.—By A. Darier, of Paris. Translated by Sydney Stephenson, M. B., F. R. C. S. Reprinted with a chapter on Chemotherapy and Salvarsan. Illustrated. Oc-

tavo, 460 pages. Cloth, $4.00 postpaid. P. Blakiston's Son & Co., 1012 Walnut St., Philadelphia, Publishers.

Ophthalmic Surgery.—A Handbook of the Surgical Operations as Practiced at the Clinic of Hofrat Prof. Fuchs, Vienna.—By Dr. Josef Meller, Privatdocent and First Assistant K. K. II University Eye Clinic, Vienna. *Second Edition.* Revised and enlarged. Edited by William M. Sweet, M. D., Prof. of Diseases of the Eye, Philadelphia Polyclinic. With 173 illustrations, some in colors. Octavo. Cloth, $3.50 postpaid. P. Blakiston's Son & Co., 1012 Walnut St., Philadelphia, Publishers.

A Text-Book of Ophthalmology in the form of Clinical Lectures.—By Dr. Paul Roemer, Greifswald. Rebman Co., New York.

Refraction and Visual Acuity.—By Kennert Scott, M. D., Edinborough.—Rebman Co., New York.

The Treatment of Shortsight.—By Prof. Dr. J. Hirschberg, Berlin. Rebman Co., New York.

FOODS (Diet and Feeding.)

Fatty Foods. Their Practical Examination. —By E. Richards Bolton, F. C. S., Consulting Analyst and Technical Chemist; and Cecil Revis, Chief Chemist, Messrs. Welford and Sons, Ltd., London. Small octavo. Cloth, $3.50 postpaid. P. Blakiston's Son & Co., 1012 Walnut St., Philadelphia, Publishers.

Food in Health and Disease.—By Nathan S. Davis, Jr., A. M., M. D., Professor of the Principles and Practice of Medicine, Northwestern University Medical School, Chicago. *Second Edition.* Thoroughly revised and rewritten. Contains much new material. Octavo, 461 pages. Cloth, $3.50 postpaid. P. Blakiston's Son & Co., 1012 Walnut St., Philadelphia, Publishers.

Infant Feeding.—By Clifford G. Grulee, A. M., M. D., Assistant Professor of Pediatrics at Rush Medical College, Attending Pediatrician to Cook County Hospital. Octavo of 295 pages, illustrated. Philadelphia. and London: W. B. Saunders Company, 1912. Cloth, $3.00 net.

Diet for the Sick. A Comprehensive Manual on Feeding in Disease.—Written and Compiled by H. Edwin Lewis, M. D. *Second Edition.* Revised. 160 pages. Cloth bound, price $1.00. American Medical Pub. Co., 84 William St., New York City.

GENITO-URINARY AND SKIN DISEASES.

Diseases of the Genito-Urinary Organs and the Kidney.—By Robert H. Greene, M. D., Professor of Genito-Urinary Surgery at the Fordham University, New York; and Harlow Brooks, M. D., Assistant Professor of Clinical Medicine, University and Bellevue Medical College. *Third Revised Edition.* Octavo of 639 pages, 339 illustrations. Philadelphia and London: W. B. Saunders Company, 1912. Cloth, $5.00 net.; half morocco, $6.50 net.

Compend of Genito-Urinary and Venereal Diseases, and Syphilis.—By Charles S. Hirsch,

M. D., formerly Jefferson Medical College Hospital, Philadelphia. *Second Edition*. With colored frontispiece and 74 other illustrations. 12 mo, 378 pages. Cloth, $1.00 postpaid. P. Blakiston's Son & Co., 1012 Walnut St., Philadelphia, Publishers.

Essays on Genito-Urinary Subjects.—By J. Bayard Clark, M. D., Assistant Genito-Urinary Surgeon to Bellevue Hospital; Consulting Genito-Urinary Surgeon to the Elizabeth General Hospital, etc. 12mo, 182 pages. Half extra muslin, $1.25 net. Wm. Wood & Co., New York.

A Treatise on Diseases of the Hair.—By George Thomas Jackson, M. D., Professor of Dermatology, College of Physicians and Surgeons, and Charles Wood McMurtry, M. D., of the College of Physicians and Surgeons, Columbia University, New York. Octavo, 366 pages, with 109 illustrations and 10 colored plates. Cloth, $3.75 net. Lea & Febiger, Philadelphia and New York.

Sexual Impotence.—By Victor G. Vecki, M. D., Consulting Genito-Urinary Surgeon to the Mount Zion Hospital, San Francisco. *Fourth Edition, enlarged*. 12mo of 394 pages. Philadelphia and London: W. B. Saunders Company, 1912. Cloth, $2.25 net.

The X-Ray Treatment of Skin Diseases.—By Dr. Frank Schultz, Berlin. Rebman Co., New York.

Diseases of the Skin and the Eruptive Fevers.—By Jay F. Schamberg, M. D., Professor of Dermatology and the Infectious Eruptive Diseases, Philadelphia Polyclinic. *Second Edition*. Octavo of 573 pages, illustrated. Cloth, $3.00 net. W. B. Saunders Co., Philadelphia.

Compendium of Diseases of the Skin.—By L. Duncan Bulkley. Based on an Analysis of Thirty Thousand Consecutive Cases with Therapeutic Formulary. Cloth. *Fifth Edition*. 286 pages. 1912, Paul B. Hoeber, New York. $2.00 net.

The Therapy of Syphilis.—By Dr. Paul Mulzer, Berlin. This book enlightens the profession as to the present position of modern specific therapy, shows what was formerly accomplished and demonstrates the development of the present day. $1.50. Rebman Co., New York.

GYNECOLOGY AND OBSTETRICS.

Practice of Gynecology. For Practitioners and Students.—By W. Easterly Ashton, M. D., LL. D., Professor of Gynecology in the Medico-Chirurgical College of Philadelphia. *Fifth Edition, thoroughly revised*. Octavo of 1,100 pages, with 1,050 original line drawings. Philadelphia and London: W. B. Saunders Company, 1912. Cloth, $6.50 net; half morocco, $8.00 net.

A Text-Book of Practical Gynecology.—By Edward E. Montgomery, M. D., Professor of Gynecology, Jefferson Medical College, Philadelphia, etc. *Fourth Edition*. Rearranged, thoroughly revised and in part rewritten. 589 illustrations, 3 in colors. Octavo, 879 pages.

Cloth, $6.00 postpaid. P. Blakiston's Son & Co., 1012 Walnut Street, Philadelphia, Publishers.

Pathology and Treatment of Diseases of Women.—By Prof. Dr. A. Martin and Dr. Ph. Jung, Griefswald. Rebman Co., New York.

Practical Text-Book of the Diseases of Women.—By Arthur H. N. Lewers. Cloth, *Seventh Edition*. 540 pages, 258 illustrations, 13 colored plates, 5 plates in black and white. $4.00 net. Paul B. Hoeber, New York City.

Guide to Midwifery.—By David Berry-Hart, M. D., etc., Edinburgh. A succinct and modern account of the facts of Obstetrics. $6.00. Rebman Co., New York.

Obstetrics: Including Related Gynecological Operations.—By Barton Cook Hirst, M. D., Professor of Obstetrics in the University of Pennsylvania. *Seventh Revised Edition*. Octavo of 1,013 pages, with 895 illustration, 53 of them in color. Philadelphia and London: W. B. Saunders Company, 1912. Cloth, $5.00 net; half morocco, $6.50 net.

The Practice of Obstetrics.—By J. Clifton Edgar, M. D., Professor of Obstetrics and Clinical Midwifery, Cornell University Medical Department, New York City. *Fourth Edition*. In parts rewritten and thoroughly revised. With 1,316 illustrations, 46 figures in colors. Octavo, 1,084 pages. Cloth, $6.00 postpaid. P. Blakiston's Son & Co., 1012 Walnut St., Philadelphia, Publishers.

Obstetrics.—By Joseph B. De Lee, M. D., Professor of Obstetrics in the Northwestern University Medical School, Chicago. Large octavo of 1,075 pages, with 921 illustrations, very many in colors. Philadelphia and London: W. B. Saunders Co., 1912.

PRACTICE OF MEDICINE.

(Including General Medicine, Internal Medicine, Pediatrics, Etc.)

Auto-Intoxication and Dis-intoxication.—By Dr. G. Guelpa, Paris. This is an account of a New Fasting Treatment in Diabetes and other Chronic Diseases, with an introduction by the Translator, F. S. Arnold, B. C., etc. (oxon), and a chapter on the Use of the Method in the Treatment of Morphine Addiction by Oscar Jennings, M. D., Paris. $1.25. Rebman Co., New York.

The Diseases of Children. A Work for the Practicing Physician. *Second Edition*.—Edited by Professor M. Pfaundler, Professor of Children's Diseases and Director of the Children's Clinic at the University of Munich, and Professor A. Schlossmann, Professor of Children's Diseases and Director of the Children's Clinic at the Medical Academy in Düsseldorf. English translation, edited by Henry L. K. Shaw, M. D., Albany, N. Y., Clinical Professor, Diseases of Children, Albany Medical College, Physician in Charge St. Margaret House for Infants, Albany, and Linnaeus E. Lafetra, M. D., New York, N. Y., Instructor of Diseases of Children, Columbia

University, Chief of Department of Diseases of Children, Vanderbilt Clinic, Assistant Attending Physician to the Babies' Hospital; with an introduction by L. Emmett Holt, M. D., Professor of Pediatrics, Columbia University, New York, N. Y. Fifth volume published 1912, which completes the set. J. B. Lippincott Co., Philadelphia. Five volumes. Imperial Octavo, 500 pages each, 90 full-page plates, 775 text illustrations, 72 in colors. Cloth, $5.00 per volume.

A System of Clinical Medicine, Dealing with the Diagnosis, Prognosis and Treatment of Disease for Students and Practitioners.—By Thos. Dixon Savill, M. D., Lond. *Third Edition;* thoroughly revised. Octavo, 969 pages; sumptuously illustrated by four full-page plates in color and by 170 engravings in the text. Muslin, $7.00, net; half morocco, $8.00 net. Wm. Wood & Co., New York.

New Aspects of Diabetes, Pathology and Treatment.—By Prof. Dr. Carl von Noorden, Professor of the First Medical Clinic, Vienna. Translated by Walker Hall, Prof. Pathology, University College, Bristol, England. Published by authority of New York Post-Graduate Medical School. E. B. Treat & Co., 241-3 West 23rd Street, New York. 8vo. 160 pages, diagrams and tables. $1.50 net.

The Treatment of Infantile Paralysis.—By Oskar Vulpius, M. D., Professor Extraordinary at the University of Heidelberg. Translated by Allan H. Todd, M. D., B. S., B. Sc. With introduction by J. Jackson Clarke, M. B. (Lond.) F. R. C. S. Octavo, 328 pages, illustrated by 243 original engravings. Muslin, $4.00 net. Wm. Wood & Co., New York.

Wheeler's Handbook of Medicine.—By William R. Jack, M. D., B. S. C., Assistant Physician to the Western Infirmary of Glasgow. *Fourth Edition.* 12mo, 543 pages, illustrated. Flexible muslin, $3.00 net; flexible morocco, $3.25 net. Wm. Wood & Co., New York.

Internal Medicine.—By David Bovaird, Jr., A. B., M. D., Associate Professor of Clinical Medicine in Columbia University, and Associate Visiting Physician of the Presbyterian Hospital, New York City. Octavo, 600 pages, 7 colored plates and illustrations. Cloth, $5.00. J. B. Lippincott Co., Philadelphia.

An Introduction to the Study of Infection and Immunity. Including Serum Therapy, Vaccine Therapy, Chemotherapy and Serum Diagnosis.—By Charles E. Simon, M. D., Professor of Clinical Pathology and Experimental Medicine, College of Physicians and Surgeons, Baltimore. Octavo, 296 pages, illustrated. Cloth, $3.25 net. Lea & Febiger, Philadelphia and New York.

Immunity. Methods of Diagnosis and Therapy, and Their Practical Application.—By Julius Citron, University Clinic of Berlin. Translated and edited by A. L. Garbat, M. D., German Hospital, New York City. 27 illustrations and 2 colored plates. Octavo, cloth $3.00, postpaid. P. Blakiston's Son & Co., 1012 Walnut Street, Philadelphia.

Diseases of the Liver, Gall-Bladder and Bile-Ducts.—By Humphry Davy Rolleston, M. A., M. D. (Cantab.), F. R. C. P. Senior Physician, St. George's Hospital; Physician, Victoria Hospital for Children, Chelsea; formerly Fellow of St. John's College, Cambridge. 8vo, 811 pages, $9.00 net; with 7 colored plates and 108 figures in the text. (The Macmillan Company).

The Practice of Medicine.—By Frederick Taylor, M. D., F. R. C. P. Consulting Physician to Guy's Hospital; Examiner in Medicine at the University of Cambridge and at the Queen's University, Belfast, etc. *Ninth Edition.* Large octavo, 1121 pages, illustrated with 8 plates and 67 text cuts. Cloth, $6.00 net. (The Macmillan Company).

Diseases of the Mouth. (Syphilis and Similar Diseases of the Mouth.)—By Prof. Dr. F. Zinsser, Cologne. $7.00. Rebman Co., New York.

Pellagra.—By George M. Niles, M. D., Professor of Gastro-enterology and Therapeutics in the Atlanta School of Medicine, Atlanta, Georgia. Octavo of 253 pages, illustrated. Philadelphia and London: W. B. Saunders Company, 1912. Cloth, $3.00 net.

Practical Treatment. In three volumes.—By 82 eminent specialists. Edited by John H. Musser, M. D., Professor of Clinical Medicine, University of Pennsylvania; and A. O. J. Kelly, M. D., late Assistant Professor of Medicine, University of Pennsylvania. *Volume III.* Octavo of 1,095 pages, illustrated. Philadelphia and London: W. B. Saunders Company, 1912. Per volume: cloth, $6.00 net; half morocco, $7.50 net.

Sprue: Its Diagnosis and Treatment.—By Charles Begg, M. B., C. M. Edinburgh. Formerly Medical Officer Chinese Imperial Maritime Customs and H. B. M. Medical Officer, Hankow, China. 120 pages, illustrated by eight full-page plates. Muslin, $2.00 net. Wm. Wood & Co., New York.

Diseases of the Stomach, Intestines, and Pancreas.—By Robert Coleman Kemp, M. D., Professor of Gastro-intestinal Diseases, New York School of Clinical Medicine. *Second Edition, revised and enlarged.* Octavo of 1021 pages, with 388 illustrations. Philadelphia and London: W. B. Saunders Company, 1912. Cloth, $6.50 net; half morocco, $8.00 net.

An Index of Treatment.—By eighty-three writers. Edited by Robert Hutchison, M. D., F. R. C. P., Physician to London Hospital and Assistant Physician to Hospital for Sick Children, Great Ormond Street, London; and H. Stansfield Collier, F. R. C. S., Surg. to St. Mary's Hospital; Joint Lecturer on Surgery in St. Mary's Hospital Medical School; Surg. to the Hosp. for Sick Children, Gt. Ormond St., London. Revised and edited to conform to American practice by Warren Coleman, M. D., Prof. of Clinical Medicine and Instructor in Therapeutics, Cornell University Medical College; Visiting Physician to Bellevue Hospital, New York. Octavo, 1067 pages, illustrated.

Price, muslin, $6.00 net; half-morocco, $7.00 net. Wm. Wood & Co., New York.

Recent Methods in the Diagnosis and Treatment of Syphilis. The Wassermann Reaction and Ehrlich's Salvarsan, "606."—By C. H. Browning, M. D., Lecturer on Bacteriology in the University of Glasgow, and Ivy McKenzie, M. D., Director, Western Asylums' Research Institute, Glasgow. Octavo, 293 pages. Cloth, $2.50 net. Lea & Febiger, Philadelphia and New York.

A System of Treatment.—Edited by Arthur Latham, M. A., M. D. Oxon., F. R. C. P. Lond. Physician and Lecturer on Medicine, St. George's Hospital; and T. Crisp English, M. B., B. S. Lond., F. R. C. S. Eng. Senior Assistant Surgeon, St. George's Hospital, assisted by 187 eminent contributors. In four royal octavo volumes, 5,296 pages, 1,000 illustrations, bibliographies and a *New Method of Indexing* for Quick Reference. Sold only in sets by subscription, per volume, cloth, $6.00; half-morocco, $7.50. (The Macmillan Company).

MATERIA MEDICA AND THERAPEUTICS.

Materia Medica and Therapeutics, Including Pharmacy and Pharmacology.—By Reynold Webb Wilcox, M. A., M. D., LL. D., Professor of Medicine (Retired) New York Post-Graduate Medical School, etc. *Eighth Edition.* Thoroughly revised. Octavo, 843 pages; cloth, $3.00 postpaid. P. Blakiston's Son & Co., 1012 Walnut Street, Philadelphia, Publishers.

The Essentials of Materia Medica and Therapeutics for Nurses.—By John Foote, M. D. J. B. Lippincott Co., Philadelphia. 12mo, 194 pages; cloth, $1.25 net.

A Manual of Pharmacy for Physicians.—By M. F. DeLorme, M. D., Ph. G., Lecturer on Pharmacy and Pharmacology, Long Island College Hospital, New York. *Third Edition.* Revised and enlarged, 19 illustrations, 12mo, 229 pages. Cloth, $1.25 postpaid. P. Blakiston's Son & Co., 1012 Walnut Street, Philadelphia, Publishers.

Commercial Pharmacy.—By D. Chas. O'Connor, Author of "Training the Future Drug Clerk;" Ex-President Fitchburg Druggists Association, Fitchburg, Mass.; Member Massachusetts State Pharmaceutical Association; Member National Association of Retail Druggists. J. B. Lippincott Company, Philadelphia. Octavo, 400 pages, 16 illustrations. Cloth, $2.50. The direct object of this book is to provide a text and reference book.

Pharmacology. The Action and Uses of Drugs.—By Maurice Vejux Tyrode, M. D., formerly Instructor in Pharmacology, Harvard University Medical School. *Second Edition.* Revised and enlarged. Octavo, 297 pages. Cloth, $1.50 postpaid. P. Blakiston's Son & Co., 1012 Walnut St., Philadelphia, Publishers.

A Text-Book of Pharmacology and Therapeutics.—By Horatio C. Wood, Jr., Professor of Pharmacology and Therapeutics in the Medico-Chirurgical College; Physician to the Med-

ico-Chirurgical Hospital; Second Vice-Chairman of the Committee of Revision of the United States Pharmacopeia. J. B. Lippincott Co., Philadelphia. Octavo 400 pages, 50 illustrations. Cloth, $4.00.

A Text-Book of Practical Therapeutics, with Especial Reference to the Application of Remedial Measures to Disease and their Employment upon a Rational Basis.—By Hobart Amory Hare, M. D., Professor of Therapeutics and Materia Medica, Jefferson Medical College, Phila. *New (14th) Edition,* thoroughly revised. Octavo, 984 pages, with 131 engravings and 8 colored plates. Cloth, $4.00 net. Lea & Febiger, Philadelphia and New York.

Therapeutics, Materia Medica and Pharmacy. Including the physiological action of drugs, special therapeutics of diseases and symptoms, the modern materia medica, official and practical pharmacy, minute directions for prescription writing, incompatibility, antidotal and antagonistic treatment of poisoning, and over 650 prescriptions and formulae. *Twelfth Edition.* Revised and enlarged. By Samuel O. L. Potter, M. A., M. D., M. R. C. P. (Lond.) Octavo 972 pages. Cloth, $5.00 postpaid. P. Blakiston's Son & Co., 1012 Walnut St., Philadelphia, Publishers.

Sahli's Tuberculin Treatment. Including a Discussion of the Nature and Action of Tuberculin and of Immunity to Tuberculosis.—By Hermann Sahli, Professor of Medicine in the University of Berne; Director of the Medical Clinic. Translated from the Third German Edition by Wilfred B. Christopherson, with a Prefatory Note by Egbert Morland, M. D., and B. Sc. (Lond.) M. D., (Berne). Octavo, 200 pages; muslin binding, $3.00 net. Wm. Wood & Co., New York.

Vaccine Therapy, Its Theory and Practice.—By R. W. Allen, M. D., B. S. (Lond.), Late Clinical Pathologist to the Mount Vernon Hospital for Diseases of the Chest; Late Pathologist to the Royal Eye Hospital; Late Gull Student of Pathology, Guy's Hospital. *Fourth Edition.* Revised, completely rewritten and greatly enlarged. Small octavo 444 pages. Cloth, $3.00 postpaid. P. Blakiston's Son & Co., 1012 Walnut St., Philadelphia, Publishers.

NERVOUS DISEASES.

Brain and Spinal Cord. A Guide for the Study of the Morphology and the Fibre-Tracts. —By Emil Villiger, M. D., of the University of Basle. Translated from the Second German Edition, with additions, by George A. Piersol, M. D., Sc. D., of the University of Pennsylvania. Octavo, 288 pages, 224 illustrations, many in colors. Cloth, $4.00. J. B. Lippincott Co., Philadelphia.

Compendium of Regional Diagnosis in Affections of the Brain and Spinal Cord.—By Robert Bing, University of Basle. $2.50. Rebman Co., New York.

Mind and Its Disorders.—By W. H. B. Stoddart, M. D., F. R. C. P., Assistant Physician to Bethlem Royal Hospital, London. *Second*

Edition, Revised and Enlarged. 74 illustrations (6 in colors). Octavo 534 pages. Cloth, $4.00 postpaid. P. Blakiston's Son & Co., 1012 Walnut Street, Philadelphia, Publishers.

Psychological Medicine. A Manual of Mental Diseases.—By Maurice Craig, M. A., M. D., F. R. C. P., Physician and Lecturer in Psychological Medicine, Guy's Hospital. *Second Edition.* Revised. With 27 plates containing 90 figures (46 in colors). Octavo. Cloth, $5.00 postpaid. P. Blakiston's Son & Co., 1012 Walnut Street, Philadelphia, Publishers.

Psychanalysis.—By A. A. Brill, Ph. B., M. D., Clinical Assistant in Psychiatry and Neurology at Columbia University Medical School. Octavo of 575 pages. Philadelphia and London: W. B. Saunders Company, 1912.

Hypnosis and Suggestion.—By W. Hilger, Magdeburg. Nature, action, import and position in Hypnosis Suggestion amongst Therapeutic Agents is emphasized. $2.50. Rebman Co., New York.

PATHOLOGY (Including Bacteriology, Etc.)

Elementary Bacteriology and Protozoology. For the Use of Nurses.—By Herbert Fox, M. D., Director of the William Pepper Laboratory of Clinical Medicine in the University of Pennsylvania. 12mo, 237 pages, with 67 engravings and 5 colored plates. Cloth, $1.75 net. Lea & Febiger, Philadelphia and New York.

Clinical Bacteriology and Haematology for Practitioners.—By W. D'Este Emery, M. D., B. Sc., (Lond.), Clinical Pathologist to King's College Hospital. *Fourth Edition.* With 10 plates containing 62 figures, some in colors, and 50 other illustrations. Octavo 283 pages. Cloth, $2.00 postpaid. P. Blakiston's Son & Co., 1012 Walnut Street, Philadelphia, Publishers.

General Bacteriology.—By Edwin O. Jordan, Ph.D., Professor of Bacteriology in the University of Chicago and in Rush Medical College. *Third Edition, thoroughly revised.* Octavo of 623 pages, fully illustrated. Philadelphia and London: W. B. Saunders Company, 1912. Cloth, $3.00 net.

Pharmaceutical Bacteriology. With special Reference to Disinfection and Sterilization.—By Albert Schneider, M. D., Ph. D., California College of Pharmacy, U. S. Dept. of Agriculture, etc. 86 illustrations. Octavo. Cloth, $2.00, postpaid. P. Blakiston's Son & Co., 1012 Walnut St., Philadelphia, Publishers.

Pathogenic Bacteria and Protozoa.—By Joseph McFarland, M. D., Professor of Pathology and Bacteriology in the Medico-Chirurgical College, Philadelphia. *Seventh edition, thoroughly revised.* Octavo of 878 pages, 293 illustrations, a number of them in colors. Philadelphia and London: W. B. Saunders Company, 1912. Cloth, $3.50 net.

Further Researches Into Induced Cell-Reproduction and Cancer. Vol. II.—By H. C. Ross, J. W. Cropper, and E. H. Ross. Illustrated. Octavo. Cloth, $1.00, postpaid. P.

Blakiston's Son & Co., 1012 Walnut St., Philadelphia, Publishers.

The Cause of Cancer. Being Part III of Protozoa and Diseases.—By J. Jackson Clarke, M. B., F. R. C. S., Senior Surgeon to the Hampstead and North-West London Hospital, and Surgeon to the Royal National Orthopedic Hospital. Octavo, 102 pages, illustrated by colored frontispiece and by eight full-page plates containing sixty figures. Muslin, $2.50 net. Wm. Wood & Co., New York.

Recent Advances in Haematology. Being the Dr. James Watson Lectures for 1910.—By Walter K. Hunter, M. D., D. Sc., Fellow of the Royal Faculty of Physicians and Surgeons, Glasgow, etc. Octavo, with a colored plate. Muslin, $2.25 net. Wm. Wood & Co., New York.

Tumors of the Jaws.—By Charles L. Scudder, M. D., Surgeon to the Massachusetts General Hospital. Octavo of 391 pages, with 353 illustrations, 6 in colors. Philadelphia and London: W. B. Saunders Company, 1912. Cloth, $6.00 net; half morocco, $7.50 net.

A Treatise on Tumors. For the Use of Physicians and Surgeons.—By Arthur E. Hertzler, M. D., of Kansas City, Mo., Assistant Professor in Surgery in the University of Kansas. Octavo, 728 pages, with 538 illustrations and 8 plates. Cloth, $7.00 net; half Persian morocco, gilt top, de luxe, $9.00 net. Lea & Febiger, Philadelphia and New York.

A Text-Book of Pathology. For Students of Medicine.—By J. George Adami, M. A., M. D., LL. D., F. R. S., Professor of Pathology in McGill University, Montreal, and John McCrae, M. D., M. R. C. P. (Lond.), Lecturer in Pathology and Clinical Medicine in McGill University; formerly Professor of Pathology in the University of Vermont. Octavo, 759 pages, with 304 engravings and 11 colored plates. Cloth, $5.00 net. Lea & Febiger, Philadelphia and New York.

The Clinical Pathology of Syphilis and Parasyphilis and its Value for Diagnostic and Controlling Treatment.—By Hugh Wansey Bayly, M. A., etc., Pathologist of the London Lock Hospital; Clinical Pathologist to the National Hospital for the Paralyzed and Epileptic; Assistant in the Bacteriological Department of St. George's Hospital. 12mo, 202 pages, illustrated by numerous cuts and tables and by three plates. Muslin, $2.25 net. Wm. Wood & Co., New York.

SURGERY.

Surgical After-Treatment.—By L. R. G. Crandon, M. D., Assistant in Surgery at Harvard Medical School, and Albert Ehrenfried, M. D., Assistant in Anatomy at Harvard Medical School. *Second edition, practically rewritten.* Octavo of 831 pages, with 264 original illustrations. Philadelphia and London: W. B. Saunders Company, 1912. Cloth, $6.00 net; half morocco, $7.50 net.

Anesthetics and Their Administration. A Text-Book for Medical and Dental Practitioners and Students.—By Sir Frederic W. Hewitt, M. V. O., M. A., M. D., Cantab., Anesthetist to His Majesty the King, Physician-Anesthetist to St. George's Hospital, Consulting Anesthetist to the London Hospital, Late Anesthetist to the Charing Cross and Royal Dental Hospitals of London. *Fourth Edition*, prepared with the assistance of Henry Robinson, M. A., M. D., B. C. Cantab., Anesthetist to the Royal Samaritan and Cancer Hospitals. Octavo, 676 pages, with 71 illustrations. Price, $5.00 net. (The Macmillan Company).

Surgery of the Brain and Spinal Cord.—By Prof. Dr. Fedor Krause, Berlin. Vols. II and III. They deal with Epilepsy, Neoplasmata of the Brain, the Frontal Brain, the Central Region, the Temporal Lobe and the Region of the Island of Reil, the Neoplasmata of the Parietal Lobe, the Occipital Brain, and the Anterior Fossa of the Skull. Symptomatology and Neoplasmata of the Base of the Brain and in the Contiguous Regions are then taken up. Neoplasmata of the Base of the Brain, Prognosis in the Extirpation of Cerebral Tumors. Intracranial suppuration, Metastatic Processes and Cerebral Injuries follow. The rest is devoted to the Surgery of the Spinal Cord. The complete work contains 122 color figures on 60 plates, 9 half-tones and two plates, and 199 illustrations in the texts, 17 of which are colored. Complete in three volumes, over 1,100 pages, $20.00. Rebman Co., New York.

Deformities, Including Diseases of the Bones and Joints. A Text-Book of Orthopedic Surgery. *New Edition* by A. H. Tubby, M. S. Lond., F. R. C. S. Eng. Surgeon in Charge Orthopedic Department, Westminster Hospital; Lecturer on Clinical and Orthopedic Surgery in the Medical School; Surgeon to the Royal National Orthopedic Hospital; Consulting Surgeon to the Seven-Oaks Hospital for Hip Disease, etc. In two volumes. Large octavo, 1,750 pages, illustrated with 70 plates and over 1,000 figures, of which nearly 400 are original, and by notes of 54 cases. Sold in sets only. Cloth, $16.00. (The Macmillan Company).

Duodenal Ulcer.—By B. G. A. Moynihan, M. S. (London) F. R. C. S., Senior Assistant Surgeon at Leeds General Infirmary, England. *Second edition, enlarged.* Octavo of 486 pages, illustrated. Philadelphia and London: W. B. Saunders Company, 1912. Cloth, $5.00 net; half morocco, $6.50 net.

Surgery of Deformities of the Face, Including Cleft Palate.—By John B. Roberts, A. M., M. D. Octavo, profusely illustrated by 273 engravings in line and half-tone. Muslin, $3.00 net. Wm. Wood & Co., New York.

A Practical Treatise on Fractures and Dislocations.—By Lewis A. Stimson, B. A., M. D., LL. D., Professor of Surgery in Cornell University Medical College, New York. 930 pages, with 459 engravings and 39 plates. Cloth, $5.00 net. Lea & Febiger, Philadelphia and New York.

The Treatment of Fractures by Mobilization and Massage.—By James B. Mennell, House Surgeon and Casualty Assistant, St. Thomas'

Hospital, London, with an introduction by Dr. J. Lucas-Championnière, Chirugien Honoraire de L'Hotel Dieu, Membre de L'Académie de Médicine, Président de la Société Internationale de Chirugie, etc. 8vo, 458 pages, with 67 half-tone illustrations. Price, $5.00 net. (The Macmillan Company).

Infections of the Hand. A Guide to the Surgical Treatment of Acute and Chronic Suppurative Processes in the Fingers, Hand and Forearm.—By Allen B. Kanavel, M. D., Assistant Professor of Surgery, Northwestern University, Medical Department; Professor of Surgery, Post-graduate Medical School and Hospital, Chicago. Octavo, 447 pages, with 133 illustrations. Cloth, $3.75 net. Lea & Febiger, Philadelphia and New York.

Surgical Handicraft. A Manual of Surgical Manipulations, Minor Surgery, etc.—By Walter Pye, F. R. C. S. Revised and re-written by W. H. Clayton-Greene, F. R. C. S., Assistant Surgeon in Charge, Out-Patients, St. Mary's Hospital. *Sixth Editon.* Revised and enlarged. Octavo, about 700 pages, 400 illustrations and plates. Cloth, $4.00 net. New York: E. B. Treat & Co., 241-3 West 23rd St.

The Immediate Care of the Injured.—By Albert S. Morrow, M. D., Adjunct Professor of Surgery in the New York Polyclinic. *Second Edition, Revised.* Octavo of 354 pages, with 242 illustrations. Philadelphia and London: W. B. Saunders Company, 1912. Cloth, $2.50 net.

Hare-Lip and Cleft-Palate.—By James Berry, B. S. (London) F. R. C. S., Senior Surgeon to the Royal Free Hospital, and T. Percy Legg, M. S. (Lond.) F. R. C. S., Surgeon to the Royal Free Hospital, London. 242 illustrations, octavo. Cloth, $4.00 postpaid. P. Blakiston's Son & Co., 1012 Walnut St., Philadelphia, Publishers.

The Course of Operative Surgery.—By Prof. Dr. Victor Schmeiden (University of Berlin). *Second Enlarged Edition*, with a foreword by Prof. Dr. A. Bier. Translated and edited by Arthur Turnbull, M. B., M. A. Large octavo, profusely illustrated by 435 beautifully executed illustrations in black and color, almost all original. Muslin, $4.00 net. Wm. Wood & Co., New York.

Surgical Operations.—By Dr. Friedrich Pels-Leusden, Berlin. 668 illustrations in the text. $7.00. Rebman Co., New York.

Text-Book of Operative Surgery.—By Dr. Theodor Kocher, Professor of Surgery and Director of the Surgical Clinic in the University of Bern. Authorized translation from the *Fifth German Edition* by Harold J. Stiles, M. B., F. R. C. S. Edin., Surgeon to the Chalmers Hospital, Edinburgh; Surgeon to the Royal Edinburgh Hospital for Sick Children; Lecturer on Applied Anatomy, University of Edinburgh; and C. Balfour Paul, M. B., F. R. C. S., Edin., Assistant Surgeon, Royal Edinburgh Hospital for Sick Children. In two super-royal octavo volumes, containing 415 illustrations, many in color. Uniform in price and binding with Allbutt & Rolleston's System of Medicine. Sold only by subscription; per volume, cloth, $6.00; half morocco, $8.00. (The Macmillan Company).

The Surgery of Oral Diseases and Malformations. Their Diagnosis and Treatment.— By George V. I. Brown, M. D., D. D. S., Oral Surgeon to St. Mary's Hospital and to the Children's Free Hospital, Milwaukee; Professor of Oral Surgery, Southern Dental College, Atlanta, Ga. Octavo, 740 pages, with 359 engravings and 21 plates. Cloth, $6.00 net. Lea & Febiger, Philadelphia and New York.

Lateral Curvature of the Spine, and Round Shoulders. Their Cause, Prevention and Cure by Gymnastic Exercise.—By Robert W. Lovett, M. D., Assistant Professor of Orthopedic Surgery, Harvard Medical School. *Second Edition*, 171 illustrations. Octavo, 203 pages. Cloth, $1.75 postpaid. P. Blakiston's Son & Co., 1012 Walnut Street, Philadelphia, Publishers.

A Manual of Surgical Treatment.—By Sir W. Watson Cheyne, M. B., F. R. C. S., F. R. S., Professor of Surgery in King's College, London; and F. F. Burghard, M. D., F. R. C. S., Teacher of Practical Surgery in King's College, London. Five octavo volumes, containing about 3,000 pages, with about 900 engravings. Per volume, cloth, $6.00 net. Lea & Febiger, Philadelphia and New York.

MISCELLANEOUS.

An Introduction to the Study of Adolescent Education.—By Cyril Bruyn Andrews, M. D. $1.50. Rebman Co.; New York.

Gould and Pyle's Cyclopedia of Practical Medicine and Surgery. A concise reference book of Medicine, Surgery, Materia Medica, Therapeutics and the varied specialties. *Second Edition, thoroughly revised and enlarged* by R. J. E. Scott, M. A., B. C. L., M. D., Attending Physician to the Demilt Dispensary, New York, etc. Including articles by 93 special contributors, with 653 illustrations, large square octavo, 1,400 double-column pages, two volume edition. Cloth, $14.00; half morocco, $17.00, or in one volume, cloth, $12.00; half morocco, $14.00.

Cyclopedia of American Medical Biography. —By Howard A. Kelly, M. D., Professor of Gynecologic Surgery at Johns Hopkins University, Baltimore. Two octavo volumes averaging 525 pages each, with portraits. Philadelphia and London: W. B. Saunders Company, 1912. Per set: Cloth, $10.00 net; half morocco, $13.00 net.

A Practical Medical Dictionary.—By Thos. Lathrop Stedman, A. M., M. D. *Second Edition. Revised and enlarged.* 4to, 1,046 pages, illustrated. Flexible red morocco. Thumb-indexed, $5.00 net; plain edges, $4.50 net. Wm. Wood & Co., New York.

International Clinics.— Edited by Henry W. Cattell, A. M., M. D., Philadelphia, Pa., with the collaboration of William Osler, M. D.; Oxford; John H. Musser, M. D., Philadelphia; Frank Billings, M. D., Chicago; Charles H. Mayo, M. D., Rochester, Minn.; A. McPhedran, M. D., Toronto; Thomas M. Rotch, M. D., Boston; John G. Clark, M. D., Philadelphia; J. W. Ballantyne, M. D., Edinburgh; James J. Walsh, M. D., New York; John Harold, M. D., London; Richard Kretz, M. D., Vienna; with regular correspondents in Montreal, London, Paris, Berlin, Vienna, Leipsic, Brussels, and Carlsbad. J. B. Lippincott Co., Philadelphia.

The International Medical Annual, 1912. A Year Book of Treatment and Practitioner's Index. Thirtieth year of issue.—By a staff of thirty-three contributing editors. New York: E. B. Treat & Co., 241-3 West 23rd St. Complete in one volume, octavo, 700 pages, fully illustrated by plain colored and stereo plates. Cloth, $3.50 net.

Pathfinders in Medicine.—By Victor Robinson. Published by Med. Review of Reviews Co., $2.50.

Principles of Hygiene. For Students, Physicians and Health Officers.—By D. H. Bergey, M. D., First Assistant, Laboratory of Hygiene, and Assistant Professor of Bacteriology, University of Pennsylvania. *Fourth edition, thoroughly revised.* Octavo of 529 pages, illustrated. Philadelphia and London: W. B. Saunders Company, 1912. Cloth, $3.00 net.

Personal Hygiene. Proper Living upon a Physiologic Basis.—By Eminent Specialists. Edited by Walter L. Pyle, M. D., Assistant Surgeon to the Wills Eye Hospital, Philadelphia. *Fifth Edition, Revised and Enlarged.* 12mo. of 516 pages, illustrated. Philadelphia and London: W. B. Saunders Company, 1912. Cloth, $1.50 net.

Aids to Tropical Hygiene. (Student's Aids Series).—By Major R. J. Blackham, D. P. H., London, R. A. M. A. 12 mo, 198 pages. Flexible muslin, $1.25 net. Wm. Wood & Co., New York.

Tropical Medicine and Hygiene.—By C. W. Daniels, M. D. Part III. Diseases Due to Protozoa and Other Vegetable Parasites, to Dietetic Errors and of Unknown Causation. Octavo, illustrated. Uniform in style with Parts I and II. Extra muslin, $3.00 net. Wm. Wood & Co., New York.

Massage and the Original Swedish Movements. Their Application to Various Diseases of the Body.—By Kurre W. Ostrom, from the Royal University of Upsala, Sweden, etc. *Seventh Edition, revised and enlarged*, 118 illustrations. 12mo, 216 pages. Cloth, $1.00.

Medical Gymnastics and Massage. For the Treatment of Disease, Deformity and Injury. —By Fredk. F. Middleweek, L. R. C. P., L. R. C. S., Director of Mechano-Therapeutics and Massage, West End Hospital for Nervous Diseases. With an introduction by J. Arvedson, Stockholm. 12mo, 75c. net. Wm. Wood & Co., New York.

Honan's Handbook to Medical Europe. A Ready Reference Book to the Universities, Hospitals, Clinics, Laboratories and General Medical Work of the Principal Cities in Europe.—By James Henry Honan, M. D., Rush Medical College, Chicago, etc. Contains maps of Berlin, Edinburgh, London, Paris. 12mo, 269 pages. Cloth, $1.50 postpaid. P. Blakiston's Son & Co., 1012 Walnut St., Philadelphia, Publishers.

The Complete Handbook for the Hospital Corps of the U. S. Army and Navy and State Military Forces.—By Charles F. Mason, Lt.-Col. Medical Corps, U. S. Army. *Third Edition.* Octavo, 610 pages, profusely illustrated. Muslin, $4.00 net. Wm. Wood & Co., New York.

Medical Service in Campaign. A Handbook for Medical Officers in the Field.—By Major Paul Frederick Straub, Medical Corps, General Staff, U. S. Army. *Second Edition.* With 2 plates and 13 other illustrations. 12mo, flexible leather, gilt edges, round corners, $1.50 postpaid. P. Blakiston's Son & Co., 1012 Walnut St., Philadelphia, Publishers.

Collected Papers by the Staff of St. Mary's Hospital (Mayo Clinic) for 1911. Octavo of 603 pages, illustrated. Philadelphia and London: W. B. Saunders Company, 1912. Cloth, $5.50 net.

A Collection of Papers (Published Previous to 1909).—By William J. Mayo, M. D., and Charles H. Mayo, M. D. Two octavo volumes, averaging 550 pages each, illustrated. Philadelphia and London: W. B. Saunders Company, 1912. Per set, cloth, $10.00 net.

What to Do in Cases of Poisoning.—By William Murrell. Cloth, *Eleventh Edition,* 283 pages, 1912. Paul B. Hoeber, New York. $1.00 net.

State Board Examinations, Questions and Answers, of the United States and Canada.—A practical work giving authentic questions and authoritative answers in full that will prove helpful in passing state board examinations. Reprinted from the Medical Record. *Fourth Edition.* Thoroughly revised; every question answered in full. 12mo, 827 pages. Muslin, $3.00 net. Wm. Wood & Co., New York.

The Surgical Clinics of John B. Murphy, M. D., at Mercy Hospital, Chicago. Volume I, Number I (February). Octavo of 133 pages, illustrated. Volume I, Number II (April), octavo of 157 pages, illustrated. Volume I, Number III (June), octavo of 174 pages, illustrated. Volume I, Number IV (August), octavo of 154 pages, illustrated. Volume I, Number V (October), octavo of 155 pages, illustrated. Volume I, Number VI (December), octavo of 155 pages, illustrated. Philadelphia and London: W. B. Saunders Company, 1912. Published bi-monthly. Price per year: paper, $8.00; cloth, $12.00.

The Pituitary Body. Clinical States Produced by Disorders of the Hypophysis Cerebri.—By Harvey Cushing, M. D., Associate Professor of Surgery, The Johns Hopkins University; Professor of Surgery (elect), Harvard University. J. B. Lippincott Co., Philadelphia, Pa. Octavo, 450 pages, 350 illustrations. Cloth, $5.00.

Medical Vade Mecum in German and English.—By B. Lewis, with preface by Dr. A. Politzer, Imperial Royal Professor of Aural Therapeutics, University of Vienna. *Second Edition.* Octavo, 574 pages. Cloth, $5.00 postpaid. P. Blakiston's Son & Co., 1012 Walnut St., Philadelphia, Publishers.

The Collected Works of Christian Fenger, M. D.—Edited by Ludvig Hektoen, M. D., Professor of Pathology at Rush Medical College. Two octavo volumes averaging 525 pages each, illustrated. Philadelphia and London: W. B. Saunders Company, 1912. Per set: Cloth, $15.00 net; half morocco, $18.00 net.

ETIOLOGY AND DIAGNOSIS.

The Diagnosis of Gall-stones.[1]—The symptoms produced by gall-stones will vary considerably in their intensity, in their variety, and in their importance, and they will correspond very closely to the lesions which they represent. Unfortunately the clear cut, classic picture of gall-stone colic is rare rather than common, and unfortunately, too, the public and the majority of the medical profession hold the mistaken view that the less severe symptoms which are usually found do not point to serious danger and do not necessarily call for surgical relief. There has been a mistaken idea in minds of our profession that in the majority of cases gall-stones do not cause symptoms. This is not so, for it is equally true that a gall-stone is always doing more or less harm and that a gall-stone will always produce more or less well marked symptoms. The fact that they are so frequently overlooked is owing to indifference on the part of the patients and to ignorance on the part of their physicians.

Some cases present classic text-book pictures; in these the diagnosis is simple. The cardinal symptoms are acute, violent pain coming on suddenly, usually at night; this pain is stabbing, lancinating in character, and it radiates to the back and right shoulder. There is usually tenderness, sometimes very acute, in the region of the gall-bladder. Frequently there is vomiting, and if the attack lasts for a day or two there may be jaundice. The attack may be ushered in with a chill, or there may be a succession of chills. Such cases present but little difficulty in diagnosis.

[1] Parker Syms, M. D., *New York Med. Jour.,* Nov. 9, 1912.

The vast majority of cases are not manifest by a severe and characteristic attack, and diagnosis is not forced upon us, but it should always be made if we pay attention to the whole picture of the cases and if we hold the view that chronic indigestion and dyspepsia are not normal conditions. In the majority of cases the gall-stones are at rest and are not causing active and violent irritation. The gall-bladder and bile ducts are chronically but not acutely inflamed. Symptoms will correspond to these conditions and will be those of a slight localized irritation or a slight inflammation of a chronic type and of a slightly disturbed function on the part of the digestive tract. They are mostly those of a chronic dyspepsia, not violent in character. Such patients will have sour eructations, belching of gas, and a sense of fullness and tension after eating. They may have slight pains, slight tenderness, and rigidity at the Mayo-Robson point. They usually suffer from constipation. These are the cases where diagnosis is certainly not easy. In some the diagnosis must be inferred. These patients should be carefully watched, and if their symptoms are sufficient to disturb their health, to undermine their nervous system, or make useless or unhappy their lives, they should certainly be operated upon, assuming that they have had careful hygienic treatment without success.

Let us consider the correlation of certain diseases of the stomach, the biliary tract, and the appendix. There are many cases which present symptoms of dyspepsia or chronic indigestion in which it would be impossible to say whether the lesion is in the appendix, in the bile passages, in the pylorus, or duodenum. These cases are to my mind of the utmost importance, and yet the vast majority of them are neglected by the medical profession. They are cases in which there is a vague sense of distress in the right upper quadrant of the abdomen, acidity of the stomach, eructation, and belching of gas, slight tenderness over the region of the gall-bladder, a sense of distension or upward pressure, sometimes irregular looseness of the bowels, usually constipation. Now, if such patient does not show an active attack of appendicitis with localized pain, tenderness, and rigidity, or a classic attack of gall-stone colic with a violent pain radiating to the back or shoulder, with vomiting, chills, and jaundice, or the positive evidence of gastric or duodenal ulcer made up of violent pain, vomiting, and hemorrhage, if such a patient does not show such a positive and unmistakable evidence of one of these conditions, he is almost invariably neglected by his physicians; and yet every such case of incurable indigestion is due to one of these three diseases, namely, peptic ulcer, gall-stones or chronic appendicitis. And every one of these patients should be cured. Gastric and duodenal ulcers may be cured by a medical treatment in a certain proportion of patients; when they are not thus cured and permanently cured they should have surgical relief. Chronic appendicitis and gall-stones are never cured by any except surgical means.

TREATMENT.

Treatment of Corneal Ulcers.[1]—In the treatment of corneal ulcers it is first necessary to remove the cause which is frequently some foreign particle such as coal dust, chips of steel, emery dust, etc., or there may be displaced cilia scratching the cornea, the palpebral conjunctiva may be roughened; in some paralyses the lids may fail to close properly and permit injury to the cornea by dust, wind, etc., in which instances the eyeball should be protected by some form of pad. A suppurating tear sac should receive appropriate treatment.

As a general rule bandages should not be used in treating corneal ulcers but the eye is protected by eye shades, smoked glasses or some form of eye-pad. When the cornea has perforated or threatens to perforate, a bandage is indicated; a copious discharge is a contra-indication to the use of a bandage. Small abrasions of the cornea simply require the use of some mild antiseptic, as a 4 per cent. boric acid solution, and will usually heal over in a short time.

For cleansing the eye, many antiseptic washes have been used, but we believe it is not so much the antiseptic used which furnishes results as the thoroughness with which the cleansing is done. A freely discharging eye would require more frequent attention than one with a scanty discharge; the former might require irrigation every hour to keep it clean; as a general rule, cleansing every three hours will suffice. Strong antiseptics are objectionable; either hydrarg. bichlorid (1-10,000) or a 3 per cent. solution of boric acid forms a most efficient eye-wash. After cleansing the eye, we instil a solution of atropin sulphate.

Atropin sulphate is almost indispensable in the treatment of corneal ulcers; one drop of a 1 per cent. solution is dropped into the eye every three or four hours to keep the pupil dilated; it acts favorably by preventing or breaking up posterior synechia; in some cases it is used oftener at first, and at times even the pure crystal is used by the surgeon; after dropping in the atropin, we should carefully wipe off the lids to prevent an absorption of any excess of the drug which may cause poisoning in susceptible cases. In cases with glaucoma or total posterior synechia, the use of atropin is contraindicated. In cases with increased tension or threatened rupture we may alternate the use of atropin with eserin sulphate ½ grain to 1 grain to the ounce, continuing the use of the former as the tension lowers. Some surgeons favor the use of eserin in marginal ulcers with threatened perforation as being less likely to produce anterior synechia.

Another valuable adjunct is dionin; it has decided analgesic and curative properties in corneal ulcers, it seems to hasten repair by opening up the lymph spaces in the cornea, permitting a freer flow of lymph to the parts;

[1] C. A. E. Lesage, M. D., Dixon, Ill., *Ill. Med. Jour.*, Nov., 1912.

in the later stages it assists in clearing up the cornea; it can be used in the form of solution or ointment, 5 to 10 per cent.; some surgeons employ the drug in powdered form. The ointment will be found a convenient form of administration; it produces a chemosis of the conjunctiva at times alarming to the patient, but it is this very reaction that is beneficial; it is used at first two or three times daily, depending on the reaction produced, and later, as repair progresses, the interval of application is lengthened. In the severer forms of ulcers we apply hot applications; cloths wrung out in hot water and frequently changed, are applied to the eye for 20 minutes to one-half hour, every two or three hours.

Urethral Drainage.[1]—Persson's paper is exceedingly interesting and the method outlined has much to commend it. The author's conclusions will give an excellent idea of the points presented.

1. Suitable drainage in the urethral canal is indicated in the treatment of urethritis, because it provides for rapid elimination of pathogenic bacteria and their products.

2. Sterile drainage is of great value as a diagnostic means to determine the presence of gonococci in doubtful cases.

3. Antiseptic drainage serves the same purpose in the urethral canal as applications of gauze in surgical treatment of wounds.

4. Drainage material used in the urethra must be absorbent in character, without which property it is useless.

5. Lactic ferments are indicated in the treatment of chronic urethritis, because these bacteria when properly used have germicidal effects on the offending organism in the urethra.

6. Certain lactic ferments produce under favorable conditions bacterial products which increase the activity of cells with which they are brought in contact, thus promoting the absorption in this instance of the perigranular infiltration that is the characteristic pathological factor in chronic urethritis.

7. The requirements necessary for success are, first, a proper method of application by which drainage may be introduced without discomfort to the patient, and, second, the use of an emollient substance which acts as a lubricant without making the drain nonabsorbent and in which the desiccated ferment finds a favorable medium for development.

8. This medium must be prepared with the aim in view of preventing the natural death of the ferment by neutralizing the excess of lactic acid when this reaches a point where it acts destructively to the organisms which produce it.

9. This medium must also contain elements in the presence of which the lactic acid organism produces a large amount of enzymes, or that bacterial product which causes increased local cellular activity and induces formation of bacteriotropic substances.

10. These requirements are not difficult to fulfill, and we are rewarded for our labors with much gratifying results in an unexpected percentage of cases.

The Treatment of Hemoptysis.[1]—The first indication is to reduce blood-pressure. As hemoptyses are sometimes preceded by a sense of tightness in the chest or by the presence of blood-streaked sputum, it may be possible to prevent their occurrence by insisting on absolute rest and by the administration of a drug—such as the nitrites—with the view of decreasing vascular pressure. Either of the following may be used:

℞	Gm. or c.c.
Sp. nitroglycerin .... 1|	M xv
Aquæ ....60|	or ʒ ij

M. S. Dose: ʒ j.

℞	Gm. or c.c.
Sodii nitritis .... 1|	gr. xv
Aquæ ....,.60|	or ʒ ij

M. S. Dose: ʒ j.

A teaspoonful of either of the above may be given every four hours for two or three days.

More commonly, perhaps, the patient receives no warning and the physician is summoned to treat an active hemorrhage. In the presence of this condition the indications are three in number: to secure absolute physical rest, to quiet the fears of the patient, and to lower the blood-pressure, attempting in this manner to favor the formation of a clot, which is nature's method of checking hemorrhage. This means that the patient must be put to bed and all unnecessary movements on his part must be avoided; he is not allowed to get up to attend to the demands of nature, nor is he allowed to talk. A comfortable position should be assumed: usually the semi-recumbent posture (with one or two pillows under the head) is best; and the patient should be assured in a few words that there is little cause for apprehension. Frazer's practice is to break one of the little "packages" of amyl nitrite, holding it for several minutes under the patient's nostrils. The patient should also receive atropin gr. 1/50 hypodermically, and this dose may be repeated two or three times within the next twenty-four hours. In place of atropin, nitroglycerin may be administered hypodermically in doses of gr. 1/100, repeated at short intervals, at first every half hour or hour, for three or four doses, later less frequently. After vasodilation has been obtained, more permanent effects may be secured by the use of sodium nitrite, gr. j, every three or four hours. Morphin, although used considerably in hemoptysis, should not be resorted to as a routine measure. It is indicated if the cough be troublesome, but its field of greatest usefulness is in those cases in which excessive nervous irritability exists. It is customary, at the onset of a hemorrhage, to place a light ice-bag over the precordium, with a view to quieting the heart's action.

---

[1] G. H. Perssons, M. D., *New York Med. Jour.*, Nov. 30, 1912.

[1] T. Frazer, Asheville, N. C., *Med. Record*, Nov. 9, 1912.

There is no specific diet for patients with hemoptysis; but the amount given should be small and fluid in character (milk in small quantities and egg-albumen are suitable); especially is it necessary to restrict the diet during the first twenty-four hours. While depletion through the intestines by means of catharsis has been advised and is theoretically indicated, it is better to wait twenty-four hours before attempting to move the bowels on account of the exertion which this action imposes on the patient. Also examination of the chest should not be undertaken, or should be restricted to auscultation; under no circumstances should percussion be practiced. As to the length of time that a patient who has had an hemoptysis should stay in bed, there exists considerable difference of opinion; it is safer to insist on rest in bed for twenty-four to forty-eight hours after the expectoration of post-hemorrhagic clots has ceased.

Weak Labor Pains.[1]—Fries, after using hypophysis extract on many patients suffering from labor pains that were diminished in frequency or were of short duration or too weak in force, says: 1. The hypophysis extract is entirely reliable and harmless for increasing the frequency, duration, and power of labor pains, giving good service in the first and second stages of labor when there is no insurmountable obstacle to delivery and when no indication for the immediate evacuation of the uterus is present. 2. In the afterbirth period its action is unreliable and not as good as the ergot preparations. 3. It is not reliable for terminating abortions or for inducing premature labor. 4. The induction of labor and its progress are successful in direct proportion to the nearness of the mother to term. The duration of labor is decidedly increased. 5. The preparation has no toxic action and can be combined with drugs acting on the heart and with the ergot preparations without compromising the action of the latter. It is injected without discomfort and has no local action. 6. The use of hypophysis extract in general practice is most desirable because a series of operative procedures which are not indifferent to the mother may be dispensed with, in particular, the so-called "luxury" forceps. 7. The extract has proved its efficacy as a tonic after gynecological operations. Its action on the urinary tract is unreliable.

SOCIETY PROCEEDINGS.

THE EASTERN MEDICAL SOCIETY OF THE CITY OF NEW YORK.

Stated Meeting, December 13th, 1912.

Executive Session.

The Executive Session was devoted to the hearing of the annual reports of the officers

[1] A. Fries, M. D., *Deutsche Med. Woch.*, Sept. 12, 1912.

and standing committees and to the election of officers.

Dr. Joseph Barsky was elected president of the Society for the ensuing year, the remaining officers and committeemen being elected as announced in the report of nominations in the last issue of AMERICAN MEDICINE.

The newly elected president was escorted to the chair and addressed the Society as follows: *Mr. Chairman and Members of the Eastern Medical Society:*

Although my election was neither a surprise nor unexpected, nevertheless, at the present moment, I am so overcome with emotion that I can hardly find words to appropriately express my feelings and to thank you adequately for the honor conferred upon me in choosing me as your presiding officer for the ensuing year.

Gentlemen, I consider it an honor, a great honor, and a privilege to be the representative of an organization which is composed of men most eminent in their profession and noted for their devotion to duty, earnestness and sincerity of purpose.

I am well aware that this great office involves a correspondingly great responsibility, a responsibility which it would have been utterly impossible for me to assume, since I possess but limited abilities, were it not for the fact that my predecessors in office, men of executive power, scientific attainments and untiring energy, have brought our Society to such an exalted position that little else remains for me to do but to follow in their footsteps and maintain our Society in its present enviable position. Nor do I consider this an easy task, for I am convinced that the Eastern Medical Society, which has accomplished so much good and scientific work in the past, stands second to no other society in this great city of ours.

Permit me, gentlemen, to avail myself of the present opportunity to tender you my sincerest thanks, which are but poor return for your kindness and for the many courtesies I have received from you. I assure you that I appreciate them very highly and that I shall endeavor to do all in my power to deserve your confidence and retain your friendship.

Scientific Session.

The Scientific Session was devoted to the Annual Oration by Prof. Joseph C. Beck, of the College of Medicine of the University of Illinois, on "The Pathological Significance of Chronic Suppurations of the Nose, Throat and Ear, with Demonstration of Specimens by Lantern."

Dr. Beck's paper was discussed by Drs. M. J. Ballin, Otto W. A. Schirmer, Jacob Weinstein, Otto Glogau, Israel Grushlaw, Martin Cohen, Charles J. Imperatori, Julius W. Weinstein, and S. J. Kopetsky.

After adjournment of the Scientific Session, the members and guests of the Society enjoyed the usual collation at the Cafe Boulevard.